EMT-Basic Field Care:

A Case-Based Approach

EMT-Basic Field Care:

A Case-Based Approach

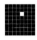

American College of
Emergency Physicians®

Chief Editor
Jon R. Krohmer, MD, FACEP
Medical Director
Kent County EMS
Grand Rapids, Michigan
and
Associate Professor
Section of Emergency Medicine
College of Human Medicine
Michigan State University
Grand Rapids, Michigan

Contributor
Loren Marshall, BA, MICP
Treeline Writers Group
Anchorage, Alaska

With Special Thanks to
Lawrence D. Newell, EdD, NREMT-P
President, Newell Associates, Inc.
Educational Consultants
Ashburn, Virginia
and
Faculty, Paramedic Education
Department of Health Technologies
Northern Virginia Community College
Annandale, Virginia

with 605 *illustrations*

Mosby

St. Louis Baltimore Boston Carlsbad
Chicago Minneapolis New York Philadelphia Portland
London Milan Sydney Tokyo Toronto

Mosby
Dedicated to Publishing Excellence

Editor in Chief: Andrew Allen
Acquisitions Editor: Claire Merrick
Mosby Developmental Editor: Tamara Myers
ACEP Developmental Editors: Susan Magee and Emma Kiewice
Project Manager: Linda McKinley
Senior Production Editor: Julie Eddy
Book Design Manager: Judi Lang
Cover Design: Scott Tjaden
Illustrations by: Jeanne Robertson and Nadine Sokol
Photography by: Rick Brady

Note to the Reader
The author and publisher of this book have made every effort to ensure that the drug dosages and patient-care procedures presented in this text are accurate and represent accepted practices in the United States. It is the reader's responsibility to follow patient-care protocols established by a medical direction physician and to remain current in the delivery of emergency care, including the most recent guidelines set forth by the American Heart Association and printed in their textbooks.

The scene photographs in this text were taken during past emergency responses. Therefore they may depict some patient-care activities that do not accurately represent the current practice in prehospital emergency care.

The American College of Emergency Physicians makes every effort to ensure that the contributors to College-sponsored publications are knowledgeable authorities in their fields. Readers are nevertheless advised that the statements and opinions expressed in this publication are provided as guidelines and should not be construed as College policy unless specifically referred to as such. The College disclaims any liability or responsibility for the consequences of any actions taken in reliance to those statements or opinions.

Mosby, Inc.
A Harcourt Health Sciences Company
11830 Westline Industrial Drive
St. Louis, Missouri 63146

Printed in the United States of America
Composition by Top Graphics
Printing/binding by Von Hoffmann Press

International Standard Book Number 0-8151-0100-7

99 00 01 02 / 9 8 7 6 5 4 3 2 1

ABOUT THE AMERICAN COLLEGE OF EMERGENCY PHYSICIANS

The American College of Emergency Physicians (ACEP) is the oldest and largest national medical specialty organization representing physicians who practice emergency medicine. With approximately 20,000 members, the College is the leading source of continuing education for emergency physicians and is the primary information resource for developments in the specialty.

ACEP exists to support quality emergency medical care and believes that emergency medical services (EMS) and prehospital medical care are integral components of emergency medical care. The College strives to provide meaningful support and leadership to the EMS industry by developing and promulgating policies to improve the quality of prehospital care, by promoting effective EMS organizational development, and by maintaining active outreach and liaison programs with various organizations and federal agencies.

A highly visible manifestation of the College's commitment to EMS is its annual sponsorship of EMS Week. This national campaign is designed to educate the public about the EMS system and injury prevention, to demonstrate to the public how to recognize and respond to a medical emergency, and to show appreciation for the contributions of every member of the EMS team.

About the Chief Editor

Jon R. Krohmer, MD, FACEP, started working in EMS over 20 years ago as a street provider. The Medical Director for Kent County EMS, Dr. Krohmer is currently the president of the National Association of EMS Physicians and the 1998 recipient of the American College of Emergency Physicians' EMS Award for outstanding contributions in EMS. He is board certified in emergency medicine and serves as an Associate Professor at Michigan State University.

About the Contributor

Loren Marshall, BA, MICP, has been a licensed paramedic since 1981. He worked 12 years for the Anchorage, Alaska Fire Department, first as a street paramedic and then as a training officer. He is now a freelance editor and writer, working on EMS and other medical and general topics.

ACEP TEXT REVIEWERS

Barbara Aehlert, RN
Southwest EMS Education, Inc.
Glendale, Arizona

Jonathon Best, NREMT-P
National Association of Emergency Medical Technicians
Stratford, Connecticut

Shelly Breeding, NREMT-P
American Medical Response
Beth Israel Deaconess Medical Center
Boston, Massachusetts

Will Chapleau, EMT-P, RN, TNS, CEN
Chairman PHTLS
EMS Coordinator
Emergency Medical Education
St. James Hospital
Chicago, Illinois

Robert Fines, NREMT-P
Director
Emergency Medical Services Program
Department of Health
Pierre, South Dakota

Mary Golub, RN, EMT-P, I/C
Regional EMS Coordinator
SWM Systems
Grand Rapids, Michigan

Jeffrey R. Grunow, MSN, NREMT-P
Department of Emergency Medicine
Carolinas Medical Center
Charlotte, North Carolina

Michael Gunderson, NREMT-P
Rural Metro Corp.
Scottsdale, Arizona

Stephanie Harrison
Emergency Medical Services
Glendale Community College
Glendale, Arizona

David B. Horowitz
Coordinator
Fire Academy
South Technical Education Center
Boynton Beach, Florida

Leroy B. Krueger, RN, NREMT-B
EMS Curriculum Specialist
Rapid City Regional Hospital
Rapid City, South Dakota

M. Jeanne Mason, RN, BSN, MA, EMT-A I/C
Professor
Nursing and Fire Science
Community College of Rhode Island
Providence, Rhode Island

Jim Moshinskie, PhD, EMT-P
Assistant Professor of Emergency Medicine
Texas A & M College of Emergency Medicine
Waco, Texas

Peter Pons, MD, FACEP
Research Coordinator
Denver Health Medical Center
Denver, Colorado

John Eric Powell, BS, NREMT-P
Paramedic Instructor
Center for Health Sciences
Roane State Community College
Knoxville, Tennessee

Adam Ray, BM, EMT
EMS Educator
Office of Emergency Medical Services
Pennsylvania State University
University Park, Pennsylvania

Norman W. Rooker, EMT-P
City of San Francisco Fire Department
EMS Division
San Francisco, California

Mick J. Sanders, BS, MSA, EMT-P
Training Specialist
Bureau of Emergency Medical Services
St. Charles, Missouri

Bruce Smith, BS, NREMT-P
EMS Education Coordinator
Emergency Medical Services Education
Illini Mobile Intensive Care Program
Black Hawk College
Silvis, Illinois

PHOTO SHOOT PARTICIPANTS

Zach Billings
Geoff Krohmer
Axel John Roest
Erin Lee Brach
Lyndsi Bremer
Rachael Systsma
Jessica Lynne English
Adam Merritt
Polly Krohmer
Cynthia L. Fairbrother
Jennifer Roche

Plainfield-Rockford Fire:
Todd Lane, FF, EMT-P

Rockford Ambulance:
Timothy E. Dickman, EMT-P
Jim Rinehart, EMT-P, I/C
Eric G. Nelson, EMT-P
Brett M. Laitila, EMT-P
Mark L. Prefontaine, EMT-P
Marcia MacGraw, EMT-P
Robert Peterson, Jr., EMT-P

AMR:
Michelle Bray, EMT-P
Laura Stanley, EMT-P
Jerry Systsma, EMT-P
Kelly Molenda, EMT-P
Gary Lindquist, EMT-P, I/C
Tom Beison, EMT-P, I/C
Jason Quinn, EMT-P
Anne Leach, EMT-P
Duane Yocum, EMT-P
John Kroblen, EMT-B
Elizabeth Byers, EMT-B

Kentwood Fire:
Tim Maday, FF, EMT-B
Russell W. Boersma, FF, EMT-B
Michael Hipp, FF, EMT-P, I/C
Nancy M. Shane

Kent County EMS:
Paul Brach, EMT-P, I/C
Jon Krohmer, MD
Linda Haan, EMT-P
Jim Klock, EMT-P

Life EMS:
David Burgess, EMT-B
Brenten D. Walker, EMT-P
Mary Gerger, EMT-B
Barbara Burney, EMT-P
L. DeMoor, EMT-P
Cari Hildebrandt, EMT-P
Kenneth W. VanHall III, EMT-P
Jon E. Thomas, NREMT-P
Patrick J. Hatch, EMT-P
John M. English, EMT-P
Jeane Grys, EMT-P

Northwest Ambulance:
Tony Curran, EMT-B
Christopher C. Bouwens, EMT-P, I/C
Jamie D. Balcom, EMT-P
Michelle R. Walker, EMT-P, I/C

Wyoming Fire:
Mark Rinks, FF, MFR
Vance Owen, FF, EMT-P
Joseph A. Jones, FF, EMT-B
Dirk Ubbink, FF, EMT-B

YWCA:
Patricia A. Haist, MSW

We Would Also Like to Thank:
Miramar Fire-Rescue Department
Prince Georges County Fire Department
Anne Arundel County Fire Department,
Emergency Medical Services

This book is dedicated to Polly, Geoff, and Beth for their love and support of my "EMS Blood Type," for joining me on calls, for being "victims" in courses, and for brightening my life immeasurably; to Mom and Dad for serving as wonderful personal role models; and to the staff of Kent County EMS and the personnel and agencies in our system for allowing me to do what I love to do.

JK

FOREWORD

Because we see the flashing lights of ambulances every time we look in the rearview mirror, hear emergency vehicle sirens, have the numbers 9-1-1 ingrained in our minds, and watch weekly television programs glorifying the emergency department, it is easy for EMTs to forget that organized emergency medicine is a young profession.

In 1966, the National Academy of Sciences published *Accidental Death and Disability: The Neglected Disease of Modern Society* and revolutionized the way we manage injury in America. The authors of that document pointed out that soldiers wounded in the battlefields of Vietnam had a better chance of survival than average Americans injured just minutes away from their local hospital. Inadequate training for ambulance personnel was a central problem. Indeed, at the time, morticians—armed with little more than a hearse—provided 50% of America's ambulance service. Preparing a nationally standardized training curriculum was, therefore, a top priority.

A new federal agency in the U.S. Department of Transportation (DOT) accepted the challenge and in 1971 introduced the first National Standard Curriculum for Emergency Medical Technicians: the *EMT Ambulance.* My career in emergency medicine began as a member of this first wave of EMTs trained using DOT's standards. I quickly learned that there are few things more rewarding than serving your community by responding to their calls for help. In fact, a crayon drawing from a young girl we saved still hangs on my office wall some 25 years later.

The EMT-Basic course presented in this textbook, based on the 1994 National Standard Curriculum, is the latest version of DOT's original standard. The current EMT-Basic curriculum, developed through a consensus process that included leaders from every aspect of EMS, stands as a yardstick for how far we have come in the 3 decades since *Accidental Death and Disability.* When I was an EMT, calling the hospital required a bag of nickels for the closest pay phone. Now we are exploring technology that connects physicians with EMTs in the field through live, interactive video. But the future of EMS involves much more than just new technology; it will be built on the knowledge and skills of the nation's emergency medical technicians.

I am certain that the next 30 years hold even more promise. The *EMS Agenda for the Future* and its companion, the *EMS Agenda for the Future: Implementation Guide,* lay out a road map of where we have been, where we are going, and how we are going to get there. The road map's legend is simple: EMS will continue to serve as the community's emergency medical safety net, catching the sick and injured who fall between the cracks of our social support systems. EMS is the linchpin tying our communities' public health, public safety, and health care systems together, and emergency medical technicians are its backbone.

This is an exciting time for EMS. Remember, each day and everything you do is another step toward our future. Invest your time wisely. I commend you on your decision to become an EMT.

Ricardo Martinez, MD
Administrator
National Highway Traffic Safety Administration
U.S. Department of Transportation
Washington, D.C.

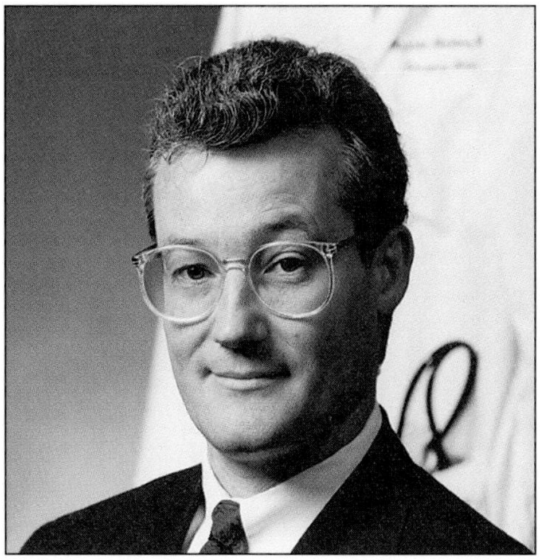

PREFACE

For many of you, this is the beginning of your education that will allow you to care for patients in your local EMS system. For some, you are expanding on earlier education and increasing your knowledge to provide a higher level of emergency medical care. For others, this is the initial step to attain your goal of becoming a paramedic or other health care provider and having increased work responsibility. Regardless of the reason, the education you are beginning now will be exciting and is very important.

The care provided by members of the emergency medical services (EMS) system is an important component of the entire health care community. Many patients access health care through the EMS system and they often do it at a time when they are under significant stress from an illness or injury. They are frightened and concerned about what is happening to them. Other patients use EMS system resources as their access to primary care. You will provide life-saving care to some patients and will experience a great sense of satisfaction upon delivering the patient to the hospital. For many other patients, you will provide fairly routine care and you may not experience the same energizing or rewarding feelings. Rest assured that the knowledge you gain and the services you will provide will be appreciated by all your patients and the community. And you will derive great personal satisfaction from performing your job well. You will be caring for patients of all ages, demographics, and social status. You will see babies born and you will be with patients as they die. You will have the truly unique opportunity to see people at their best and at their absolute worst.

It may be helpful to remind yourself that most patients you care for have no knowledge or understanding of medicine. Generally, that lack of knowledge increases their anxiety about medical problems or questions. Regardless of the reason why your patients call for help, you will be in a position to significantly affect their health and their lives. And for that reason you should feel honored and you must be well prepared. You have an important responsibility that will be with you throughout your career—on a daily basis, when you are on duty, as well as when you are off duty. Your family, friends, neighbors, and strangers will depend on you to help them in time of need.

Emergency medicine is a young yet constantly evolving specialty in medicine. Although emergency medicine is only 30 years old, there have been significant advances in the quality of care available to those experiencing acute emergencies. Prehospital, or out-of-hospital, care via the EMS system has also evolved significantly over those 30 years. Many medications and techniques that are used today were not known years ago or, if they were, were not considered for prehospital use when many of us began our careers in EMS. Care that you as an EMT are now able to provide had formerly been restricted to use by paramedics or physicians. I suspect that the next 30 years will see even more significant advances in the prehospital care EMTs will be able to provide.

This text is based on the 1994 revision of the Department of Transportation (DOT), National Highway Traffic and Safety Administration (NHTSA) EMT-Basic curriculum. This revision of the curriculum incorporated very important additions to the focus, knowledge base, and care you are able to provide as an EMT-Basic. You will be given an excellent foundation upon which to assess and care for the many medical problems that you will face. There are established limits to the care an EMT-Basic can provide, and so you will not be taught everything there is to know about general medicine and acute emergencies. This is an important point for you to realize and understand. It is just as important for you to know what you *do not* know as it is for you to know what you *do* know. It is important for you to realize that you will not be expected to know "everything." For that reason, you have other resources to turn to, such as other health care providers, instructors, paramedics, pharmacists, respiratory therapists, social workers, nurses, physicians, and others. As you continue your education and as you function as an EMT-Basic, it will be vitally important for you to learn to use those resources and to feel comfortable about the need to turn to them as necessary.

It is your responsibility to be familiar with the state laws, rules, and regulations that govern your activities as an EMT-Basic. This information will be covered as part of your education. You are also responsible for understanding the medical protocols, policies, and procedures under which you operate. Just as there is a medical director for your training program, there will be a medical director for your EMS system or your agency. Often, that medical director will be an emergency physician. In some cases, the medical director may be trained in another acute-care medical specialty. I would encourage you to use your medical director as a resource for education on a regular basis. In addition, you should access on-line medical direction physicians for any questions you have when caring for a patient. The opportunity to obtain an "ED Consult" via radio or telephone should never be viewed as a reflection of lack of knowledge on your part . . . rather, it is a required part of the system.

Every attempt has been made to include accurate, up-to-date information in this text regarding current medical care. We acknowledge, however, that there are some variations that exist around the country. If you note conflicting information between the material presented here and what you hear in your training program or in your EMS system, clarify that information with your instructor or local medical director.

Because medical care is constantly evolving, your education will not end at the completion of this course and when you successfully pass your state examination. Medical education is a constant process. It is likely that you will be required by the state regulatory agency to complete regular continuing education to maintain your knowledge and skills. In addition to attending continuing education programs, I would encourage you to regularly read EMS literature, journals, and texts. Even review this text occasionally after you have completed your initial training to refresh and deepen your understanding and knowledge.

As this text is being published, there is great interest in the EMS community about looking toward the future and how EMS personnel will fill the needs of the general population. The recently published *EMS Agenda for the Future* outlines a path for future growth in EMS. The NHTSA also has on-going projects for developing an EMS *Education Agenda for the Future* and an *EMS Research Agenda.* You will certainly hear more about those initiatives during your education.

It is exciting to think about the opportunities you will have to care for those in need and about the effect that you will have on the lives of many people. They are rare opportunities that not many people will have. Good luck and enjoy!

Jon R. Krohmer, MD, FACEP

PREFACE TO THE STUDENT

With the publication of *Paramedic Field Care,* ACEP has established a reputation for providing innovative and better ways to teach emergency care, using methods that create the best possible training environment for prehospital care givers. ACEP, as a result of the feedback from *Paramedic* and continuing research, has developed an approach to teaching that involves a more interactive text.

Most effective learners already know that the best way to take in new material is to be able to read or hear it and then interact with it. Other texts offer opportunities for reading and hearing new material—you may remember experiences that involved reading lengthy texts or listening to lectures and memorizing facts. This new text attempts to take you a step further and involve you in the material.

Knowledge of what to do in emergency situations is important, but to treat your patients, you will also need to learn the physical skills essential to an EMT. You will discover detailed skills training with step-by-step instruction throughout *EMT-Basic Field Care,* accompanied by full-color illustrations and photographs. Your instructor will train you in these skills as they are used in your community.

Before you begin your training, you might want to take a moment to familiarize yourself with what *EMT-Basic Field Care* has to offer.

Open this text to any chapter and you will notice that it begins with a list of *Objectives.* The objectives cover the U.S. DOT EMT-Basic curriculum and are divided into three groups: learning objectives, skills objectives, and attitude objectives. Learning objectives outline the information presented in each chapter that you should understand and remember. Skills objectives cover techniques you will be required to perform by the national curriculum. Attitude objectives cover subjects and issues you may need to explore and understand to work well as an EMT. These objectives will help you focus on the material you should be comfortable with when you have completed the chapter.

Key Terms follow the objectives. As a medical professional, an important part of your job is communicating precisely with patients, dispatchers, physicians, and others. All of the key terms describe concepts, techniques, organizations, and skills you will need to know. When you begin each new chapter, you may want to take a moment and read over these terms.

Every chapter also includes *It's Your Call* boxes, which present case scenarios based on material covered in the chapter. These cases continue through the chapter with a conclusion at the end of the chapter and are developed to match the presentation of the material, allowing you to immediately apply the material to a real-world situation. As you progress through your EMT training, you will find it useful to challenge yourself with the questions in these case scenarios and test yourself against them. Additional, challenging case scenarios are also given in the workbook, which accompanies this text.

You will notice that many of the chapters have *Sidebars* in them. These sidebars contain information that is not part of the national core curriculum but will prove invaluable as you begin your career as an EMT. Subjects covered include signs of gang activity, ambulance operations, additional patient lifting and moving techniques, pulse oximetry, seizures, Alzheimer's disease, commonly prescribed medications, and more.

A *Summary* concludes each chapter. This concise recap describes and pulls together the important points in each chapter. You may actually find it useful to read the summary before you begin to read the chapter. The summaries may help you keep track of the bigger picture.

After you read the chapter, you may want to take advantage of the *References* and *Suggested Readings* to get more detailed information on supporting materials and the research behind the material you have just read. Not only will this acquaint you with other publications that are available but also will give you the opportunity to look at the current advances and issues in your field.

Now that you are familiar with the features of each chapter, you may wish to look at the *Contents* at the beginning of the book. Sections 1, 2, and 3 of the text set the stage for your EMT-Basic education. They include information on your level of involvement in emergency care systems and build a foundation of knowledge that covers modes of communication; the medical, legal, and ethical aspects of your work; your own well-being; the ambulance; the basics of human anatomy; your interactions with patients; and more.

Section 4 provides information on assessing patients and recognizing priority patients. It covers information on assessing the patient and the injury, taking a focused patient history, and performing physical examinations on conscious and unconscious patients. As you read through these chapters, remember that patient assessment is a skill you will use every day in your chosen profession. Appropriate treatment for your patient starts with good patient assessment skills.

With the basics covered, Sections 5, 6, and 7 move forward to present the essential skills necessary to recognize and manage your patients' airway problems and medical and trauma emergencies. The chapters in these sections address administering medications, assessing and caring for respiratory and cardiovascular problems, and dealing with altered levels of consciousness, poisoning, environmental and behavioral emergencies, pregnancy and childbirth, and different types of trauma patients.

Sections 8 and 9 cover some of the modifications and special care necessary to assess and care for pediatric, elderly, and disabled patients or other patients with special needs.

Finally, you will find a wealth of refresher and reference information in the *Appendixes.* You can use the *National Registry of Emergency Medical Technicians (NREMT) Skills Sheets* in Appendix A to check your knowledge and ability to perform the necessary EMT-Basic skills. Appendix B, *Cardiopulmonary Resuscitation (CPR),* is an extensive article to help you brush up on your basic life support skills. Appendix C, *The Baseline Vital Signs* table, should help you feel comfortable with patient assessment as it is currently covered in the national curriculum.

The *Glossary* and *Index* will help you find material anywhere in the text and keep definitions for new terms at your fingertips.

EMT-Basic Field Care: A Case-Based Approach is the product of an ongoing commitment to innovation in the classroom. You have chosen a worthy profession, and it is our goal to provide a text to prepare the finest EMTs. We wish you all the success you seek and the care your patients deserve when you begin your new career as an EMT.

ACKNOWLEDGMENTS

It amazes me how many people are involved in pulling together a project like this. I would like to acknowledge and thank all of the people who have participated on the team to bring this EMS text to completion.

ACEP has long played an important role in EMS medical oversight and education. This text, combined with ACEP's *Paramedic Field Care: A Complaint-Based Approach,* demonstrates the College's continued dedication to EMS, promotion of quality out-of-hospital care, and interest in EMS education. Their continued support is greatly appreciated.

The ACEP staff has been a joy to work with. Susan Magee, ACEP's initial managing editor for this text, kept this project and me in line. Her leadership, guidance, educational experience, and humor were what kept me going, and she taught me more than I wanted to know about the development of a project such as this. After Susan's departure from ACEP, Emma Kiewice very capably stepped in to keep the activities moving forward. Don Kerns and Rick Murray provided very valuable counsel and input into the book. Tammy Case and Denise Fechner provided critical editorial and administrative assistance. They are all real friends and professionals.

Although Peter Pons, MD, FACEP, is not ACEP staff, we have had the opportunity to work on many ACEP projects together. His initial work on this text, and then his guidance and support, were very timely, appropriate, and much appreciated.

The EMS professionals at Mosby, Inc. have obviously been instrumental in bringing forth what we feel is a quality product. Claire Merrick, in her directed and yet very loving manner, led the initial support and guidance for this project. Kellie White and Jeanne Murphy guided everyone through the transition from Maryland to Missouri. Nancy Peterson, Carla Goldberg, Jennifer Roche, and Tamara Myers have all worked tirelessly in guiding us through the developmental, writing, and production processes. Their work in educating me and keeping us focused is greatly appreciated. Thanks also to Linda McKinley and Julie Eddy for their care of the manuscript through production; to Judi Lang and Scott Tjaden for their designing expertise; and to Derril Trakalo for listening to what EMS educators had to say.

Rick Brady's talents as a medical photographer are impressive. His ability to direct a photo shoot and get so much done in such a quality and professional manner was extremely helpful. His talent and attention to detail are amazing. Thanks are also owed to Jeanne Robertson and Nadine Sokol for lending their considerable talents to this project. They are truly an incredible illustration team.

My appreciation to Loren Marshall for his significant contributions to the development and refinement of this product. Larry Newell was also extremely important to the initial development and drafting of the text. Thanks to you both.

To the governing body and staff of Kent County EMS, thank you for allowing me to pursue this project. Jim Klock, Mary Golub, Michelle Knapp, and Paul Brach were very helpful in providing guidance and feedback in keeping us "street" honest and appropriate in our approach. Their help with administrative support and coordinating the photo shoot (in addition to serving as simulated "patients") was immensely helpful. My thanks also to the prehospital agencies and personnel in our system for all their help with photos, equipment, and suggestions and for allowing us to use some of our system's components throughout the text.

There are many colleagues who provided great support and encouragement on this project. I particularly appreciate the wisdom of Bob Domeier, Bill Fales, Bob Swor, and Rick Hunt when I'd call them and ask, "What do you think about .....?"

Finally, I am extremely grateful to my family, Polly, Geoff, and Beth for their love and support in all of the EMS projects on which I've worked and for their tolerance, patience, and understanding.

Jon R. Krohmer, MD, FACEP

Contents

SECTION 2

Emergency Medical Services Operations 88

SECTION 3

Foundations of Emergency Medical Care 134

SECTION 4

Patient Assessment 200

SECTION 5

Airway Management 236

EMT-Basic Field Care:

A Case-Based Approach

Section 1

Introduction to Emergency Care

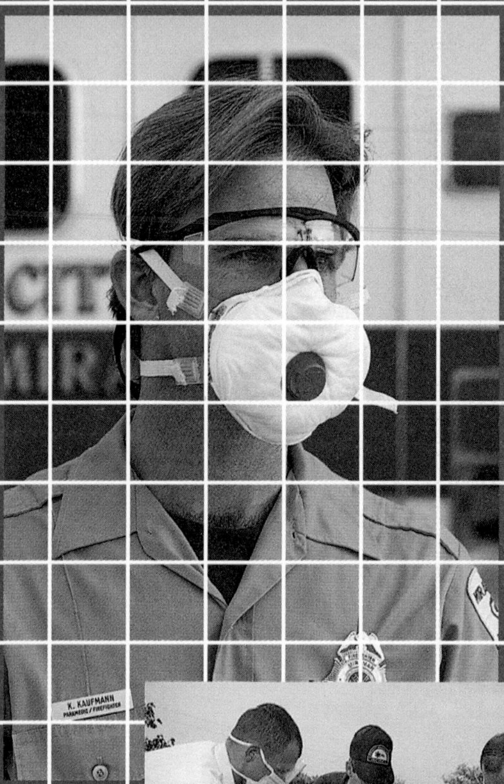

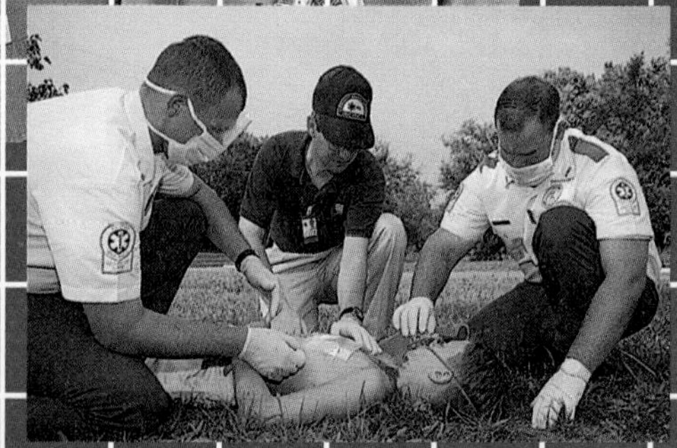

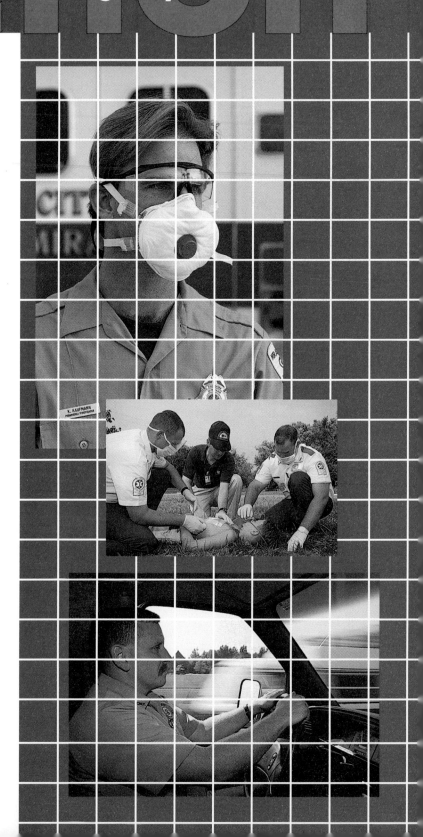

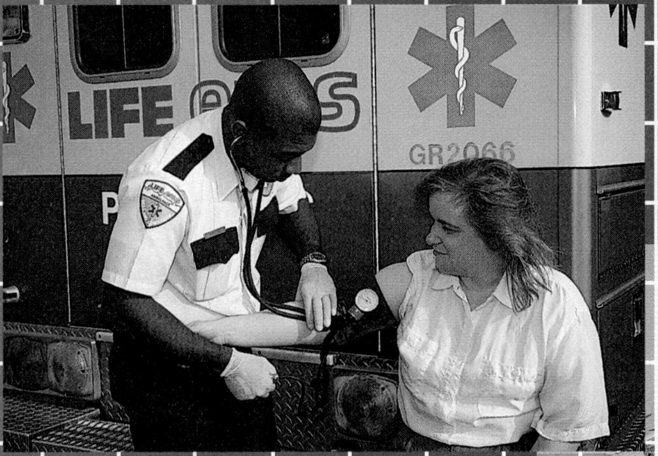
LIFE
GR2066

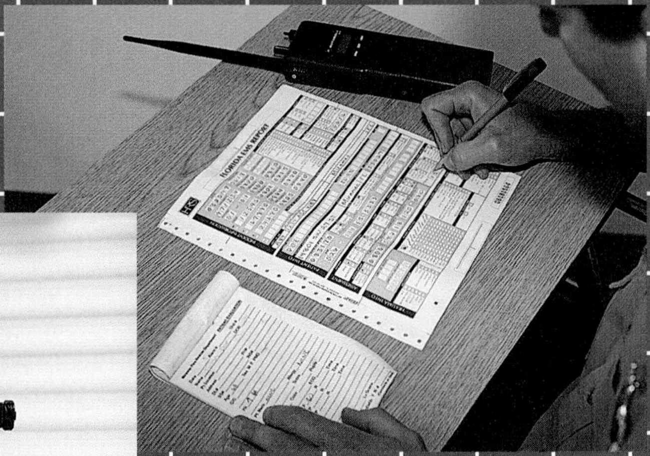

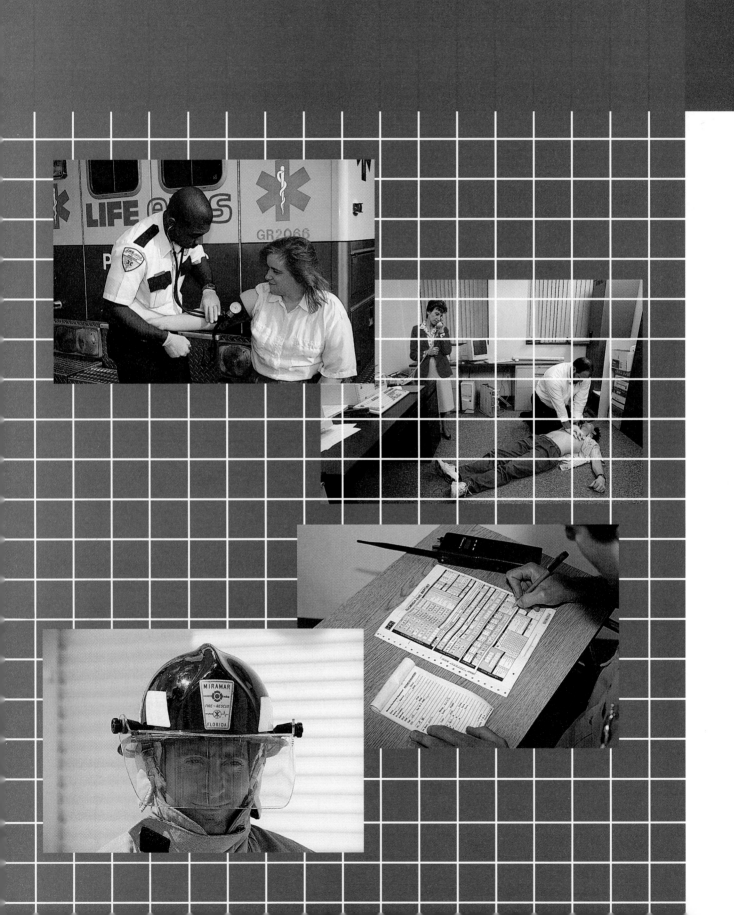
MIRAMAR
FIRE-RESCUE
FLORIDA

Chapter 1
The Emergency Medical Services System

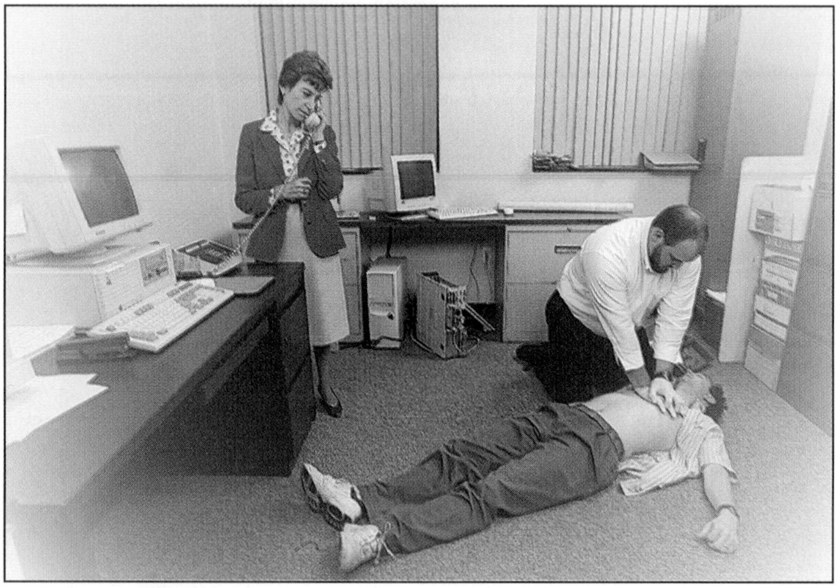

Knowledge Objectives

As an Emergency Medical Technician (EMT-Basic), you should be able to:

OBJECTIVES

1. Define the purpose of the emergency medical services (EMS) system.
2. Describe the five basic components of the EMS system.
3. Describe the various methods used to access the EMS system.
4. Differentiate an EMT-Basic from other levels of EMTs.
5. Identify seven desirable personal characteristics that will help you perform your job.
6. List seven responsibilities of an EMT-Basic.
7. Describe your role and responsibilities related to personal safety, crew safety, and patient safety.
8. Define *medical direction* and discuss your role in the process of interacting with physicians providing medical direction.
9. Describe the components of medical direction: on-line and off-line vs. prospective, concurrent, and retrospective.
10. Explain the purpose of protocols in EMS systems.
11. Identify specific laws, statutes, rules, or regulations in your state regarding the EMS system.
12. Define *quality assurance* and *quality improvement* and discuss your role in the process of maintaining a high-quality EMS system.

Attitude Objective

As an EMT-Basic, you should be able to:

1. Assess your personal feelings, traits, and conduct as an EMT.

KEY TERMS

1. **Emergency Medical Services System:** A network of resources, including medical facilities, personnel, and equipment necessary to provide care to victims of injury or illness. It includes five basic elements: patient and bystander access, emergency medical dispatch, first responder care, emergency medical technician care, and hospital care.
2. **Emergency Medical Technician:** A person who has successfully completed a state-approved training program consistent with the Department of Transportation's (DOT) national curriculum and successfully passed the certification examination. The three levels of EMTs recognized by DOT are Basic, Intermediate, and Paramedic.
3. **Enhanced 9-1-1:** An advanced form of telephone communication that routes emergency calls to the appropriate answering point; it enables a call taker to immediately know the phone number and location of the caller and to identify the appropriate response units (police, fire, rescue) to send to the emergency scene.
4. **Medical Direction (Medical Oversight):** Oversight by a supervising physician of all patient-care–related activities provided by EMTs. This oversight has two forms: on-line (direct or concurrent) and off-line (indirect; also called *prospective* and *retrospective*). Another common previously used term is *medical control.*
5. **Medical Director:** A physician who has accepted the responsibility to oversee the patient-care–related activities provided within an EMS system. This person is responsible for developing the standards (policies, procedures, and protocols) for system operation.
6. **Protocols:** Written directives from the medical director that provide a standardized approach to common patient problems and a consistent level of care for the different levels of EMTs. They include standing orders.
7. **Quality Assurance:** A process designed to continually monitor and measure the quality of clinical care provided within a system. Objective data such as response times, adherence to protocols, and survival rates are used to document the effectiveness of the system.
8. **Quality Improvement:** A process that continually reevaluates the EMS system. It takes the information obtained through the quality-assurance process, analyzes it, implements corrections, and reevaluates the process to determine if the corrections were effective.
9. **Standing Orders:** The portion of protocols issued by the medical director that authorizes EMTs to perform certain patient-care activities in specific situations without communicating directly with a physician for further medical direction.

IT'S YOUR CALL

A 9-1-1 call comes in from a cellular car phone. The caller says that there has been a serious motor-vehicle collision on one of the most dangerous stretches of road in the state. Police are the first to arrive at the scene and contact the emergency dispatcher. Information is relayed to the responding units: "Two-vehicle head-on collision on Route 15, just north of the 410 bypass. Four occupants are injured, and one occupant has been ejected from the vehicle."

Several emergency vehicles quickly respond: an ambulance, staffed by you and a paramedic, an engine company, and a heavy rescue squad truck. From another area of town, a command vehicle meets the oncoming vehicles and you proceed out of town on a back country road.

From the command unit, an officer evaluates the information and requests an additional ambulance. He also asks the dispatcher to check on the availability of air medical support from the regional Level I trauma center located 35 miles away.

Units arrive at the scene and chaos quickly turns into a well-organized rescue effort. Law enforcement personnel have closed the road and rerouted traffic. Gas leaking from one vehicle is quickly controlled by the fire department. Damaged vehicles are stabilized and rescue specialists begin to remove metal from one vehicle to gain access to the trapped passengers.

The helicopter is en route and expected to land in 5 minutes; a landing zone is being established in a nearby field. One seriously injured patient has been removed from the wreckage. Your team works feverishly to keep him alive as your unit heads toward the landing area to transfer him to more advanced medical personnel.

Additional patients are being removed from the vehicles. Another ambulance has arrived and a neighboring community is helping by sending an additional one. On-scene medical personnel communicate with emergency department staff and receive medical direction from the supervising physician. The dispatcher maintains lines of communication with the emergency personnel at the scene, the local hospital, the air medical communications center, and the trauma center.

After your patient is in the air, you return to the scene to help with the removal and care of the remaining patient. From dispatch time to removal of this last patient from the wreckage, 49 minutes have elapsed. The patient is transferred by ground ambulance to a local hospital, as were two others. One patient has been flown to the trauma center with serious injuries and is being further evaluated. Though the life-and-death struggle continues, the well-coordinated response of EMS professionals has given the victims a better chance of survival and recovery.

Has the EMS system always functioned in such an efficient manner? How did the system develop into what it is today? What safeguards are in place to help maintain a quality EMS system? How do you, as an EMT, fit into today's modern EMS system?

As an EMT, your primary responsibility is providing care for victims with serious injuries or illnesses requiring rapid emergency care. For critically ill or injured patients to survive, they will need your best efforts. This ability to adequately care for them is a direct result of the evolution of the modern day EMS system, a system that just 30 years ago did not even exist. Advances in EMS training and equipment have enhanced communications, improved the care provided, developed stronger working relationships between field personnel and emergency department personnel, and resulted in the development of regional specialized care facilities.

This chapter looks at the evolution of the EMS system. It helps you gain a better understanding of the professional development that has occurred over the years and the tiered structure that now exists for modern day EMS systems.

The History of Emergency Medical Services

A Look at the Past

The earliest structured emergency medical services began during Napolean's campaigns in the 1790s. Jean Larrey became the first physician to try to save the wounded during, rather than after, a battle. Using horse-drawn litters, the wounded were quickly removed from the battlefield and taken to a location away from the fighting where Larrey and other physicians could provide medical care.[6]

The 1860s saw the emergence of the first hospital-based ambulance services in Cincinnati and New York; horse-drawn carriages transported surgeons to emergency scenes.[11] A decade later, a more advanced communications system was being used to summon ambulances: lay people in New York reported accidents to law enforcement personnel, who used telegraph signals to notify the nearest hospital.[10]

In the 1900s wars contributed to the modernization of the EMS system. Both world wars, the Korean War, and the Vietnam War produced advances in medical care for those wounded in battle. These advances came in the form of more rapid patient assessment and evacuation of the wounded to surgical units. Throughout this period emphasis was placed on extending higher quality hospital care to the field. This period saw the emergence of the concept of uninterrupted patient care, begun promptly by medics at the scene and continued throughout transport to a hospital.

EMS Comes of Age

By all accounts the modern era of EMS began with the 1966 publication of a "white paper" by the National Research Council of the National Academy of Sciences. This paper, *Accidental Death and Disability: The Neglected Disease of Modern Society,* criticized the quality of emergency care provided by hospital emergency departments and ambulance attendants, as well as the quality of the communications systems in use at that time.[7]

In response to this report the federal government passed the National Highway Safety Act, which led to the establishment of the National Highway Traffic Safety Administration (NHTSA) within the Department of Transportation (DOT). NHTSA was given the challenge of developing EMS standards and aiding states to upgrade prehospital emergency care. Through grant money provided to each state, NHTSA funded program development, ambulance purchases, communications centers, and other EMS system improvements. In fact, the training course that you are now attending was originally developed by DOT and revised through the years in response to changes necessary for improving patient care.

Additional federal assistance came in the form of the 1973 National Emergency Medical Services Systems Act. This act was intended to be the primary effort for establishing and improving EMS systems throughout the United States. At that time the Department of Health, Education, and Welfare (now the Department of Health and Human Services) provided funding to develop regional EMS organizations. The goal of these organizations was to plan, implement, and coordinate EMS-system development throughout regions, breaking down city and county boundaries that were hindering the full development of EMS systems. More than 300 regional organizations were identified, but most were not fully funded or well organized.

Since 1973, individual states have taken more control of their EMS systems. The 1981 Consolidated Omnibus Budget Reconciliation Act (COBRA) changed the process by which EMS programs are funded. Instead of providing funds for regions, grant money became available to individual states. These grants provide funds for feasibility studies, system planning, implementation, initial operation, and system expansion and improvement.[4] Unfortunately, this act also resulted in a reduction of the total amount of funds available for EMS activities.

The evolution of the modern era of EMS has not been without challenges. One of the more significant challenges was getting communities to accept new levels of care providers. Through continued efforts by local, state, and federal government agencies, as well as media influence, a new EMS system gained acceptance and continues to evolve today. Gone are the days when funeral directors serving as ambulance attendants transported victims in hearses to local hospitals or morgues because they were the only ones who had vehicles equipped to transport patients lying down.

Standards have been established by NHTSA that define a well-structured EMS system and promote professionalism in EMS. Among these are NHTSA's Technical Assistance Program Assessment Standards. These 10 standards are provided to state EMS regulatory agencies and include the following:

1. Training: Those acting as the primary attendants to patients on ambulances must be trained (certified) to at least the EMT-Basic level. This training must meet the minimum standards identified in the DOT training curriculum.
2. Regulations: Laws must be in place that identify the lead state EMS agency and coordinate regulations, policies, and procedures throughout the state.
3. Transportation: Emergency vehicles must be licensed to ensure safe operation and availability of necessary emergency ground and air equipment.
4. Medical direction (oversight): A process must be in place in which supervising physicians ensure the quality of patient-care activities within the EMS system.
5. Resource management: There must be centralized coordination of resources that enables all individuals to have the same basic quality of care, including equal access to emergency care and treatment by competent individuals during transport to a medical facility.
6. Facilities: Appropriately staffed and equipped ambulances must ensure the delivery of the critically ill or injured in a timely manner to the closest facility appropriate for their needs.
7. Communications: A system establishing a broad range of communications, including universal access to the emergency number (9-1-1) and effective communications within EMS agency ambulances, dispatch centers, hospitals, and other jurisdictions for mutual aid must be in place.
8. Public information and education: Efforts must be made to inform the public about the important role they play as the first link in the EMS system, how and when to access the system, and how to help prevent and care for injuries.
9. Trauma systems: There must be a coordinated plan for the development of a trauma system, including patient-care protocols, guidelines for use of the trauma system, collection of pertinent data, and determination of the cause(s) of death.
10. Evaluation: A program must be in place that ensures the overall quality of the EMS system. This includes identifying areas of excellence and areas of weakness within the system and implementing a plan to improve and maintain the system's overall quality.

Team EMS

The modern EMS system works because of the coordinated efforts of people and resources; each individual does a job as part of a team. Through the coordinated efforts of local, state, and federal agencies, EMS systems continue to become more efficient by decreasing response times, providing better patient care, and rapidly identifying those patients with critical injuries or illnesses that need immediate, specialized care. There are more than 16,000 EMS agencies in the United States, with more than 750,000 paid and volunteer personnel. Each year these individuals treat and transport approximately 28 million patients, resulting in out-of-hospital medical expenses of more than 5 billion dollars[3] (Box 1-1).

BOX 1-1 Staggering Statistics

Since its conception, reliance on EMS community services has continued to grow. Listed below are statistics that reveal the scope of EMS services.

Ambulance services (includes EMS agencies, profit and non-profit, private and public, from 1995 census)	17,000
EMS providers (approximately)	815,000
EMTs (approximately)	506,000
Percentage of EMS volunteer personnel (approximately)	80%
Emergency nurses (approximately) (active and board-certified)	75,000
Emergency physicians (approximately) (active and board-certified)	14,275
Emergency departments (1993)	4,791
Emergency department visits (1994)	99,911,108
Percentage of visits by children (under 15 years of age)	24%
Percentage of visits by elderly (over 65 years of age)	15%
Deaths due to unintentional injury (1996)	93,400
Annual number of disabling injuries from unintentional injury (approximately)	18 million
Medical expenses due to unintentional injury	$74.6 billion

From ACEP 1998 EMS Fact Sheet. *The Vital Link;* 1998 Emergency Services Week Campaign Planning Kit, Dallas, American College of Emergency Physicians.

The **emergency medical services system** can be viewed as a network of community resources, including hospital and out-of-hospital facilities, personnel, and equipment that are necessary to provide care to victims of injury or illness. Another way to view it is as a series of links in a chain (Figure 1-1). There are five basic elements of the EMS system that serve as links in the chain:

1. Patient/bystander access
2. Emergency medical dispatch
3. First responder care
4. EMT care
5. Hospital care

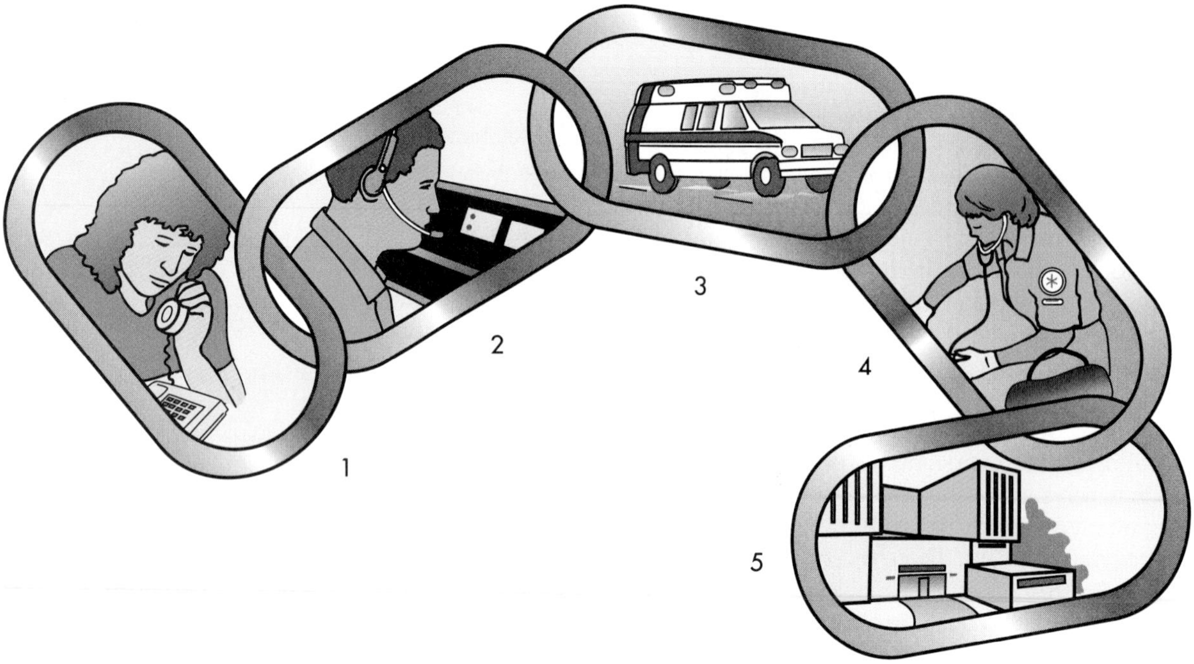

Figure 1-1

The five basic links in the EMS chain are (1) patient/bystander access, (2) emergency medical dispatch, (3) first responder care, (4) emergency medical technician care, and (5) hospital care.

Just like a chain, which is only as strong as its weakest link, the EMS system depends on the strength of each of its links. A weakness in any one link, such as a patient who delays accessing the EMS system for severe chest pain, could be disastrous. Likewise, the failure of a dispatcher to provide an ambulance crew with the correct location of a person having a serious breathing problem could result in an unnecessary death.

Patient and Bystander Access

The first link in the EMS system is citizen response—the initial action of individuals recognizing an emergency and deciding that there is a need for EMS. This response may come from the actual patient or from family members, friends, coworkers, or other bystanders. While awaiting the arrival of more highly trained individuals, bystanders may provide some form of basic care, including comforting the patient, helping to control bleeding, or performing cardiopulmonary resuscitation (CPR) (Figure 1-2). The most critical part of the citizen response is getting someone to realize the severity of a situation and overcome any reluctance to act. This includes calling for help without delay. This is particularly true of situations such as chest or abdominal discomfort that may be confused with indigestion.[8] National efforts by the Department of Health and Human Services and community efforts by organizations such as the American Heart Association, American Red Cross, and local EMS agencies can help educate citizens about when and how to access the EMS system.

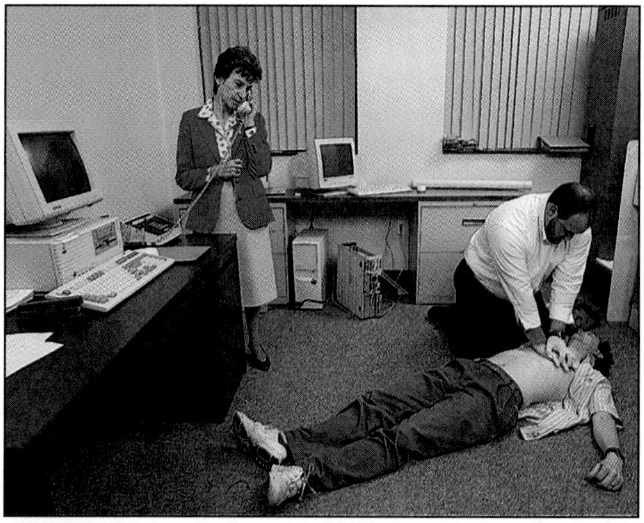

Figure 1-2

While a bystander calls a more highly trained individual, another bystander performs cardiopulmonary resuscitation (CPR).

Once the decision is made to call for help, communication lines are established between the patient or bystander and the dispatcher. For most people in the United States, the emergency phone number is 9-1-1. In

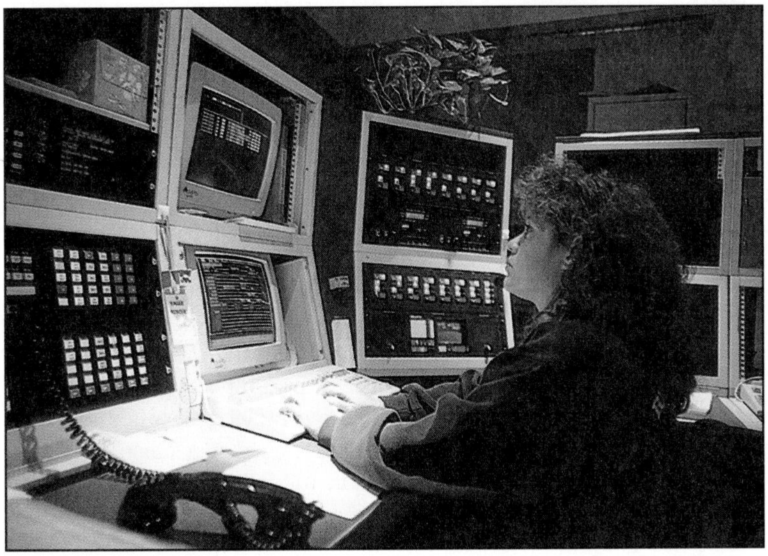

Figure 1-3

The enhanced 9-1-1 system immediately identifies a caller's location and phone number. This system enables the emergency medical dispatcher (EMD) to dispatch emergency personnel to the location even if the call is disconnected or the caller cannot communicate for some reason.

1968 the American Telephone and Telegraph Company (AT&T) announced the availability of this single national emergency number for any public safety agency and community that wished to use one common number to access emergency services. Since its beginning, the concept of calling 9-1-1 has become widely known. It is now estimated that about 78% of the U.S. population, mostly urban areas, has access to 9-1-1.[9]

A more recent advance in communications is **enhanced 9-1-1** (Figure 1-3). This system provides immediate information that identifies the location of the caller and the caller's telephone number. If the call is disconnected or the caller is unable to communicate with the dispatcher for any reason, the emergency personnel can still be dispatched to the location. It can also identify the primary and secondary responders for the location of the call to facilitate the rapid dispatch of the appropriate agencies. There are about 195 cities with populations over 100,000 that have enhanced 9-1-1 services.[9]

In communities without 9-1-1, a local seven-digit phone number or operator assistance must be used to reach emergency services. Some communities still have separate numbers for fire, EMS, and law enforcement. Unfortunately, this can be confusing and may result in delays in dispatching the proper resources to the ill or injured patient.

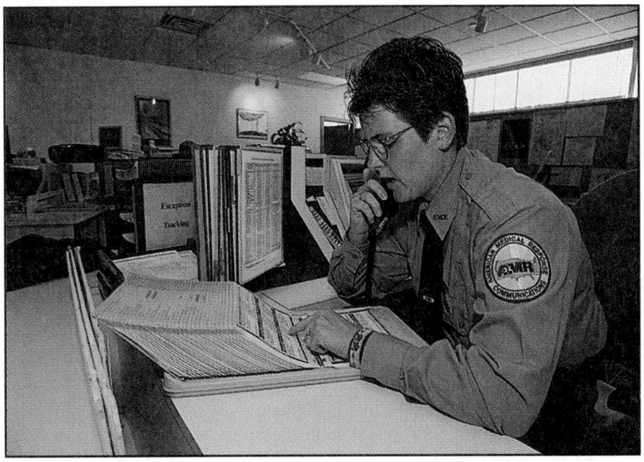

Figure 1-4

Today's EMDs are being trained to coach callers in performing CPR and other basic life-saving care while waiting for EMS personnel to arrive on-scene.

Emergency Medical Dispatch

Over the years, dispatchers have had to respond to a growing number of emergency calls. In some cases, callers ask for instructions on how they can help the patient. To help dispatchers provide this service, EMS systems have established training and certification for emergency medical dispatchers (EMDs). Dispatchers are being trained to rapidly and accurately gather information from the caller, dispatch the appropriate resources, and provide prearrival (sometimes referred to as *post-dispatch*) instructions on how to provide care for the patient until EMS personnel arrive, including how to perform CPR (Figure 1-4). This standardized training contributes to the safe, efficient performance by the dispatcher and enhances the medical dispatching function.

First Responder Care

The first person to arrive at an emergency scene is called the **first responder.** Traditionally, first responders have been law enforcement personnel and firefighters. More recent developments have seen a growing number of industrial response team personnel become first responders. To be first responders these individuals must have satisfied a specific level of training according to DOT. The medical training that these individuals receive is minimal (approximately 40 hours), focusing on identifying and caring for life-threatening emergencies. Because of the nature of their work, first responders are often close by and frequently have basic medical supplies, such as bandages to care for bleeding. Sometimes first responders will continue to assist more advanced personnel upon their arrival by providing patient information and helping to prepare the patient for transport to a medical facility (Figure 1-5).

Emergency Medical Technician Care

Since the development of the first EMT training program in 1969, there have been changes in the levels of EMT training over the years. There are currently three levels of **emergency medical technicians** defined by DOT:

1. EMT-Basic
2. EMT-Intermediate
3. EMT-Paramedic

The **EMT-Basic** is the mainstay of EMS, comprising more than 75% of all EMTs throughout the country.[3] Training for EMT-Basics is more comprehensive than the training needed for first responders. The training that you are now taking to become an EMT is based on a revised National Standard Training Curriculum developed by DOT in 1994. This training program involves a minimum of 110 hours and includes classroom, clinical, and field experiences. Within this training you will learn about the function of the human body, how to assess a patient to determine the general nature of the problem, and how to provide care for a patient, including controlling bleeding, administering oxygen, and moving a patient in a safe and efficient manner. This new curriculum also offers the opportunity for training in more advanced techniques that were once limited to more highly trained EMTs, including advanced airway management and the administration of select medications. Upon successful completion of your training, you will be eligible to take an examination and be certified by your state to provide ambulance care for persons with a variety of illnesses and injuries.

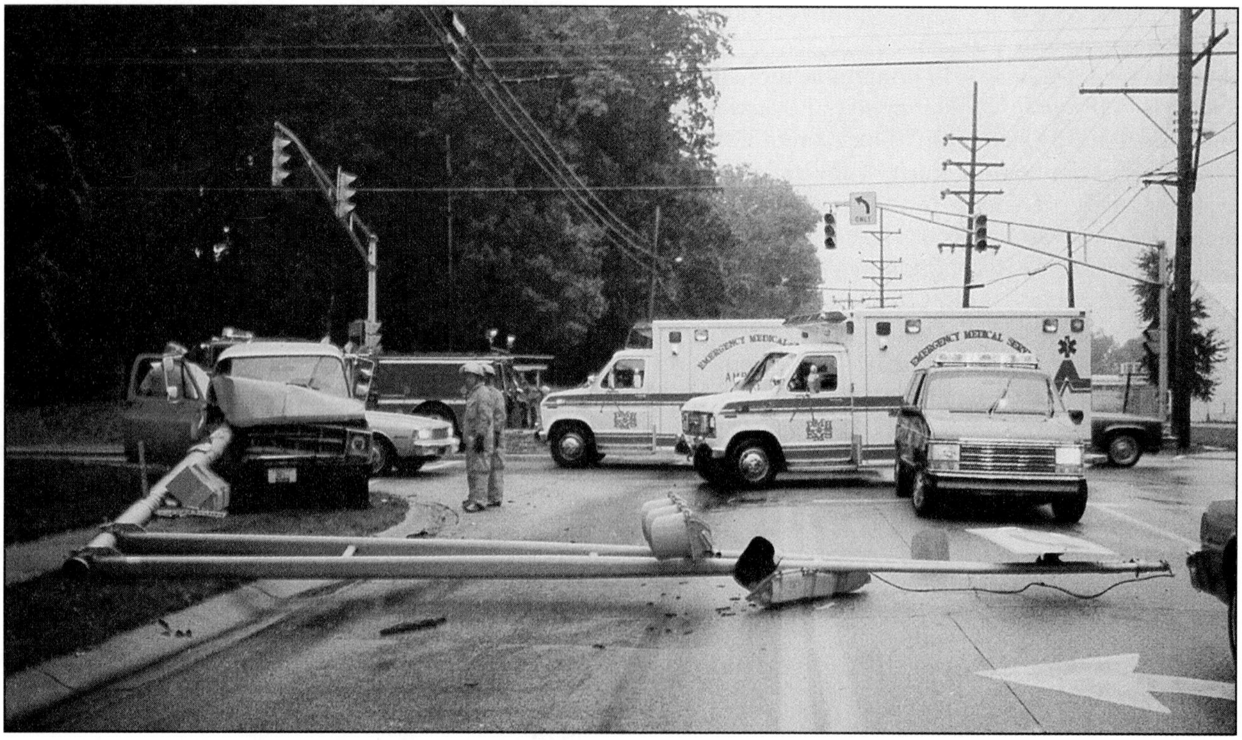

Figure 1-5

First responders and advanced life support personnel on the scene of a motor-vehicle collision.

EMT-Intermediate is the next higher level of EMT training. At this level, additional training is provided in advanced life-support skills such as intravenous (IV) access, advanced airway skills, and medication administration. This level of training meets the needs of many communities, because some EMS systems cannot afford the sophisticated equipment and training required for higher-level paramedic care. Many states have also modified this level to meet their specific needs. Approximately 12% of EMS providers are trained at the EMT-Intermediate level.[3]

The **EMT-Paramedic** is trained to perform even more advanced skills, such as interpreting difficult heart rhythm disturbances, administering more medications, and performing invasive airway and resuscitation procedures. Like the EMT-Intermediate, paramedics also make up about 12% of all EMS providers.[3] Some states have licensed prehospital nurses who routinely provide advanced life support in the prehospital setting.

Hospital Care

Regardless of their level of training, all out-of-hospital care providers have the same common goal of transporting a patient to a hospital so that he or she can be evaluated by a physician. Once an ambulance arrives at a hospital, patient care is turned over to more advanced medical personnel in the emergency department. There are more than 6,400 hospitals with emergency departments in our present health care system, providing care for the majority of emergencies. More than 800 of these hospitals are trauma centers that are prepared to handle patients with varying degrees of injury.[2]

There are four different levels of trauma centers. Levels I and II are the most advanced, staffing surgical teams 24 hours a day. Trauma centers at these levels can handle many of the most complicated injuries, such as gunshot and stab wounds, serious motor-vehicle collisions, drownings, and critical burns. Patients with less severe injuries or illnesses can be adequately cared for at Level III or IV trauma centers. In some areas of the country, all of these facilities and the out-of-hospital agencies work together to provide care in a coordinated trauma system. Many of these trauma systems incorporate air medical services to rapidly transport patients from areas where ground transport is not possible or where prolonged ground transport would delay the necessary advanced care that the critical patient needs. Other areas of the country are developing these types of structured trauma systems.

Other hospitals within EMS systems provide other specialized types of care, such as burn care. There are approximately 130 burn units in the United States[2] to which patients are transferred after they are first evaluated and stabilized in the emergency department. In some extreme situations, patients are sent directly to the burn unit.

Other specialty centers include the more than 80 hospitals that house poison control centers to assist callers with common poisoning problems that are handled over the phone without the assistance of out-of-hospital providers.[1] They also serve as a resource for other health care providers who treat patients who are poisoned or have overdosed.

With the patient at the hospital, emergency nurses and physicians, as well as radiology, laboratory, and respiratory technicians, take over patient care. The first member of the hospital team to see the patient is usually a nurse. The nurse may request updated information about the patient, such as any changes in the patient's condition during transport. The nurse will then quickly reevaluate the patient and follow a set of hospital procedures for patient care.

Many emergency departments are staffed by physicians specially trained in the practice of emergency medicine. The physician reevaluates the patient and provides further care to stabilize or resolve the condition. More extensive procedures and diagnostic tests are done in an effort to determine the exact nature of the patient's problem (Figure 1-6). If the patient requires additional care, the emergency physician involves the appropriate medical specialist, such as a cardiologist, neurologist, or surgeon. In this manner, the patient-care continuum is maintained, providing the patient with the best quality care for the specific problem.

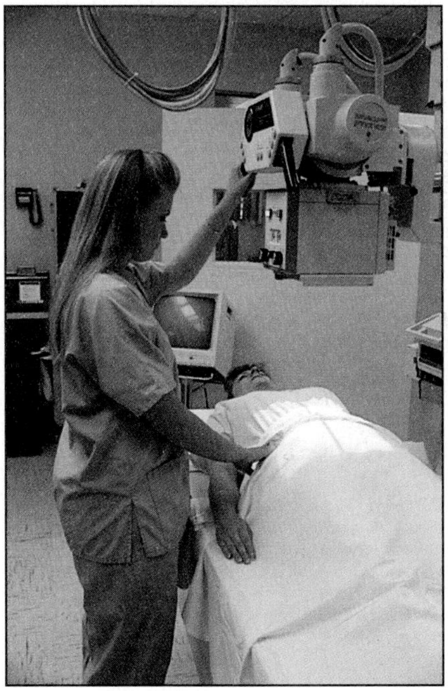

Figure 1-6

Diagnostic procedures such as radiography may be performed in the hospital emergency department to better determine the exact nature of a patient's problem.

Air medical transport has been used throughout military history for the evacuation of those injured in battle and for the transport of other soldiers and civilians. The success of air medical transport in the military, coupled with the development of regional trauma systems throughout the United States, has led to the enhanced use of air medical transport. Because the time from the onset of a serious injury to the time that a patient receives definitive care is critical for survival, minutes saved can result in an improved outcome. Helicopter transport (Figure 1-7, *A*) can mean the difference between life and death for critically ill or injured patients, especially if the local system does not have advanced life-support providers or, in the case of trauma patients, the distance to a Level I trauma center is too far. Consider air transport if environmental conditions allow, if it would enhance patient care, as allowed by local protocols.

Each year approximately 150,000 air medical transports are performed. About one third of these transports are done from accident scenes.[2] Transporting the ill or injured within about 150 miles of the air ambulance program is usually done by helicopter. However, airplanes (Figure 1-7, *B*) are often used for longer distance transports, for convalescing patients, and for organ deliveries.

A

B

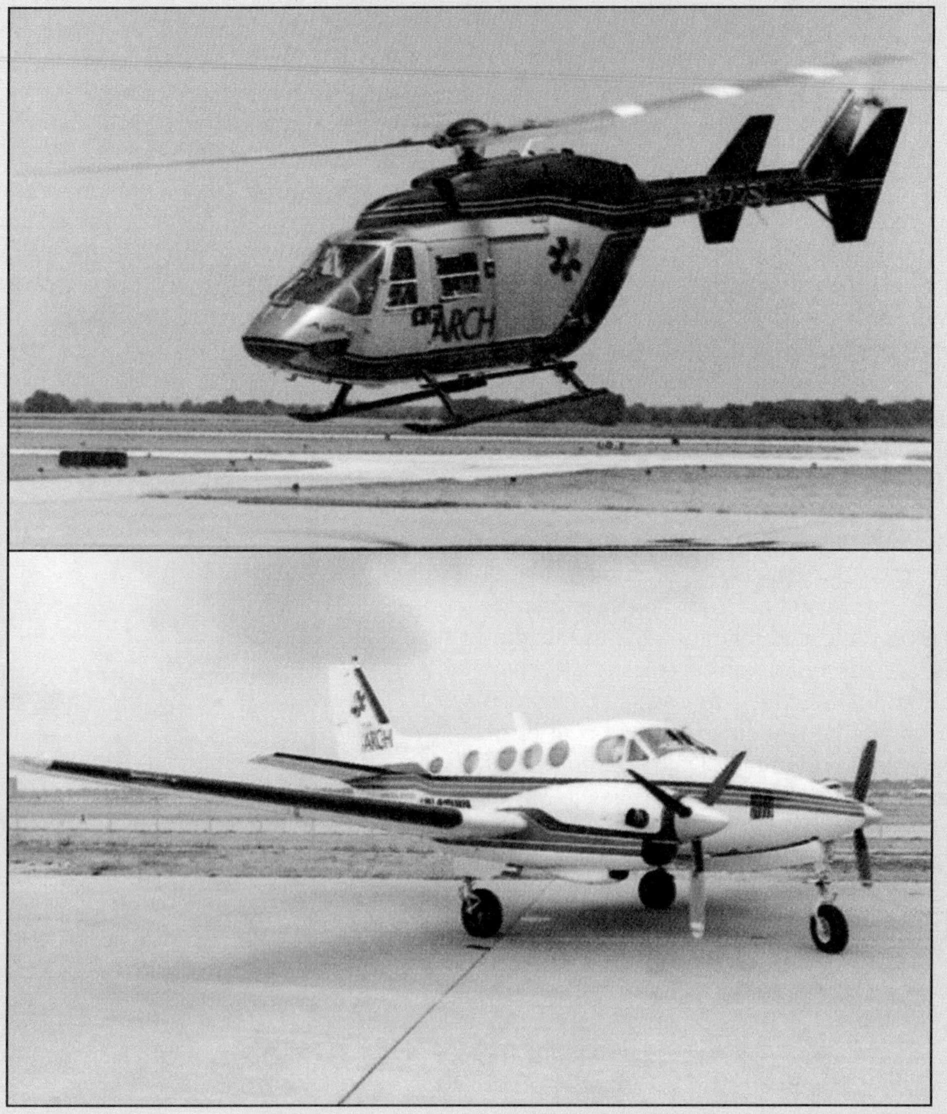

Figure 1-7

Air medical transport may be used if environmental conditions allow and if it would enhance patient care. **A,** Rotary-wing aircraft. **B,** Fixed-wing aircraft.

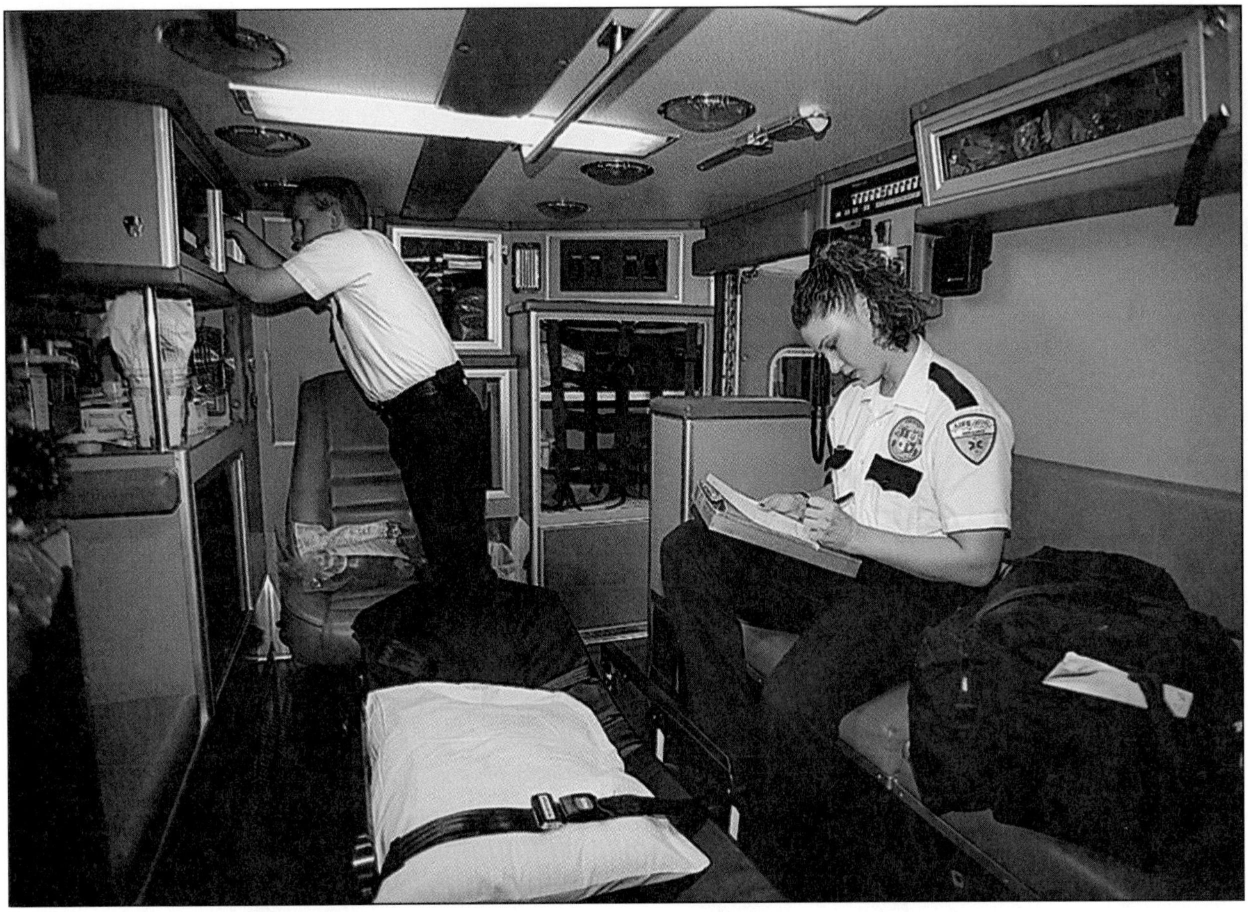

Figure 1-8
Everyday tasks: Equipment preparation.

Your Role on the EMS Team

As an EMT-Basic you must possess certain traits and skills. Each person brings individual characteristics to the EMS team that help make the team stronger. Among these are a desire to deliver quality patient care, set high personal standards, and exhibit respect for your profession. Remember that you and your profession will be constantly scrutinized by the public. By maintaining the most professional image possible, you can gain both the respect and admiration of the public and your peers.

Roles and Responsibilities of the EMT

Though you may not always think about it, people are trusting you with their lives, which is the biggest responsibility of all. One way to look at your specific responsibilities is to consider what tasks you must perform in a typical day as an EMT. These include the following:

- Maintaining safety: The importance of safety cannot be overemphasized. You are responsible for your personal safety and the safety of crew members, patients, and bystanders. Safety begins with an examination of the emergency vehicle that you will be using (Figure 1-8). Check both the vehicle and the medical equipment to make sure everything is functioning properly. Examine your personal clothing and gear to ensure everything you need is present and working as expected. Be certain to have and use personal protection equipment to help prevent disease transmission. Find out if there are any special road hazards that you should avoid during the shift, such as road closings or construction zones.
- Responding to the call: When you are dispatched to a call, proceed without delay to your unit. Verify the location, notify the dispatcher that you are responding, and operate the vehicle in a safe manner (Figure 1-9). While en route, consider the possible equipment and supplies you may need. As you approach the scene, consider potential dangers such as fires, explosions, unstable structures or vehicles, violent patients, animals, and environmental conditions. When at the scene, position the vehicle appropriately so that it protects the patient, allows easy access, and provides for personal and crew member safety.
- Assessing the patient: To provide the best care for the patient you must first try to find out the nature of the

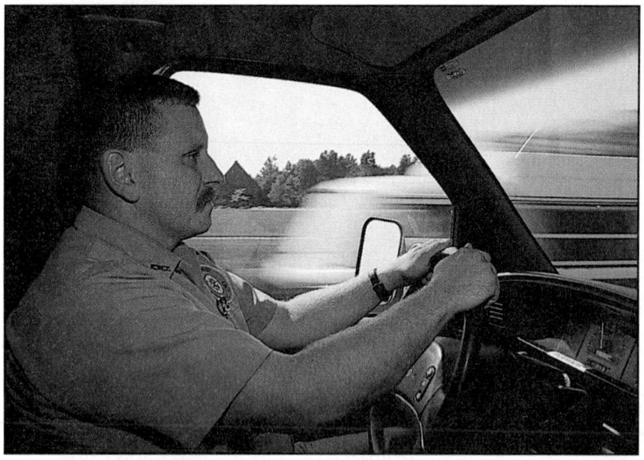

Figure 1-9

Everyday tasks: Responding to the call.

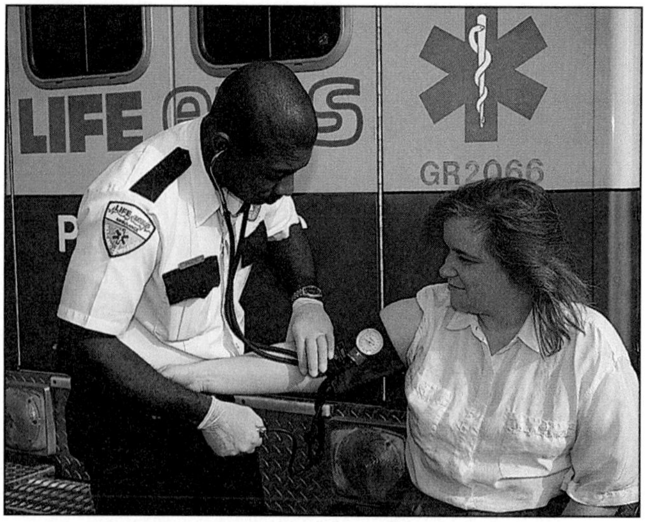

Figure 1-10

Everyday tasks: Assessing the patient.

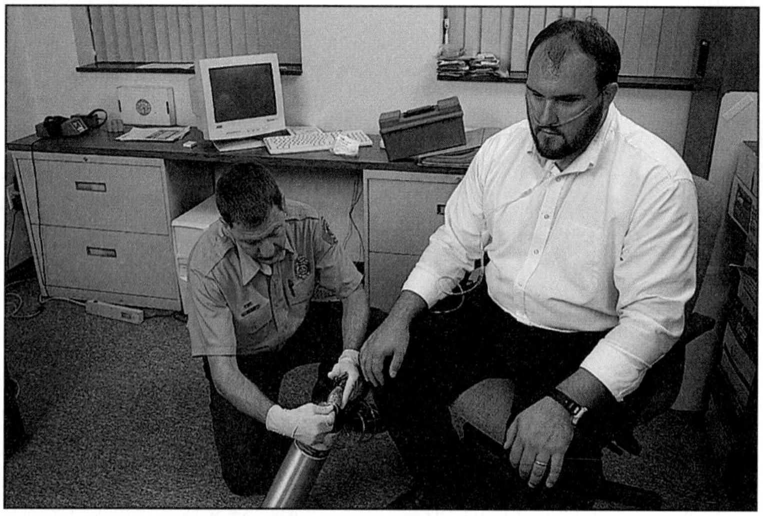

Figure 1-11

Everyday tasks: Providing patient care.

patient's primary problem (Figure 1-10). By using your senses and following a step-by-step approach, you will be able to quickly determine any life-threatening conditions and provide care. If there are no immediate threats to life, a more detailed assessment can be done to help determine the care that will be needed.

- Providing patient care: Patient care will differ based on what you determine the problem to be. Patient care includes everything from providing emotional support and helping the patient find a comfortable resting position, to controlling bleeding, performing CPR, using an automated defibrillator, and administering medications (Figure 1-11). Patient care also means speaking on behalf of the patient. It is your responsibility to address patient needs and bring concerns to other providers, including hospital staff. You are an advocate for the best interests of the patient.
- Moving the patient: Moving the patient often requires you to lift and carry the patient. Safety plays an important role here. If you lift improperly or without the necessary help of others, you could be injured. If you cannot support the patient's weight and drop the patient, then additional injury could occur to the patient. Your partner could also be injured in the process of lifting or moving the patient improperly (Figure 1-12).
- Transporting the patient: You are responsible for transporting the patient to the appropriate medical facility in a safe and efficient manner. This means abiding by

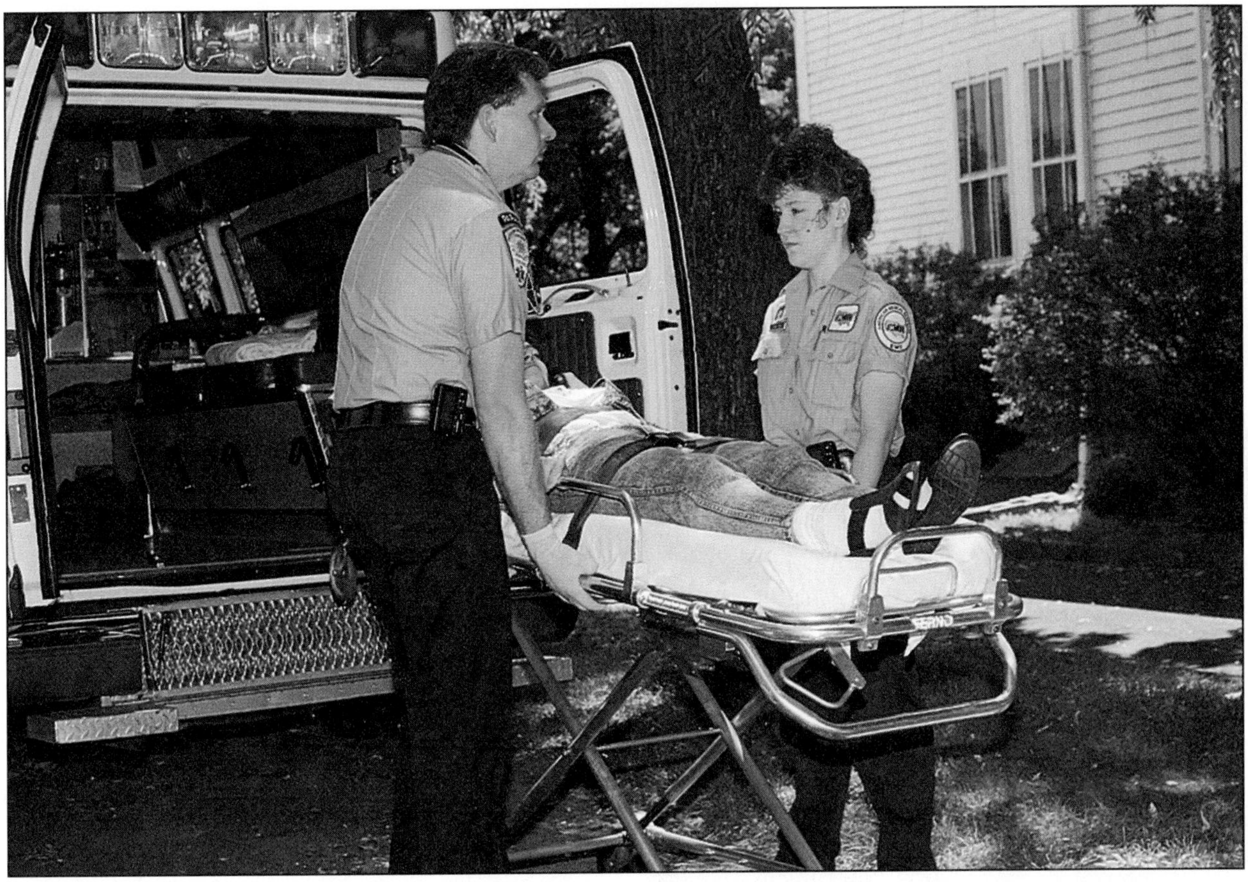

Figure 1-12
Everyday tasks: Moving the patient.

emergency driving laws while operating the vehicle. The patient must be properly secured in the ambulance so no injury will result while en route to the receiving facility (Figure 1-13).

- Transferring patient care: Once you reach the hospital you will turn over patient care to more highly trained personnel. The information you gather about the patient's condition and information about what care you provided are also turned over. Normally, a short briefing of your findings is given to a nurse or physician (Figure 1-14). Once the patient is turned over to the hospital staff, you are released from your patient-care responsibilities.
- Record keeping: The golden rule of documentation is "If it is not written down, it did not happen." Following this principle will help you present a clear and concise account of what you found during your assessment, the care you provided, and any changes that occurred during transport. The patient-care report that you complete is a legal record (Figure 1-15). These records are kept for varying lengths of time, depending on your state regulations. This information is also important for data collection and reporting and for purposes of assessing the quality of the care being provided by your agency.

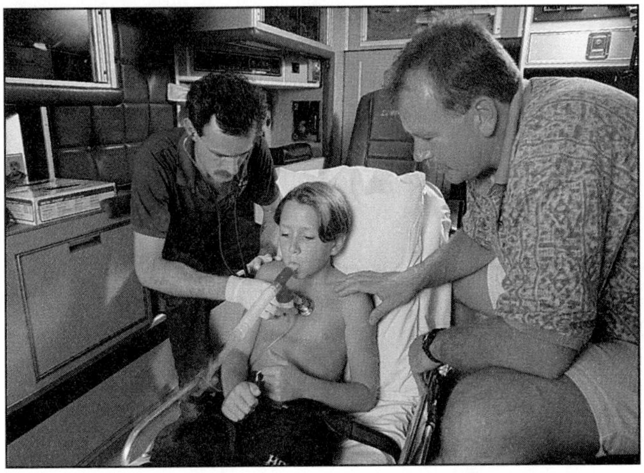

Figure 1-13
Everyday tasks: Transporting the patient.

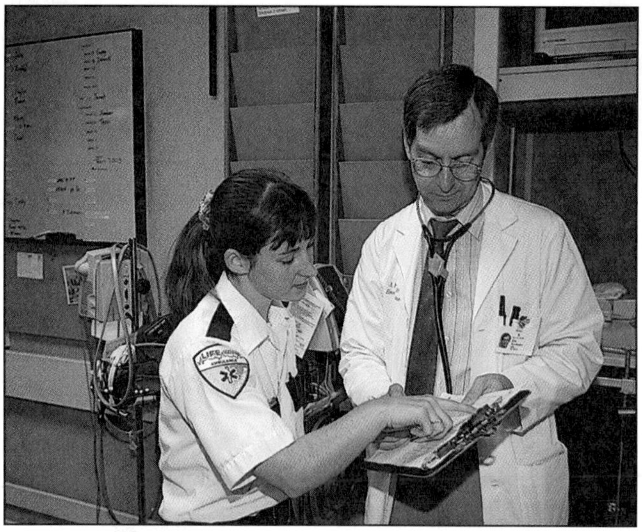

Figure 1-14

Everyday tasks: Transferring patient care.

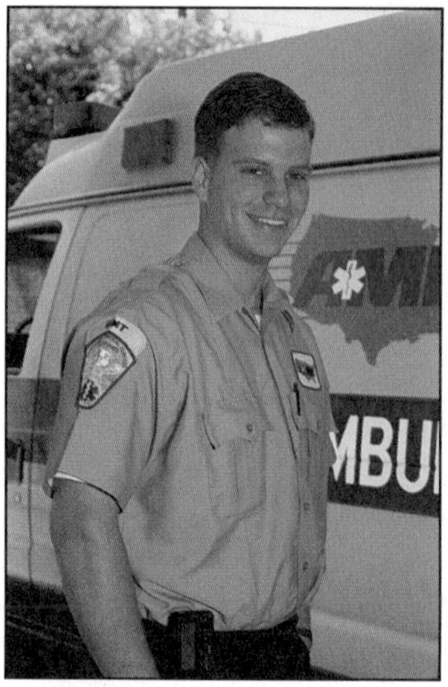

Figure 1-16

Keeping yourself and your uniform neat and clean is important to presenting a professional appearance.

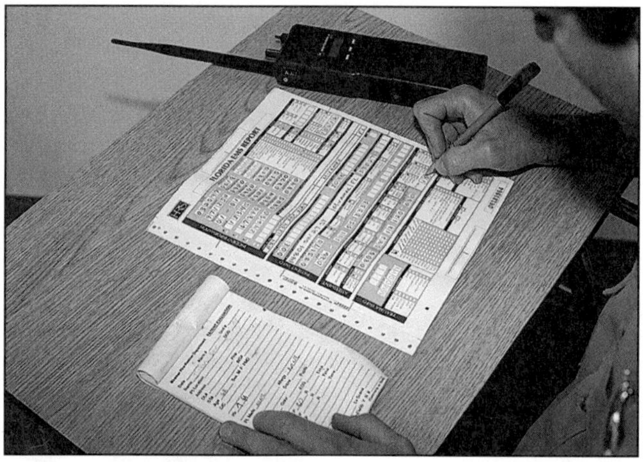

Figure 1-15

Everyday tasks: Record keeping.

Personal Characteristics

Certain personal characteristics will enhance your ability to fulfill the responsibilities of an EMT:

- Maintaining a professional attitude: A professional appearance inspires confidence (Figure 1-16). Keeping yourself neat and clean presents that professional image and decreases the likelihood of disease transmission. But beyond outward appearances, you must also exhibit a caring and professional attitude. Being compassionate and understanding of the patient's needs and fears are important characteristics. When speaking to patients and crew members, keep calm and stay under control. People pick up on your anxiety. Talk in a normal tone and make eye contact whenever possible. Remember, you are serving the public, and the first impression you make may be a lasting one.
- Maintaining ethics: Ethics are standards designed by a particular group for honorable behavior appropriate for and expected of members of that group. As an EMT you are bound by a code of ethics. You have an ethical responsibility to your patients, yourself, and your EMS colleagues as part of the group. As you perform your job you will find yourself confronted with situations that present moral dilemmas. How you act in such situations will depend on your personal values and beliefs. Legally, you must provide the best possible care. Ethically, this care includes providing for the emotional and physical well-being of the patient.
- Maintaining good health: Proper exercise and nutrition contribute greatly to your performance. Because heavy lifting is a part of your job, you will need to have the physical ability to do the tasks. Equally, the stress associated with your job can sometimes become difficult to handle. You can help manage physical, mental, and emotional stress by taking care of your body, which may mean adjusting some personal habits. To stay attentive, you should not consume alcohol within 8 hours of duty. You should also try to get adequate rest. When you are tired, you are not physically or mentally prepared to function at your full potential.
- Expanding your education: Without ongoing education, your skills and knowledge will deteriorate quickly. To overcome this you should participate frequently in crew or agency training sessions, as well as formal educational programs offered through colleges, hospitals, and independent training organizations. Lectures, videos,

scenario role-playing, demonstrations, and conferences are all examples of ways you can participate in continuing education. Your certification as an EMT will expire in several years, at which time you may have to attend refresher training or demonstrate ongoing education.

Additional traits that will help you function as an EMT are resourcefulness, leadership, and honesty. An EMS professional who has a balance of all of these personality characteristics is more likely to have a lengthy career and advance to other levels.

Medical Direction

One element of EMS systems that has been undergoing change in recent years is that of medical direction or medical oversight for EMT-Basics. Supervision of care provided by EMT-Intermediates and Paramedics has existed for many years. However, it is only recently that EMT-Basics have begun working under a medical director. Most states are now adopting this recommendation of the 1994 EMT-Basic curriculum revision. Appropriate medical direction is important for continuing development of EMS systems.

A **medical director** is a physician who provides **medical direction,** or medical oversight, of the patient care that you and others within your EMS system provide. You operate as an extension of the physician because the physician cannot be on every call that you run. The medical director and other supervising physicians are significant players in the efforts of your EMS system to improve and maintain the highest possible standards of patient care. These physicians put their trust in you to operate in a safe and effective manner, provide the best possible care, and adhere to protocols that have been established for you. Medical direction is most frequently classified as either on-line or off-line direction. However, it may also sometimes be classified as either prospective, concurrent, or retrospective (Box 1-2).

On-line medical direction (also called *concurrent medical direction*) is communication directly with a physician at a hospital or on-scene to receive patient-care orders. For example, you may wish to administer medication to a patient who is experiencing an allergic reaction. To give the medication, you may need to contact a physician at the hospital to get approval. You should never hesitate to contact a physician for medical advice when faced with situations that are confusing; it will always benefit the patient.

Off-line medical direction (also called *prospective* and *retrospective medical direction*) refers to the activities of medical oversight that occur before (prospective) and after (retrospective) you provide patient care. Your medical director, working with members of the EMS system, develops written protocols, policies, and procedures

BOX 1-2 Medical Direction Activities

Prospective (Off-Line)

1. Initial education
   - Prehospital personnel
   - Hospital personnel
2. Protocol, policy, and procedure development
   - Establish protocols that clearly define patient-care activities
   - Establish guidelines for initial education and continuing education
   - Establish guidelines for a quality improvement (QI) program
   - Develop straightforward standing orders based on critical presentations requiring clear or immediate interventions
3. System "privileging" process
4. Total quality management process
5. Political process

Concurrent (On-Line)

1. On-line
   - Involves EMS medical director, other physicians, nurses, and EMS personnel
   - Emphasizes the team nature of the EMS system
   - Promotes discussion among EMS and hospital personnel about the patient's assessment findings, care, and impending arrival at the emergency department
2. On-scene
   - EMS personnel and EMS system personnel

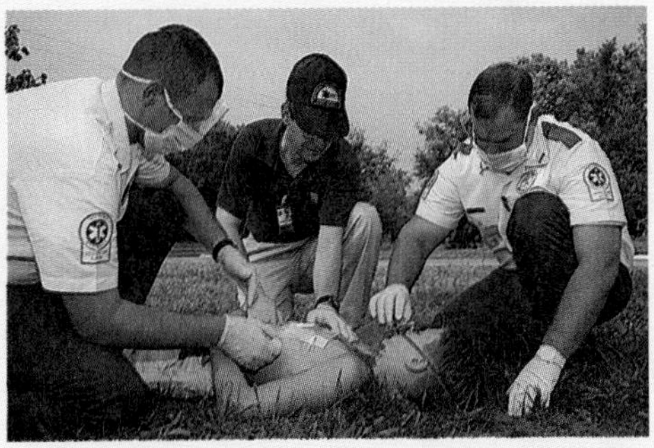

EMS medical director on-scene.

Retrospective (Off-Line)

1. Total quality management
2. Special run review; routine run review and random run review
3. Continuing education and remedial education
4. Counseling and disciplinary process (using due process)

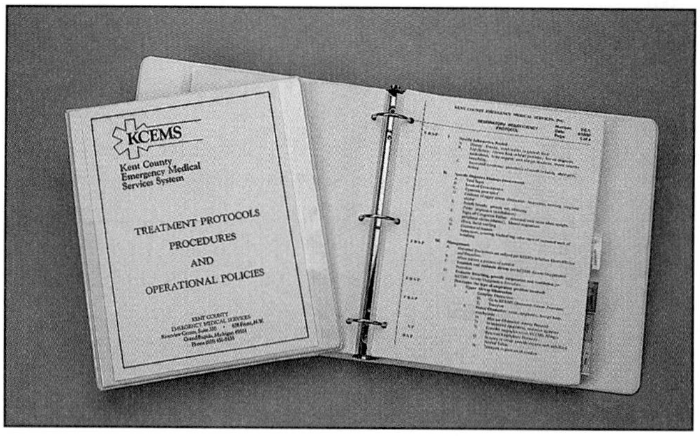

Figure 1-17

Binder containing treatment protocols, procedures, and operational policies for EMTs, developed by your medical director and members of the EMS system.

that guide the patient-care activities of your agency. **Protocols** provide a standardized approach to common patient problems and a consistent level of care for EMTs (Figure 1-17). These protocols identify what particular patient-care activities should be done in certain situations. **Standing orders** are a component of those protocols that define what care you can provide before contacting a supervising physician. For example, you will likely have standing orders to administer oxygen to a patient who is experiencing chest pain and difficulty breathing. This type of treatment occurs as a result of off-line medical direction. In this case you are allowed to provide a certain level of care without contacting a physician for approval.

Your protocols also indicate when it is necessary to contact the physician for further orders to proceed with patient care. Protocols vary among EMS systems, so it is important to regularly review the protocols governing your particular system. Your instructor will be able to inform you about your local policies and protocols. These protocols will reflect any statutes and regulations established locally or within your state. You will learn more about statutes and regulations in Chapter 2.

Another component of off-line medical direction is maintenance of the overall quality of the system (a component of retrospective medical direction). This is accomplished by establishing a system for run critique, patient-care report review, patient follow-up, continuing education, and skill review and practice.

Quality in EMS

Maintaining an efficient EMS team requires more than just initial training. Certification as an EMT-Basic should only be considered a starting point in your EMS career. Much more can be done by you and other team members to keep your system functioning at a level that enables the public to receive the highest quality care possible. The terms *quality assurance* and *quality improvement* are often used to reflect methods of reviewing the system's performance to ensure that medical care is being provided at the level desired.

Quality assurance (QA) is a process designed to continually monitor and measure the quality of clinical care provided within a system. QA uses objective data such as response times, adherence to protocols, and survival rates to document the effectiveness of the care provided. **Quality improvement** (QI) is a process that looks at the overall care provided by the EMS system. It takes the information obtained through QA, analyzes it, makes corrections, implements the corrections, and reevaluates to see if the corrections were effective.

Through QA and QI, system-wide performance reviews can be completed, identifying both the strengths and the weaknesses within the present system. If problems are identified, then a plan is put in place to correct those problems. Correction efforts are continually monitored to determine when a problem has been adequately resolved. Some specific aspects of QA and QI include the following:

- Routine peer review of patient care
- Clear documentation of any problems identified
- Gathering input from all personnel involved in patient care
- Gathering input from patients
- Using scientific data to help solve problems
- Putting processes in place to resolve system problems
- Making decisions based on facts
- Evaluating the success of quality-improvement efforts
- Providing feedback to the individuals providing care
- Recognizing, rewarding, and reinforcing good performance

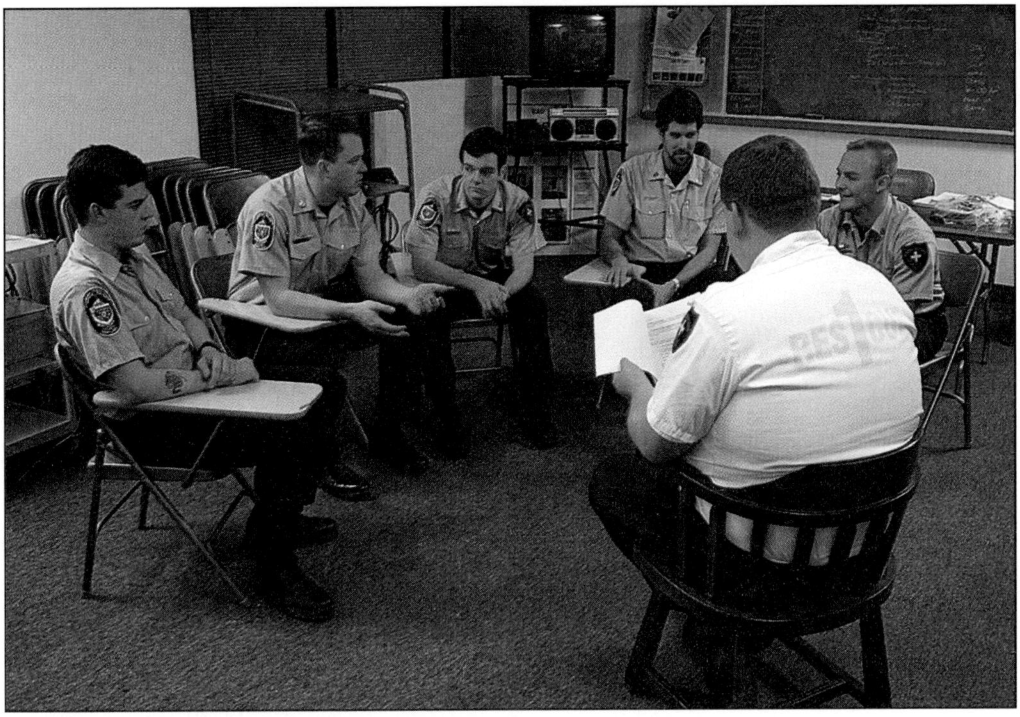

Figure 1-18

Some EMS systems use run review as part of the QA process. Run review involves analyzing calls with members of your crew and determining what went well, what could have gone more smoothly, and what improvements can be made for future calls.

Your Role in Quality Improvement

As an EMT you play a pivotal role in improving and maintaining the quality of your EMS system. Because the goal of an effective quality program is to empower field personnel to be responsible for their actions and for the success of the system as a whole, you have a great deal to offer. There are several specific ways that you can help work toward higher quality care. These include:

- Documentation: Clear, thorough data collection, such as that recorded on a patient-care report, is an excellent source of information. The patient-care report is a legal document for communicating what you noticed at the scene and any care that was provided. If the report is incomplete, then it will be of limited use when trying to make decisions about specific issues. An incomplete or inaccurate form may also be a cause for liability if you are involved in a future lawsuit. Likewise, a complete form may assist in defending the care provided if it is questioned.
- Run review: You should take the opportunity to review each call you run, especially if the call went either exceptionally well or poorly. Review the call with other members of your crew. Avoid placing blame on any individuals for things that did not go well. Instead, think of it as a larger issue that has to be resolved by the team. Have others review the run and offer opinions. In some systems an internal peer review process is used to look at all calls that the agency has (Figure 1-18). However, in other systems the volume of calls does not allow review of every call. In these cases, the peer reviewers look at a sample of calls to identify any noticeable trends.
- Quality improvement: As you become more experienced, you should consider participating on any QI committee your agency may have. Even those just completing EMT training have much to offer. For example, a system problem may be the result of inadequate training during initial EMT training or during the orientation to local policies and procedures. As a new EMT you can provide valuable information about the recent training experience that may help identify ways to correct deficiencies.
- Gathering feedback: Gathering information on the quality of care from peers, patients, and hospital staff can help make you a better EMS provider. Whether done formally or informally, this type of feedback can strengthen your skills and help you avoid future problems. In some systems patient follow-up is done by contacting recent patients and asking them to comment on the quality of the care they received. Additionally, your system may have periodic meetings with hospital staff to discuss the strengths and weaknesses they have ob-

IT'S YOUR CALL
CONCLUSION

After returning from this motor-vehicle collision, you complete your paperwork and discuss the call with others who were on the scene, focusing on both the strengths and weaknesses of the call. While most things went well, you identify a few items that could have gone better. It seems that your time on-scene was longer than you might have expected. There were some unique problems involving the safe removal of the patients from the wreckage, but there were other issues that affected scene time. Exploring this further with representatives of your QI committee, you note that there were some minor communication problems with the neighboring jurisdiction that was summoned to lend support and with the air medical team trying to pinpoint your landing zone. You believe the combination of these problems contributed to the lengthened scene time.

It is discovered that your radios were not on a compatible frequency to enable easy communications. Was this an isolated incident, or is this a system issue that requires attention? After discussing the issue with the communications center, your medical director, and local EMS and fire advisory council, new policies are written and training is provided to orient personnel to new radio procedures that are designed to help resolve the problem. A process is also put in place to monitor future calls to see whether these new efforts work adequately.

served during the normal course of receiving patients from your agency.

- Preventive maintenance: One of the first tasks you will be assigned when you arrive at your station for duty is to check the operation of the vehicle and medical equipment on your ambulances. Poorly functioning or missing equipment will prevent you from providing the quality care that is expected. Ambulance checklists are an excellent QA tool because they enable you to document the status of the units when you conduct your check. In Chapter 4 you will learn about the type of equipment on your ambulance and how to keep it functioning at peak performance.
- Continuing education: Continued training will keep you abreast of new developments in the field, and the quality of care you provide can be maintained at the expected level. Without ongoing education, your skills and knowledge will deteriorate quickly. Even among professionals who perform routine skills such as CPR, significant skill deterioration has been noted within as little as 3 months if not regularly performed.[5]
- Maintain your skills: You should practice your skills frequently in training sessions, not just on calls. Work on skills that you may not use often. This should be done with other members of your crew, if possible. This way you can work as part of a team on a simulated patient injury or illness. Patient scenarios that incorporate the need for specific skills like caring for broken bones, controlling bleeding, correcting breathing problems, performing CPR, or using an automated external defibrillator are excellent opportunities for refreshing your skills.

SUMMARY

When you become an EMT you take on many responsibilities. Top among these is the responsibility to provide the best possible patient care in all situations. This is done in a manner that provides for your safety and the safety of those around you. You become a member of a team, one that performs under the scrutiny of the public. Through your medical director, standards have been established to enable you to be successful at your job. These standards provide you with a means of caring for a variety of patients in many emergency situations. Through off-line medical direction, you can provide care without the need to contact the hospital for orders. In some cases, however, it is appropriate to contact the hospital. The physician on duty will be able to provide you with further instructions. This on-line communication will help you provide quality care.

For your EMS team to perform at peak levels, there must be a system in place to monitor performance, report results, and correct weak elements. This includes the concepts of QA and QI. Working with your medical director, hospital staff, communications division, and other out-of-hospital providers, you can play an important part in maintaining a quality system and contributing to your professional development.

REFERENCES

1. **American Association of Poison Control Centers:** *Membership directory*, 1994, Washington, American Association of Poison Control Centers.
2. **American Hospital Association:** *Hospital statistics 1994-1995,* Chicago, 1994, American Hospital Association.
3. **Cady G, Scott T:** EMS in the United States: a survey of providers in the 200 most populous cities, *J Emerg Med* 20:76, 1995.
4. **Consolidated Omnibus Budget Reconciliation Act of 1981,** Public law 97-35, August, 1981.
5. **Curry C, Gass B:** Effects of training in cardiopulmonary resuscitation on competence and patient outcome, *Can Med Assoc J* 137:491-496, 1987.
6. **Major R:** *A history of medicine*, Springfield, Md., 1954, Charles C. Thomas Publisher.
7. **National Academy of Sciences, National Research Council:** *Accidental death and disability: the neglected disease of modern society*, Washington, DC, 1966, National Academy of Sciences.
8. **National Institutes of Health, U.S. Department of Health and Human Services:** *Patient/bystander recognition and action: rapid identification and treatment of acute myocardial infarction*, Washington, DC, 1993, National Institutes of Health.
9. **National Institutes of Health, U.S. Department of Health and Human Services:** *9-1-1: Rapid identification and treatment of acute myocardial infarction*, Washington, DC, 1994, National Institutes of Health.
10. **Rideing WH:** Hospital life in New York, *Harpers New Monthly* 57:171, 1878.
11. **Stewart RD:** The history of emergency medical services. In Kuehl A, editor: *EMS medical directors handbook*, St Louis, 1989, Mosby.

Chapter

Legal and Ethical Issues

2

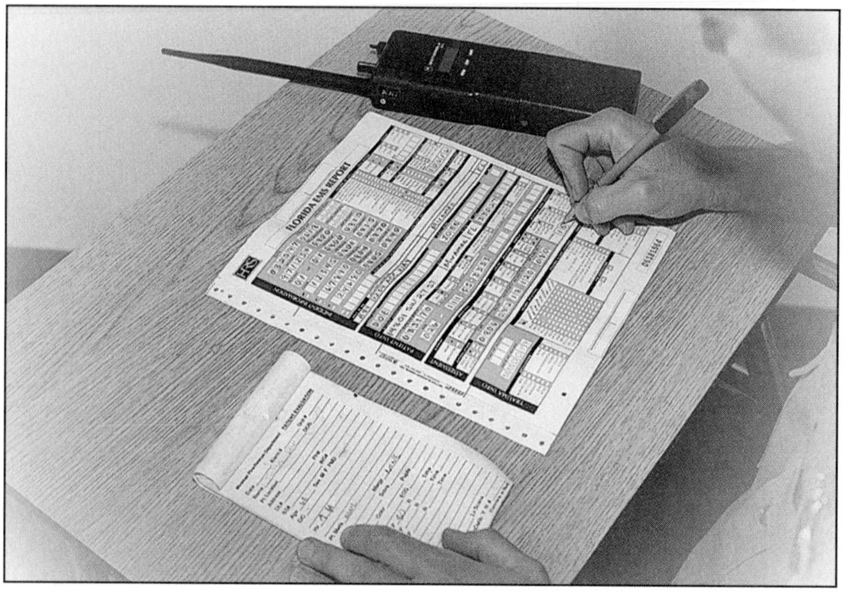

Knowledge Objectives

As an EMT-Basic, you should be able to:

OBJECTIVES

1. Describe the basic structure of the legal system.
2. Describe the standard of care as it pertains to you as an EMT.
3. Define *negligence* and describe the four elements that must be present to prove it.
4. Define your scope of practice.
5. Identify six situations that require you to report specific problems encountered on the job.
6. Explain the importance, necessity, and legality of patient confidentiality.
7. Define the types of consent and explain how consent is obtained.
8. Differentiate between expressed and implied consent.
9. Identify the steps you should take if a patient refuses care.
10. Define what constitutes abandonment.
11. Differentiate between assault and battery and describe how to avoid each.
12. Describe the conditions under which the use of force, including restraint, is acceptable.
13. Explain the purpose of advance directives relative to patient care.
14. Describe the actions you should take to preserve evidence at a crime or accident scene.
15. Discuss your responsibilities relative to resuscitation efforts for patients who are potential organ donors.

Attitude Objectives

As an EMT-Basic, you should be able to:

OBJECTIVES

1. **Describe your feelings regarding patient rights.**
2. **Describe your personal commitment to protecting the confidentiality of your patients.**
3. **Describe your personal feelings about withholding or stopping cardiopulmonary resuscitation (CPR).**
4. **Describe your personal feelings about the value of advance medical directives.**

KEY TERMS

1. **Abandonment:** Terminating patient care, without the patient's consent, at a time when there is a need for continued care by the EMT.
2. **Advance Medical Directive:** A person's written statement of preference relative to receiving medical care (e.g., do not perform CPR).
3. **Confidentiality:** The duty of the EMT not to disclose information revealed by the patient during care.
4. **Expressed Consent:** A patient's verbal or written consent to accept treatment; requires informed consent.
5. **Implied Consent:** Consent granted by virtue of law for a patient who is unconscious or otherwise unable to communicate a desire to receive medical care or who is a minor patient.
6. **Informed Consent:** Patient consent indicating that he or she has been informed of, understands, and agrees to receive the care to be rendered.
7. **Negligence:** Failure to act in a reasonable manner that thus results in harm to another person. There are four components that must be present for negligence to be proved.
8. **Scope of Practice:** Defined medical actions that are allowed to be performed by a licensed or certified health care provider.
9. **Standard of Care:** The level of care expected of the EMT based on education, laws, court decisions, local protocols, policies, and procedures.

IT'S YOUR CALL

On a cool, rainy evening, a vehicle traveling at high speed is involved in a roll-over collision, coming to rest upright in a ditch. Upon your arrival, bystanders state that the driver is on the floor of the vehicle. You determine that the patient, a 33-year-old male, is conscious, lying face down on the floor, complaining of a headache and back pain. He does not remember much about the collision. He is able to move his limbs without pain.

You recognize the need for further patient evaluation at the scene and rapid transport to the hospital. Because of the rain, you feel that it would be easier to perform a more thorough examination in the dry environment of the ambulance. The car is dismantled to allow easier access to the patient. Your protocols call for this patient to be fully immobilized, face up on a backboard. Every attempt your team makes to carefully immobilize this patient results in greater pain. The patient states that he is most comfortable lying face down.

Finally, you are able to remove the patient and place him supine on a backboard. As this is done, the patient suddenly experiences severe back pain and numbness in his legs. He continues to experience these symptoms during transport to the hospital and upon admission to the emergency department.

Nearly 6 months later, you receive notice from a lawyer representing the patient. The patient is suing you, your partner, your ambulance company, and the city that employs the ambulance company. He alleges that your actions were negligent, resulting in additional injury, prolonged hospitalization, and ongoing medical problems that may never resolve. He questions your actions on the evening that you provided care for him. He wants to know whether your actions were common practice and within established guidelines for proper patient care. He is questioning the initial training you received as an EMT, as well as any training you may have received from your employer. People are going to try to prove that you violated established protocols for patient care. You are going to have to respond to allegations that there were more appropriate ways to care for this patient. What do you think? Were your actions appropriate, or did you fail to follow reasonable guidelines for care?

Your role as an EMT is unique. It is a mixture of training and personal actions, which are guided by protocols that enable you to provide appropriate emergency care in a variety of out-of-hospital settings. To better understand your role as an EMT, you need to understand the medical, legal, and ethical parameters of your job. A thorough understanding can lead you to a more fulfilling career as a health care professional.

Understandably, you may be concerned about the possibility of being involved in a future lawsuit; public servants are increasingly frequent targets for lawsuits. Lawsuits against out-of-hospital emergency care providers have resulted primarily from collisions involving the operation of emergency vehicles. Claims involving patient care tend to occur more frequently in cases of spinal injury, heart problems, intoxicated patients, and nontransport decisions. Fortunately, lawsuits against EMTs are not as frequent as those against personnel at more advanced levels. In addition, lawsuits are rarely successful if you follow some general guidelines. Awareness of the legal principles that guide your actions can help you prevent future legal action. This chapter addresses the legal principles that concern the emergency care that you will render.

The Legal System

Legal systems have always been an important part of civilized society. A legal system is a set of laws and the structure to support and administer those laws as adopted by a particular society. The legal system in the United States helps resolve conflicts and punish individuals who violate the law. As our society becomes more complex, there will be increasingly greater reliance on the legal system to guide proper conduct.

Sources of Law

There are several sources of law in the U.S. These include federal and state constitutions, regulations by legislative bodies, and decisions of federal and state courts. This means that there are many separate lawmaking governmental groups: the states and territories and the federal government.

Constitutional law is a form of law based on the U.S. Constitution and each state's constitution, which is subject to compliance to the federal Constitution. An important aspect of constitutional law is that no state may enact a law that denies a person the protection, rights, and privileges established by the U.S. Constitution. Some specific provisions of the U.S. Constitution, which are important legal principles pertaining to EMS, can be found in the Fourteenth Amendment. These include the rights of a patient to privacy, to refuse medical treatment, and to be free from racial discrimination. In addition, EMTs have procedural protection (due process) that must be afforded if disciplinary action is being used. For example, an employee has the right to a hearing before he can be dismissed from service.

Other forms of law include statutes, ordinances, and resolutions. Statutes are established by Congress, the legislative branch of the federal government, and state legislatures. Ordinances and resolutions are often enacted by municipalities, counties, and cities. These local laws are subject to the higher laws of state and federal statutes and constitutions. This means a local law may impose more restrictive conditions than those set by federal or state law but cannot be in conflict with or more lenient than the conditions established by state or federal law.

A governmental agency, such as a state EMS office, exists as a result of a statute. This statute establishes the agency and defines its structure, power, and responsibilities. Among the powers of an agency is the authority to create **regulations.** These regulations establish the means by which the agency operates and fulfills its responsibilities. For example, a statute that empowers an EMS agency to certify persons as EMTs may include regulations on the specific procedural steps, forms, and length of certification that apply in that particular state.

Regulations have the authority of law, but if they conflict with the state statute, the statute overrides. Some state statutes are very detailed and lengthy with little left to regulations. Other states have more general statutes with very detailed regulations. Only the legislature can change a statute; however, regulations can be created and changed by an agency after a public hearing.

Another form of law is **common law,** also known as *case law* or *judge-made law.* Common law results from the acceptance of customs and norms in our society over time. These norms are reflected in the decisions of judges and help set precedent for similar future court cases. It is important to remember that common law can change over time. A precedent that is appropriate today may not be appropriate 10 years from now as societal values change.

The ability of common law to change is important for EMS. There are very few federal statutes or precedents in common law that directly apply to out-of-hospital emergency medical care. So there is also some uncertainty as to how a court may interpret EMS-related statutes or the actions of an EMT. As EMS changes, there will also be changes in common law, and new precedents will be established.

The Judicial System

The American legal system is divided into two areas: criminal and civil. Criminal law refers to crimes, which are acts committed or omitted in violation of a public law. A criminal case is prosecuted by an attorney for the government on behalf of the people of the community. Violation of these laws can result in fines, imprisonment, or both.

Civil law (also known as *tort law*) is private law that governs any two persons or entities, such as corporations. Tort is a legal term used in civil law; it refers to civil claims involving any wrongful act or injury done by a private person in a careless or reckless manner against another person or his or her property, resulting in injury or damage. A claim of negligence is a tort action.

The major difference between a crime and a tort is that a crime is an offense against the state in which the state prosecutes the individual, whereas a tort is a civil (private) wrong in which the wronged person must bring a civil lawsuit against the individual in an attempt to recover damages.

One form of civil law is administrative law. This pertains to a governmental agency's authority to enforce pertinent regulations and statutes of the agency. As an EMT, you are granted a certificate by a state agency. Any violation of the conditions and provisions of the certificate are typically reviewed in an administrative proceeding in front of an administrative law judge. If there is evidence of a violation of the provisions of the certificate, such as fraud in obtaining the certificate or substandard patient care, the certificate may be revoked. It is important to remember that certification as an EMT entitles you to perform out-of-hospital emergency care, but that you will only retain your certification as long as you comply with your state regulatory standards.

Legal Accountability

There are several legal claims that can be brought against you as a result of your professional conduct. At the onset of any civil action, the **plaintiff** has to prove that you (the **defendant**) failed to provide proper care and that your actions resulted in injury. In most jurisdictions, the mere occurrence of an error or poor outcome does not prove that care was improper. Two important legal principles are standard of care and negligence.

Standard of Care

The public expects a certain level of performance from prehospital personnel. This level is often referred to as the **standard of care**—the level of care expected of the EMT, based on education, laws, court decisions, and local protocols, policies, and procedures. EMTs are not held to the same standard of care as physicians, nurses, or paramedics. The standard of care for EMTs is based on the training guidelines developed by the U.S. Department of Transportation (DOT) and by the states and municipalities in which they serve. In this manner, the standard of care is fairly consistent across state lines.

As an EMT you are expected to act in accordance with state laws and regulations and the **medical direction** provided through your local EMS agency. The medical direction that you receive will be incorporated into a set of local protocols, policies, and procedures that you must follow. The standard of care is subject to change, however, because of research and field experiences that improve patient outcome. Because of this, the knowledge and skills that you learn initially must be maintained to continue practice within the standard of care. This can be accomplished by frequent continuing education and recertification training.

Negligence

Negligence is the failure to follow a reasonable standard of care, resulting in damage to another. A person could be negligent either by acting wrongly or failing to act at all. The plaintiff must establish four elements to prove negligence:

1. Duty to act
2. Breach of duty
3. Damages
4. Proximate cause

A closer look at each element will help better illustrate negligence. First, it must be proven that the defendant (EMT) had a **duty to act.** An EMT is usually obligated to render care to a patient because of his position of employment or membership with an EMS agency. An EMS agency, such as a private ambulance company that contracts to provide ambulance service for a city, has a legal obligation to provide emergency medical care to the citizens of that community.

Certification as an EMT does not by itself create a duty to act. The duty to act is linked with the agreement to provide care as part of an EMS agency. Consequently, in most states, an off-duty EMT does not have a legal obligation to render aid to a stranger. The exception to this is if a state statute requires a person to render aid in emergency circumstances.

The plaintiff must also prove that the defendant breached the duty to act. A **breach of duty** occurs if the defendant fails to act as a reasonable person would have acted under the same or similar circumstances. An EMT is expected to anticipate whether or not his or her actions would result in harm to a patient. For example, as an EMT you have a duty to properly apply a cervical collar to a patient with a possible spinal injury because this is the standard of care. It is reasonable to assume that failure to properly apply the collar could result in harm to the patient. Similarly, there is a duty to examine the patient and stabilize the spine before attempting to move the patient. If you fail to perform this, you may have breached your duty.

The third element of negligence is **damage.** For negligence to be proven, some type of injury must have occurred. It could be loss of limb or life, injury to reputation or character, or mental anguish suffered by an individual. Compensation for damages must be written within the law. The courts generally award the plaintiff money to cover damages such as loss of limb, pain and suffering, or reimbursement of medical expenses.

The final element of negligence is **proximate cause,** referring to the relationship between the breach of duty and the damages. Simply stated, there must be a cause-and-effect relationship between the breach of duty and the damage suffered by the plaintiff; the breach of duty must have caused the injury. Sometimes the cause is obvious, as when a patient is dropped from a stretcher and suffers back pain that was not initially present. Other times the cause is not as obvious and not as easily linked to the actions of the EMT. Consider the case of a patient in a motor vehicle collision who claims that the failure of the EMT to properly administer oxygen resulted in greater damage to the patient. In this situation it would be necessary to know the extent of the initial injury. It would also be necessary to prove that the failure to properly administer oxygen contributed to the extent of the injury.

When determining whether a person's actions have been negligent, the courts consider the specific facts of each case. For example, factors such as the physical environment and the degree of cooperation of the patient are considered. The standard of care is then judged by what a reasonable person with similar experience and training would have done under the same circumstances or similar circumstances.

Laws Affecting EMTs

You are able to function as an EMT because of statutes that help guide your actions. These statutes help ensure that quality care is provided and may act as safeguards to help protect you in your profession. You are not authorized to practice medicine. Instead, a physician delegates certain procedures that you can perform. This practice of delegation forms the basis for the first provision to be reviewed—the scope of practice.

Scope of Practice

Every state has statutes that provide for an EMS regulatory body and describe the licensure or certification of EMTs. These statutes also identify the specific medical procedures and functions that an EMT can perform. State regulations require that only persons meeting certain qualifications are granted licensure or certification to provide those medical procedures in an out-of-hospital setting.

Your actions as a health care provider are subject to the scope of practice. **Scope of practice** is defined as legally authorized medical acts that may be performed within established state law. EMTs are allowed to engage in limited medical care, usually delegated by physicians designated to supervise out-of-hospital emergency care. You often operate under the direction of a specific **medical director** who provides supervision and oversees the out-of-hospital EMS system in which you function. As explained earlier, placing EMTs under the umbrella of medical direction is still a new concept for some states.

The scope of practice for EMTs varies somewhat from state to state. EMTs may perform certain advanced procedures, such as automated external defibrillation or the administration of select medications, if there are protocols established for those procedures. It will be your responsibility to have a clear understanding of your scope of practice. Acting beyond or in violation of these statutory provisions may constitute an unauthorized practice of medicine. This could be a source of civil liability and administrative action by the state EMS lead agency. For this reason you must be thoroughly familiar with the scope of practice allowed in your own state.

Emergency Driving

Driving an emergency vehicle in an emergency mode presents a number of dangers, even under the best of conditions (Figure 2-1). The use of red lights and sirens is in-

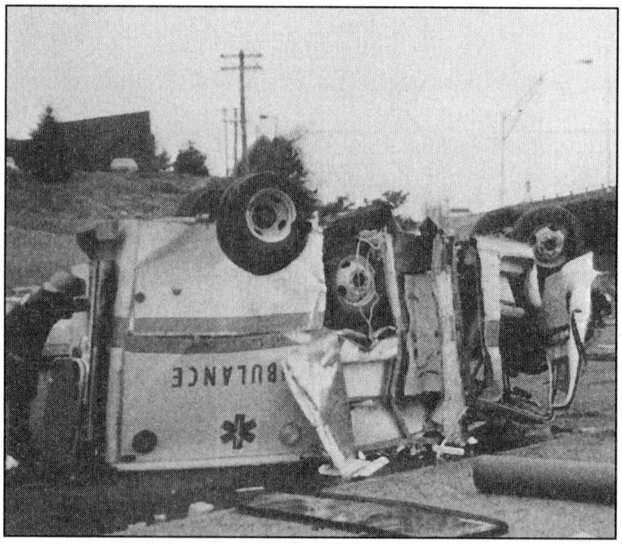

Figure 2-1

Most lawsuits against EMTs have resulted from collisions involving the operation of emergency vehicles. Even under good conditions, driving an ambulance presents a number of dangers.

tended to provide emergency vehicles special use of the roadway. It is important to note, however, that this does not automatically grant EMS providers the right of way. Never operate the vehicle in an emergency mode unless there is an emergency. When operating an emergency vehicle, you may be allowed to exceed the speed limit in limited situations. State statutes often allow an authorized emergency vehicle to be exempt from speed limits, parking restrictions, and traffic signals. But the operator of an emergency vehicle must always exercise caution when operating a vehicle in an emergency mode (Figure 2-2). In some states the operator of an ambulance is held to a standard of extreme caution, not just reasonable care.

Liability may be established if any of the following occur:

- Emergency driving contributes to the injury of a patient or other persons.
- The driver of the ambulance fails to exercise care in driving, such as failure to stop before proceeding through an intersection.
- The operator is driving too fast for weather conditions.

Emergency driving is increasingly becoming subject to criticism because there is some question that operating a vehicle in emergency status to or from a call improves patient outcome. Because different states allow different exemptions and place different responsibilities on drivers of emergency vehicles, you must know your state statutes pertaining to emergency driving.

Reporting Requirements

Most states have statutes that require reporting certain problems or conditions, including any of the following circumstances:

- Suspected child abuse
- Suspected spouse abuse
- Suspected elder abuse
- Infectious diseases
- Sexual assault
- Animal bites
- Violent acts (gunshot wounds, stabbings)
- Death from any cause

Failure to report observations or knowledge of such situations can result in civil and criminal liability. The person who reports such matters needs to have a reasonable suspicion that the event occurred and must make the report in good faith. Most states require you to report cases of suspected child abuse and will grant immunity from civil liability to those persons reporting child abuse in good faith.[8]

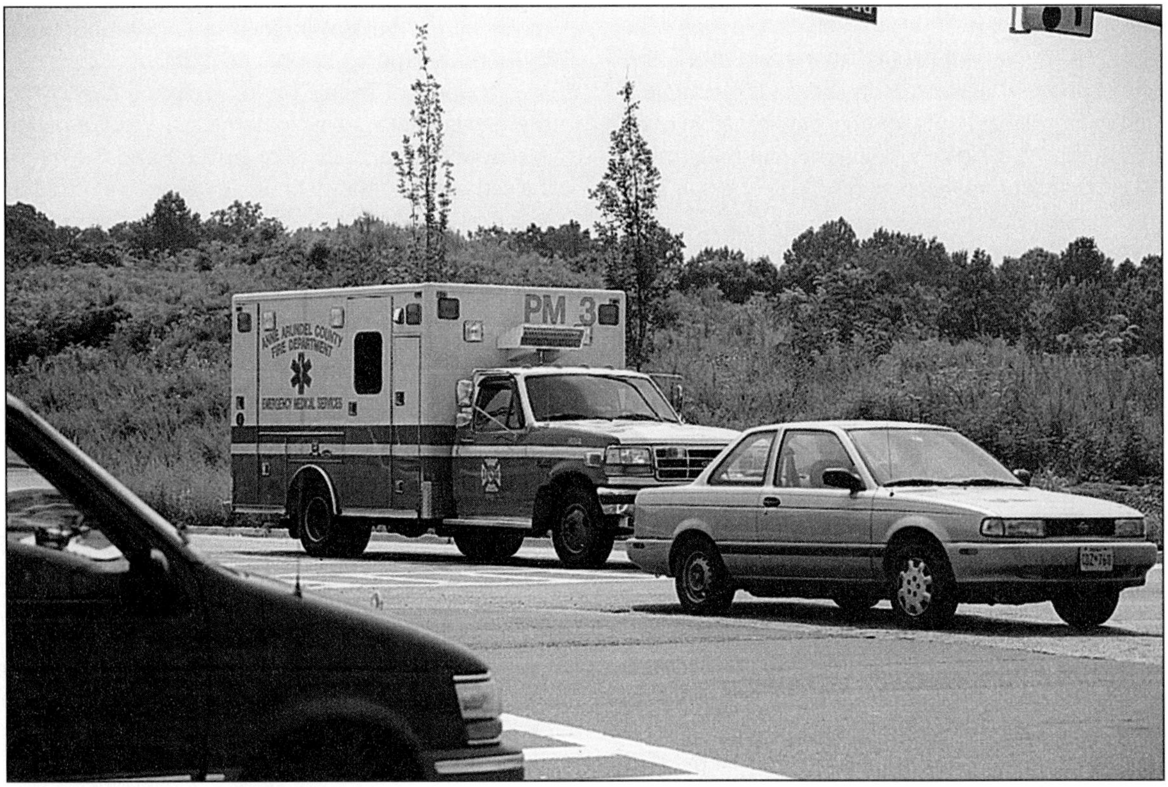

Figure 2-2

Operators of emergency vehicles must always exercise caution while driving.

Protection for the EMT

There are different state statutes that offer EMTs some form of protection against liability. The concept of the **Good Samaritan Law** has been incorporated into state statutes as an incentive for bystanders to provide medical assistance to injured victims. To encourage people to provide help, the victim is not allowed to seek damages from injuries caused by careless actions that may have worsened the victim's condition. In addition, the person rendering care is not entitled to seek payment for the services rendered.

A layperson and in some states a health care worker (e.g., EMT) who is under no obligation to help can claim protection under the Good Samaritan Law when rendering assistance, as long as the care provided is appropriate to the circumstances. In most states, Good Samaritan provisions only provide protection when services are free. Some states, however, provide alternative liability protection if the paid, on-duty EMT renders care outside of a hospital or physician's office. Others specifically state that you are entitled to immunity whenever acting under the supervision of a medical director. The immunity for off-duty EMTs is covered by Good Samaritan legislation.

Governmental immunity is a form of protection from liability that is afforded to the publicly employed EMT. It is actually designed to protect government entities from the negligent actions of their employees. Not every state provides this immunity, and the statutes that exist are subject to limitations. For example, the statute may only protect employees when using specific equipment; operation of a motor vehicle is not usually covered. The doctrine generally does not protect an off-duty EMT.

One limitation in almost every immunity statute is that immunity is provided only for acts performed in good faith. Actions that you know will cause harm are considered reckless or intentional acts and will likely result in liability.

Infectious Disease. Every health care provider should be alert to the risks of infectious disease transmission. Since the increased awareness of bloodborne infectious diseases such as hepatitis B and human immunodeficiency virus (HIV), many statutes have been enacted pertaining to the testing, sharing of information, and management of patients and rescuers involved with patients with infectious diseases. The Ryan White Act of 1990 is a federal law that requires health care facilities to notify an emergency responder who transports a patient to the facility if it is discovered that the patient is infected with a communicable disease.[11] Many states have enacted statutes that pertain to reporting confirmed exposure to infectious diseases. EMS personnel, firefighters, and law enforcement personnel may be authorized by state statute to request a patient's infectious status or to request testing of patients transported by ambulance if there is reason to believe that a significant bloodborne exposure has occurred. This is to be done in a confidential manner to protect the rights of the patient and the health care provider.

Patient Relationship

You are responsible for forming a positive relationship with your patient whenever possible. This means asking for permission to provide care, protecting confidential information, and respecting a patient's wish to refuse treatment.

Confidentiality

Working as an EMT, you will be told very personal information by patients; this information is considered privileged. The manner in which you use and protect a patient's medical information is of critical importance. It does not matter if this information comes directly from the patient, from others, or from a written record on transfer documents. You have an obligation to protect medical information about a patient. **Confidentiality** refers to the patient's right to expect that what he or she tells you in trust will not be disclosed. The medical information you acquire and document in a written report should not be revealed to persons not involved in the patient's care unless the patient authorizes disclosure.

However, there are circumstances when it is appropriate for you to share the patient's medical information. You may disclose medical information to other EMS providers and hospital staff who are responsible for the patient's care. Confidential medical information should be disclosed if it will help personnel assess and manage the patient's medical needs. This is also true of statements made by the patient indicating an intention to harm either another person or his or her self.

A claim of **invasion of privacy** can be brought if there was disclosure of information about a patient with a reasonable expectation of privacy and if that disclosure caused harm to the patient. An example would be the release of a patient's diagnosis of an infectious disease to anyone other than those caring for him, causing the patient to suffer embarrassment or loss of employment. The plaintiff does not need to prove any malicious intent on the part of the person who released the information. Instead, the claim of invasion of privacy is based on the unauthorized release of confidential or private information. Release of the patient care report to a patient's employer without a subpoena or permission of the patient could give rise to such a claim.

Consent

Consent is the verbal or written acceptance of medical treatment. In the U.S. individuals have the right to accept or refuse medical treatment. This right has been recognized as a constitutionally protected interest since 1914.[10] In a nonemergency situation the patient is allowed to decide whether or not to accept or reject medical treatment. In a life-threatening emergency other principles of law define how consent is granted. Understanding these principles and the different forms of consent is important to avoid liability.

Forms of Consent

The same principles of consent that are applied to the medical profession are generally applied to the out-of-hospital emergency care setting. There are several forms of consent that you should be familiar with, including:

- Informed consent
- Expressed consent
- Involuntary consent
- Implied consent

Informed consent is patient consent indicating that he or she understands and agrees to the care that is going to be rendered. The patient must receive sufficient information that a reasonable person would need to make an informed decision. Otherwise the patient's consent may be considered invalid. The extent of information that must be provided varies with the circumstances of the patient encounter. Usually, informed consent requires that the patient be aware of:

- The nature of the injury or illness
- The intended treatment and risks associated with that treatment
- The danger of refusing treatment

Once the patient understands what treatment will be provided and the consequences of accepting or refusing such treatment, the patient can give informed consent to continue.

Expressed (actual) consent is voluntary, verbal, or written patient consent that indicates a willingness to accept treatment. The patient is seldom asked to sign a written consent form in out-of-hospital care. Instead, he or she verbally expresses consent.

Another form of consent is **involuntary consent.** In a case of involuntary consent, permission to provide care is granted by the authority of law, regardless of the patient's desire. Examples of situations in which this type of consent applies are:

- Individuals being held for mental health evaluation
- Mentally or physically incompetent persons for whom a guardian has been appointed
- Persons under alcohol treatment orders
- Prisoners in need of treatment

Most states have enacted laws that authorize police or other professionals, such as physicians, psychologists, or social workers, to place people under involuntary treatment holds (such as alcohol treatment orders or mental health evaluations). These laws are subject to important conditions and limitations. There must be facts—not speculation or unfounded fear—that the patient is dangerous to his or her self or others. The patient may be held involuntarily until evaluated by a physician. Immunity is usually afforded to persons who act in good faith when using these statutes to take a person into custody involuntarily, including the EMT who complies with a police order. You should seek medical direction from your supervising physician in cases where you may need involuntary consent.

The final form of consent is **implied consent,** which presumes that an unconscious or mentally impaired person would consent to lifesaving treatment if he or she could do so. In such circumstances, common law provides for treatment to be rendered despite the absence of the patient's expressed consent. Implied consent is extended to situations involving children; the law assumes that parents or guardians would want lifesaving care provided to their children, if they could not be reached.

IT'S YOUR CALL
CONTINUED

In the case study at the beginning of this chapter, the plaintiff claimed that you and your team were negligent while providing care. Are the four components of negligence present?

Let's look at the case study again. It is clear that you had a duty to act. It is also clear that the patient suffered further injury while under your care. What is not clear, however, is whether you breached your duty. According to your training and local protocols, the patient should be placed in an immobilization device, transferred, and secured to a backboard in a face-up position. You did what you had been trained to do. You moved the patient cautiously while removing him from the vehicle. You removed as much of the car as possible to gain access to the patient, but did you fully live up to the standard of care? What other options were available?

Special Situations

In addition to the various types of consent, there are several unique situations that could create liability for an EMT.

Minors. The patient's age must also be considered when trying to obtain consent. An adult may give consent to medical treatment, but the age at which this can occur varies from state to state. In Alabama, for example, a person age 14 or older may consent to medical treatment. But in most states, 18 is the age of consent.[2] Legally, the minor is considered to lack the capacity to consent to or refuse care. It is generally believed that a minor cannot understand the consequences of such a decision. Most states allow only the parent or legal guardian to give consent on behalf of the child (Figure 2-3). Either parent can consent; however, if the parents are divorced, usually only the custodial parent may provide consent.

Some states also allow a person who is a minor but married or in the armed services to consent to treatment as an adult. An unmarried, teenage mother is generally

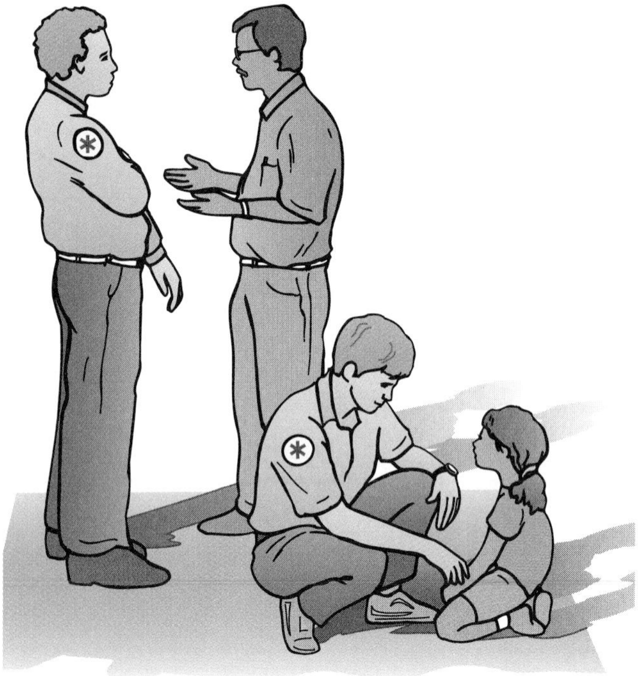

Figure 2-3

In a non–life-threatening situation, consent to provide care for a child must first be obtained from the child's parent or legal guardian.

allowed to consent to treatment for her child. Minors living on their own without financial dependence on their parents are also considered adults. In some states, college students who are minors are considered adults for purposes of medical treatment, even if they are still financially dependent on their parents. In each of these situations minors are said to be *emancipated* for the limited purpose of consenting to medical treatment.

The determination of **emancipation** can be difficult. There may be a court document acknowledging emancipation, but more likely there is not. This leaves you in the position of questioning the individual and collecting as much information as possible to verify the minor's status. In most jurisdictions, if minors misrepresent their age or emancipation status but consent to and receive treatment, the courts will not permit them or their parents to subsequently deny the consent. However, if you allow a minor to refuse treatment and then leave the scene without leaving the minor in the custody of police, social services, or another legally recognized surrogate parent, you will likely be questioned about your actions.

You should never refuse to evaluate an ill or injured child because the parent is not present. If a child is found unattended it would be inappropriate to leave the child stranded merely because the child's condition is not life-threatening.[14] Always protect the best interests of the child. In this way your actions are likely defensible.

Most states have legislation that prohibits an adult guardian from denying a child emergency medical treatment and consider such conduct to be child abuse, child neglect, or criminal negligence unless that refusal is based on religious beliefs. In such a case, a court order is required before care can be provided. While guardians are typically allowed to make treatment decisions for the child, including refusal of treatment, this is only good until the refusal threatens the life of the child.

Refusal of Care. Some patients, even those who clearly need emergency care, may refuse your help. We presume that an adult is competent to make decisions regarding medical treatment. This means the patient can understand the consequences of various treatment options, consider alternatives, and choose to accept or reject treatment.[10] In most situations you will be able to determine the patient's ability to provide consent and can either begin patient care or honor the patient's refusal. However, there may be circumstances in which the patient's decision-making capacity is not obvious. In these situations you should act in accordance with your protocols for managing consent situations. Because of the complexity of such situations you should involve physician input whenever possible. EMTs should not make this decision independently. By approaching consent matters in a systematic fashion, you are less likely to make mistakes (Box 2-1).

Question the patient to determine if he or she is alert, oriented, and able to adequately hear what you are saying. Next, verify that the patient understands the information by asking why he or she is refusing treatment. This may help you evaluate the ability of the patient to think rationally or logically. For example, if a patient says he or she can arrange to be taken to the hospital by calling a friend for a condition that is not immediately life-threatening, this reasoning seems appropriate. On the other hand, if he or she is not able to move without assistance and there is no telephone available, such an option is not logical or reasonable, and the patient's decision-making capacity appears to be impaired. Questioning the patient's decision to refuse care may reveal underlying issues of fear, money, religion, confusion about the decision, or lack of understanding of the situation.

Essential documentation in patient refusal situations includes:

- The patient's physical signs and symptoms, including vital signs, and description of the scene
- Information from the caller (if not the patient) or reason EMS was contacted
- Summary of the options discussed with the patient (transport by ambulance, private car, or other means)
- The patient's stated reason for rejecting treatment or transport
- The information given to the patient regarding the risks and consequences of not receiving treatment or transport to the hospital
- Your observations or patient statements indicating the patient understands the risks and consequences

- Instructions or direction from the medical control physician about the patient's refusal
- The patient's signature, if possible, acknowledging an understanding of the information that has been communicated to the patient

Clarifying the situation for the patient may change the patient's decision. Talk to the patient in simple words that are easily understood. Factors such as alcohol use, age, medications, anxiety, illness, injury, language barriers, and intelligence all must be considered when evaluating the patient's decision-making capacity.

Refusal of care is particularly difficult when the patient is unable to make medical treatment decisions and does not have a life-threatening injury. The state of Florida allows EMS personnel to take patients into protective custody for medical or psychiatric evaluation. Most states only allow for this when the patient is a minor, legally incompetent, or mentally ill. Some states allow physicians to exercise control in limited circumstances if patient consent is not obtainable. Therefore you need to know your local protocols and contact your supervising physician for advice. You should also contact law enforcement personnel for assistance with these patients.

There may simply be times when a competent adult insists on refusing treatment even though he or she is seriously ill or injured. If you are unable to convince such a person of the need for medical care after repeated attempts, you should honor the request. In such situations you should seek medical direction, request the assistance of more advanced EMS providers, and document the circumstances in writing. This documentation should include witnesses' statements with signatures and addresses.

Nontransport Decisions. Situations in which nontransport decisions are made should be carefully reviewed. It is often alleged that the EMT failed to assess the patient adequately or failed to adequately warn the patient of the risks of not being transported to a hospital.

Whenever possible, document your observations and findings while you are still at the scene. This will provide the most reliable information if your actions are questioned later. Taking the time to document information also allows additional time to observe the patient. Patients can change their minds about transport. If you are overly eager to leave the scene, the patient is not likely to perceive the need to seek medical treatment. Reassure the patient that changing his mind is acceptable.

Document your assessment findings, the need for further medical care, and the patient's stated reason for refusing transport. Inform the patient that EMS can be accessed at any time should the patient change his or her mind. Attempt to have the patient sign a waiver on the patient care report or a separate patient refusal sheet stating that he or she is refusing assessment, treatment, or transport (Figure 2-4). This is helpful because it gives objective information about the patient. The ability of the pa-

BOX 2-1 Dos and Don'ts of Patient Care Refusal

Dos

Conduct yourself in a professional and compassionate manner. To do this you must:

- Be courteous to patients who reject an offer of treatment or transport.
- Try to determine the reason(s) the patient does not accept the treatment or transport by ambulance. Patients may be frightened by contact with emergency personnel, worried about expense, or deny the urgency of the situation.
- Evaluate the patient sufficiently to determine the urgency or seriousness of the patient's condition.
- Assess the patient's ability to understand the medical condition and the information you communicated.
- Determine if the patient is capable of accessing assistance or taking actions for his or her own well-being (e.g., reaching a telephone, safely driving a vehicle).
- Encourage appropriate medical follow-up or access to EMS if the patient feels he or she needs medical assistance.
- Be familiar with and act consistent with your own agency protocols and local and state laws.
- Summon advanced life-support personnel whenever necessary.
- Contact your on-line physician when there is any question.
- Document the reasons for patient refusal; have the patient sign the refusal documentation.
- Obtain a witness' signature when possible.

Don'ts

Besides those things that you must do, there are also things that you should *not* do:

- Do not ignore clues to potentially serious injuries or illnesses, such as abnormal signs and symptoms, or statements of family or witnesses.
- Do not insult or embarrass a patient for refusing to accept treatment.
- Do not assume a patient who is intoxicated has no other injuries or medical needs.
- Do not ignore protocols and input from your medical control physician.

AGENCY	UNIT #		MEDCOM NUMBER
NAME		ADDRESS	DATE / DAY
PATIENT PHONE / AGE / D.O.B.		SEX M ☐ F ☐ / RACE / SSN _ _ _ – _ _ – _ _ _ _	COMPLAINT NO.
INCIDENT LOCATION	CODE	DISPATCH/"CHIEF COMPLAINT"	REPORTING POLICE DEPARTMENT

STATUS	TIME	BLOOD PRES.	PULSE RATE	PULSE QUAL.	RESP. RATE	RESP. QUAL.	SKIN	PUPILS	GCS E(4)	GCS V(5)	GCS M(6)	AVPU	PO_x	PRTY

COUNTY

TWP/CITY/VILLAGE

EST. TIME — INCIDENT T.O.C.

Dispatch

En route

Arr. Scene

Arr. Patient

Dep. Scene

Arr. Hosp.

MED. HX. ALLERGIES

CURRENT MEDS.

NARRATIVE

FORM COMPLETED BY: #

MECHANISM OF INJURY FACTORS:

- ☐ Ejected from Vehicle
- ☐ MVA w/Fatals at Scene
- ☐ Extrication > 20 Minutes
- ☐ Major Vehicle Damage
- ☐ Unrestrained
- ☐ MCA without Helmet
- ☐ Fall > 6 Feet
- ☐ Not Applicable

I.V. SITE: ______ # ATTEMPTS ______ BY # ______ EST. BY # ______ SIZE ______ TIME ______ RATE ______ TOTAL INFUSED ______

DRUGS	DRUG	TIME	DOSE	ROUTE	MEDIC #	AUTH (SO,MC,POS)

MEDICAL CONTROL PHYSICIAN

PAGE ____ OF ____

AMBULANCE PERSONNEL	No./Level	OTHER AGENCY PERSONNEL	No./Level
1.		1.	
2.		2.	
3.		3.	
4.		4.	

OTHERS WITH DIRECT PT. CONTACT

Name	Phone No.

RELEASE OF LIABILITY
REFUSAL TO CONSENT TO TREATMENT

I, the undersigned, have been advised that medical assistance on my or the patient's behalf is necessary and that my refusal to allow such assistance may result in death or endanger my or the patient's health. I have been advised of and fully understand the nature of the risks I am taking by refusing medical assistance. I assume all responsibility for the consequences of my decision.

I hereby release ______________________________ and any and all persons employed by or responding with them from any and all liability which arises now or may arise in the future from the consequences of this refusal of emergency medical care and/or transportation to the hospital. This liability is binding on anyone acting on my behalf, personally or on behalf of my estate. This release is signed in consideration of the fact that I have: (Please check appropriate box or boxes)

☐ refused emergency medical care offered to me or the patient

☐ refused transport to a medical facility which was offered to me or the patient

☐ refused transport to the nearest hospital after being advised that the welfare of the patient required prompt emergency care

WITNESSED BY:

PATIENT SIGNATURE OR IF A MINOR, PARENT OR LEGAL GUARDIAN

Signature ______________________

Address/Phone ______________________

Signature ______________________

Address/Phone ______________________

____

Address ______________________

Age of Pt. ______________________ Ambulance Dept. No.

Figure 2-4

EMS refusal of care/transportation form.

Name:________________________________ Age:________ Date:______________

Location of Call:________________________________ Report #:______________

A. Assessment of Patient (Complete each item, circle appropriate response)

1. Oriented to: Person? Yes No Place? Yes No Time? Yes No Situation? Yes No
2. Altered level of consciousness? Yes No
3. Head injury? Yes No
4. Alcohol or drug ingestion by exam or history? Yes No
5. Vital Signs obtained Yes No
6. EMS Treatment indicated Yes No
7. EMS Transport indicated Yes No

B. Medical Control

Contacted by: ____ Phone ____ Radio at _____ hours

____ Unable to contact (explain in comments section)

____ Contact not indicated

Orders:

____ Indicated treatment and/or transport may be refused by patient.

____ Use reasonable force and/or restraint to provide indicated treatment.

____ Use reasonable force and/or restraint to transport.

Other orders or information: ________________________________

C. Patient Advised (Complete each item, circle appropriate response)

Yes No Seek medical care on own.

Yes No Recontact EMS if condition worsens.

Yes No Medical treatment/evaluation needed.

Yes No Ambulance transport needed.

Yes No Further harm could result without medical treatment/evaluation.

Yes No Transport by means other than ambulance could be hazardous in light of patients' present illness/injury.

D. Disposition

____ Refused all EMS services.

____ Refused transport, accepted field treatment.

____ Refused field treatment, accepted transport.

____ Released in care or custody of self.

____ Release in custody of law enforcement agency.

Agency: ______________________ Officer: ______________________

____ Released in care or custody of: ____ Relative ____ Friend

Name: ______________________ Relationship: ____________

Yes No Patient provided with EMS Refusal Information Sheet.

Yes No Patient would not accept EMS Refusal Information Sheet.

E. Comments: (Use back of page if additional space is needed)________________________________

____

____

Signature of Provider ______________________________ Date ______________

Signature of Supervisor ______________________________ Date ______________

Figure 2-4, cont'd

Sample of a Kent County EMS patient refusal check list.

tient to follow commands, hold a pen, and write his or her name is an indication of the patient's mental state. However, if the patient staggers when standing, is unable to hold a pen without dropping it, and cannot find the signature line on the page, the refusal may not be appropriate.

Abandonment. Another claim that can arise from the patient relationship is that of abandonment. A patient generally has the right to terminate the services you are providing at any time. You have a duty to continue providing care until relieved of the responsibility by the patient or another medically qualified person or until care is no longer needed. If you stop rendering care without the patient's consent when there is still a need for treatment, this is **abandonment.**

While the burden of proof is on the patient to prove abandonment occurred, you will inevitably have to explain why you stopped providing care. How this is managed is important. For example, a patient who is in the ambulance and abruptly decides not to be taken to the hospital cannot simply be left on the highway. The patient relationship must be terminated in a reasonable manner while considering the patient's well-being.

False Imprisonment. Detaining a person without consent can lead to a lawsuit claim of **false imprisonment** based on the intentional and unjustifiable detention of a person against his or her will. It can only arise if patients know they are being detained. Situations in which the patient is unaware of the surroundings and is unable to provide informed consent or refusal provide some justification for transporting a patient to a hospital for evaluation.

Assault and Battery. Failure to obtain a patient's consent to treatment can result in a claim of assault or battery, either of which can create civil and criminal liability. **Assault** is an act that intentionally places a patient in fear of immediate bodily harm without consent. **Battery** is touching a patient without consent. A claim of battery may arise if you inappropriately use force or restrain a patient. Do not perform any procedure if the patient expresses unwillingness or expressly denies permission. Claims of assault and battery are generally avoidable if you clearly communicate your intentions to the patient and obtain cooperation before proceeding with any assessment or treatment.

Use of Force

Improper use of force can also be a source of criminal or civil liability for the EMT. The use of force is allowed only in situations in which there is a reasonably perceived immediate risk of harm. You should avoid the use of force unless absolutely necessary. If you believe a patient is going to injure you, move to safety and summon law enforcement personnel. If you are unable to do this, you may use the necessary force to restrain the patient from

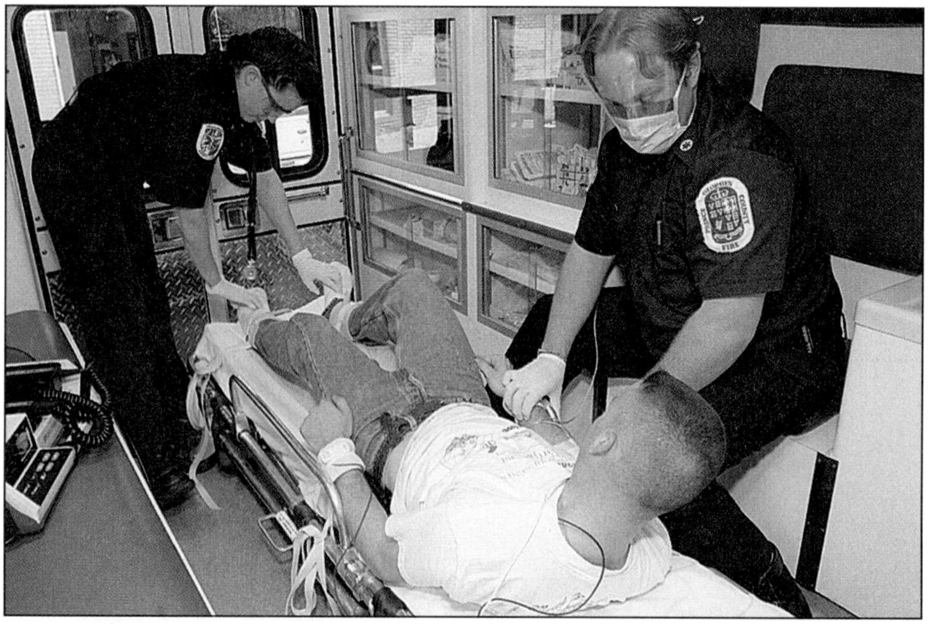

Figure 2-5

Continually monitor any patient placed in restraints to ensure adequate circulation, breathing, etc. Restraints should only be used when the patient's aggressive movements could cause harm to the patient, the EMS provider, or a bystander.

causing harm. The amount of force allowed is only that which is necessary to prevent such harm or subdue the aggressive behavior. Any greater use of force is considered excessive.

Use of Restraints

You may have to consider using restraints as a means of patient protection in very limited circumstances. Restraining a person without justification can give rise to a claim of assault and battery. Restraints should only be used when the patient's behavior warrants the restriction of movement to protect the patient or the EMS provider. Consider the following questions before placing a patient in restraints:

- Are restraints necessary or are there other alternatives?
- What type of restraints are suitable?
- How long will the patient be restrained?
- Does the patient have any injuries or illnesses that could worsen while restraints are used?

Situations where restraints might be appropriate include:

- Patients with behavioral problems
- Patients under police arrest or detention
- Patients exhibiting overt acts of violence (Police should accompany the patient in the ambulance.)
- Patients who try to injure themselves

Never lose sight of the risk to the patient from the misuse of restraints. Continually monitor a restrained patient to ensure that adequate breathing and circulation are not impaired in the extremities (Figure 2-5) or that the patient's condition does not deteriorate in any way. If the patient has a spine condition such as scoliosis (curvature of the spine), caution must be used when applying physical force to avoid further injury. Sometimes simple restraints with the use of pillows to limit movement and protect the patient can be effective for transport. Document the type of restraint applied, circulation checks, the time restraints were applied, and the reason for use.

You can be subjected to liability if the use of restraint contributes to the extent of a patient's injuries. To minimize the likelihood of this occurring, act reasonably. Avoid overly aggressive behavior (physical or verbal) when restraining the patient. Consider the relative size of the patient, the availability of others to assist, the type of behavior known or reasonably anticipated, and the likely consequences of using restraints. You should always receive training in the use of restraints before applying them.

Transporting Patients

Transporting a patient from one point to another can sometimes be a legal dilemma for the well-meaning EMT. The delivery of patients to a hospital should be a medical decision, not complicated by financial or other considerations. Issues sometimes surface when a patient needs hospital transport from a physician's office. For example, you may be called for a routine transfer to the hospital. Upon your arrival you note that the patient's condition is not stable, but the physician insists that you hastily transport the patient to a distant hospital instead of a closer facility. In this situation the patient's well-being may be compromised.

You are accountable to your EMS medical director and other supervising physicians. If you bypass the closest facility, you—not the private physician—can be blamed for negligent actions. Exercise judgment and when necessary seek medical direction to decide if a patient's condition warrants transport to a different facility or if a patient should be accompanied by Advanced Life Support (ALS) personnel. You can also use the medical control physician to interact with the private physician if necessary.

A federal law, commonly referred to as *anti-dumping* legislation, was enacted in response to hospitals that transferred indigent patients without providing necessary emergency care. The statute is part of the 1986 Consolidated Omnibus Budget Reconciliation Act (COBRA).[5] It requires hospitals with emergency departments to evaluate any patient who enters the emergency department and prohibits hospitals from transferring unstable patients or patients in labor unless the patient is first stabilized as much as possible. It mandates that necessary life-support measures accompany the patient during the transfer.

The law applies if a patient is considered unstable because of any emergency medical condition. Substantial fines may be assessed against a hospital and a physician who violates the law. They also risk losing federal reimbursement funding for Medicare patients. Because it affects emergency department decisions to accept and transfer patients, EMS providers may feel the effects of the statute and its enforcement (Box 2-2).

The issue of patient destination is complex; you should have local protocols that guide you to the most appropriate destination. Sometimes a patient may express a preference regarding his or her destination, which could further complicate the issues surrounding transport. Depending on your EMS system and the patient's condition, you may transport a patient to the nearest hospital, the most appropriate hospital, or the patient's preferred hospital. Follow your protocols, use your best judgment, and seek medical direction.

Bystander Interference

Another difficult situation that you may encounter is when a well-meaning person at the scene insists on participating in patient care. Even though this person's intentions may be good, he or she may sometimes interfere with your patient care. If this person was helping the patient before your arrival, it is understandable that he or she may feel an obligation to remain involved or even in control.

BOX 2-2 COBRA

The Consolidated Omnibus Budget Reconciliation Act (COBRA) received considerable attention in a 1991 law case involving Chicago paramedics who were instructed by a hospital base station to transport a child in cardiac arrest to a hospital that was not the closest hospital.[7] The child died, and the mother claimed that the closest hospital was negligent in directing the paramedics to the more distant hospital. She also alleged violation of COBRA on the basis that the prehospital provider's communication with the base station was sufficient contact with the emergency department to constitute a violation of the law.

The final court ruling was that the base station was distinct from the emergency department and that for purposes of this law, base station contact was not the same as coming to the emergency department.

In another court ruling, EMS providers honored a patient's choice to be transported to the hospital that he preferred, though they thought it was in the patient's best interests to be taken to a different hospital, a trauma center. They contacted their base station and received approval. The patient developed complications and later had to be transferred to the trauma center. The base station that approved the transport was not found to be negligent for honoring the patient's wishes.[13]

In yet another case, the court ruled that a patient did not have a right under the Constitution to be taken to the hospital of her choice by a county ambulance service.[15]

Maintain a professional attitude when encountering bystander interference. Remember that few people, including private physicians, understand the scope of practice of an EMT and the link to a medical director and EMS system. This can cause misunderstanding and conflict.

Sometimes the bystander providing care is a physician. The American College of Emergency Physicians (ACEP) has published a position statement that addresses the issue of a physician intervening in out-of-hospital emergency medical care.[1] The statement suggests that control of a medical emergency scene should be the responsibility of the individual in attendance who is most appropriately trained and knowledgeable in providing out-of-hospital care.

If a private physician is present and willing to accept responsibility for the patient's care, you should follow his or her orders as long as they are consistent with your local protocols. Properly document orders from the intervening physician. Never comply with any orders that exceed your scope of practice. Whenever there are questions, you should contact your medical director because he or she is still ultimately responsible for the patient that you are caring for. If there is any disagreement between the physician at the scene and the on-line physician, take orders from the on-line physician and place the two physicians in radio or telephone contact.

If on-line medical direction does not exist, you should relinquish responsibility for patient care when the physician has:

- Been properly identified
- Agreed to assume responsibility
- Agreed to document the intervention in a manner acceptable to the local EMS system
- Agreed in advance to accompany the patient to the hospital if required

The potential liability in situations where bystanders intervene must be kept in perspective. The bystander will be held accountable for his or her actions, but may be able to assert Good Samaritan status and be immune from negligent actions. You on the other hand will be held accountable for your actions, possibly without any available immunity protections. Cooperation and communication between you and any person intervening in patient care should eliminate potential conflict. If the person becomes a danger to the patient's well-being, you should invoke control measures such as requesting the assistance of police and/or an EMS supervisor. Your EMS system should have written policies that address these situations and provide you with guidance.

Resuscitation Issues

Considerable emphasis is placed on EMS providers saving lives. Resuscitation efforts require EMS providers to use all of their skills. Sometimes these efforts work and the patient is resuscitated. Many times, however, the resuscitation is unsuccessful.

A principle of law honored in our country is that adults of sound mind have the right to decide what is done to their bodies. This includes the right to decide what if any life-saving treatment is rendered, even if the result may be death. This right has been upheld by the courts even in situations in which the patient or the patient's guardian petitioned a court to withdraw life-saving treatment, allowing the patient to die.

The verbal wishes of a spouse or other family members regarding the patient's resuscitation preferences are not necessarily binding. If a patient is competent to make medical treatment decisions, the consent of others is not generally relevant or necessary.[9] If the patient is unconscious or incompetent, the family may be given the authority to make treatment decisions.[3]

Withholding or Stopping Resuscitation

As part of your responsibilities you are expected to provide resuscitation efforts. The only time this is not true is when there are valid medical or legal reasons to withhold or stop these efforts or when obvious signs of death are present. Your decision to withhold or stop resuscitation should be based on defined protocols or on-line medical direction. You must not make decisions about resuscitation based on personal beliefs.

If the patient desires, resuscitative efforts may be withheld if the medical condition is terminal, incurable, and death appears to be imminent or in situations in which treatment is of no benefit to the patient's condition.[6] In such cases a physician may order that cardiopulmonary resuscitation (CPR) be withheld when the patient suffers cardiac arrest or that CPR be discontinued once EMS personnel can validate a Do Not Resuscitate (DNR) order. Laws regarding this vary from state to state.

Advance Medical Directives

Most EMS providers have heard of *living wills*. While the term is commonly known, the document itself can be very complex and may be interpreted differently. Living wills are one form of **advance medical directives,** which are the patient's written statements of preference for medical treatment to be administered or withheld at some time in the future (Figure 2-6). Usually these documents become effective when the patient is comatose or unable to express medical treatment preferences. In addition, these documents sometimes appoint another person to make necessary medical treatment decisions on behalf of the patient (medical surrogate or durable power of attorney for medical decisions).

Many states have recognized these documents but have restricted the circumstances for their use. For example, the document may only apply to the hospital setting, or may not become operative unless the patient has a terminal, incurable condition. Directives can appear in a variety of formats, such as preprinted forms or handwritten documents. Advance medical directives can be honored in the out-of-hospital setting if allowed in your state.

Do Not Resuscitate Orders

One type of advance medical directive is a **Do Not Resuscitate (DNR)** or **Do Not Attempt Resuscitation (DNAR)** order, also referred to as a *No-CPR order* (Figure 2-7). A DNR order is commonly understood to mean that when the patient stops breathing or no longer has a pulse, CPR is not to be started.

A DNR order is usually written by the patient's physician in the patient's medical chart in a hospital or nursing home. The DNR order should be written by the physician only after consulting the patient. If the patient is unable to communicate his or her desires because of illness, the physician may consult with family members or durable power of attorney for medical care to determine the patient's treatment desires.

Patients may document their own DNR orders.[4] Although a physician typically writes a DNR order, there is nothing preventing a patient from documenting treatment choices regarding CPR. However, the written concurrence of a physician helps verify that the patient's refusal of life-saving treatment was done with the consultation and understanding of the outcome of such refusal. Because EMS personnel are instructed to identify valid DNR orders according to state policies, a self-written DNR may not be recognized. States have different statutes that govern out-of-hospital DNR orders (Box 2-3).

Whenever possible, you should act according to the patient's preferences. If there is any reasonable question as to the patient's wishes, attempt resuscitation as you would for any other patient until ALS personnel arrive or until your medical control physician can be contacted.

Organ Donation

Organ and tissue transplantation is a widely accepted medical procedure. In the course of your work you may encounter a patient who expresses a desire to be an organ donor. This notice requires a signed legal document indicating this intent. In many states individuals carry a separate donor card or the information is noted on the reverse side of a patient's driver's license (Figure 2-8). A potential donor should not be cared for any differently than any other patient. Your role is to identify the patient as a potential donor, communicate this information to your medical control physician, and provide care to maintain the organs in a viable state.

Death in the Field Setting

As an EMT it is very likely that you will witness the death of patients in the field. The legal aspects of out-of-hospital death are not simple. The authority of an EMT to determine that a person is dead should not be confused with the certification of death that a physician or coroner may legally issue. Any person can give an opinion as to

BOX 2-3 Do Not Resuscitate Orders

Considerations for Accepting a Prehospital DNR Order or Other Advance Medical Directives:

- There must be a clearly valid prehospital DNR order present with the patient (often kept at the patient's bedside, on the patient's medical chart, or on bedroom door).
- The patient's primary physician may be present to communicate the patient's resuscitation preferences.
- If the patient is unable to communicate treatment preferences, carefully examine the document to be certain that any restrictions on the use of CPR apply to the current situation.
- If the patient is conscious, determine if he or she is competent and informed as to the likely result of the DNR status.

LIVING WILL
DECLARATION

This declaration is made this __________ day of ____________________ ,19 ____ (month, year).
I, ____, being of sound mind, willfully and voluntarily make known my desires that my moment of death shall not be artificially postponed.

If at any time I should have an incurable and irreversible injury, disease, or illness judged to be a terminal condition by my attending physician who has personally examined me, and has determined that my death is imminent except for death delaying procedures, I direct that such procedures which would only prolong the dying process be withheld or withdrawn, and that I be permitted to die naturally with only the administration of medication, sustenance, or the performance of any medical procedure deemed necessary by my attending physician to provide me with comfort care.

In the absence of my ability to give directions regarding the use of such death delaying procedures, it is my intention that this declaration shall be honored by my family and physician as the final expression of my legal right to refuse medical or surgical treatment and accept the consequences from such refusal.

Signed ______________________________

City, County and State of Residence ____

The declarant is personally known to me and I believe him or her to be of sound mind. I did not sign the declarant's signature above for or at the direction of the declarant. At the date of this instrument I am not entitled to any portion of the estate of the declarant according to the laws of interstate succession or to the best of my knowledge and belief, under any will of declarant or other instrument taking effect at declarant's death, or directly financially responsible for declarant's medical care.

Witness ______________________________

Witness ______________________________

Figure 2-6

Example of a living will.

Kent County Emergency Medical Services, Inc
DO NOT RESUSCITATE ORDER

I have discussed my health status with my physician, ___________________. I request that in the event my heart and breathing should stop, no person shall attempt to resuscitate me. This order is effective until it is revoked by me. I am aware that I can revoke this order at any time by simply expressing my request verbally or in writing to my caretaking family, physician, or designated patient advocate.

Being of sound mind, I voluntarily execute this order, and I understand its full import.

______________________________ ______________

(Declarant's signature) (Date)

____

(Type or print declarant's full name)

______________________________ ______________

(Signature of person who signed for declarant, if applicable) (Date)

____

(Type or print full name)

______________________________ ______________

(Physician's signature) (Date)

____

(Type or print physician's full name)

ATTESTATION OF WITNESSES

The individual who has executed this order appears to be of sound mind, and under no duress, fraud or undue influence. Upon executing this order, the individual has (has not) received an identification bracelet.

______________________ ______________________

(Witness Signature) (Date) (Witness Signature) (Date)

______________________ ______________________

(Type or print witness's name) (Type or print witness's name)

THIS FORM WAS PREPARED PURSUANT TO, AND IS IN COMPLIANCE WITH, THE MICHIGAN DO-NOT-RESUSCITATE PROCEDURE ACT.

Figure 2-7

Example of a DNR order.

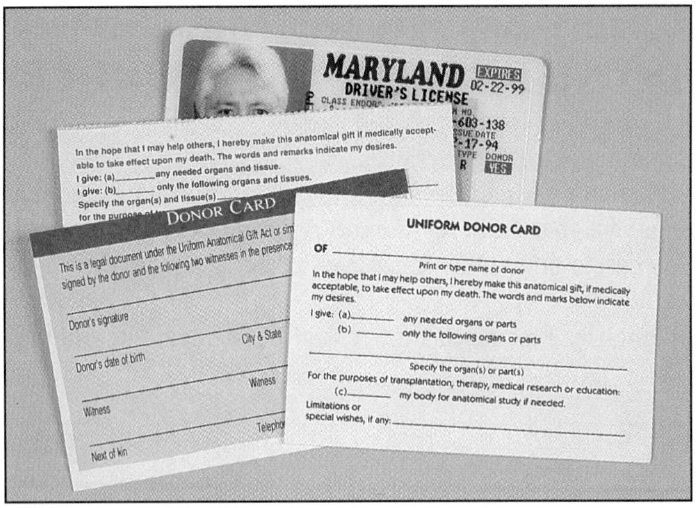

Figure 2-8

An individual's intent to be an organ donor requires a signed legal document. This may be in the form of a donor card or it may be on the back of the individual's driver's license.

whether or not a person appears to be dead, including an EMT. Obvious signs of death in which resuscitation efforts can typically be withheld are:

- Decapitation (head removed)
- Dependent lividity (pooling of blood, appearing as discoloration of the skin, in lower areas of the body)
- Rigor mortis (stiffening of the body's muscles)

If you encounter the apparent death of a patient in the field, you should at least do the following:

- Request the assistance of an ALS provider if available.
- Contact medical direction, if required by protocol.
- Document the observations and findings at the scene, as well as contact with dispatch and medical direction.
- Notify appropriate authorities (police, medical examiner, or coroner).
- Do not disturb the body or scene except as necessary to verify death.
- Be courteous and respectful to family, witnesses, and bystanders.

You must remain professional in your actions and statements and be sensitive to bystanders who may be distraught or confused.

Crime and Accident Scenes

The nature of EMS work can involve working in crime and accident scenes such as assault, domestic disputes, multiple-vehicle collisions, or suicide attempts. When confronted with such scenes, you need to take precautions to ensure that the scene is not unnecessarily disturbed or potential evidence destroyed. An example of physical **evidence** at a crime scene is a shirt that has a hole in it where a gunshot wound occurred. The location of the hole on the clothing and the condition of the fabric may be important in determining the position of the patient and the assailant when the injury was sustained, which is often critical in the prosecution of homicide charges.

Evidence from a crime scene is more useful if it is left intact so that forensic specialists can examine it. If clothing has tears, avoid the tear when cutting away the clothing to evaluate and treat the patient. Placing paper bags on a patient's hands can be important in preserving evidence of gunpowder burns. The sooner such protective measures are implemented, the more reliable the information will be at a later date. If you have to begin resuscitation, note the position of a patient before beginning your efforts.

You should also be aware of potential evidence at accident scenes. The simple fact that a car ignition was on in a vehicle found at the bottom of an embankment might help establish that the vehicle was being driven at the time of the accident. The direction that multiple vehicles were traveling, skid marks, the type of impact, and the injuries that occurred are all worth documenting.

Here are a few general guidelines to follow at a crime or accident scene:

- Maintain your own personal safety.
- Send as few personnel as necessary into the scene.
- Disturb as little as possible in any potential crime scene.
- Exit and enter the scene by the same route.

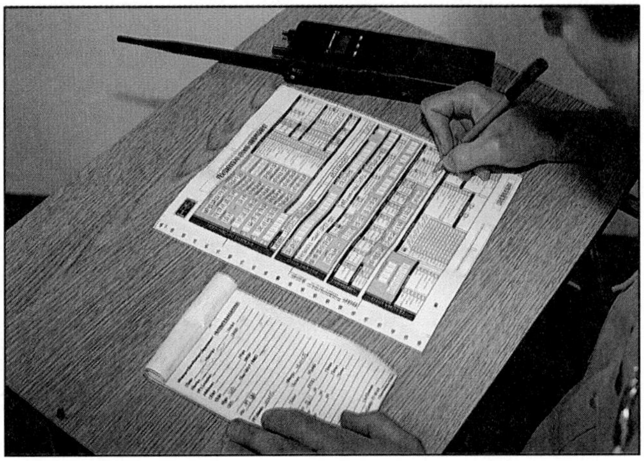

Figure 2-9

Proper documentation on a patient care report is essential to ensure that you followed all protocols for proper patient care and to protect you from possible future lawsuits.

- Inform appropriate law enforcement personnel if objects had to be moved or altered in the process of patient care.
- Adequately document pertinent information on the patient care report.

Documentation

Regardless of the circumstances surrounding a call, it is important to adequately document what you saw and heard, communication with medical direction, requests for special assistance, and the treatment you provided to the patient.[12] Proper documentation can help minimize future legal problems. The rule of documentation is simple: If it was not written down, it did not happen. Be certain to complete your agency's patient care report adequately (Figure 2-9).

When writing your report, make your narrative concise and describe unique situations carefully. Write your report clearly, reviewing it to be certain that it is logical. When documenting patient refusal, sign the report and get a signature from another EMS provider or other responsible person. Remember that you may have to read your report in court at some point in the future. Because it is unlikely that you will be able to recall all of the facts of a particular call, your written report will be a legal document that can help you present the facts clearly.

Besides your legal responsibility for accurate documentation, you also have an ethical responsibility. There are few circumstances that accept inaccurate information. While there may be a time when you record incomplete information because of environmental conditions, there

IT'S YOUR CALL
CONCLUSION

The patient in the case study claims you had a duty to provide care that included communicating with other professionals about this unique situation. You did not attempt to summon more advanced medical personnel or an EMS officer to the scene. You also did not contact medical direction for advice. In addition, the patient overheard you talking to other providers about options for care including transporting the patient face down and contacting the receiving hospital for orders. While it may not have made a difference in the outcome, the question remains: Did you do everything within your scope of training to care for this patient?

Even though the patient care that was provided was consistent with local protocols, the patient overheard the discussion about options and realized that you did not seek the advice of your supervising physician. These points are going to be made clear to the court. The case in question was settled out of court and the insurance company paid an undisclosed amount to the plaintiff for damages.

is no justification for purposely falsifying information. For example, if you only took one set of vital signs during the course of patient care, then only one set of vital signs should appear on the run sheet. Similarly, if you are unable to determine an accurate blood pressure, because of the noise or other environmental conditions, do not guess at this figure. Instead, communicate with another EMS provider that you could not attain this reading. This is also true of the care you provide. Do not state that you completed a procedure if it was not performed. Do not cover for others who may try to document false or misleading information. In such situations your actions could cause ALS personnel or hospital staff to think that a patient's condition is different from what it really is.

Similarly, you should not mislead a patient into thinking his or her condition is anything other than what you know it to be. Advising a patient to sign a waiver because you do not want to make the trip to the hospital is inexcusable. Therefore always take the time to accurately reflect what you saw and did, and any changes in your patient's condition.

SUMMARY

It is important for you to understand how competing and complex legal issues often affect patient care. States have varying laws that affect how EMTs function, including Good Samaritan laws, motor-vehicle laws, and reporting laws. The public expects a certain level of performance from EMS personnel. This standard level of care is what you must live up to when performing your job. If you had a responsibility to your patient, failed to meet the standard of care, and injury occurred, you may be found negligent in your actions. To help avoid the likelihood of a lawsuit, always perform your job to the level that you were trained. Never exceed this level, and do not function beneath this level.

The law is still evolving in some areas, such as DNR orders. The rights of patients and the broad range of laws that pertain to EMS providers must be considered when providing patient care. A single ambulance call can involve emergency driving statutes, confidentiality, consent, constitutional rights, scene management, and legal documentation. There is no substitute for a basic understanding of the legal issues and on-going training to stay abreast of evolving legal and ethical issues.

REFERENCES

1. **American College of Emergency Physicians:** ACEP policy statement: direction of prehospital care at the scene of medical emergencies, *Ann Emerg Med* 23:1145, 1994.
2. **Alabama Revised Statute,** 22-8-4.
3. ***Cruzan v Director.* Missouri,** 110 S.Ct. 2841 (1990).
4. ***Deel v Syracuse Veterans Administrative Medical Center,*** 729 F. Supp. 231 (N.D.N.Y. 1990).
5. **Emergency Medical Treatment and Active Labor Act,** 42 U.S.C.A., Section 1395dd, et seq., as amended by the Omnibus Budget Reconciliation Acts of 1987, 1989, and 1990.
6. **Fox E, Seigler M:** Redefining the emergency physician's role in do-not-resuscitate decision-making, *Am J Med* 92:125, 1992.
7. ***Johnson v University of Chicago Hospitals,*** 982 F.2d 230 (7th Cir. 1992).
8. **Maine Revised Statute Annotated,** 22-4011.
9. **Miller RD:** *Problems in hospital law*, Rockville, Md., 1990, Aspen Publishers, Inc.
10. ***O'Brien v Cunard S.S. Co.,*** 154 Mass. 272, 28 N.E.2d 266 (1981).
11. ***Ryan White Comprehensive AIDS Resource Emergency Act of 1990,*** Public Law 101-381.
12. **Selden BY, Schnitzer PG, Nola FX:** Medico-legal documentation of prehospital triage, *Ann Emerg Med* 19:547, 1990.
13. ***Smith v East Medical Center,*** 585 So.2d 1325 (Ala. 1991).
14. ***White v Rochford,*** 592 F.2d 381 (1979).
15. ***Wideman v Shallowford Community Hospital Inc.,*** 826 F.2d 1030 (11th Cir. 1987).

Chapter 3

The Well-Being of the Emergency Medical Technician

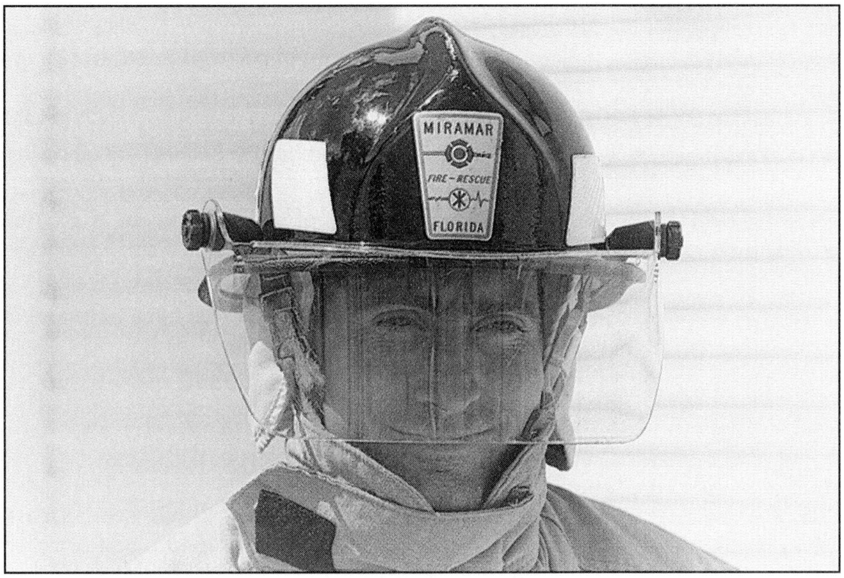

OBJECTIVES

Knowledge Objectives

As an EMT-Basic, you should be able to:

1. Describe how the body prevents and combats infection.
2. List four routes for disease transmission and give an example of how each can occur.
3. Describe how each of the following diseases is transmitted and the precautions that should be taken to prevent their transmission:
   - Hepatitis A
   - Hepatitis B
   - Human immunodeficiency virus (HIV)
   - Tuberculosis
   - Meningitis
   - Herpes simplex 1
   - Measles, mumps, and chicken pox
4. Describe how the Ryan White Act and the Occupational Safety and Health Administration (OSHA) Bloodborne Pathogen Standards assist in protecting you.
5. Describe the importance of body substance isolation (BSI) practices to prevent the transmission of airborne and bloodborne pathogens.
6. Identify at least eight guidelines for personal protection against disease transmission.
7. List the personal protective equipment necessary for the following situations:
   - Exposure to bloodborne pathogens
   - Exposure to airborne pathogens
   - Exposure to hazardous materials
   - Rescue operations involving fire, water, and ice
   - Violence
8. Identify the possible emotional reactions that someone may experience when faced with stressful situations such as death and dying.
9. Discuss the five stages in the grieving process.
10. Explain how to help a patient's family members deal with death and dying.
11. Identify the signs and symptoms of stress that may be exhibited in each of the following four categories: physical, mental, emotional, and behavioral.

OBJECTIVES

Knowledge Objectives, *cont'd*

12. **Identify the possible reactions that the EMT's family may exhibit due to their limited involvement in the activities of the EMT.**
13. **Identify three lifestyle changes that can be made to help you cope with stress.**
14. **Discuss the importance of critical incident stress management.**
15. **Describe the services provided by a comprehensive critical incident stress debriefing team.**

Skill Objectives

As an EMT-Basic, you should be able to:

1. **Given a scenario involving possible exposure to a communicable disease, demonstrate the use of appropriate personal protection equipment and how to properly remove and dispose of the equipment.**
2. **Properly clean and disinfect equipment used to provide patient care.**
3. **Complete appropriate documentation relative to any exposures that may occur in the course of providing patient care.**

Attitude Objectives

As an EMT-Basic, you should be able to:

1. **Assess your beliefs and practices regarding disease transmission and the use of personal protective equipment.**
2. **Serve as a role model for other emergency medical service (EMS) personnel in regard to maintaining a healthy lifestyle.**
3. **Advocate the benefits of working toward a goal of achieving and maintaining physical and emotional well-being.**
4. **Describe how you might feel if you have to inform a family member/friend of a patient's death.**

KEY TERMS

1. **Acquired Immune Deficiency Syndrome (AIDS):** The end condition resulting from infection with the human immunodeficiency virus (HIV), characterized by serious, often multiple infections.
2. **Bacteria:** One-celled microorganisms responsible for spreading disease. They are not dependent on other organisms for life, so they can live outside of the human body. Bacteria cause diseases such as meningitis and tuberculosis. Antibiotics are used to help destroy bacteria.
3. **Bloodborne Pathogens:** Microorganisms present in human blood and body fluids that can cause disease in humans. Infectious materials contained in other body fluids (saliva, tears, etc.) are generally included in this grouping.
4. **Body Substance Isolation (BSI):** A form of infection-control practice that is designed to prevent infections transmitted by direct or indirect contact with infected blood or body fluids. It assumes that all body fluids and substances are potentially infected.
5. **Communicable Disease:** An infectious disease that can be transmitted from person to person; also called a *contagious disease.*
6. **Critical Incident Stress Debriefing (CISD):** A team approach to counseling individuals who have been involved in a particularly stressful incident.
7. **Decontamination:** The process of cleaning a person's body, equipment, or other materials after exposure to hazardous materials.
8. **Direct Contact Transmission:** The transmission of disease by touching another person's infected blood or other body fluids or inhaling airborne particles infected with a disease-causing agent.
9. **Hazardous Materials Incident:** An incident involving the release of hazardous substances into the environment.
10. **Hepatitis:** A serious viral infection of the liver; caused by several different viruses, of which hepatitis B virus (HBV) is potentially the most serious.
11. **Human Immunodeficiency Virus (HIV):** The virus that destroys the immune system (the body system used to fight off infections) and causes AIDS.
12. **Immune System:** A complex body system designed to prevent and combat infection.
13. **Indirect Contact Transmission:** The transmission of disease through indirect contact, such as contact with an object that was contaminated by an infected person.
14. **Infectious Disease:** Any disease that invades the body as a result of a pathogen.
15. **Meningitis:** Inflammation of the membranes surrounding the brain and spinal cord, caused by either bacteria or viruses. Meningitis can cause serious consequences, including death, if not treated promptly.
16. **Pathogen:** A microorganism, such as bacteria or a virus, that causes disease.
17. **Placards:** Signs placed on vehicles, railroad cars, and storage facilities indicating the presence of hazardous materials.

18. **Ryan White Comprehensive AIDS Resources Emergency Act:** Federal legislation that allows EMS personnel, in the event that they may have been exposed to a communicable disease, to determine if they have been exposed to an infectious disease while providing care.
19. **Tuberculosis:** A respiratory system infection caused by bacteria.
20. **Universal Precautions:** A form of infection-control practice that assumes that all human blood and certain body fluids are handled as if they were known to be infectious for HIV, HBV, and other bloodborne pathogens.
21. **Vaccination:** A specific substance containing weakened or dead pathogens that is introduced into the body to build resistance against a specific infection.
22. **Virus:** Microorganisms responsible for spreading many diseases, including the common cold. They depend on other organisms to live and grow. Hepatitis B virus and HIV are the two most serious viruses of concern to EMTs.

IT'S YOUR CALL

At 1:15 AM you are dispatched to a call for an injury from a fall outside a local bar. You have been to this location before for routine calls like someone falling off a barstool or slipping on the steps exiting the building. You remember reading about how the area has been the target of increasing crime and violence over the past few months. You notice increased graffiti on the building walls as you near the scene. Upon arriving, you park the ambulance about a block away and are led to a male patient lying in an alley. It is dark and you do not have a flashlight with you. You think about going back to the ambulance to get one and moving the ambulance closer so that you would have the benefit of its lights. As you follow the blood trail leading you to the patient, you notice people "hanging out," seemingly watching your actions. They do not appear to be concerned with the patient, but something does not seem right. You notice a gaping wound in the right side of the patient's chest. He utters, "Look what they did to me!" and then he loses consciousness.

Your partner examines the patient further and you focus on providing immediate care. The patient no longer has a pulse and you begin CPR. As you bare the patient's chest, you are nearly stuck in the hand by an uncapped needle protruding from the patient's pocket. You and your partner recognize that this patient needs advanced life support (ALS) care and prepare to call for the assistance of a medic unit. Almost immediately, however, a scuffle ensues. Several of the men that you passed earlier are fighting. The fight momentarily distracts you from calling for ALS assistance.

You begin to realize what is happening. You observe that the patient's jeans, shirt, and red and black bandanna are the same as those worn by some of the men involved in the fight. You realize that you may be caught in the middle of a gang fight and no longer feel that the scene is secure. You want to retreat but feel an obligation to remain with your patient.

By now more people are involved in the fight. You suddenly feel a weight on your shoulder. It is only there for a brief second as a deafening sound rings out. As you turn toward the sound, you see that it is the arm of an assailant firing a handgun in the direction of your patient. Another shot rings out. The assailant shouts, "Let him die!" and quickly disappears into the crowd. You suddenly notice that your partner was caught in the crossfire. Struck in the head while providing care, he now lies motionless on the pavement.

Only minutes earlier, you were responding to what you thought would be a routine call. Now caught in the middle of gang violence, you are no longer a rescuer but a victim. You struggle to help your partner. The feelings of satisfaction and happiness you normally feel when providing care are replaced with feelings of fear, disbelief, pain, sadness, and anger. In a split second, your partner lies dying. The patient you were called to assist is dead. What should have been done before approaching the patient? Should you have recognized a potentially dangerous situation? Now your physical and emotional well-being are being threatened.

Because of the many potential dangers associated with an EMS response, personal well-being is extremely important. You may find yourself confronted with situations involving a physical threat from things like hazardous materials, communicable diseases, environmental hazards, traffic hazards, and violence. Besides these threats to your physical well-being, you will also encounter many threats to your emotional well-being. These include witnessing death and dying, dealing with large-scale incidents or those that demand otherwise lengthy or dangerous on-scene time, and having someone you know injured in the line of duty.

One of your more important responsibilities is to maintain your own well-being. Injury or illness in the line of duty or related to your job can be devastating. This chapter examines some of the common causes of injury and illness to EMTs and identifies ways to help safeguard your health.

The Physical Well-Being of the EMT

Disease Transmission

In 1847, an obstetrician noticed that the death rate from infection was four times greater when his patients were treated by medical students. Further investigation revealed that the students were dissecting human bodies in the anatomy lab and then providing patient care in the hospital without first properly washing their hands.[11] This discovery established the field of infectious diseases and identified the importance of hand washing with disinfectants to prevent the spread of disease.[2]

Over the years, infection-control practices have gained popularity as a result of the occupational hazard associated with the transmission of life-threatening bloodborne diseases. Examples of these diseases include HIV and *hepatitis B virus* (HBV).

OSHA is a branch of the federal government responsible for safety in the workplace. Federal law requires all states to follow federal OSHA regulations or to develop their own OSHA plans that are at least as stringent. In 1991, OSHA issued its final regulations on exposure to bloodborne pathogens, which went into effect in early 1992. This legislation was designed to protect healthcare workers against disease transmission while at work.[9,10] These regulations attempt to minimize or eliminate the likelihood of disease transmission by using a combination of engineering and work practice controls. Engineering controls include the use of equipment such as puncture-resistant containers and mechanical needle recapping devices for sharp objects. Work practice controls reduce the likelihood of exposure by modifying the behavior of the person performing the task. An example of a work practice control is always wearing gloves before making contact with any patient.

Infections

Diseases are transmitted through **hosts,** individuals or animals capable of supporting life of another organism. A microorganism is a plant or animal that is too small to be seen with an unaided eye. A **pathogen** is a microorganism that can cause disease. When pathogens enter the body they can sometimes overpower the body's natural defense mechanism, causing infection. Infection is the growth of a disease-producing organism in a suitable host. An **infectious disease** is one that is caused by a pathogen. A **communicable disease,** also called a *contagious disease,* is an infectious disease that can be spread from person to person. Serious communicable diseases include tuberculosis, hepatitis, and HIV. Because of your frequent contact with patients, your primary concern as an EMT is to protect yourself from communicable diseases. Most diseases are caused by one of six types of pathogens (Figure 3-1):

- Bacteria
- Viruses
- Fungi
- Parasites
- Protozoa
- Rickettsia

Bacteria are small, one-celled organisms that do not depend on other organisms for life and can live outside the human body. They are responsible for some common infections, such as ear and throat infections, but also for more severe infections like tuberculosis and meningitis. Antibiotics, such as penicillin and erythromycin, are effective at killing or inhibiting the growth of most bacteria.

Viruses are microorganisms smaller than bacteria that are reponsible for many diseases, including the common cold. Unlike bacteria, viruses depend on other organisms to live and grow. They are more difficult to treat because viruses live within body cells and any medication would have to selectively kill only the infected cells, leaving the healthy cells unaffected. At the present time there are few medications that effectively fight viral infections. This is part of the dilemma facing researchers as they try to find a cure for AIDS.

Fungi are another type of microorganism that includes molds and yeast. You will most often see fungi infections in the form of skin irritations, such as athlete's foot and ringworm.

Protozoa are microorganisms responsible for the transmission of diseases such as malaria, through the bites of mosquitoes, and dysentery, from unsanitary food and water.

Parasites are microorganisms that vary greatly in size, from as small as bacteria to much larger intestinal worms. Parasites are much more common in developing nations than in the United States and can cause intestinal infections, anemia, and respiratory and circulatory problems.

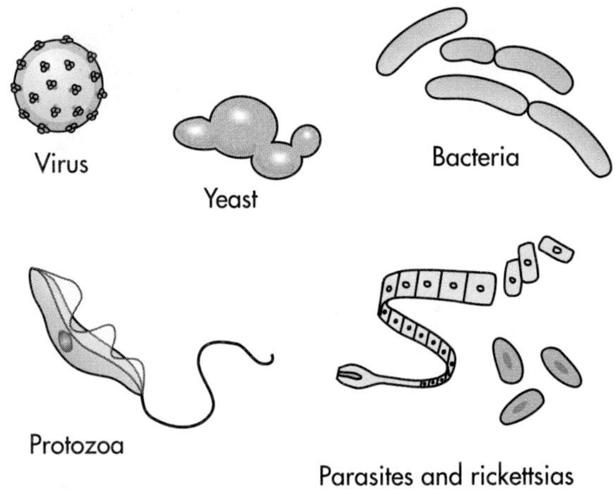

Figure 3-1

Viruses, bacteria, protozoa, yeast (fungi), and parasites and rickettsias are the six most common disease-causing pathogens.

Rickettsia are microorganisms spread through the bites of ticks and lice and are responsible for Rocky Mountain spotted fever and typhus. These diseases are fairly rare in the United States.

Natural Defenses

Human skin is particularly effective in preventing disease. As long as the skin is intact, most pathogens cannot enter. However, cuts or scrapes, regardless of size, reduce the effectiveness of skin as a barrier to prevent infection. In addition, pathogens can easily enter the body through the mucous membranes of the mouth and nose. Once inside the body, the immune system must go to work.

The **immune system** is the body's natural defense mechanism to prevent or overcome infection. It is a complex system that relies on several mechanisms, especially **white blood cells** (leukocytes), for protection. White blood cells circulate throughout the bloodstream identifying pathogens. One way this is done is by identifying the proteins that most pathogens have on their surfaces. When present in the body these proteins, called **antigens,** elicit an immune response to suppress or kill them. Some white blood cells release protein complexes of their own, known as **antibodies,** which weaken or destroy the pathogens.

In addition to the immune system response, the lymphatic system also helps fight disease. The **lymphatic system** acts as a separate circulatory system, filtering out inactivated or dead pathogens and producing more antibodies. The spleen is the primary organ of the lymphatic system and is responsible for filtering out blood cells and forming other cells that make antibodies.

Routes of Transmission

For a disease to be transmitted, three conditions must be present:

- The pathogen must be present in sufficient quantity.
- The person must be susceptible to the pathogen.
- The pathogen must enter the body through the correct entry site.

If any one of these conditions is absent, then transmission cannot occur. For example, a patient may have a bloodborne disease such as hepatitis, but if the pathogen is not present in sufficient quantity in the exposed blood, or if you take precautions to avoid any blood contact, then the pathogen cannot be transmitted to you. Communicable diseases are transmitted through four different routes:

- Contact (direct/indirect) transmission
- Airborne transmission
- Vehicle transmission
- Vectorborne transmission

Contact transmission can be either through direct contact or indirect contact. **Direct contact transmission** occurs when **bloodborne pathogens** are transmitted to an uninfected person through unprotected contact with an infected person's blood or other body fluids. Such exposure often occurs through skin breaks in the uninfected person. **Indirect contact transmission** occurs without person-to-person contact; for example, when an uninfected person touches an object, such as soiled linen, equipment, or vehicle surfaces, that has been contaminated by the body fluids of an infected person. **Airborne transmission** refers to diseases that are spread by tiny droplets when a person exhales, coughs, or sneezes. **Vehicle transmission** refers to the transmission of disease through vehicles such as food and water. **Vector transmission** occurs when a human, animal, or insect transmits a pathogen through a bite. Table 3-1 describes each of these routes and associated diseases that are commonly transmitted.

Diseases that Concern EMTs

There are many different diseases that might affect you. The communicable diseases that you are most likely to encounter are those transmitted through blood, other body fluids, and air. Airborne diseases such as the common cold are easily transmitted. While the common cold may be an annoyance, it is short-lived and rarely has any

TABLE 3-1 Transmission of Common Communicable Diseases

Route	Diseases	Incubation period
Contact (direct/indirect)	Hepatitis B, HIV	Weeks, months, years
	Herpes 2, Herpes-zoster	Days to a few weeks
Airborne	Tuberculosis, Pneumonia, Meningitis, Chicken Pox, Measles, Mumps, Herpes 1	Days to a few weeks
Vehicle	Hepatitis A and E, Salmonella, Staph	Hours, days to a few weeks
Vectorborne	Rabies, Lyme Disease, Tetanus	Days to weeks

serious consequences. Other airborne diseases such as tuberculosis, however, can be extremely serious, with debilitating effects. Bloodborne diseases such as hepatitis B and HIV are extremely serious, causing prolonged illness and death.

Hepatitis. Hepatitis is a viral infection causing inflammation of the liver. There are five well-documented types of hepatitis infection—A, B, C, D, and E. The three most serious types of hepatitis viruses in the United States are the hepatitis A virus (HAV), hepatitis B virus (HBV), and hepatitis C virus (HCV). Each of these types produces similar problems in the liver. **Hepatitis A** is a common type of hepatitis in the U.S.[7,12] It is acquired by the ingestion of contaminated food or drink or through the oral-fecal route. Hepatitis A is the only form of hepatitis that does not lead to chronic liver disease or make the infected person a long-term carrier of the infection.

Hepatitis B is a more serious type of hepatitis, resulting in destruction of the liver. It is estimated that approximately 12,000 health care providers acquire hepatitis B each year and about 250 die from the disease.[8] This is more deaths than are caused by any other communicable disease. HBV is found in blood, saliva, semen, and vaginal secretions. It is a hardy virus, capable of living outside the body for many days, either in the form of a body fluid or dried up on the surface of your equipment. This makes the disease a significant threat to all healthcare providers. Hepatitis B is the only form of hepatitis for which a vaccination is available. A **vaccination** is a specific substance containing weakened or dead pathogens that is injected into the body to cause the body's immune system to build resistance (antibodies) to specific infection. Administered in three doses over a 6-month period, the hepatitis B vaccine provides protection for 5 to 7 years. The Centers for Disease Control and Prevention, as well as OSHA, recommend that all EMS personnel receive the vaccination.[7-10]

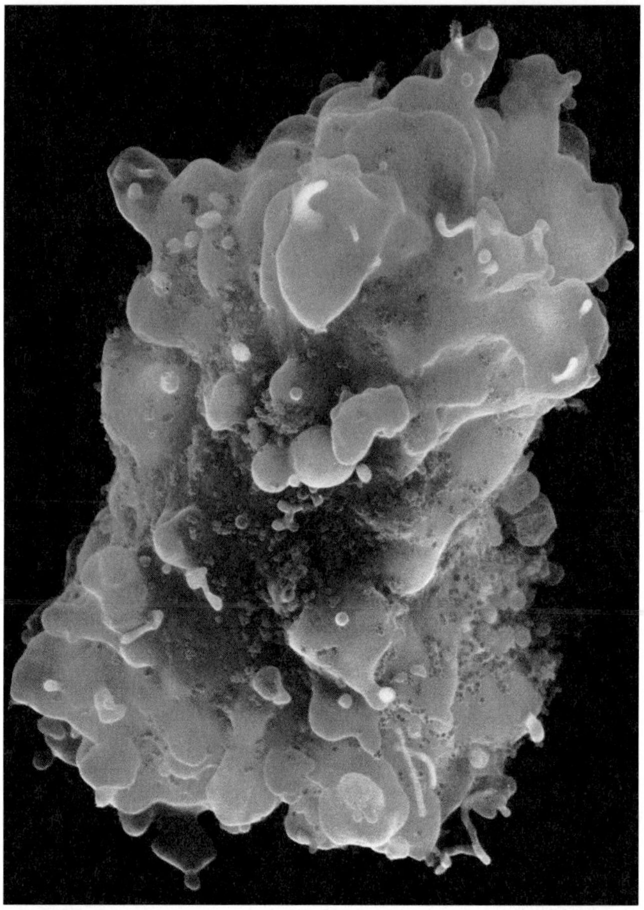

Figure 3-2

HIV, the virus that causes AIDS, is very small. It is released from infected white blood cells and quickly infects neighboring cells. More than 200 million individual viruses can fit on a typed period on this page.

Hepatitis C is also a bloodborne virus that causes problems similar to HBV. Although it was once thought to be confined to contaminated blood during transfusion, it is now being seen as a sexually transmitted disease as well, though this is uncommon.[3,12]

Regardless of the type of hepatitis, patients present with a general ill-looking appearance that includes a yellow discoloration of the skin, known as *jaundice*. Patients may complain of fever, weakness, nausea, abdominal pain, and urinary problems. In the most severe stages, the infection results in extensive liver damage that may lead to death.

Human Immunodeficiency Virus. Human Immunodeficiency Virus (HIV) was first identified in 1981 (Figure 3-2). Since that time, it has become a worldwide epidemic.[8,12] HIV is transmitted through body secretions, including blood, semen, vaginal secretions, and cerebrospinal fluid. It can be transmitted by direct contact with

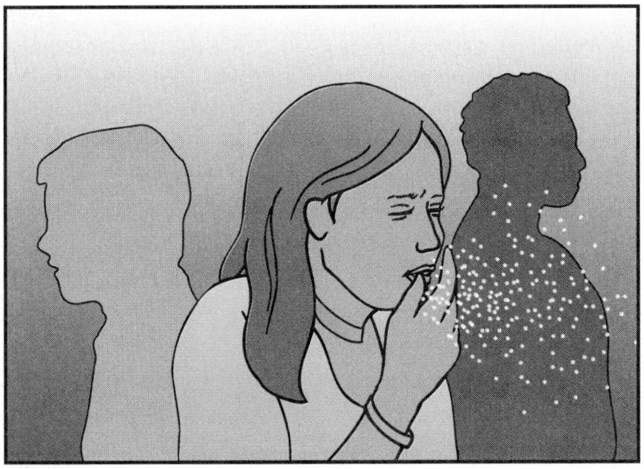

Figure 3-3

The bacteria that causes tuberculosis is highly contagious and can be spread through airborne pathogens when an infected person coughs, sneezes, or even exhales.

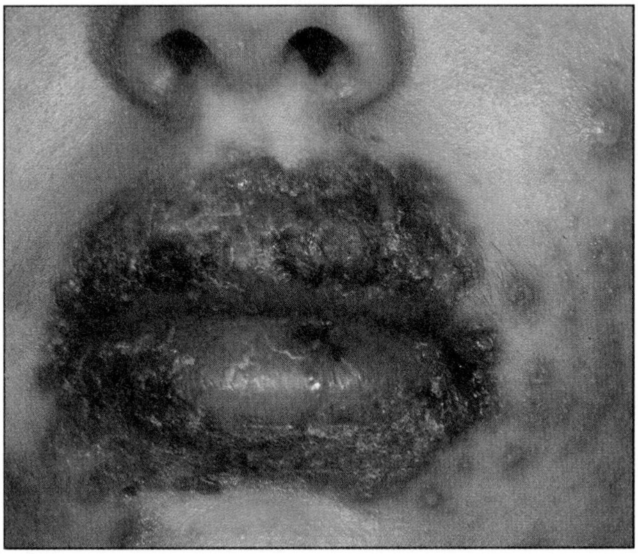

Figure 3-4

HSV-1 is usually associated with oral infection, that is, sores around and in the mouth.

infected blood or other body fluids through mucous membranes and open wounds, from mother to fetus across the placenta, and during intercourse.

Persons who test positive for HIV will likely progress through various stages of complications resulting from the gradual failure of the body's immune system. In later stages the patient is vulnerable to opportunistic infections such as *Pneumocystis carinii* pneumonia, tuberculosis, and tumors, including Kaposi's sarcoma. These are called **opportunistic infections** because they usually only occur when the patient's immune system is compromised. Once these conditions have developed, the patient is defined as having **Acquired Immunodeficiency Syndrome (AIDS).** The average time from HIV transmission to serious AIDS complications is approximately 10 years.[3,8] Patients can be infected with HIV and not know it for several years. Because there is no known cure for HIV/AIDS, EMS personnel are encouraged to follow precautions to prevent HIV transmission. These precautions are presented later in this chapter.

Tuberculosis (TB). Tuberculosis is a disease that is caused by bacteria in the air (Figure 3-3). It is contagious, and transmission usually occurs within a household or in crowded and poorly ventilated living conditions. It normally affects the lungs, but can also infect lymph nodes, vertebrae, kidneys, and other organs. It is estimated that TB accounts for more than 1 million deaths worldwide each year.[5] After the turn of the century, TB continually declined in the United States until 1985, when the trend was reversed as a result of HIV infection. It is estimated that up to 40% of those now infected with TB are also infected with HIV.[5] Signs and symptoms of TB include a cough, weakness, weight loss, and fever with night sweating.

Meningitis. Meningitis is an inflammation of the membranes that surround the spinal cord and brain. There are two primary types of meningitis: bacterial and viral. Bacterial meningitis is the more severe of the two and must be treated promptly with antibiotics. Bacterial meningitis is usually acquired through airborne transmission and contact with respiratory secretions, such as discharge from the nose and throat of infected persons. Viral meningitis is less severe and is often contacted through the oral-fecal route.

The signs and symptoms of meningitis vary depending on the age and health of the patient. Generally they include weakness, a sore or stiff neck (due to irritability of the meninges), fever, and headache. Infants may exhibit vomiting, poor feeding, and a high pitched cry.

Herpes. The **herpes simplex virus 1 (HSV-1)** is highly contagious and transmitted by direct contact. The virus enters the body through a break in the skin or mucous membranes. HSV-1 commonly causes a cold sore or fever blister and appears around the mouth (Figure 3-4). Once the primary infection has occurred, the virus lies dormant in sensory nerves until stimulated again.

Another form of the virus is herpes simplex virus 2, which is more likely to cause sores in the genital region. HSV-2 is a sexually transmitted disease that has increased dramatically in frequency in the United States. The symptoms of HSV-1 and HSV-2 infection can be treated, but the virus never goes away so reinfection is common.

The herpes zoster virus can cause two types of disease patterns. In childhood it causes chickenpox. It also causes a condition called *shingles*, which can occur at any age but is most likely to be seen in older adults. Shingles occurs in persons who have previously been exposed to the zoster virus and have usually had chickenpox. The virus lies dormant until it reactivates to cause shingles. It usually begins with a very painful rash that is usually seen on the face, neck, or chest. As the rash spreads, pus-type lesions develop. The rash forms scabs after 1 to 2 weeks, with the whole process from appearance of the rash to scabbing lasting approximately 3 weeks.

Childhood Diseases. It is likely that you will come in contact with a child who is experiencing a childhood disease such as measles (Figure 3-5), mumps, or chickenpox (Figure 3-6). These diseases are highly communicable and spread through direct and indirect contact with respiratory secretions. Most people have been vaccinated against mumps and measles. The vaccine for the prevention of chickenpox was made available in 1995.

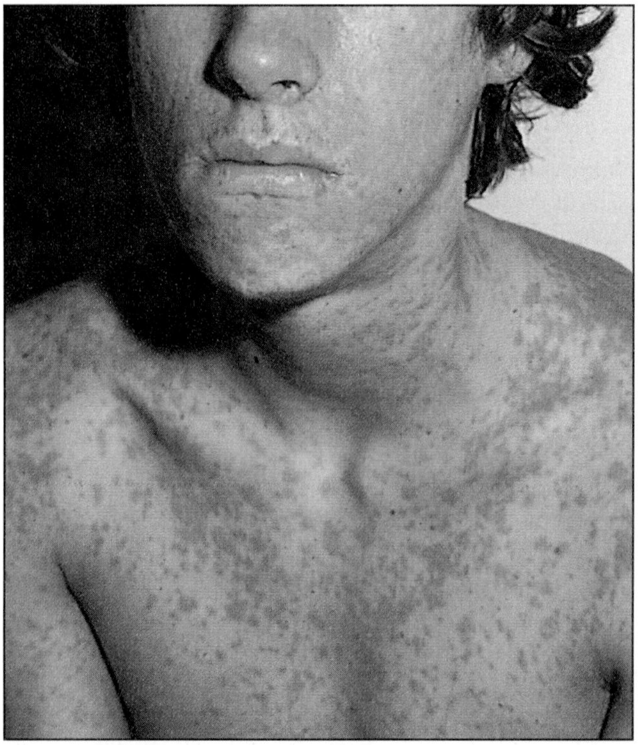

Figure 3-5

Measles, also called rubeola, is a viral disease once common among children before vaccinations against the disease became standard practice.

Infection Control Legislation

The HIV epidemic has generated fear of infection among emergency medical personnel. In the past, some agencies developed nonresponse policies for victims with known or suspected communicable diseases. Others refused to provide on-scene care or to transport a patient exhibiting high-risk behaviors for potential infections. Such policies are medically unjustified and are now illegal. Refusal to care for such patients raises issues of patient abandonment and civil rights violations. In addition, the Americans with Disabilities Act (ADA) specifically classifies HIV infection and tuberculosis as disabilities. Failure to provide care for such individuals may constitute discrimination against a person with a disability.

The **Ryan White Comprehensive AIDS Resources Emergency Act** of 1990 is a federal act that helps protect EMS personnel. Finalized in 1994, this act lists the notification requirements if EMS personnel have been exposed to a potential infectious disease while providing patient care. It requires the appointment of a "designated officer" by each employer of EMS personnel to coordinate communication between hospitals and the EMS agency to gather information in the event of a potential infectious exposure. States may establish their own laws regarding EMS personnel and infectious diseases, but the Ryan White Act is the basis for the law. If states establish their own laws, those laws must be at least as stringent as the federal legislation.

Notification of a communicable disease exposure can occur in several ways. If a transported patient is diagnosed as having a disease that could have been transmitted via the airborne route, the hospital automatically notifies the EMS agency's designated officer. This notification is to occur within 48 hours of the diagnosis. This automatic

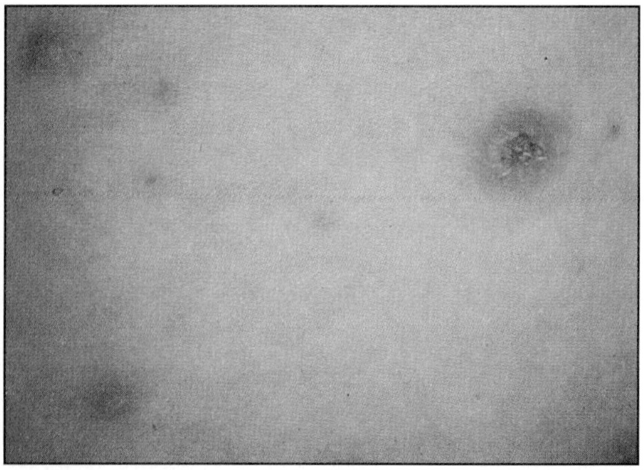

Figure 3-6

Chickenpox is a highly contagious viral disease that causes lesions all over the body. It usually occurs in childhood.

notification is important because you are not likely to know that a patient you cared for had an airborne disease such as TB.

The procedure is slightly different for bloodborne exposure. Because the hospital may not routinely diagnose a patient with HIV or hepatitis B, you must initiate the request if you have been exposed to a patient's blood or other body fluids. This request is initiated through the designated officer, who forwards the request to the hospital if he or she believes that an exposure occurred and disease transmission was possible. The hospital must gather information and report the findings to your designated officer within 48 hours. He or she will then report the findings to you. In some cases the findings will be inconclusive because the patient may have already been discharged or may refuse to allow the hospital to draw blood to confirm the presence of a bloodborne disease.

EMS personnel employed by state or local governments and those employed by private hospitals or EMS agencies can find protection under this act and related OSHA guidelines. Unfortunately, it currently does not apply to volunteer organizations.

It is important to remember that for a disease to be transmitted, there must be an exposure. For example, even if you care for a patient who is HIV positive, unless there is exposure, such as unprotected contact with the patient's blood or a needle stick injury, you cannot become infected.

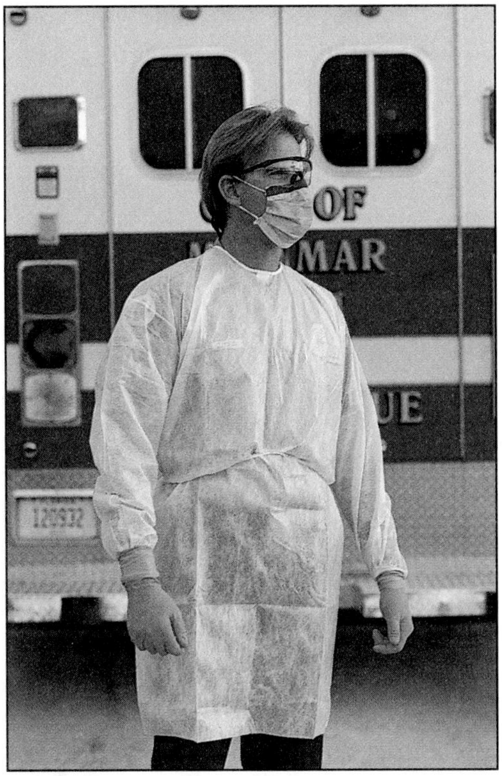

Figure 3-7

PPE should include gloves, a mask, goggles, and a gown.

Preventing Disease Transmission

In March 1992 the OSHA Bloodborne Pathogen Standard went into effect. This standard requires employers of EMS providers to take measures to protect their employees who are likely to be exposed to blood and body fluids as a routine part of their job.[10] The components of this standard include:

- Creating an exposure control plan that minimizes the likelihood of exposure through the use of engineering- and work-practice controls. These controls include the use of equipment such as puncture-resistant containers and mechanical needle recapping devices and practices such as wearing gloves designed to reduce the likelihood of exposure. This plan must be updated at least annually.
- Providing the opportunity for employees to receive vaccination against HBV at no cost to the employee and at a reasonable time and place.
- Promoting and ensuring the use of universal precautions and body substance isolation (BSI) precautions. This includes making available to employees all necessary personal protective equipment (PPE), including gloves, masks, goggles, gowns, and resuscitation equipment, at no cost to the employee (Figure 3-7).
- Developing a system for easy identification and disposal of contaminated material. This includes placing contaminated materials in appropriately labeled containers or bags and disposing of them properly with other contaminated materials.[6]
- Offering infection control training. This training must be provided at the time of initial employment and at least annually thereafter.
- Establishing a system for reporting an exposure and for postexposure treatment.
- Maintaining a record-keeping system that includes updates in policies and protocols, exposure control plans, employee training, employee medical records with vaccinations, and postexposure follow-up care.

The concept of universal precautions was originally used to protect against contact with blood and body fluids of patients who had a known or suspected disease. The problem with this approach was that it was not possible to know the infectious status of most patients being treated outside of a hospital. Another problem was that these precautions only applied to blood or body fluids that contained visible blood.[9]

More recently, the concept of **body substance isolation (BSI)** has come into favor. Although the term *BSI* is often used interchangeably with *universal precautions* by the EMS community, BSI is generally used to refer to protection from any and all body fluids and substances. **Universal precautions** refers to protection against blood and selected body fluids. It is important that EMS personnel ensure that they protect themselves from potential contamination from any body substance, whether it be blood, other body fluids, or respiratory secretions.

Guidelines for personal protection against disease transmission include:

- Vaccinations: Get vaccinated against the HBV. This is a three-shot series administered over a 6-month period. In the event of an exposure, a blood test (titer) may determine your current level of protection, and if necessary a booster will be provided. You should also be sure to be vaccinated against tetanus, a potentially fatal infection of the central nervous system. It most frequently results from injury in which a wound is contaminated with dirt, feces, saliva, or other microorganisms.
- Testing for the presence of diseases: Tuberculin purified protein derivative (PPD) testing should be done periodically to verify the absence of tuberculosis exposure.
- Masks: Wear masks when caring for a patient suspected of having an airborne disease or in cases in which there is a likelihood of body fluids splattering.
- Respirators: Wear high-efficiency particulate air (HEPA) respirators during ambulance transport or when working in confined areas with patients diagnosed or suspected of having a serious airborne disease (Figure 3-8).
- Resuscitation devices: Use resuscitation devices to provide a barrier between you and the victim's exhaled air and respiratory secretions during ventilation and clearing the airway.
- Air circulation: Use rear-compartment exhaust fans and open appropriate ambulance windows to allow outside air to circulate for patients with diseases that can be transmitted through the airborne route.

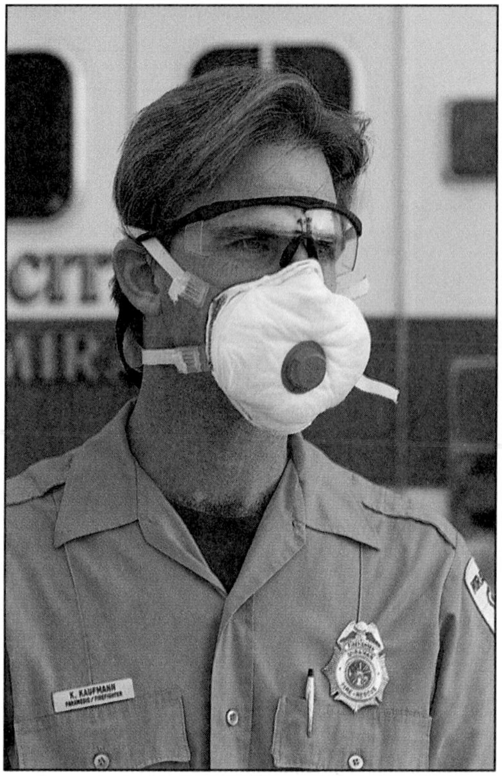

Figure 3-8

HEPA respirators can help prevent transmission of airborne pathogens.

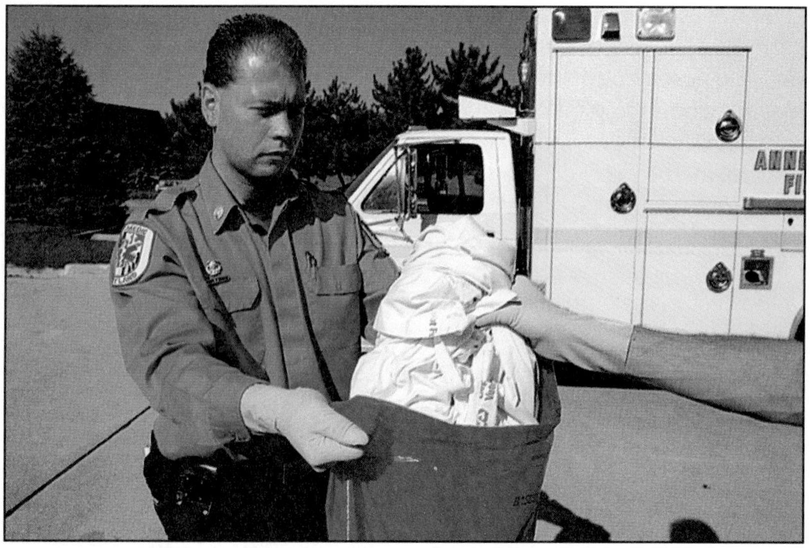

Figure 3-9

Wear gloves when placing contaminated laundry in labeled, leak-proof bags.

- Disposable gloves: Wear disposable latex gloves anytime contact with body fluid is likely. If caring for more than one patient, change gloves between patients.
- Eye protection: Wear eye protection such as goggles with side-shield protection or full face shields whenever there is a chance of body fluids splattering on your face.
- Clothing: Wear protective clothing such as disposable gowns or aprons when caring for patients with severe bleeding. If the uniform your employer provides gets soiled, it should be immediately changed and laundered at the station, not taken home to clean.
- Hand washing: Wash your hands with soap and water immediately after providing care. If soap and water are not readily available, use an antiseptic hand cleaner.
- Linen: The linen used to care for the patient should be changed immediately after use. Contaminated linen should be placed in labeled, leak-proof bags or containers and not sorted or rinsed before laundering (Figure 3-9).
- Equipment clean up: Patient-care equipment or ambulance surfaces should be decontaminated according to the manufacturer's recommendations. This usually involves cleaning with soap and water and then disinfecting with an EPA-approved chemical germicide or with chlorine bleach diluted 1:100 to 1:10 with water. Commercial disinfectants must be labeled as *tuberculocidal* to kill resistant strains of tuberculosis. (See Table 3-2 for guidelines for preventing disease transmission.)

TABLE 3-2 Guidelines for Preventing Disease Transmission

Activity	Gloves	Gown	Mask*	Eyewear
Controlling spurting blood	yes	yes	yes	yes
Controlling minor bleeding	yes	no	no	no
Childbirth	yes	yes	yes	yes
Suctioning, clearing airway	yes	yes	yes	yes
Advanced airway procedures	yes	no	yes	yes
Handling blood tubes	yes	no	no	no
Giving injections	yes	no	no	no
Measuring blood pressure	yes	no	no	no
Taking temperature	yes	no	no	no
Handling contaminated instruments	yes	yes	yes	yes
Cleaning ambulance after call	yes	no	no	no

*Protective face shields can serve as both mask and eyewear protection.
Modified from United States Fire Administration, National Fire Academy, Emmittsburg, Md, 1993.

Motor-Vehicle Collisions

When you respond to a motor-vehicle collision, there are many different safety factors you must consider, including:

- Traffic hazards
- Vehicle fire
- Hazardous materials
- Utility poles
- Unstable vehicles

Traffic Hazards

Whenever you are responding to a call that involves motor vehicles, approach the scene carefully. Observe the traffic pattern and decide the best way to approach and position your ambulance. Collisions almost always produce traffic hazards, especially if the collision results in vehicles in the roadway. This can result in secondary collisions as onlookers fail to pay adequate attention to their driving. Others may attempt to get around the collision by operating their vehicle in an unsafe manner on the soft shoulder of the roadway or in oncoming lanes.

The absence of any opposing traffic as you approach the scene may indicate that vehicles have created a blockade at the scene of the collision. Your ambulance, with its flashing lights, will serve as a form of traffic control. Position your vehicle about 50 feet away from the site of the collision. If your ambulance is facing oncoming traffic, turn off your headlights but keep other emergency lights on. Carefully exit the vehicle and be aware of any moving vehicles. Wear bright clothing or a reflective vest that can be easily seen day or night. Position reflectors or flares about every 10 to 20 feet behind your ambulance to help slow and divert traffic (Figure 3-10). The number of reflectors or flares you will need will depend on the speed of the oncoming traffic. The faster the traffic, the more flares or reflectors you will need to position over a longer stretch of roadway.

Vehicle Fires

Fortunately, vehicle fires are rare. If you find a vehicle on fire, always summon the fire department. Extinguishing vehicle fires is the responsibility of those who have been specially trained and have the necessary equipment and protective clothing to do the job. If you have the necessary protective gear and a 15- to 20-pound class A, B, or C dry-chemical fire extinguisher, you can suppress most small vehicle fires, including electrical, upholstery, and fuel components. If you are trained to extinguish a fire in the engine compartment, attempt to open the hood at least partway. Whenever possible, stand near the front windshield and with the wind at your back, and direct the spray under the hood.

Hazardous Materials

Sometimes seemingly simple incidents become major events because the vehicle involved released a hazardous

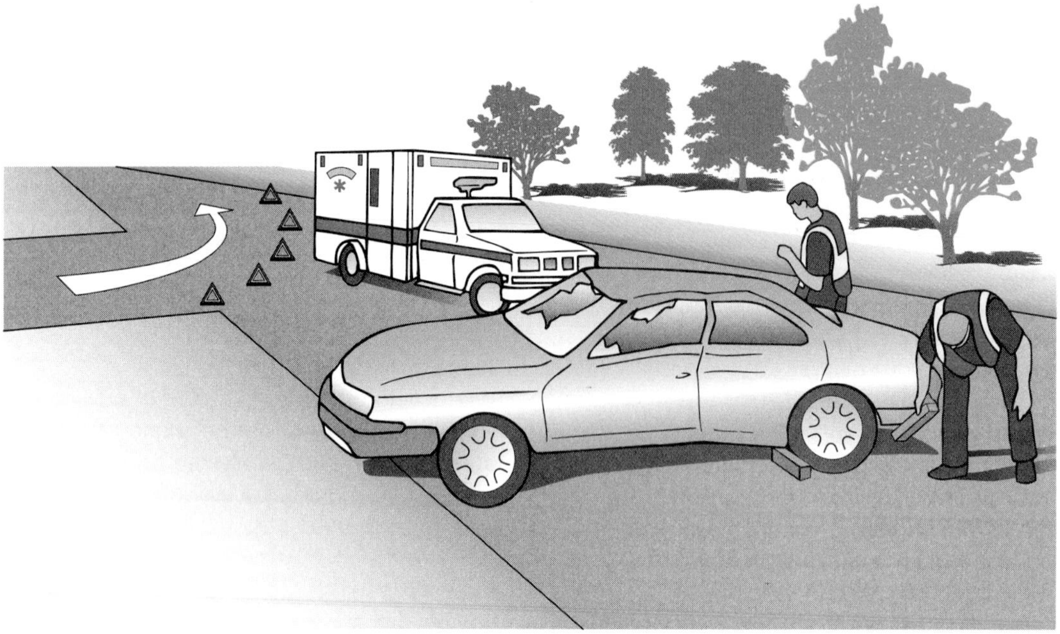

Figure 3-10

The use of reflectors helps divert traffic and makes your ambulance more visible in traffic.

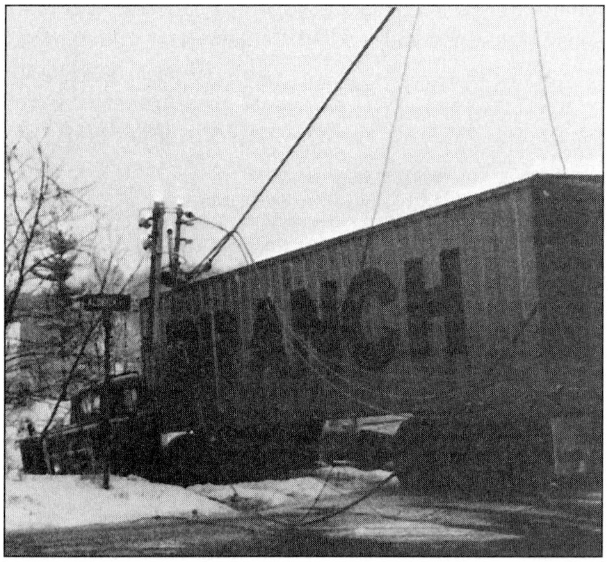

Figure 3-11

Downed electrical wires and damaged utility poles present significant risks on an emergency scene.

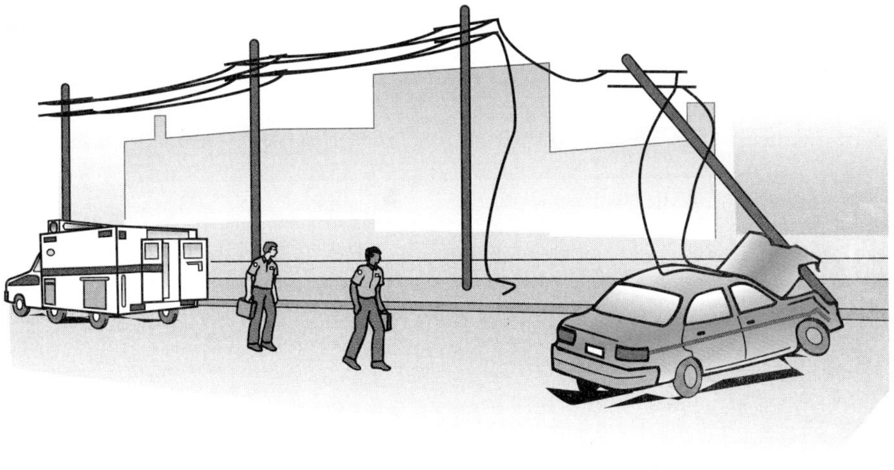

Figure 3-12

Upon arrival at a scene with downed electrical wires, park your ambulance at least two spans away from the damaged pole and do not approach the scene until the power company has deactivated the wires.

material. It is important to approach any scene in such a way as to allow you to take in the whole picture. Try to identify any placards that indicate hazardous materials before you get near or enter the vehicle to provide patient care. More detailed information on hazardous materials precautions is presented later in this chapter (see p. 57).

Utility Poles

If a vehicle is involved in a collision with a utility pole, damage to the pole may result, posing a significant threat to your safety (Figure 3-11). If a damaged utility pole results in downed electrical wires, you will need to position your ambulance in a safe location to avoid the possibility of electrocution. To do this, look at the span of wires between the poles. Park the ambulance at least two spans away from the damaged pole (Figure 3-12). Contact the power company and provide them with the location of the incident and if possible the identification number from the intact poles. This will help them rapidly deactivate the wires so that you can approach the scene and provide patient care.

Unstable Vehicles

Once you are able to approach a vehicle, you must be certain that it is stable and will not move when you enter it. Sometimes vehicles are found on their side, roof, or with wheels off the ground. Other times, the vehicle may be found on a slope. These vehicles pose a threat to both rescuers and victims. Besides being unstable, they may also result in fuel spills and ruptured fuel tanks.

Vehicles need to be stabilized before you begin to provide care. In some instances, this only involves placing the vehicle in "park," turning off the ignition, and setting the emergency brake. Sections of wood called **chocks** can be placed against the tires to further limit any movement should the brake fail. Other sections of wood called **cribbing**, airbags, and jacks can be used to stabilize vehicles found on their side or roof (Figure 3-13). All of these techniques require additional specialized training for you to function effectively.

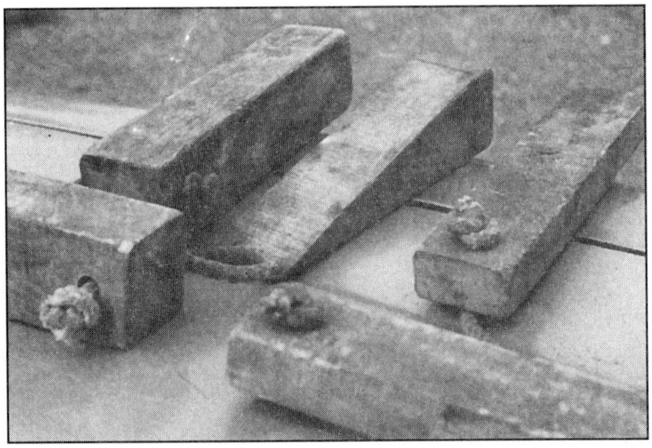

Figure 3-13

Chocks and cribbing help stabilize vehicles to prevent vehicle movement when you are providing patient care.

Violence

Another significant danger that you may face as an EMT is violence. Violent situations may erupt as a result of behavioral problems, domestic violence, or gang-related violence. While the violence may not be directed toward you, you could easily become an indirect victim caught in the middle of an altercation. As gang membership across the United States continues to grow, so does gang-related

KILLIN' COLORS

Once considered the good guys who assisted others and saved lives, EMTs, like other authority figures, are increasingly viewed by gang members with anger and distrust. Gangs are not limited by racial, ethnic, social, or economic groups. They are no longer just an urban phenomenon. Gangs are increasing in numbers as members travel swiftly to new markets to recruit new members, participate in criminal activity, confront rivals, and claim new "turf."

The psychologic bond that holds gangs together is a sense of belonging and a belief in the concept of "strength in numbers." Many gang members view other members of the gang as family. This bond is defined through an evolving, ritualistic use of hand signals, language, graffiti, behavior, and dress. When responding to a call, EMS personnel have to be acutely alert for potential violence. Protecting yourself is paramount in gang territory. In gang-infested areas you are likely to treat victims of prostitution scams, drug users, victims of violent gang initiation rites, and gang members gunned down for any number of reasons.

Being street-smart in the 1990s has taken on a whole new meaning. Careful, constant attention to your surroundings can help ensure your personal safety and may even save your life! Being aware of your surroundings in regard to gangs means recognizing gang dress—commonly referred to as *colors*—gang symbols, and gang slang. Learn the different colors of gangs in your area. Common gang slang includes:

Term	**Meaning**
Banger	Members with responsibilities for fighting rival gangs
Bust	To shoot at someone
Colors	Article(s) of clothing denoting gang affiliation
Dis	Disrespect
Dog	Law enforcement personnel
Gat	A semi-automatic handgun
Gauge	Shotgun
Home boy/girl	Local gang member
Jacked	Killed
Pawn	New recruit or young gang member
Posse	Gang
Raggin'	Displaying gang colors
Server	Drug dealer
Smoked	Killed
Slippin'	Not being aware of your surroundings
Thrillin'	Involvement in gang activities

In addition to gang slang, gang symbols are also unique to specific geographic areas; however, some of the more common symbols include the following:

Symbol	**Meaning**
187, 13, and M	Murder
AK	Anybody killers, referring to a gang philosophy that if you are on their streets and in their way, you may be killed.
⌖ ◉	Cross hairs of a gun sight or a bull's eye indicate that a gang or gang member is targeted for violence. A name or gang colors in the middle indicate who the target is.
	Crossing out names represents a dispute between gang "turf ownership" or that the person or gang has been targeted for violence.
CK$$$	Indicates the name of a gang that is trafficking drugs, and the profitability of the activity.
☺	A smiley face with a hole in the head and a particular gang color indicates that a member of that gang has been murdered.
Trigger	This term, accompanied by a gang member's street name, indicates a gang's "shooter."
Tombstone, RIP	Either symbol is used in conjunction with a gang member's name to indicate the member has been killed.

Being street smart also means following some basic street rules when entering areas frequented by gangs:

- Wear protective body armor, if issued by your agency, whenever entering dangerous areas.
- Request a law enforcement escort according to your protocols.
- Operate with a buddy system—one of you watch the patient, while the other watches the surroundings.
- Plan your entrance and exit route in advance.
- Plan and rehearse any special signals to be used to alert potential danger.
- Never get yourself cornered; always have a way out.
- Enter the area without your lights and siren.

IT'S YOUR CALL
CONCLUSION

As you will recall from the scenario at the beginning of the chapter, you were attempting to provide care for a patient who was a victim of gang violence. An assailant appeared and attempted to take the life of the patient and your partner. This is a tragic situation that may have been avoided by taking some precautions before approaching the patient.

- En route to the scene you should have asked for or been provided with additional information from your dispatcher about the actual nature of the call. While the dispatcher might not have any additional information, it never hurts to ask.
- Consider the graffiti. It may be an indication of gang activity in the area.
- Consider the location of your patient. In this case you should have asked where the patient was located before entering a dark alley.
- Position the ambulance in close proximity to the patient. If the ambulance had been positioned closer to the scene and your scene lights turned on, the lighting may have discouraged an additional attack.
- Follow your instincts. If something does not look or feel right as you arrive, do not approach immediately. If you are already approaching the patient, withdraw from the scene or take immediate action to correct a problem.
- At the first sign of assault or serious injury, you should summon law enforcement and ALS personnel (if available).
- Always be acutely aware of your surroundings.

violence toward EMS personnel. Gang-related violence also increasingly involves firearms, with young males being the primary perpetrators.[1]

Regardless of the reason for the violent behavior, there are steps that you need to be aware of to help defuse violent situations. Never enter a violent situation to provide care. Wait until law enforcement personnel arrive to secure the scene. Recognizing a potentially violent situation is an important first step in avoiding violent confrontation. The signs of a possibly violent situation include:

- Fighting, threats, or shouting
- Knowledge of previous violent behavior by the patient
- Visible weapons
- Body language suggesting confrontation
- Apparent intoxication or other drug use

Be prepared for any potential threat. If you encounter a violent patient, family member, friend, or bystander, or if you work in an area in which violence is likely, take steps to protect yourself. Wear proper shoes with nonslip surfaces. These can come in handy if you have to move quickly. Some EMS agencies issue body armor for personnel who work in high-risk areas. Always keep your portable radio with you. It is your means of immediate communication should you need to summon assistance. With your partner, determine how tasks will be split up. Either you or a partner should assume the responsibility of being an observer, responsible for the safety of the EMS team.

Remember that your first and often most appropriate response when confronted with a potentially violent situation is to withdraw from the immediate area. Immediately notify dispatch of the situation. Reassess the scene from a distance to determine if it has become safe to approach. If it is not safe or if you are not sure, stay in a safe area until law enforcement personnel advise that you can proceed. If you are unable to retreat from the immediate area and must attempt to control a violent person, try to assume a nonthreatening posture and talk in a straightforward manner and a normal tone of voice. Attempt to reason with the person. If this does not work you may have to defend yourself. Only use the force necessary to subdue the person or to get the opportunity to flee to a safe area.

Environmental Hazards

The environment itself can present many different threats to EMS personnel. Fire, water, ice, lightning, and other electrical hazards are some of the dangers faced by rescuers. Some environmental hazards can cause unstable footing, making rescuers susceptible to injuries from falls. Other times, natural hazards such as bees, snakes, and animals can pose dangers.

Fire

The common hazards found in a fire environment include smoke, heat, inadequate oxygen, and toxic gases. Smoke is comprised of particles of carbon and tar, which irritate the respiratory system, especially the lungs. The heat given off by the fire can cause burns to the skin and the respiratory tract during inhalation. Toxic gases can be irritating, poisonous, or can deprive the victim of oxygen. One gas present in every fire is carbon monoxide. This colorless, odorless gas is responsible for more fire deaths

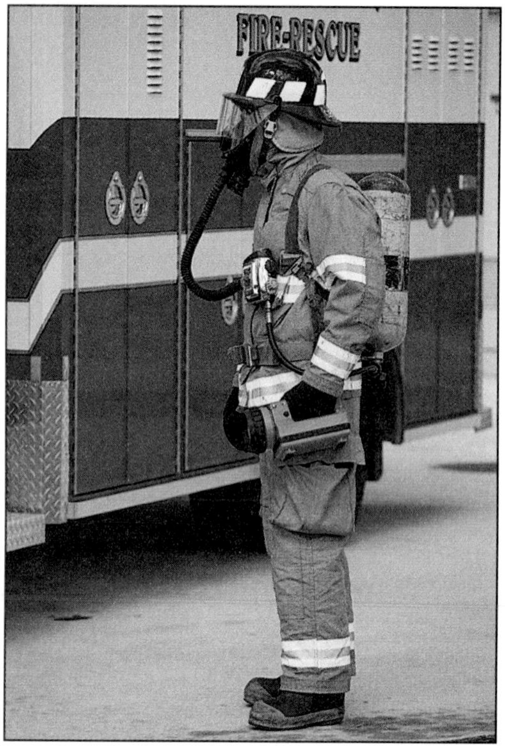

Figure 3-14

Proper protective gear for a fire includes SCBA, heat- and flame-retardant pants and coat, a helmet, gloves, steel-toed boots, and proper lighting.

each year than any other by-product of combustion.[13] This deadly gas blocks the ability of oxygen to get to the cells, resulting in toxic effects. Cyanide is another deadly gas that is created when plastics are burned.

The basic rule of fire suppression is not to enter a fire without proper equipment, training, and support personnel. The proper equipment includes the following (Figure 3-14):

- Self-contained breathing apparatus (SCBA)
- Heat- and flame-retardant turnout gear
- Head, hand, and foot protection
- Adequate lighting

If you are ever in a building that catches fire, evacuate immediately. Under normal conditions, you will only have a few minutes before the heat, flames, and smoke could overcome you. If you are providing care for a patient in a structure when a fire begins, withhold additional care and find the fastest acceptable exit for you and your patient. As you exit the building, check to see if doors are hot to the touch. If they are, do not open them. Instead, find another route of escape. Whenever possible stay close to the floor to avoid rising smoke and fumes.

Water and Ice

Swift moving water is treacherous and is often associated with flash floods, hurricanes, and low-head dams. Never venture into water or onto ice without the necessary training and safety equipment such as personal flotation devices, boats, polypropylene ropes, and wet suits. Moving water is deceptive. You will likely underestimate its force and be knocked off balance if you attempt to cross even water that is only knee high. Because you cannot see the bottom, you will not likely know the real depth of the water. Because ice varies in thickness and strength as a result of moving water, wind, and vegetation, ice is equally as dangerous.

Electricity

Anytime you suspect that an electrical hazard exists, you should stay back until the power is disconnected. Notify the fire department and power company of downed power lines, and always assume the lines are energized. Do not touch any metal fence, metal structure, or body of water in contact with a downed wire. Only attempt to move wires if you absolutely have to, and then, only with a nonconductive pole.

Hazardous Materials Incidents

Hazardous materials are common and a special risk for responding personnel. There are many toxic substances easily capable of causing death even with brief exposure. Many of these materials are transported by truck across interstate highways or by train. If you are responding to a known **hazardous materials incident,** you should position your ambulance at a safe distance upwind, and use

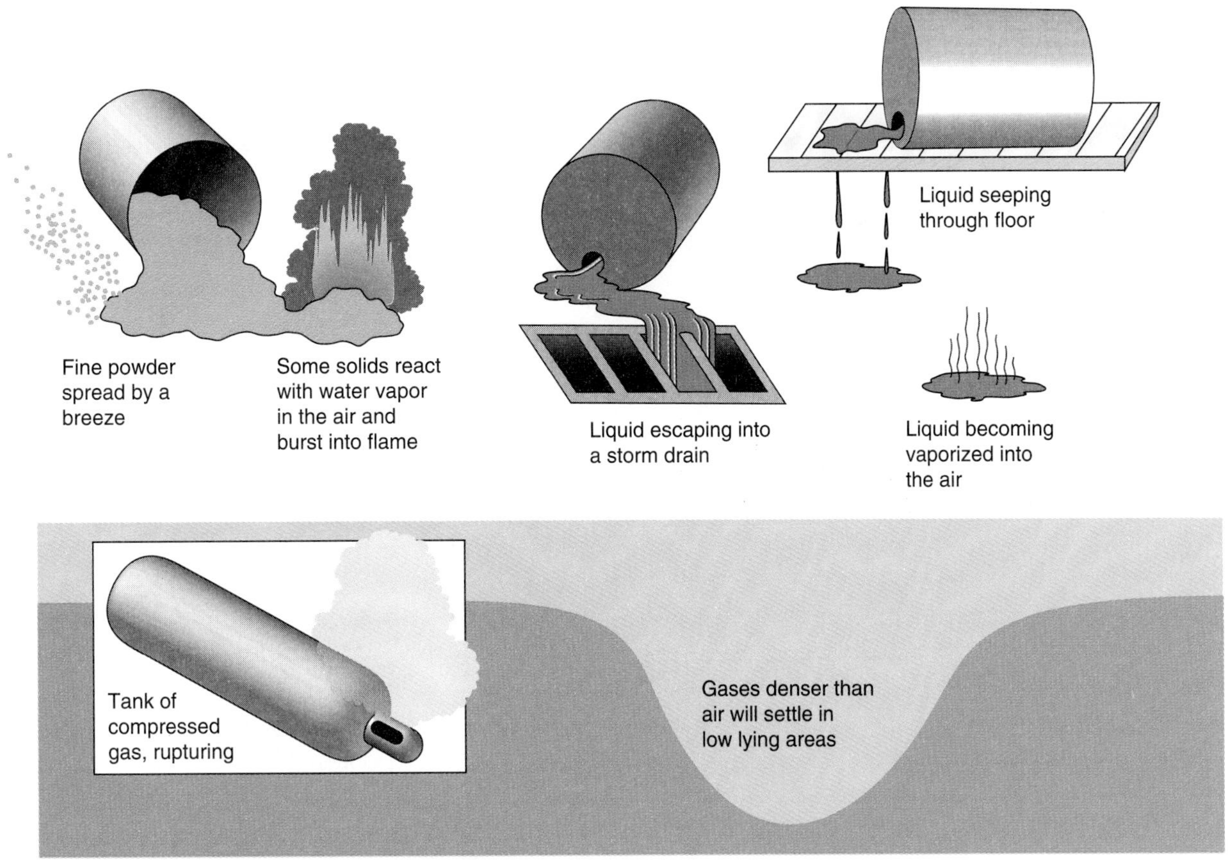
Fine powder spread by a breeze
Some solids react with water vapor in the air and burst into flame
Liquid escaping into a storm drain
Liquid seeping through floor
Liquid becoming vaporized into the air
Tank of compressed gas, rupturing
Gases denser than air will settle in low lying areas

Figure 3-15

You should look for signs of hazardous materials upon arrival on-scene. Hazardous materials can be in the form of a powder, liquid, solid, or vapor.

binoculars to evaluate the scene. Look for clues of a hazardous materials incident which include (Figure 3-15):

- Placards
- Clouds of vapor
- Spilled liquids or solids
- Disrupted containers, cylinders, or transport tanks

Placards are signs placed on vehicles, storage facilities, or railroad cars indicating the presence of hazardous materials. These placards have specific coded colors and numbers that help identify the substance(s) and the potential danger level and determine the best way to resolve the problem (Figure 3-16). These colors and numbers are listed in the U.S. Department of Transportation reference book, *Hazardous Materials: The Emergency Response Handbook*. In the event that further information is needed about a particular hazardous material, you can call hotline telephone numbers for agencies that can assist you 24 hours a day (Box 3-1).

Before entering a "hot zone," hazardous materials teams will put on specialized suits with SCBA (Figure 3-17). The individuals on these teams have been specially

BOX 3-1 Hazardous Materials Emergency Phone Numbers

CHEMTREC	Washington, DC	800-424-9300	24-hour hotline, toll free
		202-483-7616	24-hour hotline
REAC/TS	Oak Ridge, Tenn	615-482-2441	24-hour hotline

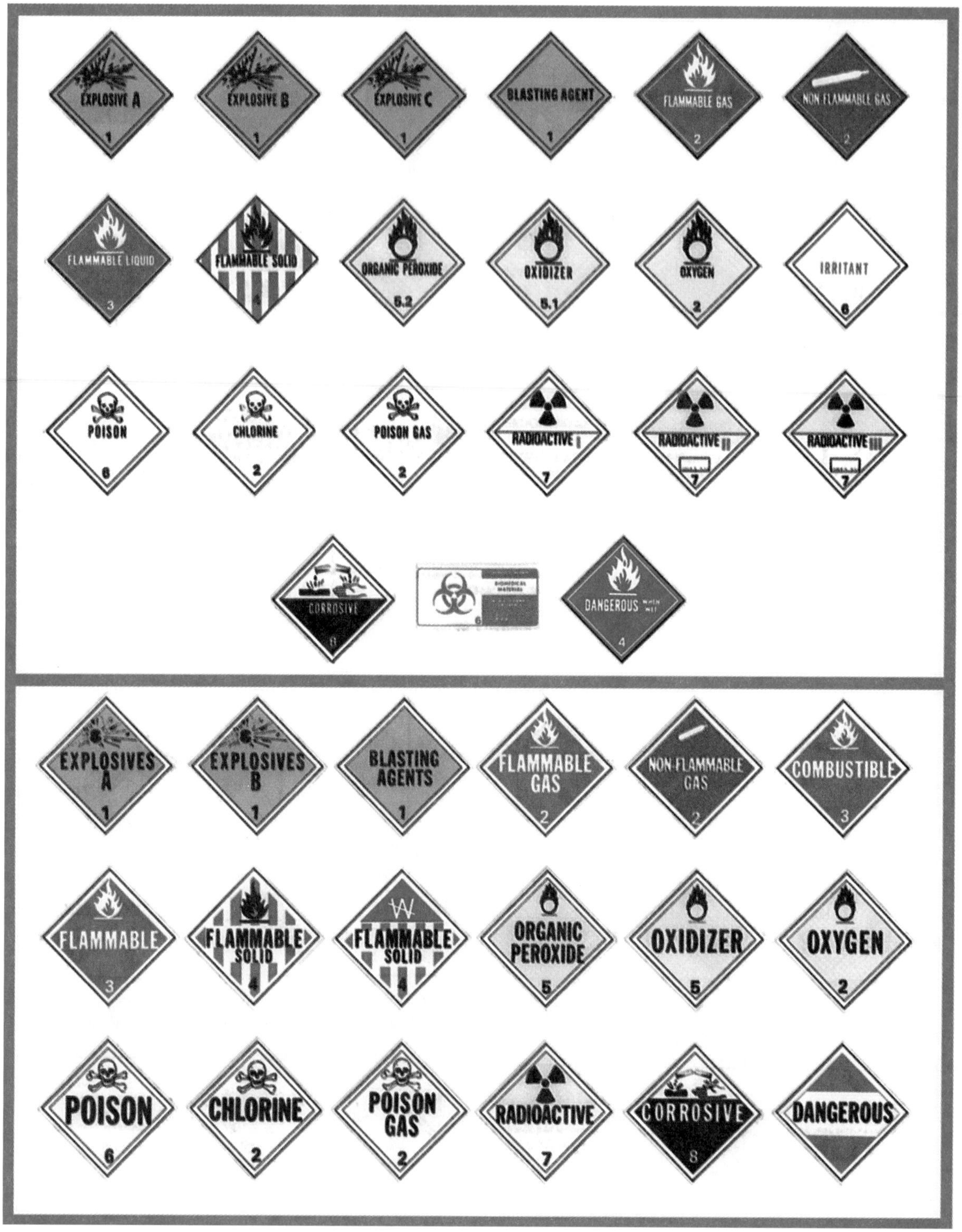

Figure 3-16

Warning placards are coded with colors and numbers to help you identify the substance and its level of danger.

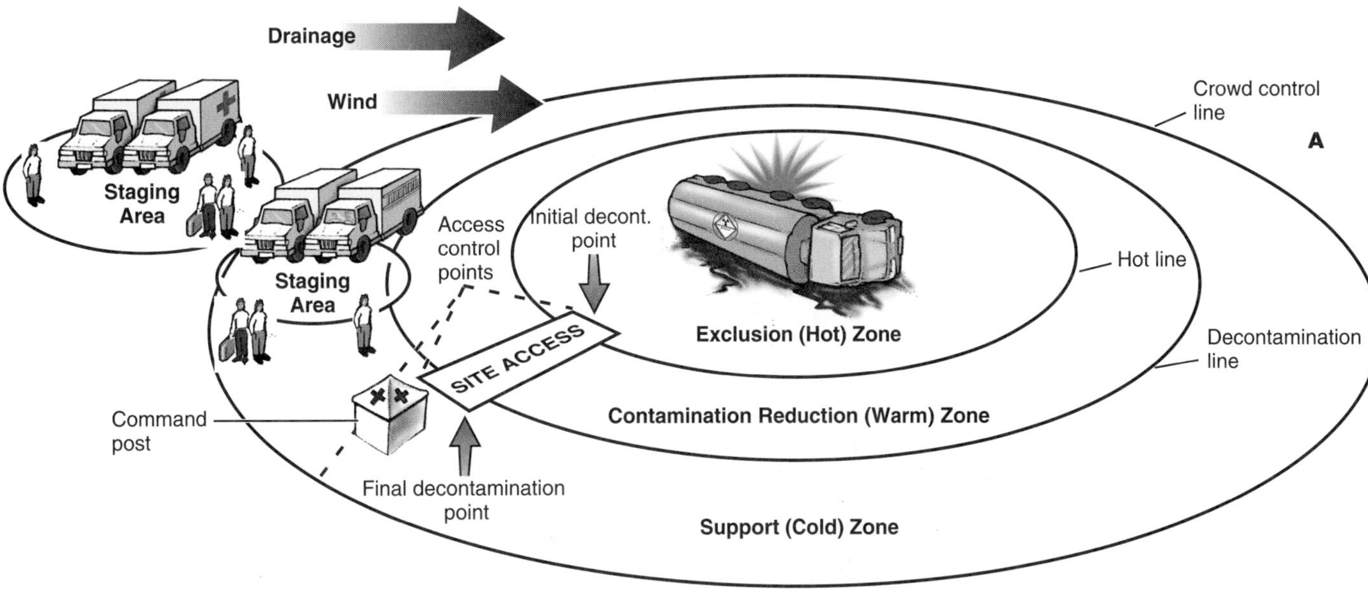

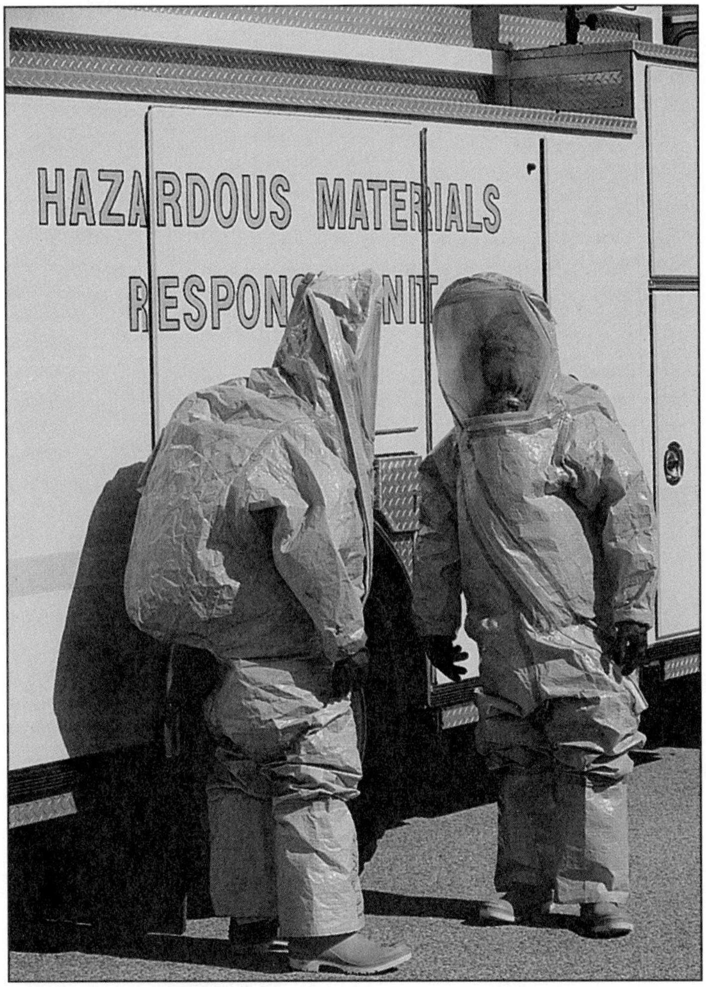

B

Figure 3-17

A, "Hot zones" should only be approached by hazardous materials teams who have special training and equipment. All others should stay in a safe location and should not provide patient care until all victims have been removed to a safe area and decontaminated. **B,** Responders in Class A personal protection equipment.

trained to deal with incidents of this type. Unless you have been specially trained, you should remain at a safe location away from hazardous materials. A safe location is usually one that is upwind and uphill from the incident. You will not have the opportunity to provide care for the patient until after he or she has been removed and decontaminated. **Decontamination** is the process of cleaning the hazardous substances off the patient's body. If not properly decontaminated, the patient will contaminate your ambulance, the hospital emergency department, and all those who come in contact with the patient.

Unsafe Structures

During your career you are likely to find patients in unsafe places such as trenches, sewers, mines, wells, silos, and buildings. If you are faced with a situation where the walls of a building or the sides of a trench are unstable, DO NOT ENTER! These areas will need to be shored up before you can reach the patient and begin providing care.

People trapped or injured in confined spaces present challenging situations. You should not enter areas that involve confined spaces, such as wells, sewers, and silos without the proper training and equipment. Confined spaces must be considered one of the more hazardous environments that you could face because of the diminished concentration of oxygen and higher concentration of toxic substances (e.g., methane, sulfides) in the air in those spaces. These areas require the use of SCBA and devices to measure the safety of the air.

Protective Clothing for the EMT

Besides the specialized clothing needed for situations like hazardous materials incidents and water rescue, you should possess some basic items that will provide general safety for you in other situations. The protective clothing that you should have includes:

- Puncture-proof gloves: These are firefighters' gloves that help protect your hands and arms from sharp objects, such as broken glass, and exposure to hot and cold surfaces.
- Helmet: Head and face protection is necessary anytime there is a chance of falling or flying objects. Firefighter helmets are frequently used because they provide this type of protection (Figure 3-18).
- Eyewear: Helmets are made so that faceshields can be attached. A full face shield will provide you with protection for your eyes and face. However, they are cumbersome and loose fitting, so debris may still be able to strike your eyes at certain angles. Safety goggles are also available. These form-fitting goggles provide excellent protection for your eyes.
- Turnout gear: This includes a heavy duty turnout coat and pants. These are designed to provide protection for your body.
- Footwear: Because of the risk of objects being dropped on your feet, or ankle injuries occurring, high-top, steel-toe work shoes are recommended. They provide excellent ankle support and the maximum protection for your toes.

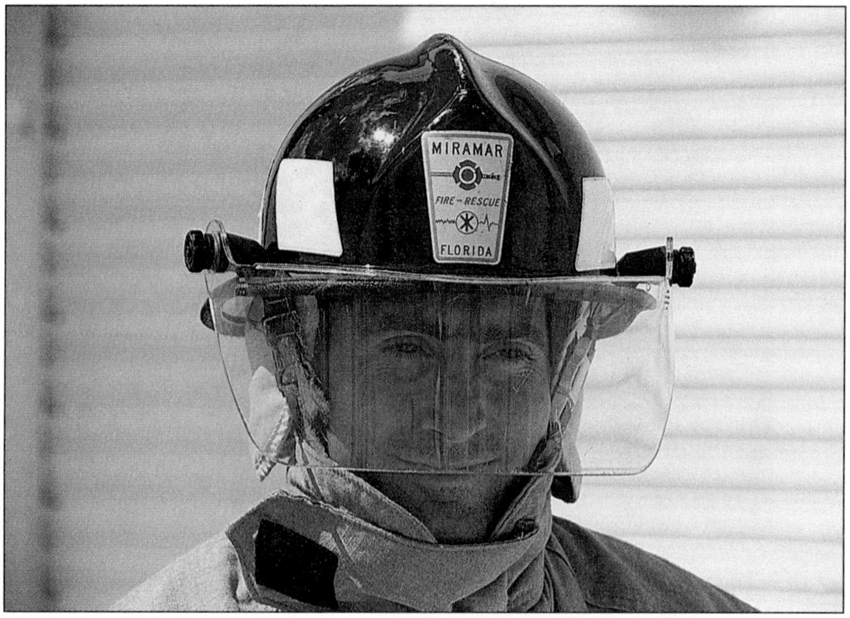

Figure 3-18

Firefighter helmets provide good protection from any falling or flying objects that might hit the head or face.

Emotional Well-Being of the EMT

There are few professions that involve more emotional stress than the life-and-death situations that you are likely to encounter as an EMT. Death and dying are an unfortunate part of EMS and result in high levels of stress for EMS personnel.

Death and Dying

Your reaction to death and the dying patient reflects your own beliefs and fears. It is natural to feel uncomfortable about discussing this subject with the dying patient or family members. As you gain more experience, these discussions will become easier for you. Because the patient and family are experiencing many emotions during a terminal condition or at the time of a death, it is important to understand these emotions.

The Grieving Process

A dying patient and his or her family members experience a grieving process that has several identifiable stages:

- Denial: This first stage is experienced by most dying patients and those anticipating or mourning the death of a loved one. It is a defensive mechanism used to create a buffer between the shock of dying or witnessing death and having to deal with it. It is a temporary stage that involves refusing to accept the inevitable death resulting from a terminal condition or the unexpected death of a loved one.
- Anger: Anger in the form of aggressive verbal or physical behavior marks the second stage of the grieving process. In this stage the patient or family members are dealing with the question "why?" They are often expressing their frustration at not being able to accept the event or do anything about it. You may be the recipient of this anger. Do not take the anger or insults personally. Be tolerant, empathetic, and use good listening skills.
- Bargaining: This is a defensive mechanism used by the patient that involves an "agreement" in exchange for an extension of life.
- Depression: At this stage the patient is saying goodbye to the things and people that he or she has known and loved. It is a stage marked by sadness and despair over things not accomplished. The dying patient is usually silent and unwilling to communicate with others.
- Acceptance: This final stage of the process is one in which the dying patient accepts the inevitability of death and admits to being ready to die. The patient often has only one fear: to not die alone. The patient is often able to accept the situation before family members, who may not accept the death for weeks, months, or even years.

Dealing With Death and Dying

Treat a dying patient in a dignified manner, respecting his or her wishes for privacy. Do not falsely reassure the patient, but let the patient know that everything that can be done to help will be done. Try to comfort the patient and when appropriate use a reassuring touch.

Though you are seldom involved in the patient's final acceptance of death, you are likely to witness the reactions of family members experiencing the death process. Denial is common among those who do not recognize the seriousness of the situation. Guilt is also common among those who feel they should have done more. This is especially true of parents experiencing the death of their child. When it is necessary to inform family members of the death of a loved one, use a gentle, but direct approach. Use the words *death* or *dead* when expressing the patient's condition. Avoid phrases such as *passed away* or *not with us any longer*. Be compassionate and take time to answer questions that family members may have. If the family asks for a priest or chaplain, assist them in making the appropriate contact.

The Needs of the EMT

Death is hard for anyone to deal with, and EMS personnel are no different. Just because you are an EMT, you are not exempt from the emotions that others experience. Although you attempt to do your job in a professional manner without becoming overcome by emotion, the feelings associated with death and dying are sometimes overwhelming. You may find it difficult to suppress these emotions while providing patient care.

You can expect to feel some of the same emotions that family members feel as they grieve. These reactions are normal. You should attempt to discuss these feelings as soon as possible after the incident. You may find that this helps lessen the emotional burden.

Stress

By their nature, emergencies are stressful events. Some of the incidents that tend to be the most stressful are:

- Death and dying, especially when children or coworkers are involved.
- Multiple casualty incidents.
- Rescues, whether failed or successful.
- Resuscitation efforts, whether failed or successful.
- Abuse and neglect of children or elders.
- Domestic violence.
- Major trauma, including amputations.

From the time that the call is dispatched, you become involved in the event. As you provide care for a patient, you experience some of the pain and stress of the patient and in some severe cases, the bystanders. Often, the longer the event, the greater the stress. EMS providers assisting with the 1995 Oklahoma City bombing experienced great stress as they attempted to rescue survivors and deal with the death of hundreds of others. Events such as this can produce noticeable stress responses.

You may think of stressful incidents only as those that result in death, but lengthy rescue operations that are successful can produce just as much stress. Another factor that may produce stress is your work schedule, which can disrupt family time. It can be difficult to plan other activities because of shift work. Family members may not understand your passion for your profession. This lack of understanding can cause frustration because of your desire to share work-related happenings. You and your family members may sometimes feel alone and depressed, because of the inability to share experiences that may be stressful to you.

Recognizing Stress

One of the most common symptoms of stress is anxiety. This is often defined as a feeling of apprehension and is common in EMS because of the unknown outcome of some of the patients that you will be caring for. It can be caused by internal conflicts, such as unhappiness with a career choice or the inability to meet personal expectations. It can also be caused by external conflicts with colleagues, supervisors, and spouses.

Outward signs of stress include changes in physical, emotional, mental, and behavioral responses. Box 3-2 provides a detailed list of the signs and symptoms of stress that fall into these four categories. These signs and symptoms should alert you and others close to you that there is a potential problem.

BOX 3-2 Signals of Stress

Physical	Emotional
Chest pain	Anger
Heart rhythm abnormalities	Denial
	Fear
Difficulty breathing	Feeling of being overwhelmed
Nausea and vomiting	Panic reactions
Profuse sweating	
Sleep disturbances	
Mental	**Behavioral**
Confusion or disorientation	Changes in eating habits
	Crying episodes
Decreased level of awareness	Hyperactivity
	Withdrawal and isolation
Indecisiveness	Increased alcohol or tobacco use
Distressing dreams	
Memory problems	Loss of interest in work or sex
Poor concentration	

Coping With Stress

There are several different ways to cope with job-related stress. Because each individual has a particular way to deal with stressful situations, different coping strategies are needed. Some individuals cope with stress by increasing work activity. Others look to family and friends to laugh or talk through stressful situations. Besides these positive ways to cope with stress, however, some individuals may develop negative habits, such as drug use and withdrawal.

Managing stress effectively begins with recognition of the signs and symptoms of stress. Once this has been accomplished, you can begin to use strategies to help manage the stressful situations in your life.

Lifestyle Changes. The most effective way to deal with stress is to make a positive change in your personal and professional lifestyle. This involves a wellness approach to mind and body that includes:

- Developing a healthy diet. Reducing sugar, caffeine, and alcohol will sometimes reduce stress because it helps decrease hyperactivity and sleep disturbances. Avoiding fatty foods and increasing your consumption of carbohydrates will help minimize the risk of cardiovascular disease.
- Exercising regularly. Proper exercise will help you maintain the proper muscle development necessary for your physically demanding profession. Exercise aids in the metabolism of foods, provides an outlet for the physical demands of stress, and helps you to relax and rest easier. Aerobic exercises such as jogging, biking, or swimming burn off calories and help prevent cardiovascular disease.
- Relaxing. Relaxation exercises are a form of focused meditation that help reduce stress by helping the body relax. Deep breathing is a relaxation exercise best done in a quiet environment. However, relaxing with family and friends, changing your work shifts, or requesting assignment in a less busy area may also help you reduce stress.

In addition to these techniques, stress intervention can include professional peer counseling and group discussions and the pursuit of activities or hobbies outside of work. By balancing your lifestyle between work, recreation, family, and health, you will be better able to cope with the stress in your life.

Critical Incident Stress Management

Critical incident stress debriefing (CISD) was originally developed in the 1970s to assist emergency personnel who had been exposed to significant incidents.[4] Since that time, CISD has been expanded to a broader-based management approach that provides assistance to anyone who may have had a particularly stressful call.

Critical incident stress management (CISM) involves a team approach, based on a partnership of mental health professionals and peer group support. This team helps emergency personnel express their feelings toward a particular call or situation that had a strong emotional effect. It is important to remember that a stress debriefing is not an investigation, interrogation, or psychiatric assessment; and all information discussed is confidential.

CISM is an open discussion that encourages participants to talk about any fears or reactions that they have had after a call. The timing of a debriefing session is important and ideally should be held within 24 to 72 hours after an incident. It is important to note that CISM is not confined to events involving the death of others. Even a successful large scale rescue effort can cause tremendous stress for the rescuers. CISM leaders and mental health personnel evaluate the information and offer suggestions to help overcome the stress brought on by the situation. In this manner, CISM allows for group support and the opportunity to determine if someone needs additional assistance. There are 10 services that a comprehensive CISM team provides[4]:

1. Preincident stress education. This is designed to educate the EMS provider about the stress involved in specific situations, what to expect, how to cope, and how CISM will help.
2. On-scene peer support. CISM team members provide support on the scene to those involved in the incident in an effort to begin the process that may follow in a larger group session.
3. One-on-one support. Sometimes the EMS provider will be more comfortable discussing feelings in a more intimate setting. One-on-one support is designed to assist individuals who feel this is more appropriate for them.
4. Disaster services support. In the event of a disaster, CISM teams bring their valuable training to assist those working the disaster, as well as those who may have been victims of the disaster.
5. Defusings. A defusing session is often a small group session, limited only to those most directly involved in the most stressful aspects of the incident. It is usually held within the first few hours of the incident (Figure 3-19). For example, the first rescue teams working the Oklahoma City tragedy were defused immediately at the end of their shift in which they were searching for survivors inside the structure.
6. Debriefing. A debriefing is a larger group meeting for the purpose of discussing feelings that were present at the time of the incident and after the incident.
7. Follow-up services. Attendees will be contacted within 24 hours after a debriefing to determine if they need additional support and referral.

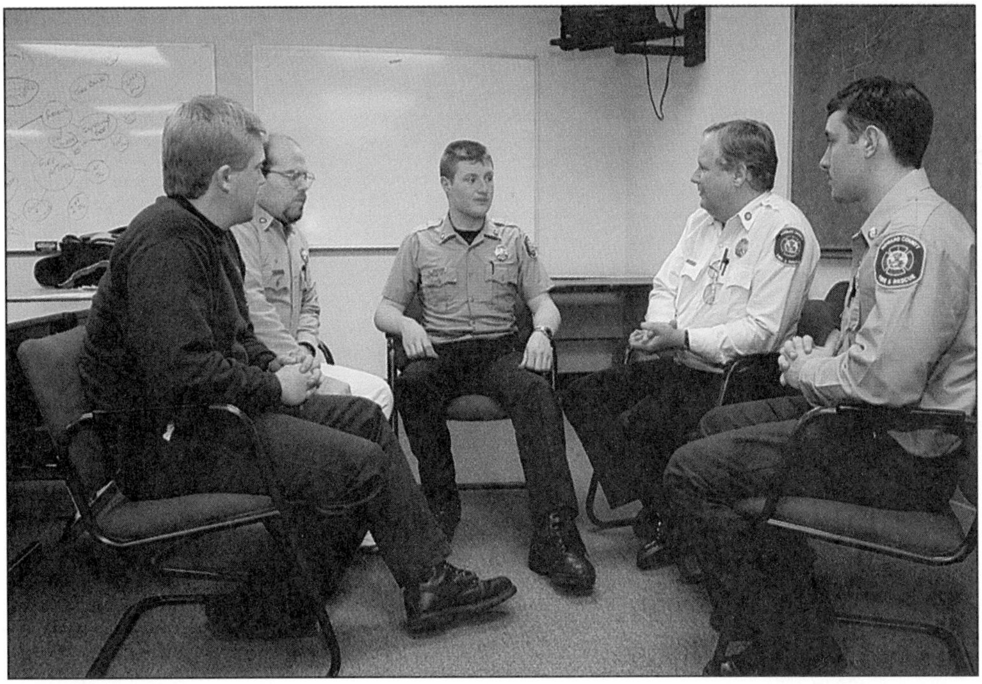

Figure 3-19

Defusing sessions should be held within a few hours of the incident and should be limited to workers who were involved in the incident.

8. Spouse and family support. It is important that loved ones understand what EMS personnel are going through and that they be counseled to help the provider cope with the incident.
9. Community outreach. Because of the devastating effect that a particular incident can have on the people of a local community, outreach programs are used to help those directly and indirectly involved to cope with the incident. Examples include CISD teams helping students cope with the death of classmates or workers coping with the loss of a colleague.
10. Wellness initiatives. A comprehensive approach to managing critical incident stress may sometimes include establishing wellness centers and community activities to help individuals relieve tension, anxiety, fear, and anger. These initiatives could include periodic stress evaluations, seminars on stress reduction, pastoral services, and additional counseling.

These and other stress-management approaches are valuable resources to EMS personnel and the local community as a whole in understanding and coping with the stress produced by emergency situations.

SUMMARY

Maintaining your well-being is extremely important to your overall satisfaction and job success. If you become injured in the line of duty or are responsible for someone else's injury, there are now additional patients that need attention. It is unlikely that you can effectively provide care for others if you are injured or ill. Whenever you arrive at the scene of an emergency, take the time to assess the dangers, identify the need for additional resources, and when necessary retreat to a safer area. By following these guidelines, you can minimize the likelihood of injury from violent situations, motor-vehicle collisions, and environmental factors such as fire, water, and ice.

Illness can come in many forms, such as disease transmission. Be well informed of your agency's policies and protocols for avoiding disease transmission and reporting exposures. If you think you have had an exposure, report it immediately. Follow universal precaution practices with all of your patients so that you can prevent the spread of communicable diseases. Use appropriate clothing and equipment to protect you against illness and injury.

Illness can also result from job-related stress. Emergencies create stressful situations that are not always easy to identify or cope with. For this reason, professional assistance is available to the EMS personnel in the form of comprehensive stress-management efforts that include CISD. Follow the strategies presented in this chapter to help reduce the stress associated with the demanding EMS field.

REFERENCES

1. **Atkinson WK:** Dodging bullets: gang violence and EMS, *J Emerg Med Serv* 18:55, 1993.
2. **Crowe SJ:** *Halstead of Johns Hopkins,* Springfield, Md., 1957, Charles C. Thomas Publisher.
3. **Gerberding JL, Henderson DK:** Management of occupational exposures to bloodborne pathogens: hepatitis B virus, hepatitis C virus, and human immunodeficiency virus, *Clin Infec Dis* 12:79, 1992.
4. **Mitchell J, Bray G:** *Emergency services stress,* Englewood Cliffs, NJ, 1990, Brady.
5. **United States Department of Health and Human Services, Centers for Disease Control:** *Draft guidelines for preventing the transmission of tuberculosis in health care facilities,* 52810-854, ed 2, Washington, DC, 1993, Federal Register.
6. **United States Department of Labor, Occupational Safety and Health Administration:** *Hazardous waste operations and emergency response,* standard 1910.120, Washington, DC, 1990, Occupational Safety and Health Administration.
7. **United States Department of Health and Human Services, Centers for Disease Control:** Protection against viral hepatitis: recommendations of the immunization practices advisory committee, *Morbidity and Mortality Weekly Report,* 39:RR-2, 1990.
8. **United States Department of Health and Human Services, Centers for Disease Control:** Guidelines for the prevention of transmission of human immunodeficiency virus and hepatitis B virus to health care and public safety workers, *Morbidity and Mortality Weekly Report,* 38:S6, 1989.
9. **United States Department of Labor, Occupational Safety and Health Administration:** *Occupational exposure to bloodborne pathogens: final rule,* 29 CFR Part 1910.1030, Washington, DC, 1991, Federal Register.
10. **United States Department of Labor, Occupational Safety and Health Administration:** *Enforcement procedures for the exposure to bloodborne pathogens,* standard 29 CFR Part 1910.1030, Washington, DC, 1992, Occupational Safety and Health Administration.
11. **Wenzel R:** *Handbook of hospital acquired infections,* Boca Raton, Fla, 1981, CRC Press.
12. **West K:** *Infectious disease handbook for emergency care personnel,* ed 2, Cincinnati, 1994, American Conference of Governmental Industrial Hygienists, Inc.
13. **Worsing RA:** *Basic rescue and emergency care,* Park Ridge, Ill, 1990, American Academy of Orthopaedic Surgeons.

SUGGESTED READINGS

1. **Meade DM, Relf RH:** When colors kill, *Emerg Med Serv* 21(1): 20-26, 1992.

Chapter 4

Ambulance Operations

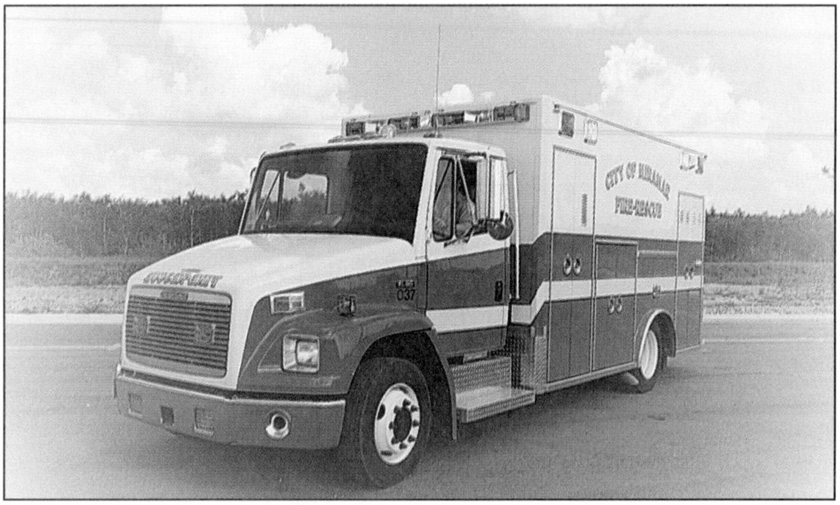

Knowledge Objectives

OBJECTIVES

As an EMT-Basic, you should be able to:

1. Identify the standard ambulance equipment needed to respond to an emergency.
2. List the phases of an ambulance call.
3. Identify the characteristics of a good emergency vehicle operator.
4. Describe the general provisions in the law governing the operation of emergency vehicles with regard to:
   - Speed
   - Audible warning devices
   - Visual warning devices
   - Parking
   - Right-of-way
   - Turning
5. Describe factors that contribute to unsafe driving conditions.
6. Identify the dangers posed when:
   - Using escorts or during multiple vehicle responses
   - Approaching intersections
7. Explain the meaning of the legal phrase *operating an emergency vehicle in a manner that provides for the safety of all others.*
8. Identify what information is essential for a dispatcher or call-taker to obtain from the caller to allow for appropriate dispatch of EMS resources.
9. Describe how the following factors can adversely affect your response to a call:
   - Weather
   - Day of the week
   - Time of day
   - Road construction
   - Other vehicular traffic, including school buses
10. Differentiate between the various methods of transferring a patient to an ambulance based on injury or illness.
11. Explain the importance of adequate preparation of the ambulance before receiving a call.
12. Differentiate among the following terms:
    - Cleaning
    - Disinfecting
    - Sterilizing

Attitude Objectives

As an EMT-Basic, you should be able to:

OBJECTIVES

1. **Express your feelings about the importance of having an ambulance in proper working condition and with the necessary equipment and supplies to respond to a call.**
2. **Advocate the need for transferring accurate patient information to other health care providers in a timely manner.**
3. **Serve as a role model for others when checking and restocking an ambulance before working a shift and after every call.**

KEY TERMS

1. **Ambulance:** Emergency vehicle used to treat and transport ill or injured patients to medical facilities.
2. **Defensive Driving:** Driving in a manner that considers factors affecting safe vehicle operation and incorporates practices that will minimize the likelihood of a collision.
3. **Emergency Vehicle Operator Training:** Specialized training for persons who will be driving emergency vehicles, such as an ambulance, to assist them in operating the vehicle in a safe manner.

IT'S YOUR CALL

Weather reports indicate that a severe winter storm is approaching rapidly, and there are forecasts for heavy snow and ice. Neighboring counties have reported power outages and treacherous road conditions. Suddenly, multiple vehicle collisions are reported. Ambulances are dispatched from points all over the county.

You and two partners have just started to inspect your ambulance, when you are dispatched to provide help for a patient lying unconscious with a head injury in her vehicle. As you near the scene, you turn down a side street, only to find that it has been closed for repair and traffic is being rerouted. You think it odd that you had not heard anything about this street being closed, but you realize that you had not had time to check with the dispatch center or your own station's road status board.

After a few additional diversions, you finally arrive at the scene. It took significantly longer than normal to reach the scene, but you are still the first emergency vehicle to arrive. You attempt to maneuver the ambulance behind the damaged vehicle, but a patch of ice causes your vehicle to lose traction on the road. Your vehicle begins to slide, but you are able to control it and bring it to a stop. Unfortunately, two of the wheels are in deep snow near the patient's vehicle. As you exit the ambulance, you hope that the oncoming traffic will see the flashing lights of your vehicle in the diminishing visibility caused by the winter storm.

The three of you approach the patient's vehicle and gain access with little difficulty. The patient is now conscious but disoriented and very cold. As you work to control the patient's bleeding and prepare her for transport, one of your partners tells you that there is only one blanket on the ambulance to help warm the patient. As you prepare to remove the patient from the vehicle, you suddenly hear the sound of a horn. You watch as an oncoming vehicle slides out of control, barely missing your ambulance and coming to rest in a ditch. You may now have an additional injured person. Traffic continues to proceed down the road. Your ambulance is likely stuck in the snow and it is unlikely that you will be able to transport any patients.

You are now faced with the dilemma of correcting problems that possibly did not need to occur in the first place. Looking back at the call, can you identify some of the problems that could have been avoided? What specific steps could have been taken?

Responding to an emergency situation requires that you make sure your emergency vehicle is appropriately equipped and properly functioning before you need to use it. It requires that you and other emergency medical service (EMS) personnel be adequately trained to respond to and locate a variety of calls under a variety of environmental conditions. Operating the vehicle in a safe manner helps ensure your safety and the safety of other crew members, other drivers, and pedestrians. If you do not maintain the vehicle in proper working condition and fail to operate it in a safe manner, you could be involved in a motor-vehicle collision, could fail to get to a scene because of mechanical failure, or could lack the proper supplies or equipment needed to care for a patient.

This chapter provides an overview of emergency vehicle operations, including the different phases of ambulance operations:

- Call preparation
- Dispatch
- Response
- Arrival
- Transfer to the ambulance
- Transport to a receiving facility
- Turning a patient over to a receiving facility
- Returning to service*

*The DOT curriculum separates returning to service into two segments: en route to station and postrun.

Each phase is critical to the effective operation of an ambulance. The importance of the information presented in this chapter cannot be overstated. All of your training will not help you save a life if you cannot get to the scene in a safe and efficient manner with the right equipment necessary to provide the best possible care.

The Evolution of the Ambulance

Ambulances have changed over the years in design and purpose. From its conception, the ambulance has been used to transport patients to the hospital (Figure 4-1). While it still serves this original purpose, the modern ambulance is much more than simply a mode of transportation to the hospital. Instead it functions as a mobile emergency care facility, taking equipment and supplies to the patient (Figure 4-2). It was not until 1974 that federal specifications for ambulances were developed by the General Services Administration for the Department of Transportation. These specifications known as *KKK-A-1822* standardized ambulance design to allow for medical care both on scene and en route to the receiving hospital. These specifications defined three types of ambulances:

- Type I: This is a conventional ambulance with a truck cab and chassis, upon which a modular ambulance body is mounted. There is no passageway for individuals to move between the patient compartment and the cab (Figure 4-3).

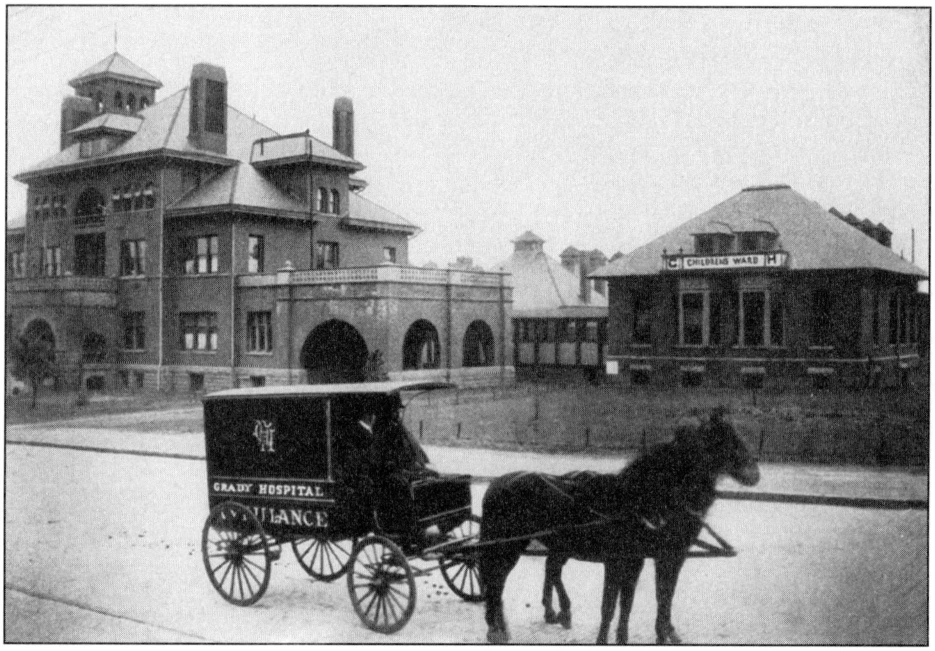

Figure 4-1

Originally, ambulances were not equipped to provide the patient care of today's ambulances. Their primary function was transporting patients to hospitals.

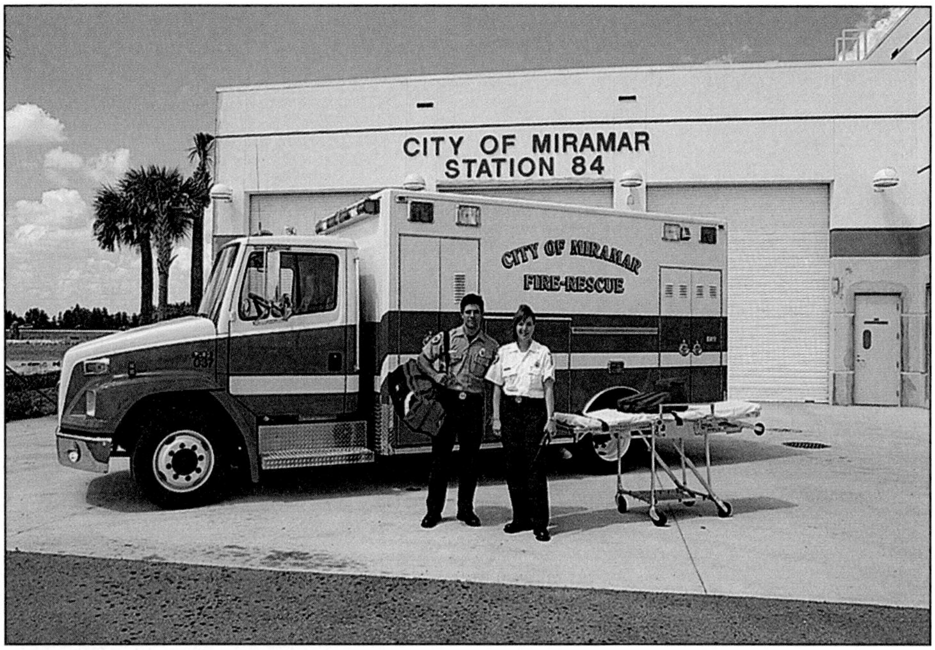

Figure 4-2

Modern ambulances are equipped to provide much more than transportation. The equipment and crew on board today's ambulances provide reliable life support and medical care while en route to the hospital.

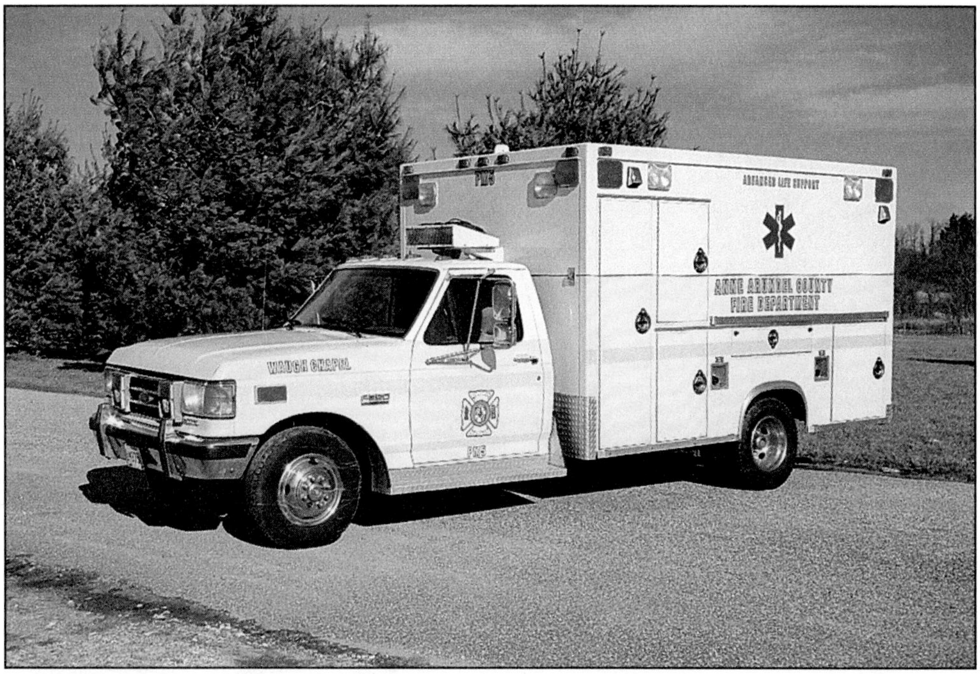

Figure 4-3

Type I ambulances have separate cab and patient compartments; there is no access to the patient compartment from the driver's compartment.

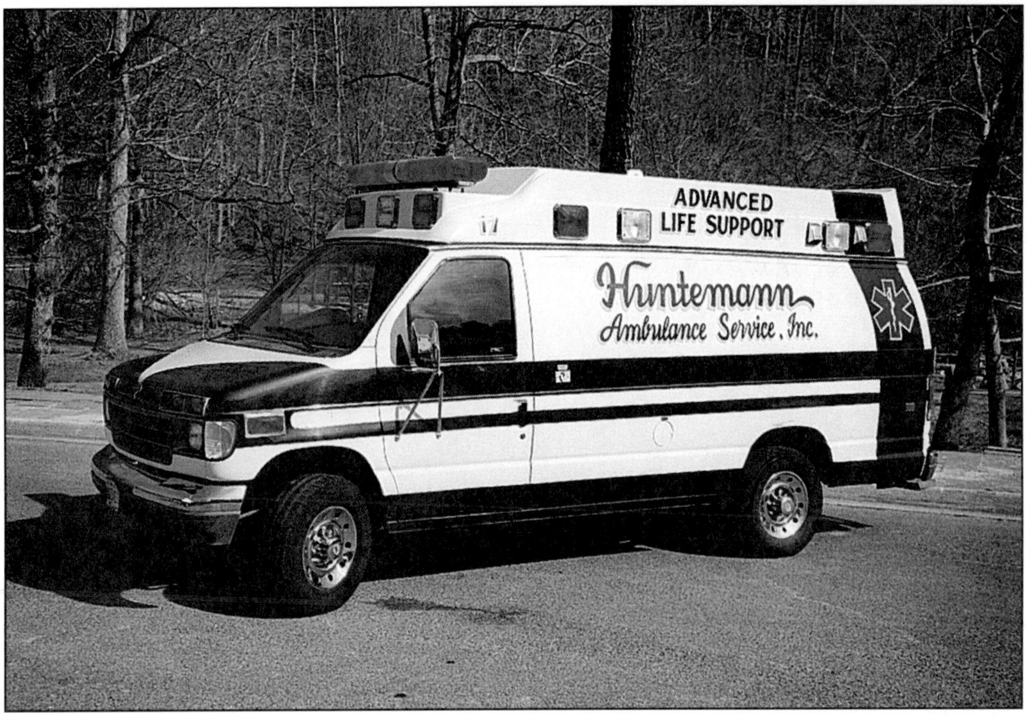

Figure 4-4

Type II ambulances are conversion vans with the driver and patient compartments in one unit; there is access between the driver and patient compartments.

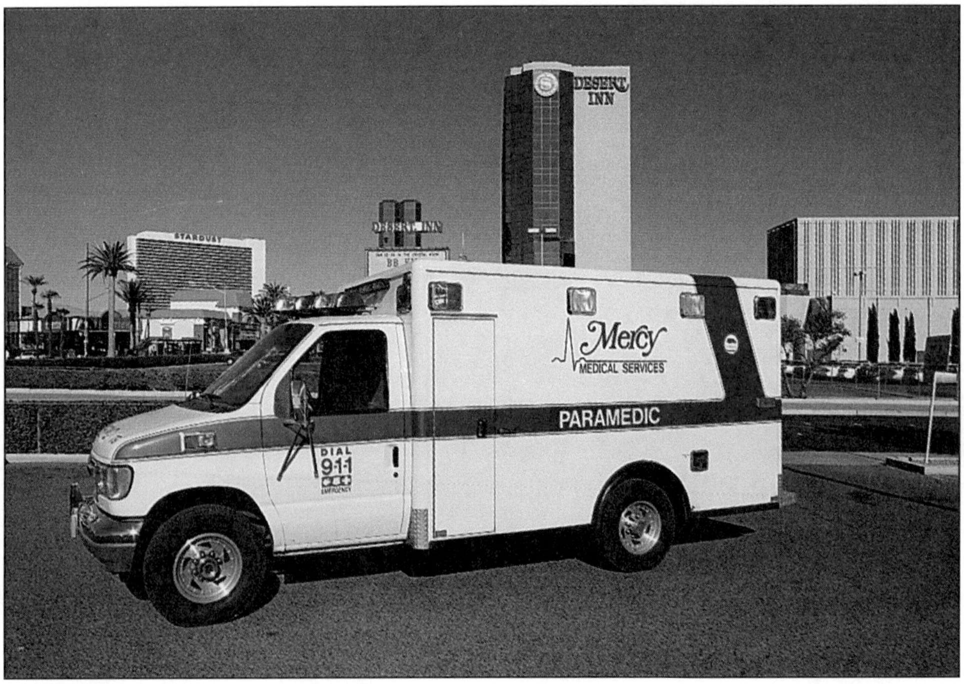

Figure 4-5

Type III ambulances are specialty vans that allow easy access between the driver and patient compartments.

- Type II: This is a standard van in which the cab and body are one unit, allowing access from the front to the rear of the vehicle (Figure 4-4).
- Type III: This unit is a specialty van in which the cab and body are one unit, allowing easy access from the front to the rear of the vehicle (Figure 4-5).

Other types of ambulances have emerged over the years as well. These include specially designed vehicles that serve as mobile critical care units or neonatal intensive care units. Because of the growing demands for more equipment and services, such as specialty rescue and advanced life support, some ambulances are being made with a heavier chassis that is stronger, more durable, and allows greater storage area. Some vehicles have special equipment installed on the chassis to allow for easier loading and unloading of patients.

Besides specifications for ambulance design, states have requirements for equipment and supplies to be carried on all emergency vehicles. National organizations have also established guidelines for equipment and supplies to be carried on ambulances. The American College of Surgeons' Committee on Trauma has established a recommended standard set of equipment for all basic life support ambulances. The American College of Emergency Physicians has similar guidelines for equipment and supplies for both basic and advanced life support vehicles.[1] These guidelines are used as resources by individual state EMS offices to establish regulations regarding the necessary equipment and supplies for ambulances.

Preparing for a Call

As you arrive at the station for duty, one of your first priorities is to check your vehicle to ensure that it holds all the supplies and equipment needed for personal safety and patient care. Some EMS systems have ambulances with varying configurations for holding supplies and equipment. You must be familiar with the storage areas for all of these items regardless of the differences in ambulance configurations.

Inspecting the Ambulance

Being adequately prepared for a call means that the equipment and supplies are easily accessible and in proper working order. Equipment and supplies should be placed in the ambulance according to their importance and need. For example, oxygen equipment should be immediately available near the patient's head. Items that are not often used, such as restraints, could be placed in an area that is not immediately accessible, such as within a cabinet away from the patient.

You should have a means of documenting that the vehicle has been checked and stocked appropriately for service. Many agencies use an ambulance checklist for this purpose. Some checklists are more thorough than others. They are often designed according to the location of the supplies and equipment in the vehicle. This makes it easy to determine if the right equipment and supplies are in the proper location.

Checklists must be functional, meaning that you must not only check to see that the necessary equipment is present but also that it is in proper working condition. Liability becomes a real concern if your equipment fails to function when you need it. Becoming thoroughly familiar with your agency's ambulances will enable you to rapidly locate and operate the necessary equipment or retrieve the needed supplies in an emergency.

Nonmedical Equipment and Supplies

The nonmedical equipment and supplies that you should have available on your ambulance include personal-safety items, warning devices, map books, and tools needed to gain access to patients under special situations. The nonmedical equipment and supplies on your ambulance will vary according to the responsibilities that you may have. For example, some ambulance agencies only provide patient care; other ambulance agencies may also be responsible for rescue operations. A typical equipment list may include items such as:

- Turnout gear for each crew member, including gloves, eyewear, coat, and helmet
- Portable radio
- U.S. Department of Transportation *Emergency Response Guidebook*
- Spotlight/floodlight
- Binoculars
- Map books
- Jumper cables
- Flares/reflectors
- Wheel chocks
- Utility rope
- Tools for accessing patients, including a center punch, prybar, Biel tool, hammer, and flat head axe
- Triage tags, tarps, and incident logs for use with multiple-casualty incidents
- Command/identification vests
- Clipboards with patient-care reports
- Personal flotation device
- **Self-contained breathing apparatus** (SCBA) (optional)
- Disposable tyvek suits (optional)

Medical Supplies and Equipment

The medical supplies and equipment that you should have on your ambulance include those items needed for:

BOX 4-1 Medical Equipment and Supplies for Ambulances

Personal Protection

- Disposable latex, vinyl, or other synthetic gloves in various sizes
- Protective eyewear, such as eye shields or goggles with side protectors
- Gown for large exposure to body fluids
- Face masks, including HEPA masks
- Sharps containers for the vehicle and portable ALS kit
- EPA-registered disinfectants for cleaning
- Biohazard bags for labeling and disposal of infected waste materials
- Bags for labeling and disposal of trash
- Bags for labeling used linen for laundering
- Disposable emesis bags or basins
- Bedpan/urinal
- Patient restraining devices

Patient Assessment

- Stethoscope
- Blood pressure cuffs of various size
- Penlight
- Thermometer
- Scissors

Airway and Breathing Management

- Oropharyngeal and nasopharyngeal airways of various sizes
- Suction unit, including a fixed mechanical unit and portable mechanical or manual unit
- Oxygen masks and nasal cannulas of various sizes
- Fixed and portable oxygen delivery systems
- Spare portable oxygen cylinders
- Oxygen regulators
- Resuscitation masks with air-diverting valves
- Disposable bite stick
- Bag valve masks of various size
- Oxygen-powered ventilation device (optional)
- Automatic transport ventilator (optional)
- Pulse oximetry (optional)

Resuscitation

- Automated external defibrillator (AED)
- Mechanical chest compressor

Wound Care

- Sterile gauze pads of various sizes, including multitrauma dressings
- Occlusive dressings
- Self-adhering roller bandages in various sizes
- Adhesive strip bandages
- Hypoallergenic tape of various sizes
- Sterile burn sheets or commercial burn kit
- Irrigation fluid, such as normal saline and water
- Ring cutter

Muscle and Bone Injury

- Splints of various sizes and types, including padded rigid splints, air splints, vacuum splints, and wire splints
- Backboards for spinal immobilization
- Rigid cervical collars of various sizes
- Head immobilizer, either commercially available or rolled blankets
- An extrication device
- Straps of various sizes for securing a patient to a backboard
- Pneumatic anti-shock garment (PASG) for immobilizing pelvic injuries
- Chemical cold packs
- Tongue depressors for finger injuries
- Triangular bandages for slings and binders

Medical Emergencies

- Activated charcoal for poisoning
- Disposable cups for oral administration of poisoning medications
- Instant glucose for diabetic problems
- Constricting bands for snakebite injuries

Childbirth

- Obstetrical kit, including umbilical cord clamps, bulb syringe, receiving blanket, infant caps, and sanitary napkins

Patient Transport and Comfort

- Pillows and pillow cases
- Sheets and blankets
- Wheeled stretcher capable of conforming to various positions and heights
- Reeves stretcher
- Folding chair
- Scoop stretcher
- Child safety seat

- Personal protection against communicable disease
- Patient assessment
- Airway and breathing management
- Resuscitation
- Wound care (including burns)
- Muscle and bone injuries
- Medical emergencies
- Childbirth
- Patient transport
- Advanced life support equipment (if applicable)

Box 4-1 provides a detailed list of the medical supplies and equipment needed for each of these areas. The types and amounts of supplies to be carried are mandated by individual states.

Vehicle Maintenance

Preventive maintenance is critical for proper functioning of the ambulance. Because of the constant workload that the ambulance is subjected to, it is important to service the vehicle regularly. EMS agencies may use their own mechanic or contract with an outside source to maintain the ambulance. However, proper daily maintenance is necessary to ensure that the vehicle operates safely and efficiently. It also helps reduce the cost of major servicing if the vehicle were to breakdown.

Most EMS agencies use a checklist for daily maintenance, allowing you to ensure that the vehicle is properly functioning and to document that you have completed a thorough check of the unit. Begin checking the ambulance by inspecting the outside of the vehicle. Inspect the body of the vehicle for any significant damage that would result in the vehicle operating in an unsafe manner. This could include a damaged section that extends beyond the normal wheel well, restricts wheel movement, or causes failure of warning lights or sirens. Check the tires for proper inflation, excessive wear, punctures, or shards of debris. Examine and clean mirrors and windows to make certain that vision is not restricted. Check to see that the turn signals, headlights, brake lights, and warning lights and sirens are in working order. Be sure that all windows and doors can open, close, and lock appropriately. Open all external compartments and make certain the equipment and supplies that are supposed to be in the compartment are there. Wash the vehicle if it is dirty.

Check under the hood. Visually inspect the belts. While the vehicle is cool, check the level of the fluid in the cooling system. Fill fluids to the normal level if they are low. Examine hoses and clamps to be sure there are no obvious leaks. Check other fluids, including oil and brake, power steering, battery, and battery cables, if possible (Figure 4-6).

Inside the cab check all gauges, especially fuel. Fuel the vehicle properly if it is lower than what your agency recommends. Some agencies require refueling whenever the gauge indicates that the fuel tank is half empty. In some vehicles this means filling more than one tank. Be certain to fill the ambulance with the proper type of fuel. Check to see that the parking brake is functioning. Turn on the windshield wipers and washers to confirm proper

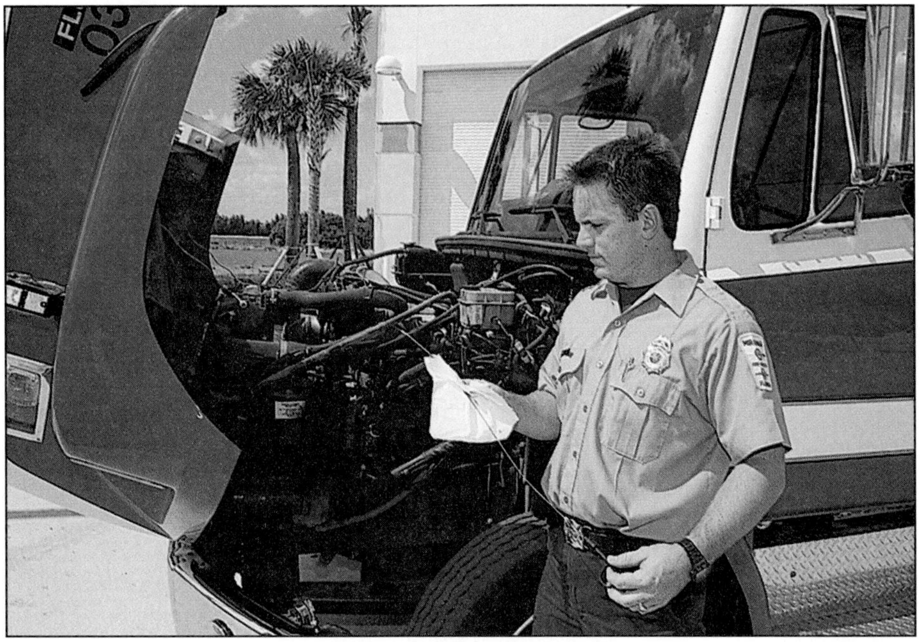

Figure 4-6

Checking engine fluids is an important part of checking over the ambulance in preparation for a call.

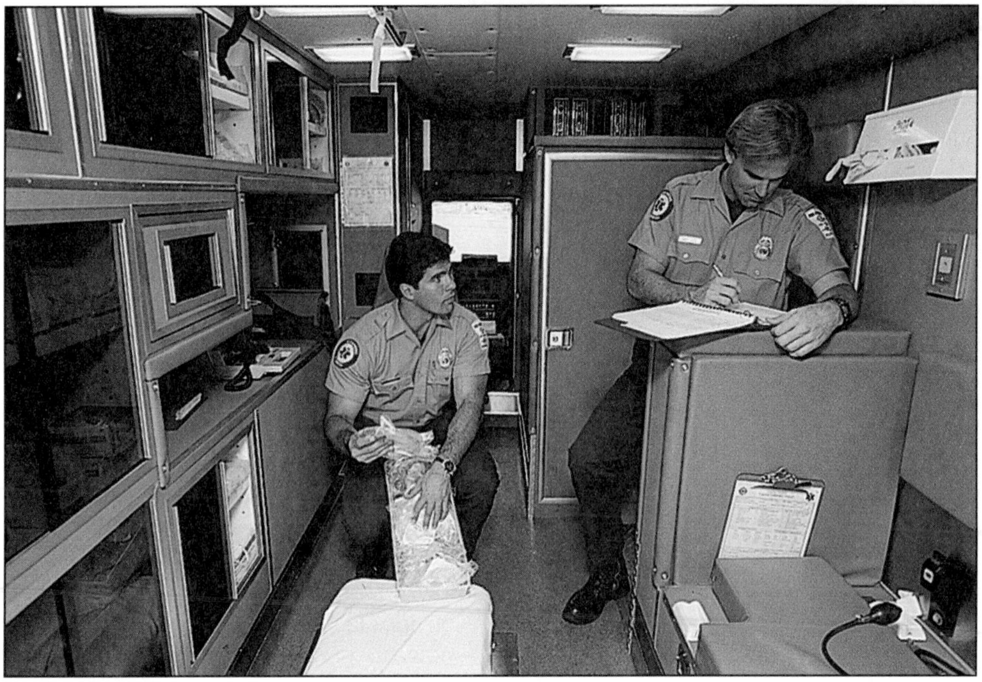

Figure 4-7

It is helpful to work with a partner when checking ambulance supplies and equipment against the ambulance checklist.

operation. Check your communication equipment to make sure that both the portable and mobile radios are functioning normally. Examine the operation of the heating and cooling systems in both the cab and patient compartments. Check to see that all necessary map books are present in the cab. This should include any agency map books for directions to the scene from the station, as well as city or county map books providing grid coordinates.

Check to see that all of the equipment and supplies in the patient compartment are present, in proper working condition, in adequate quantity, and in the assigned location (Figure 4-7). Secure all compartments to avoid having items fall on the floor or patient. Check the stretcher to see that it is locked into place and that the locking device is working properly.

When you have finished inspecting and correcting any vehicle deficiencies, document your findings on the vehicle check sheet or status board. Notify supervisors of any problems that you could not correct, because they could jeopardize the safe operation of the vehicle. The vehicle may need to be placed out of service until the problems can be corrected.

Staffing the Ambulance

Operating an ambulance means that you have adequate staff to provide patient care and drive the ambulance. At least one EMT is needed at the level at which the ambulance is licensed. Many agencies operate with more than one EMT. Some agencies operate with two basic-level EMTs minimally. Some pair an EMT-Basic with an advanced life support (ALS) technician, such as a paramedic. Others may use first responders to drive the ambulance with one or more EMTs on board the ambulance. The staffing of your agency's ambulances will depend on the availability of personnel, their certification or licensure level, and what is required by state law.

When preparing for your shift, determine who will be driving the ambulance and who will be responsible for patient care. The person handling patient care usually rides in the passenger seat and is responsible for:

- Locating the incident in the map book
- Providing directions to the driver
- Handling radio communications with the dispatch center
- Acting as another set of eyes for the driver to ensure safe arrival at the scene

As you begin your shift, check to see that all roads are still accessible for ambulances and that there are no unusual traffic problems or detours created by road repairs. This can be done by reviewing posted memorandum from other crews or officers or by contacting your dispatch center. If there are road closures or access problems, you should be aware of alternate routes to bypass the problem. Knowing the road conditions while you are on duty will help you avoid any sudden problems, which may result in delayed response times.

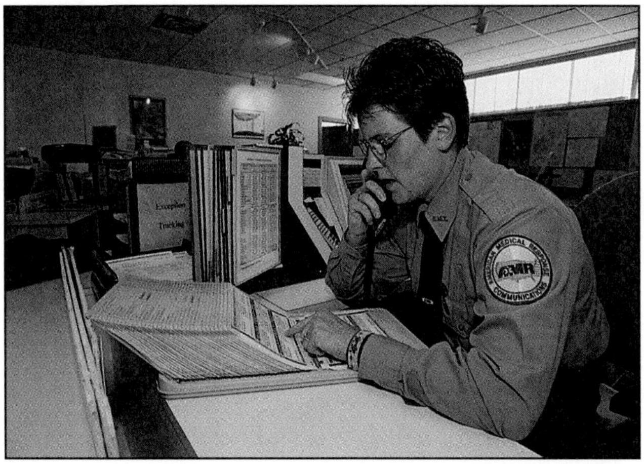

Figure 4-8

The dispatcher providing instruction to the caller.

Dispatch

The dispatcher listens to and asks questions of those who call with emergencies, dispatches an ambulance with the appropriate level personnel to handle the call, and relays critical information to the responding ambulance crew. Dispatchers can also provide instructions to the caller on what to do while waiting for EMS personnel to arrive (Figure 4-8). The dispatch center is staffed 24 hours a day, 365 days a year. Personnel trained as dispatchers may have been certified as emergency medical dispatchers. When dispatching a call, the information the dispatcher will get from the caller includes the following:

- Location of the incident
- Call-back number
- Type of incident
- Number of patients
- Severity of problems
- Other pertinent information (e.g., unsafe scene)

When initially dispatching a call, the dispatcher often provides only the basic information needed for the ambulance to proceed to the scene. The following is an example of an initial dispatch:

"Ambulance 15, respond to an injury from a fall, 410 West Sterling Road."

Responding to the Call

As you prepare to leave the station, make sure that all crew members are on board and wearing seat belts. Carefully pull the vehicle out of the bay and proceed safely with the appropriate lights and sirens once you are certain of the directions to the scene.

Communicating with the Dispatch Center

Notify the dispatch center that you are responding and obtain confirmation that they received your transmission. Once you communicate that your unit is responding, the dispatcher may provide additional information about the circumstances of the incident, such as:

"Injury from a fall, 410 West Sterling Road, map page 42, sector 12. Ambulance 15 responding at 16:45. Ambulance 15, this call came from a neighbor who states that an adult male patient fell from a ladder, injuring his knee and ankle. Patient is conscious but unable to walk."

You and other crew members will be better able to prepare mentally for this call based on the additional information provided by the dispatcher. If you need clarification on the nature or location of the incident or if you need more information, the dispatcher may be able to assist you. (Additional information about the communication systems and equipment that you will be using is covered in more detail in Chapter 5.)

Locating the Incident

To help you locate the incident, your agency may have a specialized map book that provides detailed directions from your station to the scene. This specialized map book will have the streets in your primary area in alphabetical order with directional arrows, or the names of the roads indicating right or left turns, when responding from a fixed location (e.g., a station). In some states, general community map books are available that indicate streets and grid coordinates. When using these map books, you often have to look up the street name in the index, which will provide you with the page and grid coordinate in the map book where the street is found. These books can also be helpful when trying to communicate the location of the landing zone to air medical personnel, if they have the same map book.

Responding to a call at night is significantly different from responding to the same type of call during the day. While locating a main street will not be any different, finding an individual location at night is often more difficult. Using your vehicle's spotlight will help you find the right address.

Some EMS systems use a system status management (SSM) plan for positioning ambulances to respond to calls. This plan considers how call volume changes throughout the day and week. Based on a review of run location and frequency information, ambulances will be moved to various locations to service the areas likely to have a greater need during certain times. This means that you may be on the road with your ambulance or be positioned somewhere other than your main station at different times of the shift so that you can respond more quickly to a call.

Safe Vehicle Operations

Operating an emergency vehicle safely requires that you be knowledgeable in four areas:

- Characteristics of good ambulance operators
- Laws regarding ambulance driving (vehicle operations)
- Use of warning devices
- Use of defensive driving techniques

If you are planning to operate an ambulance, you may be required to attend an approved **emergency vehicle operators training** course. This course includes both classroom and road training and is designed to make you a more knowledgeable and defensive vehicle operator.

Characteristics of Good Emergency Vehicle Operators

Operating an emergency vehicle requires that you be a good driver. Characteristics of good emergency vehicle operators include:

- Physical fitness: Any impairment that you have that would jeopardize your ability to safely operate an ambulance must be corrected. For example, if your vision is impaired, corrective lenses are needed for safe operation of the vehicle.
- Mental fitness: This is very important because the vehicle you will be operating will be moving at a high rate of speed under stressful conditions. Coping appropriately with stress will help keep you mentally healthy. Never operate an emergency vehicle while fatigued, ill, or under the influence of any drug, especially alcohol, or medication that would impair your ability to respond properly.
- Confidence in your ability to operate the vehicle in an appropriate manner.
- Tolerance of other drivers even if they show reluctance to yield the right-of-way to your vehicle. People will react differently when they see and hear your vehicle with its warning lights and sirens.
- Adherence to any restrictions on your license, such as wearing corrective lenses.
- Knowledge and observance of the laws governing the operation of emergency vehicles.
- Operation of the vehicle in accordance with the design characteristics of the vehicle for such things as speed, turning radius, height restrictions, and weight.

Knowing the Law

One important facet of your training is learning the laws within your state that govern the operation of emergency vehicles. The operator of an emergency vehicle is often provided certain exemptions from the law with regard to the operation of the ambulance. These exemptions often involve vehicle speed, turning, passing, proceeding through red lights, direction of travel, and parking. You are granted some exemptions when operating the vehicle on your way to a call and while transporting the patient to the hospital, as long as you are using warning devices and operate the vehicle in a safe manner. However, these same exemptions do not apply during nonemergency situations.

The law requires the driver to operate the vehicle in a manner that provides for the safety of others. To drive an emergency vehicle you must possess a current driver's license and, in many agencies, complete specific training for the vehicle. If you fail to operate the vehicle in the proper manner, you are subject to ticket, arrest, and lawsuits in the event of negligence. Specifically, the law allows you to:

- Proceed through stop signs and red lights with caution. In most states, this means coming to a complete stop before proceeding through the intersection.
- Exceed the speed limit. States often set a limit on how many miles per hour the driver is allowed to exceed the speed limit.
- Pass in no-pass zones as long as this is done with caution. One limitation on this exemption applies to passing a school bus. You must wait for the bus operator to secure all children and then indicate that it is acceptable for you to proceed by turning off the red lights on the bus.
- Proceed against traffic with caution. This means that you can disregard directional signs, as long as you do so with caution and only during emergency situations that require you to do so. For example, you are allowed to go against traffic on a one-way street, if traffic and/or collisions have blocked your entry from the other end.
- Park your vehicle in a manner that otherwise might be unacceptable, as long as it does not endanger others or damage property.
- Drive your vehicle on surfaces normally restricted from vehicular traffic. For example, if the ground is firm enough, you may be able to drive your ambulance onto a golf course to access a patient.

Using Warning Devices

One controversial topic concerning the operation of ambulances is whether warning devices, such as lights and sirens, are really necessary. Most references indicate that the use of lights and sirens rarely contributes to patient outcome, does not save significant time, and are more likely to lead to accidents than when ambulances do not use lights and sirens, as in nonemergency mode.[2] In some cases, however, the few minutes saved can be critical to the outcome of the patient. For this reason, warning devices including headlights, beacons, flashers, horns, and sirens are commonly used by EMS systems across the country.

AMBULANCE ACCIDENTS: FACT OR MYTH?

1. Fact Myth Most ambulance accidents and fatalities occur in the daylight hours.
2. Fact Myth Most ambulance accidents and fatalities occur on wet roadways.
3. Fact Myth Most ambulance accidents and fatalities result from inclement weather, including rain, sleet, fog, and snow that impairs visibility.
4. Fact Myth Most ambulance accidents and fatalities occur while traveling on curved segments of roadway.
5. Fact Myth Most ambulance accidents occur where traffic signal devices are present.
6. Fact Myth Collisions with pedestrians are the most frequent type of ambulance accident.
7. Fact Myth Ambulances operating in an emergency mode are more than twice as likely to be involved in an accident than those operating in nonemergency mode.
8. Fact Myth Most ambulance fatalities occur on roadways with speed limits of 55 mph or greater.
9. Fact Myth Most ambulance accidents involve another vehicle striking the ambulance.
10. Fact Myth Most ambulances involved in fatal accidents have only minor-to-moderate damage.

LET'S SEE HOW YOU DID:

1. **Fact.** Most accidents and fatalities occur in the daylight hours. You are more than twice as likely to be involved in a fatal ambulance accident in the afternoon, than you are late at night.
2. **Myth.** The vast majority of accidents occur on dry roadways.
3. **Myth.** Only approximately 25% of all accidents occur during inclement weather.
4. **Myth.** Most accidents occur on straight segments of roadway.
5. **Fact.** Most accidents occur at intersections where some form of traffic signal device is in operation.
6. **Myth.** Nearly 85% of ambulance accidents involve other motor vehicles.
7. **Fact.** More than 50% of ambulance accidents happen while driving in an emergency mode.
8. **Myth.** More than two thirds of all fatalities occur on improved roads at speeds less than 50 miles per hour.
9. **Myth.** In most ambulance accidents, the ambulance struck another vehicle or object.
10. **Myth.** Most ambulances involved in fatal accidents are disabled, with approximately 90% requiring towing service.

The use of warning devices does not always mean that a motor vehicle operator or pedestrian will see or hear your emergency vehicle. Warning lights used during daylight hours do not stand out as much as they do at night. Some motorists will not hear your siren until you are within 100 feet of them. They may not have the ability to react as quickly as you might like, or they may not readily yield the right of way. For this reason, you must remember that you cannot always rely on your warning lights for people to see you. Lights and sirens only ask drivers to yield the right-of-way, they do not guarantee right-of-way.

Most states regulate the use of warning devices. Also, many EMS agencies develop policies for the use of warning devices. You should be aware of your agency's policy governing the use of these devices.

Some states require the use of a siren whenever the ambulance is operating in an emergency mode. Others restrict its use. Drive with caution and try to remain calm whenever using a siren. This is not always as easy as it seems because continuous use of a siren can increase anxiety, which could have a detrimental effect on the driver, crew, and patient. It could cause the driver to operate the vehicle at a speed faster than normally accepted. For patients, use of a siren may cause a heightened sense of a serious condition and make them more anxious about the situation.

Visual warning devices, combined with audible devices, provide you with the best chance of being noticed by other motorists and pedestrians. These visual devices include your vehicle's headlights, beacons, and flashers. Whether day or night (Figure 4-9, *A* and *B*), the headlights should be on when you are operating the ambulance. Lights located in the front of the ambulance, on the roof of the cab, and on the patient compartment all help make your vehicle more easily seen, even through the rearview mirrors of motorists ahead of you. But like the audible warning devices, you must also be familiar with your agency's policy on the use of visual warning devices.

Calls other than emergency calls should be considered a routine response. For example, you may be dispatched as a public service for a person locked out of a vehicle, or you may be transporting a patient with only a minor injury to a receiving facility. In nonemergency situations such as these, warning devices are not necessary, and you must follow all laws regarding normal driving.

A

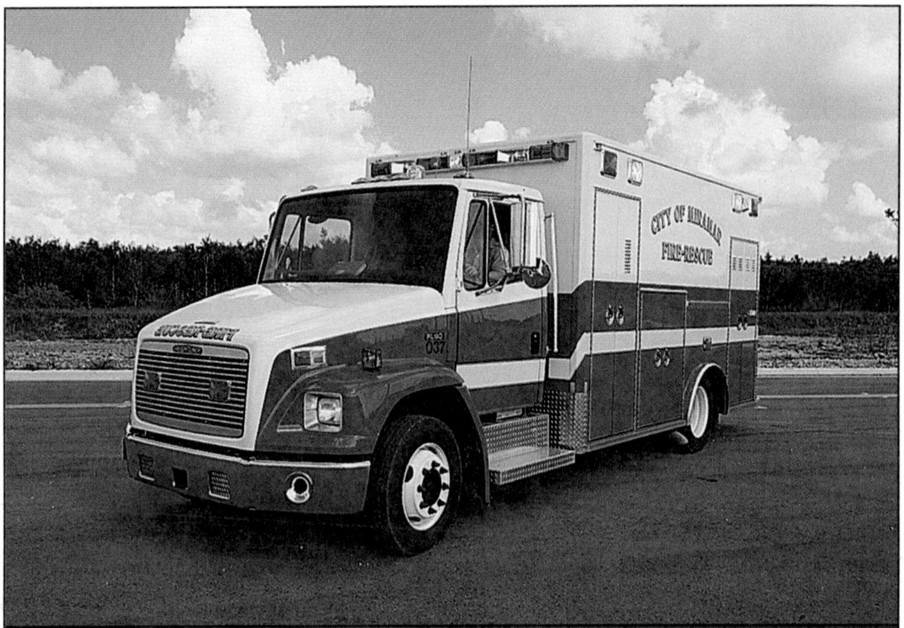

B

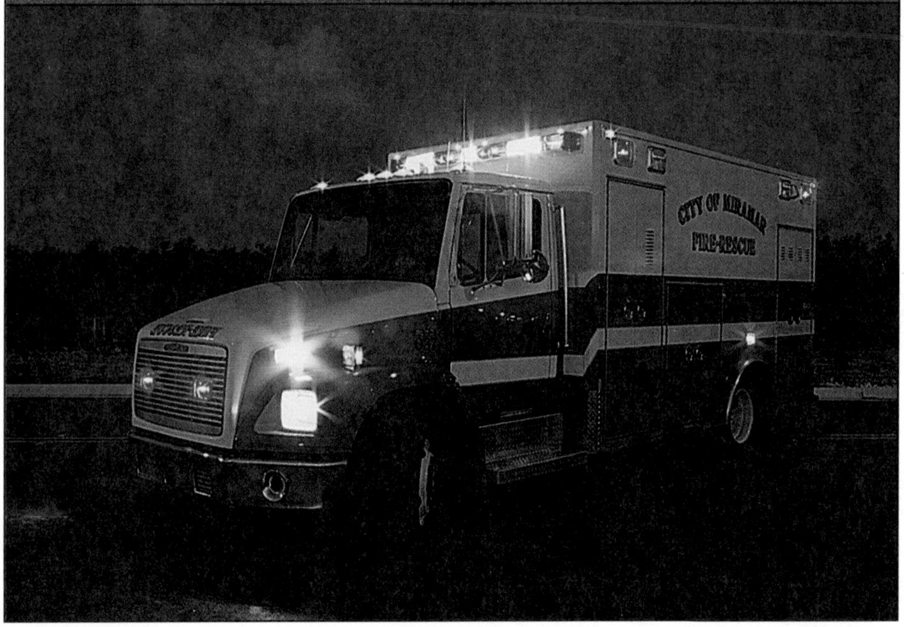

Figure 4-9

When operating an ambulance, be aware that your visual warning devices are less noticeable to other drivers during the day **(A)** than they are at night **(B).**

Defensive Driving

According to the National Highway Traffic Safety Administration, EMS vehicles are involved in more than 15,000 accidents each year. This same agency reports that 100 EMS providers and 300 civilians died in ambulance-related accidents in the 10-year period between 1984 and 1993.[3] In New York, 1,412 ambulance accidents occurred over a 4-year period, accounting for injuries to 1,894 ambulance occupants.[2] Another study looked only at fatal ambulance crashes in America over a 4-year period and reported that 109 crashes resulted in 126 deaths.[4]

Defensive driving is the best way to avoid accidents. Just because you are operating an ambulance does not mean that everyone will immediately yield the right-of-way to you. Instead, be prepared for those who will not see you coming and will not yield. In this manner, you can drive according to state law, in a safe and efficient manner. If you are responding to motor-vehicle collision, consider that one likely reason you are responding in the first place is because of hazardous road conditions that others were unprepared for.

Be aware of factors that could affect your driving, such as:

- Weather conditions that may result in slippery surfaces and reduced visibility
- Traffic conditions that vary according to day and time, such as rush hour or vacation weekends
- Obstacles that impede response, such as train crossings, bridges, tunnels, construction work, road repair, school or hospital zones, and other vehicles that you must yield to, such as school buses

Intersections are especially dangerous areas, accounting for many accidents. Motorist and pedestrian traffic is heavier at intersections, and sight and hearing may be limited. For this reason, it is always smart to approach all intersections with extreme caution, slowing or stopping your vehicle until you are certain that oncoming traffic recognizes that you are in an emergency-response mode and comes to a stop. Your partner can help check traffic for you on his or her side of the vehicle. Road conditions and the speed of travel also contribute to accidents. Because reduced traction is difficult to detect, it is imperative that the driver proceed cautiously to compensate for any error in judging the road condition. It is often recommended that the speed at which an emergency vehicle can travel be restricted. In some states this is restricted to 10 miles over the speed limit. Under inclement conditions it is generally recommended that you reduce your normal speed by 25% for rain, 50% for snow, and 75% for ice. If you are using chains or cables for snow and ice conditions, you should be aware of any recommendations by the vehicle manufacturer or procedures in place by your local agency as to how fast the vehicle should be operated. On newer vehicles with automatically deployed chains, operating the vehicle at too fast a speed can cause the chains to become disengaged, damaging your vehicle and creating an unsafe situation.

Take special caution during escorted and multiple-vehicle responses. In an escorted response, the ambulance is led by another vehicle, often a police vehicle. If the driver of the ambulance follows too closely, he or she may not be able to stop without striking the lead vehicle, should that vehicle make a sudden stop. If other motorists do not see the following vehicle, they may think that they only need to yield to the lead vehicle. Consequently, motorists may pull back into traffic lanes as the lead vehicle goes by, causing a collision with the following vehicle. A similar problem also exists for multiple-unit responses. To help eliminate the problems associated with escorted and multiple-vehicle responses, you should always maintain a safe distance between the lead and trailing vehicles. This way motorists will have a better chance to see multiple emergency vehicles approaching.

Finally, good defensive driving techniques involve the same driving skills you use to stay safe in your car, including slowing down before you start into a curve, signaling when you are making turns, properly positioning your wheels and engaging your parking brake when leaving the vehicle, reducing your speed in inclement weather, and obeying all laws that apply to the operation of emergency vehicles in your state.

Arriving at the Scene

When you approach the scene, try to take in the whole picture. Determine where the patient is located and where you should position your vehicle. Turn off any audible warning devices that may have been used en route to the scene. Notify the dispatch center that you are on the scene. If the patient is at a residence, park your vehicle in front of the residence in a manner that allows easy access to the patient compartment. With the parking brake engaged, check both mirrors before exiting the vehicle. This way you and your partner can avoid being struck by an oncoming vehicle as you open the doors. EMS personnel in the front of the vehicle also have a responsibility to those riding in the patient compartment. Notify any additional EMS personnel when it is safe to exit the vehicle. Because their view is restricted, they may not always know when the vehicle is parked and when it is safe to exit.

Responding to motor-vehicle collisions poses certain inherent dangers. Consider the flow of traffic and the lighting. In dark areas it is always advisable to wear a brightly colored reflective vest while outside the vehicle (Figure 4-10). When parking the ambulance, position it on the same side of the road as the incident, approximately 50 to 100 feet in front of or behind the collision (Figure 4-11). Avoid having your vehicle stick out into the lane of traffic. Where you park depends on the type of

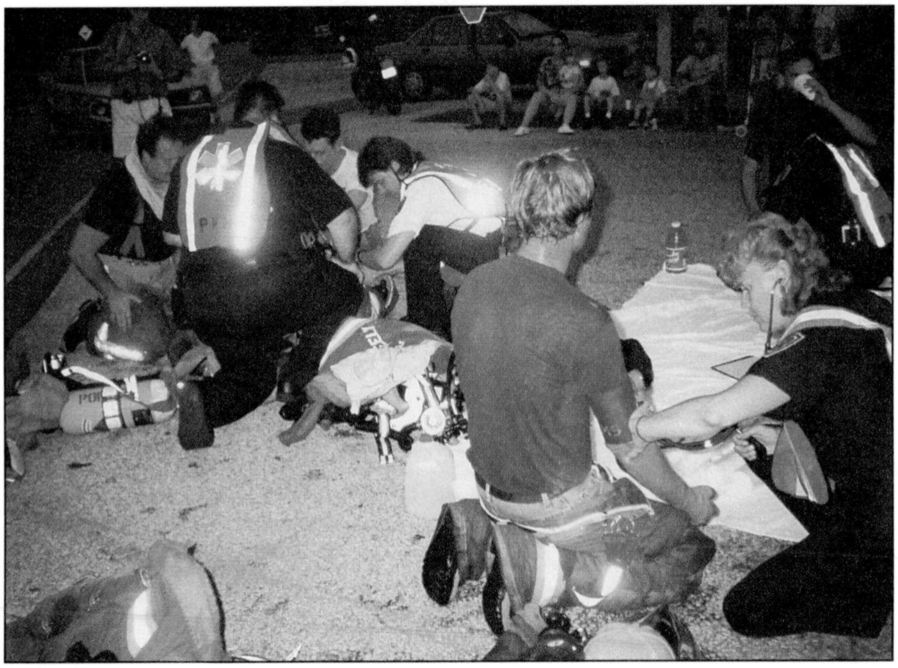

Figure 4-10

Because of darkness at the scene, EMS personnel wears a brightly colored reflective vest.

danger present and whether other emergency vehicles are already present. As a general rule, if you are the first to arrive, position your vehicle behind the collision. Create a safe working area by placing flares or reflective cones or triangles behind your vehicle. This way oncoming traffic will be aware that there is an accident ahead. When using flares, be certain that there is no leaking fuel that could come in contact with the flares. If another emergency vehicle, such as a police car is already on the scene, park in front of the collision. This generally makes transferring the patient to the ambulance and departure of the ambulance somewhat easier.

Exceptions to these general rules exist when there is a dangerous situation such as a vehicle fire, downed power lines, a hazardous material spill, or violence. In such cases, you should park the ambulance upwind to avoid exposure to fire, smoke, or hazardous materials. You will also need to park your vehicle away from the danger zone created when power lines are involved. The danger area usually extends one span beyond each intact pole and to the sides for a distance that the downed wires could reach.

Size up the scene. If you note leaking fuel or another type of spill, notify the dispatch center of the need to contain the spill. If the leak is only radiator fluid or a minor fuel leak, you can proceed to approach the patient. If the leak is severe or if you are uncertain of the nature of the spill, do not approach. Look at the position of any vehicles and try to determine how they came to rest in that position. This may assist in determining the patient's mechanism of injury and can help determine the type and extent of the injuries the occupants may have suffered. Do not attempt to reach any patients if the vehicles are unstable. For example, a vehicle on its side or dangling over a guard rail could change position while you are attempting to provide care. Before providing care, make certain that the vehicle is stabilized. Chapter 7 provides detailed information on how to stabilize vehicles.

As you prepare to assess the patient, be sure to use the necessary body substance isolation (BSI) precautions. Determine how many vehicles are involved and how many patients may need help. Summon additional personnel as soon as possible to avoid any delay in getting additional resources to the scene. If there are multiple patients, begin sorting the patients according to the severity of their problems. This process, known as **triage,** helps ensure that those patients in need of urgent care receive it ahead of others with lesser injuries. Chapter 6 provides detailed information on triage.

Once you have rapidly assessed the patients, you will have a better idea of the severity and complexity of the situation. This will enable you to determine the need for additional medical assistance, including possible helicopter transport for the most serious patients. In all cases your actions at the scene must be well organized and directed toward the goal of transporting the patient as rapidly and efficiently as possible. You will learn more about scene assessment and safety in Chapter 6.

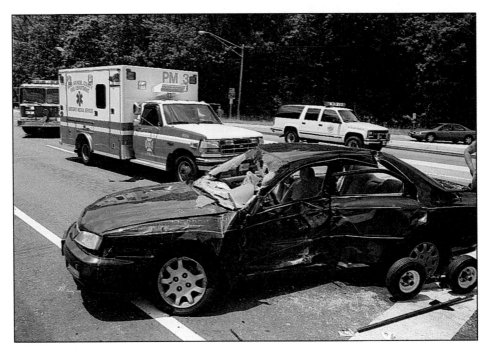

Figure 4-11

Upon arrival on-scene at a motor-vehicle accident, position your ambulance between on-coming traffic and the emergency scene to provide a safety barrier for crew and accident victims.

IT'S YOUR CALL
CONCLUSION

As you may recall from the case study presented at the beginning of the chapter, several problems occurred while en route to the scene and even after arrival at the scene. These problems included a lengthy response time because of a detour. By checking for any memorandums posted at the station or by checking with the dispatch center, you may have learned about the detour. By reducing speed and watching carefully for icy areas, you could have kept the vehicle under control and avoided sliding into deep snow. Remember that besides driving at a slower speed, snow and ice may require the use of chains or cables to prevent this type of accident. Because of the deteriorating visibility, additional warning devices such as reflectors or flares could have been placed to alert oncoming traffic of the need for caution. This would have provided motorists more time to react. Because you were uncertain of the status of your vehicle, you should have alerted dispatch to the need for an additional ambulance and possibly even the need to close down a section of the roadway until the scene could be made safe.

Finally, the quality of the patient care being provided could be considered substandard because of the failure to adequately stock the ambulance with the necessary supplies, such as blankets. By being more attentive when checking the ambulance and bringing the supply issue to the attention of the crew that just completed their shift, you will be able to easily avoid this deficiency in the future.

Transferring the Patient to the Ambulance

Once the patient has been initially cared for at the scene, he or she needs to be transferred to the ambulance. The type of device you use to help move the patient to the ambulance will be based on the condition of the patient. For example, a patient with a medical emergency, such as a breathing problem, will likely be transferred to the ambulance in an upright position by means of a wheeled stretcher (Figure 4-12). A patient who has sustained a fall and is complaining of back or neck pain should be secured to a backboard first and transferred to the ambulance on the stretcher in a horizontal position (Figure 4-13). A major consideration in taking the time to secure patients using **extrication** devices is whether the patient's condition is stable enough to warrant the time it takes to apply the device and straps, or whether the patient needs rapid transport. You will learn more about making these decisions in later chapters on patient assessment.

Regardless of the device being used, lifting and moving the patient requires that you follow general guidelines for your personal safety and the safety of your partner and the patient. In some cases the patient's weight or the route to the ambulance will require the assistance of several EMS providers to lift and move the patient. Do not be afraid to summon additional personnel to assist in moving the patient. Lifting and moving techniques and the use of equipment to transfer patients are discussed in detail in Chapter 7.

As you transfer the patient to the ambulance, consider what you can do to help improve the patient's level of comfort. This may be as simple as applying sheets and blankets to a patient. A sheet may be all that is needed in warm weather, whereas a sheet and multiple blankets may be needed when it is cold. Some patients are allergic to wool, so it is always better to place a sheet on the patient first when using wool blankets. When applying straps to secure the patient to a device for transfer to the ambulance, be sure that the straps are secure but not too tight.

Once in the ambulance, check that the stretcher is locked in place and the patient is secured to the stretcher. You may need to remove some blankets or clothing to gain access to the patient for further assessment. Adjust the temperature control of the patient compartment so that the patient remains comfortable. While the temperature may not be the most comfortable for you, the patient's level of comfort is the higher priority.

Transporting the Patient

As you prepare to depart the scene with your patient, check to see that you have all of the equipment that was used at the scene. This would include the portable radio, clipboard with patient care report, and medical supply kit. Also be sure that the patient's personal items have been placed in the ambulance.

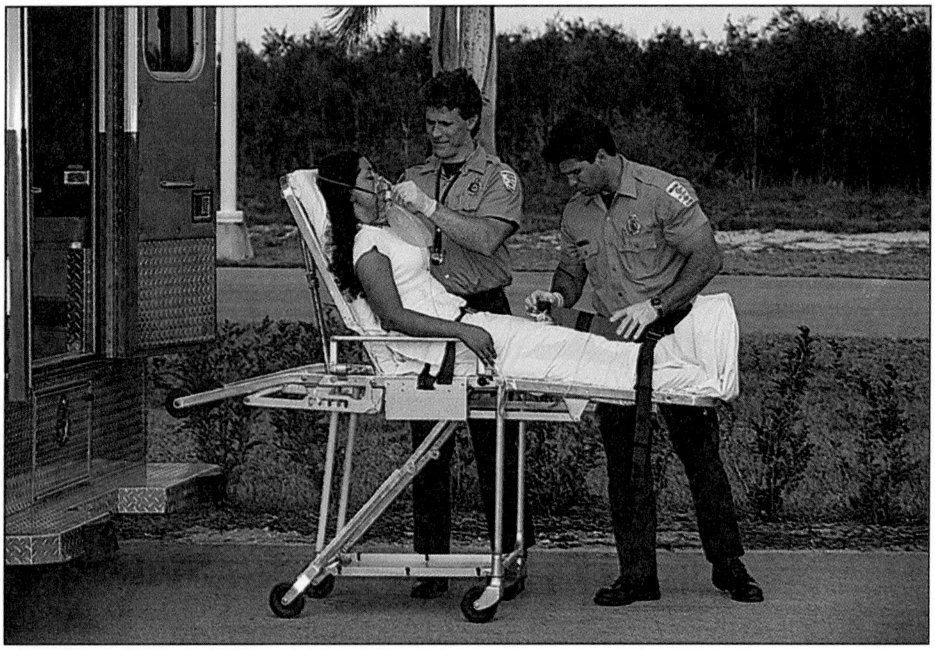

Figure 4-12

Patients with breathing problems are often best transferred to the ambulance in an upright position.

Next check to see that the person providing care for the patient is prepared to depart. Personnel may be performing procedures that require a slight delay before departing. It is also preferable for personnel in the patient compartment to be seated, wearing seatbelts whenever possible, as you depart the scene. Before departing the scene, make sure that you know which hospital will be receiving the patient, and your best route of travel. Consult with other EMS personnel and your map books if you are uncertain of the route of travel. Notify the dispatch center that you are departing the scene with your patient. Advise dispatch of the receiving hospital and the status of your unit (i.e., emergency or nonemergency transport).

In some areas the dispatch center will relay basic information for you to the hospital, such as the patient's age, chief complaint, nature of the problem, treatment provided, and estimated time of arrival. In other areas you may have to communicate this information directly to the hospital. This is usually the responsibility of the person providing patient care. Chapter 5 provides detailed information on communication with the receiving facility.

Patient care en route to the hospital includes reassuring the patient, reassessing the patient's condition, providing additional care, recording the findings, and completing the patient care report. If the patient becomes uncomfortable and the condition allows, you may be able to help reposition him or her in order to alleviate the discomfort.

On rare occasions it is necessary to restrain violent patients. This is best accomplished at the scene, where additional personnel are available to assist in applying the restraints. If restraints were placed on the patient before departure, do not remove them during transport unless it is absolutely necessary (e.g., improper positioning compromising the patient's circulation or making breathing difficult). However, once released, the patient could become violent again, which could result in injury to the patient and the EMS providers.

Special Considerations

There are several special considerations that you should be aware of when transporting patients. These include transporting children, using air medical transport, and interfacility patient transports.

Transporting Children

Children can become frightened at the thought of traveling in an ambulance. Have a parent or other adult guardian travel with the child, whenever possible. Some EMS agencies keep toys available to help comfort children. Secure the child to the stretcher and seat the adult guardian nearby with the appropriate safety restraint. Your agency may have car seats for securing young children. You can ease a child's fear by gaining his or her trust. Talk in a calm, positive, reassuring manner. Do everything you can to reduce or eliminate the child's fears.

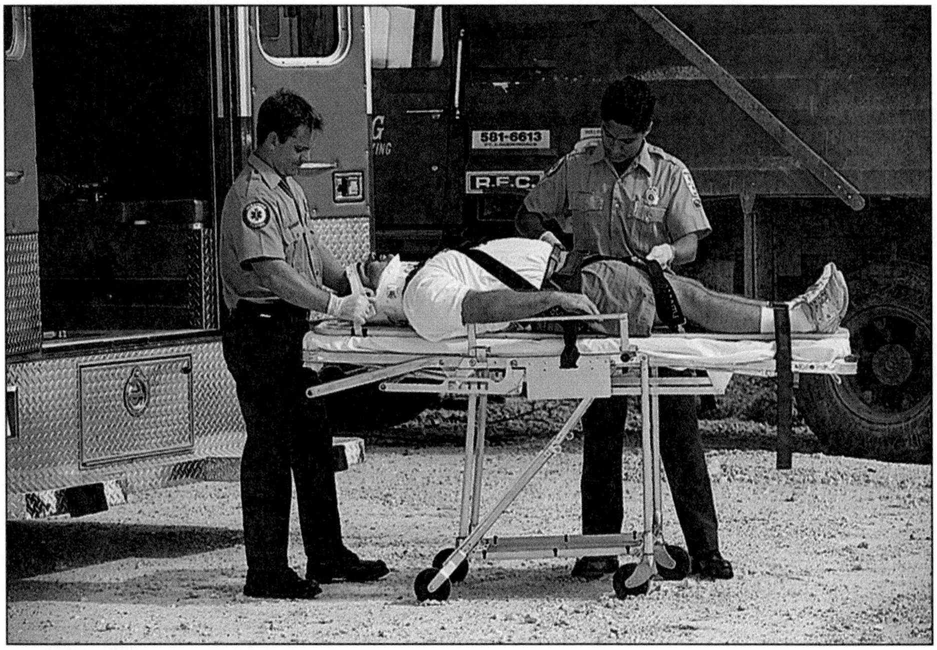

Figure 4-13

Patients with back or neck injuries should be secured to a backboard and transferred to the ambulance in a horizontal position.

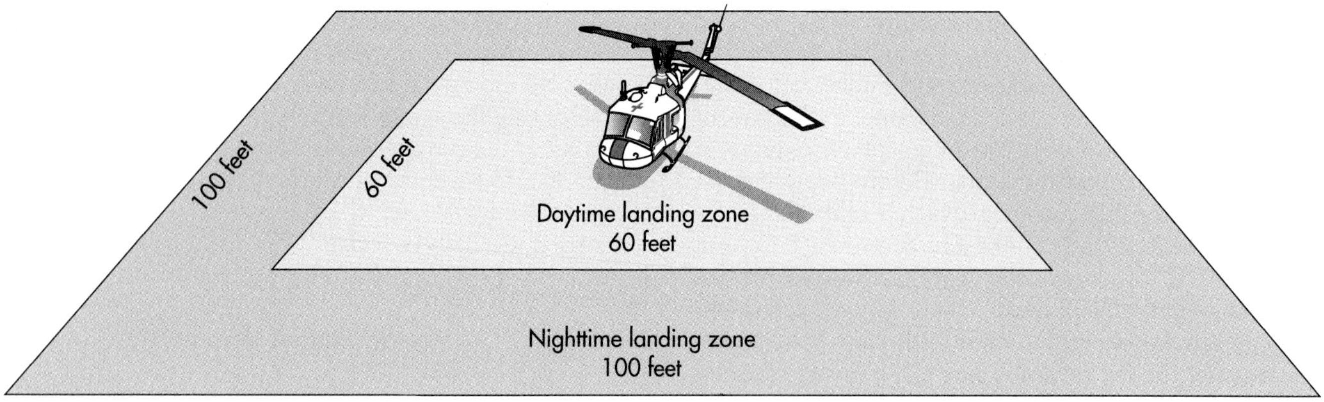

Figure 4-14

Because of the reduction in visibility at night, nighttime landing zones for helicopters should be at least 100 feet by 100 feet; daytime landing zones may be slightly smaller.

Air Medical Transport

Helicopters are used for two primary reasons: rescue situations and specialized medical care. For medical situations, the use of an air medical transport may provide specialized medical care resources and expedite the transport of a severely ill or injured patient. Generally, you are requesting not only the vehicle but also the medical care resources of the crew on the helicopter. For rescue situations the helicopter may be able to reach a patient more quickly and with less danger to rescuers than an ambulance. The helicopter may also be able to get to a patient who is otherwise inaccessible by ground vehicles.

You should have local protocols to follow regarding the procedures for requesting a helicopter for transport. In some areas the senior medical person or incident commander on the scene has the authority to call for air medical resources. In other areas the request for those resources must be funneled through the physician providing medical direction. He or she will authorize the use of a helicopter based on the information provided about the patient's condition. If a helicopter is dispatched, information must be given to the pilot about the location of the landing zone. This often includes map grid coordinates and major landmarks such as intersections and structures. Information should also be given to the medical crew so that they know how to best prepare for that patient on arrival at the medical facility.

Establishing a Landing Zone. A landing zone is a safe area in which the pilot will land the helicopter. It should be set up in an area free of obstructions, such as power lines, trees, or structures. This may be a field or roadway near the scene. If you are providing for the care of the patient, you will need additional personnel to establish the landing zone. To set up a landing zone, remember these guidelines:

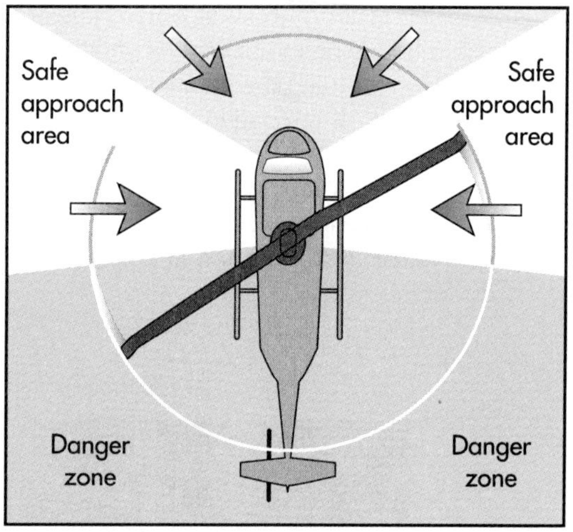

Figure 4-15

Approaching a helicopter from the rear is dangerous because you are out of the pilot's line of sight.

- The size of the landing zone is usually a minimum of 100 feet by 100 feet (Figure 4-14).
- The landing surface should be relatively flat (less than an eight-degree slope).
- The area should be free of obstructions.
- The area must be clearly marked. Visual warning devices such as chemical light sticks, flares, or vehicles positioned in the corners of the landing zone with only their rotating lights on are used to mark the area.
- Do not direct headlights or spotlights toward the helicopter as it is landing. This may temporarily blind the pilot on approach. The pilot and crew will be able to see your emergency lights and the outlined landing zone without additional lighting.

TRICKS OF THE TRADE

Even under the best of situations, mechanical failures seem to occur. If your agency has a good vehicle maintenance program, fewer problems will occur. Sometimes, however, these seemingly mechanical problems are actually due to operator error. Here are some tips that may help you avoid problems or quickly overcome them if they do occur.

TURN SIGNAL MALFUNCTION
If you are trying to merge lanes in heavy traffic at night, and your turn signal suddenly fails to work, flash your side scene lights. Motorists normally get the idea and yield to your vehicle.

BRAKE MALFUNCTION
If your brakes fail to function and you need to slow down the ambulance, downshift gradually to lower gear 2 and then to 1, in this order. The transmission will help slow the vehicle. Gently apply the parking brake. If you have air-brakes and the parking brake fails to disengage, try pumping the brake pedal.

VEHICLE LEAKING FUEL
Most often this is due to overfilling the tank(s) and/or not securing the cap. This is sometimes worsened by parking the vehicle on ground that causes it to sit sideways and allow more fuel to escape.

ELECTRICAL FAILURE
Large scale electrical system failure is very rare. The first place to start is to make certain that the vehicle is turned on. Next, check the circuit breakers to see that the breakers are all engaged.

PORTABLE RADIO FAILURE
Everyone will likely experience this at some time in their EMS career. First, check to see that the radio is on. Next, check to see that the volume is turned up. Continue by checking to see that you are broadcasting and monitoring on the proper channel. Try replacing the battery with a fully charged one.

VEHICLE IDLES FAST OR STALLS WHILE PARKED
If your vehicle idles fast, check the vehicle for a "high idle switch" that may still be engaged. Similarly, if you have a high idle switch, engage it in cold weather to avoid the vehicle stalling while parked.

- Keep all personnel, equipment, and bystanders out of the landing zone.
- Do not approach the helicopter until the pilot advises it is safe to do so.
- Always stay in the pilot's line of sight, approaching the helicopter from the front. NEVER approach a helicopter from the rear (Figure 4-15).
- Wait for the helicopter crew to exit and come to you.
- Wear protective gear, including a helmet, and stay in a crouched position when approaching the helicopter.
- Secure your patient and protect him or her from flying debris as the aircraft lands.
- Always approach from the down-hill side when a helicopter is parked on a hillside.

You will need to become familiar with your local protocols for the use of helicopters and how to establish a safe landing zone. Many air medical programs conduct helicopter orientation programs and landing zone classes.

Interfacility Transport

There are a number of instances when you may be called to transport a patient from one care facility to another. Among the important points to consider is making sure that you have the properly trained personnel and the equipment necessary to care for the patient's condition. If you are going to be responsible for interfacility transfers, your agency should see that you receive the appropriate training to successfully assume the responsibility for patient transport. If you have not had the appropriate training before the request for transport, you should not do the transport. Inform the transferring physician that you are not adequately trained to manage the patient's complex condition. Generally, a patient who requires ALS procedures, such as intravenous lines, medications, and cardiac monitoring, should be cared for by ALS personnel. As you learned in Chapter 2, COBRA requires specially trained personnel, sometimes hospital personnel, to accompany critical patients during interfacility transfers.

The Receiving Facility

Notify the dispatch center when you arrive at the hospital. Remove the patient from any fixed devices within your ambulance, such as oxygen. Use portable devices for transporting the patient into the hospital. Wheel the patient into the emergency department and wait until the staff assigns a bed or other area to the patient, either within the emergency department or elsewhere in the hospital.

With the patient transferred to the hospital bed, provide the hospital staff with an overview of the patient's condition and the care you provided. Do not abandon your patient without being certain that hospital staff are aware of the patient's condition and are prepared to take over care.

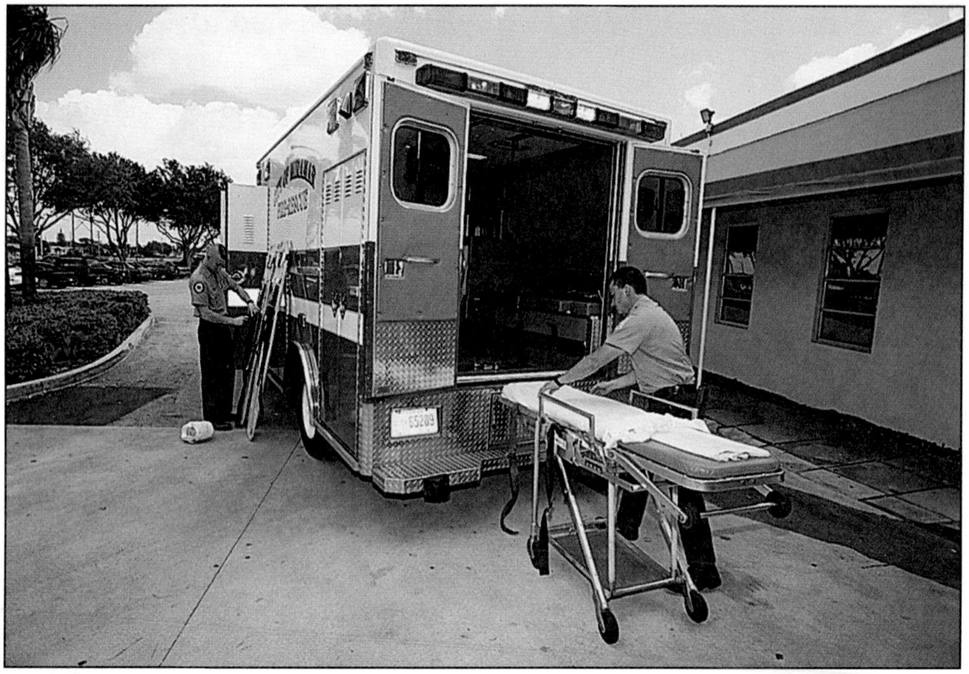

Figure 4-16

Take the time to replace linens and do a thorough cleaning of the ambulance and all equipment between emergency calls.

Before departing, clean yourself, your equipment, and your ambulance properly. Because you may receive another call at any time, it is important to have your vehicle ready for service as soon as possible. This includes removing any soiled articles, such as gloves, and washing your hands thoroughly. Dispose of used supplies and clean any used equipment. You will also need to clean the patient compartment and dispose of any linen, trash, and biohazard waste according to your agency's policies. Sweep and mop away dirt, mud, and water that may have been tracked into the patient compartment.

Disinfect the patient compartment, as well as all nondisposable equipment with an EPA-approved disinfectant or a 1:100 bleach solution. Place new sheets, pillowcases and blankets on the wheeled ambulance stretcher (Figure 4-16). If your clothing was contaminated, remove it as soon as possible and place it in a properly labeled biohazard bag for transport to the station for cleaning.

Restock your ambulance with the necessary equipment and supplies according to your agency's policies. In some situations you may have to wait until the hospital can release the equipment to you (e.g., backboards). If you leave the hospital without the proper equipment, you should notify the dispatch center that your unit is out of service because of inadequate equipment. Once you get to the station, replace this equipment.

Completing Your Report

Before leaving the hospital, complete your patient-care report and provide a copy to the hospital staff. If you are completing an interfacility transport, turn over any additional reports such as the patient's chart including lab reports and x-ray results. In some areas, you will be required to obtain the signature of the attending physician or charge nurse before leaving a copy of the report with the hospital. This is sometimes the case if you performed advanced skills, such as administering medication. Double check the accuracy and thoroughness of the report. Remember that this written document will be a permanent record of your patient care. Some areas require that additional information be provided regarding patient care. For example, if you used an automated external defibrillator for a patient in cardiac arrest, you may be required to leave a tape recording from the call and complete a questionnaire regarding the use of this device, as part of an overall system quality-improvement effort.

Some calls can cause great stress for you and other EMS providers. You may want to discuss the call in private with crew members or with the attending physician in an effort to reduce some of the stress you are experiencing. As a new EMT you may experience greater stress than veteran EMTs. It is not uncommon to want some reassurance that you did what was expected and provided the best care possible.

Returning to Service

Once you have completed the tasks of transferring the patient, cleaning and restocking the ambulance, and completing the patient care report, you are once again ready for service. Notify the dispatcher that you are available and are departing from the hospital. Also notify dispatch if your ambulance is not available for service (e.g., a shortage of personnel or equipment or mechanical failure of the vehicle).

Once you are back at your station, notify dispatch. Complete any cleaning or restocking of supplies. Sanitize the patient compartment if that has not been done already, and change any soiled clothing that you may still be wearing. Clean your clothing as soon as possible. Deposit soiled linens in the appropriate container. Replace oxygen cylinders, including both portable and fixed cylinders that may be low on oxygen. Check to make sure that your vehicle is adequately fueled. Clean the ambulance exterior as necessary. Complete any unfinished report forms and file the reports in the appropriate place. If you did not have adequate time to debrief personnel immediately after the call, do it now before another call. This way you can be sure that your ambulance and crew are ready to function adequately when dispatched. If your unit was placed out of service for any reason, notify dispatch as soon as it is back in service.

SUMMARY

Responding to an emergency requires that your ambulance is functioning properly and that you are aware of your agency's policies for operating the ambulance. There are several different phases of ambulance operations, from preparing for a call, to returning to service following a call. Throughout each of these phases, you are expected to function in a professional manner that provides for your personal safety, as well as the safety of your crew, other EMS personnel, the patient, and bystanders.

Follow the guidelines provided in this chapter for safe vehicle operations. These guidelines start with knowing and abiding by the laws governing the operation of an emergency vehicle in your state. You should also recognize the personal characteristics needed to operate an emergency vehicle properly, including being familiar with the various warning devices on your vehicle and how and when to use them. Utilize defensive driving techniques whenever you are behind the wheel. Remember that you can never rely on other motorists to do the "right thing." Therefore, you are the one that must make the decisions so that you can get to and from the emergency scene in a safe and expedient manner.

There are several special considerations for patient transport. When transporting children, remember that they are often scared and require a great deal of support. Whenever possible, transport the child with his or her adult guardian to help reduce the fear and anxiety. Secure children in car seats whenever necessary. If you need to summon a helicopter (air medical resources), follow your local protocols and prepare the landing zone appropriately. Always take the necessary safety precautions when operating near a helicopter. Provide the air medical crew with necessary patient information.

Once you have arrived at the hospital and patient care has been turned over to hospital staff, you must prepare your ambulance for service. This includes cleaning and disinfecting equipment and surfaces, and restocking supplies. It also means debriefing personnel, analyzing the call. This way you can be sure that your ambulance and crew are ready to function adequately when dispatched to another call. Double check that your patient care report is complete and leave a copy with the hospital staff. Notify dispatch that your unit is ready for service. Complete any final paper work or cleaning and restocking tasks.

REFERENCES

1. **American College of Emergency Physicians:** Equipment for ambulances, *Ann Emerg Med* 26: 403, 1995.
2. **Elling R:** Dispelling myths on ambulance accidents, *JEMS* 14(7):60-64, 1989.
3. **National Highway Traffic Safety Administration,** National Center for Statistics and Analysis: *Fatal accident reporting system: 1988-1993,* Washington, D.C., 1993, NHTSA.
4. **Pirrallo R, Swor RA:** Characteristics of fatal ambulance crashes during emergency and non-emergency operation, *Prehosp Disaster Med* 9:125, 1994.

Section 2

Emergency Medical Services Operations

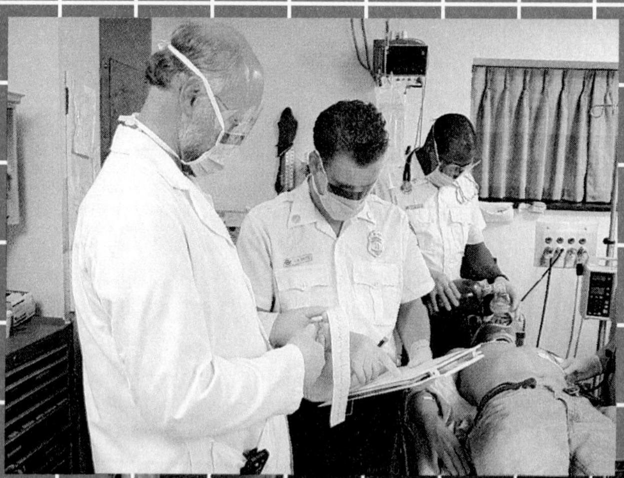
 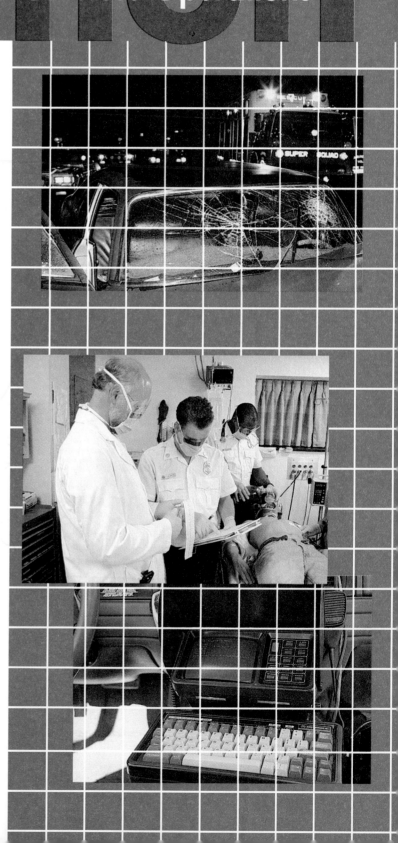

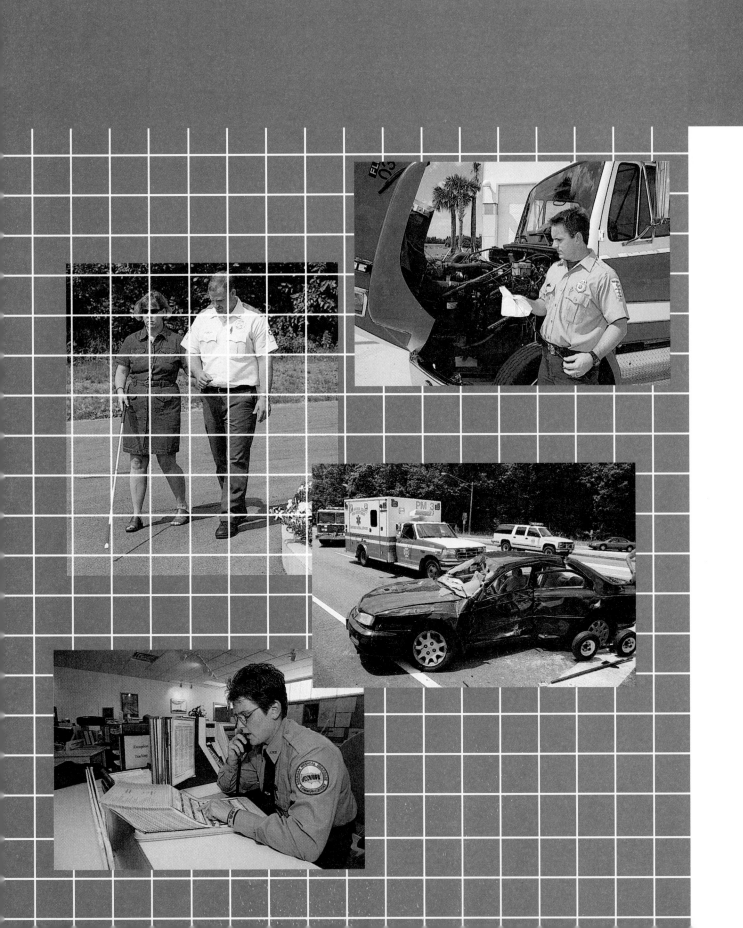

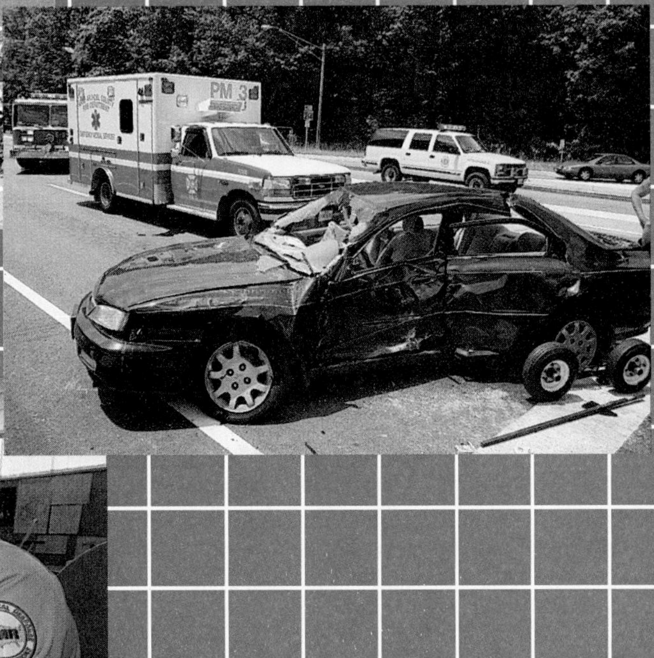
PM 3

Chapter 5

Communication and Documentation

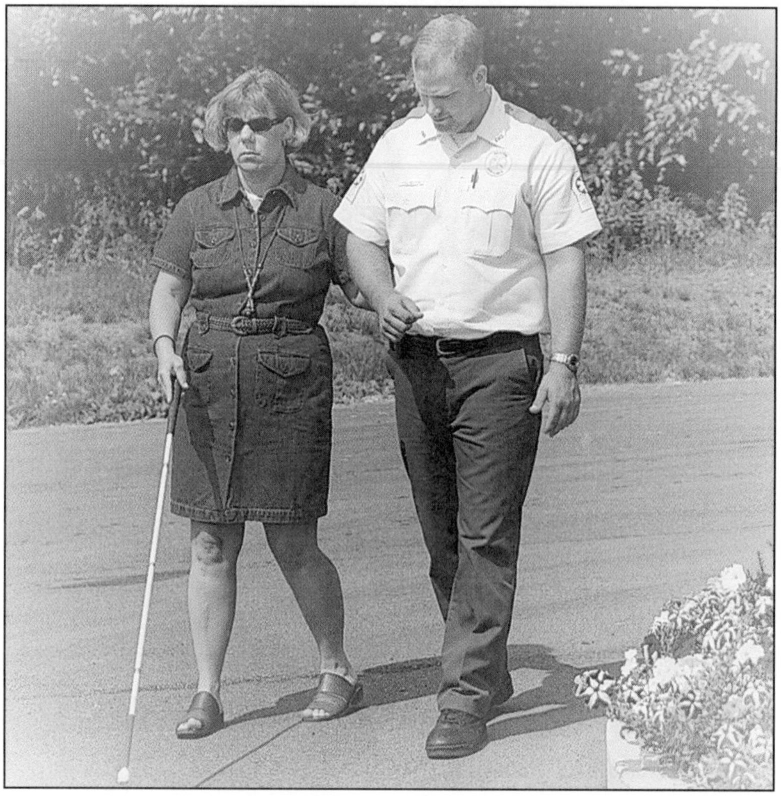

Knowledge Objectives

As an EMT-Basic, you should be able to:

OBJECTIVES

1. Describe the components of a communication system.
2. List the proper methods of initiating, providing, and terminating a radio call.
3. List the essential components of a verbal medical report.
4. Outline the sequence for relaying patient information to a hospital or dispatch center.
5. Describe six interpersonal communication skills that should be used to enhance communication with patients.
6. Describe the correct radio procedures to be used in the following phases of a call:
   - Responding to the scene
   - Arriving at the scene
   - Transporting to the hospital
   - Arriving at the hospital
   - Returning from the hospital
   - Arriving at the station
7. Describe methods used to communicate effectively with the following special populations:
   - Children
   - Elderly
   - Hearing impaired
   - Visually impaired
   - Developmentally disabled
   - Non-English speaking
8. Describe the sections of a patient care report.
9. List the essential elements that should be contained in a patient care report.
10. Describe the proper way to document patient refusal of treatment or transportation.
11. Describe how to correct an error properly on a patient care report, either before or after it has been submitted.

OBJECTIVES

Skill Objectives

As an EMT-Basic, you should be able to:

1. **Simulate an organized, concise radio transmission.**
2. **Provide a verbal report to advanced life support (ALS) personnel arriving on the scene.**
3. **Provide a verbal medical report to hospital staff.**
4. **Accurately complete a patient care report.**

Attitude Objectives

As an EMT-Basic, you should be able to:

1. **Describe your feelings about using interpersonal communication techniques when speaking with a patient.**
2. **Explain why it is important to communicate accurate patient information to hospital staff.**
3. **Evaluate your own feelings about the importance of thorough documentation and the consequences of falsifying information on a written report.**

KEY TERMS

1. **Base Station:** A fixed station, such as a hospital or dispatch center, containing equipment necessary for radio transmission and reception; equipment includes at least a transmitter, transmission lines, antenna, and receiver.
2. **Duplex:** A mode of radio transmission in which simultaneous two-way communication takes place using two separate frequencies to transmit and receive.
3. **Interpersonal Communication Skills:** Skills used to enhance verbal communication, including the proper use of eye contact, body language, verbal language, and attentive listening.
4. **Multiplex:** A mode of radio transmission that enables voice and other data to be transmitted simultaneously on the same frequency.
5. **Patient Care Report:** A written report summarizing vital patient and administrative information; a medical-legal document.
6. **Portable Radio:** A hand-held, low-power device that allows for radio communication when responders are away from the ambulance.
7. **Repeater:** A radio base station that receives a low-power radio transmission on one frequency and retransmits it over another higher-power frequency to increase the range of the broadcast.
8. **Simplex:** A mode of radio transmission in which transmission and reception occur on the same frequency, limiting communication to one direction at a time.
9. **Telemetry:** Radio or telephone transmission of converted electronic signals; sometimes used by ALS personnel to transmit heart rhythm findings.
10. **Ultra High Frequencies (UHF):** Radio frequencies that perform well in the presence of large physical obstacles, such as skyscrapers, but are not as effective as very high frequencies (VHF) over long distances.
11. **Very High Frequencies (VHF):** Radio frequencies that perform well over long ranges but are more prone than UHF to interference from large physical obstacles.

IT'S YOUR CALL

It is that time of year when changing weather patterns stir up heavy storms. An exceptionally severe storm has generated a series of tornadoes that struck a neighboring community. You are dispatched along with other units to provide mutual aid for this community, which has just declared a disaster situation. As you depart your jurisdiction, your dispatch center advises you to switch to another channel to receive instructions. As you do so, you hear static and what seems to be multiple units indicating their arrival on a scene where a school building is on fire. The static continues and then the channel goes silent.

As you continue on a rural road, debris is scattered about and several large trees have fallen across the roadway, blocking your direct route to the scene. Fearing more detours, you attempt to notify the local dispatch center to check if they have additional information about alternate road conditions. After repeated unsuccessful attempts, you switch back to your primary channel and contact your own county's dispatch center. However, they are experiencing the same problems in making contact.

You assume that the local emergency operations center (EOC) has been activated according to standard disaster procedures, but you are also unable to contact the EOC. Are you left unable to communicate with the dispatch center or with the incident command on the scene? Are there other ways to communicate? How can you alert the local dispatch center and incident command of your situation? Will you be able to communicate with hospitals later in the incident?

We rely heavily on the ability to communicate as part of our daily routine. In EMS, communication is a critical link that holds the team together. From the time you depart for a call until you report back at your station, you are communicating. The system will not work properly without the ability to communicate with your dispatch center, other units responding to the scene, and the hospital.

Many of your professional actions will depend to a great degree on effective communication, whether it is verbal, written, or electronic. This could be face-to-face communication with a patient or colleague, or a phone relay through your dispatch center with a poison control center 50 miles away. This chapter examines the variety of ways in which you will communicate as part of your job, including notifying the dispatch center that your unit is responding to a call, talking to your patient, and completing the patient care report documenting the call.

Verbal Communication

To function effectively in EMS, you must be able to adequately communicate with others, including patients and their families and your coworkers. Additionally, possessing a working knowledge of the basic components of any communication system will help you prevent interruptions in your communications with others. For example, being away from your vehicle while caring for a patient requires that you remember to take some form of portable communication device with you, such as a portable radio or cellular phone. Without it, you may waste time returning to the ambulance to summon additional personnel or resources or to contact the hospital to provide a patient care report.

Communication Systems

There are several important components of a communication system. Some systems allow for minimum communication, while others provide state-of-the-art, high-tech communications resources. Included among these components are:

- Base stations
- Mobile radios
- Portable radios
- Repeaters
- Cellular phones
- Digital equipment

Your EMS system will have some or perhaps all of these components. You will need to learn the specific features of your particular system.

Base Stations

Base stations are usually the principal fixed stations for transmitting and receiving information for EMS communications and patient information (Figure 5-1). The dispatch center and the hospital's emergency department are examples of base stations. Depending on the community, there may be only one base station used to dispatch police, fire, and ambulance personnel. In other areas, multiple independent base stations may be in use. Using powerful radios with effective antennas, a base station operator can communicate with field personnel at great distances.

Mobile Radios

Mobile radios are those permanently mounted in vehicles. Because they operate at lower power than base stations, their range is limited to about 15 miles over average terrain. Mountainous terrain and urban buildings will decrease this range, while transmission over water increases

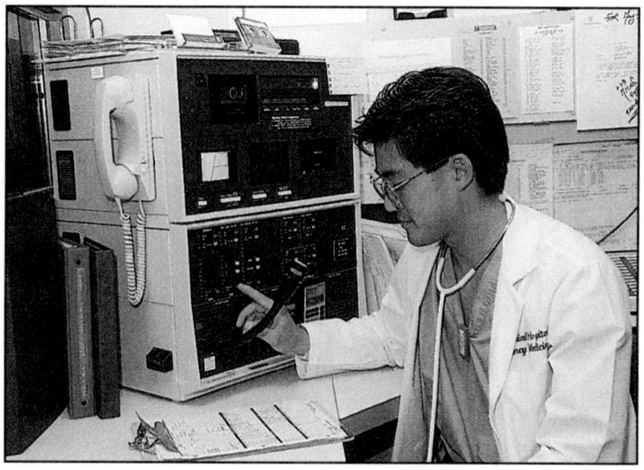

Figure 5-1

A base station is the hub of hospital communication in an EMS system.

it. Mobile radios can be either single- or multichannel, depending on the needs of the EMS system.

Portable Radios

Portable radios allow a user who is away from a fixed station or vehicle to transmit and receive effectively (Figure 5-2). These hand-held units have even less power than mobile radios, limiting the distance over which they will operate. Like mobile radios, portables can have single or multiple channels. These radios operate on batteries that require periodic recharging.

Repeaters

A **repeater** is a device that receives a low-power transmission on one frequency and retransmits it at a higher power on another frequency. Because of the low-power output of mobile and portable radios, a repeater is often necessary to boost the signal. Repeaters can be either fixed or mobile; many EMS systems use both to achieve the necessary communication over large areas (Figure 5-3).

Cellular Phones

Cellular phone use is increasing among EMS systems, particularly because its multichannel capability can help create a link between EMS personnel and hospitals (Figure 5-4). Some agencies have opted for cellular phone use as their primary means of hospital communication. Others rely on

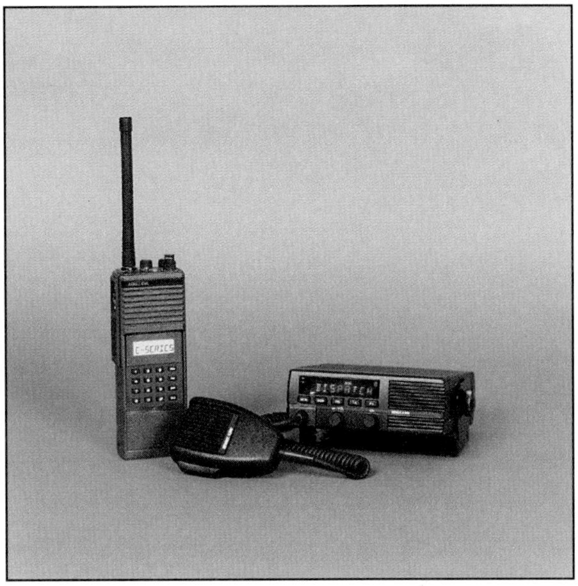

Figure 5-2

A portable radio (left) and a vehicle-mounted two-way radio.

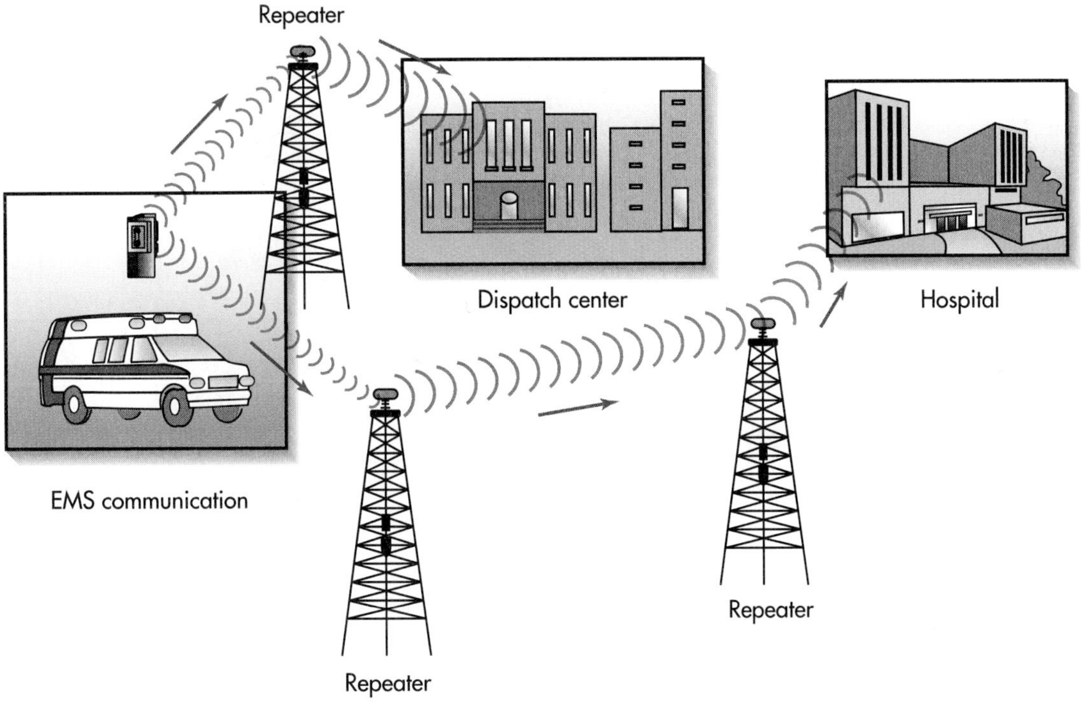

Figure 5-3

Repeaters aid in EMS communications by receiving low-power transmissions (e.g., from mobile or portable radios) and retransmitting them at a higher power to hospitals or dispatch centers.

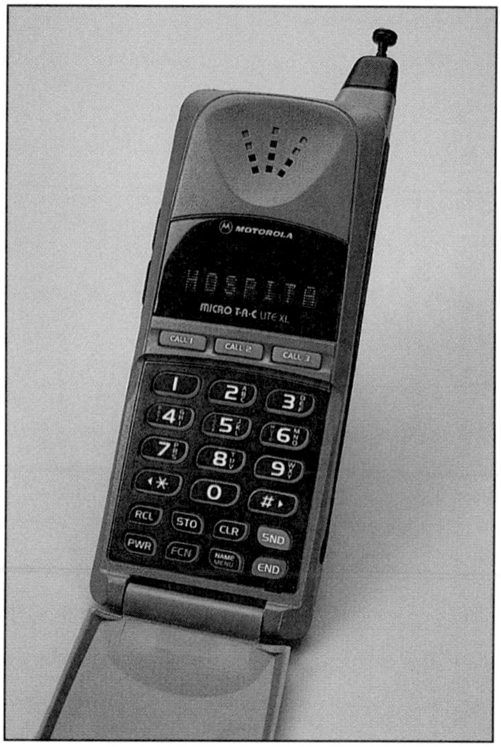

Figure 5-4

An example of a cellular phone used in EMS systems.

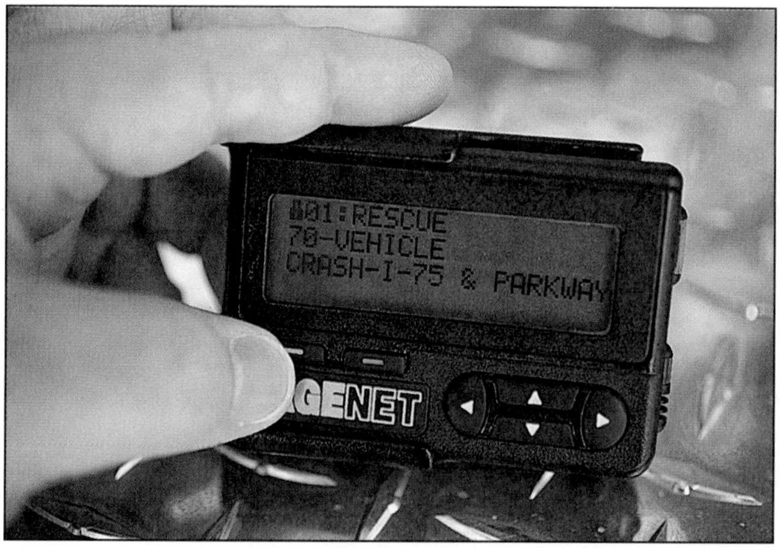

Figure 5-5

Alphanumeric pagers can relay dispatch information when verbal communication is not possible or is too slow.

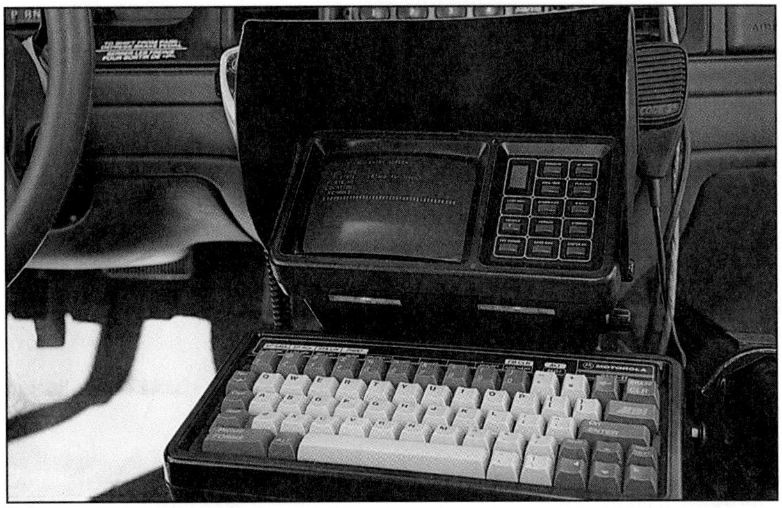

Figure 5-6

Computer units are used to facilitate dispatch activities.

cellular phones as a back-up system. There are disadvantages to using cellular phones. Although phones are inexpensive and monthly rate charges are often reduced for EMS agencies, cellular technology does not allow for priority access or for monitoring by other units that may need to respond. There are also still some geographic areas where cellular service does not work well.

Digital Equipment

Although EMS providers rely heavily on verbal communication through radios, digital signals are also used to alert providers and transmit information. Digital signals are transmitted rapidly and can possibly allow quicker communication than radios and cellular phones. There are several different forms of digital signals. Some EMS systems use pagers or audible tone systems to alert EMS providers to respond to a call. Alphanumeric pagers can be used to provide more detailed written messages (Figure 5-5). Some agencies use computer units (Figure 5-6) to facilitate dispatch activities. These mobile data terminals (MDTs) receive dispatch information and written messages in electronic data bursts rather than voice transmissions. MDTs also log response times and can interact with computer-aided dispatch programs to help monitor response time components and communicate written messages.

Telemetry is a specialized type of radio transmission. It encodes electronic signals into audible signals and transmits them over a radio or telephone. The receiver decodes the transmission back to the original electronic signal. This is how ALS personnel can send a tracing of the heart's electrical activity, known as an electrocardiogram (ECG), to the hospital for analysis by a physician.

IT'S YOUR CALL
CONCLUSION

In the scenario presented previously, tornadoes have disrupted radio communications with a neighboring jurisdiction. You and other units have been detoured as a result of weather conditions but are unable to relay this information to the neighboring dispatch center. With the radios inoperable, you search for another way to contact the center. Your dispatchers advise you that they are unable to contact the neighboring dispatch center over standard phone lines. Because local cell sites have been damaged, the cellular system is overloaded and your back-up attempt with a cellular phone is also unsuccessful. What about paging? Could your dispatch center send a voice or digital message to key individuals in the neighboring county responding to the scene? It is possible, but the phone lines will be critical and dispatch must have the appropriate numbers.

There are still other alternatives. If you can make contact with law enforcement officers, they may be able to relay information. Many EMS systems include organized groups of amateur radio operators in their disaster plans and exercises. Making use of this resource may require face-to-face contact with one of these operators, but it can be a valuable tool when it is available. A citizen's band (CB) radio in a private vehicle could also offer a link to local responders, although it may not be as effective as a preplanned strategy involving organized radio operators.

Finally, remember to consider hospitals as communications resources. They usually have backup systems to work around power outages and are often linked to public safety agencies and other hospitals. Because they will play a central role in the incident after triage begins, it is doubly useful to keep them in mind early on.

Radio Communication

Your ability to communicate with others depends on the power of the weaker of the two radios and the mode of operation of the radios. Base stations and radios operating with repeaters have a greater range and clearer transmission quality than portables do. For this reason, depending on your location, you may be able to clearly hear your dispatcher at times that he or she may not be able to hear you. Likewise, two ambulances in different areas may both be able to hear and respond to the dispatcher, but lack the ability to communicate directly with each other. Remember that even small changes in location can affect transmission. For example, higher ground with fewer obstacles allows for better transmission and reception than valleys with numerous obstacles.

Effective radio communication requires that you follow some general rules and practice communications procedures frequently. Some EMTs do not have the opportunity to use the radio often, which could result in poor radio reports. Some of the more common radio communication problems that occur in various stages of the incident can be avoided if you know what to look for (Box 5-1).

Modes of Operation

There are four primary operation modes in use in EMS communication systems:

- One-way
- Simplex
- Duplex
- Multiplex

The one-way mode is generally used for alerting someone; a pager is an example. This allows for communication in one direction only. In **simplex** mode, transmission and reception occur on the same frequency, restricting the user to transmitting and then waiting for a response. This is the

BOX 5-1 Guidelines for Proper Radio Communication

- Be sure the radio is on and the volume is properly adjusted.
- Reduce background noise whenever possible.
- Speak slowly, clearly, and in a normal tone.
- Hold the microphone about 3 inches from your mouth.
- Keep your transmission concise.
- Avoid the use of "ten codes," slang, or abbreviations that are not known system-wide.
- Make sure your frequency is available before transmitting.
- Key the microphone for 1 second before beginning to talk. This avoids cutting off your first few words.
- When discussing a patient, use objective statements regarding your findings. Do not try to offer a diagnosis of the problem.
- Avoid using a patient's name.
- Avoid informal, unprofessional phrases or unnecessary phrases such as *be advised, thank you,* or *you're welcome.*
- Pronounce each number of a multiple digit number. For example, "Medic 153" is transmitted "Medic one, five, three."
- Never use profanity or statements that could be considered slanderous.
- Do not use the radio for anything other than EMS-related business.
- Consider using an alternate channel to talk with other units, thereby keeping the main channel free for emergency traffic.
- Always take your portable radio with you.
- Turn on the repeater when removing your portable radio.
- Be sure your battery charger is on when replacing your portable radio.

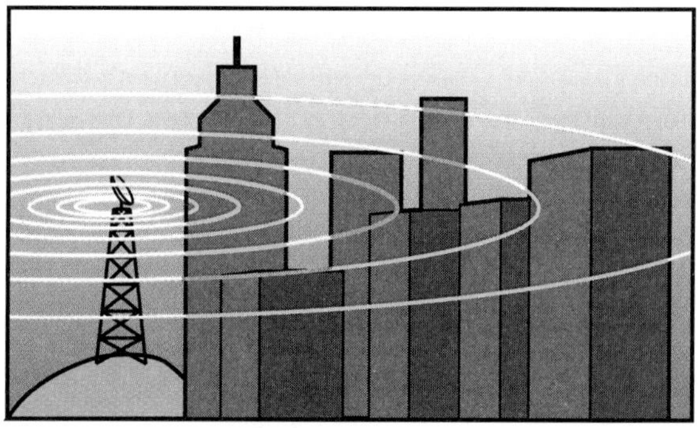

Figure 5-7

Although UHF has a limited range, it is good for use in urban areas because it can withstand interference from electricity and large objects such as buildings.

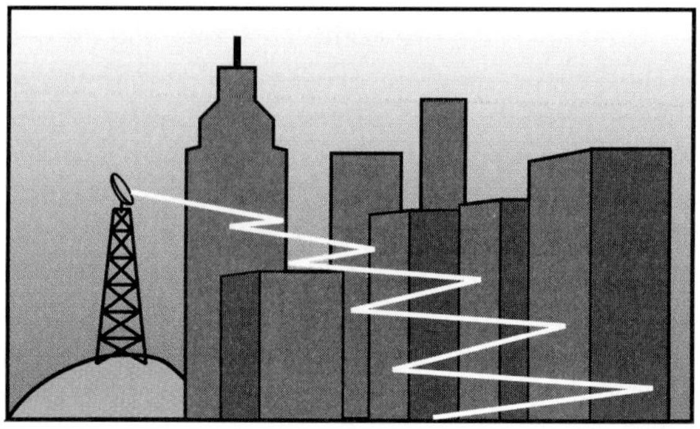

Figure 5-8

VHF performs well over long ranges, but is more susceptible than UHF to electrical and structural interference. It is best used in rural areas.

most common form of dispatch system in use today. A third mode is called **duplex,** which uses two frequencies, thereby allowing simultaneous two-way communication, as on a telephone. **Multiplex** enables voice and other data to be transmitted simultaneously on the same frequency. This mode is used most frequently by ALS providers to send telemetry to the hospital at the same time they are talking with hospital staff.

Frequencies

The Federal Communication Commission (FCC) has designated several different radio frequencies **(Med channels)** for use by EMS and public safety personnel. These include the **ultra high frequency (UHF)** and **very high frequency (VHF)** bands.

Although they have a limited range, UHF frequencies are often used in urban areas because of their ability to provide excellent communication even when confronted with large objects such as buildings (Figure 5-7). UHF frequencies are also less susceptible than VHF to electrical interference. VHF signals generally have a greater range than UHF signals but are subject to more interference from physical structures (Figure 5-8).

The FCC has also made frequencies available for what is called *trunked* radio technology. Trunking features the use of multiple frequencies that are allocated via computer technology on a moment-to-moment basis by the equipment itself. This helps reduce frequency crowding problems and frees dispatchers and field personnel from having to make some of the decisions about frequency choices.

Communicating With the Dispatch Center

Your dispatch center is the link for vital information. Dispatchers respond to a call for help by summoning EMS units to assist and by providing additional information as those units respond.

Initial Dispatch

In some systems, dispatchers trigger alert tones to notify personnel of the need to respond. Other systems use a simple radio dispatch followed by information about the nature and location of the call. As a third method, voice pagers can be used to dispatch EMTs.

An increasing number of dispatch centers now have computer-aided dispatch (CAD) systems, which are computer-based programs that facilitate dispatching activities, time recording, and record keeping. Some agencies can also link directly to the 9-1-1 system, allowing immediate access to the caller's address and phone number. This feature is known as enhanced 9-1-1 (see Chapter 1). Mobile data terminals are available that enable EMTs to view the same information on a computer screen in the ambulance. The terminal may include a printer that provides a hard copy of the data.

If you are unsure of the dispatched address, contact the dispatcher and clarify the information. Do not depart until you are sure where you are going. Incorrect address information can waste valuable time.

From the point that the original call comes in, the dispatch center is responsible for recording incident times, including:

- Call received
- Ambulance dispatch
- Ambulance response
- Scene arrival
- Arrival at patient
- En route to the hospital
- Hospital arrival
- Available for service
- Arrival back at the station

Responding to the Call

Once you are certain of the location of the call, notify the dispatcher that you are responding. Start by making sure that your mobile radio is on. When you are certain the channel is clear from other transmissions, key the microphone. Speak clearly and in a normal tone, with your mouth several inches away from the microphone. Provide your unit number and the status of your unit. For example, "Dispatch, Medic 6-2 is responding."

Once you are en route, the dispatcher may provide additional information, including more patient information, potential hazards, or the status of other responders such as law enforcement personnel.

Arriving at the Scene

Communicate with your dispatcher when you arrive on the scene. It is important for the purposes of accuracy that you report upon actual arrival at the incident and not while you are still approaching. If you are the first unit on-scene, you will need to communicate additional information, including:

- The exact location of the patient. This is especially important if the patient location is different from that originally dispatched.
- Hazards. These may include hazardous materials, downed power lines, trees, or other debris obstructing access.
- Establishing incident command. If it is necessary to declare an incident a multiple casualty incident or disaster situation and establish a command center, then dispatch should be notified of this decision.
- Scope of incident. It is important to notify the dispatch center of the specifics of the incident. For example, if you were dispatched for a motor vehicle collision, you would need to report involvement of multiple vehicles or patients. If dispatched to a structure collapse, notify incoming units of the status of the structure and the best route of approach.

- Additional resources. Other specialized personnel may be needed to assist with the incident. You may also need more EMS personnel to help, for example, with a cardiac arrest or to assist in moving a patient.
- Staging area. In large incidents, identify the point at which you want vehicles to stage (see Chapter 6 for more details).
- Alternate channel. Larger incidents mean that more units and personnel will be involved and that communication will be even more important in managing these resources. It is advisable to request an alternate channel, if available, to communicate with units responding to this incident and to avoid jamming the primary channel.

Your report should be concise but convey the necessary elements. Remember that callers do not always provide correct information, and sometimes conditions change after the call is placed. Consider the following transmission from an ambulance initially dispatched to a single motor-vehicle collision:

> *Dispatch, Ambulance 6-1 on the scene. There are three vehicles involved, one on its side. Correction on the location, this is in the southbound lane of I-79, between mile markers 26 and 27. Ice on the bridge, advise incoming units to use caution as they approach.*

This is helpful information that will be relayed to other units.

Some dispatch centers now use automatic vehicle locator (AVL) systems to track the positions of field units. Improved computer mapping technology has made this possible, along with inexpensive global positioning system (GPS) equipment. GPS uses satellites to provide accurate locations in almost any terrain.

Reporting Your Situation

The dispatch center will be monitoring your situation. You may be contacted periodically to check on your progress or just to let you know how long you have been on-scene, according to your agency's protocols. For example, the dispatcher may contact you after the first 10 minutes of your notification of arrival at the scene, or every 30 minutes during a major incident.

Once your patient has been transferred to the ambulance and you are prepared for transport, contact the dispatch center. You may have to advise dispatch of the destination hospital, the patient's age, chief complaint, and other information unique to the situation. For example:

> *Dispatch, Ambulance 6-2 is en route to Hillcrest Hospital with an 8-year-old female complaining of difficulty breathing. Parents are accompanying her. Our ETA is 15 minutes. Requesting a channel 4 patch to the emergency department.*

You will also need to advise the dispatch center when you arrive at and depart from the hospital as well as any change in your unit's status.

Communicating With the Hospital

You will communicate with hospital staff as a routine part of patient care. This communication will take place over the radio (via specific med channels) or telephone and in person when you arrive with the patient. In most cases you will provide initial verbal information over the radio about the patient's condition and the treatment you have provided, which will help the hospital staff make decisions about the room, equipment, and services that are needed. In some situations, you may also request further treatment orders.

The Medical Report

When you provide a verbal report to hospital staff over the radio or phone, make it logical, clear, and concise. This report presents the most important elements about the patient's condition. It often helps to have the patient care report or communication format guideline in front of you as you speak (Figure 5-9). Generally, the radio report is much briefer than the verbal report you will provide once you arrive in the emergency department.

When providing the verbal medical report over the radio or telephone, there are several general elements to include:

1. Unit and personal identification. *Parkview Hospital, this is EMT Phillips with Ambulance 6-2. How are you receiving this transmission?* This last question verifies that the hospital is receiving your transmission, before you proceed.
2. Receiving hospital and estimated time of arrival (ETA). *We are en route to your location with a 15-minute ETA.* It is necessary to announce what hospital you are going to, because it is possible that you may, depending on the EMS system, be receiving medical direction from one hospital while transporting the patient to another. The ETA helps receiving personnel prioritize the steps in their preparation for your patient.
3. Patient's age and gender. *We are transporting a 19-year-old male. . . .*
4. Chief complaint. . . . *with a chief complaint of pain and inability to move his right ankle or foot.*
5. Pertinent history of the present incident. *Patient was injured while sliding feet first into a base during a softball game.*
6. Pertinent past history. *Patient had surgery to repair damage to his foot approximately 2 years ago.*
7. Vital signs (level of consciousness, pulse, respirations, blood pressure, skin). *He is alert and oriented. Pulse is 90 and regular, respirations 16 and normal, blood pressure is 130/80, skin is warm and moist, and pupils are equal and reactive.* Some EMS systems encourage EMTs to shorten the transmission by stating that all vital signs are within normal limits when this is the case.

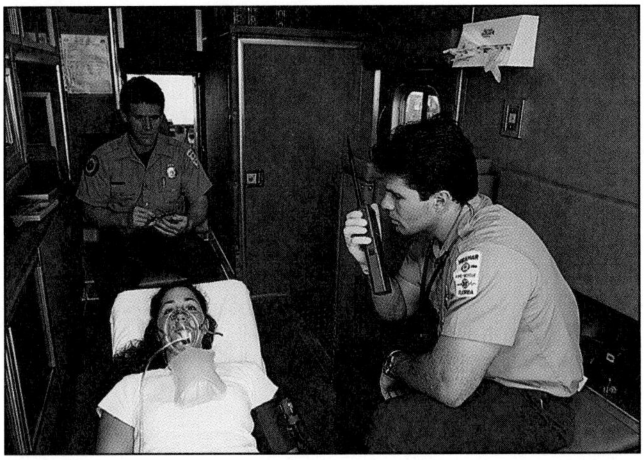

Figure 5-9

While en route with a patient, an EMT radios the receiving hospital with a verbal medical report.

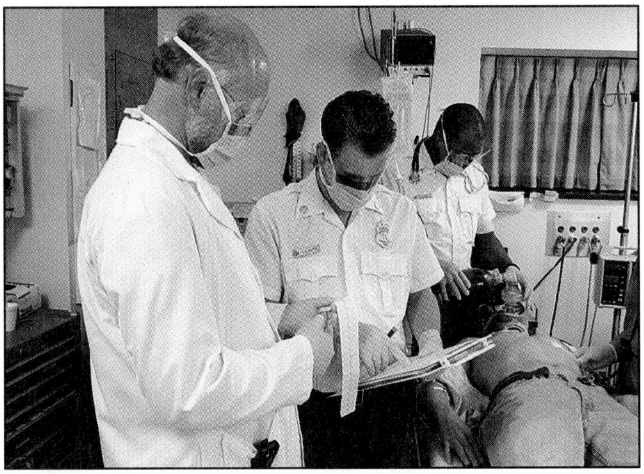

Figure 5-10

Upon arrival at the receiving hospital, an EMT updates a member of the hospital staff on the patient's condition.

8. Pertinent findings upon physical examination. *Patient's ankle is painful, swollen, bruised, and deformed. Pulses are present in his ankle and capillary refill is normal.*
9. Treatment provided. *We have splinted the ankle and applied cold compresses.*
10. Patient response to the treatment. *The patient's pain has been reduced somewhat.*
11. Further instructions or additional information. *Do you have any further orders?* If you do receive additional instructions, repeat the orders to confirm that you heard them correctly. If you did not understand the order, ask to have it repeated. If it appears to be inappropriate, question the order. The physician providing the order may have misunderstood your report, or the order could have been confused by someone relaying it to you. The hospital may also request additional information from you.

When you have completed your report, allow the hospital to terminate the call. This ensures that the staff has received the necessary information. If the patient's condition deteriorates en route to the hospital, you should call again and report the change.

When you arrive at the hospital, you will often have to briefly update your report to the nurse or physician. Introduce the patient by name. Provide the patient's chief complaint, any history that was not previously mentioned, additional treatment provided en route, and any changes in the patient's condition (Figure 5-10).

Local policy and practice will determine exactly which procedures are required to complete the transfer of care from the EMT to hospital personnel. At a minimum, this requires a good verbal report. It usually also includes leaving a copy of the written report and may involve having hospital caregivers sign that they have received the patient.

Communicating With Other Health Care Providers

You will interact with many different health care providers during your career as an EMT. These include colleagues such as other EMTs or paramedics, physicians and nurses providing patient care upon your arrival on-scene, and hospital staff in and beyond the emergency department. Likewise, you may communicate with ALS personnel who have been summoned to assist with your patient. In any of these communications it is important to provide a brief report and answer any questions.

Communicating with other caregivers can be stressful when disagreements arise about procedures or patient care. Listed below are some guidelines for handling these situations:

- Discuss disagreements away from the patient and do not let those disagreements delay urgent care.
- If specific policy, procedure, or protocol applies, explain it and try to use this to resolve the problem.
- When a situation falls outside of policy and protocol, consider the patient's best interest. This should provide quick common ground for at least a short-term agreement.
- Contact medical direction for advice on specific therapies or other issues that cannot be agreed on. Then get back to patient care and leave any remaining personal or administrative issues for discussion after the call.

Communicating With Patients

Establishing rapport with your patient is critical to the overall care that you provide. You should strive to be a caring, professional EMT and practice good "bedside manner." With all that takes place at an emergency scene, it is easy to get distracted and fail to communicate well. Make a conscious effort to remember that you are there to care for people who need your help.

Interpersonal Communication Skills

Though communication seems to occur naturally, some people still lack the necessary skills to communicate effectively. **Interpersonal communication skills** involve two-way communication with your patient. This means that you must be able to talk and listen effectively. How you say something verbally or with body language can be misinterpreted.

In face-to-face communication with a patient, follow these guidelines:

1. Maintain eye contact. This shows that you are attentive to what the other person has to say. It is important to note that some people will avoid eye contact with you, which is normal in some cultures.
2. Be aware of your body position. When speaking to someone, position yourself in front of the person and at his or her level. If your patient is a child or is lying down, this often means kneeling next to the patient (Figure 5-11), thereby presenting a less threatening position. Avoid crossing your arms or standing sideways, which can be interpreted as impersonal, disinterested, or threatening positions (Figure 5-12).
3. Speak slowly, clearly, and in simple terms. Avoid using medical terms and EMS jargon that the patient will not understand. Do not ask a patient, "Do you have any pertinent respiratory or cardiac history?" Ask instead, "Do you have any medical problems, such as breathing or heart problems?"
4. Stay calm. Patients may note any apprehension or shouting, which could heighten their fears.
5. Use the patient's name whenever possible. Show respect for the patient. For adult patients and especially for the elderly, use "Mr., Ms., or Mrs." before their last name.
6. Be honest. To gain a patient's trust, you must be honest, even if what you say may not be pleasant to hear. For example, the patient may ask whether his or her wrist is broken. Sometimes this is obvious, such as when broken bone protrudes through the skin. Other times, however, swelling may mask deformity and you will not be able to say with certainty. Give the patient your honest opinion. Likewise, if you must perform a procedure that may be uncomfortable, advise the patient before beginning. Honesty does not always mean telling everything you know or suspect; it must be applied with common sense. Blunt honesty can be cruel, and the EMT will have to use judgment about deferring questions that it is not wise to answer at the moment.
7. Listen attentively. You are the one that normally asks most of the questions. When you ask a question, listen to the complete answer before asking another question. Write down the pertinent information that the patient provides. Avoid distractions while the patient is answering.

Communicating With Special Populations

In the course of doing your job, you will encounter individuals who may have difficulty communicating. This could include children, elderly, hearing and sight impaired, developmentally disabled, and non-English speaking individuals.

Children. Children are not just small adults. They have unique needs that you must consider. Because you are a stranger, they often will not accept you even though you are there to help. This can make it difficult to communicate with children and determine what their problems are. A child fears strangers, illness, injury, and above all else, being separated from parents. In some cases, the age of the patient will make communicating difficult. However, even a child too young to speak will communicate if he or she is in pain.

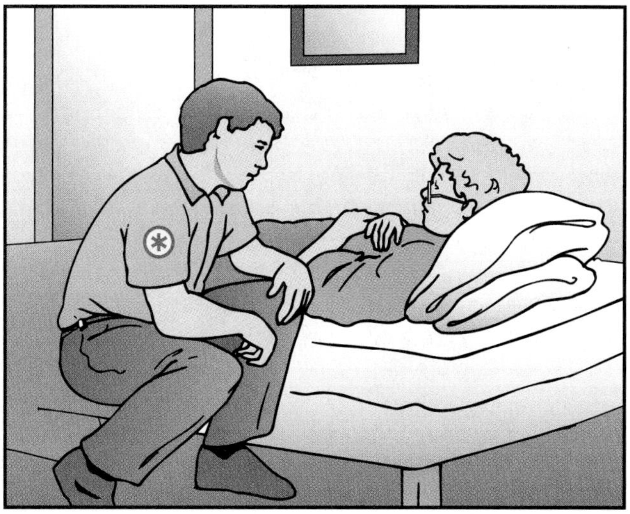

Figure 5-11

Getting down at the patient's eye level communicates a caring, non-threatening demeanor to your patients.

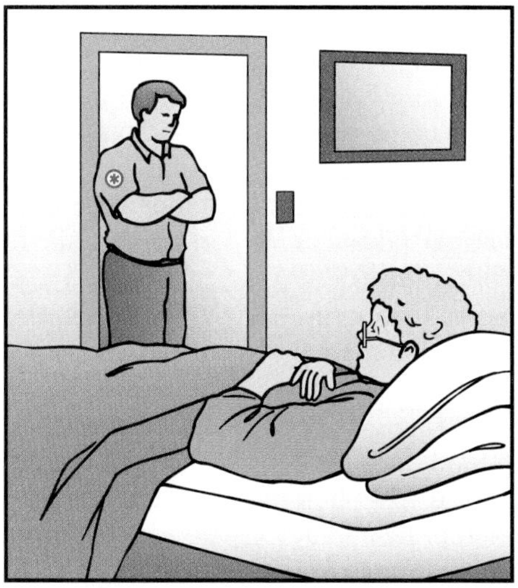

Figure 5-12

Crossing your arms, standing sideways, and standing above your patient are gestures that communicate an impersonal, disinterested, and even threatening attitude.

When attempting to communicate with a child, keep these guidelines in mind:

- Remain calm and approach the child in a gentle, friendly manner.
- Do not separate the child from his or her parents or guardians unless it is absolutely necessary. A patient sitting in a parent's lap is usually calmer and easier to treat than one sitting alone (Figure 5-13).
- Communicate directly with the child whenever possible.
- Attempt to gather information from the parent or guardian.
- Explain the procedures that you will perform. Be truthful when explaining procedures that may cause further pain. You want to gain the patient's trust, so make sure you are being honest.
- Before performing a procedure, tell the child what you are going to do and why.
- Whenever possible, *show* the child what you are going to do before doing it.

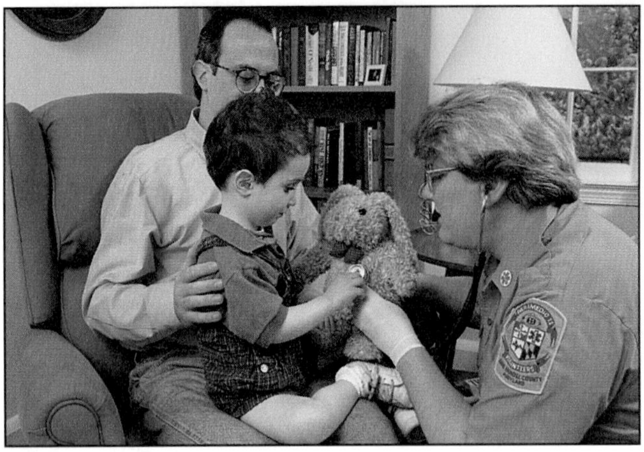

Figure 5-13

Reassuring a child with the presence of a parent and distracting him with a toy are ways to make him more comfortable with what might otherwise be perceived as a threatening situation.

- Position yourself at eye level with the child. An adult can be threatening just because of size.
- Use stuffed animals or other toys to help calm the child.
- Use simple words that the patient can understand.

Elderly. As life expectancy increases because of advances in health care, so do your chances of caring for elderly patients. The general decline in body function that occurs with age results in changes in hearing, sight, and mental capacity. These changes can affect your ability to communicate with elderly patients.

Begin by positioning yourself at eye level. Introduce yourself and ask why the ambulance was called. Use short sentences and be prepared to repeat or rephrase your questions. Geriatric patients often need more time to understand and respond than do younger patients. It may seem like they are not paying attention when they are simply trying to think about what you said and how to respond. Slowing your speech can make it easier for them to understand what you are saying. It often helps to pause and wait after you have asked a question.

Hearing Impaired. While some patients develop hearing disabilities as they age, others have this problem throughout their lives. Those with hearing impairments may be partially or completely deaf. Communicating with a person who is deaf may be a little more difficult, but it should not overwhelm you.

The patient may be able to read lips, so always face the patient and speak normally. If you know sign language or have a colleague who can sign, use this to communicate. You may want to learn some basic words or phrases in sign language, such as *name, pain,* and *sick* to help you communicate with the hearing impaired (Figure 5-14). There are numerous books and reference guides available. You can also write questions for the patient. This system is slow, but usually effective. Avoid restraining a deaf person's hands whenever possible; hands are important tools in communication.

Visually Impaired. Visually-impaired patients can either be partially or completely blind. Ask the patient whether he or she can see any images, such as shadows. Visual disabilities will not often affect your ability to communicate with the patient. Begin by introducing yourself. Advise the patient of others in the immediate area who will be assisting you. Remember that these individuals use their hands to do the work of their eyes. They may want to touch your hand or other objects around them to explore a new environment. When walking with a blind patient, have him or her hold your arm for assistance (Figure 5-15). Walk at a normal pace and alert the patient to any hazards. If the patient has a guide dog, make efforts to keep it with the patient; however, if this is not possible, try to arrange care for the animal.

Developmentally Disabled. Impairment of mental function can be caused by a previous injury or infection or by a genetic problem such as Down syndrome. In some cases, you will know that the patient is developmentally disabled because a caregiver or guardian informs you. Approach the patient as you would any other patient of the same age. Speaking in a calm, slow voice and using simple terms, try to determine the patient's level of understanding. Reassure the patient to help reduce fear and anxiety. Ask a parent or guardian to help you with communication whenever possible.

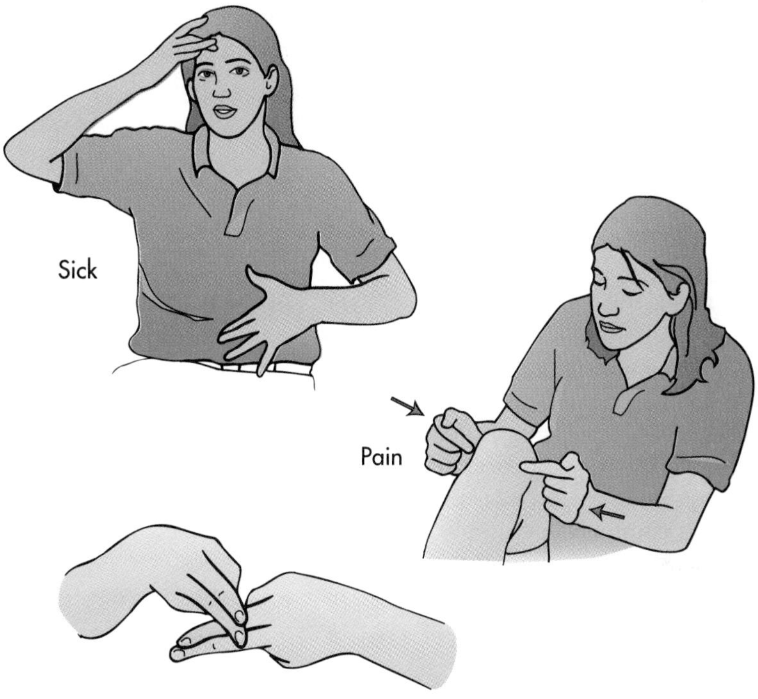

Figure 5-14
Learning sign language for some commonly used terms can help in communication with hearing impaired patients.

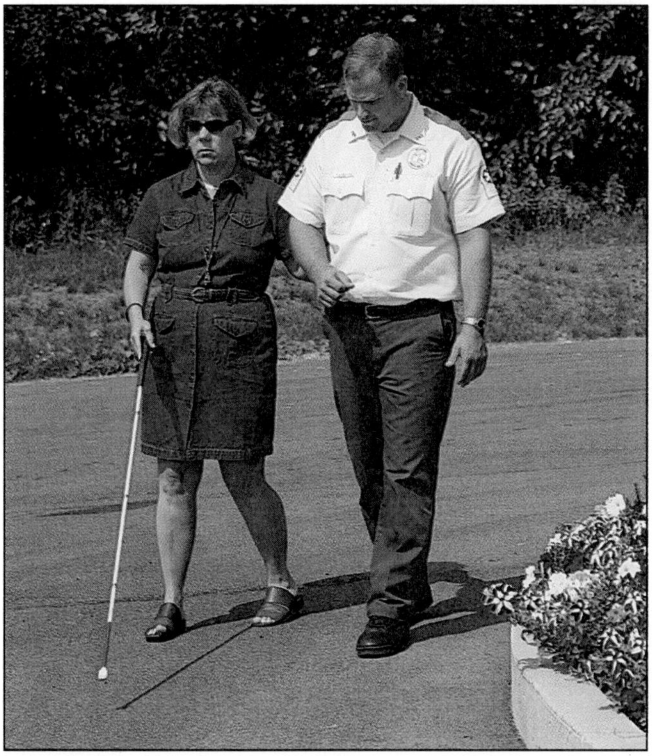

Figure 5-15
An EMT giving his arm for assistance to a visually-impaired patient.

Although not developmentally disabled, patients with mental or emotional disturbances also present challenges to clear communication. Chapter 20 discusses behavioral topics in more depth.

Non-English–Speaking Patients. There are a significant number of individuals in the United States who do not speak English fluently or who do not speak it at all. This is especially true for certain segments in large urban areas. When working with non-English–speaking patients, try to use simple words and small phrases to determine how much English a person understands. As with elderly patients, it helps to slow your own speech and allow longer pauses than usual for answers to questions. Point to parts of the body while asking questions. Learning a few key words in a second language likely to be encountered in your area can help you communicate more effectively. Use an interpreter whenever possible. Your service may provide reference cards or books that present standard patient examination questions in English and several other languages. By pointing to questions and answers, you and the patient can cover many of the basics even when there is no common language.

Written Communication

As presented in Chapter 2, written communication such as a patient care report is a way to document your patient's condition and your actions. This documentation is important for the continued care of the patient. Information gathered from family members about a patient's previous medical history or information about the medications given to an unconscious patient may help hospital staff resolve the patient's problem more quickly. Documentation may also be important for your legal protection should a question ever arise about the quality of care you provided.

The patient care report also provides a means of collecting and studying data that could result in improvements in your EMS system. It allows systematic review of your agency's responses to various situations and assists with billing accuracy.

The Patient Care Report

Besides the verbal medical report you provide by radio, telephone, or in person at the hospital, you also have a formal written report that must be filled out. Whenever possible, the **patient care report** should be completed before you leave the hospital. Leave a copy with the hospital and take the original and other copies back to your station to be filed. Different states, cities, and counties use different forms. Some are on paper, others are in electronic form. You must be aware of your system's reporting procedures, including:

- What information should be provided on the complete patient care report
- Whether the emergency physician or nurse needs to sign the report
- How and when to file the report
- How the information is used locally

Do not delay patient care to complete the report. It can be written after the patient has been stabilized or after transfer of care at the hospital.

SOAP: The Medical Charting Standard

Although your service's report form may not follow it exactly, you should understand the reporting method that most physicians and nurses use. The "SOAP" method divides the report into four areas that closely follow the actual sequence of assessing, treating, and monitoring the patient.

Subjective: Historical information that is reported by the patient or others, but not observed directly by the caregiver.

Objective: Physical examination data gathered through direct observation or measurement by the care provider.

Assessment: The caregiver's summary of the problem or problems being attended to. (EMTs make a general assessment, not a medical diagnosis.)

Plan: The treatment provided and any response to treatment, or other changes noted afterward.

Types of Forms

Report forms vary greatly among different jurisdictions (Figure 5-16). Most EMS agencies still use traditional paper forms with check boxes and blank areas for recording information. Other agencies are using computerized versions of these forms, which are primarily a series of check boxes. After completion the form is inserted into a scanner or reader, which automatically enters the information into a database (Figure 5-17). Still other systems use an electronic clipboard that allows the information to be entered into a portable computer. This information is later transferred into a master database.

Essential Elements

The essential elements of a patient care report fall into two general categories of information: patient and administrative (Figure 5-18). Patient information includes all pertinent information gathered about the patient from the time you first make contact until you transfer care to the hospital staff. Administrative information includes logging the times at which different events occurred and gathering statistical information about the patient. The recommended minimum data that should appear on all reports,

EMS RUN MEDICAL FORM

AGENCY	UNIT #			MEDCOM NUMBER
NAME		ADDRESS		DATE / DAY
PATIENT PHONE	AGE / D.O.B.	SEX M ☐ F ☐	RACE / SSN ___-__-____	COMPLAINT NO.
INCIDENT LOCATION		DISPATCH/"CHIEF COMPLAINT"	PRTY:	REPORTING POLICE DEPARTMENT

PHYSIOLOGIC STATUS

TIME	BLOOD PRES	PULSE RATE	PULSE QUAL.	RESP. RATE	RESP. QUAL.	PUPILS	GCS E(4)	GCS V(5)	GCS M(6)	AVPU	SKIN	PO_x	PRTY

COUNTY

TWP/CITY/VILLAGE

EST. TIME — INCIDENT T.O.C.

Dispatch

En route

Arr. Scene

(EST) Arr. Pat.-

Dep. Scene

Arr. Hosp.

DEFIBRILLATE

TIME	ECG	WATT/S	ECG	BY NO.

CPR INITIATED Yes ☐ No ☐
By: MFR ☐ Bystander ☐ PD ☐ ALS ☐ Mechanical Device ☐

AED Yes ☐ No ☐

MAST ☐ In Place ☐ Inflated

DESTINATION
Hospital ________
Diversion From: ________

CHOSEN BY
☐ Patient ☐ MEDCOM
☐ Relative ☐ Hospital
☐ EMT ☐ Physician
☐ Other ______

BARRIERS
☐ Gloves
☐ Goggles
☐ Mask
☐ HEPA
☐ Gown
☐ ______

MECHANISM OF INJURY FACTORS:
☐ Ejected from Vehicle
☐ MVA w/Fatals at Scene
☐ Extrication >20 Minutes
☐ Major Vehicle Damage
☐ Unrestrained
☐ MCA without Helmet
☐ Fall > 20 Feet
☐ Rollover

DRUG TIMES

DRUG	TIME	DOSE	ROUTE	MEDIC #	AUTH (SO,MC,POS)	DRUG	TIME	DOSE	ROUTE	MEDIC #	AUTH

Time Med Dir Contact: Est. Wt.: Blood Sugar /

AIRWAY
Basic: O2 Flow ______ L/Min @ ______ Time via: NC SFM M/RES P. MASK BVM Adj: OPA NPA $ETCO_2$ Used: Yes ☐ No ☐
Advanced: Proc: ______ Size: ______ # Attempts ______ by # ______ Est. by # ______ Time ______ $ETCO_2$ Confirmed: Yes ☐ No ☐ N/A ☐

I.V. SITE: ______ # ATTEMPTS ______ BY # ______ EST. BY # ______ SIZE ______ TIME ______ RATE ______ TOTAL INFUSED ______

I.V. SITE: ______ # ATTEMPTS ______ BY # ______ EST. BY # ______ SIZE ______ TIME ______ RATE ______ TOTAL INFUSED ______

MED. HX. ALLERGIES PT. PHYSICIAN

CURRENT MEDS

NARRATIVE

PAGE OF AGENCY PRESENT UPON ARRIVAL: MFR ☐ E-Unit ☐ Amb ☐ FORM COMPLETED BY: #

	AMBULANCE PERSONNEL No./Level	OTHER AGENCY PERSONNEL No./Level	FIRST IN EQUIPMENT
SIGNATURE	1. ______	1. ______	FIRST IN BAG ☐
Printed Name	2. ______	2. ______	AIRWAY BAG ☐ /DEFIB ☐
DEA Number	3. ______	3. ______	O_2 ☐ STRETCHER ☐
ETT Confirmed;	4. ______	4. ______	AUX COT ☐

Figure 5-16

An example of an EMS patient care report.

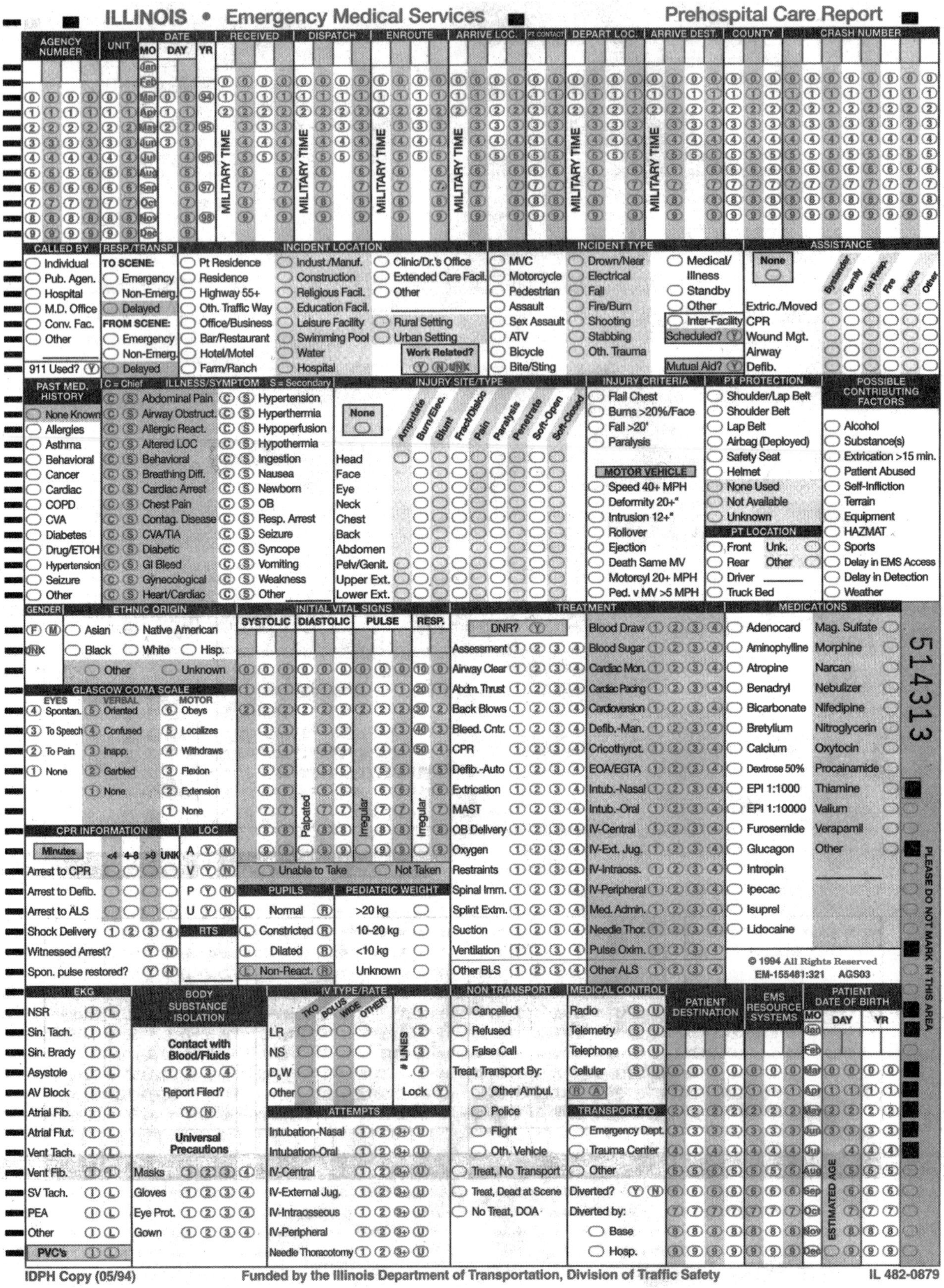
ILLINOIS • Emergency Medical Services Prehospital Care Report

AGENCY NUMBER | UNIT | DATE (MO DAY YR) | RECEIVED | DISPATCH | ENROUTE | ARRIVE LOC. | PT CONTACT | DEPART LOC. | ARRIVE DEST. | COUNTY | CRASH NUMBER

Jan Feb Mar Apr May Jun Jul Aug Sep Oct Nov Dec; 94 95 96 97 98; MILITARY TIME

CALLED BY: Individual, Pub. Agen., Hospital, M.D. Office, Conv. Fac., Other, 911 Used? (Y)

RESP./TRANSP.: TO SCENE: Emergency, Non-Emerg., Delayed; FROM SCENE: Emergency, Non-Emerg., Delayed

INCIDENT LOCATION: Pt Residence, Residence, Highway 55+, Oth. Traffic Way, Office/Business, Bar/Restaurant, Hotel/Motel, Farm/Ranch, Indust./Manuf., Construction, Religious Facil., Education Facil., Leisure Facility, Swimming Pool, Water, Hospital, Clinic/Dr.'s Office, Extended Care Facil., Other, Rural Setting, Urban Setting, Work Related? (Y) (N) UNK

INCIDENT TYPE: MVC, Motorcycle, Pedestrian, Assault, Sex Assault, ATV, Bicycle, Bite/Sting, Drown/Near, Electrical, Fall, Fire/Burn, Shooting, Stabbing, Oth. Trauma, Medical/Illness, Standby, Other, Inter-Facility, Scheduled? (Y), Mutual Aid? (Y)

ASSISTANCE: None; Bystander, Family, 1st Resp., Fire, Police, Other; Extric./Moved, CPR, Wound Mgt., Airway, Defib.

PAST MED. HISTORY: None Known, Allergies, Asthma, Behavioral, Cancer, Cardiac, COPD, CVA, Diabetes, Drug/ETOH, Hypertension, Seizure, Other

ILLNESS/SYMPTOM (C = Chief, S = Secondary): Abdominal Pain, Airway Obstruct., Allergic React., Altered LOC, Behavioral, Breathing Diff., Cardiac Arrest, Chest Pain, Contag. Disease, CVA/TIA, Diabetic, GI Bleed, Gynecological, Heart/Cardiac, Hypertension, Hyperthermia, Hypoperfusion, Hypothermia, Ingestion, Nausea, Newborn, OB, Resp. Arrest, Seizure, Syncope, Vomiting, Weakness, Other

INJURY SITE/TYPE: None; Amputate, Burn/Elec., Blunt, Fract/Disloc, Pain, Paralysis, Penetrate, Soft-Open, Soft-Closed; Head, Face, Eye, Neck, Chest, Back, Abdomen, Pelv/Genit., Upper Ext., Lower Ext.

INJURY CRITERIA: Flail Chest, Burns >20%/Face, Fall >20', Paralysis; MOTOR VEHICLE: Speed 40+ MPH, Deformity 20+", Intrusion 12+", Rollover, Ejection, Death Same MV, Motorcyl 20+ MPH, Ped. v MV >5 MPH

PT PROTECTION: Shoulder/Lap Belt, Shoulder Belt, Lap Belt, Airbag (Deployed), Safety Seat, Helmet, None Used, Not Available, Unknown; PT LOCATION: Front, Unk., Rear, Other, Driver, Truck Bed

POSSIBLE CONTRIBUTING FACTORS: Alcohol, Substance(s), Extrication >15 min., Patient Abused, Self-Infliction, Terrain, Equipment, HAZMAT, Sports, Delay in EMS Access, Delay in Detection, Weather

GENDER: (F) (M) UNK; ETHNIC ORIGIN: Asian, Native American, Black, White, Hisp., Other, Unknown

INITIAL VITAL SIGNS: SYSTOLIC, DIASTOLIC, PULSE, RESP.; Palpated, Irregular, Irregular; Unable to Take, Not Taken

GLASGOW COMA SCALE: EYES: 4 Spontan., 3 To Speech, 2 To Pain, 1 None; VERBAL: 5 Oriented, 4 Confused, 3 Inapp., 2 Garbled, 1 None; MOTOR: 6 Obeys, 5 Localizes, 4 Withdraws, 3 Flexion, 2 Extension, 1 None

CPR INFORMATION: Minutes <4 4-8 >9 UNK; Arrest to CPR, Arrest to Defib., Arrest to ALS, Shock Delivery, Witnessed Arrest? (Y) (N), Spon. pulse restored? (Y) (N)

LOC: A V P U; RTS

PUPILS: Normal, Constricted, Dilated, Non-React.; PEDIATRIC WEIGHT: >20 kg, 10–20 kg, <10 kg, Unknown

TREATMENT: DNR? (Y); Assessment, Airway Clear, Abdm. Thrust, Back Blows, Bleed. Cntr., CPR, Defib.-Auto, Extrication, MAST, OB Delivery, Oxygen, Restraints, Spinal Imm., Splint Extm., Suction, Ventilation, Other BLS; Blood Draw, Blood Sugar, Cardiac Mon., Cardiac Pacing, Cardioversion, Defib.-Man., Cricothyrot., EOA/EGTA, Intub.-Nasal, Intub.-Oral, IV-Central, IV-Ext. Jug., IV-Intraoss., IV-Peripheral, Med. Admin., Needle Thor., Pulse Oxim., Other ALS

MEDICATIONS: Adenocard, Aminophylline, Atropine, Benadryl, Bicarbonate, Bretylium, Calcium, Dextrose 50%, EPI 1:1000, EPI 1:10000, Furosemide, Glucagon, Intropin, Ipecac, Isuprel, Lidocaine, Mag. Sulfate, Morphine, Narcan, Nebulizer, Nifedipine, Nitroglycerin, Oxytocin, Procainamide, Thiamine, Valium, Verapamil, Other

© 1994 All Rights Reserved EM-155481:321 AGS03

514313

PLEASE DO NOT MARK IN THIS AREA

EKG: NSR, Sin. Tach., Sin. Brady, Asystole, AV Block, Atrial Fib., Atrial Flut., Vent Tach., Vent Fib., SV Tach., PEA, Other, PVC's

BODY SUBSTANCE ISOLATION: Contact with Blood/Fluids, Report Filed? (Y) (N), Universal Precautions, Masks, Gloves, Eye Prot., Gown

IV TYPE/RATE: TKO, BOLUS, WIDE, OTHER; LR, NS, D_5W, Other; # LINES; Lock (Y)

ATTEMPTS: Intubation-Nasal, Intubation-Oral, IV-Central, IV-External Jug., IV-Intraosseous, IV-Peripheral, Needle Thoracotomy

NON TRANSPORT: Cancelled, Refused, False Call; Treat, Transport By: Other Ambul., Police, Flight, Oth. Vehicle; Treat, No Transport; Treat, Dead at Scene; No Treat, DOA

MEDICAL CONTROL: Radio, Telemetry, Telephone, Cellular; TRANSPORT TO: Emergency Dept., Trauma Center, Other; Diverted? (Y) (N); Diverted by: Base, Hosp.

PATIENT DESTINATION | EMS RESOURCE SYSTEMS | PATIENT DATE OF BIRTH (MO DAY YR) | ESTIMATED AGE

IDPH Copy (05/94) Funded by the Illinois Department of Transportation, Division of Traffic Safety IL 482-0879

Figure 5-17

Information on scannable patient care forms can be scanned and entered into a database.

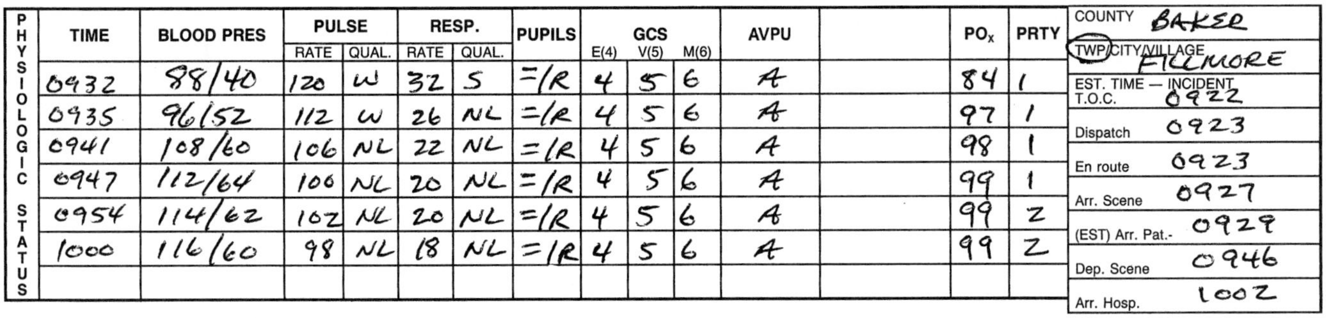

PHYSIOLOGIC STATUS TIME	BLOOD PRES	PULSE RATE	PULSE QUAL.	RESP. RATE	RESP. QUAL.	PUPILS	GCS E(4)	GCS V(5)	GCS M(6)	AVPU		PO$_x$	PRTY
0932	88/40	120	W	32	S	=/R	4	5	6	A		84	1
0935	96/52	112	W	26	NL	=/R	4	5	6	A		97	1
0941	108/60	106	NL	22	NL	=/R	4	5	6	A		98	1
0947	112/64	100	NL	20	NL	=/R	4	5	6	A		99	1
0954	114/62	102	NL	20	NL	=/R	4	5	6	A		99	2
1000	116/60	98	NL	18	NL	=/R	4	5	6	A		99	2

COUNTY	BAKER
TWP/CITY/VILLAGE	FILLMORE
EST. TIME — INCIDENT T.O.C.	0922
Dispatch	0923
En route	0923
Arr. Scene	0927
(EST) Arr. Pat.-	0929
Dep. Scene	0946
Arr. Hosp.	1002

Figure 5-18

The patient information on a patient care report lists the patient's vital signs and the times that they were taken. The administrative information lists the times that specific events of the run took place.

regardless of where you practice as an EMT, is listed in Box 5-2.

While there is now some attempt to standardize the minimum data collected across the U.S., systems differ in the additional information required on their reports. Minimum elements include:

- Response data: Includes information such as date, times, service provided, unit, crew names.
- Patient data: Patient's name, address, gender, date of birth, and age; location of the call; the type of problem, including mechanism of injury or nature of illness; care provided before EMS arrival; signs and symptoms; vital sign measurements; care provided by EMS personnel; pertinent medical history and changes in condition.
- Check boxes: Areas that allow for a means of rapidly documenting parts of the call, such as the level of care provided and how the hospital was contacted.
- Narrative: Objective and subjective information written in a narrative form. In essence you are writing a short story documenting the patient's situation and what you did to help the patient (Figure 5-19).

Use of the Narrative. The narrative is sometimes the hardest part of the report to fill out, especially for new EMTs, because they are uncertain of how much detail to provide. Several different perspectives have been offered over the years regarding the narrative. One perspective is that the narrative is used to clarify any item that may be questioned from another section of the report. For example, you will normally record vital signs every few minutes, depending on your patient's condition. But if there was a gap of 20 minutes between reported vital sign measurements, the narrative can state that extensive extrication procedures were underway to free a patient from wreckage. Special circumstances do occur, and the narrative can help explain them.

Another perspective on the use of the narrative section is that it should not repeat information already clearly available in another section. Instead it should support and be consistent with the information provided in other report areas.

A third perspective is that you should use the narrative to present information not covered elsewhere at all. For example, while you have an area on the report to record the patient's chief complaint, you may not have an area to record how the call was dispatched. You may be dispatched for an unconscious patient, only to arrive and find a patient who complains of a headache and never lost consciousness. In this case, the narrative could

BOX 5-2 Minimum Elements for a Patient Care Report

Patient Information

- Chief complaint
- Mechanism of injury or nature of illness
- Level of consciousness (mental status on a four-level scale)
- Pulse rate
- Breathing rate and effort
- Systolic blood pressure
- Skin perfusion (capillary refill)
- Skin color and temperature

Administrative Information

- Time of the incident
- Time the unit was notified
- Time of dispatch
- Time of arrival at the scene
- Time of arrival at the patient
- Time the unit left the scene
- Time the unit arrived at the destination
- Time the unit returned to service

DRUG TIMES	DRUG	TIME	DOSE	ROUTE	MEDIC #	AUTH (SO,MC,POS)	DRUG	TIME	DOSE	ROUTE	MEDIC #	AUTH
	EPI-PEN	0934	0.3mg	IM	3213	SO	N/A					

Time Med Dir Contact: 0952 Est. Wt.: 172 # Blood Sugar N/A

AIRWAY
Basic: O2 Flow 15 L/Min @ 0932 Time via: NC SFM (M/RES) P. MASK BVM Adj: OPA NPA $ETCO_2$ Used: Yes ☐ No ☐

Advanced: Proc: ______ Size: ______ # Attempts ______ by # ______ Est. by # ______ Time ______ $ETCO_2$ Confirmed: Yes ☐ No ☐ N/A ☐

I.V. SITE: N/A # ATTEMPTS ______ BY # ______ EST. BY # ______ SIZE ______ TIME ______ RATE ______ TOTAL INFUSED ______

I.V. SITE: ______ # ATTEMPTS ______ BY # ______ EST. BY # ______ SIZE ______ TIME ______ RATE ______ TOTAL INFUSED ______

MED. HX. ASTHMA / BEE STINGS ALL. ALLERGIES NKDA PT. PHYSICIAN JONES

CURRENT MEDS PROVENTIL (AS NEEDED)

NARRATIVE S: 23 YO WM CLEANING OUT STORAGE AREA OF STORE WHEN STUNG ON Ⓛ ARM BY MULTIPLE BEES. PT C/O SOB / FACIAL SWELLING / RASH & ITCHING. HAS EPI-PEN BUT DID NOT USE PTA.
O: ATF PT SITTING IN CHAIR, PALE, DIAPHORETIC, ANXIOUS, SOB. MOVING AIR WELL c̄ DIFFUSE MILD WHEEZES ALL FIELDS. MILD DIFFUSE FACIAL SWELLING / ERYTHEMA. DIFFUSE HIVES TRUNK, ARMS & LEGS. PERRL, NARES PATENT, PHARYNX W/O SWELLING. CV - TACHY LUNGS DIFFUSE WHEEZING, ABD SOFT EXT W/O EDEMA.
A: PT LAID ON FLOOR, V.S. & O_2 AS ABOVE. PT ASSISTED WITH USE OF EPI-PEN BY # 3213 IN Ⓛ LAT THIGH
PT PLACED ON STRETCHER & TRANSFERED TO UNIT - GRADUAL IMPROVEMENT IN RASH / ITCHING / SOB. O_2 MAINTAINED. REPEAT VS AS ABOVE DURING TRANSPORT. PT FEELING MUCH BETTER BY ED ARRIVAL. CARE TO ED STAFF IN RM 3

PAGE 1 OF 1 AGENCY PRESENT UPON ARRIVAL: MFR ☐ E-Unit ☐ Amb ☐ FORM COMPLETED BY: J Smith #

SIGNATURE Steve Jones MD	AMBULANCE PERSONNEL	No./Level	OTHER AGENCY PERSONNEL	No./Level	FIRST IN EQUIPMENT
Printed Name JONES	1. J SMITH	EMT-B	1.		FIRST IN BAG ☐
DEA Number	2. T JONES	EMT-B	2.		AIRWAY BAG ☐
	3.		3.		DEFIB ☐
ETT Confirmed;	4.		4.		O_2 ☐
					STRETCHER ☐
					AUX COT ☐

Figure 5-19

The narrative portion of a patient care report is a chronological account of what took place during the call.

begin with how the call was dispatched and what you initially found. For example:

> *Dispatched to chest pain. Arrived to find 55-year-old male in cardiac arrest, with bystander CPR in progress.*

A final perspective is that the narrative can be used to tell the entire story from start to finish in a concise, logical manner.

Regardless of the perspective your agency follows, the narrative must have some common elements. It must describe the incident but not draw any conclusions from it. For example, it is acceptable to write, *Bystanders state that the patient staggered out the doorway and fell onto the sidewalk, striking his head and cutting his hand on a glass bottle that he was carrying.* Upon examination you may report that, *The patient's breath had an odor of alcohol.* These are objective statements; they are measurable and verifiable.

It would not be acceptable to conclude in your report that the patient was intoxicated. This cannot be concluded without the proper test procedures (e.g., breathalyzer, urine test, blood test), and the patient could file a complaint or consider a legal action against you. Box 5-3 shows the contrast between a useful and uninformative narrative.

BOX 5-3 Narrative Reporting Samples

Example A below illustrates a well-summarized patient report that quickly gives the reader the main points. Its brevity would also make it an ideal radio report on a crowded EMS frequency.

Example A

The patient is a 52-year-old male complaining of chest pain, shortness of breath, and heaviness in his left arm. He reports no cardiac risk factors. He is awake and alert, his pulse is regular, and his other vital signs are within normal limits. His skin is pale and diaphoretic, and his lung sounds are clear.

Example B

The patient had chest pain for 3 hours, and no other problems. His lungs are clear. We transported to the hospital.

Example B is too brief for either a written or verbal report. The reader or listener will not understand the overall situation after the report.

Your narrative should also include subjective information that the patient provides, such as, "I feel nauseated." Also include observations on your part, such as, "The patient appeared sad, quiet, and refused to provide information; however, she acknowledged that she understood the questions."

Also include pertinent negatives in your narrative. These are items that the patient denies, such as the presence of chest pain or difficulty breathing in a patient with cardiac history, or loss of consciousness in a driver involved in a vehicle accident.

Other general items to remember when writing a narrative are:

- Limit the use of codes and abbreviations to those accepted by your system.
- Write or print legibly, with correct spelling.
- Use medical terminology correctly.
- Include important observations about the scene, such as details about mechanism of injury.
- Document the incident thoroughly. Remember the golden rule of EMS documentation: "If it wasn't written down, it didn't happen."

A thorough report provides for continuity of care from the time you arrive and assume patient care until you transfer care to more qualified personnel. It should include any changes in the patient's condition over time. Therefore document the time and the findings each time you reassess the patient's vital signs. This report allows other health care providers a mechanism to review the patient's condition and response to care over time.

Special Situation Reports

Some situations require that you modify your report or complete additional forms and file them with the proper authorities. These situations can include those involving the following:

- Patient refusal
- Correcting errors
- Multiple casualty incidents
- Violence or abuse
- Contagious diseases

Patient Refusal. As discussed in Chapter 2, an adult has the right to consent to or refuse both treatment and transport. A refusal is sometimes called a decision "against medical advice," or AMA. Before accepting the patient's refusal, attempt to assess the patient's competence to make an informed, rational decision. (Chapter 2 also discusses competence in more detail.) The effects of an injury or illness could limit the patient's ability to think logically. Inform the patient why he or she should be evaluated in the emergency department and list the possible consequences of not doing so. Encourage the patient to be evaluated by a physician. If the patient refuses your help, advise the patient about other care alternatives. Consult your supervising physician, as directed in local protocols.

EMS REFUSAL OF CARE/TRANSPORTATION FORM

AGENCY: METRO — UNIT #: 162 — MEDCOM NUMBER: 98 - 21759

NAME: CINDY DUNLAP — ADDRESS: 675 WEST OAK 29172 — DATE: 8/20/98 — DAY: TH

PATIENT PHONE: 541-7924 — AGE: 30 — D.O.B.: 6/9/68 — SEX: M ☐ F ☒ — RACE: B — SSN: — COMPLAINT NO.: 8-8-280

INCIDENT LOCATION: BRIDGE @ STOCKING — CODE — DISPATCH/"CHIEF COMPLAINT": BIKE VS CAR — REPORTING POLICE DEPARTMENT: SPD

STATUS TIME	BLOOD PRES.	PULSE RATE	PULSE QUAL.	RESP. RATE	RESP. QUAL.	SKIN	PUPILS	GCS		PO$_x$	PRTY
1730	142/88	92	NL	18	NL	W/D	=R	15		98	3
1746	136/70	74	NL	16	NL	W/D	=R	15		—	3

COUNTY: BAKER — TWP/(CITY)/VILLAGE: STANTON

MED. HX.: Ø — ALLERGIES: Ø

CURRENT MEDS.: Ø

NARRATIVE
C: INJURED Ⓛ FOREARM
H: 30 YO BF RIDING BIKE WHEN Ⓛ FOREARM STRUCK BY CAR MIRROR PT HELMETED - FELL TO GROUND W/O OTHER TRAUMA ⊖ LOC - C/O ONLY Ⓛ FOREARM PAIN ⊖ NUMBNESS
A: A/OX3 NO HEAD TRAUMA ⊖ NECK/BACK/CHEST/ABD PAIN OR TEND. Ⓛ FOREARM OBV. DEF; M/P/S INTACT.
Rx: Ⓛ FOREARM SPLINTED ELBOW → HAND. PT REFUSED TRANSPORT - HUSB ARRIVED TO TRANSPORT TO HOSP.

FORM COMPLETED BY: J Smith

EST. TIME — INCIDENT T.O.C.	1712
Dispatch	1713
En route	1714
Arr. Scene	1722
Arr. Patient	1722
Dep. Scene	1800
Arr. Hosp.	—

MECHANISM OF INJURY FACTORS:
- ☐ Ejected from Vehicle
- ☐ MVA w/Fatals at Scene
- ☐ Extrication > 20 Minutes
- ☐ Major Vehicle Damage
- ☐ Unrestrained
- ☐ MCA without Helmet
- ☐ Fall > 6 Feet
- ☐ Not Applicable

I.V. SITE: N/A # ATTEMPTS ____ BY # ____ EST. BY # ____ SIZE ____ TIME ____ RATE ____ TOTAL INFUSED ____

DRUG	TIME	DOSE	ROUTE	MEDIC #	AUTH (SO,MC,POS)
N/A					

MEDICAL CONTROL PHYSICIAN: S. JONES, MD — Steve Jones, MD

PAGE 1 OF 1

NOTE: PT & HUSBAND ADVISED TO CALL US BACK IF NEEDED. J Smith

AMBULANCE PERSONNEL	No./Level
1. J. SMITH	EMT-B
2. T. JONES	EMT-B
3.	
4.	

OTHER AGENCY PERSONNEL	No./Level
1. N/A	
2.	
3.	
4.	

OTHERS WITH DIRECT PT. CONTACT

Name	Phone No.
G. DUNLAP	541-7924
L. GREER	SPD

RELEASE OF LIABILITY
REFUSAL TO CONSENT TO TREATMENT

I, the undersigned, have been advised that medical assistance on my or the patient's behalf is necessary and that my refusal to allow such assistance may result in death or endanger my or the patient's health. I have been advised of and fully understand the nature of the risks I am taking by refusing medical assistance. I assume all responsibility for the consequences of my decision.

I hereby release METRO AMBULANCE SERVICE and any and all persons employed by or responding with them from any and all liability which arises now or may arise in the future from the consequences of this refusal of emergency medical care and/or transportation to the hospital. This liability is binding on anyone acting on my behalf, personally or on behalf of my estate. This release is signed in consideration of the fact that I have: (Please check appropriate box or boxes)

- ☐ refused emergency medical care offered to me or the patient
- ☒ refused transport to a medical facility which was offered to me or the patient
- ☐ refused transport to the nearest hospital after being advised that the welfare of the patient required prompt emergency care

WITNESSED BY:

Signature: George Dunlap
Address/Phone: 675 West Oak 541-7924
Signature: L Greer #762 SPD
Address/Phone:

PATIENT SIGNATURE OR IF A MINOR, PARENT OR LEGAL GUARDIAN

Address

Age of Pt. — Ambulance Dept. No.

Figure 5-20

Example of a patient refusal form that is part of the patient care report.

REFUSAL OF SERVICES

I hereby refuse the emergency medical services and/or transportation offered and advised by the above named service provider and its emergency personnel, ______________ hospital, and the emergency medical and nursing personnel from said hospital giving directions to the service provider. I understand that my refusal may jeopardize the health of the patient, and hereby release the above named parties from any and all claims of liability in connection with my refusal.

Signature of Patient or Legally Authorized Representative

Signature of EMT/Field RN

Witness

Date

Figure 5-21

Example of a separate patient refusal form statement.

If the patient refuses treatment or transport after multiple attempts to explain the need, document this refusal. This is done on a patient refusal form, which may be part of your patient care report (Figure 5-20) or may be a separate form (Figure 5-21). Have another member of your crew listen while you explain what the refusal form means. Have the patient sign the form, sign it yourself, and have someone else sign as a witness. This could be another member of your crew, a family member, police officer, or bystander.

If the patient refuses to sign the form, have a witness note this while signing. In the narrative section of the report, detail the circumstances surrounding the patient refusal. Explain that you discussed the following items to confirm that the refusal was an informed one:

- The consequences of refusing either treatment or transport
- Alternative methods of obtaining care
- Your willingness to return if the patient had a change of mind

On the patient care report or on a separate refusal form, include your findings, the care you provided, the additional care you wished to provide, and if possible, the reason for the refusal.

Error Correction. Everyone makes a mistake from time to time when writing a report. The key in minimizing the number of mistakes you make is to take your time and think through the incident. Then read the report, and when possible, have another member of your crew check it before you turn it over to the hospital.

If you discover an error before the report is turned in, draw a single line through it, correct it, and initial it (Figure 5-22). If the error is discovered after the report has been submitted, you generally should not make a change or correction on the original form. You should usually use a separate form, which is then attached to the original. This should have the date of the correction and your signature or initials. If the error involved information that was omitted, you should complete an addendum form with the additional information. Date and sign the form and attach it to the original report.

The worst thing you could do is intentionally falsify a report. This could include making up vital signs, reporting a procedure that was not performed, or failing to report a procedure that was performed, whether performed correctly or incorrectly. This could lead to suspension or revocation of your EMT certification. It could also result in legal action.

Multiple Casualty Incidents (MCI). When an incident involves many patients, there may not be time initially to document all of the patient information. You may have to rely on other forms, such as triage tags. These are tags placed on patients by a team that rapidly assesses and classifies patients into categories that define the urgency of care based on the severity of the illness or injury. Your local disaster plan should have guidelines to follow in the event of an MCI. Chapter 6 provides more information on the process of triage and the use of triage tags.

Other Special Situations. There may be other situations that require you to complete supplemental forms, documenting a specific situation. One of these involves exposure to an infectious disease. Others could involve personal injury report forms, reports for suspected abuse, and referrals to social service agencies. Become familiar with the requirements of your agency regarding reporting special situations.

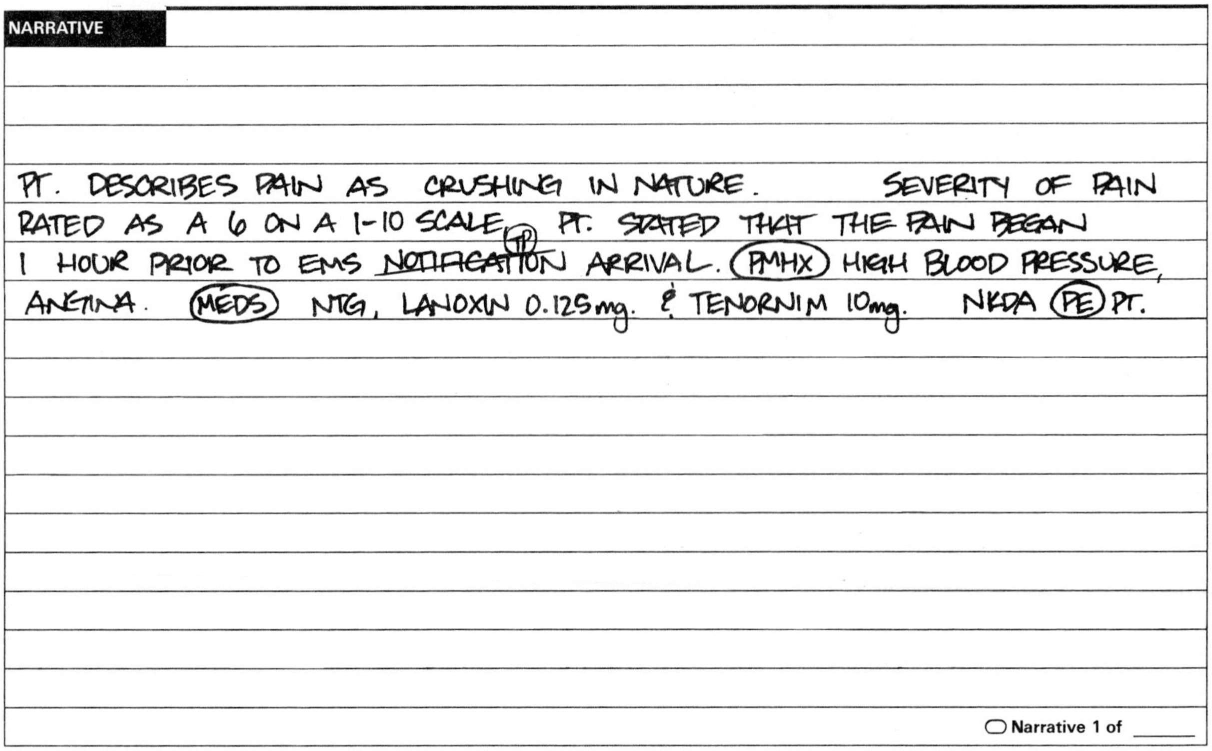

NARRATIVE

PT. DESCRIBES PAIN AS CRUSHING IN NATURE. SEVERITY OF PAIN
RATED AS A 6 ON A 1-10 SCALE. PT. STATED THAT THE PAIN BEGAN
1 HOUR PRIOR TO EMS ~~NOTIFICATION~~ (TP) ARRIVAL. (PMHX) HIGH BLOOD PRESSURE,
ANGINA. (MEDS) NTG, LANOXIN 0.125mg. c̄ TENORNIM 10mg. NKDA (PE) PT.

◯ Narrative 1 of ______

Figure 5-22

Correct errors on a patient care report by drawing a line through the mistake, correcting it, and initialing it.

SUMMARY

Effective communication is an essential part of every EMTs job. Whether verbal or written communication, basic guidelines exist that can help you better communicate with the dispatcher, patient, colleagues, and hospital staff. When communicating through radio or telephone, speak clearly and slowly. When speaking to a patient, use proper techniques including maintaining eye contact, positioning yourself at the level of the patient, and listening to the patient's response to questions.

If you are preparing a written report, keep it legible, concise, and focused on the most important items of the call. If you make a mistake writing the report, correct it as soon as it is noticed, according to the guidelines presented in this chapter. Under no circumstances should you ever falsify any information on the patient care report. Remember that this is a legal document; what you write can be introduced as evidence in a court of law.

SUGGESTED READINGS

1. **Augustine JJ:** Communications. In Kuehl AE, editor: *National Association of EMS Physicians prehospital systems and medical oversight,* ed 2, St Louis, 1994, Mosby.
2. **Gaull ES:** Scene communication pitfalls, *Emerg Med Serv* 21:23, 1992.
3. **Shanaberger C:** The unrefined art of documentation, *J Emerg Med Serv* 17(1):155-157, 1992.

Chapter 6

Scene Assessment

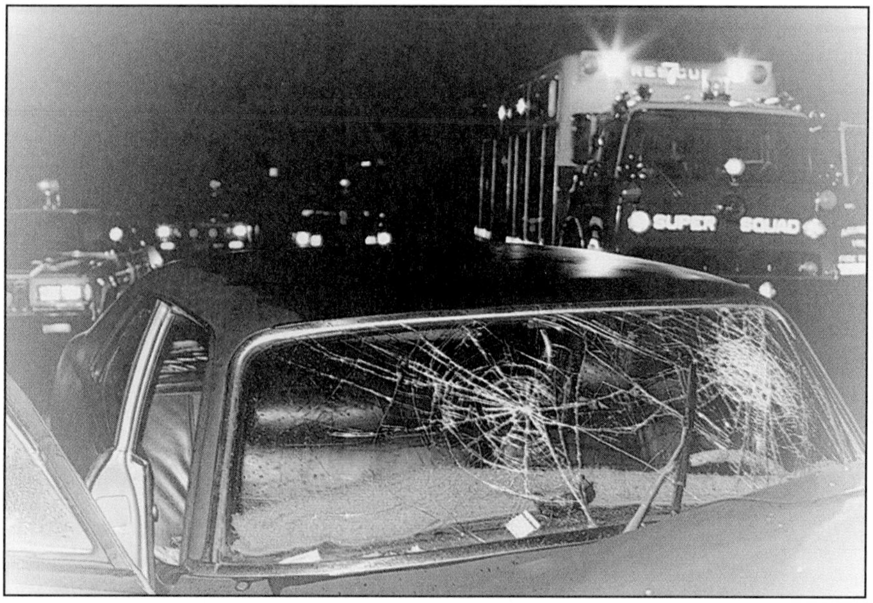

Knowledge Objectives

As an EMT-Basic, you should be able to:

OBJECTIVES

1. Identify key questions to ask as you arrive at any emergency scene.
2. Describe common potential hazards found at the scene of trauma and medical emergencies.
3. Describe how to determine if a scene is safe enough for you to approach and how to take precautions to protect yourself, patients, and bystanders.
4. Describe what is meant by *mechanism of injury* and *nature of illness* and what is the purpose of assessing them at the scene.
5. Discuss common mechanisms of injury and types of illness.
6. Explain what is meant by a multiple casualty incident and provide examples of different magnitudes.
7. Discuss why it is important to identify the total number of patients at the scene.
8. Explain the importance of identifying the need for additional assistance at the scene.
9. Identify the basic components of a disaster plan.
10. Describe the responsibilities you are likely to have as an EMT in a disaster operation.
11. Describe the basic components of the incident command system.
12. Explain the purpose of triage and name the four levels of severity classification according to the Mettag system.

OBJECTIVES

Skill Objectives

As an EMT-Basic, you should be able to:

1. **Identify potential hazards and necessary corrective actions when presented with a scenario involving injury or illness.**
2. **Perform triage on a group of patients when presented with a scenario involving an MCI.**
3. **In an exercise scenario, simulate:**
   a. **Establishing initial incident command, including identifying locations for the command post and staging area and designating or requesting a special radio frequency.**
   b. **Relinquishing command to an arriving fire or police officer.**
   c. **Setting up the medical command sector.**

Attitude Objectives

As an EMT-Basic, you should be able to:

1. **Describe your feelings about maintaining personal safety and the safety of others.**
2. **Act as a positive role model for others when assessing scene safety and taking precautions to protect yourself, patients, and bystanders.**
3. **Act as a positive role model for others when using the mechanism of injury or nature of illness in relation to a patient's condition.**
4. **Describe your personal feelings about conducting triage during an MCI.**

KEY TERMS

1. **Blunt Trauma:** External impact to the body by a mass that does not penetrate internal body areas.
2. **Confined Space:** Any enclosed structure or natural formation whose lack of open-air ventilation poses the risk of a toxic atmosphere.
3. **Critical Trauma:** Life-threatening injury; the result of blunt or penetrating trauma.
4. **Disaster:** An incident of such great magnitude that it exhausts all local resources and requires the assistance of several other jurisdictions; includes natural and man-made disasters. A disaster does not necessarily result in injuries.
5. **Disaster Plan:** A predetermined set of activities that identifies how a community will deploy its resources in the event of a disaster or mass casualty incident.
6. **Incident Command System (ICS):** A system used to manage a disaster or MCI. The system defines a chain of command that begins with the overall scene commander and includes others responsible for functions such as triage, treatment, and transportation. This is sometimes referred to as ***incident management system.***
7. **Golden Hour:** The first 60 minutes after a critical injury or illness until the patient receives definitive care in the hospital emergency department or operating room.
8. **Kinetic Energy:** The energy an object has while it is in motion. It is related to the velocity and size (mass) of the object.
9. **Mechanism of Injury:** The manner in which an injury occurs, including the force, direction of force, and areas of impact involved.
10. **Multiple Casualty Incident (MCI):** An incident, sometimes called a ***disaster,*** where the incident and number of victims overwhelms the capabilities of the EMS service or system.
11. **Nature of Illness:** The general type of illness, often described by the patient's initial complaint or the primary physical examination finding.
12. **Penetrating Trauma:** Penetration of the body by a projectile such as a bullet or by a knife or other sharp instrument.
13. **Placard:** A sign attached to a transport container or vehicle that uses text, numbers, or symbols to identify hazardous contents.
14. **Triage:** A systematic process of establishing treatment and transportation priorities in an MCI according to the severity of patient conditions.

IT'S YOUR CALL

You are dispatched to assist police with a high-speed vehicle collision. Your partner remarks that the location is on a stretch of highway notoriously traveled at excessive speeds. As you arrive, you see debris scattered in the roadway. When you exit the ambulance you notice people gathered around a vehicle in a grassy, depressed area about 30 feet off the road. You do not see tire marks indicating the vehicle's direction of travel as it left the road. Nearing the vehicle, you recognize the remains of a convertible, now crumpled around the driver. The airbag has deployed. Another patient lies outside the vehicle, about 20 feet away.

As you attempt to take in the whole picture, a number of questions go through your mind. How did the vehicle get this far from the road without leaving marks in the grass? How did the second patient end up outside the vehicle? Were both patients wearing seat belts? Did the airbag help prevent injuries to the driver? What injuries are the patients likely to have sustained?

Scene safety and the need to avoid putting yourself, crew members, patients, or bystanders in danger were discussed in Chapter 3. However, there is more to scene assessment than just avoiding dangers. The scene of a trauma or medical emergency is full of clues about what happened, whether it is the scene of a suicide, assault, vehicle collision, poisoning, or environmental emergency. Information about how the incident occurred can give you insight into the possible problems your patients may have. You can use this knowledge to direct the patient assessment.

The scene also provides an indication of the magnitude of the incident, including the number of patients and the special conditions that can influence their safety and survival. When you are the first to arrive, you are the eyes and ears for the entire EMS system. The information you gather will help the dispatch center summon adequate personnel and equipment to the scene.

Surveying the Scene

Safety Considerations

As you arrive on scene, try to take in the complete picture. Your first thought must be for the safety of you, your crew, and any bystanders. If the scene is not safe, take actions to make it so. Summon additional personnel to assist when you have incidents that involve multiple patients or require special equipment or responder training. Assess the safety of bystanders and move them if they are in danger. To help size up the situation and maintain your safety, ask yourself a series of questions as you arrive:

- Is there any fire, smoke, or vapor present?
- Are any structures or vehicles unstable?
- Are hazardous materials **placards** or other signs of toxic danger visible?
- Is anyone at the scene behaving violently?
- Do behaviors or other scene factors suggest that weapons might be present?
- Are there signs that the situation might deteriorate?
- Can the ambulance be parked in a location that avoids oncoming traffic?
- Is there more than one patient?
- What additional resources are needed?

The presence of any of these conditions requires caution.

Recognizing Potential Hazards

There are many different hazards to be aware of as you approach the scene. Specific hazards you are likely to encounter include:

- Disease transmission: Follow body substance isolation (BSI) practices in every situation, regardless of whether or not the patient is bleeding visibly. Other body fluids could pose a threat, as well as airborne contagious diseases. As you exit the ambulance, have the proper personal protective equipment (PPE) ready (Figure 6-1).

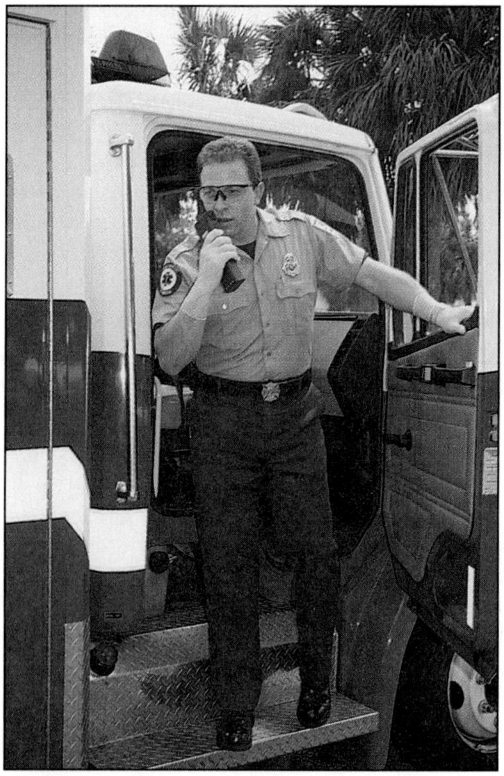

Figure 6-1

Goggles and gloves should always be worn during scene assessment and patient care to prevent disease transmission.

- Motor vehicles: A danger zone exists around every vehicle collision. Consider the risks of uncontrolled traffic or an unstable vehicle and take precautions. Precautions include positioning the ambulance properly, wearing reflective clothing, placing flares or reflectors in the roadway to divert traffic, and stabilizing the patient's vehicle before attempting to examine the patient (Figure 6-2).
- Hazardous materials: Not all hazardous materials are obscure chemicals with complex names. Fuel spilled from a motor vehicle can be a hazardous material. If a significant amount of fuel has been spilled, be cautious when using flares. Park the ambulance uphill from the fuel whenever possible. Notify dispatch and have the fire department respond to contain the spill. For other hazardous materials, position your ambulance a safe distance from the scene, preferably upwind and uphill from the scene. If you are able to see a placard identifying the substance, consult the *Emergency Response Guidebook*[1] for special information about the substance, including the parameters for establishing a safety zone. Entering the "hot zone" (dangerous, potentially contaminated area) requires specialized training and equipment that would not be readily available on an ambulance.
- Unstable structures: Buildings damaged by a motor vehicle or natural disaster should not be entered until they have been determined safe. This usually requires the assistance of specially trained personnel (Figure 6-3).
- Unstable surfaces: Water, ice, mud, and sloping terrain are common unstable surfaces. Working on hazardous surfaces requires special equipment and training (Figure 6-4).
- Fire: Never enter a fire without the necessary equipment and training to protect you from the heat and toxic fumes. This includes proper clothing, self-contained breathing apparatus (SCBA), and back-up personnel.
- Electricity: No matter what the source of the electricity, it must be turned off before you can safely approach a patient. Downed power lines do not have to be arcing or emitting sparks to be dangerous. Await confirmation from the power company or fire department that the power has been turned off.
- **Confined space:** Do not enter a well, silo, cave, or collapsed building without advance knowledge of the air quality. Many confined spaces contain toxic gases that are dangerous to rescuers. In fact, many of those who die in confined spaces are rescuers. Safely entering confined spaces is a skill that requires specialized training and equipment for monitoring the air and breathing.
- Violence: Violent behavior by anyone at the scene is cause for you to take a safe position at a distance. If you are already on the scene when violence erupts, retreat to a safer area. Notify law enforcement personnel and do not return to the scene until they advise that the scene is secure. This is especially true when weapons are present. Consider the likelihood of violence when responding to a location where you have witnessed violence previously, and be cautious of areas known for gang activity.

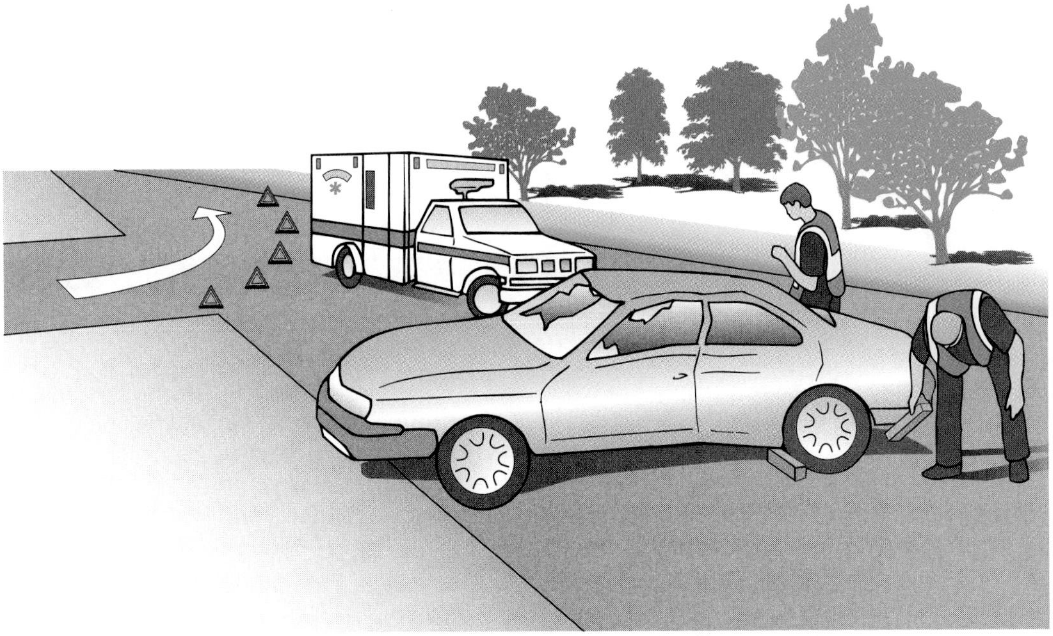

Figure 6-2

Take steps to ensure safety when called to the scene of a traffic accident. These can include some or all of the following precautions: proper ambulance positioning, using flares or reflectors to divert traffic, wearing reflective vests, and securing an unstable vehicle with chocks.

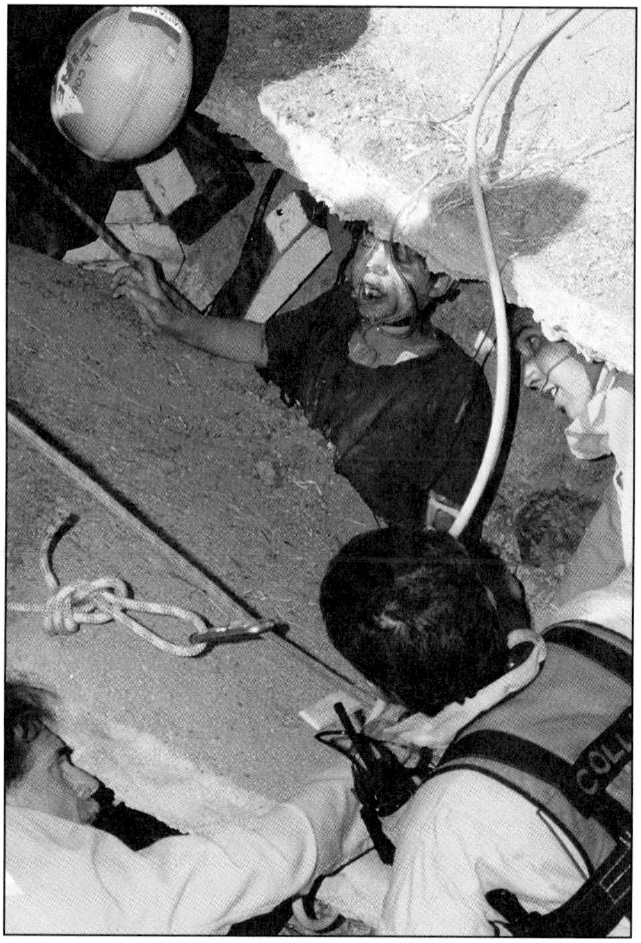

Figure 6-3

To prevent further building collapse and resulting injury to care providers, have specially trained personnel examine unstable structures before entering to provide care.

EXPECTING THE UNEXPECTED

Caution is the key word when responding to calls that may involve violent situations and therefore pose a potential danger for care providers. When responding to a call in an area in which violence may be a consideration, ensure that the scene has been secured by law enforcement personnel before your arrival. If this is not possible, attempt a rapid entry and quick departure with your patient.

Listed below are some general rules for dealing with violence:

- Stay on the scene only long enough to assess the patient quickly and make a rapid transfer to the limited safety of the ambulance.
- Try to be respectful, without compromising your position.
- If violence arises, retreat and call for help.
- Explain procedures to the patient.
- Avoid confrontation, including shouting at or touching violent persons.
- If the area is known to have a strong gang presence, learn whose "turf" you are on and who the leaders are.
- Avoid approaching the patient in the presence of members of more than one gang.
- Avoid cutting a gang member's "colors" (clothing with gang identification) while providing care.

Violence is often associated with pack behavior, in which the group displays more courage and violence than an individual would by himself. Remember that your uniform can lead people to think that you are a police officer. When you are in a gang situation or when violence seems likely for some other reason, have one crew member monitor the surroundings while the other cares for the patient. Stay aware of the environment and try to avoid confrontation.

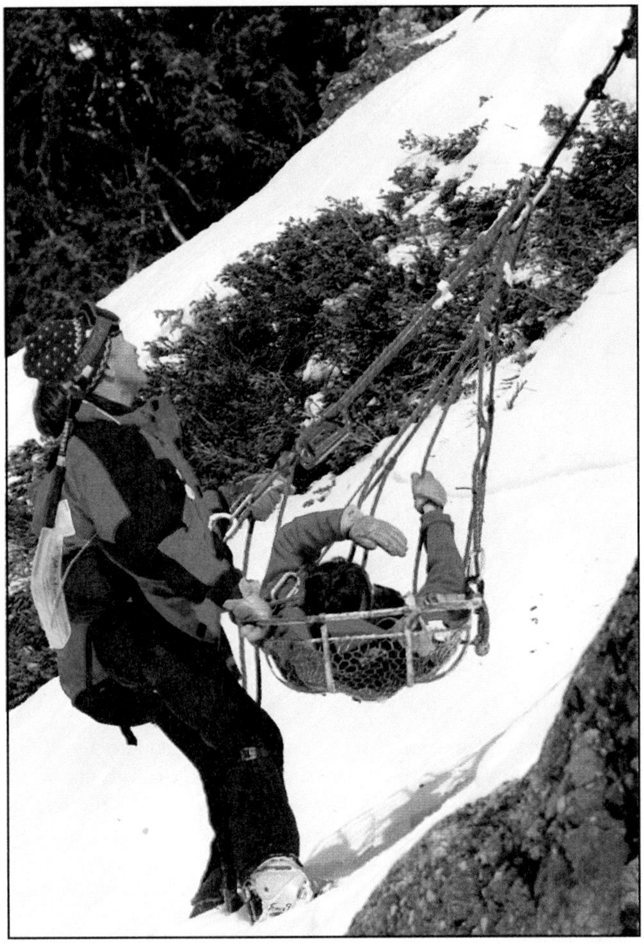

Figure 6-4

Snow and sloping terrain are considered unstable surfaces, and special equipment and training are required for rescue efforts in such environments.

Mechanism of Injury or Nature of Illness

As you look at a trauma scene, consider how the incident occurred and what forces were present. This is not always as clear as it seems. A person who has lost control of a vehicle and struck a tree could sustain head trauma from hitting the windshield. However, the loss of vehicle control may have been caused by a sudden onset of severe chest pain or a loss of consciousness resulting from a medical condition. Bystanders may be able to provide clues.

In considering the cause of the incident, also examine the forces involved, such as the speed of a vehicle, a bullet's caliber and angle of entry, or the amount and type of poison ingested.

Trauma

When you respond to a trauma call, look for clues about the exact mechanism of injury. For example, a patient who has bent the steering wheel upon impact must be considered to have potentially serious chest injuries. Similarly, a trauma patient who is found unconscious should be assumed to have a head injury until proven otherwise.

Critical trauma refers to a life-threatening injury and may be the result of **blunt** or **penetrating trauma** to single or multiple body systems. Critical trauma can be caused by:

- Vehicle collisions and vehicle-pedestrian accidents
- Falling from a height greater than three times the height of the patient
- Blast injuries
- Penetrating injuries to the head, neck, chest, or abdomen
- Fire
- Drowning

Injuries occur as a result of the transfer of energy from some external source to the body. The type of energy transferred and the location and speed of transfer determine the extent of injury. By considering the laws of inertia and the law of conservation of energy, it is easy to see how patients can be critically injured. One law of inertia states that an object in motion will stay in motion

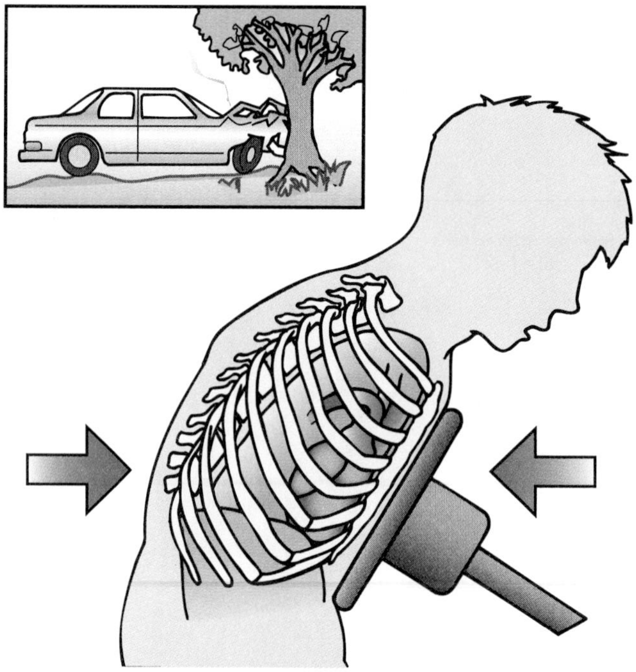

Figure 6-5

When a moving car is suddenly stopped by colliding into a stationary object, three collisions actually occur: (1) the car with the object; (2) the passenger with the inside of the car; and (3) the passenger's internal organs with other organs and the cavity walls.

until acted upon by an outside force. The conservation of energy law states that energy changes form, but cannot be created or destroyed.

Consider what happens when an unrestrained 200-lb person drives a vehicle into a stationary object at 65 mph. The vehicle stays in motion until acted upon by the pole. Mechanical energy (the vehicle moving forward) is immediately absorbed by the pole, vehicle, and driver. The resulting events can be described as a progression of three collisions: (1) the vehicle strikes the pole; (2) the body strikes the interior of the vehicle; and (3) internal organs strike each other and the walls of the cavities that contain them (Figure 6-5).

The patient's size, the velocity of the vehicle, and the rate of deceleration, all indicate that the body is going to absorb a large amount of **kinetic energy** in this process. Kinetic energy is the energy an object has while it is in motion and is related to the velocity and size (mass) of the object. The amount of kinetic energy transferred to the body in a crash of this magnitude is likely to exceed the amount that the body can withstand, leading to critical injury or death.

Mechanism of Injury

The **mechanism of injury** refers to the injury-causing external forces exerted on the patient. These forces vary according to the type of accident. An overturned vehicle on an interstate highway can result in trauma that is substantially different from a minor fender bender caused by a car backing out of a driveway. The first example has a much greater likelihood of causing serious injury because of the higher speed and the type of forces involved.

Six distinct mechanisms can result in critical injuries:

1. Rapid forward deceleration
2. Lateral impact
3. Rotational impact
4. Rollover impact
5. Rapid vertical deceleration
6. Projectile penetration

Rapid forward deceleration is common in vehicle collisions, including head-on and rear-impact collisions (Figure 6-6, *A*). Patients often strike the windshield or steering wheel, especially if the patient is not wearing a seat belt. This can result in serious head and chest injuries. Rear-end collisions are often associated with neck injuries, such as whiplash, when the head snaps back and then forward during impact (see Figure 6-6, *A*).

Lateral impacts, such as "T-bone" collisions, cause the body to be pushed sideways and the head to move in the opposite direction (Figure 6-6, *B*). This can result in serious neck injury and crushing injuries to the rest of the body as the vehicle collapses into the passenger compartment.

Rotational impact occurs when a vehicle is struck in a way that causes it to spin (Figure 6-6, *C*). The vehicle may

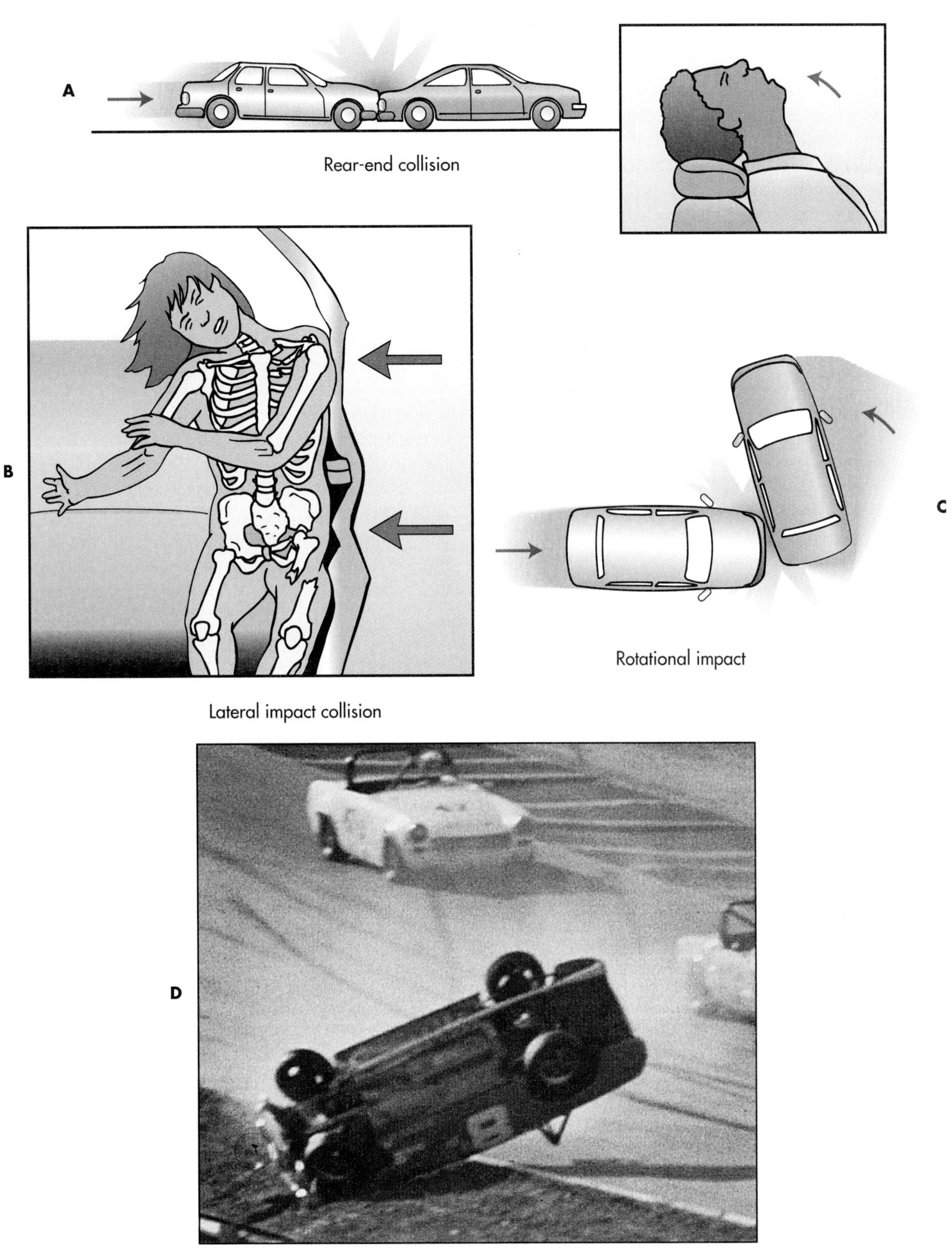

Figure 6-6

A, Rear-end collisions often result in whiplash. **B,** Lateral impact collisions can cause serious neck injury and crushing injuries. **C,** Because there are several directional changes in rotational impact collisions, multiple injuries are likely. **D,** Rollovers can result in very serious injuries, especially to any unrestrained passengers, who may be ejected out of the car.

strike multiple objects and change direction several times before coming to rest. This type of impact often results in multiple injury patterns.

Rollovers often produce the most serious injuries (Figure 6-6, *D*). Occupants can be subjected to multiple impacts, including ejection from the vehicle. Ejection is an especially high-risk factor because it can involve all six of the critical-injury mechanisms.

Upon arrival at the scene of a vehicle collision, take a few seconds to evaluate the damage to the vehicles and consider how the incident occurred. Try to determine where the patient was seated in the vehicle relative to the damage. Other clues that can enhance the assessment and management of trauma patients involved in vehicle collisions include:

- Estimated speed: Greater speed increases the injury potential.
- Skid marks: If present, they indicate that the vehicle was decelerating upon impact, reducing the kinetic energy involved. This tends to produce less serious injuries than a full-speed impact.
- Ejected patient: Whether thrown from a motorcycle or other motor vehicle, an ejected patient usually is more seriously injured than one who was restrained.
- Airbag deployment: This indicates significant impact and requires consideration of injuries associated with the airbag itself. These include facial and eye irritation caused by the chemical that inflates the airbag, and injuries to the arms, legs, and other areas that the airbag may not protect.

Generally, patients are less critically injured when airbags are deployed because the airbag dissipates the force of impact. However, remember that the success of airbags is also linked to the use of restraint belts. An airbag by itself will not adequately protect vehicle occupants. Determine if the patient was using a seat belt at the time of the collision and whether side airbags deployed in addition to the front one. If both the front and side airbags deployed, the vehicle was struck in multiple locations, as might occur in a rollover collision.

Airbags are designed to protect adult patients. However, they have been shown to potentially cause serious injury and death to children in car seats and small children (and even small adults) sitting in front seats. For that reason, those people should not ride in the front seat of cars with functioning airbags. They should ride in the rear seat, wearing seat belts. Some automobile manufacturers are considering installing switches in vehicles that deactivate the airbag if a smaller person is riding in the front seat.

As a safety issue, rescuers need to consider the possible risks of undeployed airbags. Some can be deactivated to help prevent injury by accidental deployment during extrication. Fire crews may be able to help with deactivation.

- Restraint belt use: Evaluate whether the vehicle had only lap belts or was equipped with a three point lap-and-shoulder belt system. Seat belts save many lives, but patients can still have injuries associated with their use. Bruising is commonly seen across the chest during collisions involving significant forces. Lap belts can re-

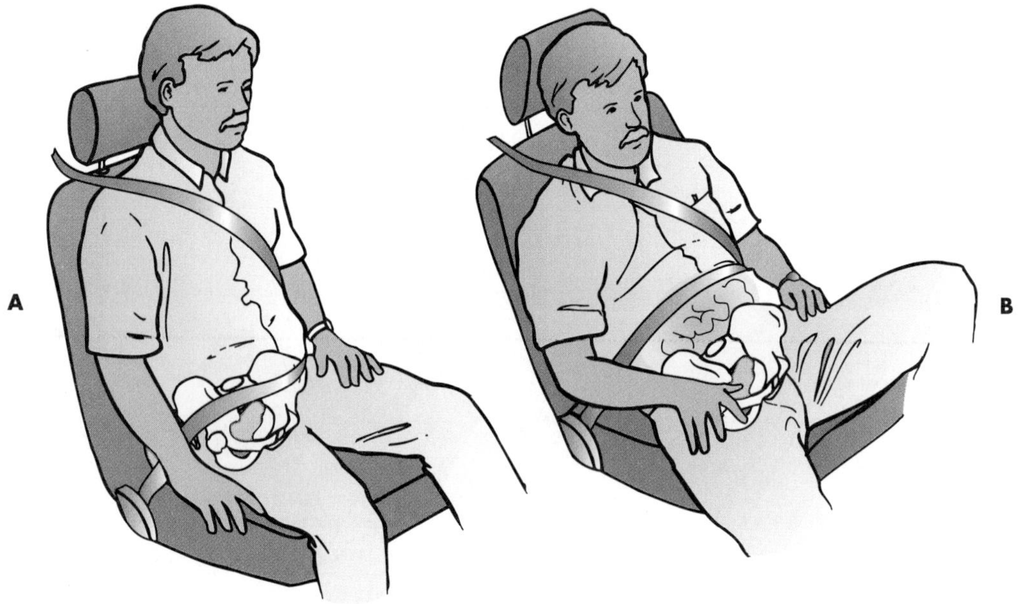

Figure 6-7

A, A properly worn seat belt sits across the pelvic bones. **B,** An improperly worn seat belt is worn high and can result in injury to abdominal organs.

sult in injury to abdominal organs if the lap belt is placed across the lower abdomen, rather than worn properly across the bones of the pelvis (Figure 6-7). Though seat restraints can cause injuries, they are usually less severe than those that would have occurred when the belts were not worn. You should also be aware that infants and small children may be more likely to be injured if their car seats are secured to the front seat in the vehicle. Some safety experts now believe that child seats should only be used in the rear vehicle seat.

- Number of collisions: Multiple damage sites on the vehicle indicate the possibility of multiple injuries to the patient. Because an airbag quickly deflates after deployment, it acts only to minimize the initial impact, not subsequent collisions.
- Broken windshield: A "spider web" type crack in the windshield could indicate direct impact from an occupant (Figure 6-8). This is a common indication of significant head injury.

Falls from a height greater than three times the patient's own height produce rapid vertical deceleration that can cause severe injuries. With small children, a fall from only twice the child's height can be serious. Adults tend to land on their feet initially and fall backwards with outstretched arms. This can lead to multiple injuries to the hands, arms, feet, legs, pelvis, and spine. Small children are more vulnerable to head injuries when they fall because their heads are the heaviest parts of their bodies. Other factors associated with the severity of the injury include the density and irregularity of the surface that the patient contacted as well as any objects struck on the way down. For example, a patient falling 15 feet onto a smooth, grassy area will not likely be injured as severely as one who falls the same distance onto an uneven, rocky surface and strikes protruding boards or metal while falling.

The most common forms of penetrating trauma are from knife and bullet penetration. The severity of a knife wound and the potential organs injured depend on the length of the blade, the angle of penetration, and the area of the body penetrated. The extent of damage caused by a bullet is based on the weapon used to fire it, the distance from which it was fired, the type of ammunition, and the area of the body struck. The damage caused by a projectile such as a bullet is proportional to the density of the tissue that it contacts. High-density tissues (bones, muscle, and solid organs such as the liver) sustain more damage than less dense organs. In addition, the bullet may change direction several times as it enters the body, deflecting off of bones. A bullet wound to the head, chest, or abdomen should be immediately classified as a critical injury.

Prearrival Considerations

A number of aspects of trauma care should be in place before the response takes place. Protocols serve as templates for trauma care and should address the issue of transport destination for the critical trauma patient. There may be specialized facilities in your area designated for critical trauma patients. Some EMS systems have transport policies that call for transport directly to a trauma

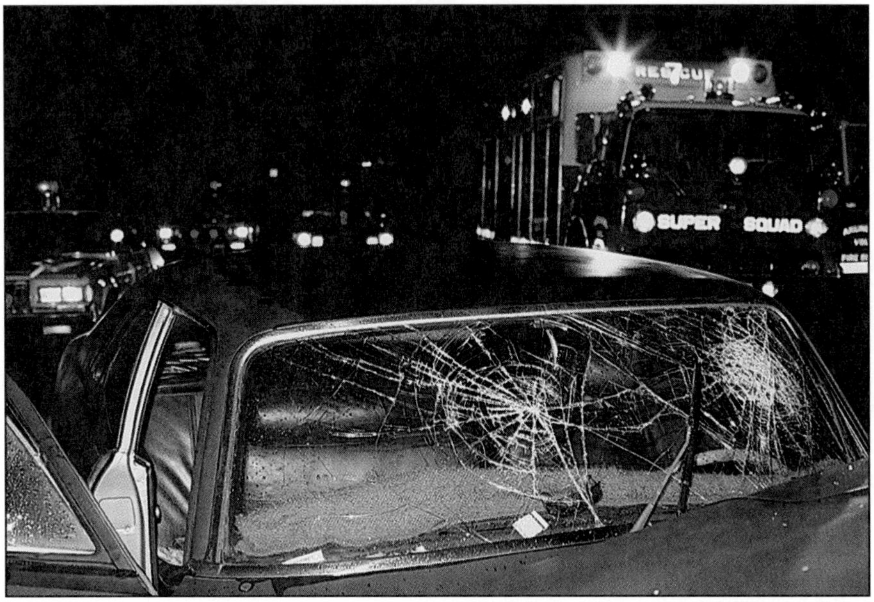

Figure 6-8

This type of "spider web" crack can result when a passenger in a vehicle directly impacts the windshield. During scene assessment this is a good indication of possible head and spine injury.

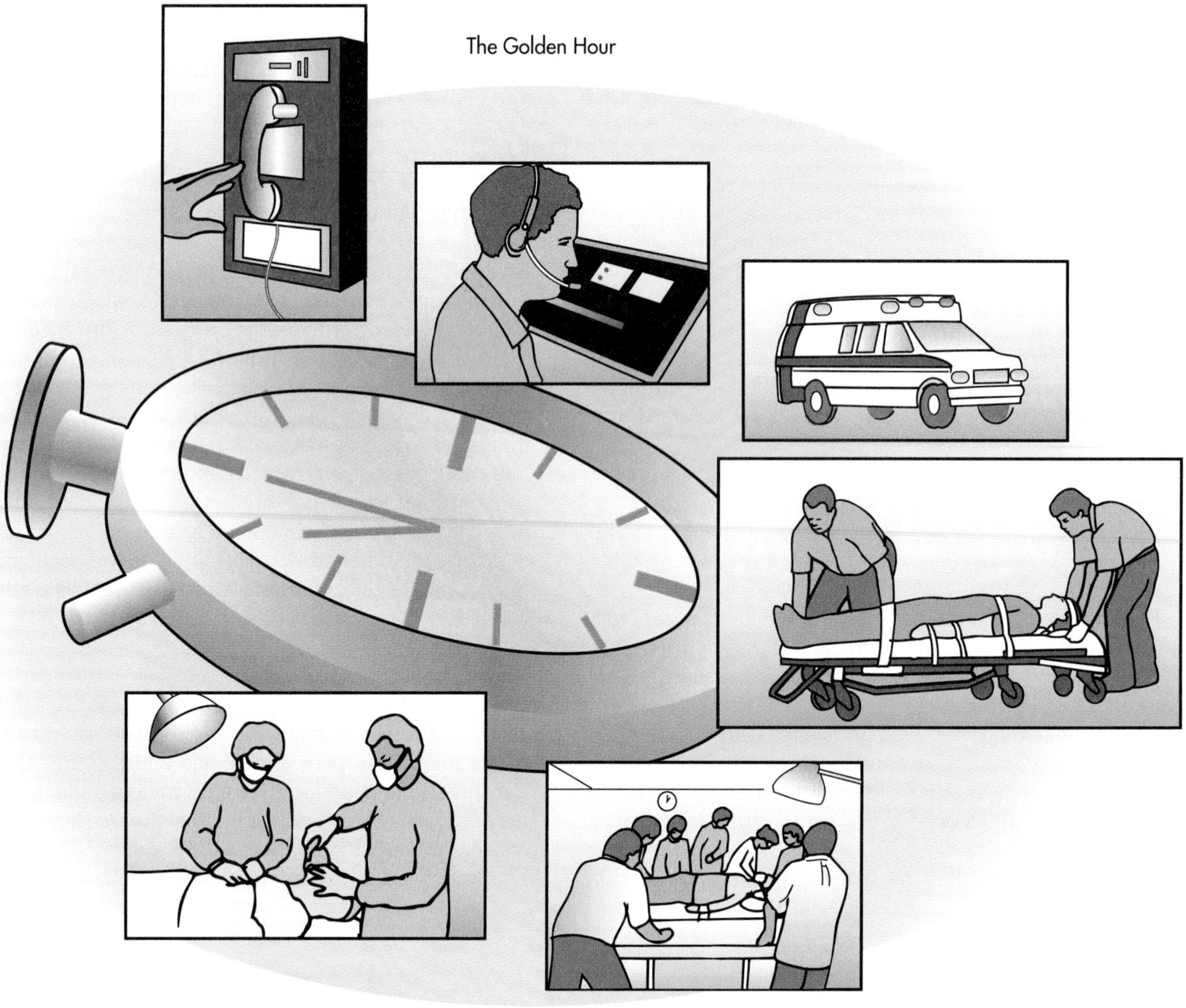

Figure 6-9

The Golden Hour in a trauma case begins at the onset of the problem and extends to definitive care at the hospital. The person who places the 9-1-1 call, the dispatcher, the EMTs, the emergency department staff, and the trauma doctors all play key roles in determining the patient's outcome.

IT'S YOUR CALL
CONCLUSION

In the scenario introduced at the beginning of the chapter, you were faced with several questions about how the vehicle collision occurred and what injuries the patients might have sustained. Because it was a high-speed accident, the vehicle careened out of control, spinning, rolling, leaving the roadway airborne, and landing in the grass. This implies significant speed. The ejection of the passenger also implies significant force and possibly an unrestrained patient who may have suffered other serious injuries while the vehicle rotated. Although the airbag was deployed, it did so on the initial impact and did not provide protection afterward.

In your assessment of the scene, based only on the mechanism of injury, you conclude that these patients likely sustained serious injuries. However, you still do not know how many people were in the vehicle. It is possible that even more were ejected or trapped underneath the vehicle. You should already be preparing mentally to care for two or more critical patients and ensuring that a thorough search is made to find any patients that are not immediately visible. Discovery of any further patients would likely require a call for additional personnel and possibly initiation of the **incident command system (ICS)** (see p. 127).

center, bypassing other hospitals. Other systems call for the rapid transport of the patient by ground ambulance to the closest hospital. If transport times are long, as is often the case in rural areas, stabilization may be done at a community hospital, with transfer later to a trauma center.

If your EMS system uses a specific trauma center for critical trauma patients, there should be a protocol for deciding which patients qualify for transport directly there. This protocol helps avoid transporting a critical trauma patient to a hospital that is not as well prepared to manage the injuries. It also minimizes the likelihood of delivering a noncritical trauma patient to a trauma center.

In addition to trauma designations, some EMS systems have specific destination protocols for patients with certain medical problems. Examples include critical pediatric patients, obstetric patients, kidney dialysis patients, and patients who have burns or require **hyperbaric** therapy. You should be familiar with these special situations in your system.

Medical Problems

In terms of scene assessment, there are some similarities between medical and trauma patients. Both medical and trauma scenes provide clues about how the incident arose. For the medical patient, this is referred to as the **nature of illness.** Look at the entire scene and try to gather information from different sources. Often the patient will be the best source. Family members or bystanders may also have valuable information; their help is especially important when the patient is unconscious or disoriented.

In addition to the information that people provide, examine the scene itself. Look for items such as:

- Medicine containers or pills lying around
- Unusual odors
- Nearby poisonous substances
- A home oxygen system that may be malfunctioning and therefore not getting adequate oxygen to a patient
- Unsanitary or abusive living conditions

Make a mental note of these and other observations at the scene that may have played a role in the patient's medical condition. Whenever possible, try to take items such as medications and poison containers with you to the hospital.

The Golden Hour

A patient may die within seconds or minutes after a critical injury or illness affecting the cardiovascular, respiratory, or central nervous systems. Even if the patient survives the initial incident, the next 60 minutes are critical. This interval of time from the onset of the problem to the beginning of definitive care is commonly called the **Golden Hour** (Figure 6-9). Although this term was once reserved for trauma patients, the Golden Hour has been applied more recently to patients with significant cardiovascular, respiratory, and neurologic problems. Although critical trauma patients often require immediate surgery, medical patients such as those experiencing a heart attack or stroke may also need special medications as soon as possible.

Trauma patients who die within this 60-minute time period often have a combination of injuries referred to as *multisystem* trauma. Heart attack patients can often have significant destruction of the heart muscle. Stroke patients experience loss of brain cells. You play a crucial role during this Golden Hour by considering the mechanism of injury or nature of illness and, in the appropriate situations, rapidly transporting the patient to the hospital for definitive care.

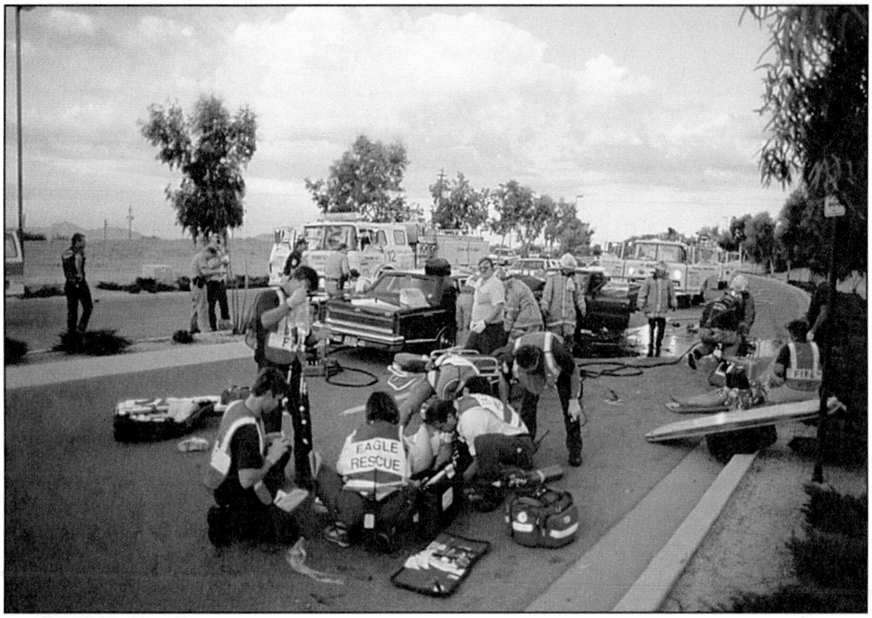

Figure 6-10

MCIs often involve the assistance of emergency workers from several different disciplines and jurisdictions.

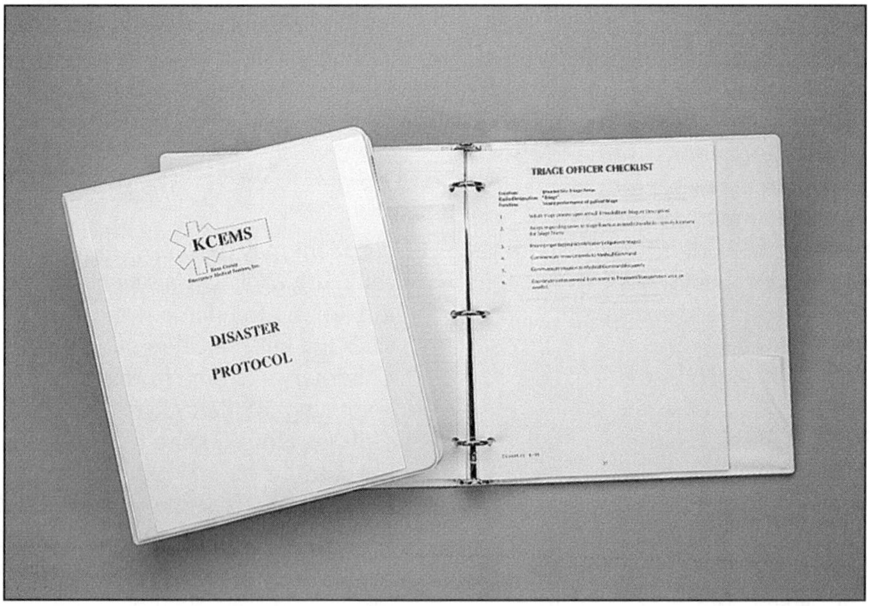

Figure 6-11

The disaster plan.

Multiple Patients

Any scene that has more than one patient is considered a **multiple casualty incident (MCI)** (Figure 6-10). An MCI can involve two patients with only minor injuries, which could probably be handled by one ambulance. However, at other times the magnitude of the incident is so great that it exhausts all local resources and requires the assistance of several other jurisdictions. This is a **disaster** situation. Disasters can be man-made (e.g., terrorist bombings and airline crashes) or natural (e.g., earthquakes, tornadoes, and hurricanes). A disaster situation can involve many injuries and deaths or none at all. Disasters that do not involve many injuries can still tax a region's food, water, utilities, health care, and other resources.

While most agencies are capable of handling small-scale incidents, larger incidents are stressful for those involved and can be frustrating and dangerous if not coordinated properly. Local disaster plans are developed to minimize the operating difficulties associated with large-scale incidents. A **disaster plan** is a predetermined set of activities that identifies how a community's resources will be used during a disaster (Figure 6-11). The plan is tailored to local needs. For example, a town in a land-locked state does not need to plan for hurricanes. The disaster plan should accurately reflect the total resources that the community has available. Overestimating these resources can result in failure of the disaster plan when it is needed. Personnel expected to respond to a disaster should fully understand the plan and its use.

The only way to adequately prepare for a disaster is to rehearse and periodically revise the disaster plan according to changes in available resources. Exercises can include "table top" simulations, in which participants talk through the disaster response, as well as actual simulated scenarios. Your agency may routinely be involved in disaster drills simulating airplane crashes, earthquakes, hurricanes, or tornadoes. The evaluation of the disaster drill is critical to future success in a real disaster. Conclusions reached in postdrill evaluations must be used to refine and update the disaster plan.

Incident Command System (ICS)

During scene assessment try to determine the approximate number of patients and the resources that will be needed to assist them (rescue teams, additional ambulances, fire department, etc.). This process will help you decide whether to activate the disaster plan. If it is necessary to do so, you will assume one of several responsibilities within the ICS. The ICS is a system used to manage an MCI. ICS was originally developed to manage large numbers of firefighters involved in major brush and forest fires. It has since been modified for use in a variety of multiple casualty situations and often involves a coordinated effort among fire, EMS, and law enforcement personnel. ICS is also called the *incident management system*, a term that may be heard more frequently in the future. ICS defines a clear chain of command that begins with an overall scene commander. The command chain also assigns responsibility for functions that must occur. One such responsibility is setting up a medical sector for activities such as triage, treatment, and transportation. One person, the medical commander or coordinator, is responsible for overseeing those functions and reporting to the incident commander.

The first EMT on the scene initiates this system by assuming temporary incident command and providing a radio report of the nature of the incident, its exact location, and the approximate number of people involved. If a disaster is declared, your dispatch center will assist in summoning the appropriate resources. Both initial command personnel and those who take over later are responsible to assess the need for extra personnel and specialized response teams (haz-mat, confined space, dive, etc.) and request that they be dispatched.

An important part of the incident commander's role is maintaining effective communication. If you are the first on the scene, notify the dispatch center that you are establishing a command post at a specific area. If appropriate, ask for an alternate radio channel for the incident. Inform responding units how best to approach the scene, where to stage, and how to locate the command post. Your communication with the dispatch center might sound something like this:

> *Communications, this is Ambulance 1-5-2 at the scene of a multiple vehicle collision involving an overturned tractor trailer. There are at least six patients, two that are entrapped with possible serious injuries. We are establishing Route 6-8-3 command.*
>
> *Dispatch four ambulances, an additional fire company, and Squad 15 for extrication. Designate an alternate channel for the incident and advise all incoming units to stage in the westbound lane at Route 6-8-3 and Dodson Road.*

As more experienced personnel arrive, you may relinquish responsibility as incident commander (or medical command) and assume responsibilities for other functions in the medical sector. Who assumes the role of incident commander will vary with the nature of the incident. It is often a senior fire officer; however, depending on the type of incident, it can also be a police supervisor or forestry officer.

The complexity of the incident will determine the number of **sectors** (also called *divisions*) needed. There are four common, primary sectors: fire, EMS, rescue, and law enforcement (Figure 6-12). A sector officer, who is subordinate to the incident commander, coordinates the activities of each sector. These sectors have predetermined tasks that help ensure a smooth operation and the safety of personnel. Each primary sector can include several subsectors, sometimes called *groups*. Subsectors that

A

B

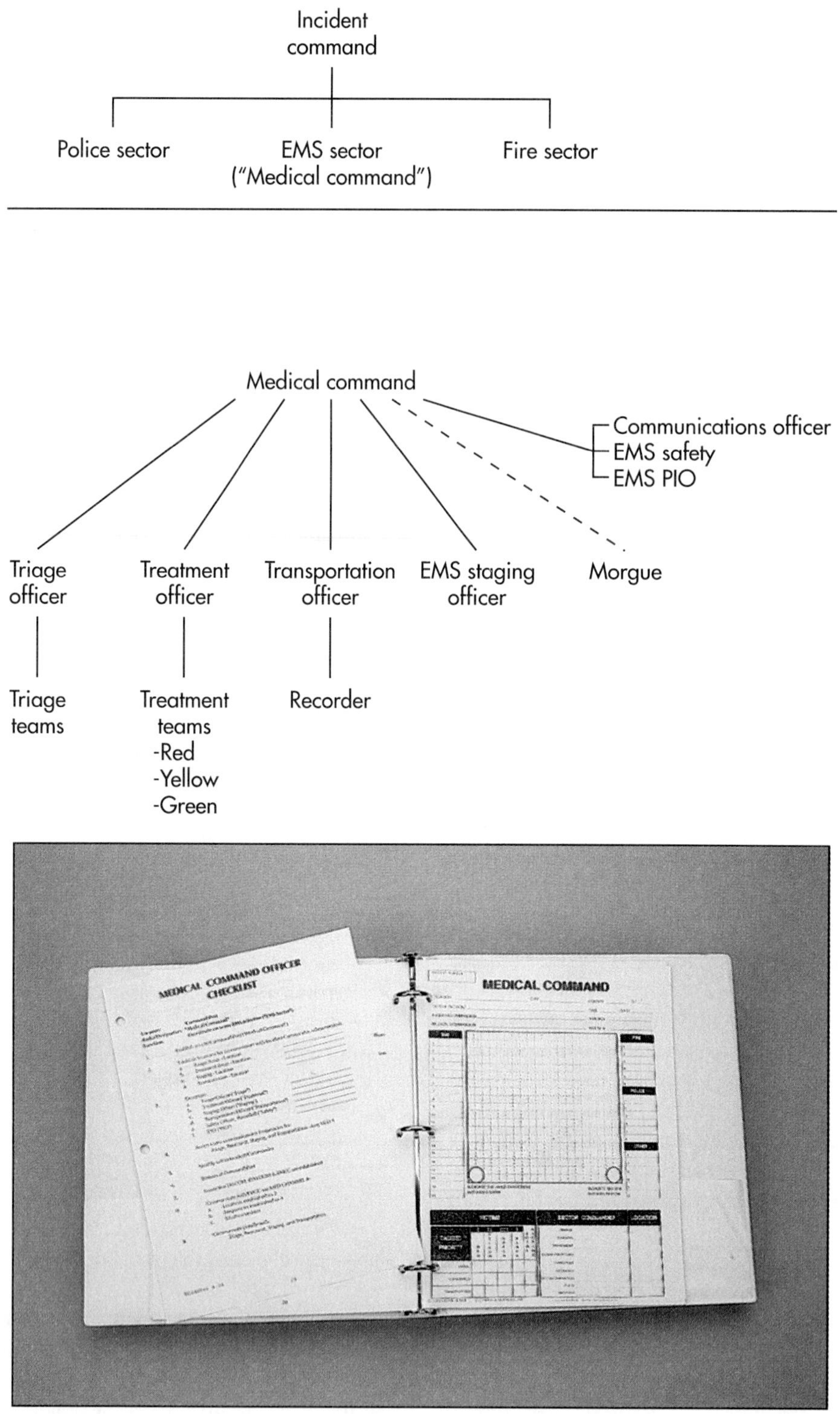

Figure 6-12

A, In an ICS, the primary sectors can be broken into several subsectors, many of which fall within the EMS sector. **B,** The disaster plan defines the roles and responsibilities of the responders.

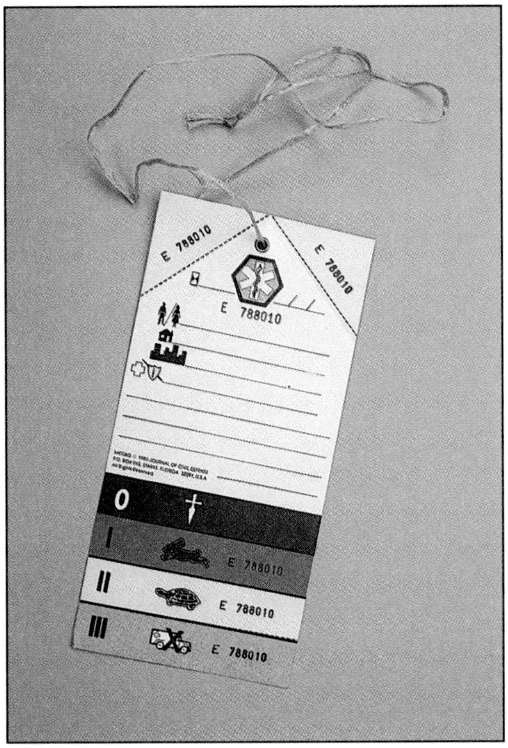

Figure 6-13

Mettag, a product used to identify and track the simple triage and rapid transport (START) method to sort patients.

frequently fall within the medical sector and thus become EMS responsibilities, include:

- Extrication: Disentanglement and removal of patients from wreckage and structures. This activity may instead be assigned to the fire or rescue sector.
- **Triage:** Rapid sorting and prioritizing of patients according to the severity of their conditions.
- Treatment: The collection point where more detailed patient assessments are conducted, treatment is provided, and the patients are prioritized for transport. Although EMS personnel do not often consider what roles hospital staff can play in the early phases of an MCI, the disaster plan may include options for hospital caregivers to respond and assist with treatment in very large incidents or in incidents that involve unusually prolonged extrication.
- Transportation: The process of calling ambulances and personnel from the staging area to transport patients in the order suggested by triage and treatment personnel. This also involves arranging patient destinations, in coordination with hospitals and other receiving facilities.
- Staging: The holding area for arriving ambulances and personnel.
- Supply: The management of extra equipment and supplies, including extrication tools and medical and comfort supplies.

To effectively use the ICS it is important to complete the responsibilities assigned to you and not stray to other sectors. If you are responding to the incident in an ambulance, report to the staging area for an assignment. Going to any other area upon arrival will only create confusion. Once your tasks are completed in the assigned sector, report this to command and move to the staging area for reassignment. If your tasks were significantly stressful, you may be assigned to a rehabilitation area before returning for additional assignments. This is an area where you can rest, replace nutrients, and have your health evaluated before returning to work.

Triage

Triage is the systematic process of establishing treatment and transportation priorities according to the severity of patient conditions. The goal of triage is to do the most good for the most patients possible using available resources. The process involves rapidly assessing patients and classifying them into several categories depending on the severity of their injuries. The majority of prehospital triage systems use a method known as simple triage and rapid transport (START) to sort patients, and a product called Mettag to identify and track them (Figure 6-13).

START begins by separating patients who can walk from those who are more seriously injured. It then proceeds to a 60-second assessment that evaluates breathing, pulse, and level of consciousness in order to divide the injured patients into three categories: immediate care, delayed care, and nonsalvageable (dead or dying). Rescuers use Mettags or some other identification system to

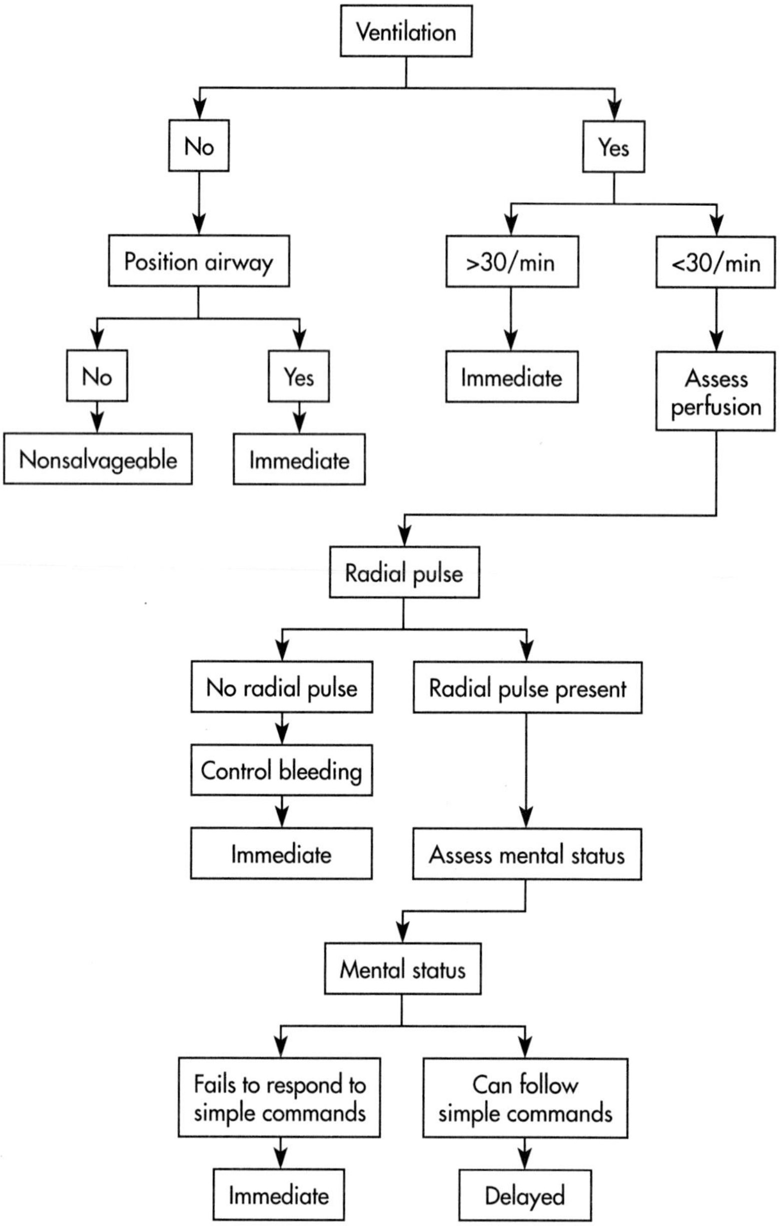

Figure 6-14

Following the specific steps in the START system can aid in the efficiency of care in an MCI.

indicate a patient's status. The order of the assessment steps in the START system are found in Figure 6-14.

The Mettag system is a four-color tag system for classifying patients according to treatment priorities. The categories are:

- Red: Immediately life-threatening but treatable conditions. These are the most critically injured patients, who could die within minutes if not treated.
- Yellow: Serious but not immediately life-threatening conditions. These less critically injured patients could suffer serious disability or die if not treated within hours.
- Green: Minor conditions that can wait for hours to days to be treated. They have non–life- or limb-threatening injuries or illnesses and are generally the last to be transported. This includes most of the patients who were separated from the seriously injured group at the beginning of the START process by the fact that they could walk.
- Black: Nonsalvageable conditions. The black designation refers to patients who are dead or dying. It may include those who still have vital signs or who might be resuscitated in a single-patient scenario, but who cannot be treated in an MCI without pulling resources away from patients with better chances of survival (Box 6-1).

The triage process and the use of triage tags allow rapid prioritization of care and transport at the scene. If possible, brief assessments should be recorded on the tag once all patients have been triaged. This will improve efficiency at the scene because each person who subsequently contacts a patient will not have to repeat the assessment.

The triaged patient is moved to the treatment area for further assessment, care, and transport. Patient conditions are constantly reevaluated. For example, a patient with a serious but non–life-threatening condition could improve with treatment or deteriorate and be reclassified. Because initial triage and tagging does not provide treatment sector workers with much specific information about patient condition, reclassifying a patient into a lower priority category after he or she is taken to the treatment area could be dangerous and is not recommended.

The process of updating hospitals about the total number of patients and the number of patients in each triage category should begin as early as possible in the triage process. Ideally, dispatchers or emergency operations center personnel will relay information until initial triage is completed and responders have arrived to take charge of treatment and transportation. At this point, direct contact between the field medical sector and receiving facilities will be more practical.

The process of triage can be stressful. It forces rescuers to respond differently from what comes naturally and from what their training would tell them to do in more routine situations. The challenge is to sort patients and apply limited resources in a way that will benefit the most patients.

BOX 6-1 Triage Priorities by Patient Condition

Triage Category	Conditions
High Priority (Red)	
Patients requiring immediate assistance and transport	Airway, breathing difficulty Uncontrolled or severe bleeding Decreased level of consciousness Severe medical conditions Shock (hypoperfusion) Severe burns
Moderate Priority (Yellow)	
Patients with serious but not life-threatening conditions that allow treatment and transport to be delayed	Burns without airway complications Major or multiple bone or joint injuries Back injuries with suspected spinal cord injury
Low Priority (Green)	
Patients with minor injuries whose treatment and transport can be delayed until last	Minor bone, joint, or soft-tissue injuries Back injuries without suspected spinal cord injury
No Priority (Black)	
Obvious death or wounds incompatible with life	Decapitation, incineration Exposed brain matter Cardiac arrest (no pulse)

Mental and Emotional Aspects of MCIs

Patients involved in MCIs can pose challenges for EMS personnel. Beyond the obvious physical conditions that you can see, patients can also be under great psychologic stress. By talking and comforting terrified patients, family members, or bystanders, you can help diffuse some of their fears and anxiety. This may help relieve some of the sorrow that they are experiencing.

Stress may also be evident among those responding to the incident. As you learned in Chapter 3, critical incident stress debriefing (CISD) is available for those affected by the incident.

SUMMARY

A thorough assessment of the scene is important for safety purposes as well as to extract valuable information about the possible condition of your patient. By recognizing potential hazards, you can either avoid or correct these hazards. Once it is safe for you to approach, examine the scene and consider the mechanism of injury or nature of illness. Use this information to guide your patient assessment and treatment. Appropriate care and transport within the Golden Hour is the primary goal.

MCIs can vary from two patients with minor problems to a full-scale disaster involving large numbers of patients. Follow local protocols regarding implementation of the ICS and the local disaster plan. ICS helps maintain good communication and a coordinated response that saves lives in disaster and MCI situations.

REFERENCES

1. **U.S. Department of Transportation:** *North American emergency response guidebook*, Washington, DC, 1996, Department of Transportation.

SUGGESTED READINGS

1. **Auf der Heide E:** *Community medical disaster planning and evaluation guide*, Dallas, 1995, American College of Emergency Physicians.
2. **Auf der Heide E:** *Disaster response: principles of preparation and coordination*, St Louis, 1989, Mosby.
3. **Bosner L et al:** Catastrophic events. In Kuehl AE, editor: *Prehospital systems and medical oversight*, ed 2, St Louis, 1994, Mosby Lifeline.
4. **Koop CE, Lundberg GD:** Violence in America: a public health emergency, *J Am Med Assoc* 267:3075, 1992.
5. **Leonard RB:** Planning EMS disaster response. In Roush WR, editor: *Principles of EMS systems,* ed 2, Dallas, 1994, American College of Emergency Physicians.
6. **Lilja GP, Madsen MA:** Medical aspects of disaster management. In Kuehl A, editor: *EMS medical directors handbook*, St Louis, 1989, Mosby.
7. **Lilja GP et al:** Multiple casualty incidents. In Kuehl A, editor: *Prehospital systems and medical oversight*, ed 2, St Louis, 1994, Mosby Lifeline.
8. **Meade DM, Councell RE, Councell PA:** When worlds collide: treating suspected gang members in the emergency department, *Top Emerg Med* 16:53, 1994.
9. **Meade DM, Relf RH:** When colors kill, *Emerg Med Serv* 21:20, 1992.
10. **Waeckerle J:** Disaster planning and response, *New Engl J Med* 324:815, 1991.

Section 3

Foundations of Emergency Medical Care

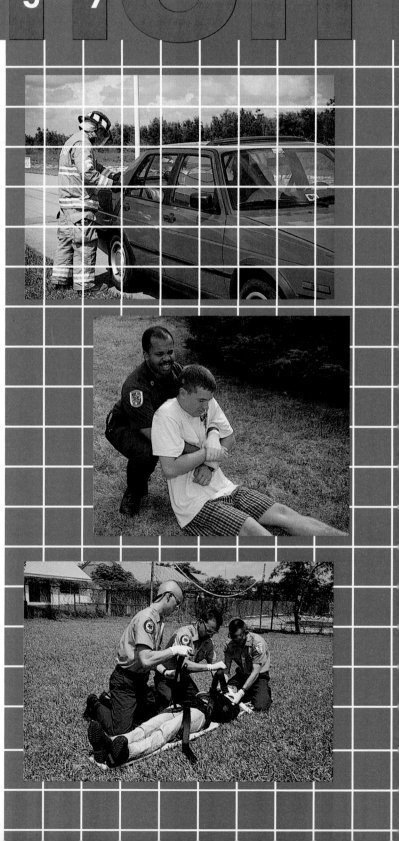

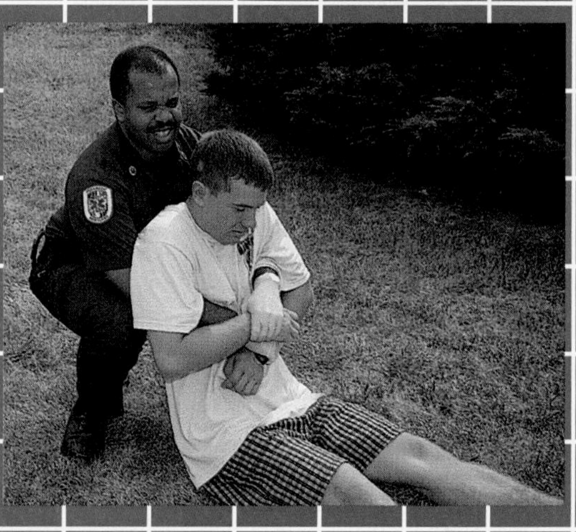

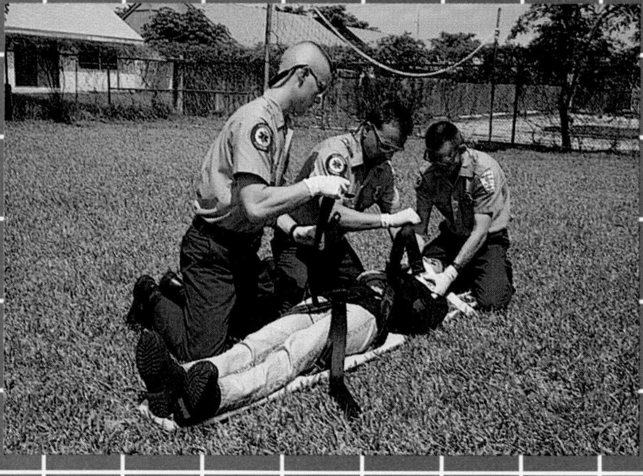

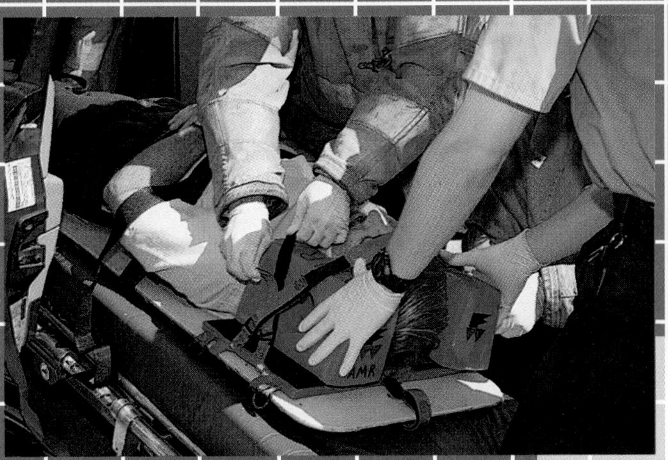
AMR

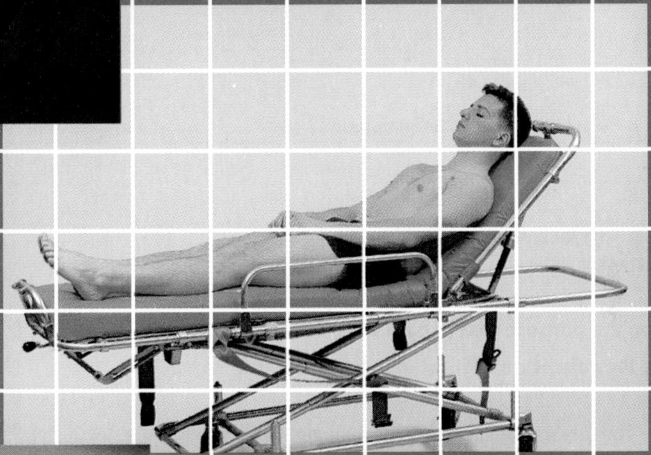

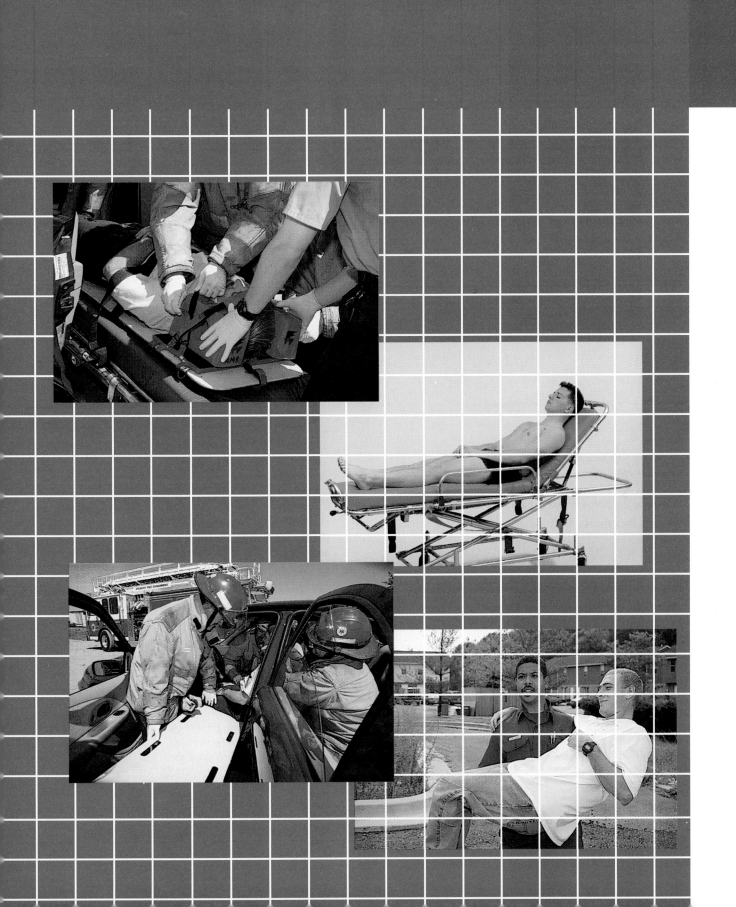

Chapter 7

Reaching, Lifting, and Moving Patients

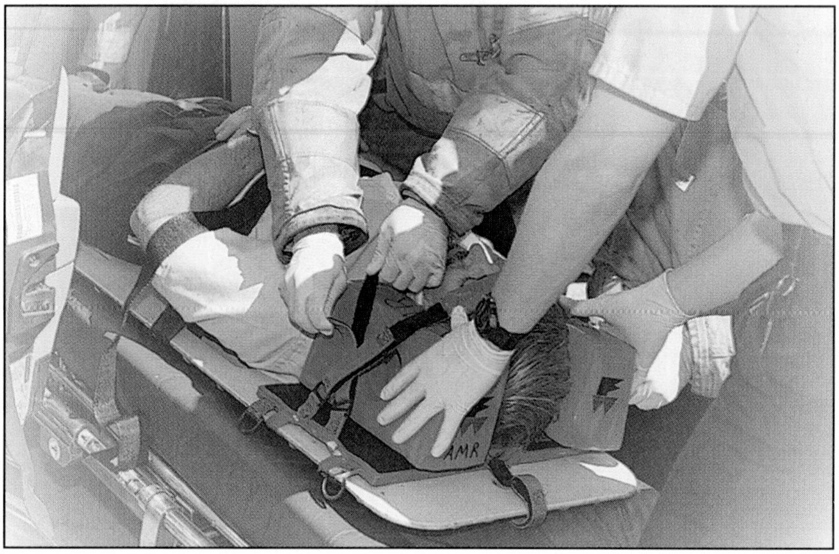

Knowledge Objectives

OBJECTIVES

As an EMT-Basic, you should be able to:

1. Describe the purpose and phases of extrication.
2. Discuss the role of an EMT-Basic in the process of extrication.
3. Identify the personal safety equipment needed for extrication.
4. List the steps to ensure patient safety during extrication.
5. Describe how to stabilize a vehicle that is:
   - Upright
   - On its side
   - Overturned
6. Evaluate various methods of gaining access to a patient.
7. Distinguish between simple and complex access.
8. Explain the importance of recognizing a specialized rescue situation and the need to summon appropriate resources.
9. Define body mechanics and why they are important when lifting and moving patients.
10. Discuss the guidelines and safety precautions for lifting and carrying patients.
11. Describe how to carry patients properly on stairs.
12. Discuss the guidelines for using one-handed carrying techniques.
13. List the safety guidelines for reaching for a patient or equipment.
14. Discuss how the safety guidelines for reaching can be applied to a situation such as "log-rolling" a patient.
15. List the guidelines for safely pushing or pulling a patient.
16. Differentiate between nonurgent, urgent, and emergency moves.
17. Describe three situations that could require the use of an emergency move.
18. Describe how to perform the rapid-extrication technique.
19. Provide four examples of nonurgent moves.
20. Identify the following patient-carrying devices:
    - Wheeled ambulance stretcher
    - Portable ambulance stretcher
    - Stair chair
    - Scoop stretcher
    - Long spine board (backboard)
    - Basket stretcher
    - Flexible stretcher

OBJECTIVES

Skill Objectives

As an EMT-Basic, you should be able to:

1. **Work with a partner to prepare, properly position, transfer, move, and load a patient into an ambulance using the following devices:**
   - **Wheeled ambulance stretcher**
   - **Portable ambulance stretcher**
   - **Stair chair**
   - **Scoop stretcher**
   - **Long spine board (backboard)**
   - **Basket stretcher**
   - **Flexible stretcher**
2. **Work with a partner to transfer a patient from a wheeled ambulance stretcher to a hospital stretcher.**
3. **Demonstrate proper body mechanics during patient lifting and moving.**
4. **Perform emergency removal of a patient from various positions and locations.**
5. **Perform the rapid-extrication technique on a trauma patient seated in a vehicle.**

Attitude Objectives

As an EMT-Basic, you should be able to:

1. **Describe your feelings about maintaining personal safety and the safety of others while gaining access to, lifting, and moving patients.**
2. **Serve as a role model for others, explaining the importance of using proper body mechanics to prevent injury when lifting and moving patients.**

KEY TERMS

1. **Backboard:** A rigid device used to support patients suspected of having head, spine, pelvic, or extremity injury.
2. **Basket Stretcher:** Commonly called a *Stokes' litter,* this is a basket-shaped device with high sides used to move patients in technical rescue situations, such as mountain, cave, or water rescues.
3. **Body Mechanics:** The way the body works when lifting and moving patients and equipment.
4. **Direct Ground Lift:** Technique requiring two or more rescuers to lift a patient with no suspected spinal injury from the ground to a stretcher.
5. **Draw-Sheet Method:** A technique used to transfer a patient between a stretcher and a bed using the bed sheet on which the patient is lying.
6. **Extremity Lift:** A lifting and moving technique for a patient without spine or extremity injury that requires two rescuers to grasp the patient under the arms and legs.
7. **Extrication:** The removal of a patient from a building, vehicle, or area of danger to a location more suitable for care and preparation for transport. The term can also refer specifically to removal from a damaged vehicle, collapsed structure, or other position of entrapment.
8. **Flexible Stretcher:** A carrying device capable of being rolled or folded.
9. **Log-Roll:** A method of rolling a supine patient onto his or her side with a minimum of spinal movement; usually performed to place a backboard under the patient.
10. **Portable Stretcher:** A lightweight folding device used to carry a patient.
11. **Power Grip:** A technique used to securely grasp an object such as a stretcher with both hands.
12. **Power Lift:** The preferred lifting position in which the rescuer squats near the object to be lifted, keeps a straight back, and uses his or her legs to lift. This technique reduces the chance of back injury.
13. **Rapid Extrication:** A technique used to quickly move a patient from a sitting position in a vehicle to a spine board for immobilization; generally used only in critical situations involving immediate danger to the patient or rescuers.
14. **Scoop Stretcher:** A rigid carrying device split lengthwise into two sections; used to lift and move a patient while minimizing movement of the spine and other areas of possible injury.
15. **Stair Chair:** A lightweight carrying device used to transport a seated patient up or down stairs.
16. **Wheeled Ambulance Stretcher:** A device with wheels and a collapsible undercarriage used to transport patients.

IT'S YOUR CALL

While en route to a motor-vehicle collision call, you are advised that two vehicles are involved. The driver of one of the vehicles appears to have only minor injuries; however, the other driver is entrapped and may be seriously injured. When you arrive along with another ambulance, you find that law enforcement personnel have established a danger zone and are rerouting traffic. With an engine company and rescue squad still on the way, you position your ambulance safely (see Chapter 4) and exit the vehicle wearing protective equipment suitable for a vehicle extrication.

As you approach the two vehicles involved in the collision, you note the mechanism of injury. It was a "T-bone" collision, with vehicle #1 striking vehicle #2 at a high speed, forcing the driver-side door of vehicle #2 into the passenger compartment and damaging the rear door on that side as well. The damage to vehicle #1 is confined to the front of the vehicle, and its airbag has deployed. The driver in vehicle #1 is already out of his vehicle and talking to police about the accident. While the other ambulance crew cares for this driver, you and your partner focus on the driver trapped in vehicle #2.

With both driver-side doors inaccessible, you need another way to get in. However, the other doors are locked, and the windows are rolled up. You are concerned about the patient and want to gain access quickly. How are you going to reach this patient? What are your alternatives? What equipment might be necessary to help you gain access, and how should it be used to prevent further injury? What other steps should be taken before you try to enter the vehicle?

In the vast majority of responses, access to patients will be easy. You will usually be able to enter buildings with little or no problem and extricate patients from them using basic equipment and techniques. However, patients trapped in vehicles pose challenges that require advanced training in extrication techniques and the use of specialized extrication tools.

This chapter discusses extrication equipment and techniques and the preparatory steps of stabilizing the vehicle and gaining access to the patient. Technical problems also arise in building collapses, outdoor recreation accidents, and other settings. This chapter presents an overview of these situations, which are often dangerous and may require specialized rescue teams.

Many of the calls to which you will respond will require you to lift and move a patient. In rare situations you will need to immediately move the patient because of dangerous conditions at the scene, such as fire or toxic substances, or because the patient's condition is deteriorating so quickly that transport to a medical facility is crucial for survival. In such cases rapid extrication is often performed with little or no equipment and may include dragging or carrying the patient to safety.

Regardless of the situation, it is important that you understand how to lift and move patients without injuring yourself, the patient, or any assisting crew members. Safe lifting and moving involve proper body mechanics. Understanding body mechanics can help reduce injuries that far too frequently interrupt—and sometimes end—EMS careers. Back injuries are the most common of these injuries that occur during improper lifting and moving of patients or equipment. Good physical conditioning and knowledge of how to position your hands and use your arms and legs can reduce your chances of injury and improve the outlook for a long and pain-free career.

Extrication

In general, **extrication** means moving a patient from an initial location to another location that is more appropriate to begin care and prepare for transport. This can refer to routine patient movement, but the term can also mean removal of a patient trapped in vehicle or building wreckage, isolated by difficult terrain, or threatened by some immediate danger (Figure 7-1).

There are several different phases of the extrication process:

- Determining the magnitude of the problem
- Stabilizing vehicles or structures or otherwise ensuring rescuer safety before entry
- Gaining access to patients
- Disentangling patients
- Immobilizing and removing patients

Your activities during the extrication process will vary and will be determined by your training and your role in the incident. You may be the EMT-Basic assigned to the ambulance and thus be limited to patient care or you may respond as a part of the rescue team performing the extrication. In this role you might handle the rescue equipment and not provide any direct patient care. Some EMS systems do not have adequate personnel for two separate responding units; therefore you could find yourself working in both extrication and patient-care roles for a single call. Remember that the type and amount of personal protective equipment (PPE) required depends on your function at the rescue scene.

Regardless of the exact role you play, it is critical that everyone involved in the extrication process communi-

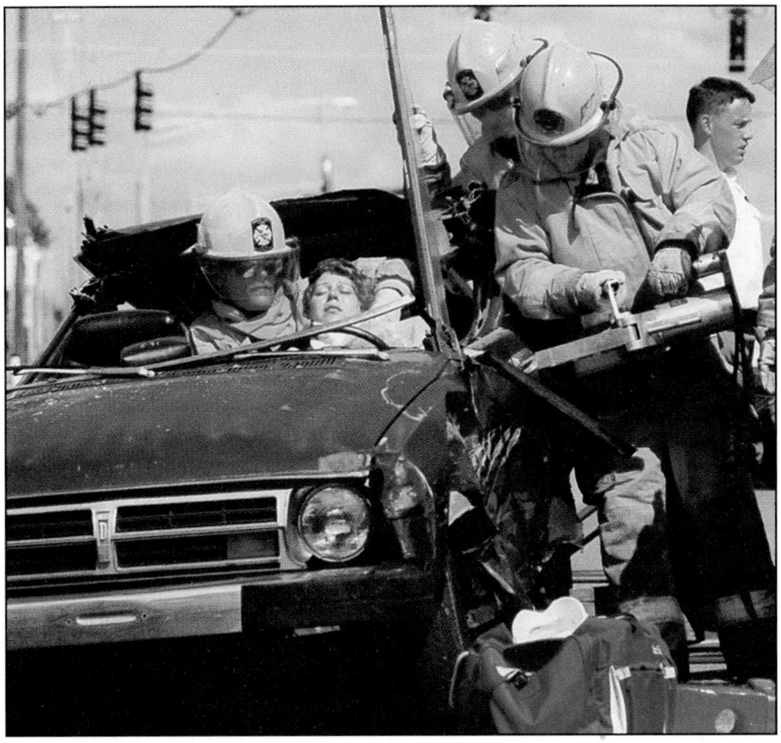

Figure 7-1

Extrication frequently refers to removing a patient from a trapped position, such as in a vehicle.

cates clearly. This is best accomplished by identifying a leader at the scene—someone who has both an understanding of patient-care priorities and a working knowledge of the extrication process. A clear chain of command helps eliminate communication problems and expedite the extrication process.

If you are attending the patient, you have a responsibility to communicate the patient's condition to others assisting you. This helps other rescuers decide the best way to remove the patient. A "load-and-go" situation is one in which the patient's condition is critical and requires immediate care. Such a situation necessitates rapid extrication, meaning that less time and equipment are used for immobilization. When the patient's condition is stable, the extrication process may take longer and involve more attention to the details of immobilization. You will also be involved in decisions about the priorities of care relative to extrication. Patient care is often given before and during extrication, although it may be delayed when immediate hazards to the patient or rescuers require rapid extrication and prevent the ability to provide care.

Extrication Supplies and Equipment

The supplies and equipment needed for extrication include those used for personal protection and those used to gain access and disentangle a patient. The items that you need will vary according to the situation.

Personal safety is always the top priority. Your PPE for a vehicle extrication may include full turnout gear with helmet and faceshield and heavy-duty gloves and clothing (Figure 7-2). Even if you are only providing patient care, it is important to protect yourself if you are in the car while other rescuers dismantle it. Latex gloves and other protective devices that help prevent disease transmission are always required when there is a chance of contact with body fluids.

In addition to personal safety, you have the patient's well-being to consider. During initial access to the vehicle and throughout the extrication process, protect the patient from broken glass, sharp metal, or other hazards. Use protective coverings such as nonflammable blankets, turnout gear, or a backboard (Figure 7-3). If the patient is conscious, explain the extrication process.

Bystanders can also be injured during extrication. They should be kept at a safe distance from the incident, outside of a clearly marked danger zone.

Other supplies and equipment are needed to help stabilize the vehicle and gain access to the patient. These include both common and specialized items used for extrication. Box 7-1 lists the different classifications of equipment used in extrication situations. Some of these items are discussed in more detail later in this chapter.

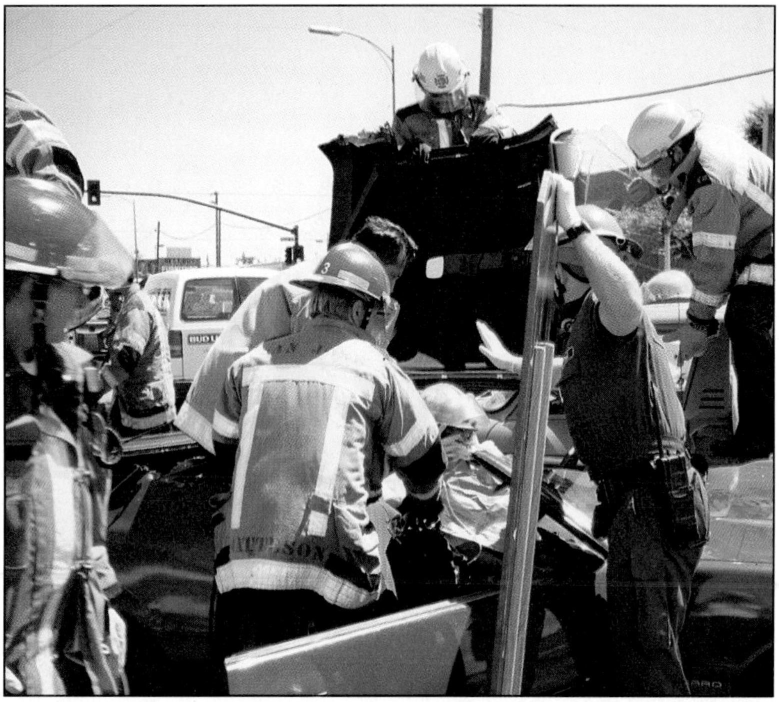

Figure 7-2

Personal safety is always a priority in an extrication. Appropriate protective equipment can vary from gloves to full turnout gear with helmets and faceshields.

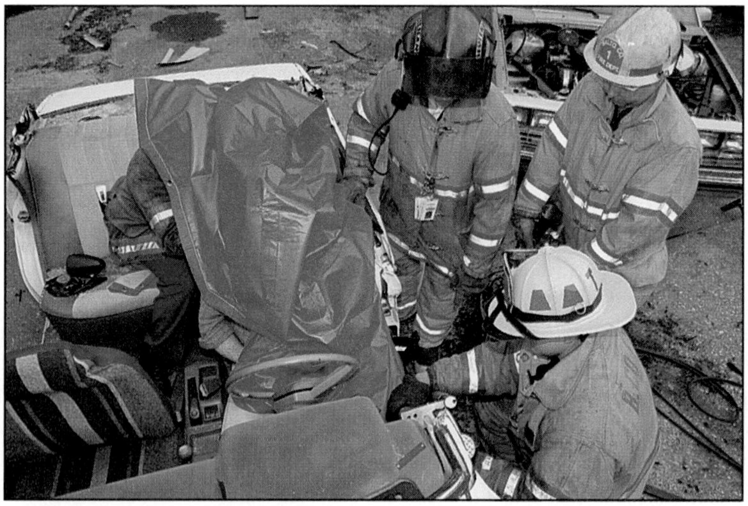

Figure 7-3

The patient will need to be protected from broken glass, sharp metal, and other hazards involved in an extrication. Protective coverings such as nonflammable blankets may prove useful.

Stabilizing Vehicles

Stabilizing a vehicle can be a simple task if the vehicle is upright and level, the transmission is intact, and the emergency brake can be applied. However, even then it is important to take additional precautions to ensure the safety of the patient and rescue personnel.

BOX 7-1 Supplies and Equipment for Vehicle Stabilization and Access

Items needed for stabilizing vehicles and gaining access include:

- Cribbing blocks of various size to help stabilize a vehicle (hardwood blocks, wedge blocks, ladder cribbing blocks, step-chock wood blocks, and hardwood cribbing blocks)
- Tools for forcible entry (hydraulic tools such as a power spreader or ram; manual tools such as a flat-head axe, halligan bar, pry bar, sledgehammer, and spring-loaded center punch)
- Cutting and disassembly tools (hacksaw, tin snips, bolt cutter, air chisel, air impact wrench, reciprocating saw, chain saw, hand saw, and electric drill)
- Manual pulling tools (hand winch, chain, and snatch-block device)
- Lifting equipment (manual lifting equipment such as a mechanical or hydraulic jack; air bag or air-cushioned rescue system)
- Rope (static kernmantle of various lengths)
- Basic hand tools (wrenches, socket set, screwdrivers, pliers, hammer, and fiberglass pike pole)

Upright Vehicle

For the most part, vehicles on their wheels can be stabilized easily, especially if they are on flat ground. When access to the inside of the vehicle is possible, basic stabilization methods include:

- Placing the transmission in "park."
- Turning off the ignition.
- Setting the parking brake.

Outside the vehicle, you can also:

- Place wheel chocks in front of and behind all tires (Figure 7-4). If these are not immediately available, use a spare tire, large rocks, or tree limbs.
- Place cribbing under the rocker panels.
- Deflate the tires by pulling the valve stems with a pair of pliers.

In normal circumstances it might seem that any one of these precautions would be adequate. However, vehicle accidents are not normal. Mechanical systems such as transmissions and emergency brakes are prone to failure, especially in damaged vehicles. Rescue procedures such

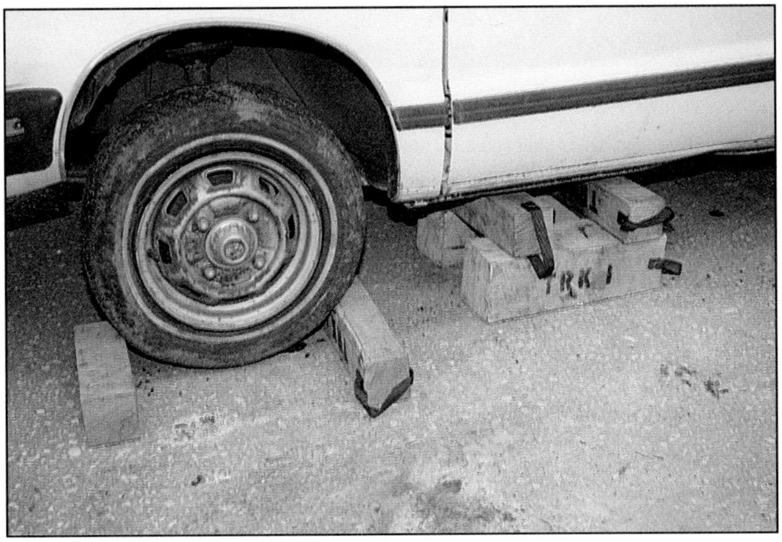

Figure 7-4

After the vehicle is in "park," with the ignition off and the parking brake set, place wheel chocks in front of and behind all tires and cribbing under rocker panels to further stabilize the vehicle.

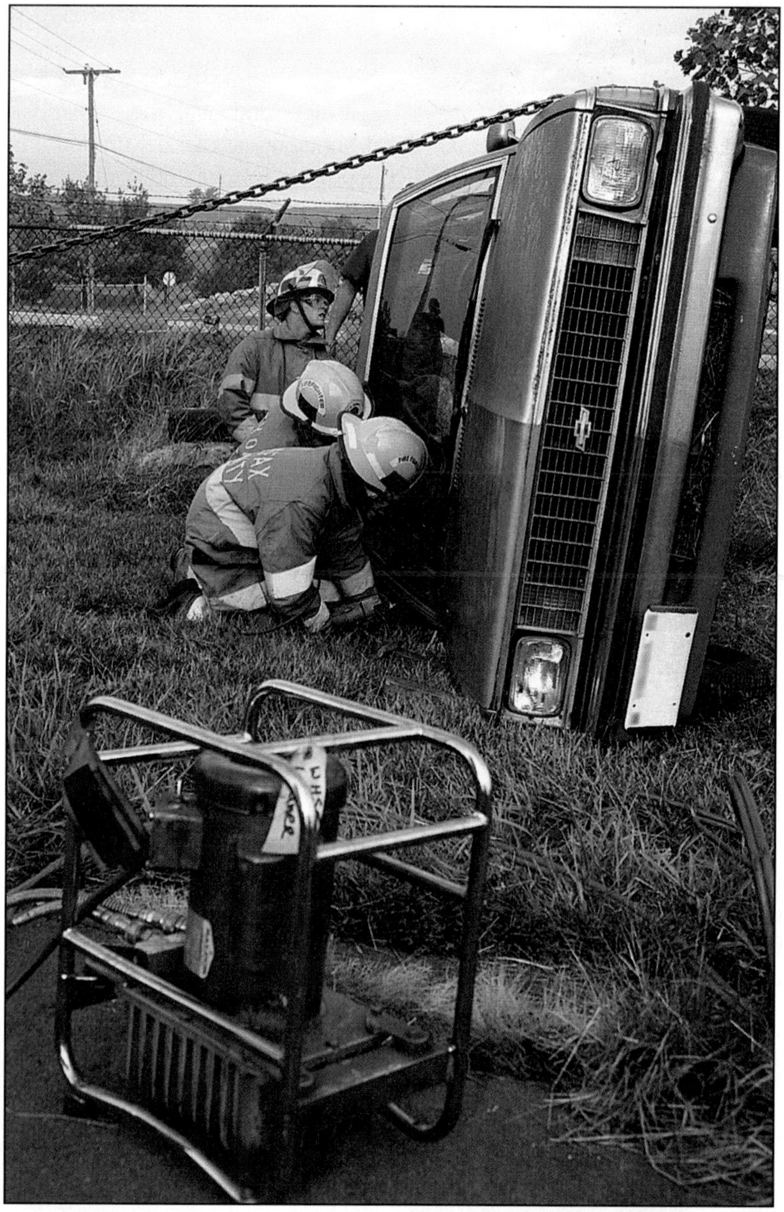

Figure 7-5

A vehicle on its side must be stabilized before rescuers attempt to gain access to the patient. This vehicle was secured with chains before rescuers moved in.

as placing wheel chocks or wooden cribbing can prove inadequate in unpredictable scene conditions. Rescuer and patient safety demands the use of as many back-up levels of vehicle stabilization in combination as is practical.

If an upright vehicle is on uneven ground, it is even more important to secure the vehicle because it can easily move. Avoid approaching the vehicle from the direction that it might move. Approach and chock the wheels from the side. If you think the vehicle may still move, use additional wheel chocks or secure a chain, cable, or appropriate rope to the frame of the vehicle and a secure anchor, such as a large tree, guardrail, tow truck, or emergency vehicle. Some emergency vehicles are equipped with cable and winch systems that are capable of actually pulling the vehicle.

Vehicle On Its Side

A vehicle on its side is extremely unstable, and not much is required to roll it. Do not attempt to gain access to the patient until the vehicle has been stabilized. Cribbing or jacks can be used; and cables, chains, or ropes can be rigged to the uppermost wheels (Figure 7-5). This is a complex task requiring special training. Do not crawl toward a vehicle on its side to attempt to set cribbing. Stay on your feet so that you can move away quickly if the vehicle should shift.

Overturned Vehicle

A vehicle resting on its roof is much less stable than it appears. The roof posts may appear to maintain the vehicle's weight, but they can collapse at any time, crushing a rescuer who is inside the vehicle or trying to enter it. As with the vehicle on its side, you must completely secure the vehicle before entering it. This is done by placing cribbing or jacks under the trunk and hood. If the roof posts have already collapsed, access through the windows or roof will not be possible. Instead, cut a hole through the side of the vehicle. (Cutting through the floor is also an option but is a more complex and risky process.) Access to a vehicle on its roof requires specially trained personnel and proper equipment.

Gaining Patient Access

The patient is not always immediately accessible. Terrain problems can complicate outdoor access, and you may have to clear debris in a structure collapse. In a vehicle the patient may be unable to unlock a door, or the doors could be crushed. How you gain access depends on the type of incident, your training, and the equipment and other resources available.

Gaining access to a patient in a damaged vehicle can be either a simple or complex situation. Until the early 1980s, vehicles were relatively easy to open. Gaining access through a locked door was simple with the use of a pry bar. However, stricter safety standards imposed on automobile manufacturers have led to more complex access situations for rescuers. Extrication of patients is now more likely to involve hydraulic tools and prolonged periods of time. Though the proper use of these tools requires specialized training, there are basic guidelines to follow whether you are operating equipment or assisting in some other way.

Simple Access

Simple vehicle access means reaching the patient without equipment or specialized training. It is surprising how often simple access is possible even when vehicle damage is dramatic. Therefore you should always look for and attempt to use simple routes of access before committing to more drastic methods. Dismantling the vehicle delays extrication and increases the risk of injury to rescuers and patients.

Once the vehicle has been stabilized, use the door handles to see if any door can be opened so you can reach the patient. If all doors are locked but a window is rolled down, reach in and try to unlock the door. If the windows are up, ask an occupant to unlock a door, if possible. If the window is open but the door will not open, enter through the window. This can be done easily if you are small enough and have the assistance of other rescuers; however, it requires proper protective gear to avoid injury from broken glass or other sharp objects.

Complex Access

If simple access is impossible, you will need basic tools or specialized equipment to enter the vehicle. You may only need to break a window with a spring-loaded center punch, a small device that is placed against a lower corner of a side or rear window to break the glass (Figure 7-6). When using a center punch, remember to use it on a window as far away as possible from the vehicle's occupants.

Because windshields are stronger than other car windows, a center punch will not break them. A flat-head axe or Glas-Master saw can make windshield removal relatively easy. Windshields are usually only removed when it is necessary to remove the roof or to displace a dashboard or steering column that is trapping the patient.

Once you gain access, you can begin to assess the severity of the patient's condition and provide initial care. Meanwhile, other rescuers will be determining whether additional access points are necessary for patient removal. Removing the patient through the access point at which you entered may not be possible. Expanding the access may include prying open and removing one or more doors, removing the roof, or pulling the dashboard or steering column away from a trapped patient (Figure 7-7). These techniques require specialized training that is beyond the scope of this text and your initial training as an EMT-Basic. Courses in basic vehicle rescue or vehicle extrication will help you become proficient in handling extrication tools and gaining access to patients in complex situations.

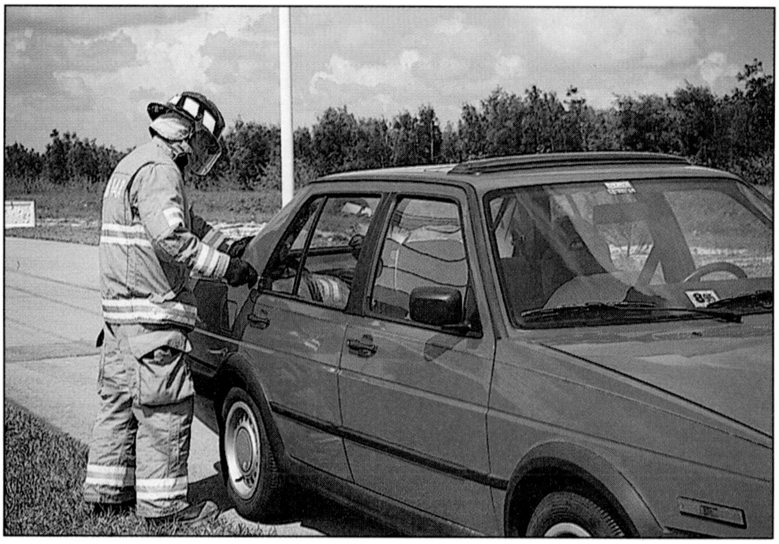

Figure 7-6

A spring-loaded center punch breaks the glass of the vehicle. To protect the vehicle's occupants it should be used on a window as far from them as possible.

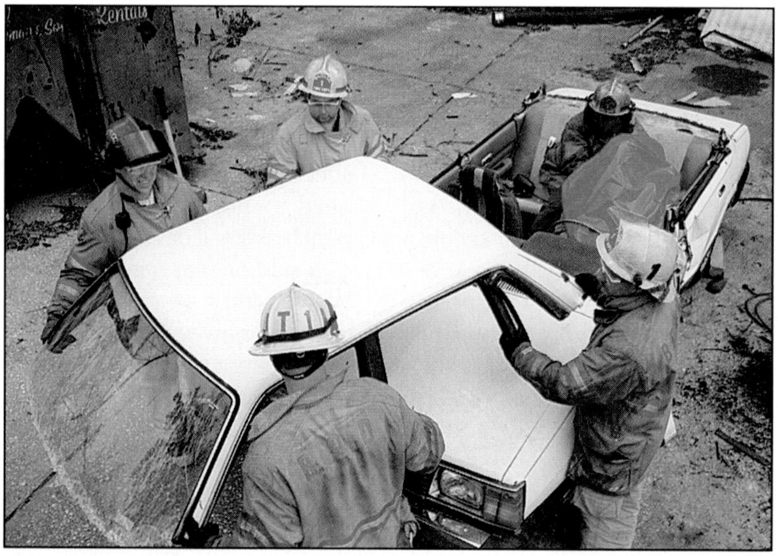

Figure 7-7

A patient cannot always be removed through the initial access point. One of the methods to expand access is removing the vehicle's roof.

IT'S YOUR CALL
CONTINUED

In the opening scenario, a driver has been trapped by a side-impact collision. Her door is crushed, and the window is shattered. The door behind her is also crushed, but that window is still intact. Immediate access through these doors is impossible, and the remaining windows are rolled up. Before attempting to gain access, you note that the car is still running. Looking through the window, you see that the transmission is still in "drive." Wearing your turnout gear, you quickly position wheel chocks and then reach through the broken window and place the transmission in "park." You turn off the vehicle but are unable to reach the parking brake. A master power door lock button is located on the driver's door, but fails to release the locks on the other doors.

Other rescuers arrive and begin to crib the car to provide better stabilization. You explain the extrication procedure to the patient, who is slumped away from the door because of the force of the collision. You place a blanket over her head before another rescuer breaks the passenger-side rear window with a center punch. That rescuer releases the door lock and enters the rear of the vehicle. He reaches forward to unlock the front passenger-side door, where you enter and begin to assess the patient. Your assessment reveals that she likely has an injury to her left hip. There are no signs of more serious injury, although the mechanism of injury calls for spinal protection and monitoring for signs of internal bleeding. A paramedic unit is on the way.

Rescue specialists work to free the patient from the wreckage. While you provide care and protect the patient from additional injury, hydraulic tools are used to remove the roof, the driver-side door, and the windshield. Because the vehicle does not have an airbag, the steering column is displaced away from the patient using a hydraulic tool. If an airbag was present, that would have to be deactivated. A paramedic arrives as you are preparing to remove the patient from the vehicle. How are you going to remove this patient without further complicating her injuries? What equipment is readily available, and how will you use it?

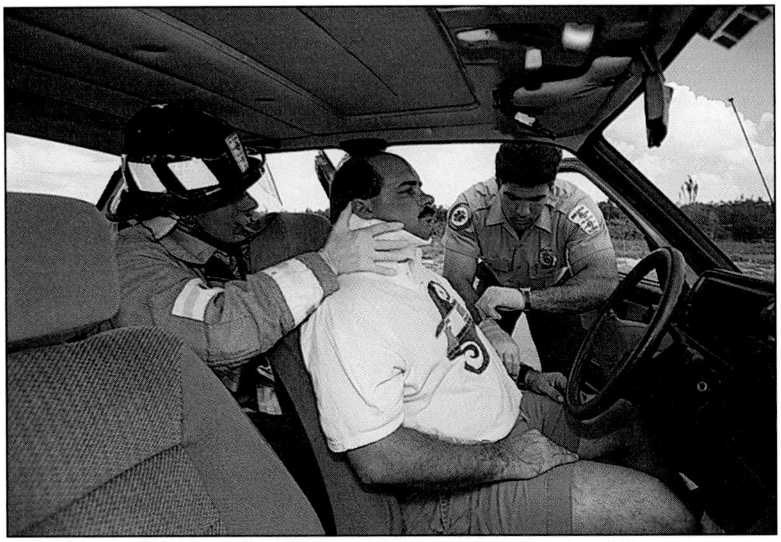

Figure 7-8

The first step in removing the patient is making sure that the cervical spine has been stabilized.

Removing the Patient

Patient removal requires strength, stamina, planning, and a coordinated effort by several rescuers. As you prepare to remove the patient from the vehicle, ensure that the cervical spine is immobilized with a cervical collar and manual stabilization (Figure 7-8). The technique for placing the head in the neutral position and measuring and applying a cervical collar are discussed in detail in Chapter 25.

In most vehicle-extrication situations, you will be able to secure the patient's head, neck, and back in an extrication device that helps minimize movement in these areas. The Kendrick extrication device (KED) is frequently used for this purpose (Figure 7-9). Short backboards are also used in vehicle extrication settings, and there are several other commercial extrication devices available similar to the KED. Application of these short spine devices is discussed in Chapter 25.

In addition to protecting the spine from further injury, you must complete an initial assessment early in your contact with a patient. Occasionally your initial assessment will reveal immediate life threats requiring rapid extrication without taking time to apply spinal immobilization equipment. These are often called *load-and-go* situations. The **rapid-extrication** technique (described on pp. 155-160) provides some support for the patient's spine but without equipment. The technique does not offer as much support as a spinal immobilization device such as the KED, but the procedure can be performed in less than 1 minute. This saves time over the 5 to 10 minutes typically needed to apply a spinal immobilization device—time that could be critical to ensuring patient survival. Rapid extrication is also appropriate when external hazards such as toxic gases or nearby fire threaten the safety of the patient.

Specialized Rescue

Vehicle extrication is not the only type of rescue that requires special training. Other areas of rescue specialty include:

- High-angle rescue: This highly technical rescue requires a thorough knowledge of ropes and anchor-setting devices, descending a rope (rapelling), ascending a rope, traversing dangerous areas, and moving patients over difficult terrain, including lowering or raising them in a basket litter (Figure 7-10).
- Trench rescue: When the dirt walls of a trench collapse and trap a patient, special methods and equipment are used to shore up the walls and create a working area in which the patient can be freed without threat of further ground collapse (Figure 7-11).
- Confined-space rescue: Confined-space rescue often presents dangerous environmental conditions that require the use of special breathing equipment and protective clothing. Because the air in confined spaces such as wells, sewers, silos, and holding tanks can be toxic, it is important to wear a self-contained breathing apparatus (SCBA) before entering. High-angle rescue tech-

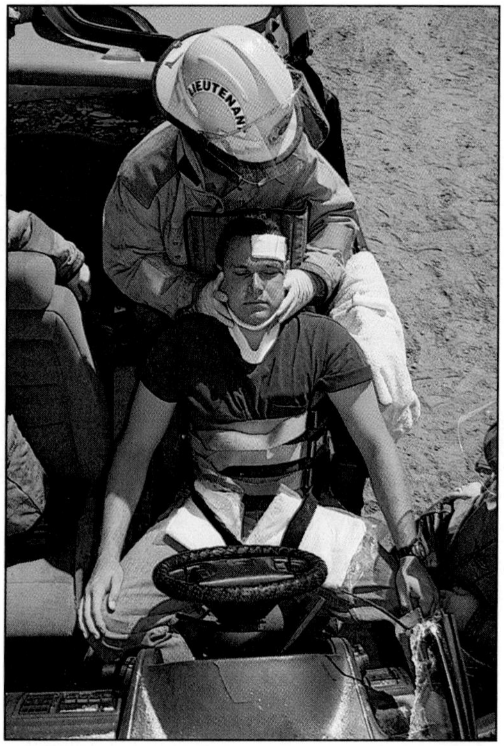

Figure 7-9

The KED is a short, vest-like device used to help immobilize patients during extrication.

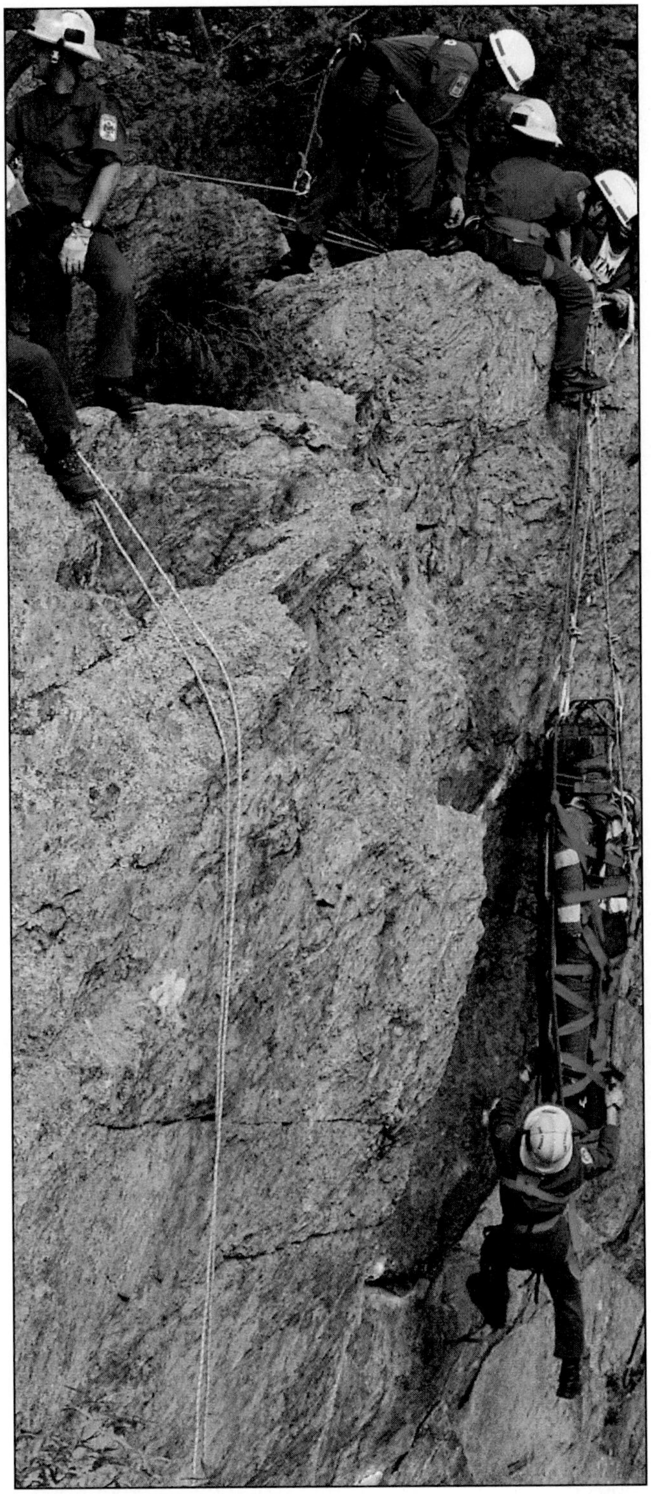

Figure 7-10

High angle rescue requires rescuers to use special equipment and techniques in moving themselves and patients over difficult terrain.

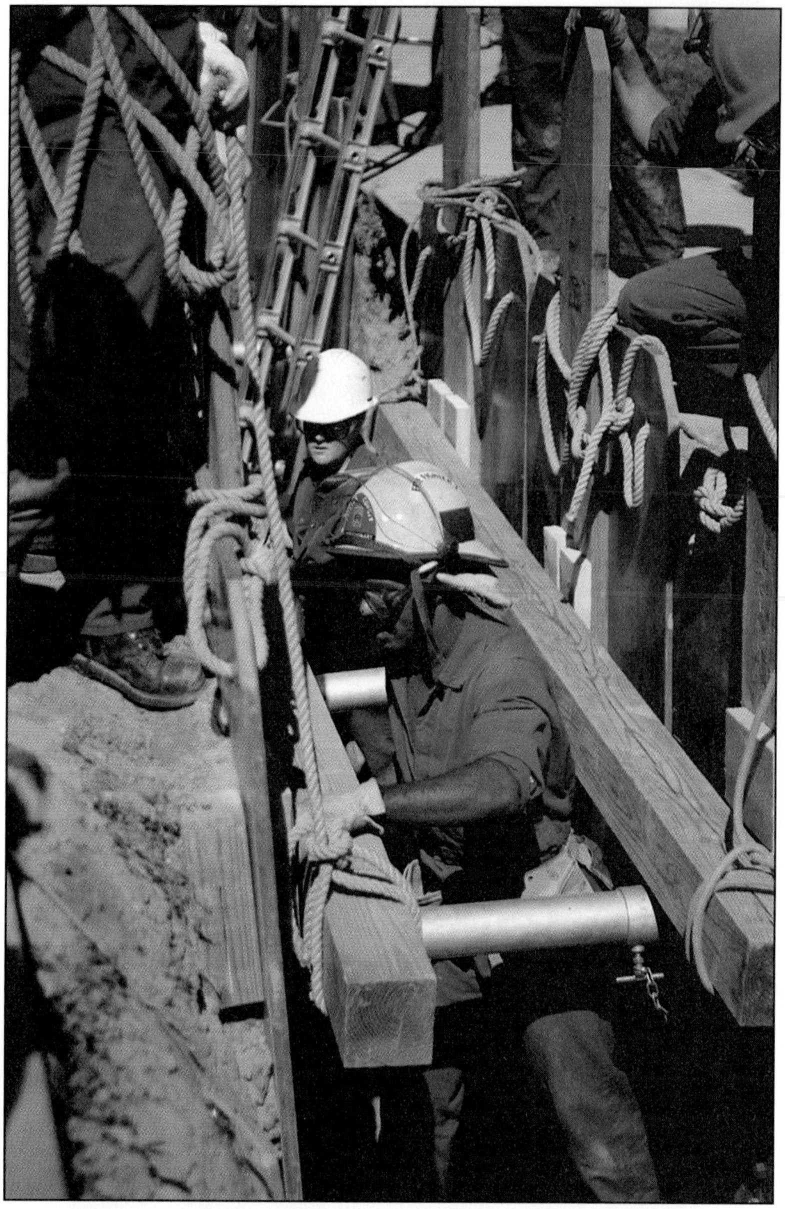

Figure 7-11

Trench rescue can involve shoring up and creating walls so rescuers can gain safe access to patients.

niques are often used to raise and lower rescuers and patients in confined-space settings (Figure 7-12).

- Hazardous-materials rescue: This type of rescue, involving chemical, biological, and radioactive hazards is increasingly common; and consequently the demands on emergency personnel to understand those hazards are growing as well. Federal regulations require a minimum awareness level for all emergency responders. Specialty response teams with advanced training and sophisticated equipment are now available in many areas.
- Cave rescue: This relatively new specialization requires an understanding of underground environments. Much of the equipment and many of the techniques used for patient removal from caves are similar to those used in high-angle rescue.
- Swift-water rescue: The force of moving water is often underestimated; it can easily sweep people away or strand them in vehicles or remote areas. Sometimes victims are trapped in the turbulent undertow caused by water cascading over rocks or concrete, such as the spillways at low-head dams. Boat operations, swimming skills, and rope-rescue techniques are important in these settings.

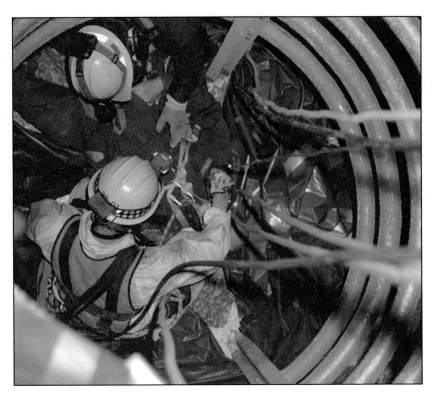

Figure 7-12

Confined-space rescue can present a number of dangers to rescuers including difficult access, a toxic environment, and a need to use special techniques to move patients.

- Wilderness rescue: Wilderness rescue requires knowledge of orienteering, mountain climbing, backpacking, high-angle rescue, and survival skills.
- Urban search and rescue: Another of the newer specialties, urban search and rescue, focuses on locating patients trapped in debris, usually after building collapses caused by explosions or earthquakes. Specialists often use a combination of techniques that includes using search dogs and high-technology electronic equipment.

Lifting and Moving a Patient

Lifting and moving patients are important procedures that are frequently performed by EMTs. Unfortunately, they are not always done correctly. Both the rescuer and patient can suffer as a result of improper lifting and moving techniques. Whether moving a patient or simply reaching for a trauma kit, attention to **body mechanics** is a constant priority. In the context of this chapter, the term *body mechanics* refers to the way the body works when lifting and moving patients and equipment. An understanding of how body movements such as twisting and leaning can contribute to injury will make you better able to perform your duties and will reduce your chances of injury.

Safety When Lifting

When you are preparing to lift a patient or piece of equipment, first consider the weight of the object. Do not attempt to lift anything that you feel is too heavy for you to handle. The amount of weight that a rescuer can safely lift will vary according to his or her strength and conditioning and the use of proper lifting techniques. If you are lifting a patient who has already been placed on a wheeled ambulance stretcher, consider the additional weight of the stretcher (as much as 70 pounds). To ease lifting, try to have another rescuer of approximately the same height lift the other end of the stretcher.

Most patient-moving equipment has a patient weight limit. Exceeding the given limit means that you will need extra assistance, and it may raise safety concerns regarding equipment failure. Even when not exceeding the safety limit, you should summon additional personnel to assist if the weight is too great for you and your partner to lift safely. Do not be embarrassed to ask for help when it will help protect the patient or prevent rescuer injury.

Lifting patients inappropriately poses a significant risk of lower back injury. When you are preparing to lift a patient or heavy equipment, communicate with your partner before lifting. Try to keep the weight of the object close to your body and avoid any type of twisting or rota-

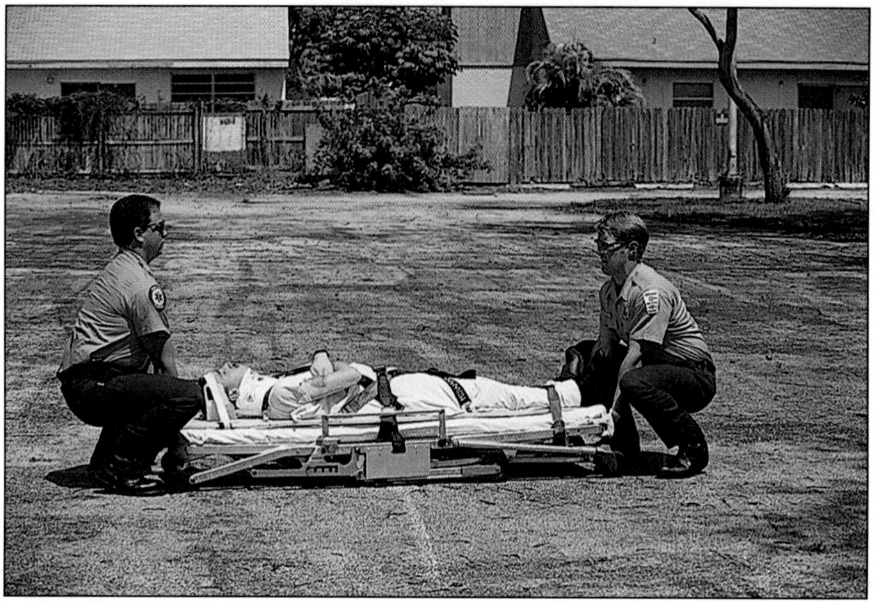

Figure 7-13

In the power-lift position, the back is straight, the head is up, and the feet are kept about shoulder width apart.

tion when lifting. Place your feet flat on the ground about shoulder width apart with one foot slightly in front of the other. Keep your head up and your back straight, avoid bending at the waist, and squat down. This position, called the **power-lift** position, enables you to keep your back straight and locked (Figure 7-13). Grasp the object, such as the stretcher rail, with a **power grip:** place your hands at least 10 inches apart with your palms under the bar facing up and your fingers completely contacting the object (Figure 7-14). Stand up, lifting with your legs and not your back (Figure 7-15). If you have to lower a stretcher or set the patient down, reverse these steps. Whenever possible, use sliding extension bars on stretchers to help avoid leaning forward while lifting.

Safety When Carrying

Generally, carry a patient only a short distance before placing him or her on a wheeled stretcher and moving to the ambulance. However, **wheeled ambulance stretchers** do not move well across uneven terrain or steps. In these situations, you will often find yourself carrying the patient and the stretcher with the help of others. When carrying a patient, you will need to follow the same precautions used for lifting. This means that you should consider the weight of the patient and any carrying device, know the limitations of your crew's abilities, communicate with each other, coordinate your movements, and use proper body mechanics. Always remember to carry the patient at a pace that the slowest person can keep up with and, whenever possible, match rescuers with partners of similar height and strength.

When carrying a patient down stairs, you should use a **stair chair** rather than a stretcher, if the patient's condition allows. If you get tired, you can easily rest without bearing a great deal of weight, unlike a wheeled ambulance stretcher. Before progressing down stairs, ask another rescuer to help steady your back and guide your steps (Figure 7-16). Although the stair chair allows for greater flexibility while moving the patient, it must be avoided if the patient has any possibility of a spinal injury or other condition that a sitting position would compromise.

Sometimes there will be several people to assist you in carrying a patient. In these situations you will likely be carrying a patient on a wheeled stretcher, long backboard, or similar device that provides many hand-holds around its edges. By positioning personnel at the sides of the patient's head and feet, each rescuer can use one hand to carry the patient. Using more rescuers is safer because the device is more balanced and there is less weight for each rescuer to bear (Figure 7-17). Coordinate your movements so that you can lift and carry the patient as a team. One-handed carrying also has risks. Keep your back locked and straight, and avoid leaning or twisting.

Safety When Reaching, Pushing, and Pulling

It is surprising how easily back injuries can occur when simply reaching for your patient or a piece of equipment. In any kind of reaching there are safe principles to re-

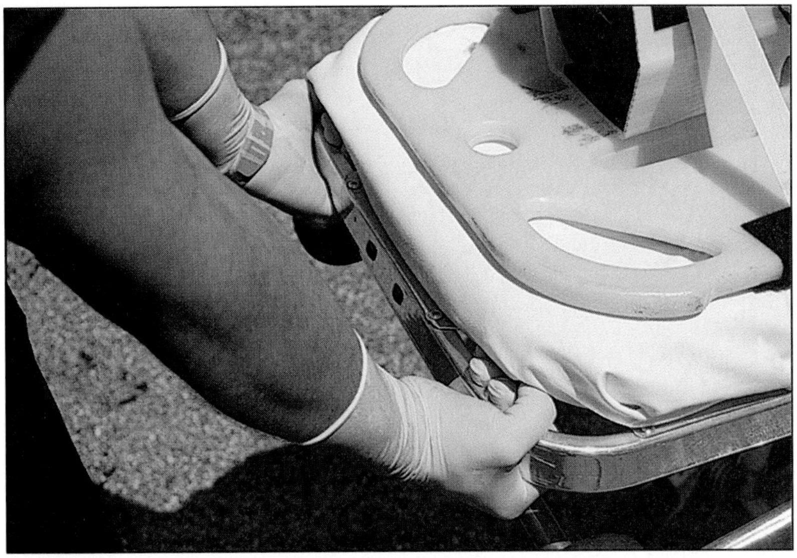

Figure 7-14

For a power grip, keep hands at least 10 inches apart, palms up, and fingers completely in contact with the object.

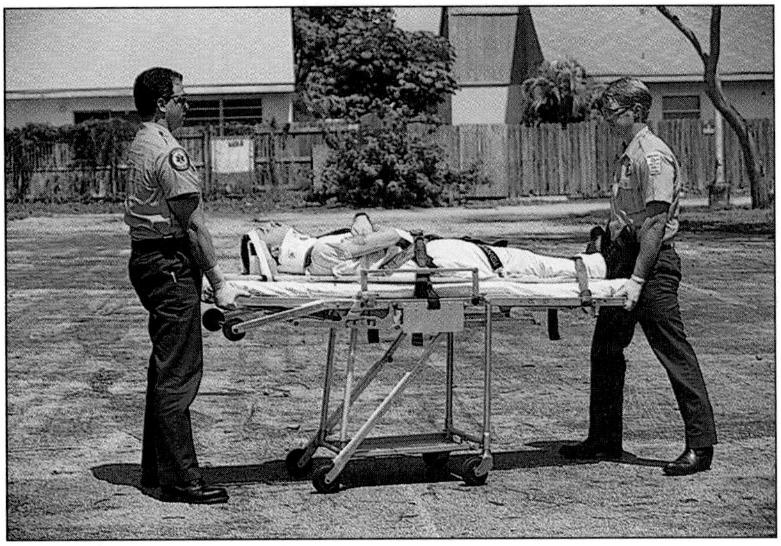

Figure 7-15

Always lift with the legs, not the back.

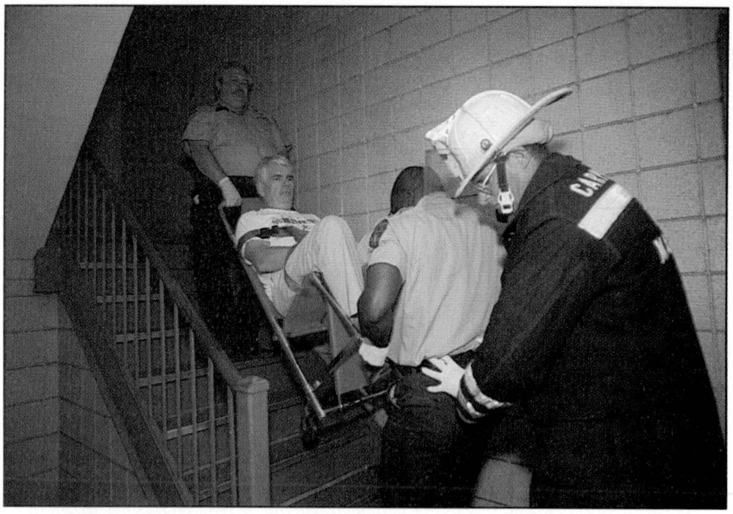

Figure 7-16

To prevent twisting and stumbling, always have one rescuer serve as a guide when using a stair chair.

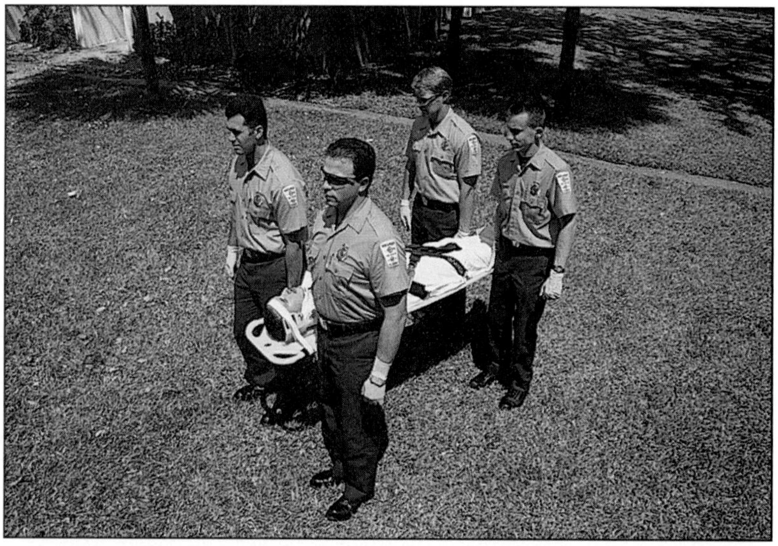

Figure 7-17

One-handed carrying lessens the weight for each individual rescuer and balances the load better, but it is still important for rescuers to avoid leaning, twisting, or lifting with their backs.

member. Injuries often occur because rescuers overreach, twist, or attempt to support the weight of an object while reaching. Follow these basic guidelines when reaching:

- Limit yourself to reaching no more than about 20 inches in front of you.
- Avoid reaching to the side or twisting while reaching.
- Avoid prolonged reaching; it will tire your muscles.
- Try not to bear much weight while reaching.
- Keep your legs flexed and stomach muscles tight.

When performing a **log-roll,** kneel close to the patient, keep your back as straight as possible while leaning over the patient, and use the strength of your shoulders and arms to roll the patient (Figure 7-18). Working around the

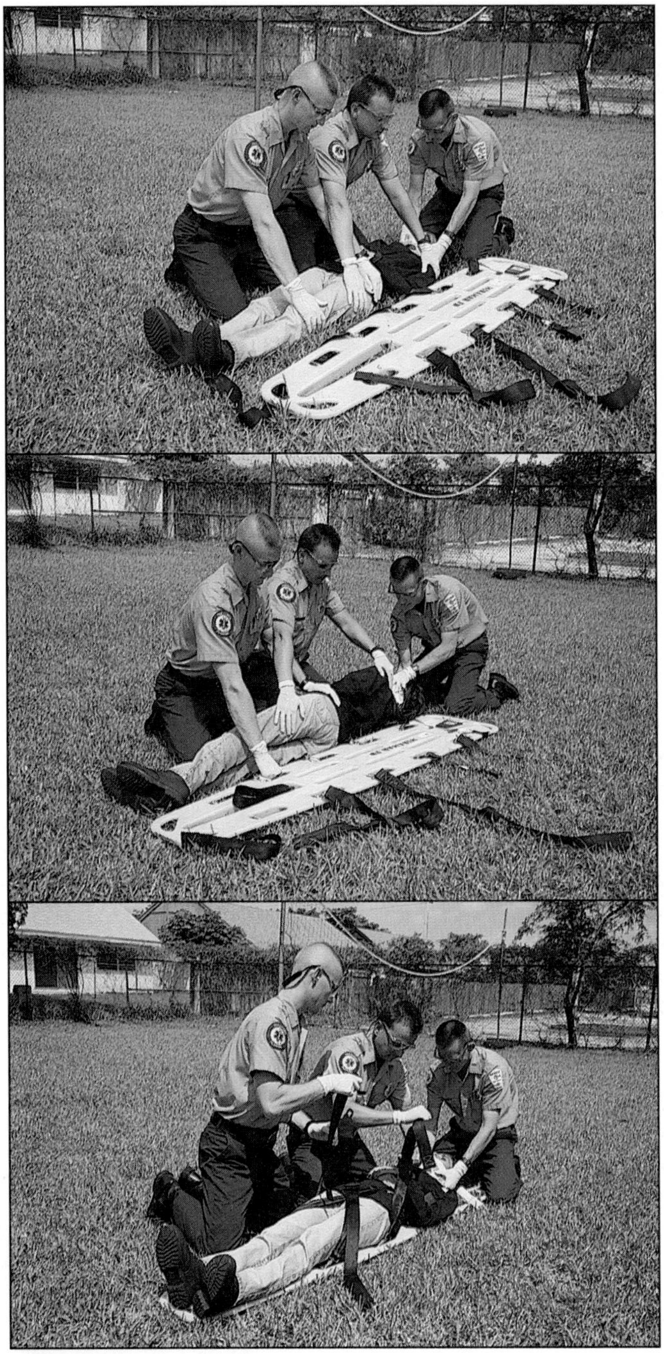

Figure 7-18

A log-roll requires rescuers to use their arms and shoulders to roll the patient.

patient in the back of the ambulance is a particularly risky process. You should squat or sit as much as possible to limit leaning over the patient from a standing position.

When it comes to a choice between pushing or pulling a stretcher, push rather than pull whenever possible. However, if you are wheeling a stretcher, someone must push while the other person pulls. Always attempt to push or pull the weight load at a height just above your waist. Avoid pushing or pulling objects above your head or below your waist. If you must push or pull an object below your waist, bend your knees and keep your back straight.

Principles of Moving Patients

In most cases, moving a patient will be done in a systematic and unhurried manner. When there is no threat to life and you can provide care safely without hurrying, the patient will be moved using a nonurgent move. If the patient's condition is deteriorating, an urgent move can be used. When there is an immediate danger to the patient or rescuers, or when the patient cannot be cared for in the presenting position or location, you may perform an emergency move.

Emergency Moves

Emergency moves should be performed whenever there is an immediate danger posed by fire, explosives, hazardous materials, flash flooding, or other uncontrollable factors that could potentially harm the patient or rescuers. An emergency move is also called for when a patient cannot receive life-saving care without being repositioned, such as a cardiac arrest patient who has collapsed in the shower.

There are several different emergency moves with which you should be familiar. Each takes into consideration the possibility that the patient may have a spinal injury. However, the need to move the patient away from immediate danger takes priority over efforts to completely immobilize the patient's spine. When performing emergency moves involving a patient with possible spinal injury, attempt to keep the patient's body in a straight line and move the patient in the direction of the long axis of the body.

Patients found lying on the ground can be dragged to safety by pulling on the patient's clothing, rolling the patient onto a blanket and pulling on the blanket, or supporting the patient under the arms and dragging the patient. Each of these emergency moves allows for some protection of the patient's spine without complete immobilization.

To perform a clothing drag, squat down at the top of the patient's head and grasp the patient's clothing around the back of the neck and shoulders. Cradle the patient's head in your arms and hands and drag the patient to safety (Figure 7-19). For a lightweight patient you may be able to reach under the patient's arms, grasp the opposite wrists, and drag the patient in a more upright position (Figure 7-20). This hold can also be used for an uncooperative patient. If a blanket is readily available, you can perform a blanket drag. Lay the blanket next to the patient and log-roll the patient onto one side. Place the blan-

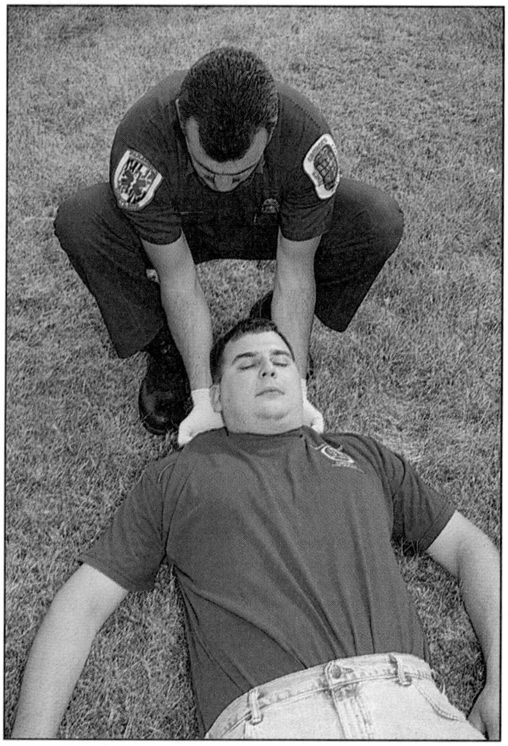

Figure 7-19

When performing a clothing drag, remember to cradle the patient's head.

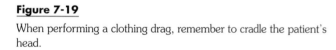

ket under the patient and roll the patient back onto the blanket, face up. Grasp the end of the blanket and drag the patient (Figure 7-21). Note that the rapid-extrication technique, described below as an urgent move, can also be used in emergency situations.

Urgent Moves

Urgent moves are necessary when a patient's condition is critical and could rapidly become life threatening. Patients who may require the use of an urgent move include those who are unconscious, having difficulty breathing, or showing signs of shock. These are referred to as *load-and-go* situations. These patients should be moved to an ambulance as quickly as possible for treatment and transport. If you do not suspect a spinal injury, move the patient in the swiftest manner possible without aggravating the problem.

Rapid-Extrication Technique. A patient who has been involved in a vehicle collision and experienced significant injuries needs urgent movement. The rapid-extrication technique is used to remove these patients from the vehicle quickly, while still providing some protection for the spine.

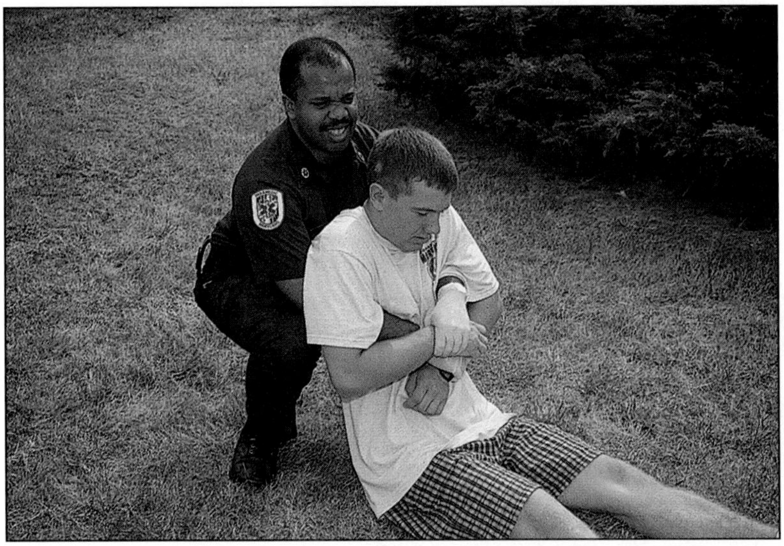

Figure 7-20

When performing a clothing drag on lighter-weight patients, it may be possible to drag the patient in a more upright position.

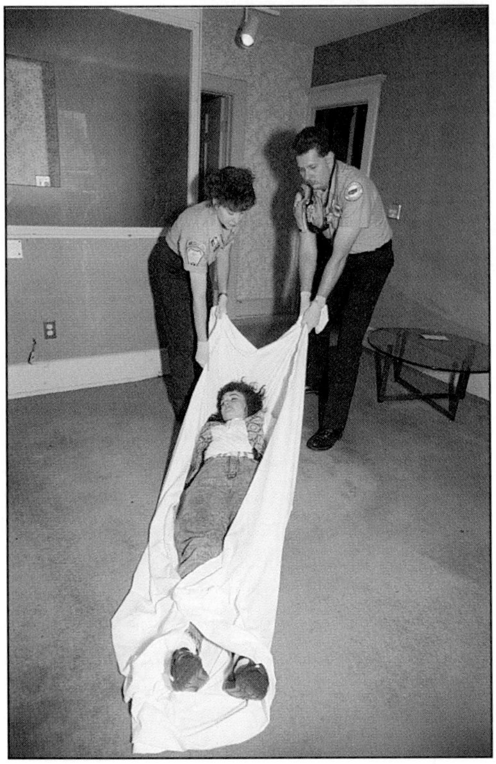

Figure 7-21

For a blanket drag, the patient will need to be log-rolled onto one side, the blanket placed under the patient, and the patient rolled back onto the blanket, face up.

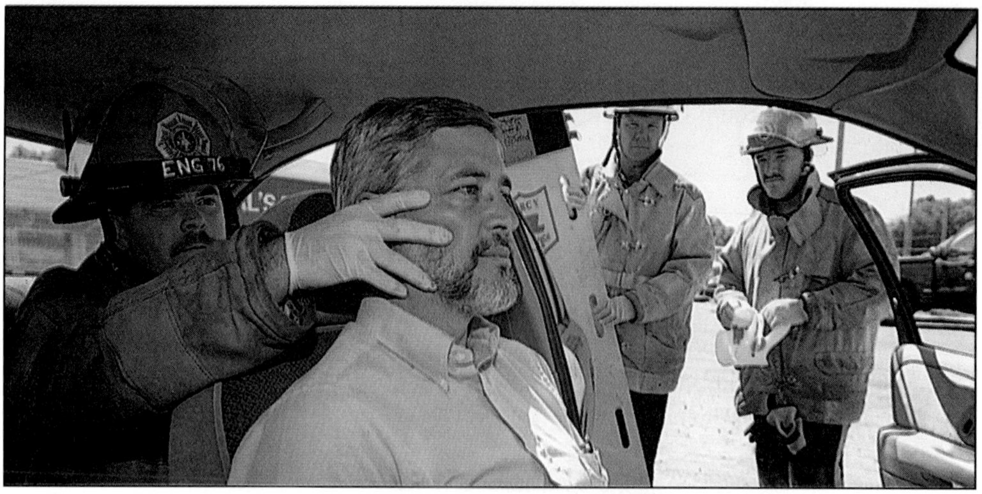

Figure 7-22

The patient's head must be stabilized in a neutral position.

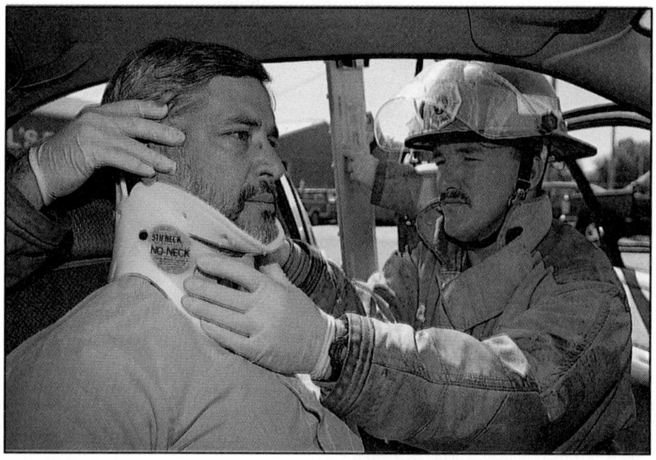

Figure 7-23

After examining the patient's neck, a second rescuer applies a cervical collar. Manual stabilization is maintained.

Three or more rescuers are needed to perform the rapid-extrication technique. The steering wheel should be tilted up, if possible, and the seat should be moved back as far as it will go. The following procedure requires three rescuers:

1. Rescuer 1 climbs into the back seat, places both hands at the sides of the patient's head, and positions the head in a neutral position, in line with the body. This is called in-line stabilization (Figure 7-22). If the back seat is inaccessible, the rescuer can stand in the doorway and perform this maneuver. However, in these instances the rescuer is beside the patient and must take extra care to ensure that the patient's head and neck are in line with the body.
2. Rescuer 2 gets into the vehicle next to the patient, examines the patient's neck, and applies a cervical collar (Figure 7-23).

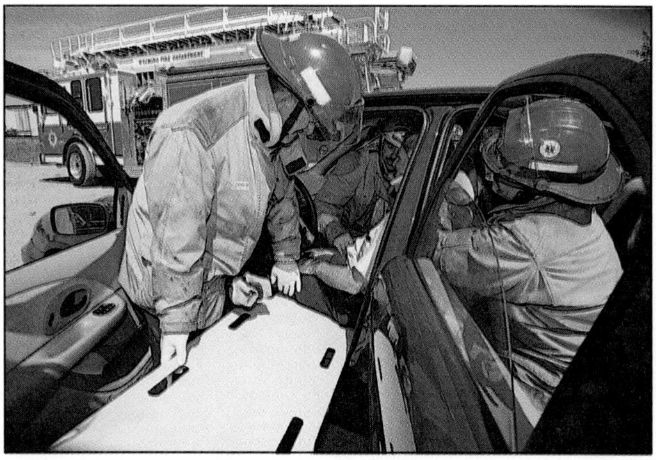

Figure 7-24

A third rescuer positions the long backboard on the seat and stretcher. It may be helpful to have another person hold the stretcher and backboard to keep them from moving.

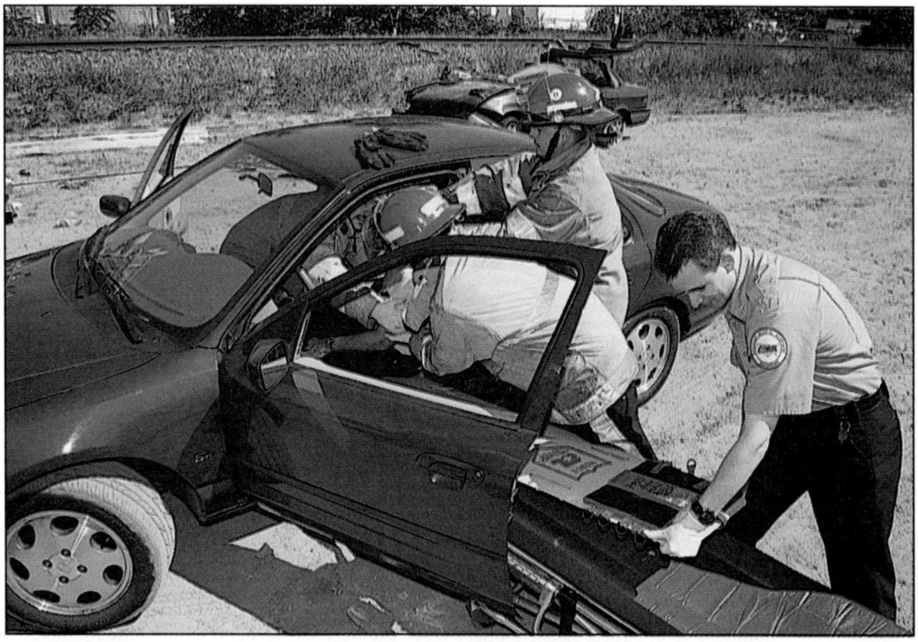

Figure 7-25

Maintaining manual stabilization, the patient is rotated 90 degrees. During this maneuver, the second rescuer will support the patient's chest and spine.

3. Rescuer 3 places a long backboard on a wheeled stretcher that has been lowered to the level of the car seat. The rescuer positions one end of the backboard on the seat (Figure 7-24) and squeezes into the doorway at the edge of the board. If available, a bystander can hold the stretcher to keep it and the backboard from moving.
4. With rescuer 1 supporting the patient's head and rescuer 3 in the doorway supporting the patient's chest and using one arm as a splint behind the patient's spine, rescuer 2 rotates the patient's legs and feet 90 degrees so that the patient's back is facing the doorway (Figure 7-25). This usually results in the extremities extending onto the adjacent seat.

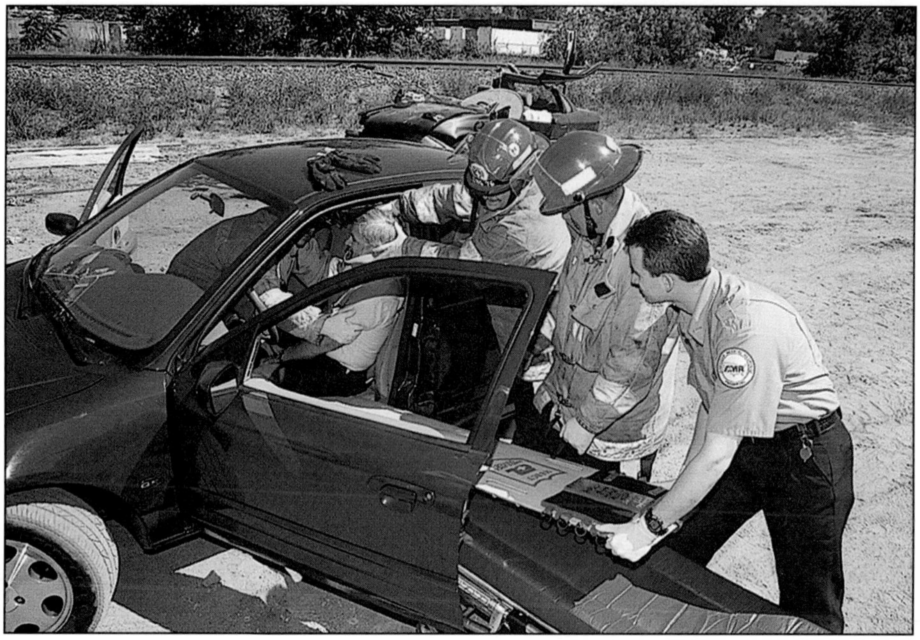

Figure 7-26

The first rescuer turns over manual stabilization to the third rescuer.

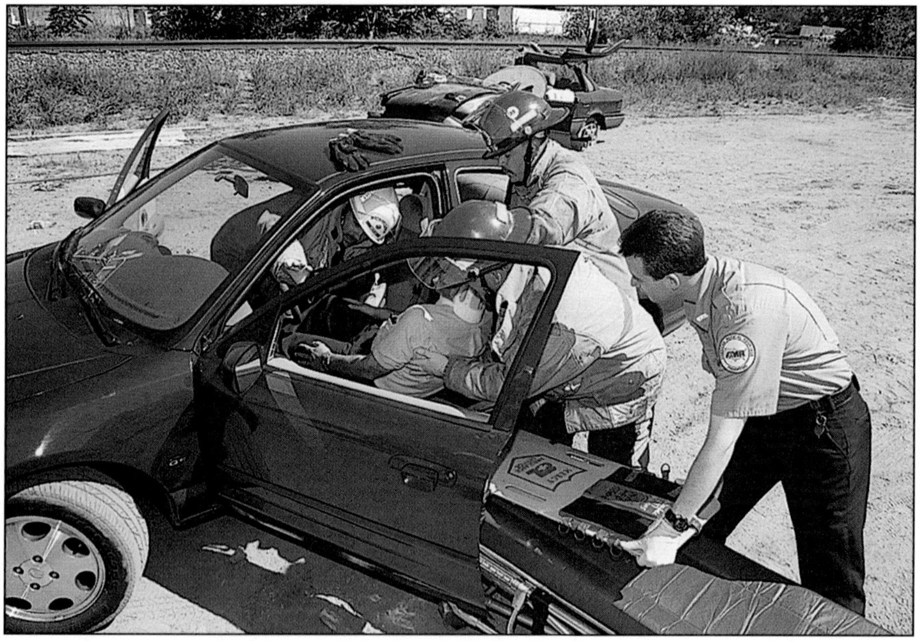

Figure 7-27

The first rescuer exits the vehicle and helps position the patient and backboard.

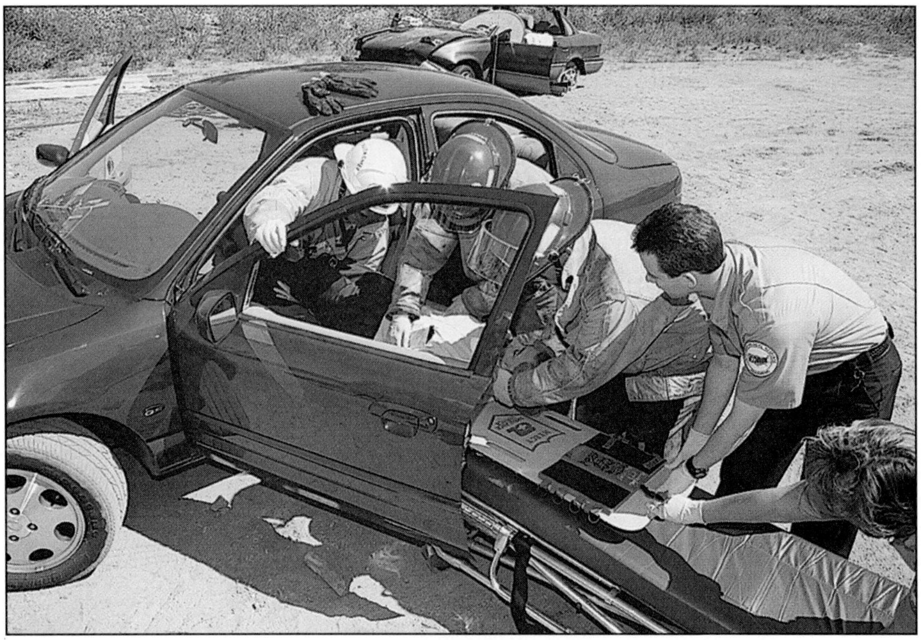

Figure 7-28

After the first rescuer has retaken manual stabilization, the patient is lowered onto the backboard.

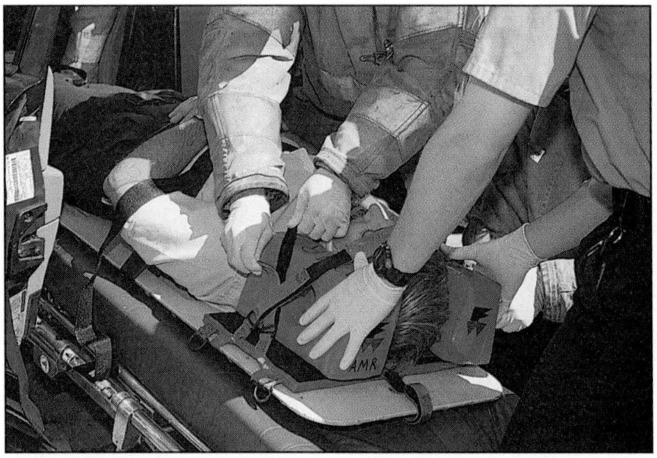

Figure 7-29

Once the patient is on the board, the body straps are fastened, followed by the head immobilizer.

5. During rotation rescuer 1 will have to turn over support of the head to rescuer 3 in the doorway (Figure 7-26).
6. Rescuer 1 exits the vehicle, comes around to the doorway, and helps position the long backboard so that the edge is against the patient's buttocks (Figure 7-27).
7. Rescuer 1 again takes control of the patient's head from rescuer 3.
8. The patient is lowered onto the backboard. Rescuer 1 keeps the patient's head in line with the body while the other two rescuers slide the patient onto the board (Figure 7-28). This is done quickly with rescuer 2 leaning across the seat, grasping the patient's hips, and helping move the patient onto the board. Throughout this lowering and sliding process, rescuer 1 coordinates the movements of all three rescuers with verbal commands and 1-2-3 counts as needed.
9. The rescuers slide the patient onto the board, fasten the body straps and the head immobilizer, lift the board onto the stretcher, secure the stretcher straps, and move the patient to the ambulance (Figure 7-29).

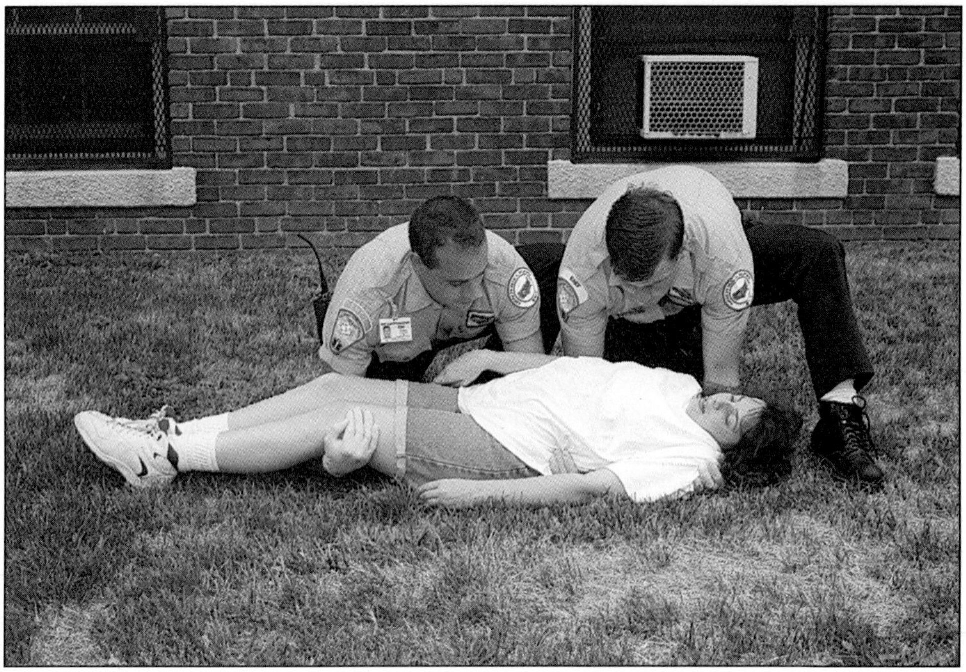

Figure 7-30

The rescuers use their arms to support the patient's head, shoulders, back, hips, and legs.

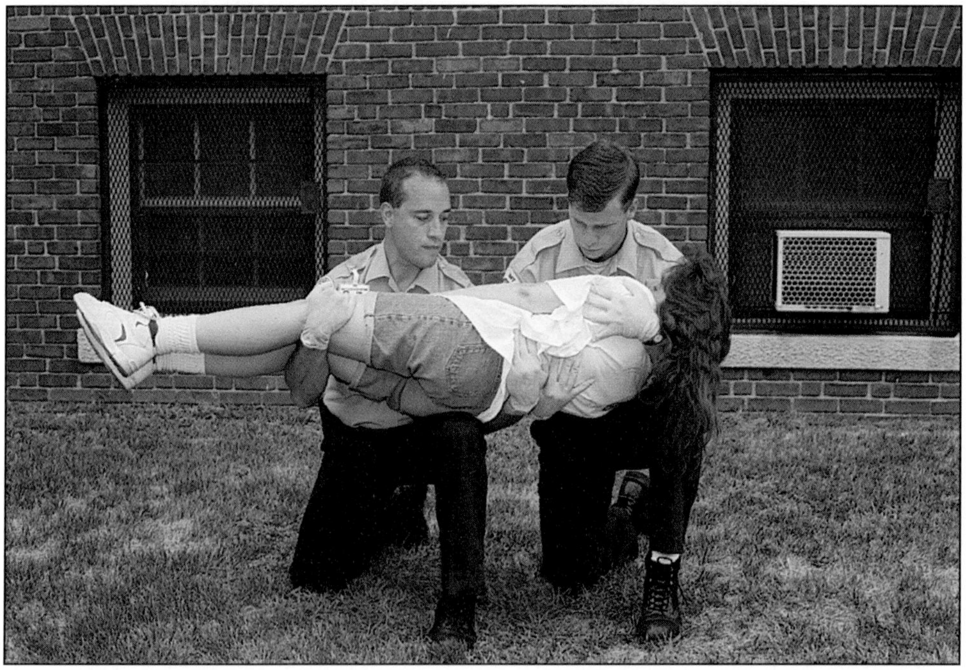

Figure 7-31

The rescuers lift the patient in unison, rolling the patient slightly towards their chests.

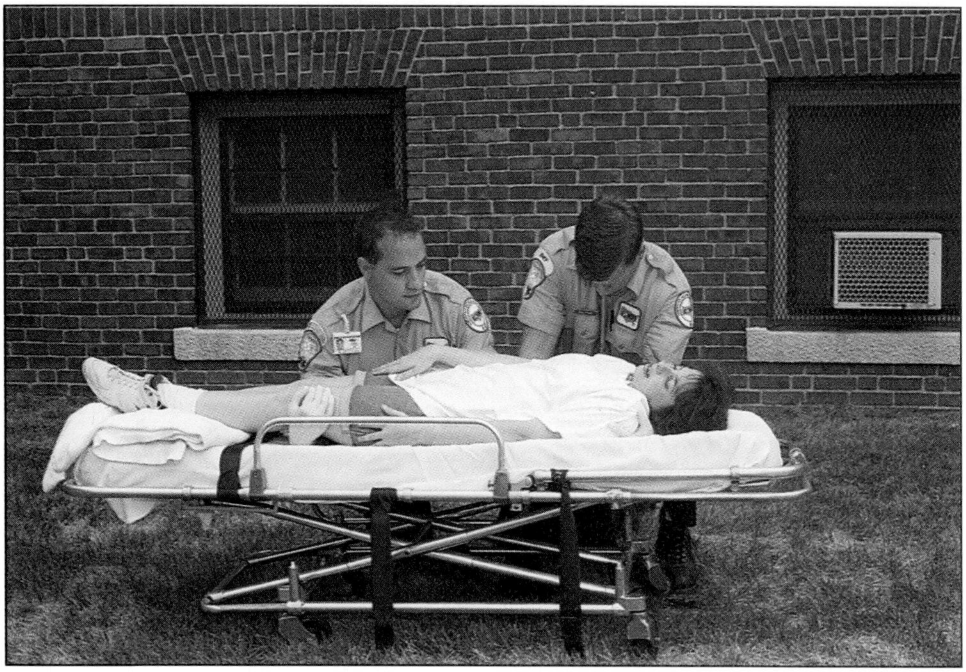

Figure 7-32
The rescuers place the patient on a stretcher.

Basic Trauma Life Support (BTLS) and Prehospital Trauma Life Support (PHTLS) courses teach modifications of this technique.

Nonurgent Moves

When there is no immediate threat to life, move the patient to the ambulance after completing an assessment and providing initial care. Nonurgent moves should be performed in a manner that minimizes the risk of injury to both the patient and the rescuers. There are several nonurgent methods for moving a patient from the ground, a bed, a chair, or a couch. Among the more common ones are the:

- Direct ground lift
- Extremity lift
- Direct carry method
- Draw-sheet method

The **direct ground lift** requires two or three rescuers to lift a patient without suspected spine injury from the ground onto a stretcher. The number of rescuers needed depends on the size and weight of the patient. The patient should be lying supine with arms folded on the chest. Rescuers kneel next to and on the same side of the patient and place their arms under the patient's body, supporting the patient's head and shoulders, back, hips, and legs (Figure 7-30). With one rescuer leading by giving commands or 1-2-3 counts, together the rescuers lift the patient onto their knees and roll the patient slightly toward their chests (Figure 7-31). They then stand together and move the patient to the stretcher (Figure 7-32).

The **extremity lift** is a two-rescuer skill that can also be used to move the patient from the ground to a stretcher, assuming the patient does not have any extremity injuries. With the patient in a seated position, one rescuer grasps the patient's legs under the knees. The second rescuer places one hand under each of the patient's arms and grasps the wrists (Figure 7-33). Together the rescuers stand and carry the patient to the stretcher (Figure 7-34).

To move a patient from a bed onto an ambulance stretcher or from a stretcher onto a hospital bed, you can use either the direct groundlift method or the draw-sheet method. The direct carry method is similar to the direct groundlift in that it requires several rescuers to place their arms under the patient and support the patient's head and shoulders, back, hips, and legs. Rescuers lift the patient directly from a bed or stretcher, roll the patient slightly toward their chests, and move the patient to the bed or stretcher.

The **draw-sheet method** requires several rescuers to be positioned on both sides of the patient. Position the stretcher at the same height as the bed and loosen the bed sheet under the patient. Rescuers grasp the sheet in the area of the patient's head, chest, hips, and legs, and slide the patient gently onto a stretcher or hospital bed

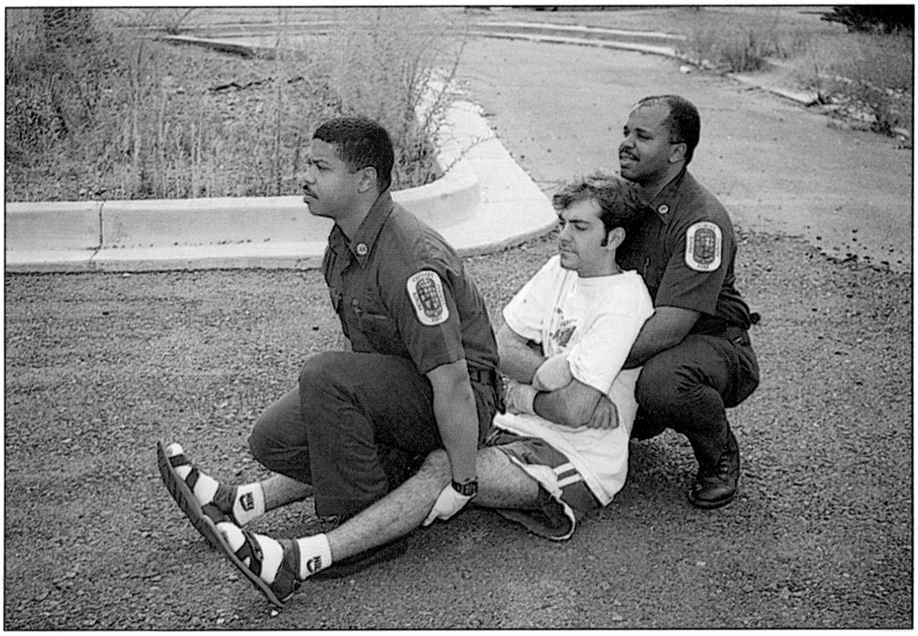

Figure 7-33

The extremity lift can be done on a patient that does not have any spinal or extremity injuries. One rescuer is positioned at the seated patient's back as the second rescuer kneels at the patient's knees.

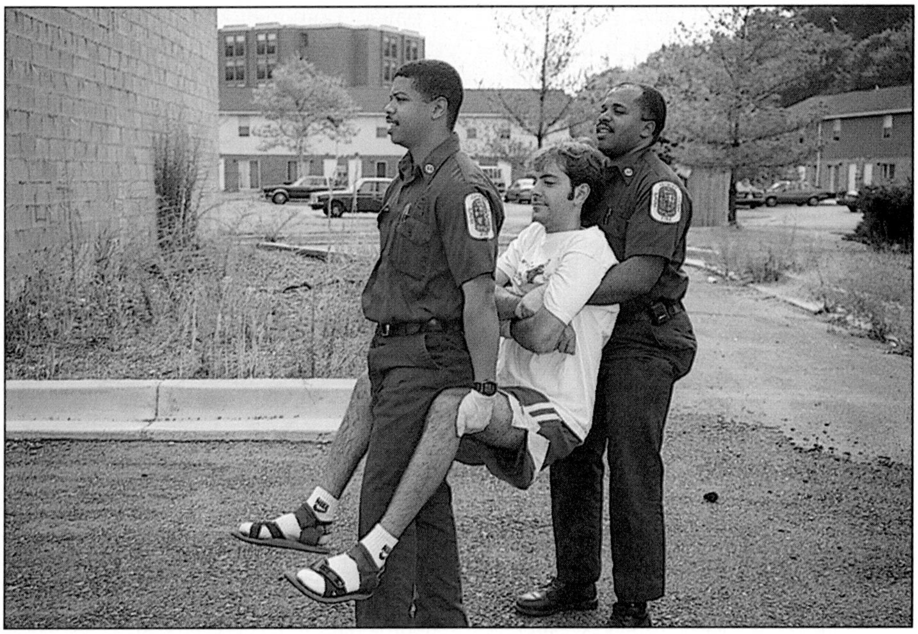

Figure 7-34

The rescuers stand together, grasping the patient's wrists and knees.

There are a variety of additional methods for moving a patient depending on the situation that you encounter. You must consider the patient's condition and weight, your strength limitations, and the number of rescuers available to assist.

CRADLE CARRY

If your patient is light, you can use a cradle carry. Support the patient under the legs and back.

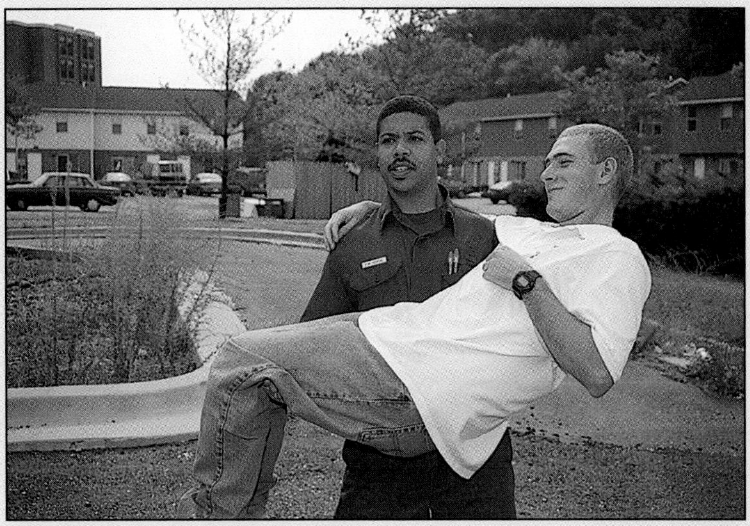

The cradle carry can be used with lighter-weight patients.

PACK-STRAP CARRY

With the patient standing and facing you, turn your back to the patient and squat down slightly. Bring the patient's arms over your shoulders and pull the patient onto your back so that the patient's armpits rest on your shoulders. Hold the patient's wrists and stand up.

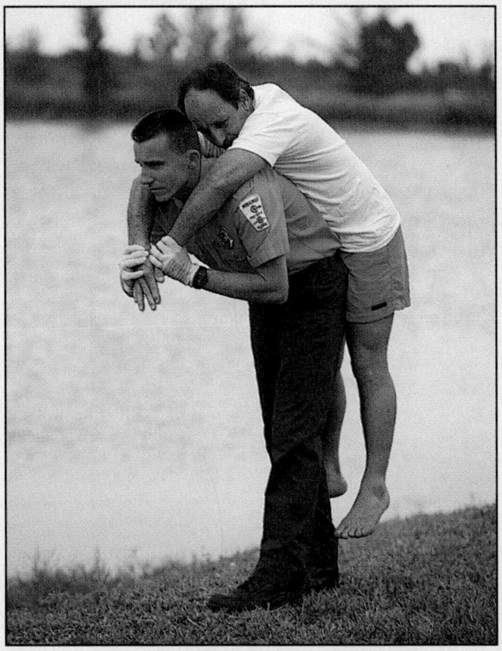

The pack-strap carry involves pulling the patient onto the rescuer's back.

WALKING ASSIST

Wrap one of the patient's arms around your neck and grasp the patient's wrist. Use your free arm to support the patient around the waist and help the patient walk to safety. If a second rescuer is available, the patient can be supported from both sides.

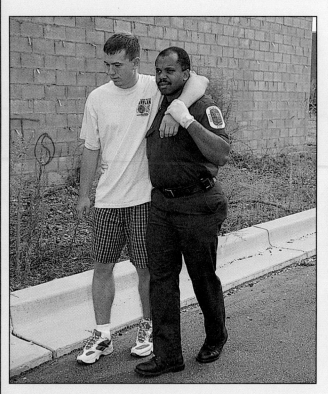

To provide the walking assist, the rescuer grasps the patient's wrist and supports the patient around the waist.

FIREFIGHTER'S CARRY

Squat down while facing the patient and have a second rescuer lower the patient face down across one of your shoulders and your back. Hold one of the patient's wrists and with your free hand reach between the patient's legs and grasp the thigh on the same side of the patient's body as the wrist you are holding. Stand up and support the patient's weight on your shoulders.

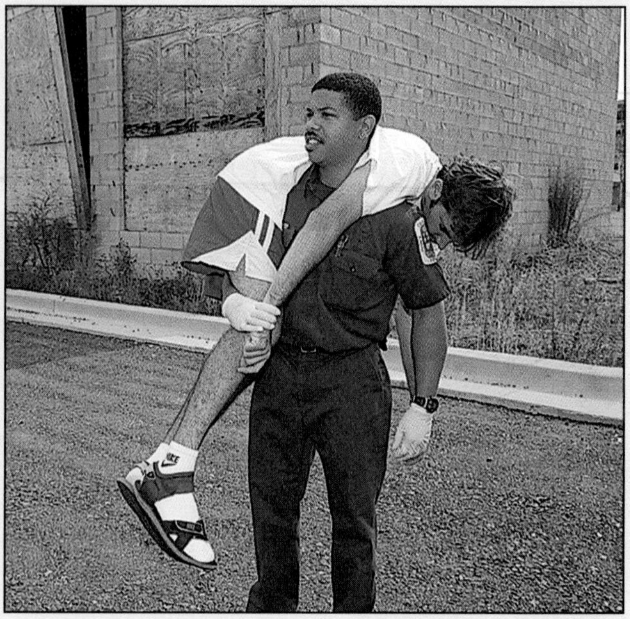

The firefighter's carry places the patient's weight across the rescuer's shoulders.

PIGGY-BACK CARRY

With the patient standing and facing you, turn your back to the patient and squat down. Place the patient's arms over your shoulders in a manner similar to the pack-strap carry. Reach back and grasp the patient's thighs. Position the patient on your back. As you stand, reach under the patient's knees and if possible grasp the patient's wrists.

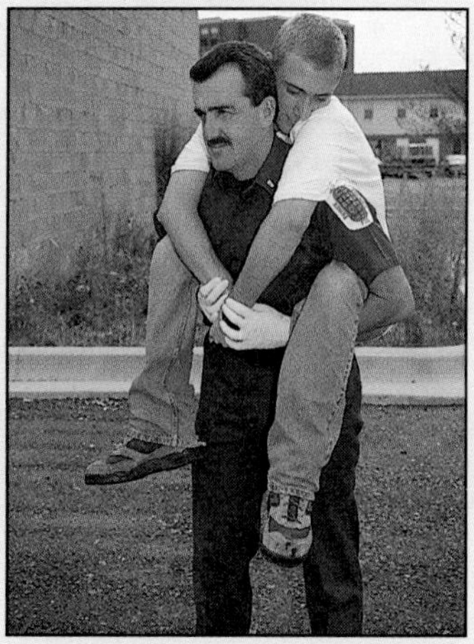

When attempting the piggy-back carry, the rescuer ideally holds the patient's wrists as well as supports his or her knees.

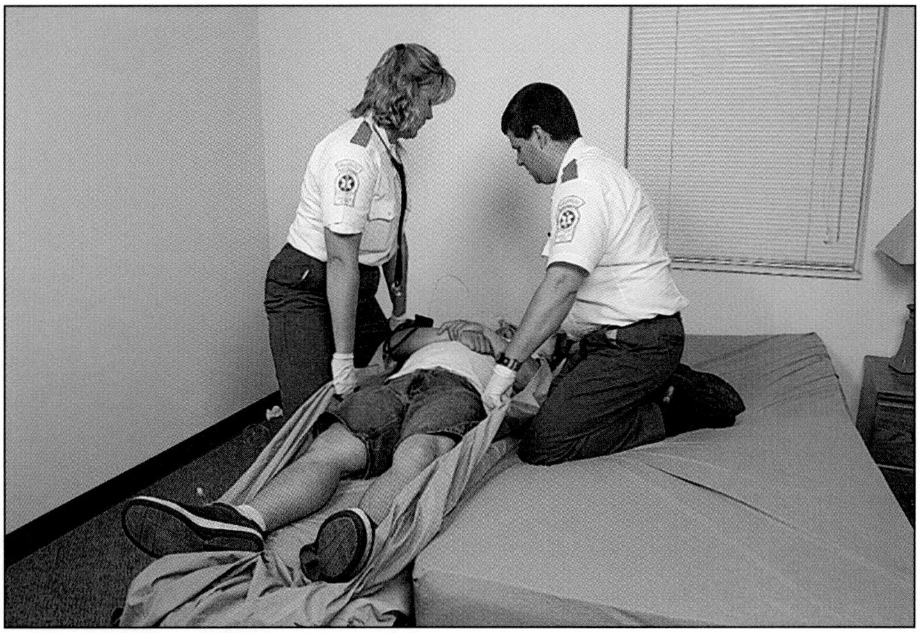

Figure 7-35
The draw-sheet method requires two or more rescuers.

(Figure 7-35). It is wise to inspect the sheet material before this move to ensure that it is in good condition and strong enough to support the patient's weight.

Patient-Carrying Devices

There are several different carrying devices that you should be familiar with, including the following:

- Wheeled stretcher
- Portable stretcher
- Scoop stretcher
- Flexible stretcher
- Basket stretcher
- Long and short backboards
- Stair chair

Wheeled Stretcher

The wheeled stretcher is the most commonly used device for carrying patients. Almost all patients who are placed in your ambulance will be on the wheeled stretcher. Because of its wheels, soft pad, ability to adjust to many heights, and ability to elevate the head and feet, the wheeled stretcher can make the job of moving patients much easier. It also provides the greatest flexibility for patient comfort (Figure 7-36). However, this device is not without limitations, including an inability to use the device over rough ground and the additional weight when lifting a patient on the stretcher.

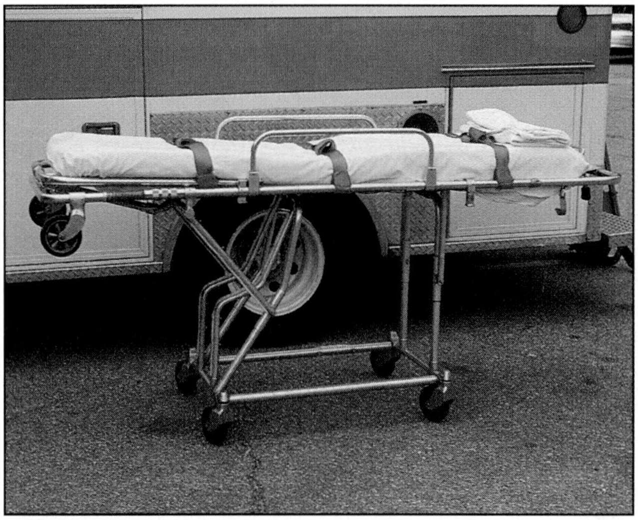

Figure 7-36
Wheeled stretcher. Because of its wheels, adjustability, and soft pad, this is most often the most convenient and comfortable kind of stretcher.

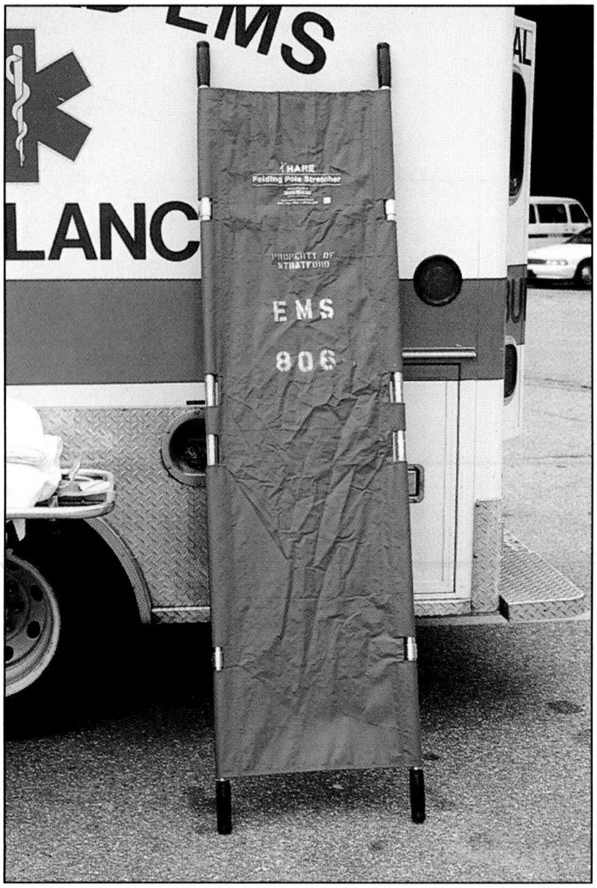

Figure 7-37

Portable stretcher. This stretcher is often used for transporting a second patient, extricating from a confined space, or moving patients involved in MCIs.

Lifting or moving a wheeled stretcher takes a minimum of two rescuers, one at the patient's head and the other at the feet. If more personnel are available, they can be positioned alongside the stretcher to help lift. To carry the stretcher over rough ground, a four-person carry is recommended.

When moving a patient into or out of the ambulance, your primary concern is safety. Once the patient is placed on the stretcher, lift the side rails and fasten the straps. Wheeled stretchers vary with regard to the type and location of patient straps, position of the release mechanism for lowering and raising the stretcher, and procedures for lifting the stretcher in and out of the ambulance. It is important that you familiarize yourself with the manufacturer's directions for the stretcher you will be using, including its weight limits. This is particularly important when the stretcher is in the "up" position. Recently, manufacturers have developed stretchers that are much easier to place in and remove from ambulances. These often allow one person to operate them, although using two rescuers is still the safest method.

Portable Stretcher

A **portable stretcher** can be used for transporting a second patient to an ambulance, extricating a patient from a confined area, and moving patients in multiple casualty incidents (MCIs) (Figure 7-37). These stretchers are made of canvas, heavy plastic, or aluminum and can be folded in half for easy storage. Straps are positioned across the patient, and the stretcher can be secured on the ambulance bench seat for transport.

Scoop Stretcher

A **scoop stretcher** can be used to pick up a patient lying flat on the ground or in a bed. This device is called a scoop stretcher because it can be separated lengthwise into two pieces, which are placed on either side of the patient and then fastened to "scoop" up the patient (Figure 7-38). The foot end of the device can be extended to adjust for the patient's height.

The scoop stretcher can be used with patients lying prone, supine, or on their side. However, because the device does not directly support the patient's back, there is controversy about its use for patients with suspected spinal injury. Some agencies suggest using it to lift a patient onto a long backboard.

Flexible Stretcher

Use a **flexible stretcher** such as a Reeve's stretcher when there is no suspected injury to a patient's spine. It is made of canvas or rubberized material with wooden slats sewn in for additional support. Handles placed at the

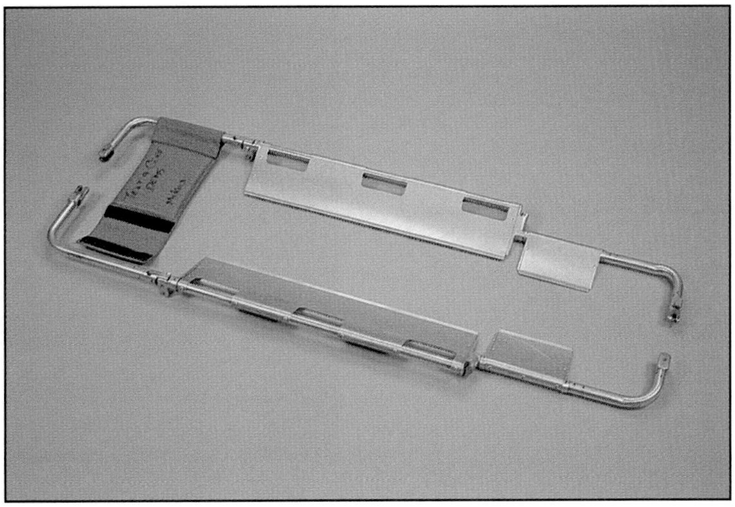

Figure 7-38

Scoop stretcher. This kind of stretcher does not directly support the patient's spine; its use is somewhat controversial.

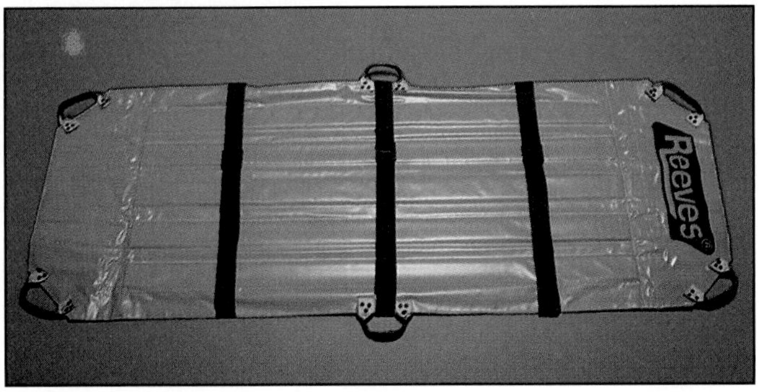

Figure 7-39

Flexible stretcher. This stretcher is ideal for restricted areas but it does not have a rigid back support and therefore should not be used with patients who may have a spinal injury.

head, sides, and feet enable multiple rescuers to grasp and carry a patient (Figure 7-39). The flexible stretcher is ideal for restricted areas and for patients who need to remain in a supine position when being carried down stairs.

Basket Stretcher

The **basket stretcher** is primarily for use in rescue situations requiring a patient to be moved from a roof or through a window, or raised out of a well or up a hill. The older basket stretchers were made of steel and wire mesh, which caused problems when the basket was being moved along rough terrain. The mesh often got caught on uneven spots and did not provide much protection for the patient. The newer models have a heavy plastic covering the steel, which provides more protection for the patient and slides over protruding objects better than the mesh basket (Figure 7-40).

Backboards

Backboards are made in different shapes and sizes. Long backboards (Figures 7-41 and 7-42) are used primarily to immobilize a patient's entire body. Anytime you suspect a patient may have a spinal injury, the patient should be placed on a long backboard. It is easily applied to a patient who is lying on a flat surface; the patient is **log-rolled** onto the board, and the straps are fastened. When log-rolling a patient with a suspected spinal injury, one rescuer holds the patient's head in line with the body

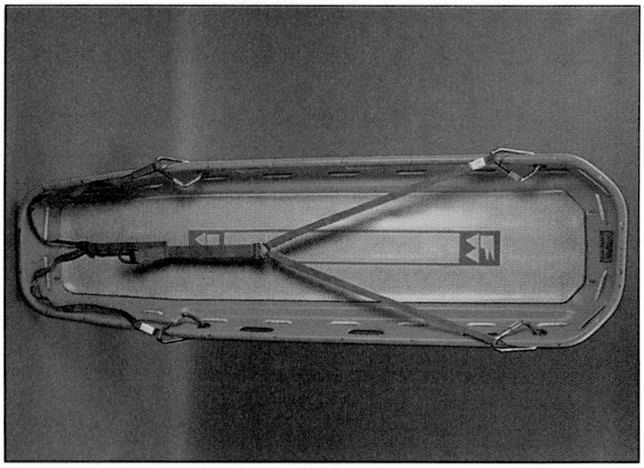

Figure 7-40

Basket stretcher. These stretchers are often used in rescue situations where the patient needs to be lowered from a higher vantage point, such as a roof, or raised from a lower vantage point, such as a steep hill.

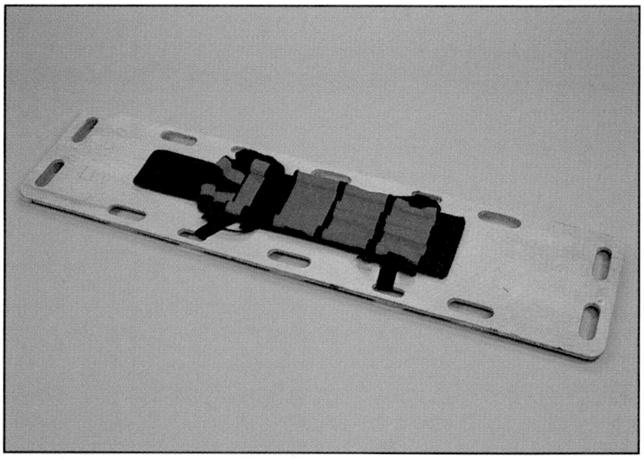

Figure 7-41

A wooden long backboard (with a pediatric backboard secured to it).

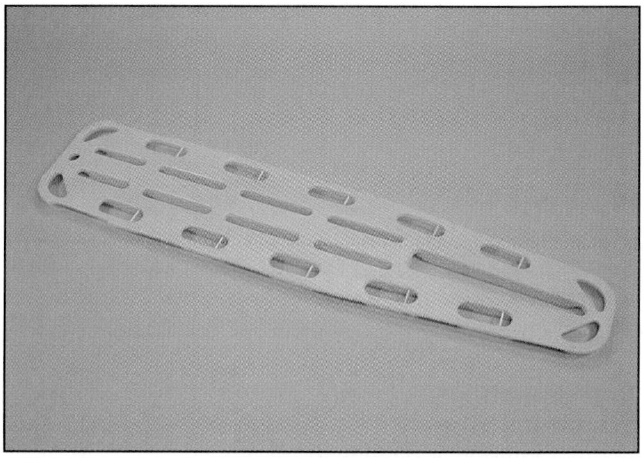

Figure 7-42

A plastic long backboard.

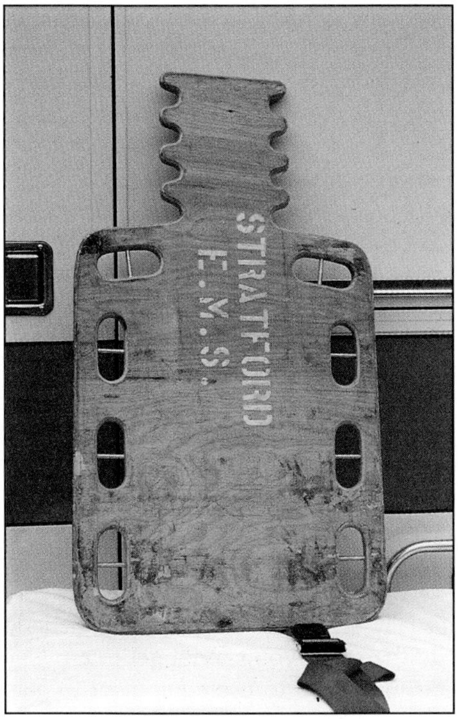

Figure 7-43
A wooden short backboard.

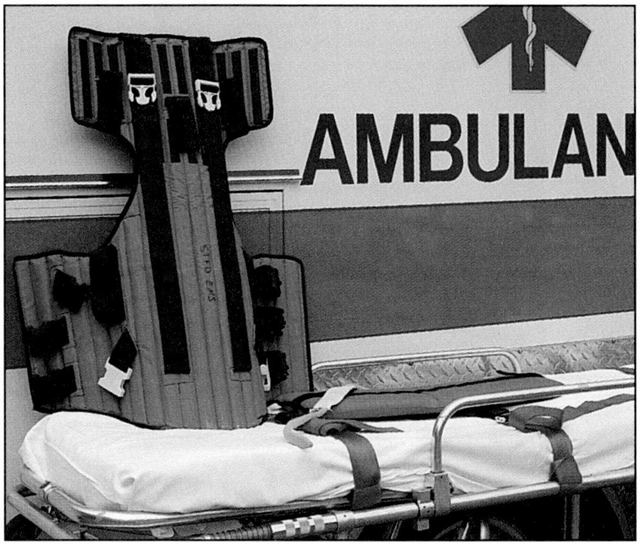

Figure 7-44
A vest-style short backboard.

while other rescuers roll the patient to the side. You will learn more about log-rolling a patient and applying a backboard in Chapter 25.

Use short backboards (Figures 7-43 and 7-44) when it is not immediately possible to place a patient on a long backboard or when you find a patient with possible spinal injuries (and no other life-threatening injury) in an upright position. This is often the case with patients who present in a sitting position, such as those injured in vehicle collisions. Short boards come in two types: wooden and vest. Wooden short backboards are the traditional type, while commercially available vest-type short boards, commonly referred to as *extrication devices*, are newer. (Wooden boards, both long and short, are falling out of favor for infection-control reasons. Damage to the finish coating can make them porous to body fluids and therefore difficult or impossible to decontaminate.) Either type of device can be used to immobilize a patient's spine during extrication. After the patient is removed, leave the device in place as the patient is secured to a long backboard. These half-length devices are the standard for immobilizing patients who present stable and in a seated position.

IT'S YOUR CALL
CONCLUSION

Your patient is ready to be removed from the vehicle. The team of vehicle extrication specialists has made it easy to work on this patient by removing several doors, the windshield, the rear window, and roof. While one rescuer holds the patient's head in line with the body, a second rescuer applies a cervical collar. The rescuers slide an extrication device into place behind the patient and secure it. They remove the patient from the vehicle through what used to be the back window, slide the backboard along the trunk, and lift it onto the wheeled stretcher. They then roll the stretcher to the waiting paramedic unit.

Stair Chair

The stair chair is the preferred device for moving patients up or down stairs or through narrow hallways. This is an excellent device for moving all patients except those with a suspected spinal injury or other condition requiring the patient to be kept in a supine position. The stair chair requires two rescuers to support the patient from the front and rear. Most stair chairs have wheels on the rear that make it easy to lean the patient back slightly and roll the chair along smooth surfaces (Figure 7-45).

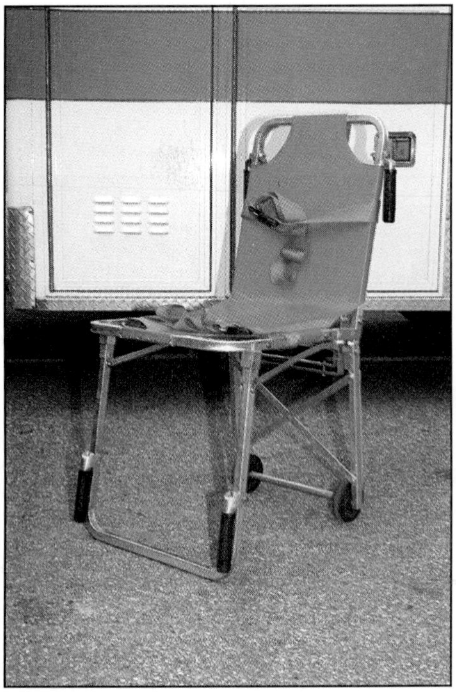

Figure 7-45

Stair chair. Although this is the preferred device for moving patients up or down stairs, it should not be used on patients with a possible spinal injury.

Patient Positioning

The position in which you transport your patient is based on the patient's condition. If you do not suspect trauma or a spinal injury, unresponsive patients should be placed on their side to allow secretions to drain from their mouth. This position is commonly referred to as the **recovery position** or *left lateral recumbent position*. If the patient vomits, the airway can be kept clear so that breathing is not impaired (Figure 7-46).

A patient with a suspected spinal injury needs to be transported on a backboard and secured well enough for the board to be turned on its side (in case of vomiting) without compromising spinal alignment. A patient showing signs or symptoms of shock should also be placed on his or her back with feet elevated 8 to 12 inches. Any patient more than 3 months pregnant should be placed on her left side, especially if she is showing signs and symptoms of shock. This will help keep the fetus from restricting venous blood return to the mother's heart. Patients with chest pain or difficulty breathing and those experiencing nausea or vomiting should be transported in the position in which they are most comfortable. For a patient with breathing difficulty, this is usually a sitting-up position. A patient with an extremity injury will be transported in a position that helps minimize movement of the injured area.

Pediatric and geriatric patients can sometimes be a challenge to immobilize when you are concerned about potential spinal injuries. If they are found in a car seat, children can often be adequately immobilized in that car seat. If not in a car seat, they require appropriate immobilization in an extrication device or on a backboard before transport. You will have to continually reassure these children. Even if there is no concern for spinal injuries, pediatric patients should be adequately restrained (usually in a car seat) when being transported. Geriatric patients should be transported in their position of greatest comfort as much as possible. This is generally sitting up as long as there is no concern for spinal injury. It may take longer to transfer older patients to the stretcher and get them secured.

SUMMARY

You will usually be able to reach your patients with little difficulty. In the event you cannot get to a patient immediately, you may need to use equipment to gain access. Whether you are breaking a window to enter a home or a car or using hydraulic equipment to cut your way to the patient, safety remains a priority. This chapter reviewed the equipment and techniques used to extricate a patient trapped in a vehicle. It discussed stabilizing vehicles found in various positions and how to gain access quickly and efficiently. Always stabilize the vehicle before attempting any type of entry.

Once you have gained access, begin to assess your patient's condition. Sometimes you will need to immediately move the patient because of dangerous scene conditions such as fire or toxic substances or because deterioration of the patient's condition calls for immediate transport to a medical facility. In these cases rapid movement is done with little or no equipment. This may include dragging or carrying the patient to safety by yourself or with the help of other rescuers.

After a rapid assessment and consideration of other factors, such as available personnel, you can make decisions about how to move the patient to the ambulance. You will usually use a wheeled stretcher. Regardless of the device used, you must be able to lift and carry the patient safely. Use proper body mechanics. Keep your back straight, the weight close to you, and lift with your legs rather than your back. Avoid reaching, twisting, or leaning. These maneuvers can cause injury if you attempt to lift an object that is too heavy. Always try to calculate the weight that you will be lifting and carrying before you begin, including the additional weight of the device used to move the patient. Back injuries are far too common because of improper techniques and failure to maintain a physical conditioning program that protects the back. By following the principles presented in this chapter, you can minimize the likelihood of injury while moving a patient.

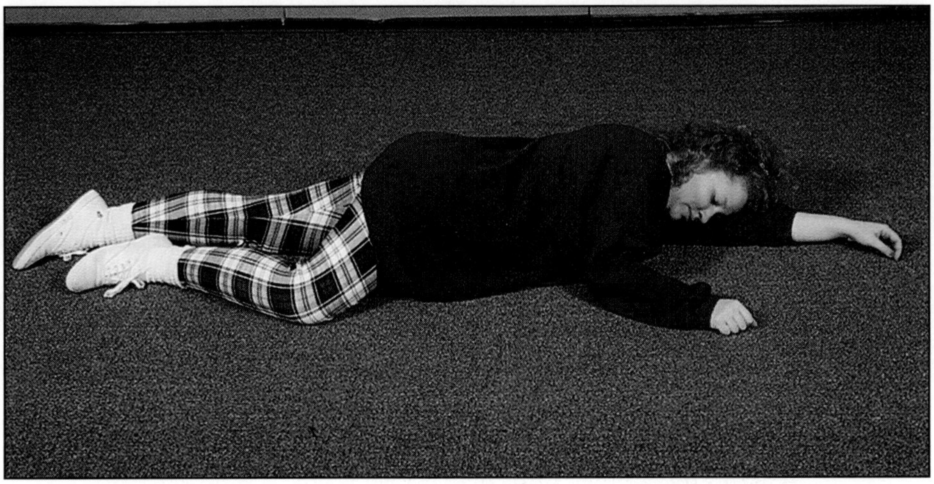

Figure 7-46

The recovery position is used to allow fluids to drain from the mouth of the patient. Patients with a suspected spinal injury should not be placed in this position.

SUGGESTED READINGS

1. **American Academy of Orthopaedic Surgeons:** *Basic rescue and emergency care*, Park Ridge, Ill., 1990, American Academy of Orthopaedic Surgeons.
2. **Campbell JE:** BTLS: *Basic trauma life support for the EMT-B and first responder*, ed 3, Upper Saddle River, NJ, 1995, Brady/Prentice Hall.
3. **Clarke D:** Why Johnny can't read a wreck, *Rescue* 8:54, 1995.
4. **Moore RE:** *Vehicle rescue and extrication*, St Louis, 1991, Mosby.
5. **National Association of EMTs:** *PHTLS: basic and advanced prehospital trauma life support*, ed 3, St Louis, 1994, Mosby.
6. **Valcourt G:** Balancing act: the tools of vehicle stabilization, *Rescue* 8:44, 1995.

Chapter 8

Understanding the Human Body

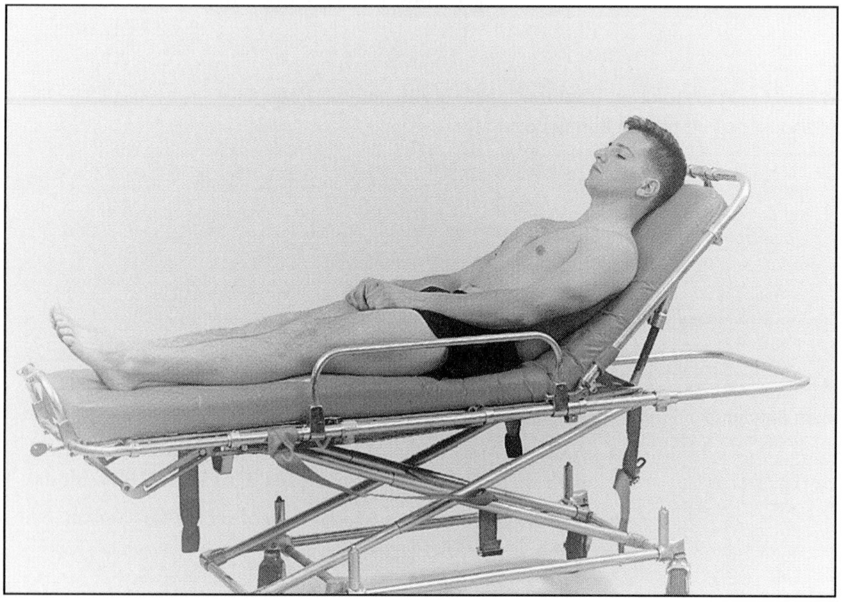

Knowledge Objectives

As an EMT-Basic, you should be able to:

OBJECTIVES

1. **Describe the following body positions: anatomic, supine, prone, lateral recumbent, Fowler's, and Trendelenburg's.**
2. **Describe the following directional terms: anterior, posterior, medial, lateral, proximal, distal, superior, inferior, midline, midclavicular, midaxillary, coronal, sagittal, unilateral, bilateral, palmar, and plantar.**
3. **Identify the five major body cavities.**
4. **Describe the anatomy and function of the following body systems: respiratory, circulatory, nervous, musculoskeletal, integumentary, digestive, endocrine, urinary, and reproductive.**
5. **Provide examples of medical or trauma emergencies that would affect each of the body systems listed above.**

KEY TERMS

1. **Airway:** The passages through which air travels to the lungs; divided into the upper and lower airways.
2. **Anatomic Position:** Standing, facing the observer, with arms at the sides and palms facing forward; an imaginary position used as standard for consistent references to locations on a patient's body and directions in relation to the body; also called *standard anatomic position.*
3. **Circulatory System:** The organs and structures that transport oxygen and other nutrients in the blood to all parts of the body.
4. **Digestive System:** The organs and structures that digest food and eliminate waste.
5. **Endocrine System:** The organs and structures that produce chemicals to help regulate the activities of other body systems.
6. **Integumentary System:** The organs and structures, especially the components of the skin, that cover the body, establish identity, retain fluid, and prevent infection.

KEY TERMS

7. **Musculoskeletal System:** The organs and structures that provide support and structure for the body, protect internal organs, and manufacture blood cells.
8. **Nervous System:** The organs and structures that coordinate the function of body systems by generating and transmitting electrical impulses throughout the body.
9. **Reproductive System:** The organs and structures involved in the conception, development, and delivery of human offspring.
10. **Respiratory System:** The organs and structures that function to bring oxygen into the body and remove waste products, such as carbon dioxide, through respiration.
11. **Urinary System:** The organs and structures that filter and excrete waste products from the body in the form of urine.

IT'S YOUR CALL

You respond to a scene with multiple patients involved in a serious bicycle accident during a triathlon. Your patient is a 20-year-old female who lost control of her bike while descending a hill at approximately 40 mph. As she fell, two other cyclists collided with her, sending all three crashing to the ground. During the assessment your patient states that she has pain in her head, chest, back, and leg. She also has numbness and tingling in her legs and feet. She has a cut on her face and on her right arm and an obvious deformity to her shoulder and knee. She is having slight difficulty breathing.

Your two partners administer oxygen, apply a cervical collar, secure her on a backboard, control bleeding, and quickly immobilize her injured extremities. You contact the emergency department and provide the staff with patient information.

It is important that you describe your patient's injuries accurately. What body systems are affected, and how is this reflected in the patient's signs and symptoms? How would you describe the location of your patient's injuries using appropriate medical terminology?

To conduct an accurate patient assessment and provide appropriate treatment, you need an understanding of the structure and function of the body. Specifically you need to understand how different body systems interact. When a person is healthy, the body systems work well together; however, when one system is affected by illness or injury, resulting problems can occur in other systems. For example, when a decrease in heart function occurs, the other body systems will initially work to compensate for that decrease. However, because body systems rely on each other, they may ultimately fail unless damage to the heart can be stopped in time.

As part of a large health care team, you will interact with other professionals who need to know what you find during your assessment and management of patients. When talking with other professionals, you must be able to describe efficiently and accurately the exact location of an abnormal finding. This requires a working knowledge of common medical terminology, including directional terms and body positions. This chapter provides an overview of important terminology, reference points, and functions of key body systems.

Anatomic Terminology

You do not have to be an expert in anatomy to describe the location of a patient's injury or illness. By knowing some key body structures and their locations and functions, you will be able to identify and describe serious conditions. Relaying this information to others involves using terms that identify the patient's position and the location of the problem.

Body Positions

The unique external features of the body serve as landmarks for structures hidden beneath the skin. When you use terms to identify parts of the body, refer to the body as if it is in the **anatomic position**—standing and facing you, with arms at the side and palms facing forward (Figure 8-1). Although a patient is rarely found in this position, it provides a standard reference for discussion of your physical findings. All directional terms that you read in this text refer to the body in this standard anatomic position.

More commonly a patient is found lying flat, either on the back in the **supine position** or on the stomach in the **prone position** (Figure 8-2). Other positions include Trendelenburg's position, Fowler's position, and lateral recumbent (recovery) position. These latter three terms most often refer to positions in which caregivers place patients for treatment purposes; they less frequently describe the way patients are found.

Trendelenburg's position refers to a patient flat on the back with the feet elevated approximately 12 inches higher than the head (Figure 8-3). **Fowler's position** also describes a patient lying on the back, but

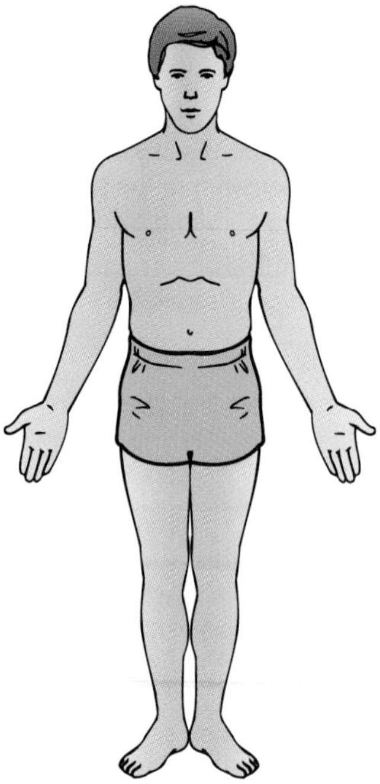

Figure 8-1

All directional terms refer to the patient in anatomic position.

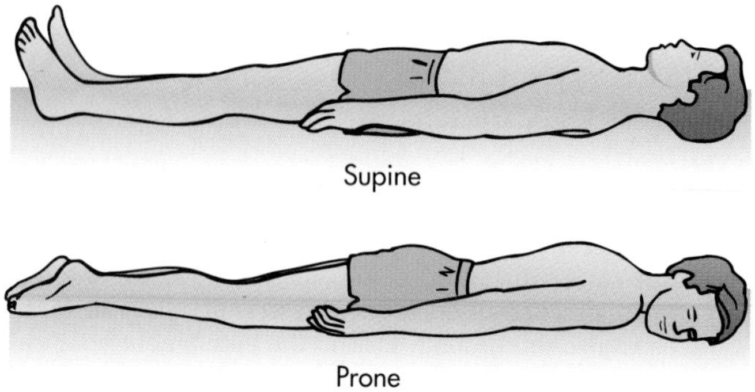

Figure 8-2

A supine patient is lying flat on the back. A prone patient is lying flat on the stomach.

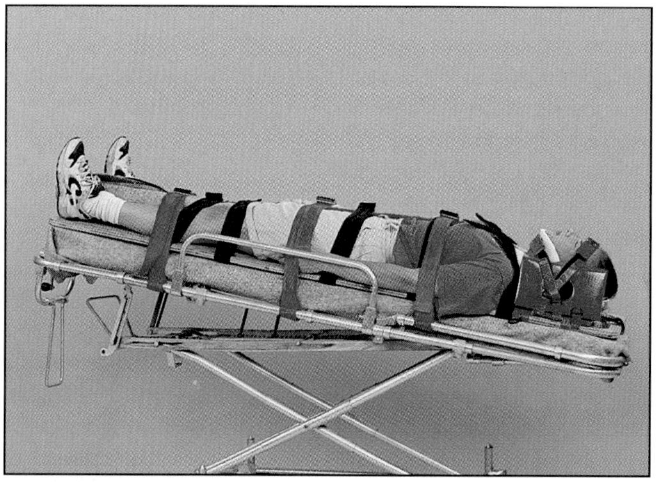

Figure 8-3

The Trendelenburg position is a common shock position for patients who need full spinal immobilization.

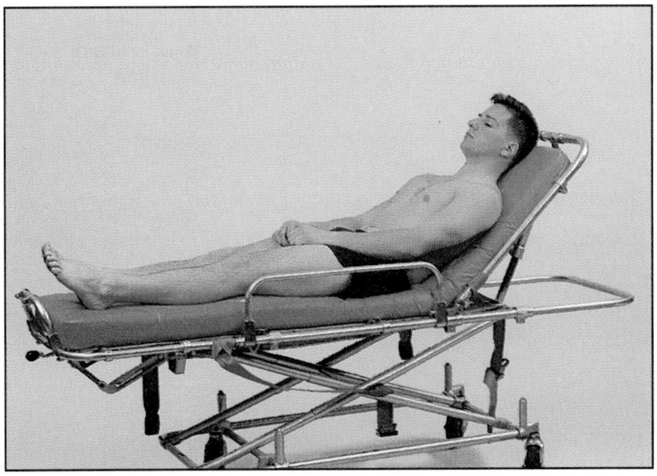

Figure 8-4

Fowler's position is often used to transport patients with general illness or minor extremity injury who do not require spinal immobilization.

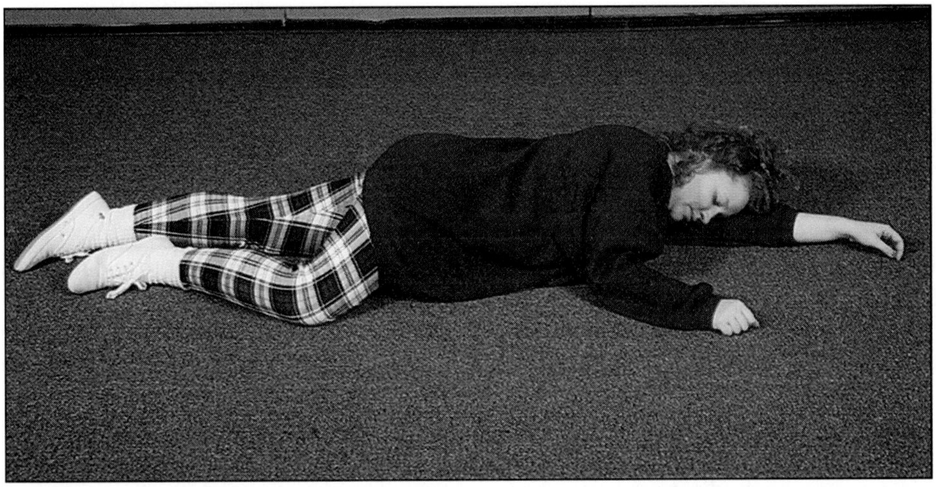

Figure 8-5

The recovery position allows fluids to drain from the patient's mouth. This position is often used with patients who are unresponsive and who are not suspected of having a spinal injury.

with the upper body elevated about 45 degrees (Figure 8-4). This position is often used to transport a patient who has general illness or minor, isolated extremity injury. Finally, the **lateral recumbent position** refers to a patient lying on his or her side (Figure 8-5). This position allows fluids to drain from the patient's mouth and is used when the patient prefers lying down or is unresponsive; it should only be used when you do not suspect the presence of a spinal injury.

Directional Terms

The body can be divided into several planes by imagining lines passing through the body (Figure 8-6). Any vertical plane running through the body from front to back is called a **sagittal plane.** An imaginary line running vertically through the center of the forehead and dividing the body into right and left halves is called the **midline.** (The midline is also known as the *midsagittal plane.*) The

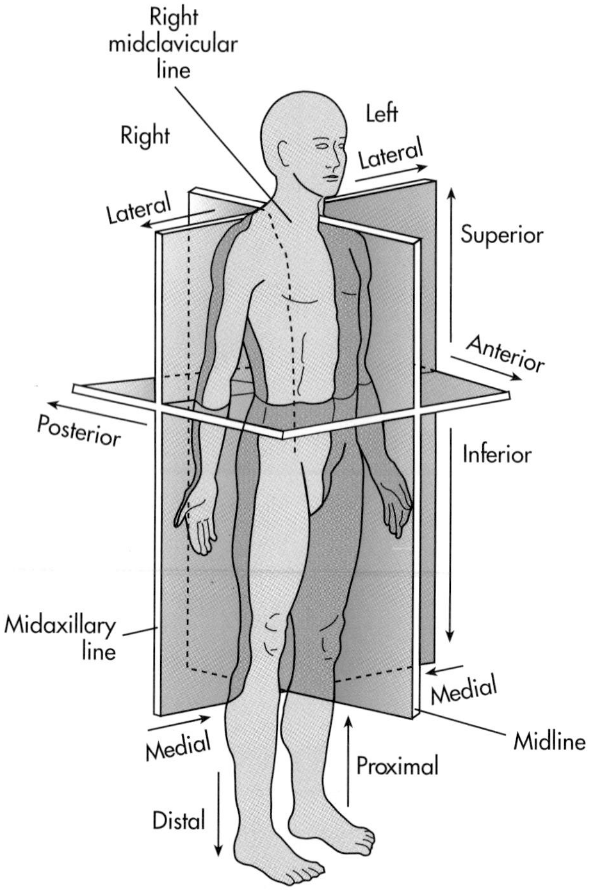

Figure 8-6

Directional terms on the body in anatomic position.

nose, trachea, sternum, and spine are examples of midline structures. When discussing a condition that affects only one side of the body, remember that you are referring to a patient's right and left sides, not your own right and left.

Structures that lie away from the midline are said to be **lateral,** while those toward the midline are called **medial.** For example, a patient's eyes are medial to the ears, and the ears are lateral to the nose. The inner side of a patient's knee is medial, while the outer side is lateral. **Unilateral** describes something found only on one side of the midline, and **bilateral** refers to both sides. When listening to breath sounds or observing the rise in a patient's chest, you might comment that breath sounds and chest movement are equal bilaterally (the same on both sides).

Other imaginary vertical lines can be drawn to divide the body into additional planes. **Midclavicular lines** are vertical lines on each side of the midline, extending downward from the center of the clavicles. Structures found along these lines include the nipples and the legs. Looking at a patient from a side view, **midaxillary lines** are vertical lines that begin at the middle of the armpits and extend downward. These lines, which form the **coronal plane,** divide the body into front and back sides. The front of the body is the **anterior** or **ventral** surface; the back is the **posterior** or **dorsal** surface.

The body can be further divided into **superior** (top) and **inferior** (bottom) halves. This is done by a **transverse** (horizontal) plane that runs through the body at approximately the level of the navel. The terms *superior* and *inferior* also describe the relative position of body parts. For example, the stomach is inferior to the heart, and the heart is superior to the pelvis.

The directional terms *proximal* and *distal* can refer to any two structures on an **extremity** (limb). Structures closer to the trunk are **proximal,** and those farther away are **distal.** The elbow is proximal to the wrist but distal to the shoulder. The palm of the hand is referred to as the **palmar** surface, and the bottom or sole of the foot is called the **plantar** surface. The back of the hand and top of the foot are called the **dorsal** surfaces.

Body Cavities

The body is divided into five major cavities (Figure 8-7):

1. Cranial cavity: Located in the head, the cranial cavity contains the brain and is protected by the skull.
2. Spinal cavity: Extending from the base of the skull to the lowest portion of the back, the spinal cavity con-

IT'S YOUR CALL
CONTINUED

You contact the emergency department and provide the staff with patient information, describing your patient's injuries as follows: *The patient complains of significant pain in her chest and back. Bruising is evident on the right lateral chest. The chest is moving symmetrically, but her respiration is rapid and shallow. Her back pain is confined to the lumbar region, and she complains of numbness and tingling in her legs and feet. The patient's right shoulder is displaced anteriorly, with bruising and swelling. She has good distal pulses in both the brachial and radial arteries. Her right patella is displaced laterally. She has limited movement of her toes, but the pedal pulse is present. She also has a 3-inch laceration at the middle forehead and a 4-inch laceration on the ventral, right forearm.*

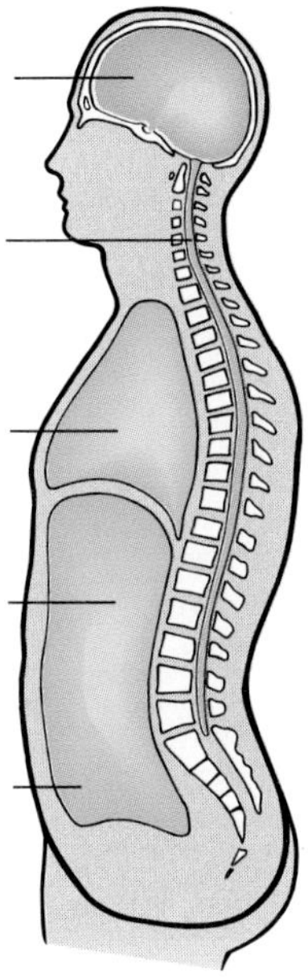

Figure 8-7

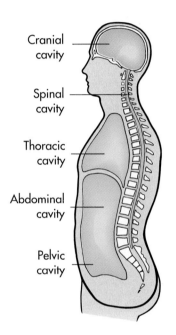

Five major body cavities.

tains the spinal cord and is protected by the spinal column.

3. Thoracic cavity: Extending from the base of the neck to the diaphragm, the thoracic cavity contains the heart, lungs, and other structures. It is protected by the rib cage.
4. Abdominal cavity: Located between the diaphragm and the pelvis, the abdominal cavity contains many important organs, including the liver, spleen, stomach, and intestines. The ribs provide some protection for the liver and spleen, but other abdominal organs have little bony protection and can be more easily injured.
5. Pelvic cavity: Located within the area that is partially protected by the pelvis, the pelvic cavity contains the bladder, rectum, and female reproductive organs.

Body Systems

The human body is a complex machine that is most easily understood by examining systems separately. The body is composed of billions of **cells,** the most basic unit of life. Similar cells work together to form **tissues.** For example, cardiac muscle cells combine to form the heart muscle, a tissue. Connective tissue is the most abundant type of tissue in the body. It includes the fibrous tissue that makes up tendons and cartilage. Other types of tissue are muscle and nervous tissue. Tissues, in turn, form organs. An **organ** is a structure that is made of two or more types of tissue. The heart, with muscle, nerves, and blood vessels, is an organ. A body system is made up of a group of organs that perform specific tasks (Figure 8-8).

Even though each body system has a specific func-

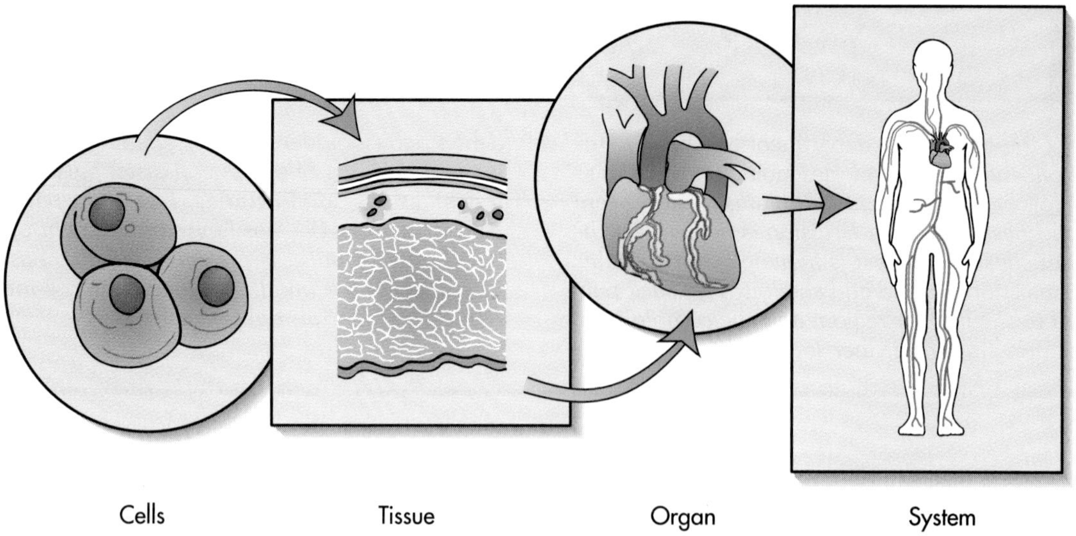

Figure 8-8
Hierarchy of body systems.

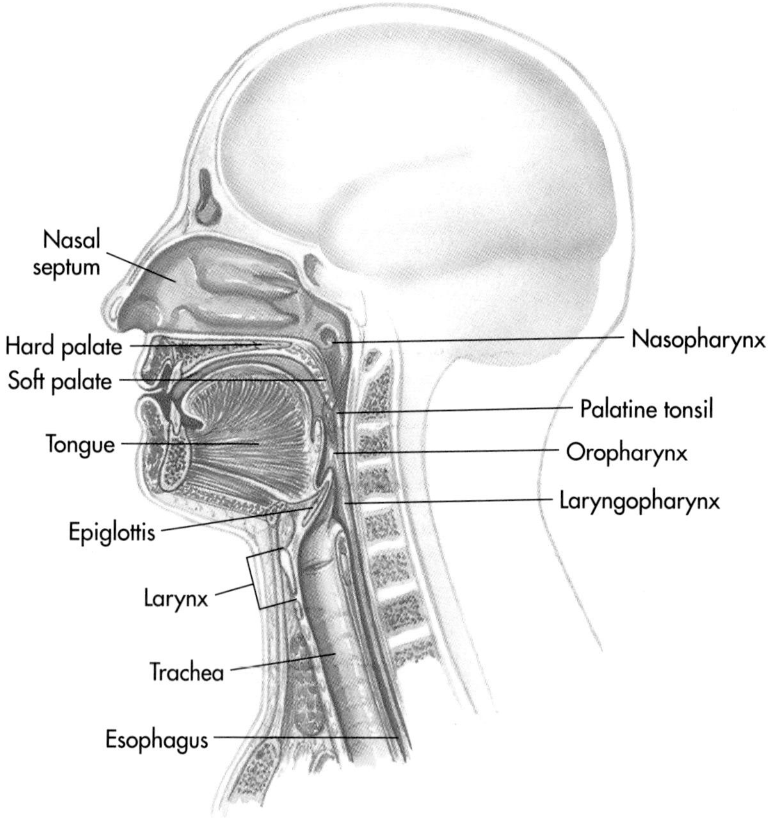

Figure 8-9
Structures of the upper airway.

tion, the systems are interdependent. If the nervous system, which contains the brain, fails to notify the respiratory system to breathe, the entire body will lack oxygen. The heart (circulatory system) is heavily dependent on oxygen and will ultimately fail to pump blood as a result of oxygen deficiency. Without enough oxygenated blood, other vital organs will also fail. Understanding how body systems rely on each other helps explain how injury or illness in one body system affects the rest of the body.

Respiratory System

The cells of the body need oxygen to convert sugar to energy. This process, called *aerobic* (with air) *metabolism,* gives off carbon dioxide as a waste product. The **respiratory system** is responsible for supplying the body with adequate oxygen and removing the carbon dioxide.

Structure and Function

The respiratory system is divided into upper and lower **airways.** The upper airway regulates air flow and helps warm, filter, and humidify the air as it proceeds to the lower airway. The upper airway begins with the cavities of the mouth and nose and extends past the **pharynx** to the **larynx** (voice box), where the vocal cords are housed (Figure 8-9). The pharynx is divided into the portion behind the nose (nasopharynx) and the portion behind the mouth (throat). The larynx is the prominent cartilage (Adam's apple) that can be felt in the midanterior neck. The lower portion of the larynx is the cricoid cartilage.

An important function of the upper airway is preventing food and fluid from entering the lungs as a person eats and drinks. The **epiglottis,** a small flap of tissue above the vocal cords and the superior portion of the trachea, closes over the trachea during swallowing, causing food to enter the esophagus. This prevents **aspiration** (inhalation) of foreign materials. In addition to generating sound, the vocal cords also have the ability to close (laryngospasm), preventing objects from entering the trachea.

The lower airway begins just beneath the larynx and extends to the **alveoli** (Figure 8-10), tiny air sacs in which the gas exchange takes place. Air enters the lower airway through the **trachea,** which divides into the two main **bronchi** that lead to the lungs. These bronchi divide into secondary bronchi, which further divide into the smallest air passages, called **bronchioles.** The bronchioles end in the alveoli. The alveoli are surrounded by thin membranes containing capillaries. Oxygen enters the blood across the cell membranes, and carbon dioxide passes out in the other direction. A chemical called **surfactant** helps prevent the alveoli from collapsing as air moves in and out.

Pleura are thin, membranelike tissues covering the outside of the lungs and lining the inside of the chest cavity (Figure 8-11). They consist of two layers: the visceral pleura (innermost; covers the lungs), and the parietal

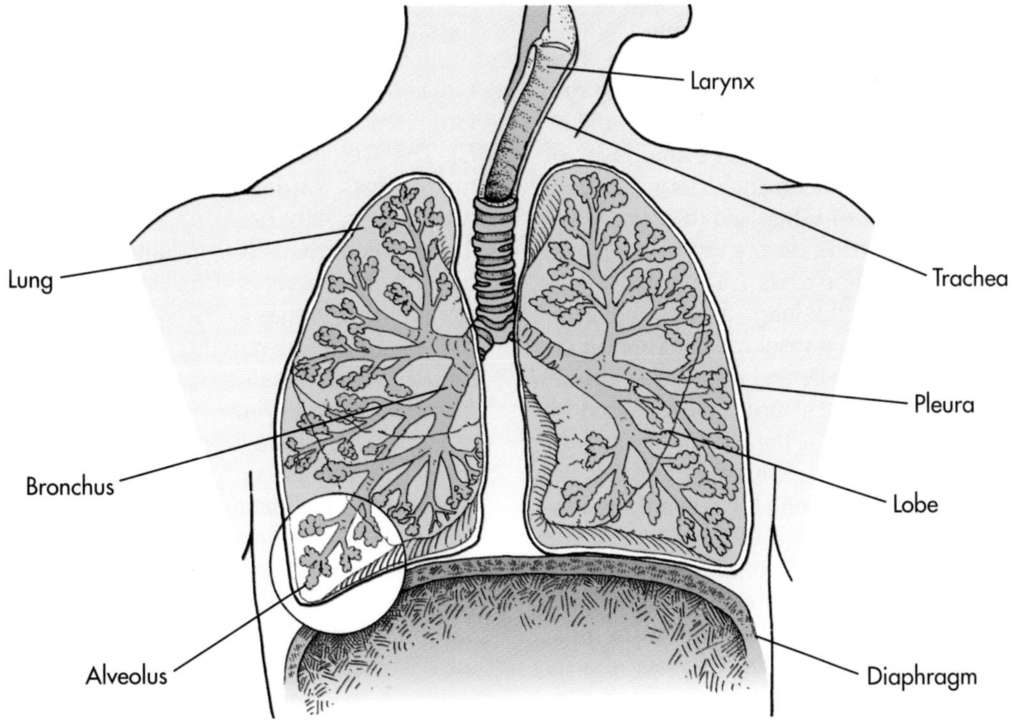

Figure 8-10

Lower airway structures.

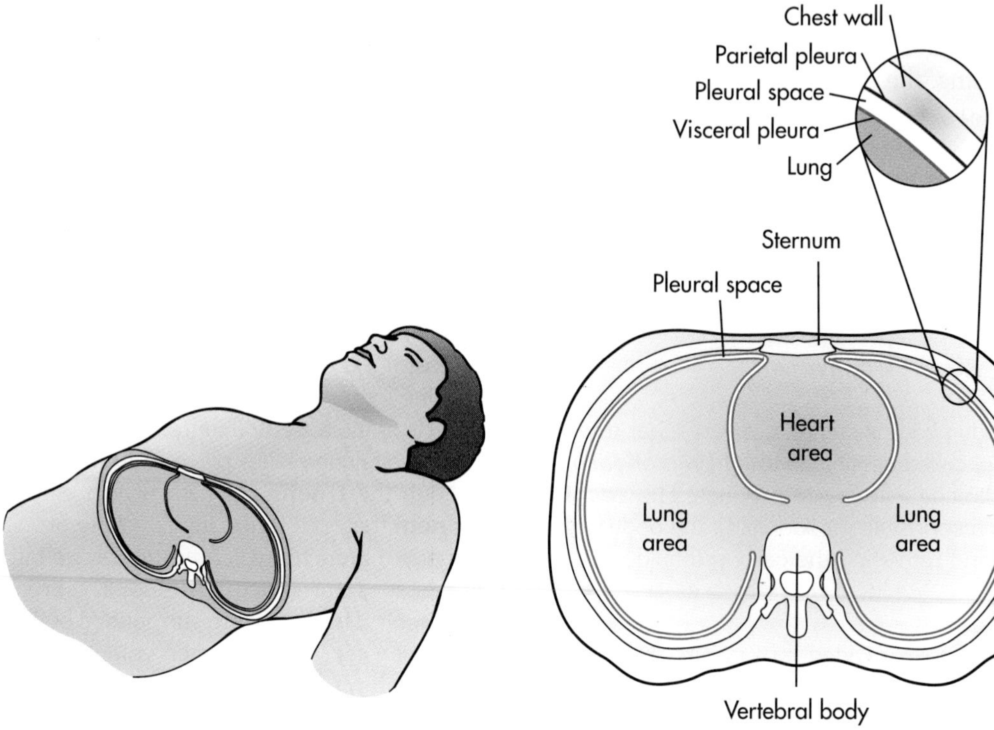

Figure 8-11

Pleural fluid between the visceral pleura and the parietal pleura allow for painless, easy movement of the chest wall and lungs during inspiration and expiration.

pleura (outermost; lines the thoracic cavity). A small amount of pleural fluid lies between these two layers and acts as a lubricant in the area known as the *pleural space.* This fluid allows for painless, easy movement of the chest wall and lungs against each other during inspiration and expiration. The pleural space is a "potential space," meaning it is normally only large enough for a thin layer of pleural fluid. However, it can develop into a larger space if trauma or disease causes air or other fluid to enter.

The process of **respiration** occurs when there is an exchange of oxygen and carbon dioxide between the cells and the blood and between the lungs and the environment. This process occurs as a result of pressure differences between the thoracic cavity and the outside atmosphere. These pressure differences are in turn caused by changes in the size of the lungs as the chest wall expands and contracts during breathing. The entire process requires coordinated interaction among the respiratory, nervous, and musculoskeletal systems.

The **diaphragm** is the large, dome-shaped muscle that separates the abdominal and thoracic cavities. When it contracts, it lowers and flattens. The *intercostal muscles* lie between the ribs and when they contract, the rib cage moves up and outward (Figure 8-12, *A*). During inspiration the muscle movement involving the intercostal muscles and the diaphragm increases the size of the thoracic cavity and causes a reduction in pressure inside the thorax. This pressure reduction is sufficient to draw air from outside the body, where the pressure is greater, into the lungs.

Conversely, during expiration the muscle movement reduces the size of the thoracic cavity, thereby increasing intrapulmonary pressure and forcing air out (Figure 8-12, *B*). The average, healthy adult breathes 12 to 20 times a minute, with a **tidal volume** (the amount of air taken in with each breath) of about 500 milliliters (approximately 1 pint). Although 500 milliliters is taken in with each breath, only about 350 milliliters of this volume is actually available for gas exchange at the alveoli. The remaining 150 milliliters remains in the trachea, bronchi, and bronchioles as "dead space"; air exchange does not take place in these passages.

The area of the brain known as the **medulla** is the primary nervous center regulating breathing. Special receptors in the medulla continuously monitor changes in the blood concentrations of oxygen and carbon dioxide. The carbon dioxide level plays the most important role in controlling respiration. If a person fails to breathe, carbon dioxide builds up. The brain responds to this increased carbon dioxide level by increasing the respiratory rate and depth in an attempt to remove the excess carbon dioxide.

Although the respiratory system is generally the same in children as it is in adults, the nose, mouth, pharynx,

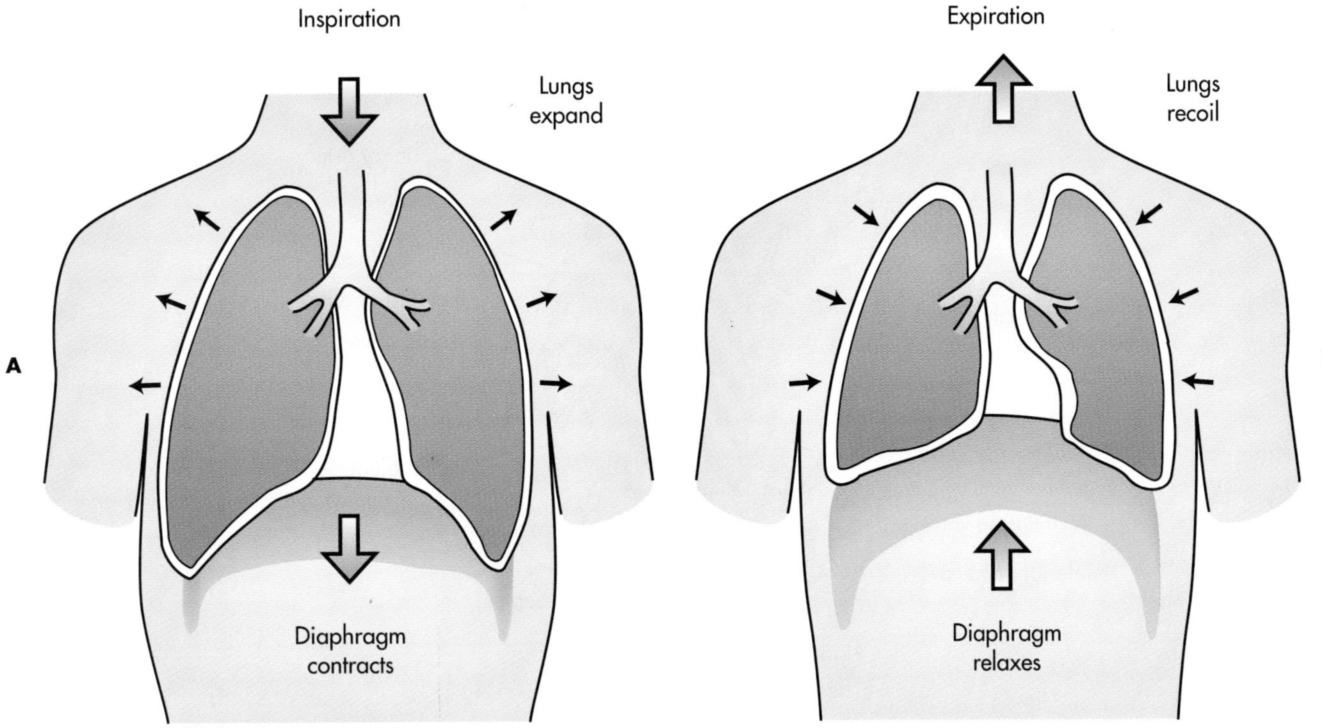

Figure 8-12

A, During inspiration, the intercostal muscles move out, causing the chest wall to expand. The diaphragm contracts downward. **B,** During expiration, the intercostal muscles move in and the diaphragm expands upward.

larynx, and trachea are smaller in a child. Another difference is that the tongue of a child is larger in proportion to the airway than an adult's tongue. For these reasons airway obstruction is more common in children; foreign objects lodged in the airway and swelling of the tissue around the larynx and trachea can both cause problems more readily in children than in adults.

Children also rely more on the diaphragm for breathing. The younger a child, the more dramatic the dependence on the diaphragm is and the more noticeable the movement of the abdomen with labored respiration. Newborns, above 3 months of age, breathe almost entirely through the nose. If an infant's nose is obstructed, the airway is also obstructed. Respiratory difficulty in children may be indicated by flaring of the nostrils and retraction of the intercostal muscles.

Problems Requiring Care

Difficulty breathing, commonly called **respiratory distress,** is the most common type of respiratory emergency that you will encounter. It often results from injury or illness but may also occur as a result of stress, anxiety, or excitement. It can be caused by conditions narrowing the airway, foreign objects obstructing the airway, or conditions affecting the nervous and musculoskeletal systems. If respiratory distress is not recognized and managed, the patient may stop breathing, a condition known as **respiratory arrest.** A number of specific medical conditions can result in respiratory emergencies (Box 8-1).

Circulatory System

Working in conjunction with the respiratory system, the **circulatory system** distributes oxygen and other nutrients through the blood to all parts of the body and removes waste products. Any disruption of the circulatory system for even a few minutes can result in death.

Structure and Function

The cardiovascular system consists of three components: the heart, blood vessels, and blood. The heart is a fist-sized muscular organ with four chambers: two atria and two ventricles (Figure 8-13). The heart has several layers of tissue. The pericardium, the outermost protective sac, itself has two layers: the visceral layer (innermost; covers the heart muscle), and the parietal layer (outermost; lines the inside of the sac). A small amount of pericardial fluid lubricates the surfaces between these two layers as they move against each other during contraction of the heart. Just under the pericardium is the epicardium, the outside layer of heart muscle. Beneath the epicardium are the myocardium (the thick muscle mass) and the endocardium (the innermost layer lining the chambers of the heart).

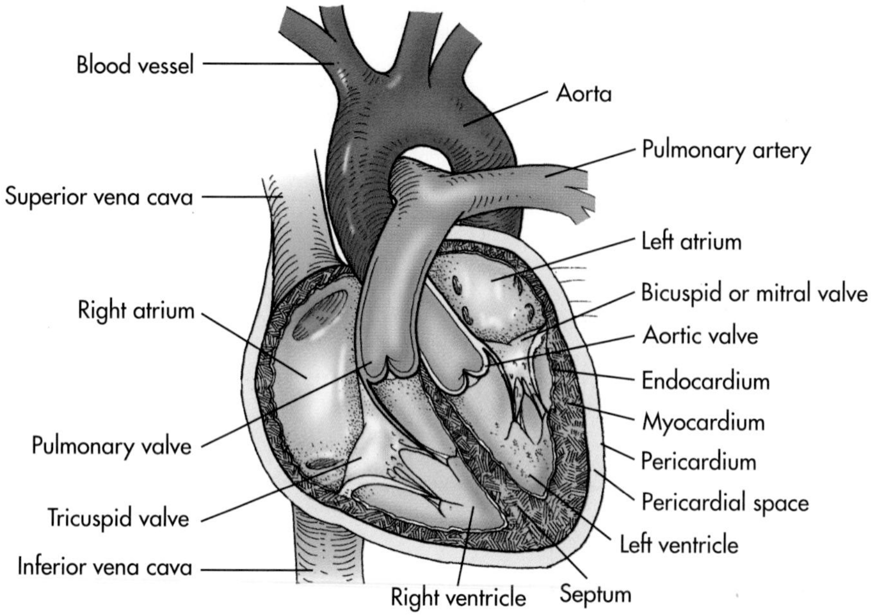

Figure 8-13

The heart is divided into four chambers.

BOX 8-1 Conditions That Can Cause Breathing Emergencies

Medical Conditions

- Airway obstruction
- Altered mental status
- Anaphylaxis
- Asthma
- Chronic bronchitis
- Croup
- Drug overdoses that cause respiratory depression
- Emphysema
- Epiglottitis
- Heart conditions such as congestive heart failure and pulmonary edema
- Pneumonia
- Pulmonary embolism

Traumatic Conditions

- Brain injuries
- Burns to the face, neck, and airway
- Cervical spine injury
- Fractured larynx
- Fractured trachea
- Pneumothorax
- Rib fractures

The myocardium is the strong muscle that forces blood throughout the body.

Blood vessels carry blood throughout the circulatory system to all parts of the body. Arteries normally carry oxygenated blood away from the heart, while veins return deoxygenated blood to the heart. Because arteries are under greater pressure than veins and contain oxygen-rich blood, arterial bleeding is bright red and spurts from a wound. Venous bleeding is a darker red and flows steadily rather than spurting.

Blood plays many critical roles, including:

- Carrying red blood cells, which contain the hemoglobin that binds with oxygen.
- Removing carbon dioxide from the tissues.
- Carrying white blood cells, which are part of the body's immune system for fighting infections.
- Carrying platelets, which aid in blood clotting.

Blood contains plasma, the fluid that acts as the transport mechanism for the blood cells and platelets. Plasma contains a small amount of dissolved oxygen; the majority of the oxygen is attached to hemoglobin in the red blood cells.

Blood leaves the heart through the major artery in the body, the **aorta.** The aorta curves around after leaving the heart and extends down through the thorax and upper abdomen. At the level of the navel, the aorta branches into iliac arteries.

The surge of blood passing through the arteries can be felt as a pulse at specific points close to the surface of the skin, where arteries pass over bones. Some of the most common points used to feel for a pulse are the:

- Carotid arteries (neck)
- Brachial arteries (arms)
- Radial arteries (wrists)
- Femoral arteries (groin)
- Dorsalis pedis arteries (feet)

As arteries move away from the heart, they branch off into smaller arterioles. These arterioles lead to *capillaries,* the smallest blood vessels in the body. It is in the capillaries that the exchange of oxygen and other nutrients for waste products, including carbon dioxide, takes place. Capillaries join together to form venules, the smallest vessels on the venous side of the circulatory system. The venules lead to larger veins, which transport deoxygenated blood back to the heart. The veins increase in size as they approach the heart; the largest are the inferior vena cava and superior vena cava (Figure 8-14).

Among the heart's four chambers, the two *atria* are located superior to the two *ventricles.* The atrial septum (dividing wall) separates the right atrium from the left. The ventricular septum similarly divides the two ventricles. Each septum contains connective tissue and muscle. Deoxygenated blood flows into the right atrium from the superior and inferior vena cava. This blood passes through a series of one-way valves in the heart; the first is the tricuspid valve between the right atrium and the right ventricle. The blood exits the right ventricle through the pulmonic valve and enters the pulmonary arteries, which carry it to the lungs. Oxygen is absorbed into the blood, carbon dioxide and other waste products are removed, and oxygenated blood returns to the heart. (Pulmonary circulation is unusual in that deoxygenated blood travels to the lungs through arteries and oxygenated blood returns to the heart through veins. This is the opposite of the general circulation in which arteries carry oxygenated blood and veins contain deoxygenated blood.)

The oxygenated blood returns to the heart through the pulmonary veins, enters the left atrium, passes through the mitral valve, and continues into the left ventricle. The oxygen-rich blood passes through the aortic valve into the aorta for distribution to the body. As the blood leaves the heart, some blood is pushed through coronary arteries to supply nutrients to the myocardial muscle. The two main coronary arteries, right and left, originate in the aorta just outside the aortic valve. These vessels have the unusual ability to develop collateral circulation, alternate pathways for blood flow in the event that one or more of the coronary arteries becomes blocked. Deoxygenated blood leaves the heart through the coronary veins, which drain into the right atrium.

Mechanical Activity. Blood will not flow freely throughout the body without some force pushing it. The heart's pumping activity depends on the coordinated efforts of the atria and ventricles during contraction and relaxation of the heart. The right and left atria contract at the same time, filling the ventricles with blood. The ventricles are at rest during this filling period, called *diastole.* The ventricles also contract together, pushing blood into the pulmonary arteries and the aorta. This period of ventricular contraction is known as *systole.*

The *stroke volume,* which is the amount of blood ejected with each contraction, is the same for each ventricle. Because the left ventricle must pump against the resistance of the entire arterial system, it is more muscular and capable of more forceful pumping than the right ventricle. The left ventricle and the arteries are a high-pressure system. In contrast, the right ventricle produces lower pressures. The average stroke volume is approximately 70 milliliters and depends on three elements:

1. Preload: The volume of blood delivered to the ventricle during diastole.
2. Contractility: The ability of the heart muscle to contract.
3. Afterload: The pressure against which the ventricles must pump.

As the amount of blood returned from the venous system to the right atrium increases, so do contractility and preload. Increased venous blood return therefore means greater stroke volume. The volume of blood ejected from the heart is also measured in terms of *cardiac output,* the amount of blood pumped in 1 minute. This is calculated as stroke volume multiplied by heart rate. The average heart beats approximately 70 times per minute, and the average stroke volume is 70 milliliters. The average cardiac output is thus 4900 milliliters (nearly 5 liters) per minute.

Blood pressure, the pressure exerted by blood flow on the walls of the arteries, is measured in millimeters of mercury (mm/Hg). The pressure in the arteries during systole is known as the *systolic blood pressure;* the arterial pressure during diastole is the *diastolic blood pressure.* Chapter 9 provides detailed information about blood pressure measurement.

Electrical Activity. To circulate blood the heart must be stimulated to contract in a coordinated manner. The heart contains special areas from which electrical impulses arise automatically. The most important area is the sino-atrial (SA) node. This generates regular electrical impulses that are conducted over the nerves in the heart to stimulate cardiac muscle cells to contract. Myocardial cells have unique electrical properties that allow for the rapid transmission of electrical impulses between cells. This process involves special connections that lie within cardiac muscle fibers. When one cell is stimulated, others react in a way that ensures a coordinated contraction. The heart's electrical system will become disturbed if areas of the heart are injured or deprived of oxygen.

A heart monitor produces an electrocardiogram (ECG), which is a tracing of the heart's electrical activity

A

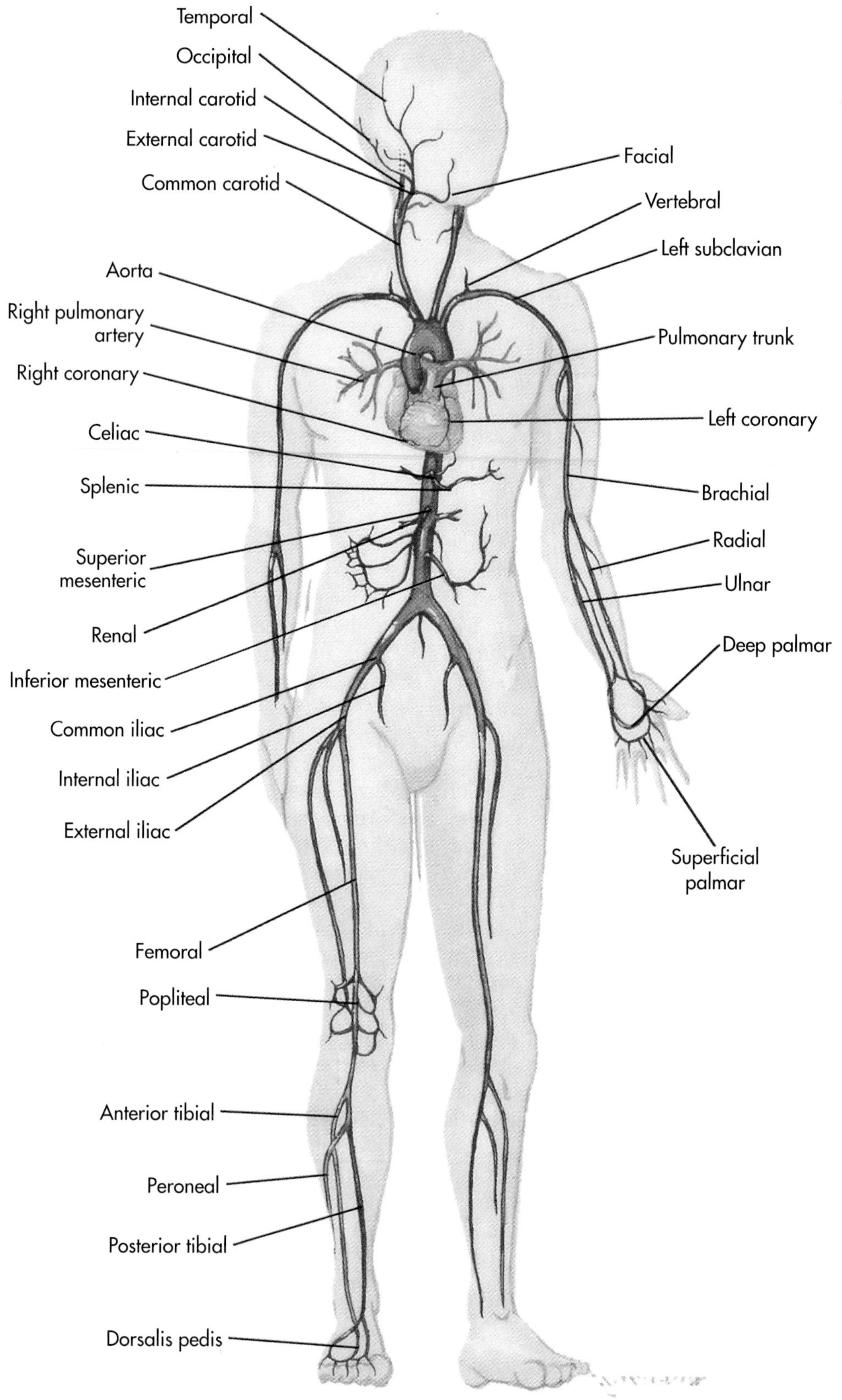

Figure 8-14

A, Primary arteries in the circulatory system.

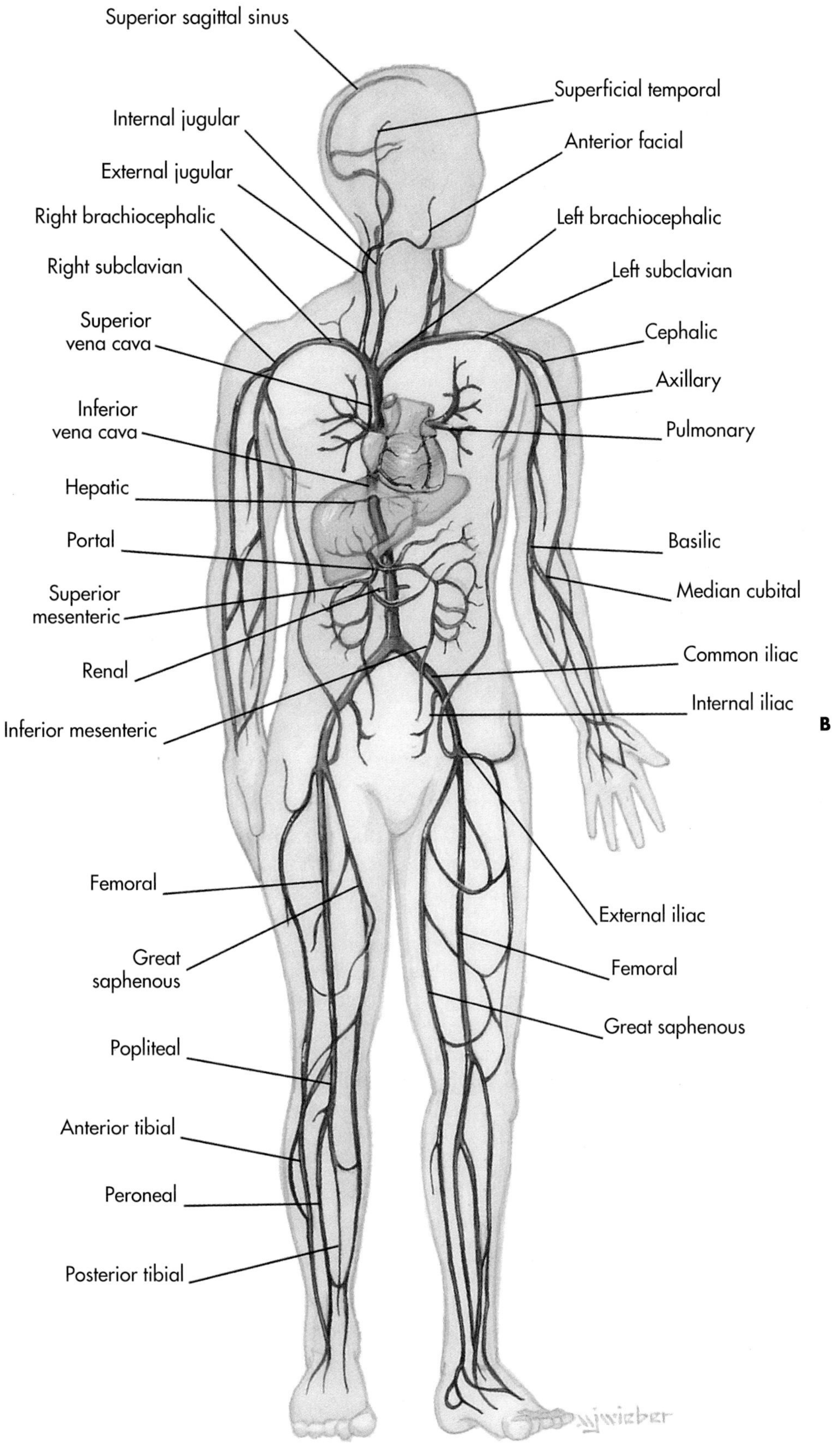

Figure 8-14, cont'd

B, Primary veins in the circulatory system.

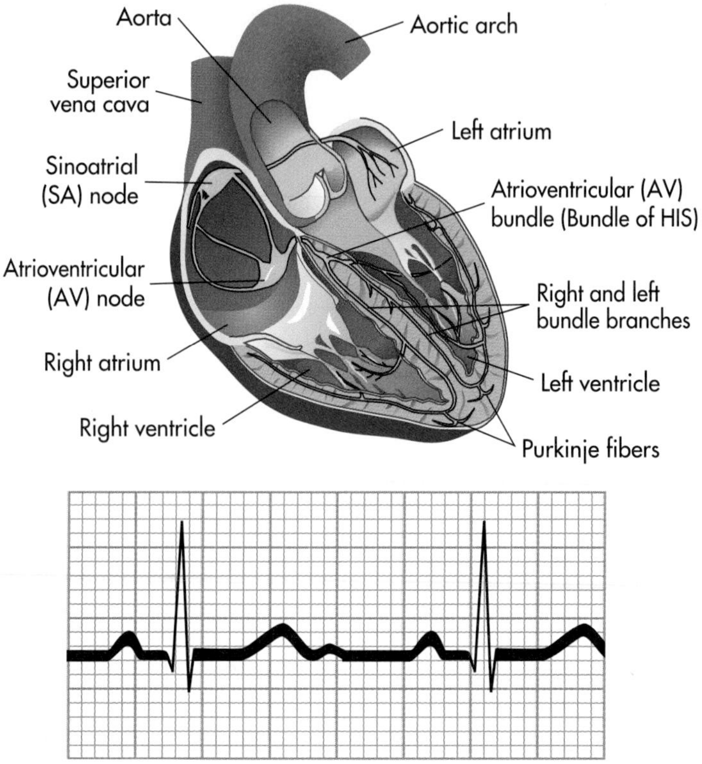

Figure 8-15

Each part of the ECG tracing is related to a certain kind of electrical activity in the heart.

during its working and relaxation phases (Figure 8-15). The ECG's shapes can be interpreted as normal or abnormal. You will learn more about the electrical activity of the heart in Chapter 15.

Problems Requiring Care

Circulatory system problems can occur as a result of several conditions. One significant problem is inadequate circulation of oxygenated blood to the vital organs, including the heart. This could result from pumping failure in the heart, from inadequate blood volume, or from a vessel blockage that impairs blood flow.

The condition in which circulation compromise causes insufficient delivery of oxygen and nutrients to the cells is known as **shock** (hypoperfusion). The body responds to shock by trying to preserve circulation to vital organs such as the heart and brain. It can do this by increasing the heart rate and force of contractions and by redistributing blood flow from noncritical organs such as the skin, skeletal muscles, and abdominal organs to more vital organs. Chapter 22 discusses this process in more detail.

Patients with cardiovascular disease may develop a build-up of material on the inside of artery walls. This condition, known as *atherosclerosis,* increases the chance of coronary artery blockage, which would compromise cardiac circulation. Severe compromise can lead to death of the heart muscle, known as a **myocardial infarction,** or heart attack. When very serious, myocardial infarctions are associated with massive damage to the left ventricle, which impairs pumping capacity.[1] **Cardiogenic shock** can develop if the heart is unable to deliver adequate circulating blood volume to perfuse the vital organs. While only approximately 5% to 10% of patients hospitalized for myocardial infarction develop cardiogenic shock, it is fatal approximately 75% of the time when it does occur.[2] In this and other types of shock, the end result could be stoppage of the heart, a condition known as **cardiac arrest.** Cardiac problems are discussed more fully in Chapter 15.

Nervous System

The **nervous system** is the most complex of all of the body systems. The ability to maintain a balanced state of function results primarily from the regulating and coordinating activities of the nervous system. This system controls all voluntary and involuntary activities of the body.

Structure and Function

The nervous system is divided into two main parts: the central nervous system and the peripheral nervous system (Figure 8-16). The **central nervous system** comprises

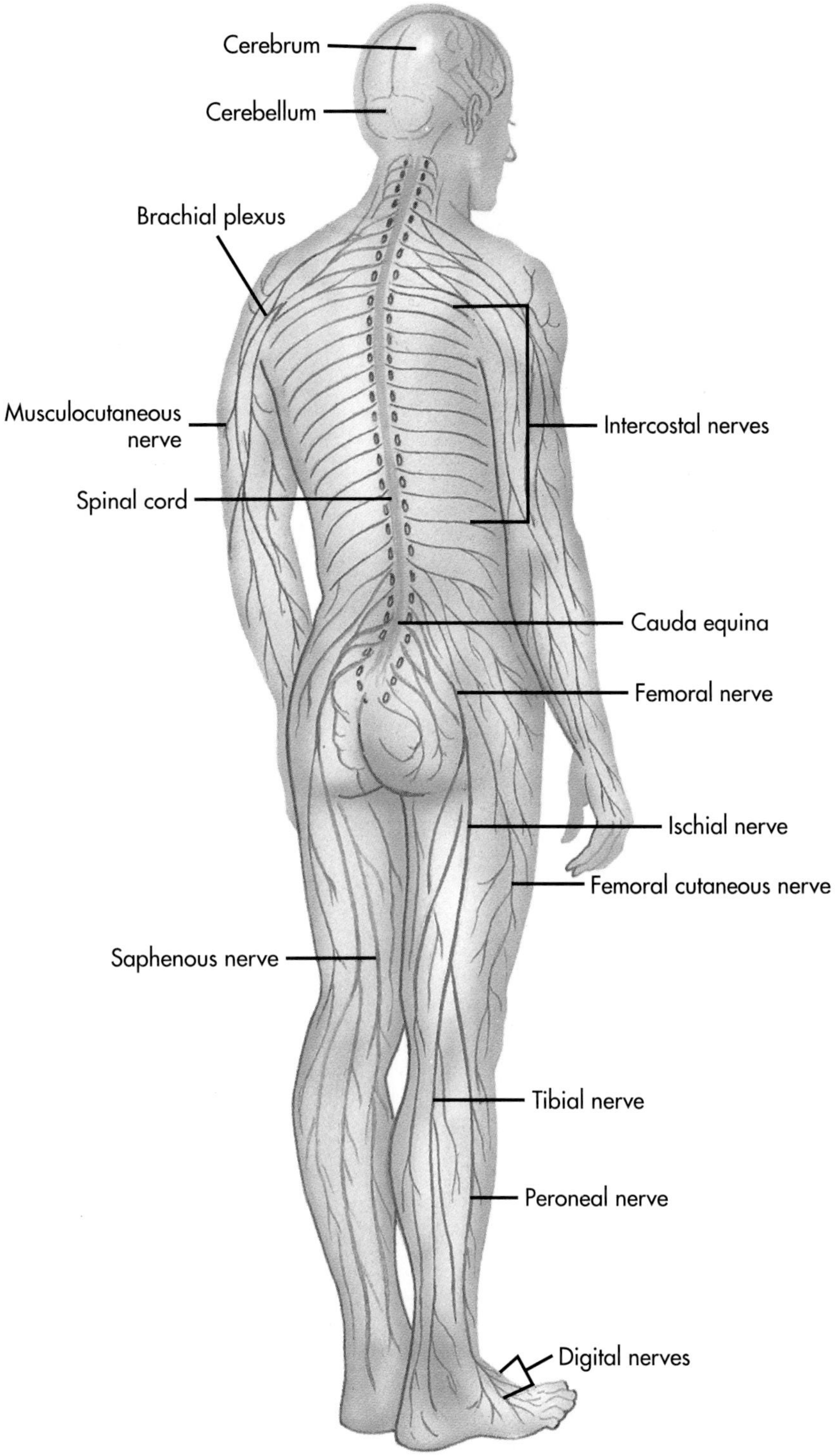

Figure 8-16

The brain and spinal cord make up the central nervous system. The peripheral nervous system consists of the motor and sensory nerves.

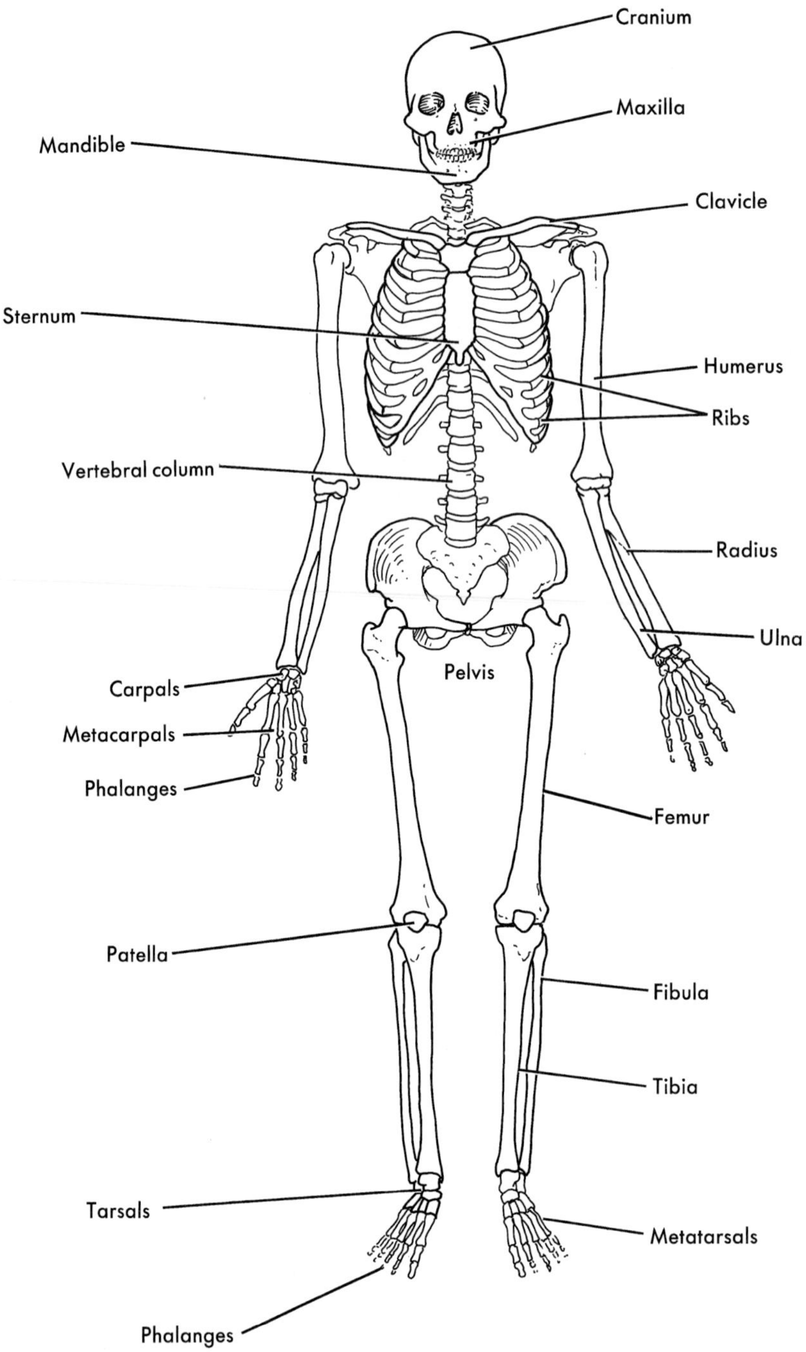

Figure 8-17

The skeleton is made up of more than 200 bones.

the brain and spinal cord. The brain, located in the cranial cavity, is the center of the nervous system. It coordinates several primary functions:

1. Motor functions (coordinated movement)
2. Sensory functions (use of the senses to gather information)
3. Autonomic functions (involuntary activities such as those managed by the digestive and endocrine systems)
4. Consciousness
5. Higher mental functions (memory, emotions, language)

The brain coordinates all body activities by receiving and transmitting information through nerves. **Nerves** transmit information as electrical impulses from one area of the body to another. The largest bundle of nerves is the spinal cord. Located in the spinal cavity and protected by the vertebrae of the spinal column, the spinal cord runs from the brain to the lower back. Nerves extend from each part of the spinal cord to create a network throughout the body.

All nerves outside the central nervous system make up the **peripheral nervous system** and are classified as either motor or sensory nerves. Sensory nerves act as "lookouts" for the body. They receive information from the environment and transmit that information through the spinal cord to special areas of the spinal cord or to the brain. The types of information transmitted include pain, pressure, heat, cold, and body position. Generally, the brain interprets the information and makes a decision about how to respond. This decision is communicated through the motor nerves, which initiate muscle movements. For example, when facial skin is exposed to cold air, sensory nerves inform the brain and the brain then triggers constriction of the skin vessels in the area, thereby reducing heat loss at the skin's surface.

The nervous system constantly interprets incoming data and makes adjustments. Some of these decisions are made consciously. However, the spinal cord can also trigger automatic reflex responses. For example, when you touch something very hot, a spinal cord reflex causes you to pull away your hand even before your brain consciously tells you that the object is hot.

Problems Requiring Care

Illness or injury that affects brain cells is particularly dangerous because brain cells cannot be replaced once they are destroyed. They rely heavily on oxygen; inadequate oxygen will quickly result in cell damage or destruction. When this happens, as in shock, the level of consciousness is one of the first things affected. This is also true of the brain's reliance on sugar. If the cells fail to get adequate sugar from the bloodstream, changes in consciousness follow quickly. The lack of oxygen or sugar can also result in seizures.

The transportation of oxygen and other nutrients to the brain can be affected by injury, such as head trauma. Blood can pool within the brain and skull, creating increased pressure in the skull or brain and restricting oxygen delivery. This too can result in altered levels of consciousness and possibly seizures.

Injury to the spinal cord can result in paralysis below the injury site or respiratory paralysis if the injury occurs in the upper cervical (neck) vertebrae (see Chapter 25). Trauma to the extremities can cause nerve damage and result in a lack of sensation or limb movement.

Musculoskeletal System

The **musculoskeletal system** provides a framework for support, protection, and movement of the body. It comprises bones, muscles, and connective tissues that include cartilage, tendons, and ligaments. It is one of the more frequently injured body systems.

Structure and Function

Bones. More than 200 bones make up the skeleton. This rigid framework gives shape to the body, protects organs from injury, enables body movement, and provides attachment points for muscles and tendons. The skeleton can be divided into two general areas: central (axial) and peripheral (appendicular) (Figure 8-17).

The central skeleton consists of the skull, mandible (lower jaw), rib cage, and spinal column. The skull is made up of 8 bones that form the cranial cavity, and 14 facial bones. The cranial bones fit together at tight joints called *sutures.* These sutures enable the bones to move slightly without breaking. The facial bones form the structure of the face. Among these are the mandible, maxilla (upper jaw), zygomatic bones (cheeks), nasal bone (nose), and orbits (eye sockets).

The spinal column is made up of 33 bones, divided into 5 regions: cervical (7), thoracic (12), lumbar (5), sacral (5), and coccyx (4) (Figure 8-18). The cervical vertebrae make up the neck, and the thoracic vertebrae form the upper and mid back. The bones of the lumbar region comprise the lower back, and the sacral bones form a joint with the pelvis. The fused bones of the coccyx make up the tail bone. These bones, called **vertebrae,** are stacked on top of one another and are separated by disks that allow movement and absorb shock. Each vertebra has a canal in its center, through which the spinal cord runs.

The thorax contains 12 pairs of ribs, which make up the rib cage. Each of these ribs attaches to a thoracic vertebra posteriorly. Ribs 1 to 10 also attach anteriorly to the sternum (breastbone). The lowest two pairs of ribs, called the *floating ribs,* are fixed to the other ribs by cartilage rather than attaching directly to the sternum. The upper third of the sternum is called the *manubrium;* the large portion in the middle is called the body of the sternum; and the lower end is the *xiphoid process,* which

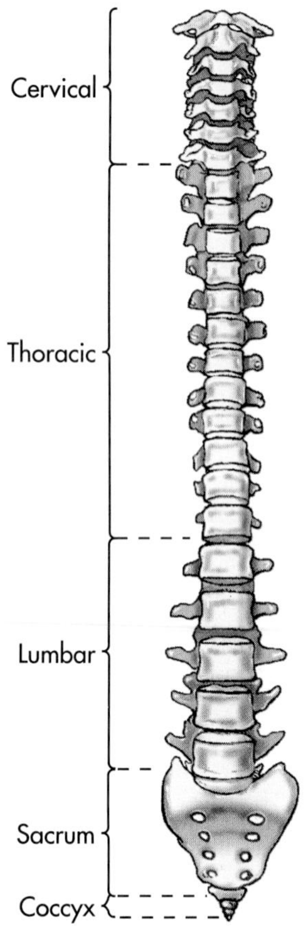

Figure 8-18

Five regions of the spinal column.

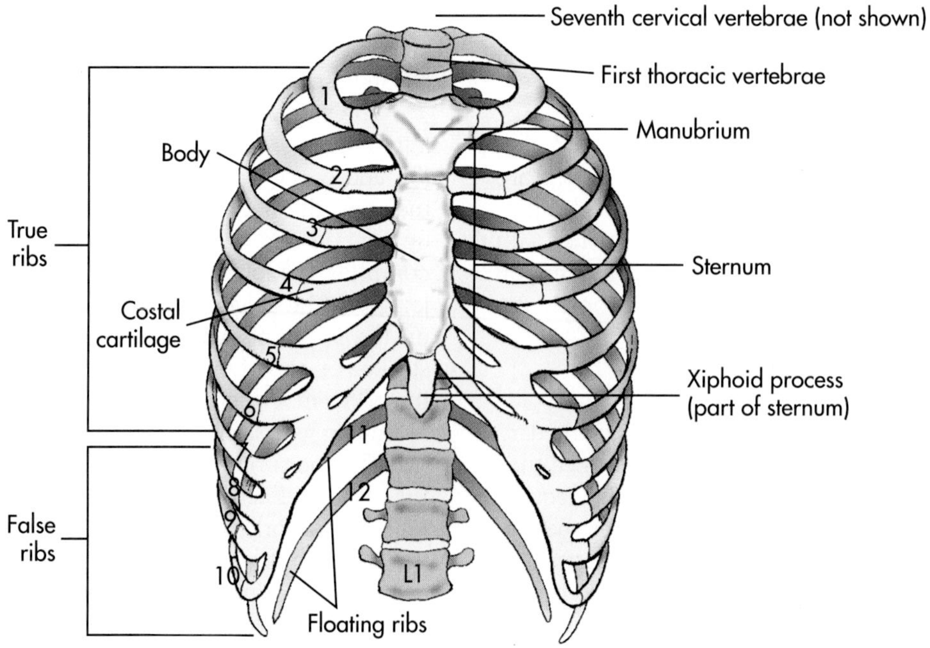

Figure 8-19

Twelve pairs of ribs make up the rib cage.

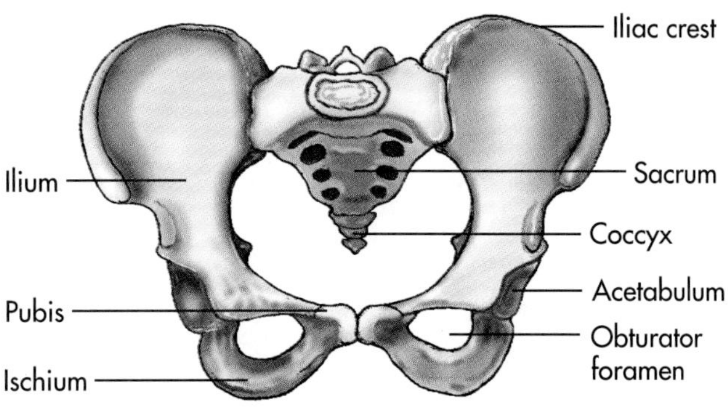

Figure 8-20

The pelvis is formed from the sacral vertebrae and additional fused bones.

serves as a landmark for hand placement during cardiopulmonary resuscitation (CPR). The rib cage provides protection for many of the body's most vital organs, including the heart, lungs, spleen, and liver (Figure 8-19).

The peripheral skeleton is made of bones that form extremities, including the arms and legs and the "girdles" that attach them to the central skeleton. The girdle for the legs is the pelvis, and for the arms it is the clavicles and scapula (shoulder girdle).

The pelvis is formed in the rear by the sacral vertebrae. Additional fused bones form the pelvic girdle. The *ischia* (singular: ischium) are the two looped "sit bones" in the posterior pelvis. The superior portions of the pelvic girdle are the *iliac crests* or wings. The pelvic bones attach in the front at the *pubic symphysis.* The socket where the leg (femur) attaches to the pelvic girdle on each side is the *acetabulum* (Figure 8-20). The pelvis provides some protection for organs such as the bladder, ureter, rectum, and female reproductive organs.

The *femur,* the bone of the upper leg, is the largest bone of the body. The proximal head of the femur meets the acetabulum in the pelvic girdle to form the hip joint. The femur extends to the knee, where it joins with the two bones of the lower leg, the *tibia* and *fibula.* The *patella* (kneecap) helps protect the structures of the knee from frontal injury. Of the two bones of the lower leg, the tibia is the largest and the main weight-bearing bone. The fibula, which does not bear weight, aids with ankle movement. Both the tibia and fibula also form part of the ankle. The distal portion of the tibia on the medial side of the leg forms the *medial malleolus* of the ankle. On the lateral leg, the distal fibula forms the *lateral malleolus.* The bones of the foot include the tarsals, metatarsals, calcaneus (heel), and phalanges (toes) (Figure 8-21).

The upper extremities begin with the bones of the shoulder girdle, the *scapula* in the rear and *clavicle* in the front. These two bones join at the acromioclavicular (AC) joint. The *humerus* is the single bone of the upper arm. It joins the scapula in the shoulder girdle and the two bones of the lower arm (radius and ulna) at the elbow.

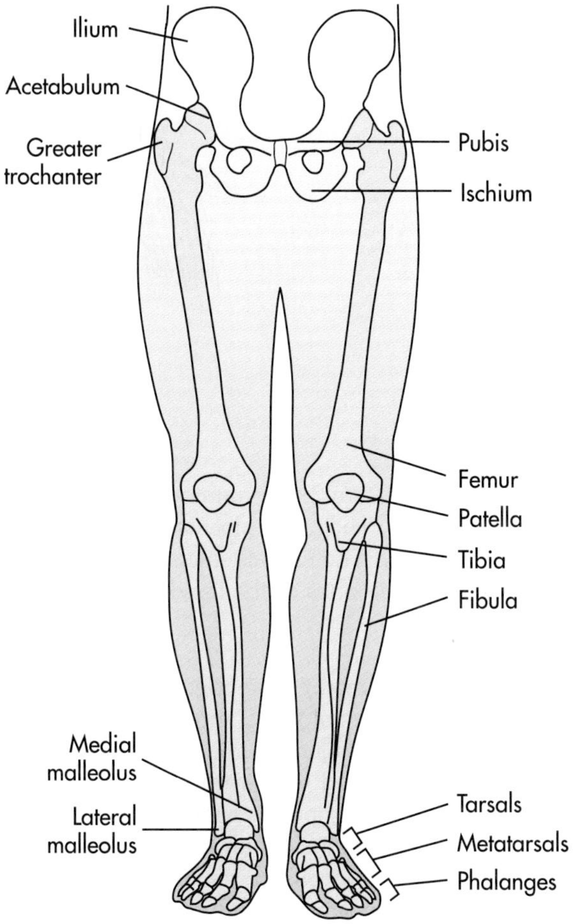

Figure 8-21

Bones of the lower extremities.

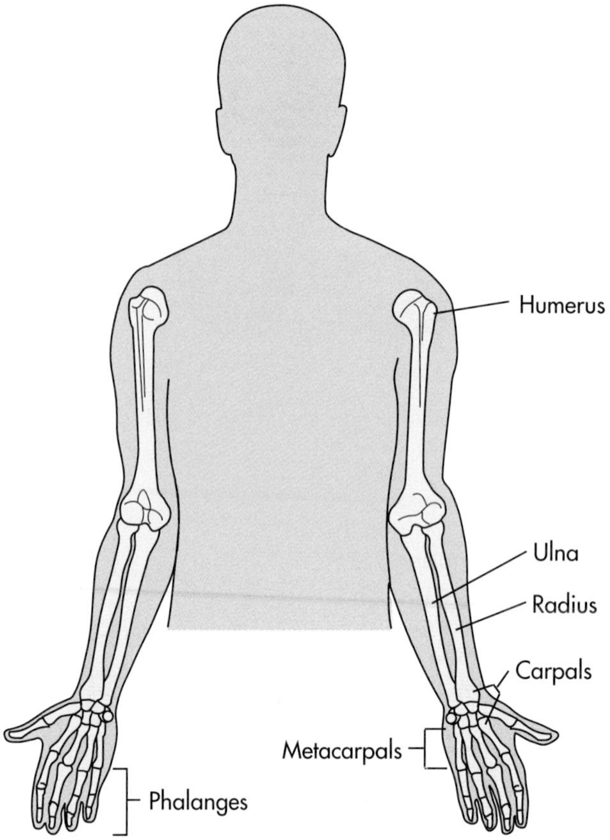

Figure 8-22

Bones of the upper extremities.

The *radius* is the lateral bone running along the thumb side of the forearm. The *ulna* is located along the medial side of the forearm. The carpals, metacarpals, and phalanges make up the bones of the hands and fingers (Figure 8-22).

Joints. Joints are formed where bones join other bones. There are several types of joints, most notably hinge and ball-and-socket joints (Figure 8-23). The bone surfaces in these joints are covered with a thin layer of cartilage, which provides for a smooth surface where the bones meet. Synovial fluid, found within the joint, helps create lubrication for easier movement. Hinge joints only permit movement in one plane and are found in the elbows, fingers, knees, and toes. Ball-and-socket joints, which allow for a greater range of motion, are found in the shoulders and hips. Bones are often held together at joints by fibrous bands called **ligaments.** Ligaments aid movement but also limit range of motion.

Muscles. There are three types of muscles: skeletal, smooth, and cardiac (Figure 8-24). Movement of body parts depends on skeletal muscles, which have the ability to contract (shorten). Skeletal muscles are voluntary muscles that are attached to bones by tendons. When these muscles contract, they provide the necessary force to move the body.

Unlike skeletal muscles, smooth muscles are involuntary. They automatically carry out many of the body's functions, such as digestion. Smooth muscles are circular and are found in the walls of tubelike structures such as the intestines, bronchi, and blood vessels. When they contract, they change the internal diameter of the tube and thus regulate the flow of substances through the tube.

Cardiac muscle is found only in the heart. Like the brain, it is extremely sensitive to decreases in oxygen, and like smooth muscle, it is involuntary. Cardiac muscle has the ability to contract on its own. This property, known as *automaticity,* enables the heart to generate and conduct electrical impulses without depending entirely on outside nervous or hormonal control.

Problems Requiring Care

Musculoskeletal injuries include fractured (broken) bones and dislocated (displaced) joints. Injuries also commonly occur to ligaments and tendons. Ligaments protecting a joint can be sprained (stretched) or torn, and tendons and muscles are subject to the same injuries. EMS providers will often not be able to determine the extent of the damage. In some situations, injuries will not look severe, but

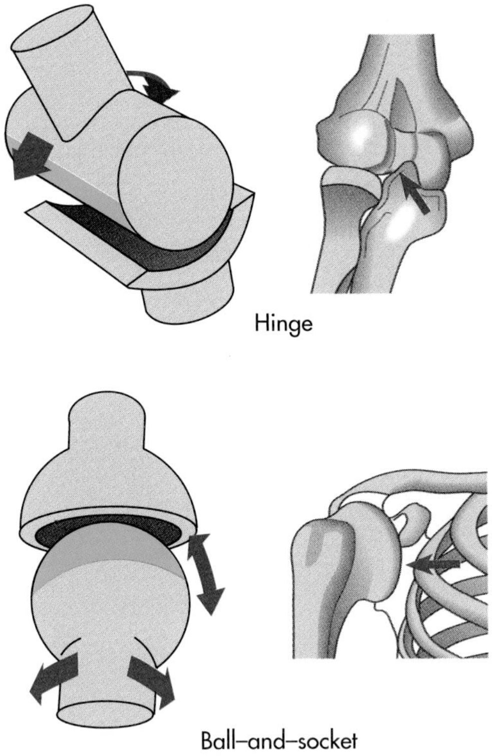

Figure 8-23

Joints are formed where bones join other bones.

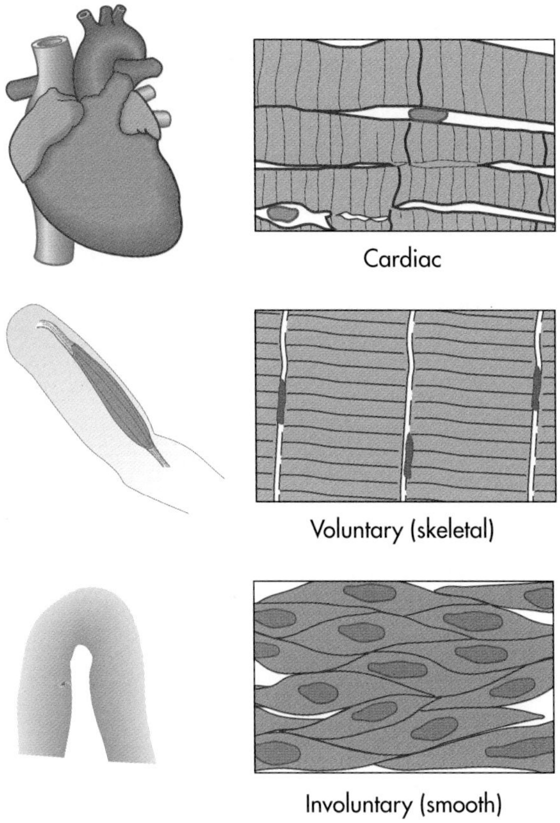

Figure 8-24

Skeletal, smooth, and cardiac muscle.

damage to nearby nerves and blood vessels can cause serious problems. For example, an injured elbow can impair circulation and nerve transmission below the point of injury, or a fractured rib could puncture a lung and cause a respiratory emergency. You will learn more about musculoskeletal injuries in Chapter 24.

Integumentary System (Skin)

The **integumentary system** is the largest system in the body. It is made up of skin, hair, nails, and glands. The skin covers the musculoskeletal system and helps protect the body from injury and invading microorganisms. It also helps retain fluids, prevent dehydration, and regulate temperature.

Structure and Function

One of the skin's most important functions is its ability to repel disease-producing microorganisms. Its tough, elastic fibers stretch easily without tearing, protecting it from injury.

The skin has three layers: the epidermis, dermis, and subcutaneous tissue (Figure 8-25). The epidermis is the outermost layer, consisting of cells that are continually rubbed away and replaced by new cells generated beneath the surface. The next layer, the dermis, is much thicker than the epidermis and is largely made up of connective tissue. The dermis also houses nerve endings that provide sensory information about touch, temperature, pain, and pressure. Hair follicles, blood vessels, and sweat and sebaceous (oil) glands are also found in the dermis. The third layer, which is composed of connective tissue and fat, is the subcutaneous tissue. This layer serves as a shock absorber, protecting underlying tissue from injury, and acts as an insulating layer that minimizes heat loss.

Blood supplies the skin with nutrients and to some degree is responsible for changes in skin appearance. When temperatures are hot, blood vessels dilate, allowing blood to circulate closer to the surface of the skin to eliminate body heat. This makes the skin feel warm and appear flushed. Because sweat glands function to maintain normal internal body temperature, they produce sweat as the temperature increases, making the skin feel moist. As this moisture evaporates, the body cools. During prolonged cold temperatures, blood vessels in the skin constrict in an effort to shunt blood to the vital organs for warmth. The skin feels cool and looks pale because less blood is circulating near the skin.

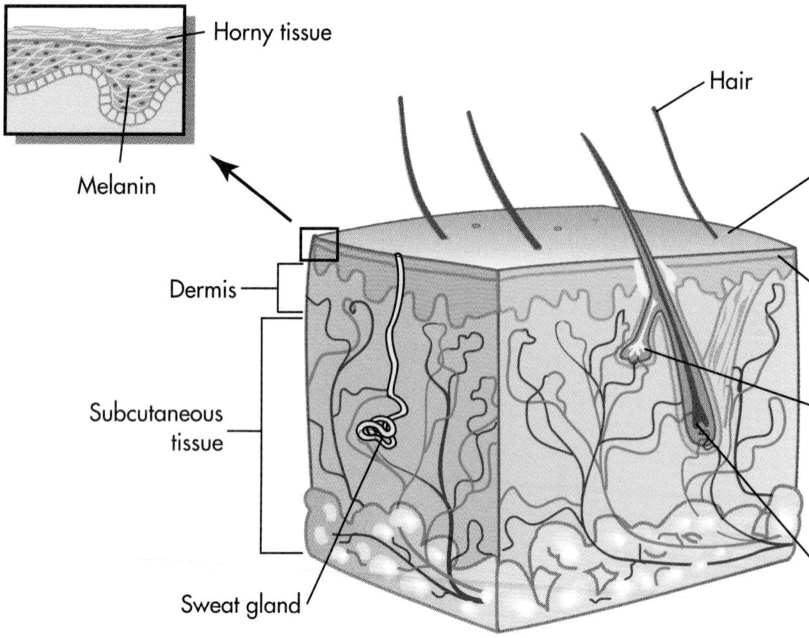

Figure 8-25

Layers of the skin.

DID YOU KNOW . . . ?

- There are more than 700 million alveoli in your lungs.
- The lungs would spread out to cover an area the size of a tennis court, while the skin would cover only 20 square feet.
- You breathe approximately 23,000 times a day, 8½ million times a year, and 630 million times in a lifetime of 75 years.
- The average heart beats approximately 100,000 times a day, 36 million times a year, and 2½ billion times in a lifetime of 75 years.
- There are more than 62,000 miles of capillaries in the body.
- Blood will travel completely through the body approximately 516,000 times a year.
- Nerve impulses can travel the length of a football field in less than 1 second.
- At birth an infant has approximately 350 bones, while an adult has approximately 200 bones.
- The small intestine is approximately 20 feet long, while the large intestine is only 5 feet long. Together they are approximately as tall as a 2-story building.
- Food spends approximately 10 seconds being chewed in the mouth, 10 seconds passing through the pharynx and esophagus, 3½ hours in the stomach, 4 hours in the small intestine, and 20 hours in the large intestine before being excreted.
- There are approximately 650 muscles in the body.
- There are more than 2 million sweat glands in the body.
- In the bone marrow, about 115 million red blood cells are generated every minute.

From Gab M: *Questions and answers: our body and science,* London, 1990, Christensen Press; and Sanders MJ et al: *Mosby's paramedic text,* St Louis, 1994, Mosby.

Problems Requiring Care

Objects can burn, cut, tear, scrape, puncture, or bruise the skin. Breaks in the skin can result in infection and loss of vital fluids. Extreme heat or cold can burn or freeze the skin. Heat-related illness can result in a breakdown in the sweat mechanism, causing the sweat glands to fail and the body to retain heat.

You will learn more about the problems that affect the skin and how to provide care for these problems in later chapters.

Digestive System

The **digestive system,** also called the *gastrointestinal system*, ingests food, transports it through the digestive tract, absorbs nutrients, and eliminates waste.

Structure and Function

Figure 8-26 shows the major organs of the digestive system. Food enters this system through the mouth and passes into the *esophagus,* where muscular contractions

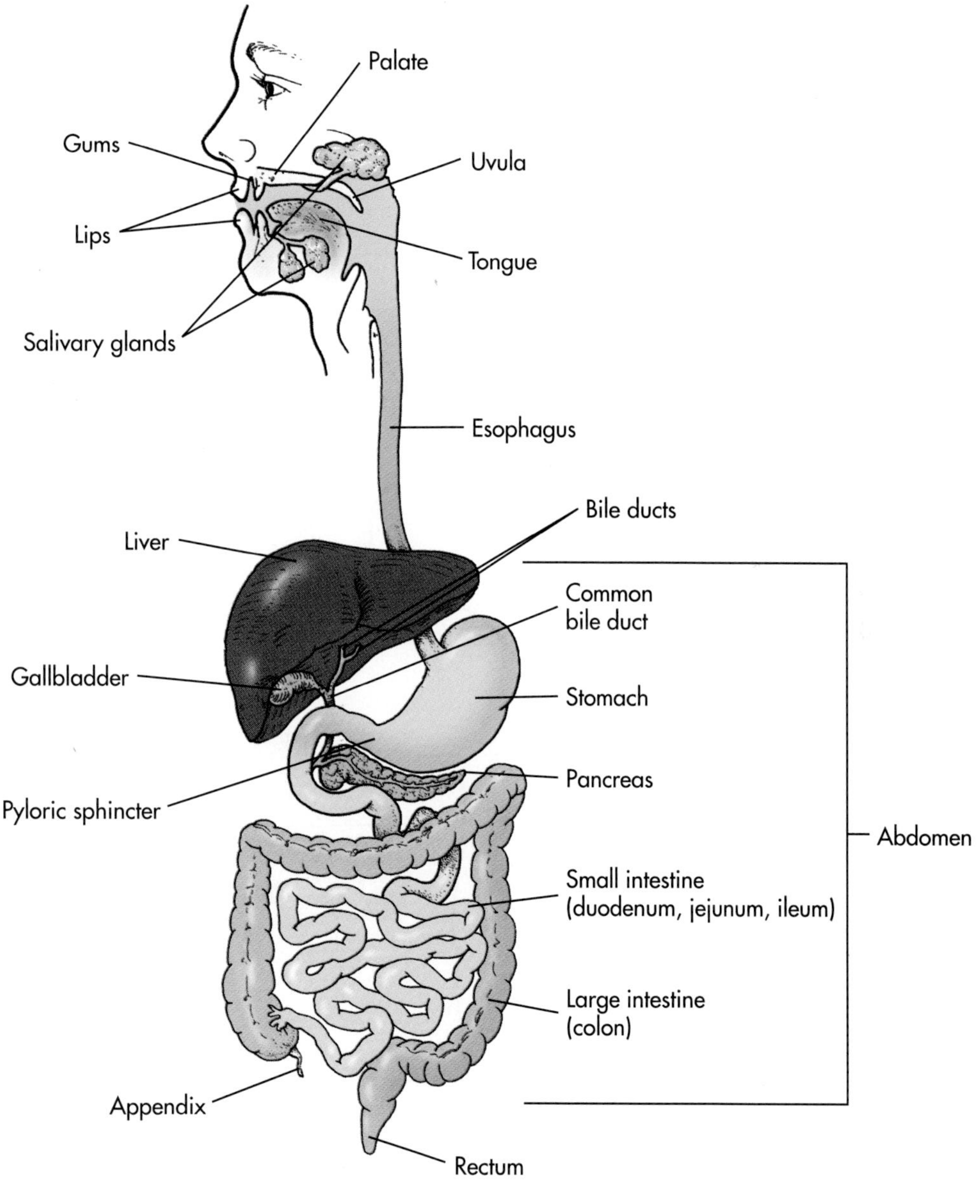

Figure 8-26

Digestive system.

push the food into the *stomach.* The stomach acts as a storage area where food is mixed with gastric secretions that help break it down. At the lower end of the stomach, food enters the first section of the small intestine, the *duodenum.* With assistance from chemicals secreted by the *liver* and *pancreas,* it is further digested and moved through the remaining small intestine (*jejunum* and *ileum*) to the large intestine *(colon).* The final absorption of water and nutrients occurs there, as does the conversion of the remaining food to feces, which is eliminated through the *rectum.*

Problems Requiring Care

Because most of the digestive organs lie in the relatively unprotected abdominal cavity, they are vulnerable to injury. Blunt or penetrating trauma can result in blood loss from damage to these internal organs. The digestive organs can also spill wastes into the abdominal cavity, which causes severe pain and may produce infection. Illness affecting the liver can be serious. Hepatitis, an inflammatory condition of the liver, can cause extended illness and is occasionally fatal.

Endocrine System

Like the nervous system, the **endocrine system** acts as a regulatory system to help coordinate the activities of other body systems.

Structure and Function

The endocrine system consists of various glands that release **hormones** (chemical messengers) into the blood (Figure 8-27). These hormones influence body functions. Two important hormones are epinephrine (adrenaline) and insulin. **Epinephrine,** secreted by the adrenal glands, helps the body respond to stressful situations. **Insulin** is produced in the pancreas and is critical for effective use of the sugar glucose that fuels the body. Among the other endocrine glands, the thyroid and pituitary glands are particularly important. The thyroid secretes hormones that regulate metabolic functions, and the pituitary produces hormones that control growth and development.

Hormones are not always maintained at a constant level within the body. Thyroid hormones are maintained in a relatively constant range; however, epinephrine is re-

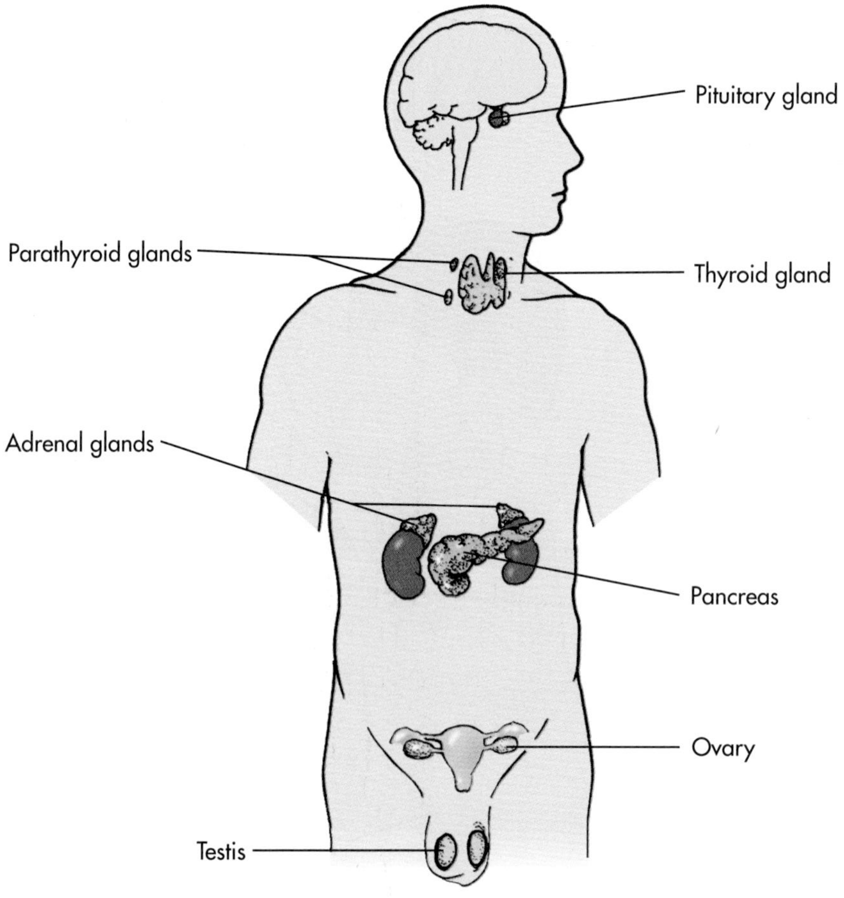

Figure 8-27
Endocrine system.

leased in large amounts in response to stressful conditions such as injury or physical exertion. Similarly, insulin is released after the body recognizes an increase in blood glucose.

Problems Requiring Care

The most frequent endocrine system emergency that EMTs encounter involves a diabetic patient who fails to balance sugar and insulin levels. Without adequate insulin, the body cells cannot absorb the glucose they need from the blood. As a result, glucose builds up in the bloodstream; and cells become starved and begin to use other sources of energy, such as fat. This results in the production of acids, which causes numerous problems with body functions. Some of the excess glucose in the blood is eliminated in the urine. Over a period of hours or days, the patient can become dehydrated and experience abdominal cramps and a decreased level of consciousness.

Too much insulin, or too little sugar, results in low blood sugar levels. This deprives the brain of the sugar it needs to function normally. It can result in a rapid onset of problems that include an altered level of consciousness and seizures. You will learn more about how to recognize and care for diabetic emergencies in Chapter 16.

Urinary System

The **urinary system** works with other body systems to help maintain an internal state of fluid and chemical balance. It does this by removing waste products and keeping fluid volume and composition constant.

Structure and Function

The urinary system consists of the kidneys, ureters, bladder, and urethra. There are two **kidneys,** located in the lower, posterior portion of the trunk on either side of the spine. The kidneys filter waste products from the blood and produce urine. The average adult produces 1 to 2 liters of urine per day. The urine is transported from the kidneys to the bladder by means of two tubelike structures called **ureters.** The **bladder** is a hollow, muscular organ lying in the pelvic cavity that holds the urine until it is ready to be excreted through the **urethra** (Figure 8-28).

Problems Requiring Care

Significant trauma to the back or pelvis can injure the kidneys or bladder, respectively. However, trauma is not the only major problem that requires care. The aging process causes significant functional changes in the kidneys. Blood flow is reduced, as is the effectiveness of filtration. This can lead to fluid and electrolyte imbalances and toxic conditions as a result of medication or drug use. Kidney stones may develop at any age; movement of these stones is very painful and often causes blood in the urine. The severe pain usually causes patients to seek medical care.

Reproductive System

The **reproductive system** consists of the organs involved in the conception, development, and delivery of human offspring. It is the system that differs most between male and female bodies. This section discusses the male reproductive system; the female system is covered in Chapter 21.

Structure and Function

The primary organs and structures of the male reproductive system are the testes (gonads), prostate gland, seminal vesicle, penis, and a number of connecting tubes or ducts (Figure 8-29). The urethra, part of the urinary system, belongs to this system as well because of its second function, which is transmission of seminal fluid to the female during sexual intercourse. The functions of all of these organs relate to the production and delivery of seminal fluid.

IT'S YOUR CALL
CONCLUSION

The mechanism of injury in your patient's bicycle accident was significant and appears to have resulted in multisystem trauma. Her obvious injuries are musculoskeletal, possibly involving broken or dislocated bones and damaged ligaments and tendons. However, these injuries could have easily caused damage to other organs. Closer evaluation of the chest reveals bruising and mild difficulty breathing. She may have broken ribs and a punctured lung. The force of the fall could also have been severe enough to injure the heart directly. Even without specific signs of cardiac injury, the circulatory system has been affected by blood loss from several wounds. It is also possible that she has injured her nervous system. Although a bike helmet can absorb some of the impact, the speed and type of collision could have resulted in significant head injury. The pain she is experiencing in her back could simply be musculoskeletal or it could represent a much more serious spinal injury.

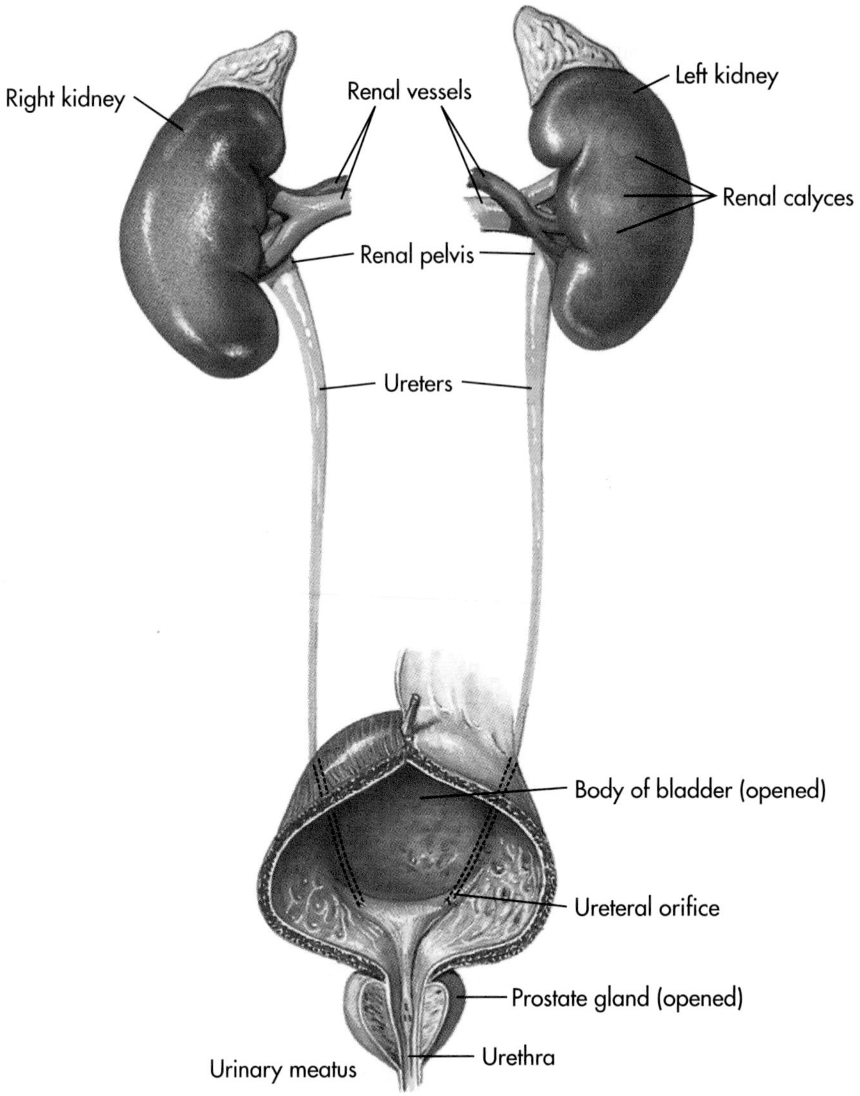

Figure 8-28
Urinary system.

Problems Requiring Care

Most emergencies involving the male reproductive system relate to trauma to the external genitals: the penis and testes. The **testes** are suspended in the scrotal sac, or **scrotum,** and, along with the penis, are subject to both blunt and penetrating trauma. A number of medical conditions can also present with genital signs or symptoms, including infections and kidney and urinary disorders. Structural problems such as hernias and prostate enlargement can also occur. Field care is limited to standard management of any threatening problems, such as external bleeding and signs of shock.

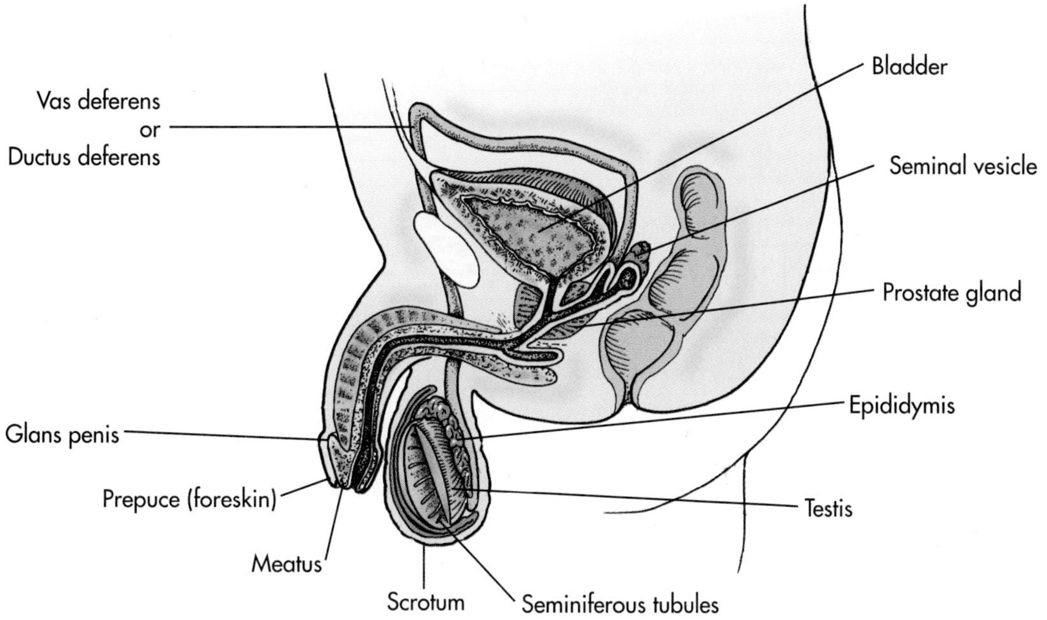

Figure 8-29

Primary organs of the male reproductive system.

SUMMARY

Your knowledge of anatomic landmarks, terminology, and body systems will help you understand how illness and injury can impair the functions of these systems. The systems you should be familiar with include the respiratory, circulatory, nervous, musculoskeletal, integumentary, digestive, endocrine, urinary, and reproductive systems.

When assessing a patient's condition, consider how injury or illness in one body system can cause changes in other systems. Part of an EMT's job is determining whether those changes are natural responses, such as increased heart rate in response to pain, or are signs of more serious problems.

In the next two chapters you will learn how to conduct a systematic body assessment to locate possible problems. Your interpretation of what you find and your ability to recognize multisystem problems will depend on your understanding of normal function.

REFERENCES

1. **American Heart Association:** Guidelines for cardiopulmonary resuscitation and emergency cardiac care, *J Am Med Assoc* 268:2177, 1992.
2. **Rappaport EM et al:** Guidelines for the early management of patients with acute myocardial infarction, *J Am Coll Cardiol* 16:249, 1990.

SUGGESTED READINGS

1. **Seeley RR, Stephens TD, Tate P:** *Anatomy and physiology*, ed 2, St Louis, 1992, Mosby.

Section 4

Patient Assessment

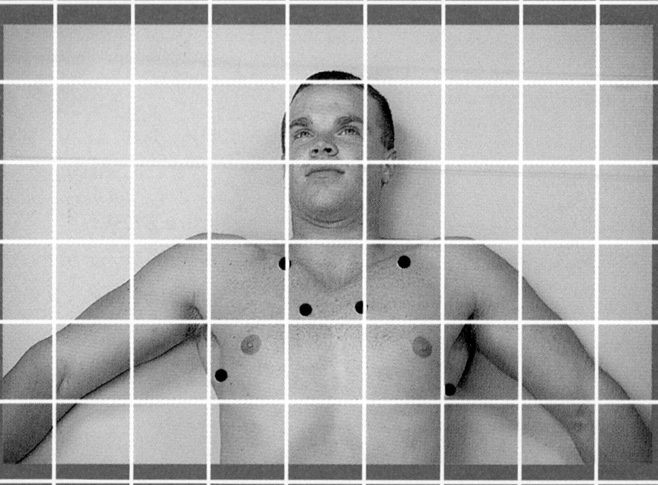

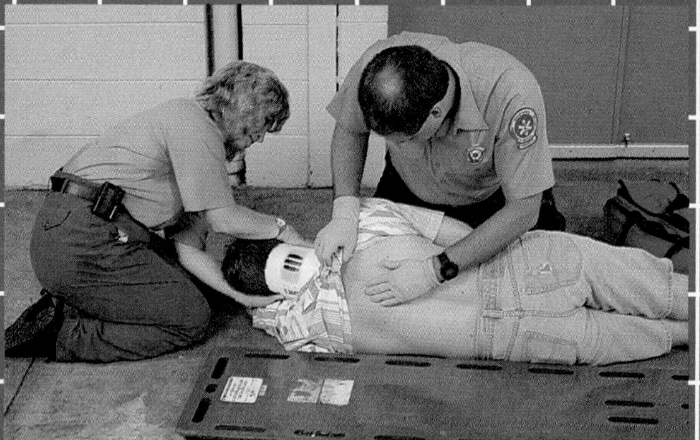

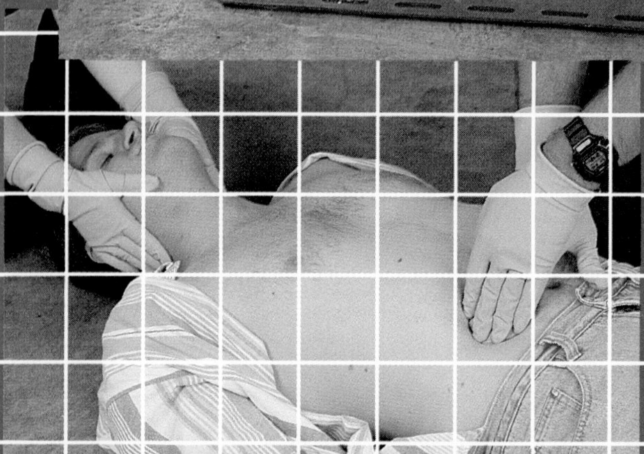

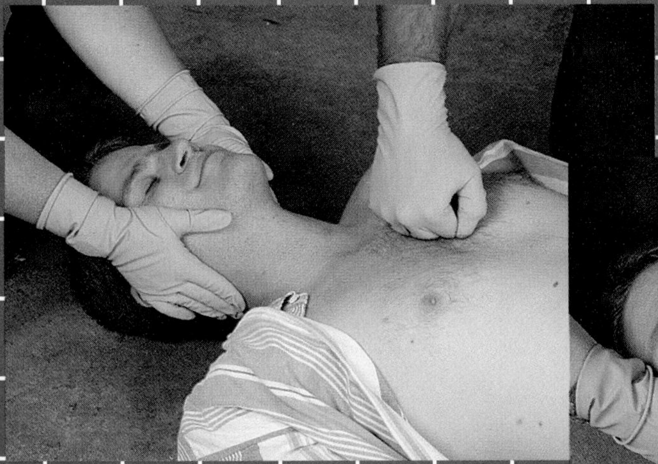
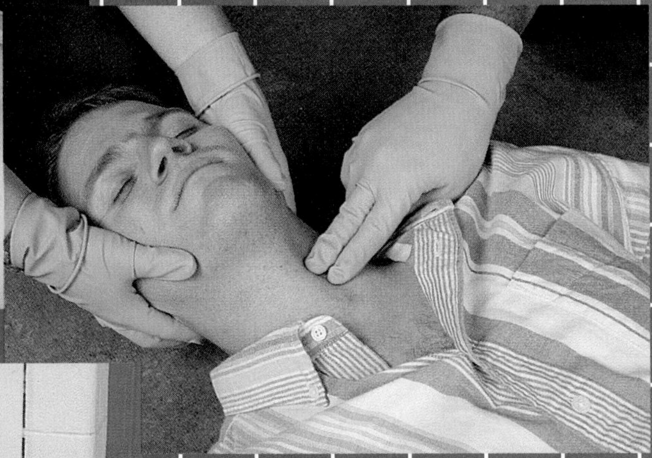
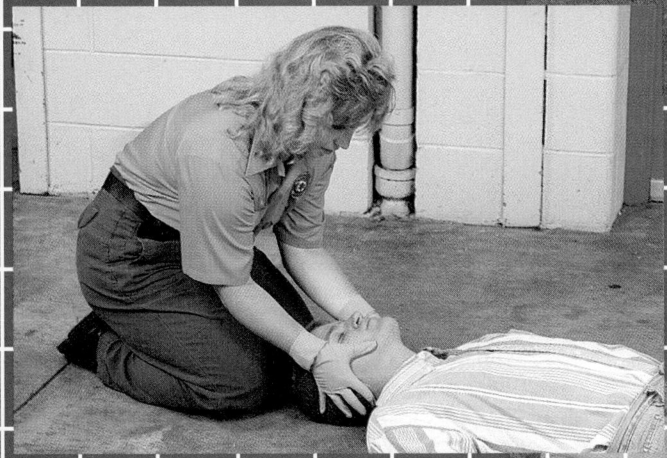
 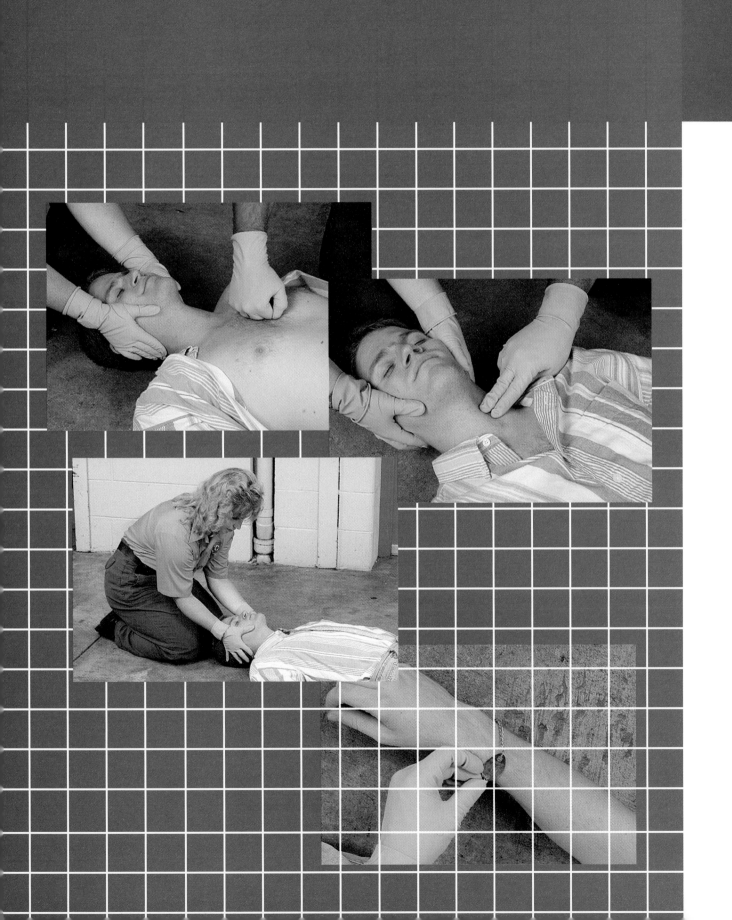

Chapter

Initial Patient Assessment

9

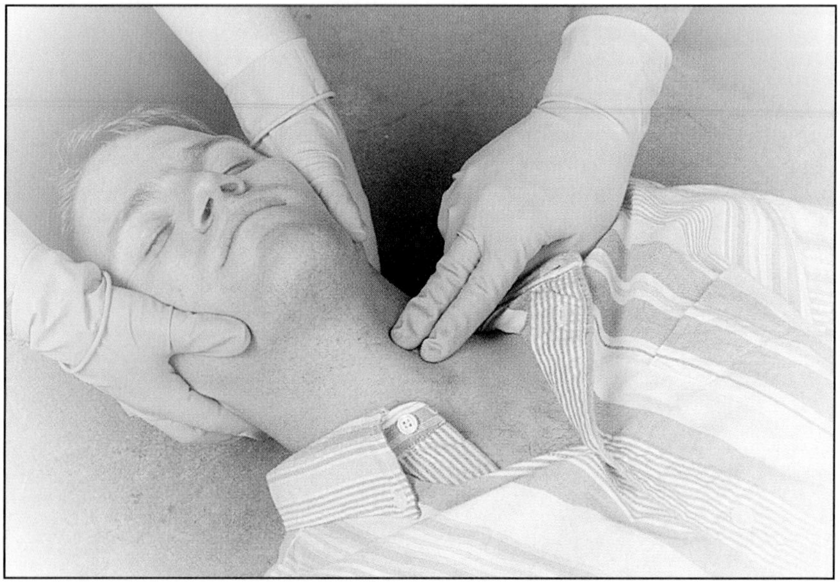

Knowledge Objectives

As an EMT-Basic, you should be able to:

OBJECTIVES

1. Explain why it is important to form a general impression of your patient's condition upon arrival.
2. Describe how to use your senses to recognize immediately life-threatening conditions.
3. Describe how to assess level of consciousness.
4. Describe how to assess airway adequacy.
5. Explain why it is important to properly manage the cervical spine in trauma patients.
6. Describe how to assess breathing rate and quality.
7. Differentiate between a patient with normal breathing and one with abnormal breathing.
8. Describe how to assess pulse rate and pulse quality.
9. Differentiate between a patient with a normal pulse and one with an abnormal pulse.
10. State the importance of assessing a patient for severe external bleeding.
11. Differentiate between a patient with normal skin conditions and one with abnormal skin conditions.
12. Describe how to assess skin capillary refill.
13. Explain the importance of prioritizing a patient for care and transport.
14. Describe how to care for each of the following life-threatening conditions:
    - Unconsciousness
    - Airway obstruction
    - Absent breathing
    - Difficulty breathing
    - Absent pulse
    - Severe bleeding
    - Inadequate perfusion

OBJECTIVES

Skill Objectives

As an EMT-Basic, you should be able to:

1. **Demonstrate how to assess mental status.**
2. **Demonstrate how to assess airway adequacy.**
3. **Demonstrate how to make quick initial assessments of the following vital signs:**
   - **Level of consciousness**
   - **Breathing**
   - **Pulse**
   - **Skin signs**
   - **Capillary refill**
4. **When given a patient scenario, demonstrate how to conduct an initial assessment and identify transport priority.**

Attitude Objectives

As an EMT-Basic, you should be able to:

1. **Describe your feelings about conducting an initial patient assessment.**
2. **Serve as a role model for others, demonstrating the importance of following a systematic plan for initial patient assessment.**

KEY TERMS

1. **Auscultation:** The use of a stethoscope to listen to sounds in the body, such as breath and blood pressure sounds.
2. **AVPU: A**lert, **V**erbal, **P**ainful, **U**nresponsive; a four-point assessment of level of consciousness based on patient response.
3. **Capillary Refill:** The time required by a capillary bed to refill after the application and release of pressure in an area such as the nail bed or finger pad. Refill time of 2 seconds or less is considered normal.
4. **Chief Complaint:** The most important, current problem as reported by the patient.
5. **Cyanosis:** Bluish discoloration of the skin caused by inadequate oxygenation of the blood.
6. **History:** Subjective information about a patient's condition, as reported by the patient.
7. **History of Present Illness (or Incident):** Information provided by a patient about the current event; begins with the chief complaint and proceeds to questions that gather more information about it.
8. **Initial Assessment:** The first phase of the patient-assessment process; used to rapidly identify and correct immediate threats to life that include consciousness, airway, breathing, and circulation problems.
9. **Level of Consciousness (LOC):** A patient's state of awareness and orientation. Initial assessment may be done on a four-point scale (see *AVPU*).
10. **Pulse:** The wave of pressure in the blood generated by the pumping of blood from the heart.
11. **Sign:** A readily observed objective indicator of a patient's condition, such as sweating or vomiting (in contrast to subjective elements; see *symptom*).
12. **Symptom:** A subjective (history) factor that is not readily observable and must be described by a patient, such as the presence and location of pain (in contrast to objective elements; see *sign*).
13. **Vital Signs:** Signs that indicate the level of function in vital body systems. Usual vital-sign measurements include level of consciousness, respirations, pulse, blood pressure, skin signs, and pupils.

IT'S YOUR CALL

You are dispatched to a call for an illness and on the way are informed that prearrival instructions are being provided to a family member because she thinks her father is not breathing. You arrive to find a crying, 16-year-old female kneeling beside her 45-year-old father.

You quickly determine that the scene is safe, take precautions against disease transmission, and begin to check the patient. The daughter says that her father began to look ill while they were out shopping, and he decided they should come home. He made it into the living room, where he collapsed on the couch. Moments later, he did not seem to be breathing.

You check to see if he is conscious, but he does not respond. You determine that this is a medical rather than a trauma emergency and move the patient to the floor.

You need to assess the patient. What should you check for and in what order?

Most patients you will encounter as an EMT will be conscious and able to provide you with information about why you were summoned. These patients will be relatively easy to assess and will be able to assist you by answering questions. However, patients with immediately life-threatening conditions may be unable to provide information. In these situations, you will not have either the time or the need to do a lengthy patient examination. Instead, you will perform the first few steps of the patient-assessment process. These first steps, the initial assessment, are the core of all patient-assessment skills. The **initial assessment** is a systematic approach to identifying the most critical conditions a patient may be experiencing.

General Patient Impression

In previous chapters, you learned about scene safety and the importance of considering the mechanism of injury or the nature of illness. As you arrive on the scene, take precautions to avoid disease transmission and consider how the incident may have occurred. In most cases, you will be able to determine if a patient has a medical or trauma problem by briefly observing the scene and the patient. Occasionally this will be less obvious. For example, when a driver has lost control of a vehicle and struck a tree, the reason for the loss of control may not be clear. The patient may tell you that it was caused by a sudden onset of severe chest pain. If the patient is unable to talk, you may be able to get helpful information from someone else or you may simply have to rely on your own observations.

As you begin to assess the patient, consider the possible mechanism of injury or nature of illness to help you form a general impression of the patient. Your general impression includes the patient's gender, approximate age and size, chief complaint, and likelihood of serious injury or illness. Rely on your sight, speech, hearing, and smell to reveal information, such as the patient's general appearance, external bleeding, vomiting, sweating, flushed or pale skin, or seizures. Your sense of smell can help identify odors such as vomit, alcohol, fecal material, or acetone (fruity) breath (sometimes found in diabetic emergencies).

Talking and listening to the patient will reveal things such as level of consciousness (LOC), presence or absence of breathing, degree of breathing difficulty, and degree of pain. The things that you can readily observe (objective findings) about the patient's condition are commonly called **signs.** Examples include vomiting or a deformed extremity. Things that are not readily observable and must be described to you by the patient (subjective findings), such as the presence and location of pain or the fact that the patient is nauseated, are referred to as **symptoms**.

Consider whether the patient's problem is medical or traumatic. Are the patient's signs and symptoms consistent with the patient's **chief complaint** and the mechanism of injury or nature of illness that you noticed upon arrival?

With this information, you can make an initial decision about transporting the patient. This is an important decision because some patients require immediate hospital care and should be transported quickly. If you are uncertain about the initial transport decision, the patient's **vital signs** can be helpful.

Vital Signs

A rapid, general assessment of vital signs can tell a great deal about a patient's overall condition and need for rapid transport. During initial assessment, the vital-signs assessment is limited to gathering quick impressions rather than taking exact measurements (Chapter 10 presents instructions for making more precise measurements). You might think of this initial vital-sign check as "semispecific." It adds more detailed information to your general impression to help you judge the severity of the patient's condition. However, it does not give the level of detail provided by vital-sign measurements.

The vital signs to check during initial assessment are:

- LOC
- Respiratory rate and quality
- Pulse rate and quality
- Skin signs

Notice that these vital signs heavily overlap with the elements of the initial assessment itself, described on p. 208. What vital signs do not include, which is critical to the initial assessment, is attention to the airway. That is discussed later in the chapter and integrates the information about vital signs into the steps of the initial assessment.

Level of Consciousness

Level of consciousness (LOC) is one of the most important indicators of a patient's overall condition. A patient's LOC can vary from being fully alert to unresponsive. The letters *A, V, P,* and *U* are used for an accurate initial description of LOC on a scale from the highest to the lowest level. These letters stand for:

A = Alert
V = Verbal stimulus
P = Painful stimulus
U = Unresponsive

Alert implies that a patient is aware of the surroundings and able to respond appropriately to questions. A person who is oriented to person, place, time, and event is said to be "alert and oriented times four." If unable or slow to respond, a patient is considered "disoriented."

Verbal refers to a patient who must be stimulated by sound in order to respond. This patient is not likely to provide complete and accurate responses.

Painful means that it requires a painful stimulus to make a patient respond. This is often done by pinching the skin on the earlobe or above the collarbone, or by rubbing the sternum (Figure 9-1). The response can be described as appropriate (patient tries to move the source of pain away) or inappropriate (patient moves some other part of the body or moans without moving).

Unresponsive describes a patient who does not respond to either verbal or painful stimulus. This is the most serious of the four LOCs.

The **AVPU** scale is a general way to get a quick impression of the patient's LOC. Chapter 10 will discuss the Glasgow Coma Scale, a more specific method that many EMS systems use to more accurately assess and document LOC.

Begin to check a patient's LOC by talking. If the patient can converse with you, much of your initial vital-sign check is done: the patient is conscious, breathing, and has a heartbeat. If the patient does not respond immediately to your voice, tap a shoulder and ask more loudly, "Can you hear me?" If there is still no response, try a painful stimulus. If this does not work, the patient is unresponsive. Note the patient's initial LOC and compare it with later assessments to identify any change in the patient's condition.

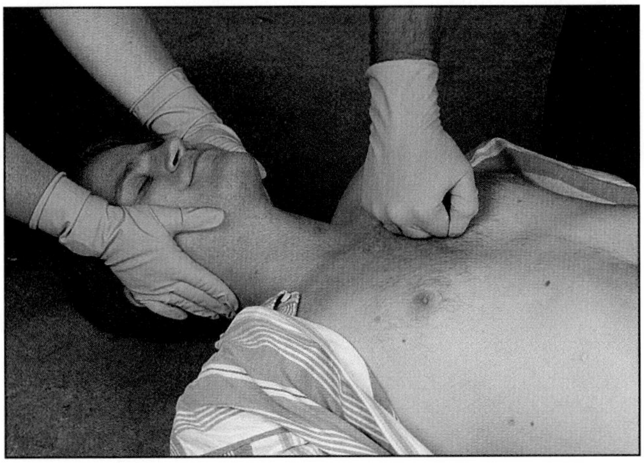

Figure 9-1

If a patient does not respond to verbal stimulus, try a painful stimulus, such as rubbing the sternum.

Respirations

If a patient is obviously breathing, observe the chest and abdomen for signs of abnormal breathing patterns or characteristics. Consider these questions:

- Is air moving? (The chest may move in an attempt to breathe, even when the airway is obstructed.)
- Is the rate very fast or slow?
- Are the respirations unusually shallow or deep?
- Does the breathing appear labored?
- Does the chest rise symmetrically (equally on both sides)?
- Is the breathing rhythm regular or irregular?
- Is there visible use of accessory breathing muscles in the neck and between the ribs (Figure 9-2) or of nasal flaring in a child (Figure 9-3)?
- Is there exaggerated abdominal motion, suggestive of heavy reliance on the diaphragm for breathing?
- Can you hear wheezing, snoring, or other abnormal breath sounds without using **auscultation?**

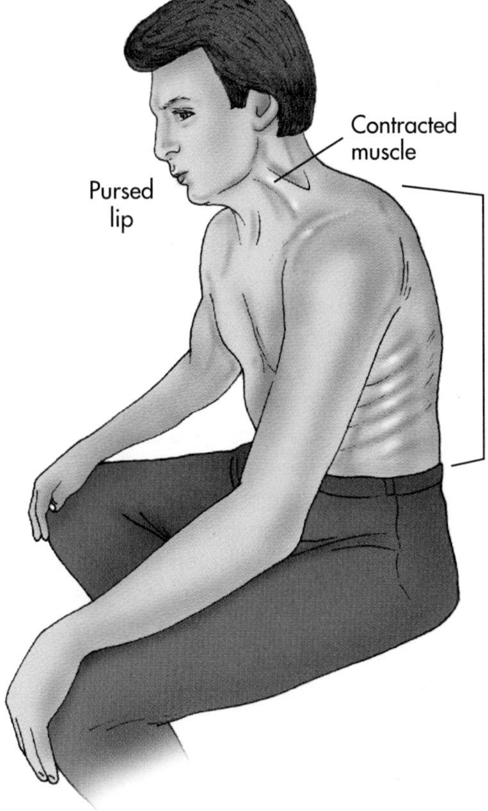

Figure 9-2

Visible accessory breathing muscles in the neck and between the ribs is a sign of abnormal breathing patterns in an adult patient.

If it is not clear whether a patient is breathing, look, listen, and feel for chest and air movement. Place your ear near the patient's mouth and nose. If the airway is not

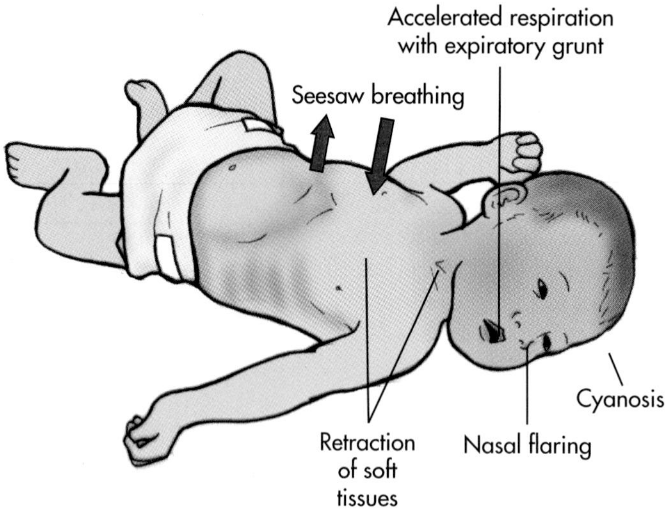

Figure 9-3

Seesaw breathing, nasal flaring, and other signs indicate abnormal breathing in a child.

open, you will have to open it. If the patient has experienced trauma, stabilize the cervical spine while opening the airway.

Note any abnormalities and continue with your rapid vital-sign check. The full picture is more likely to emerge as you add all of the findings of your initial assessment together.

Pulse

The **pulse** is the wave of pressure forced through the arterial system each time the heart contracts and forces blood through the arteries. Checking the pulse can help you determine whether circulation is appropriate. Use two or three fingertips to apply pressure to a pulse point, a spot where an artery lies close to the skin and just above a bone. The most common pulse site is the radial artery in the wrist (Figure 9-4, *A*), but pulses are also assessed at the carotid artery in the neck (Figure 9-4, *B*), the brachial artery in the arm (Figure 9-4, *C*), and the femoral artery in the groin. If you are unable to locate a radial pulse in one wrist or the brachial pulse on one arm of a child, try the other side. If it is still not present, check the carotid artery. This site is easier to find in an emergency and is the one usually assessed in unconscious patients.

Answer these questions as you palpate the pulse:

- Is the rate unusually fast or slow? (This is a quick impression only. Do not count at this point.)
- Is the pulse weak or abnormally strong (bounding)?
- Is the rhythm regular or irregular?
- If the radial pulse (brachial, for a child) is not present, can you palpate a carotid pulse?

You will notice that blood pressure is not included in the list of vital signs for this quick, initial check. However, your observations about the pulse will give you general information about blood pressure. Weak or strong pulses may indicate low or high pressure, respectively. Pulses that are absent peripherally but present in a central location are often a sign of low blood pressure.

Another quick way to estimate perfusion status is a combination of skin color and pulse assessment by compressing the fingernail beds or pads of the fingers. **Capillary refill** is the time it takes for the capillary beds to return to a pink color after being depressed and released and can also be performed on a patient's toes. Poor perfusion is indicated if it takes longer than 2 seconds for the color of the capillary bed to return to normal. There is some controversy about whether capillary refill testing is reliable in adults, but it can be used reliably in children.

Skin

Skin color, temperature, and moisture are additional indicators of patient condition. Skin is normally warm and dry to the touch. Sometimes a patient's skin may feel excessively dry, which may indicate dehydration. Cool, wet (clammy) skin often indicates a shock (hypoperfusion) state in which peripheral vessels have constricted to force blood toward vital core organs (see Chapter 22). This often occurs with pale or **cyanotic** skin.

Skin can feel cold because of the surrounding air temperature or because of shock. An exception is a trauma patient with a spinal cord injury, whose skin may be warm, flushed, and dry (see Chapter 22). Other changes in the skin are discussed in more detail in Chapter 10.

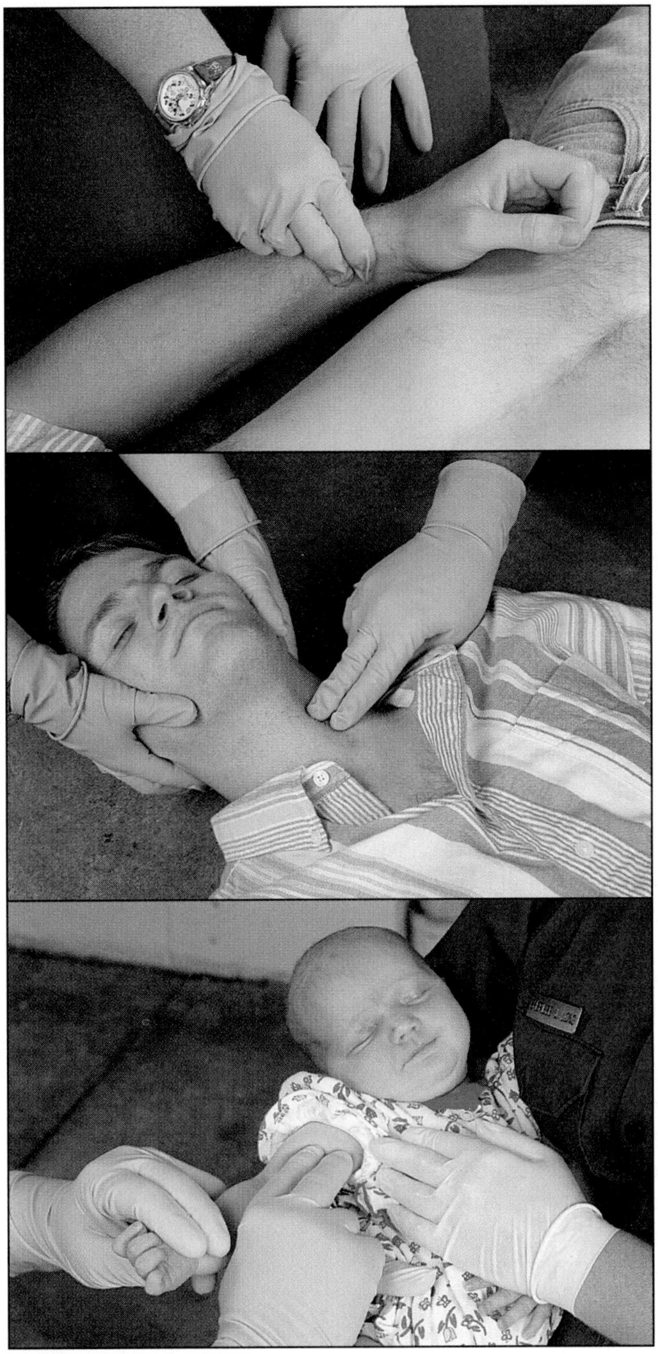

A

B

C

Figure 9-4

A, The most commonly used pulse point is the radial artery in the wrist. **B,** Carotid artery. **C,** Brachial artery.

Patient History

A main purpose of gathering patient **history** is determining a patient's chief complaint. Ask questions such as, "Why did you call for an ambulance?" An important start for a trauma patient could be, "Do you hurt anywhere?"

Because the chief complaint is a present-time matter, this and other pertinent information about the current event are called the **history of present illness (or incident).** Once the chief complaint is known, follow up with additional questions relative to this main problem. These extra questions are not part of the initial assessment, however.

Recognizing and Managing Immediate Threats to Life

Your ability to form a quick general impression and complete a rapid initial check of vital signs will enable you to identify immediate priorities. The **initial assessment** is directed at discovering life-threatening problems that require rapid intervention. Such conditions include problems with the patient's LOC, airway, breathing, and circulation, including pulse and external bleeding (Box 9-1). The initial assessment is an orderly process that checks each of these conditions; the process should be routine and should not be altered from patient to patient.

In most cases, the steps in the initial assessment will only take seconds to complete. If you arrive and hear a patient talking coherently to bystanders, your initial assessment is nearly complete. This patient is conscious, has a clear airway, is breathing, and has a pulse. You would look quickly for any severe bleeding and, finding none, could conclude that the patient's condition is not immediately life threatening. You would then be ready to proceed to the steps of the focused history and physical examination described in Chapter 10.

The initial assessment will take longer to complete if you need to intervene at any point. For example, you may arrive and find the patient not moving or talking. Assessment shows that the patient is unconscious and has vomit in the mouth, creating a potential airway obstruction. You clear the airway before checking breathing and circulation. Even if the patient has no pulse or appears to have lost a large amount of blood, you still check consciousness, airway, and breathing—and correct them as necessary—before moving to the final step, circulation. However, if there is help available, having someone else control bleeding while you proceed with the assessment sequence will accomplish all of the necessary steps in less time.

During initial assessment of a critical patient, it is enough to recognize that there is a serious problem that requires intervention, and then provide that intervention. It is not necessary to know precise vital-sign measurements to provide appropriate care. For example, in some critical cases, patients will require hospital treatments such as blood transfusions and surgical control of internal bleeding. In these settings, rapid intervention and early transport will be much more important than a detailed assessment.

BOX 9-1 Conducting the Initial Patient Assessment

1. Form a general impression of the patient, including the likelihood of a medical versus trauma problem.
2. Check the patient's LOC.
3. Check the patient's airway.
4. Check the patient's breathing.
5. Check the patient's circulation (pulse, bleeding, and skin signs).

Assessing Consciousness

As you arrive at a patient's side, begin initial assessment with a check for consciousness. If you suspect that the patient was involved in trauma to the head or neck, have someone hold the patient's head in line with the body to minimize movement and potential injury to the cervical spine (Figure 9-5).

Check the patient's LOC by introducing yourself and asking a question. If the patient does not respond immediately to your voice, tap a shoulder and speak more loudly. If there is still no response, try a painful stimulus, such as pinching the fingernail or rubbing the sternum. If this does not work, the patient is unresponsive. Any patient who responds only to painful stimulus or who is unresponsive needs constant airway attention and supplemental oxygen.

Assessing the Airway

The airway must be open for a patient to breathe adequately. It must be free of obstructions, both anatomic (the tongue) and mechanical (food, fluid, vomit, or other objects). In an alert patient, checking the airway is easy. If the patient is talking clearly or crying loudly, the airway is open. If the patient is conscious but unable to talk, cry, or cough forcefully, then the airway is likely obstructed and in need of clearing. Sometimes a patient will exhibit a high-pitched crowing sound, referred to as **stridor.** This sound is made during inhalation by partial obstruction of the upper airway. If the patient is able to cough, encourage him or her to do so. This is the body's natural way of trying to expel a foreign object.

If the airway is completely or partially obstructed with poor air exchange, you will need to perform the abdominal thrust and other procedures. In Chapter 11, basic

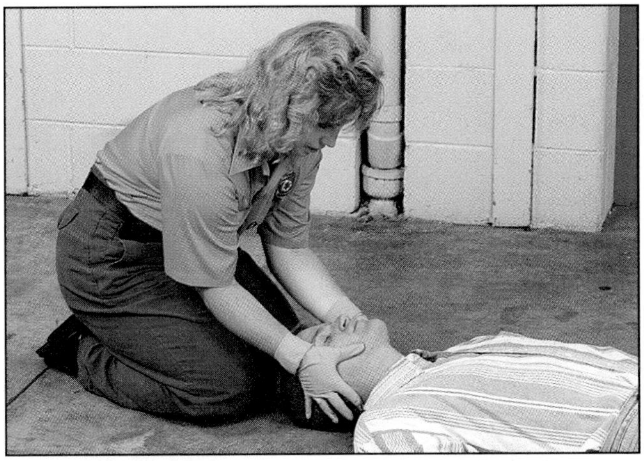

Figure 9-5

If spinal injury is suspected, maintain in-line stabilization of the head.

airway-management techniques are discussed. Clearing the airway may also require suction equipment. You should have suction ready for immediate use when approaching a patient with potential airway problems.

Assessing Breathing

As with airway assessment, a talking, coughing, or crying patient immediately tells you most of what you need to know. To decide whether a breathing patient has problems that need immediate attention, watch for signs of abnormal breathing discussed on p. 205.

In the unresponsive patient, begin by placing your ear near the patient's nose and mouth, with your eyes toward the chest; look, listen, and feel for air and chest movement. If the patient is not breathing, provide rescue breathing (see Chapter 11) and proceed to the circulation check. If the unresponsive patient is breathing, observe briefly for any signs of abnormal breathing or respiratory distress.

Assessing Circulation

Once you have assessed and corrected any airway and breathing problems, evaluate the adequacy of the patient's circulation. The term *circulation* refers here to checking the patient's pulse, skin color, and skin temperature, and doing a body-wide check for bleeding. See p. 206 for a discussion of the basic signs. When evaluating your findings, remember that what is normal varies somewhat with each patient and situation.

Pulse

A person who has just finished exercising, or one who is anxious or in pain, can be expected to have an accelerated heart rate. Likewise, a patient who has been relaxing, sleeping, or on certain heart medications is likely to have a slower heart rate.

If a patient is unconscious, check the carotid arteries in the neck. If the patient does not have a pulse, perform CPR until the automatic external defibrillator can be applied to determine the patient's heart rhythm. EMTs will learn the specifics of performing CPR in a certification course on that topic.

Cardiac arrest is not the only life-threatening circulation problem. Even in a patient with a pulse, inadequate blood flow can still be a major problem. The possible causes are numerous, including fluid loss, cardiac pumping failure, and widespread vessel dilation caused by allergic reaction or spinal injury.

If the patient has a pulse, it is important to assess its rate and quality. A rapid, weak pulse often indicates insufficient blood volume. This is also true if the radial pulse is absent but the carotid pulse is present. In each of these situations, the problem is shock. Interventions for shock include proper positioning, oxygen administration, and rapid transport. Chapter 22 presents more extensive information on shock. Checking capillary refill can also help with assessment of circulation.

Bleeding

Another problem associated with deficient circulation is severe bleeding. Whether internal or external, bleeding can rapidly make a patient's condition unstable. It is easy to determine whether a patient is bleeding externally (Figure 9-6). However, signs of internal bleeding are not as obvious and often are not identified until after the initial assessment. If severe external bleeding is present, control it with direct pressure and other techniques as needed. Rapid transportation to the hospital is important for a patient with major blood loss.

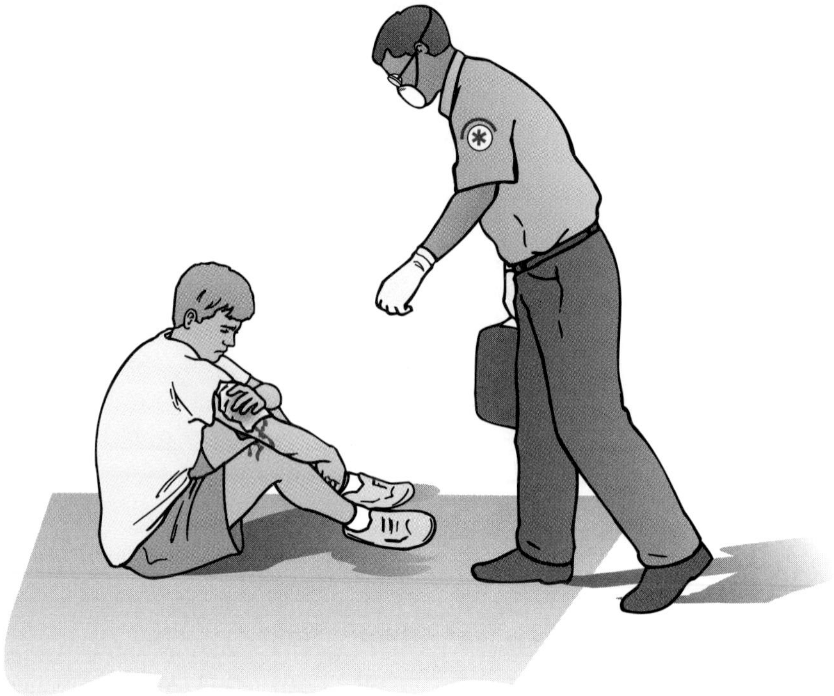

Figure 9-6

External bleeding is often easy to detect, but internal bleeding can be much more difficult.

IT'S YOUR CALL CONTINUED

Your 45-year-old patient was found on a couch in his home. You moved him to the floor after determining he was unconscious. You next check his airway, breathing, and circulation and find that he is not breathing and has no pulse. You advise the dispatch center that you have a patient in cardiac arrest and request advanced life support (ALS) assistance.

Your partner begins CPR and you quickly attach the electrodes from the automatic defibrillator. The machine analyzes the patient's heart rhythm and directs you to shock the patient. You administer the first shock and the machine reanalyzes. Your partner prepares the oxygen and pocket mask or bag-valve mask. A second shock is ordered. You administer the second shock, and the machine reanalyzes the patient's heart rhythm. It now advises you to check the pulse. You reassess and find a slow, weak pulse in both his neck and wrist. What should you check now, and what care will you provide?

Skin Assessment

A rapid evaluation of a patient's skin, including capillary refill, can also provide information about the patient's circulatory status. While palpating the pulse, you can determine the patient's skin temperature (hot, cold), color (pale, blue, red, yellow), and condition (moist, dry). Patients with cool, pale, and moist skin must be presumed to have a serious problem, often associated with hypoperfusion (see p. 206).

Recognizing Priority Patients

Patients with serious conditions affecting consciousness, airway, breathing, or circulation need quick intervention at the scene followed by rapid transport to a medical facility. These signs indicate that a patient is in trouble or soon will be if you do not act quickly.

Do not be overly influenced by injuries or conditions that are dramatic in appearance. Some of these are indeed emergencies; however, the emphasis must remain on assessing vital body systems. Concentrate on the airway, bleeding, and the clinical signs that have been discussed in this chapter.

More generally, to identify critical patients, you can look for the following:

- Poor general impression
- Unresponsiveness
- Disorientation
- Difficulty breathing
- Signs and symptoms of shock
- Uncontrolled bleeding
- Severe pain

As you study other chapters, you will learn about numerous specific conditions that pose life-threatening emergencies. You should call for ALS personnel as soon as you recognize that a patient has a serious condition. If you are able to begin transporting the patient before ALS personnel arrive, coordinate a location where they can meet you on the way.

Once the initial assessment is complete and you have stabilized life-threatening conditions, you can proceed to the next assessment phase, the focused history and physical examination. Chapter 10 presents this information.

IT'S YOUR CALL
CONCLUSION

The patient still has not responded to your efforts to arouse him and still is not breathing. Your partner opens the airway and begins to ventilate, providing high-concentration oxygen with the pocket mask. You assess the patient quickly for other problems. You note that his skin is pale, moist, and cool. His pulses remain weak. He is not bleeding externally and has no signs of injury. A paramedic unit arrives. With this additional assistance, you roll the patient onto a backboard, place him on your stretcher, and wheel him to your ambulance. En route to the hospital, the paramedic provides ALS measures while you and your partner continue to ventilate the patient and monitor vital signs. As you near the hospital, you note that his condition is improving. He begins to breathe on his own and his pulse is returning to normal.

SUMMARY

Effective assessment techniques enable you to detect and manage both medical and trauma emergencies. By systematically following initial assessment steps, you can ensure that critical patients receive appropriate, early intervention, which will increase the likelihood of patient survival.

SUGGESTED READINGS

1. **Emergency Cardiac Care Committee and Subcommittees,** American Heart Association, Guidelines for Cardiopulmonary Resuscitation, *JAMA* 2184-2198, 1992.

Chapter 10

Continued Patient Assessment

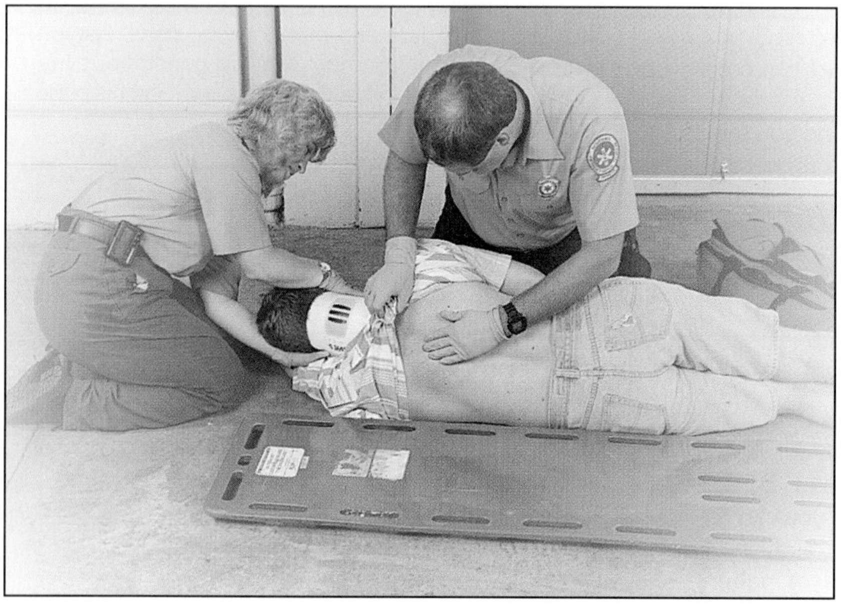

Knowledge Objectives

As an EMT-Basic, you should be able to:

OBJECTIVES

1. Discuss the purpose of the focused history and physical examination for medical and trauma patients.
2. Describe how the focused history and physical examination differs when performed on a(n):
   - Conscious trauma patient
   - Unconscious trauma patient
   - Conscious medical patient
   - Unconscious medical patient
3. Discuss the importance of reconsidering the mechanism of injury or the nature of illness when conducting the focused history and physical examination.
4. Provide examples of situations that involve a significant mechanism of injury.
5. Explain why every trauma patient with a significant mechanism of injury should receive a rapid physical examination.
6. State the areas of the body included in the rapid physical examination.
7. Describe how to perform a rapid physical examination for a trauma patient.
8. Explain when it would be appropriate to alter the order of the physical examination to provide patient care.
9. Describe how prior medical history can alter the focused history and physical examination for a responsive patient.
10. Describe the purpose and components of a detailed physical examination.
11. Differentiate between a detailed physical examination performed on a trauma patient and one performed on a medical patient.
12. List the six vital signs that EMTs assess and briefly describe the importance of each.
13. Discuss why it is important to repeat the initial assessment as part of your ongoing assessment.
14. Describe the components of an ongoing assessment and what is meant by "trending" of these components.

Skill Objectives

As an EMT-Basic, you should be able to:

OBJECTIVES

1. **Demonstrate how to perform a rapid physical examination for a trauma patient.**
2. **Demonstrate how to perform a focused history and physical examination on a patient with an isolated injury and no significant mechanism of injury.**
3. **Demonstrate how to perform a focused history and physical examination on a responsive medical patient.**
4. **Demonstrate how to perform a focused history and physical examination on an unresponsive medical patient.**
5. **Demonstrate how to assess and document mental status using the Glasgow Coma Scale.**
6. **Demonstrate how to measure respiratory rate and assess the quality of respirations.**
7. **Demonstrate how to measure pulse rate and assess the quality of the pulse.**
8. **Demonstrate how to assess skin signs.**
9. **Demonstrate how to measure blood pressure by auscultation and by palpation.**
10. **Demonstrate how to assess pupils.**
11. **Demonstrate how to perform a detailed physical examination.**
12. **Demonstrate how to perform an ongoing assessment.**

Attitude Objectives

As an EMT-Basic, you should be able to:

1. **Explain the importance of following a systematic plan for conducting a physical examination.**
2. **Recognize and respect the feelings that patients may experience during a physical assessment.**

KEY TERMS

1. **Chief Complaint:** The major problem, as stated by the patient; often the reason EMS personnel were summoned.
2. **Crepitus:** The grating vibration caused by bone fragments rubbing together or by air under the skin (subcutaneous emphysema); also referred to as *crepitation.*
3. **Detailed Physical Examination:** A thorough, methodic assessment of the patient after completion of the focused history and physical examination.
4. **Focused History and Physical Examination:** The second phase of the patient-assessment process; includes gathering pertinent information, obtaining vital signs, and completing a physical examination while focusing on the chief complaint.
5. **Ongoing Assessment:** The final step of the patient-assessment process; repeats the initial assessment and the focused history and physical examination.
6. **OPQRST:** Abbreviation used to help remember questions for gathering the history of present event (or illness); stands for **O**nset, **P**rovokes, **Q**uality, **R**adiation, **S**everity, **T**ime.
7. **Paradoxical Movement:** Movement of one part of the chest wall in opposition to the remainder of the chest during breathing; may occur when multiple consecutive ribs have been broken in more than one place (flail chest).
8. **Rapid Assessment:** Another term for the physical examination portion of the focused history and physical examination when performed on a critical medical or trauma patient.
9. **SAMPLE:** Acronym used to gather pertinent medical information from a patient; stands for **S**igns and symptoms, **A**llergies, **M**edications, **P**ast history, **L**ast oral intake, and **E**vents leading to the incident.

IT'S YOUR CALL

You are dispatched to an unconscious patient at a local business and arrive to find a 28-year-old female motionless on the floor. A bystander states that he noticed the woman stagger, caught her before she fell, and lowered her to the ground. She experienced a seizure that lasted about 1 minute. There is no additional pertinent information available.

Because the patient is unconscious, you conduct the initial assessment as if this were a trauma emergency, in case the reason for the woman's collapse was caused by a previous injury. You clear her airway of vomit before you assess breathing. She is breathing rapidly and has a strong pulse, but remains unresponsive.

Now that you have completed the initial assessment, it is time to check the patient in more detail. Where do you begin, and what should you look for? Is the patient's condition stable or unstable? How much time will you spend at the scene, and how extensive should the examination be? What about the need for ALS personnel?

In Chapter 9, you learned how to perform an initial assessment on all patients, medical and trauma, which enables you to identify and correct any immediately life-threatening conditions. This chapter deals primarily with the focused history and physical examination, which follows the initial assessment and focuses on the patient's chief complaint.

The sequence and depth of a focused assessment vary depending on how the patient presents. In an unconscious patient, it can be dangerous to assume anything about the problem. You will need to start with the basics (consciousness, airway, breathing, and circulation) and proceed to a rapid head-to-toe examination. This will ensure that you gather all available information about the patient's condition. During your assessment you could still discover a problem that would soon pose a threat to the patient. Such an instance may require interrupting the assessment to give treatment.

In a conscious patient, you are more likely to begin with at least a partial idea of what the problem is. Investigate the chief complaint, beginning with determining whether the condition is medical or traumatic. It is not always possible to make this determination, but this will enable you to focus the remaining assessment more narrowly on the areas pertinent to the current problem.

Like the initial assessment, the focused history and examination provides a simple plan that helps you determine the severity of the condition. For trauma patients, first consider the mechanism of injury; if it is significant or if the patient's mentation is altered (head injury, alcohol, drugs), conduct a rapid physical examination of the entire body, record vital signs, and obtain a brief history, if possible. This enables you to begin the proper treatment; in serious situations such as chest or abdominal trauma, this means rapid transport to a nearby trauma center with further care provided while en route. For isolated, minor injuries, it is usually not necessary to examine the entire body. Instead, you will be able to focus on the isolated injury.

For conscious patients with medical conditions, start with the nature of the illness. Next, gather information about the patient's medical history, both past and present. Depending on how many EMS providers are present, you could take the history while another provider performs the physical examination and records vital signs. For a patient with an isolated, minor illness, focus instead on the patient's chief complaint, such as chest pain or difficulty breathing. Care for what you can find to stabilize the patient, and then transport.

With the focused history and physical examination complete and care in progress for the patient's most serious conditions, you can proceed to the next phase of patient assessment—the detailed examination. This step is performed after serious conditions have been adequately cared for, usually while en route to the hospital or when there are no serious conditions. At this point, you can do a more complete physical assessment without delaying transport. You may uncover additional injuries or other information that will help the emergency physician diagnose the problem.

A systematic evaluation provides valuable clues regarding the nature and severity of a patient's condition, but initial findings represent only one moment in time. The patient's condition may change. Patient assessment is an ongoing process that you must continue until you transfer care at the hospital. If the patient's condition deteriorates, you may have to return to basic skills, such as opening the airway. This chapter focuses on the steps for conducting a continued patient assessment, including the focused history and physical examination, detailed examination, and ongoing assessment.

The Focused History and Physical Examination

The initial assessment is generally the same for both medical and trauma patients. All patients are evaluated for their level of consciousness (LOC) and adequacy of airway, breathing, and circulation. The only significant difference is that you must ensure that the neck of a trauma patient is stabilized before opening the airway. Otherwise, immediate life threats are assessed and managed in the same manner, whether medical or traumatic in nature.

After the initial assessment is complete, continue to the **focused history and physical examination,** a process designed to provide further assessment and intervention without unnecessarily delaying transport. The length of time it takes varies depending on the number of EMS providers available, but it is usually completed in only a few minutes.

The steps of the focused history and examination are similar for medical and trauma patients, but the order of the steps and the amount of emphasis that each receives are somewhat different. For example, knowledge of past medical history relative to smoking is a concern for a medical patient complaining of chest pain or difficulty breathing, but is not likely a concern for a trauma patient with chest pain. Likewise, a past history of diabetes is an important thing to know when assessing a medical patient with a diminished LOC. In the case of a trauma patient, greater emphasis is placed on the mechanism of injury.

While some medical or trauma conditions can be handled at the scene, a patient with a significant trauma or medical condition may need early hospital care. This means rapid identification of critical conditions, both actual and potential, and transport to the appropriate hospital. The phrase *load and go* has often been used to reinforce the importance of rapid transport in providing the best possible outcome for critical patients.

You should not spend more than 10 minutes at the scene for a patient with serious trauma or illness unless the patient is entrapped or you are forced to await the arrival of an advanced life support (ALS) unit. Always request ALS support if you suspect that your patient is seriously ill or injured. Local protocols may call for you to begin transport and meet ALS on the way. Because the extent of illness or injury is not always easy to identify, considering the mechanism of injury or nature of illness is important in determining the amount of time to spend at the scene.

The focused history and physical examination has four main steps:

1. Consider the mechanism of injury or nature of illness.
2. Gather pertinent information about the history of the event.
3. Obtain vital signs.
4. Conduct a physical examination.

The Mechanism of Injury or Nature of Illness

After the initial assessment, consider the possible cause of the trauma or illness and the extent of problems that could result (Figure 10-1). Use your observational skills to identify factors related to the patient's problem. If the event involved a medical emergency, determine what activity the patient was involved in immediately before the onset of the problem. Try to determine whether the patient was exposed to any harmful substances. Look for any indications of drug use, including drug paraphenalia. Ask when the patient last ate and what was eaten.

If the event involved trauma from a vehicle collision, try to determine the speeds of the vehicles. Once you have learned the approximate speeds, ask yourself a series of other questions concerning the mechanism of the injury (Box 10-1). Answers to these questions provide important information regarding possible injuries. Assume serious injuries in a patient who was ejected from a vehicle or an unrestrained occupant who was thrown across the vehicle during impact. Similarly, assume that an unconscious patient has a head injury. It is up to you to provide hospital personnel with a verbal and written picture of the scene, including the external forces applied to the patient.

If the event was an injury from a fall, try to determine:

- How far the patient fell
- What the patient landed on
- How the patient landed
- What objects the patient hit during the fall

The information you need may not be volunteered by the patient. It is also possible that you will not make the con-

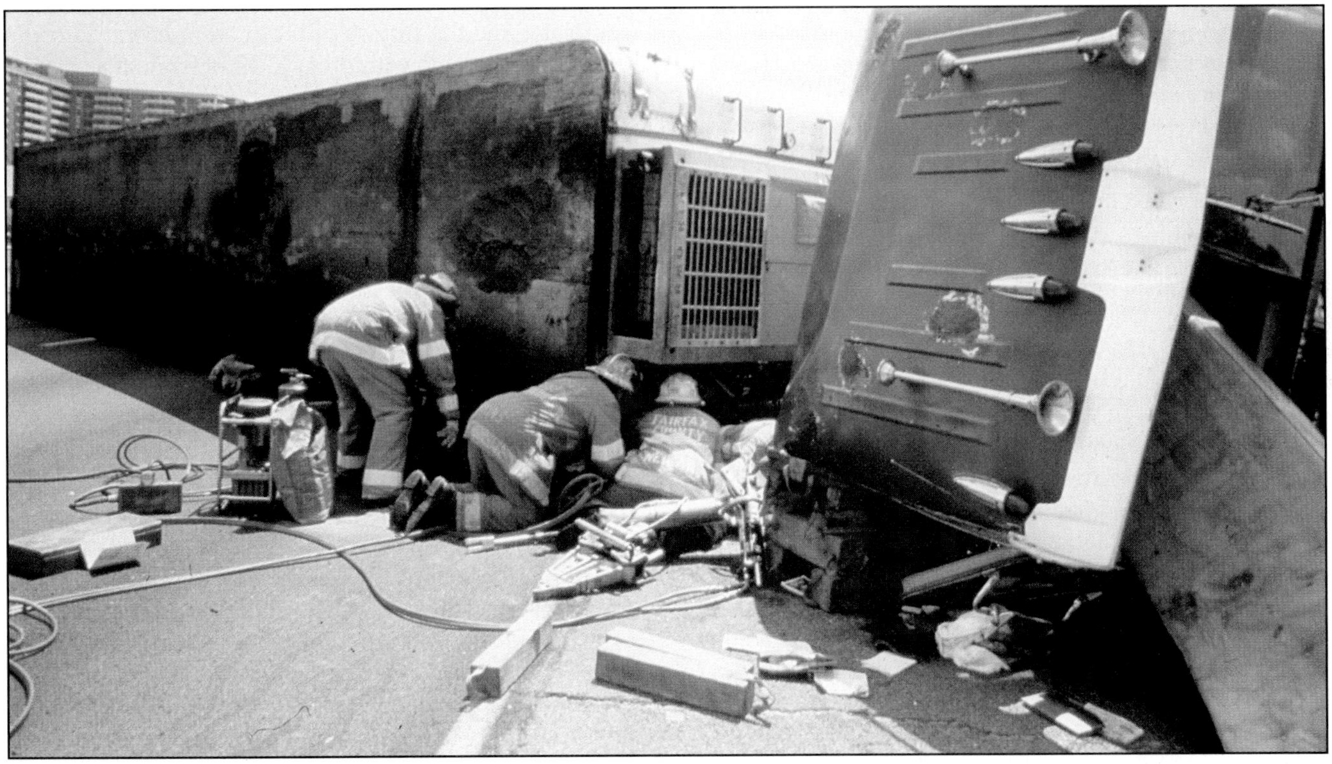

Figure 10-1

The mechanism of injury can provide a great deal of information about the extent and type of injury.

BOX 10-1 Questions Regarding the Mechanism of Injury in Vehicle Collisions

When assessing a patient involved in a vehicle collision, ask these questions:

- What was the exterior and interior damage to the vehicle? This may help identify the extent and degree of injury to the patient.
- Did the vehicle strike another moving vehicle or a stationary object? Striking another vehicle coming in the opposite direction greatly magnifies the force involved and the chance of major injury.
- Was there intrusion into the vehicle interior? Intrusion indicates that dangerous forces were involved and that the occupants could have been directly struck by the intruding objects.
- Was the windshield damaged from within, indicating that someone's head may have come in direct contact with it?
- Was the steering wheel bent, reflecting forces of impact from a victim's chest?
- Did the vehicle roll over? If so, you should expect multiple injuries, especially to unrestrained passengers.
- Was the patient ejected from the vehicle? These patients often have serious injuries requiring rapid transport.
- Was there death of another occupant in the same vehicle? This suggests forces likely to cause major injuries to others.
- Where were the occupants initially seated in the vehicle? Location relative to the point or points of impact is an important part of the mechanism of injury. Unrestrained passengers often do not present where they were sitting before impact.
- Were restraining devices used? Occupants generally suffer more severe injuries when restraints are not used. However, sometimes the restraint itself adds to the injury.
- Was the car equipped with an airbag? If so, did it function and were other restraints used?
- Airbags are most effective when used in conjunction with other restraints. Proper airbag deployment can reduce the severity of injuries resulting from frontal impact.

nection between a chief complaint and the mechanism of injury or nature of illness until continued assessment and care. Patients are sometimes afraid to talk about a situation or problem until they are in the privacy of an ambulance. Consider repeating initial questions later, worded in a different way. You should be prepared to update your report to the hospital if additional information is volunteered by the patient or is discovered at a later time.

The focused history and examination will enable you to gather all of the necessary information needed to make decisions about the general nature of the patient's problem and the care to provide. The amount of time you take to gather information and provide care can make a difference in the outcome of seriously ill or injured patients.

Gathering Pertinent Information

The patient should be the primary source of information whenever possible. However, the patient may be initially unconscious, or language barriers could limit communication. Other sources of information include what you observe at the scene and what you are told by first responders, witnesses, or bystanders.

Effective communication is essential to gathering pertinent information. The stronger your communication skills, the clearer the picture you will have about what happened. Sometimes the incident will make the patient frightened or hysterical. Patients under the influence of drugs may exhibit abusive, combative, or otherwise abnormal behavior. However, an abusive or combative patient may also be suffering from inadequate oxygen, low blood sugar, or a serious head injury. Do not jump to conclusions regarding patient behavior. Staying calm and developing a rapport may result in a more cooperative patient and a more accurate collection of pertinent information.

A conscious medical patient is the type you will encounter most commonly. While it is necessary to conduct a further physical examination of this patient, it is equally important to gather information relative to the past and recent history leading up to the event. This information is usually easily obtained from the patient. In situations involving trauma, some of this is a priority; while other information is secondary to rapid completion of the physical examination.

The most important information is the patient's chief complaint and the history of the present event. Because you will be working with other EMS personnel as part of a team, one of you can gather this information while someone else conducts the physical examination, focusing on the area of the chief complaint and determining the patient's baseline vital signs.

The Chief Complaint

The **chief complaint** is a simple statement of why EMS assistance is needed. These are complaints that cannot be seen but are felt by the patient. Normally it is a statement of what the patient is experiencing, such as dizziness, weakness, nausea, shortness of breath, or pain. What actually caused this complaint is considered later, when you gather the incident history and link it to the mechanism of injury or nature of illness. There may be times when the patient will not be able to express complaints. In these situations, a statement of what you observe will be adequate, such as "unresponsiveness."

Ask questions to determine the patient's chief complaint. The first key question that you might ask is, "Why did you call for an ambulance?" or, "What seems to be the problem today?" For a trauma patient, an important question could be, "Do you hurt anywhere?" Once the chief complaint is known, follow up with additional questions regarding the history of the event and any pain that the patient may be experiencing.

History of the Present Event

Learning and documenting how the event happened is another important part of gathering pertinent information. Sometimes the explanation the patient provides will be as concise as "I tripped on the step and twisted my ankle." In other cases, questions will need to be asked to determine if a medical problem was responsible for a traumatic event. For example, a patient who does not recall falling and injuring his or her head may have had a fainting episode caused by a circulatory problem. (In medical situations, this is sometimes called the *history of present illness,* rather than *event*.)

Ask questions about any pain that the patient reports. The letters **OPQRST** will help you remember what to ask. These letters stand for:

Onset: What were you doing when the pain began?
Provokes: Is there anything you can think of that might have caused the pain or that makes it worse?
Quality: Can you describe the pain (sharp, dull, throbbing)?
Radiation: Does the pain spread to any other areas in your body?
Severity: How bad is the pain on a scale of 1 to 10, with 10 being the worst you have ever experienced?
Time: When did the pain first begin? Has it changed since it started?

At first glance you might think these questions are only appropriate for medical patients, such as an elderly patient experiencing chest pain; however, this is not the case. For example, you are summoned to a local residence where a 17-year-old male is experiencing chest pain and difficulty breathing. In response to your questioning, the patient states that the pain had an acute onset while he was lying in bed. He further states that his chest was already sore from a high school wrestling match that had ended about an hour earlier. He states that he "had the wind knocked out of him" during the match and that the right side of his chest was injured.

In describing his present pain, he states that it is constant, hurts more on inspiration, and he cannot take a deep breath. The pain seems confined to the right side and is about an 8 on a scale of 1 to 10. Additionally, he states that the pain started to get worse about 15 minutes ago and there is nothing he can do to relieve it. The OPQRST questions could provide the necessary background information about the possible nature of the patient's problem and an underlying condition related to chest trauma and lung injury.

Past Medical History

Once you have gathered the information about the patient's present condition, including how the incident occurred and any pain the patient is experiencing, you need to gather other related information, such as past medical history. This is commonly referred to as the **SAMPLE** history. Each letter of the word *sample* stands for additional questions that you will ask.

Signs/symptoms: Have you had any other symptoms (dizziness, nausea, vomiting, diarrhea)?
Allergies: Are you allergic to any medications?
Medications: Are you taking any medications? What are they for?
Past history: Have you had this problem before? Do you have other problems?
Last oral intake: When did you last eat or drink anything?
Events leading up to the problem: How were you feeling before this problem began? Have you been doing anything different from your ordinary routine?

In some cases, the information gathered through present and past history will help you determine the probable nature of the problem. This information is often more important for medical patients than trauma patients. The SAMPLE information, like that gathered from the OPQRST questions, may be unavailable if the patient is unconscious and no bystanders knowledgeable about the patient's condition are present. In these situations, you will rely on physical findings, such as vital signs and items discovered during physical examination.

The past medical history may uncover a medical condition that could have contributed to the present incident, such as light-headedness or dizziness before a fall. This information may alert you to the presence of significant underlying medical problems and help you anticipate immediate complications. An example would be a patient with **hemophilia** (a bleeding disorder) that may require urgent evaluation even for injuries that would normally be considered minor to other patients.

Knowing what medications the patient is taking or is supposed to be taking is also important. If the medications are known but you are unable to determine exactly what they are used for, seek advice from the on-line physician, who can use that information to determine the probable medical conditions and the appropriate treatment plan. An example is the anticoagulant (blood thinner) Coumadin, which prevents sudden blockage of an artery or vein and may have been prescribed because of a past circulatory problem. This information becomes even more important if the patient will need surgery.

Obtaining Vital Signs

In Chapter 9, you learned how to do a quick, general evaluation of vital signs as part of initial patient assessment. In the focused assessment, you will refine that earlier picture by taking accurate measurements of vital signs.

It is important to record an initial set of vital signs so that you and other providers have a baseline indicator of the patient's condition. Your patient-care report should have room to record multiple sets of vital-sign measurements (Figure 10-2). Vital signs include:

- Level of consciousness (LOC)
- Respirations (and lung sounds)

EMS RUN MEDICAL FORM

AGENCY METRO	UNIT # 162		MEDCOM NUMBER 98-21732
NAME SAM ANDERSON	ADDRESS 12785 CUMBERLAND		DATE 8/19/98 DAY WE
PATIENT PHONE 423-7219 AGE 23 D.O.B. 8/3/75	SEX M☒ F☐ RACE C	SSN 216-37-9845	COMPLAINT NO. 8-8-275
INCIDENT LOCATION ANDERSON SHOES - WEST MALL	DISPATCH/"CHIEF COMPLAINT" ALLERGIC RXN	PRTY: 1	REPORTING POLICE DEPARTMENT COUNTY

PHYSIOLOGIC STATUS

TIME	BLOOD PRES	PULSE RATE	PULSE QUAL.	RESP. RATE	RESP. QUAL.	PUPILS	GCS E(4)	GCS V(5)	GCS M(6)	AVPU		PO$_X$	PRTY
0932	88/40	120	W	32	S	=/R	4	5	6	A		84	1
0935	96/52	112	W	26	NL	=/R	4	5	6	A		97	1
0941	108/60	106	NL	22	NL	=/R	4	5	6	A		98	1
0947	112/64	106	NL	20	NL	=/R	4	5	6	A		99	1
0954	114/62	102	NL	20	NL	=/R	4	5	6	A		99	2
1000	116/60	98	NL	18	NL	=/R	4	5	6	A		99	2

COUNTY BAKER
TWP/CITY/VILLAGE FILLMORE
EST. TIME — INCIDENT T.O.C. 0922
Dispatch 0923
En route 0923
Arr. Scene 0927
(EST) Arr. Pat.- 0929
Dep. Scene 0946
Arr. Hosp. 1002

DEFIBRILLATE

TIME	ECG	WATT/S	ECG	BY NO.
N/A				

CPR INITIATED: Yes ☐ No ☒
By: MFR ☐ PD ☐ Bystander ☐ ALS ☐ Mechanical Device ☐
AED Yes ☐ No ☒
MAST: ☒ In Place ☐ Inflated

DESTINATION: Hospital DWTN; Diversion From: —
CHOSEN BY: ☒ Patient ☐ Relative ☐ EMT ☐ Other ☐ MEDCOM ☐ Hospital ☐ Physician

BARRIERS: ☒ Gloves ☐ Goggles ☐ Mask ☐ HEPA ☐ Gown ☐

MECHANISM OF INJURY FACTORS: ☐ Ejected from Vehicle ☐ MVA w/Fatals at Scene ☐ Extrication > 20 Minutes ☐ Major Vehicle Damage ☐ Unrestrained ☐ MCA without Helmet ☐ Fall > 20 Feet ☐ Rollover

DRUG TIMES

DRUG	TIME	DOSE	ROUTE	MEDIC #	AUTH (SO,MC,POS)
EPI-PEN	0934	0.3mg	IM	3213	SO

DRUG	TIME	DOSE	ROUTE	MEDIC #	AUTH
N/A					

Time Med Dir Contact: 0952 Est. Wt.: 172 # Blood Sugar N/A

AIRWAY — Basic: O2 Flow 15 L/Min @ 0932 Time via: NC SFM (M/RES) P. MASK BVM Adj: OPA NPA ETCO$_2$ Used: Yes ☐ No ☐
Advanced: Proc: ____ Size: ____ # Attempts ____ by # ____ Est. by # ____ Time ____ ETCO$_2$ Confirmed: Yes ☐ No ☐ N/A ☐

I.V. SITE: N/A # ATTEMPTS ____ BY # ____ EST. BY # ____ SIZE ____ TIME ____ RATE ____ TOTAL INFUSED ____
I.V. SITE: ____ # ATTEMPTS ____ BY # ____ EST. BY # ____ SIZE ____ TIME ____ RATE ____ TOTAL INFUSED ____

MED. HX. ASTHMA / BEE STINGS ALL. ALLERGIES NKDA PT. PHYSICIAN JONES
CURRENT MEDS PROVENTIL (AS NEEDED)

NARRATIVE S: 23 YO WM CLEANING OUT STORAGE AREA OF STORE WHEN STUNG ON Ⓛ ARM BY MULTIPLE BEES. PT C/O SOB / FACIAL SWELLING / RASH & ITCHING. HAS EPI-PEN BUT DID NOT USE PTA.
O: ATF PT SITTING IN CHAIR, PALE, DIAPHORETIC, ANXIOUS, SOB. MOVING AIR WELL c̄ DIFFUSE MILD WHEEZES ALL FIELDS. MILD DIFFUSE FACIAL SWELLING / ERYTHEMA. DIFFUSE HIVES TRUNK, ARMS & LEGS. PERRL, NARES PATENT, PHARYNX W/O SWELLING CV - TACHY LUNGS DIFFUSE WHEEZING, ABD SOFT EXT W/O EDEMA.
A: PT LAID ON FLOOR, V.S. & O$_2$ AS ABOVE. PT ASSISTED WITH USE OF EPI-PEN BY # 3213 IN Ⓛ LAT THIGH
PT PLACED ON STRETCHER & TRANSFERED TO UNIT - GRADUAL IMPROVEMENT IN RASH / ITCHING / SOB. O$_2$ MAINTAINED. REPEAT VS AS ABOVE DURING TRANSPORT. PT FEELING MUCH BETTER BY ED ARRIVAL. CARE TO ED STAFF IN RM 3

PAGE 1 OF 1 AGENCY PRESENT UPON ARRIVAL: MFR ☐ E-Unit ☐ Amb ☐ FORM COMPLETED BY: J Smith #

SIGNATURE Steve Jones MD
Printed Name JONES
DEA Number
ETT Confirmed;

AMBULANCE PERSONNEL	No./Level	OTHER AGENCY PERSONNEL	No./Level
1. J SMITH	EMT-B	1.	
2. T JONES	EMT-B	2.	
3.		3.	
4.		4.	

FIRST IN EQUIPMENT: FIRST IN BAG ☐ AIRWAY BAG ☐ DEFIB ☐ O$_2$ ☐ STRETCHER ☐ AUX COT ☐

Figure 10-2

Repeat vital sign measurements often to determine any trends (see shaded area).

- Pulse
- Skin signs
- Blood pressure
- Pupils

When assessing vital signs, consider the average parameters for patients of different ages in order to recognize abnormal findings (Table 10-1). Any abnormalities in these areas should be noted and further explored once you have made a decision about patient transport. However, it is equally important to repeat your vital-sign measurements often so that you can identify any trends. You should reassess vital signs in stable patients every 15 minutes. A stable patient is one whose vital signs are within normal limits and are not changing significantly. Because of the seriousness of a patient with unstable vital signs, you should reassess this patient's vital signs frequently, perhaps every 5 minutes. Record vital signs after each measurement, noting changes after treatments (oxygen, position change, medication).

When assessing vital signs, consider the patient's activity. For example, if the patient has just finished running a distance race on a hot day, you might expect the patient to be tired, to have faster-than-normal pulse and respirations, and for the skin to be warm and damp.

Level of Consciousness

To measure a patient's LOC, refine the quick impression obtained with the AVPU (alert, verbal, painful, unresponsive) scale during the initial assessment (see Chapter 9). To do this, rate the patient's neurologic function with the Glasgow Coma Scale (GCS) (Box 10-2). The GCS measures three neurologic indicators: eye opening, verbal response, and motor response. The total points possible range from three (no response in any of these categories) to 15 (fully conscious and responsive). You should document repeated GCS assessments according to the specifics of the 15-point scale. This information may be important to hospital personnel in determining later care.

Respirations

Breathing should be virtually silent and effortless. Whether conscious or unconscious, a patient experiencing difficulty breathing will usually display obvious signs. Breathing too slow or too fast is an abnormal sign. To determine breathing rate, watch the rise and fall of the patient's chest and listen for the sound of the patient inhaling and exhaling. Count the number of breaths in 30 seconds and multiply by two. This will give you the approximate number of respirations per minute. The normal range is 12 to 20 per minute. Patients breathing less than 8 or more than 24 per minute will most likely need oxygen therapy and possibly ventilation.

Besides measuring rate, you should also examine the quality of breathing. Consider whether the patient is straining to breathe (labored respirations). Note if the patient is using accessory muscles in the neck and between the ribs to breathe, and whether the skin is pale or cyan-

TABLE 10-1 Average Vital Signs

Age	Pulse	Respirations	Blood pressure
Newborn	120-160	30-60	80 plus twice the age (systolic)
1-12 months	80-140	25-40	80 plus twice the age (systolic)
1-3 years	80-130	20-30	80 plus twice the age (systolic)
4-5 years	80-120	20-30	90/60
6-10 years	70-110	15-30	100/60
11-15 years	70-90	15-20	110/64
16 and older	60-80	12-20	120/80

BOX 10-2 Glasgow Coma Scale

Eye Opening	
Spontaneous	4
To voice	3
To pain	2
None	1

Verbal Response	
Oriented	5
Confused	4
Inappropriate words	3
Incomprehensible words	2
None	1

Motor Response	
Obeys command	6
Localizes pain	5
Withdraws from pain	4
Flexion (in response to pain)	3
Extension (in response to pain)	2
None	1

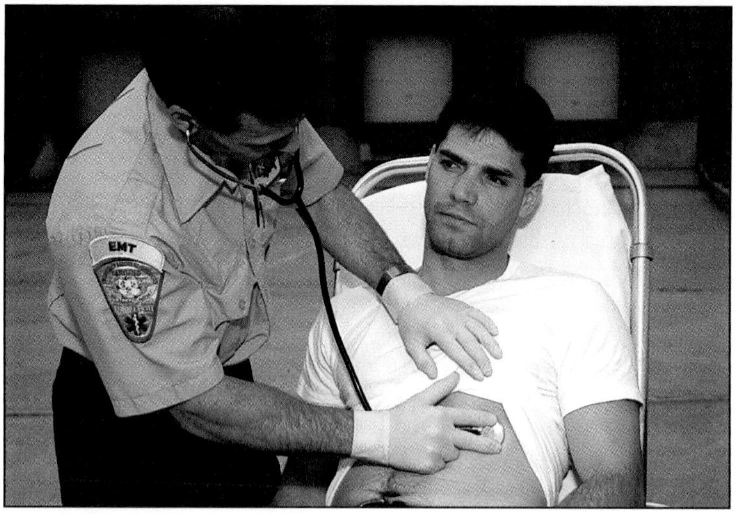

Figure 10-3

The diaphragm of the stethoscope should be held directly against the patient's skin during auscultation.

otic. Look also for signs of shallow breathing, indicated by only slight movement of the chest or abdomen. A patient with shallow respirations may have suffered a chest or abdominal injury that causes pain during breathing. Look for nasal flaring in children, another sign of respiratory distress.

Listen for abnormal sounds, which would also be a cause for concern. At a convenient point in your assessment, listen to breath sounds with a stethoscope. This is called *auscultation*. Place the stethoscope ear pieces pointing slightly forward in your ears and instruct the patient to breathe through the mouth while you listen. Hold the diaphragm of the stethoscope firmly on the patient's chest and listen carefully (Figure 10-3). Place the stethoscope directly on the skin; auscultation of breath sounds cannot be performed effectively through clothing.

There are six auscultation points on the chest (Figure 10-4). Note that the lower stethoscope placements are on the lateral rather than the anterior chest. This is in part because of the heart's position in the mid-to-left chest. Listening at a low spot on the left anterior chest would not give effective access to sounds from the lower left lobe. It is also important to listen to all four points on the back whenever possible. For each stethoscope placement, listen to at least one full respiratory cycle—inhalation and exhalation. Listen for equality from side to side, as well as diminished or abnormal sounds.

Many terms are used to describe abnormal breath sounds. Some of the more common terms include:

Crackles: Fine, moist crackling sounds caused by fluid in the smaller airways. Crackles are also called *rales*.

Rhonchi: Harsh, rattling sounds more prominent than crackles, resulting from excessive mucus or other secretions in the larger airways.

Snoring: Harsh, inspiratory and expiratory noises from nose and mouth. Often indicates an upper airway obstruction, usually from the tongue obstructing the airway of an unconscious, supine patient.

Stridor: High-pitched crowing sound, indicating a narrowing or obstruction of the upper airway.

Wheezing: High-pitched whistling or musical sounds produced by air moving through narrowed breathing passages.

When evaluating respiratory status, remember that chest movement by itself does not necessarily supply oxygen to vital organs. There must be an intact respiratory system and an open (patent) airway. You may have to maintain a patent airway as you remove any secretions with suction and assess breathing. Problems in these areas can lead to inadequate ventilation and oxygenation.

Pulse

Determine pulse rate in a manner similar to that used to assess breathing. Count the number of beats in 30 seconds and multiply by two to determine the number of beats per minute. The normal range for an adult at rest is 60 to 100 per minute. The beats should have a regular rhythm. Skipped beats result in an irregular rhythm and often indicate a heart problem. Feel also for pulse quality. You should feel a strong, steady pulse in a normal, healthy patient; a rapid, weak pulse in a patient who has lost blood and is in shock; and a bounding pulse in a patient who is frightened or who has high blood pressure.

A slow pulse in a traumatized patient can be an ominous sign, because the normal compensations for pain and blood loss tend to produce an increased rather than decreased pulse rate. A weak, slow, fast, or irregular pulse in a patient complaining of chest pain may be an indication of a heart attack.

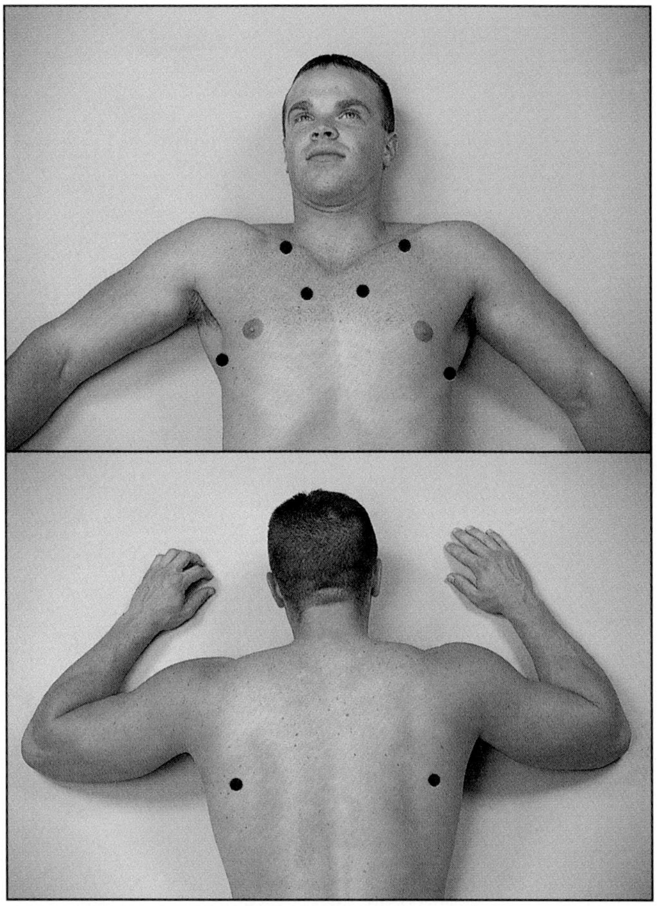

Figure 10-4

A, Common anterior auscultation points. **B,** Common posterior auscultation points.

Loss or weakening of peripheral pulses in a patient who is bleeding or dehydrated can indicate one of two things. First, as fluid loss begins, the peripheral arteries constrict in an attempt to force blood toward vital organs in the body core. This constriction reduces peripheral blood flow and may weaken the pulse. Second, as fluid loss continues, the fluid shortage has a more direct effect: there may simply not be enough blood left in the vessels to produce a strong pulse.

The body's attempt to force blood toward the core leads to the strategy of checking more central pulses if peripheral pulses are not present. If the radial pulse (brachial in a child) is absent on both sides, the carotid pulse may still be present. Because they supply the brain, the carotid arteries maintain flow when peripheral arteries shut down. (The brain gets priority as a core organ even though it lies outside the central trunk area.)

Presence of pulses can be used as a very rough way to estimate blood pressure. In adults, a radial pulse indicates a minimum systolic pressure of 80 to 90 mm Hg. A carotid pulse suggests a systolic pressure of at least 50 to 60 mm Hg.

Skin Signs

Skin color, temperature, and moisture are additional indicators of a patient's condition. Skin is normally warm and dry to the touch. (Occasionally a trauma patient with a spinal cord injury will have warm, dry, flushed skin.) Sometimes a patient's skin may feel excessively dry, which can indicate dehydration. Cool, wet (clammy) skin often indicates a shock (hypoperfusion) state in which peripheral vessels have constricted to force blood toward vital core organs. This often accompanies pale or cyanotic skin color. Cool or cold skin that is dry is more likely to be a sign of exposure to cold.

In addition to abnormal findings in skin temperature and moisture, a patient can have abnormal skin colors that include:

- Pale (white, ashen)
- Cyanotic (blue)
- Flushed (red)
- Jaundiced (yellow)

Pale skin indicates poor perfusion (low blood flow), often caused by constriction of peripheral vessels. This

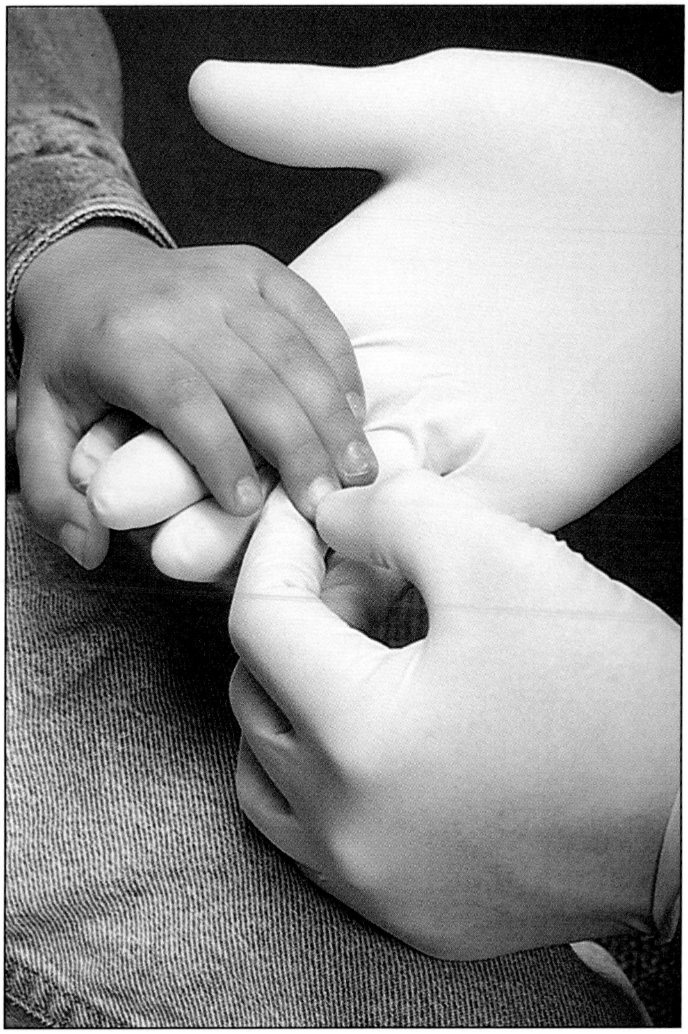

Figure 10-5

Capillary refill testing can be reliably used to check perfusion status in children.

constriction can be in response to blood or other fluid loss, exposure to cold, or extreme mental reactions, such as intense fear. Cyanosis indicates inadequate oxygenation of the blood; hemoglobin is red when saturated with oxygen and blue when it is deoxygenated. Cyanosis is usually the result of airway obstruction or a condition that compromises gas exchange between pulmonary capillaries and the alveolar sacs in the lungs.

Flushed skin may result from exercise, a heat emergency, or a type of shock caused by spinal cord injury. Jaundiced skin usually indicates a problem with the patient's liver. This could involve an infectious disease and should remind the EMT to take appropriate body substance isolation (BSI) precautions.

Dark-skinned patients may require a different approach to skin-color assessment. Check the membranes inside the mouth and eyelids, or the fingernail beds, for abnormal colors.

Another quick way to estimate perfusion status is a combination of skin color and pulse assessment by compressing the fingernail beds or pads of the fingers. **Capillary refill** is the time it takes for the capillary beds to return to a pink color after being depressed and released (Figure 10-5). This can also be done in the toes. Poor perfusion is indicated if it takes longer than 2 seconds for the color of the capillary bed to return to normal. There is some controversy about how reliable capillary refill testing is in adults, but it can be used reliably in children.

Blood Pressure

Blood pressure is the pressure of the circulating blood on the walls of the arteries during the contraction and relaxation phases of the heart. Systolic blood pressure is the pressure during contraction, and diastolic pressure reflects the pressure in the arteries when the heart relaxes and refills.

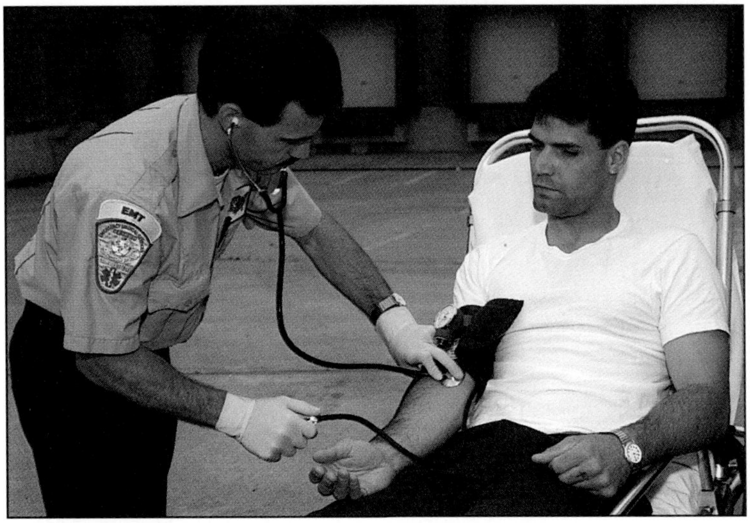

Figure 10-6

When auscultating for blood pressure, place the stethoscope on the brachial pulse site in the elbow crease, just below the lower edge of the cuff.

Auscultation is the preferred method for assessing blood pressure. This method requires the use of an inflatable cuff (sphygmomanometer) attached to the patient's arm and a stethoscope applied to the brachial artery. Because blood pressure cuffs come in various sizes to fit large, average, and small patients, you should select the proper one for your patient.

To assess blood pressure by auscultation:

1. Wrap the cuff securely around the patient's upper arm, with the lower edge of the cuff just above the brachial pulse site in the elbow crease (antecubital fossa), which is where you will place the stethoscope (Figure 10-6).
2. Close the valve attached to the bulb, and begin to squeeze the bulb. Watch the pressure gauge and continue to squeeze until the pressure reaches 200 mm Hg. At this point, the pulse is usually not heard because the cuff constricts blood flow through the artery. If you can still hear the pulse, continue pumping until the sounds disappear.
3. Open the valve slightly and allow the cuff to release pressure slowly. Listen for the return of the first sound of the pulse as it surges through the artery.
4. When sounds return, note the number on the pressure gauge. This is the systolic blood pressure.
5. Continue to listen to the pulse until it disappears or becomes muffled. The number on the gauge at this point is the diastolic blood pressure.
6. Blood pressure is recorded as the systolic pressure reading over the diastolic pressure reading (e.g., 120/80).

In some environments, such as a moving ambulance, it will be too noisy to auscultate blood pressure accurately. Under such circumstances, it is appropriate to palpate blood pressure (Figure 10-7). To take a blood pressure by palpation:

1. Apply the blood pressure cuff.
2. Palpate the patient's radial artery.
3. Inflate the cuff past the point at which the pulse disappears.
4. Slowly release the pressure in the cuff.
5. Note the point at which the pulse is first felt in the radial artery.
6. Record this finding, indicating that it is the systolic pressure only, taken by palpation (e.g., 120/p).

Many factors can affect a blood pressure reading, such as anxiety, stress, trauma, heart failure, or an inappropriately sized blood pressure cuff. Coupled with your assessment of the patient's LOC, and pulse and skin signs, blood pressure can help confirm suspected problems with circulation. Instead of regarding the measured numbers as absolutes, use your first reading as a baseline against which to compare later readings.

Like the other vital signs you record, one blood pressure measurement may not mean much. Trends, such as rising or falling blood pressure, are much more important. Some patients may be aware of their normal blood pressure and can provide this information to you to compare with your findings. Additionally, because young children can maintain normal blood pressure readings even in the presence of significant trauma or illness, blood pressure

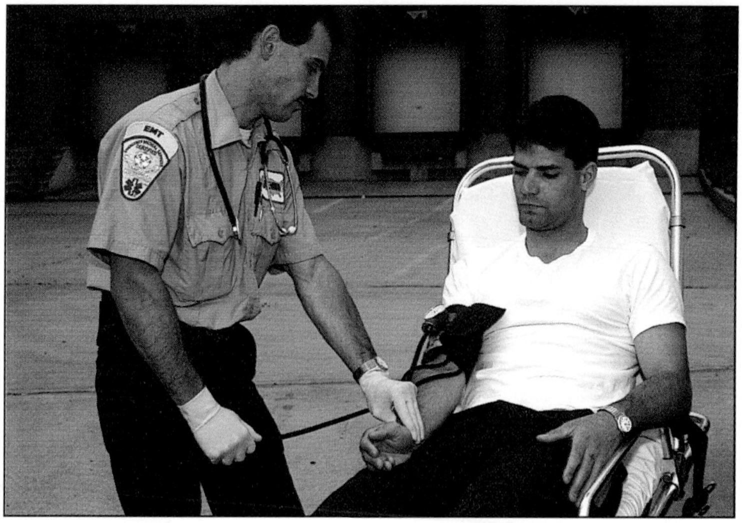

Figure 10-7

In some environments, it is appropriate to palpate a blood pressure. This will only determine systolic pressure.

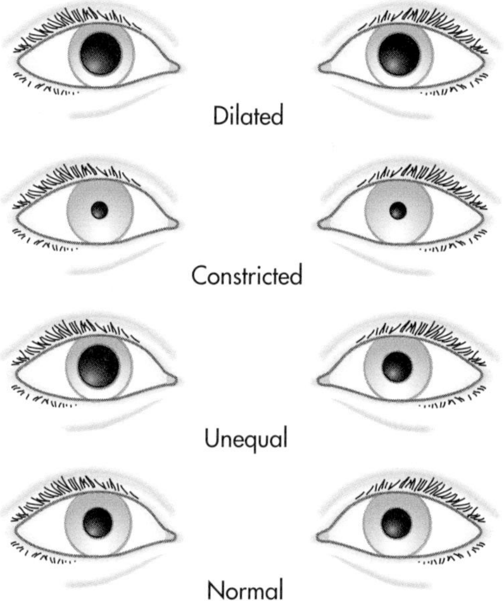

Figure 10-8

When assessing the pupils, note whether or not the pupils are equal and reactive to light.

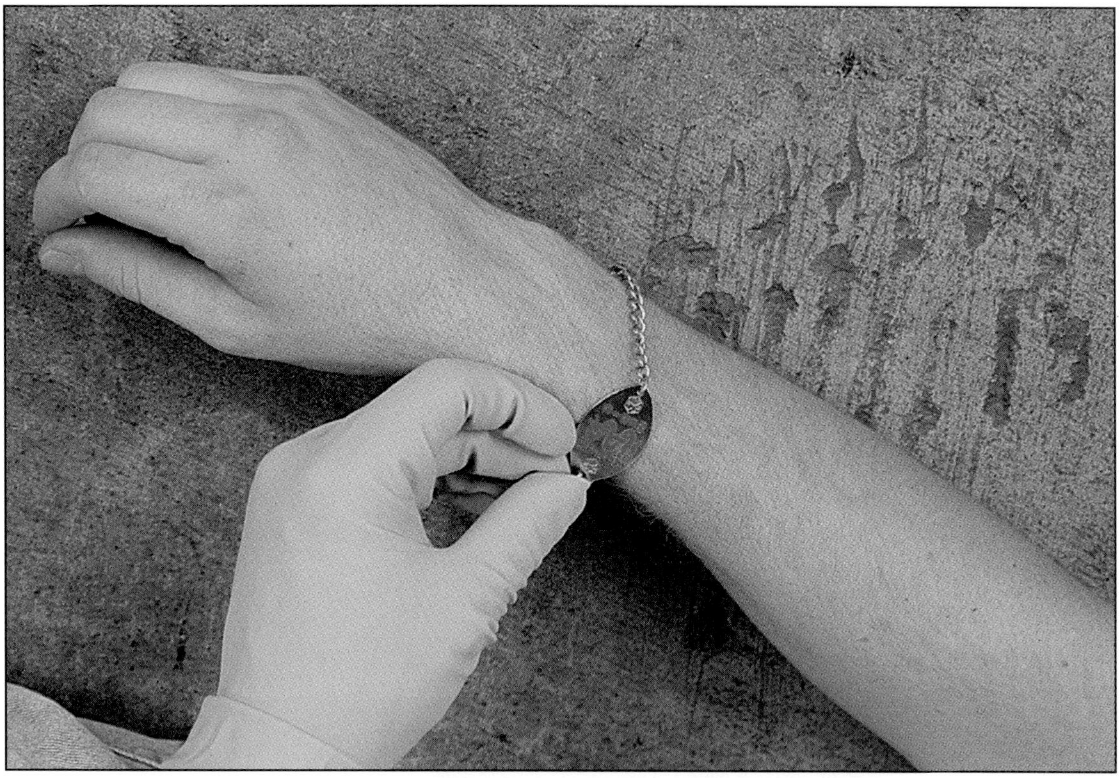

Figure 10-9

Always look for medical bracelets or necklaces. They can provide valuable information about the nature of the problem.

measurements are not taken on children less than 3 years of age. In small children, even more than in adults, you should rely more heavily on other clinical signs than on blood pressure.

Pupils

The pupils are normally symmetrical and change size together in response to changes in light or the nervous system through contraction and relaxation of the muscles controlling the iris, the colored part of the eye. Drugs, hypoxia, and strong emotions such as fear and anger are among the factors that can trigger nervous-system changes in pupil size.

In dimness or darkness, the pupils dilate (get larger), and when it gets brighter, the pupils constrict (become smaller); this action controls the amount of light entering the eyes. Pupils are also described in terms of being equal or unequal and reactive or unreactive to light (Figure 10-8). To assess the pupils, shine a penlight briefly into the patient's eyes and note the response.

The Rapid Physical Examination

How a physical examination is performed depends on whether the incident is a trauma or a medical emergency and whether the patient is conscious or unconscious. The physical examination involves a quick head-to-toe evaluation of the entire body, during which you look, listen, and feel for abnormalities. Also called the **rapid assessment,** the physical examination quickly identifies major problems. The rapid assessment is appropriate for all unconscious patients, whether the problem is medical or traumatic in nature.

A complete head-to-toe physical assessment is not necessary for a conscious patient with an isolated minor injury, such as an injured finger or hand, a cut on the arm, or a twisted ankle. Nor is it necessary for a conscious patient with a medical emergency, such as chest pain or difficulty breathing. In these situations, focus your attention on the area of the chief complaint and conduct a physical assessment of areas pertinent to that problem. For the patient with chest pain or difficulty breathing, this means examination of the neck and chest, and possibly the ankles for signs of edema. Local protocols often dictate what level of assessment is to be performed on various patients. Watch for medical alert bracelets or necklaces (Figure 10-9). These can provide clues to the nature of the problem.

Significant problems associated with trauma and medical emergencies are those affecting the head, neck, chest, and abdomen. Problems in these areas can present as unconsciousness, seizures, difficulty breathing, and pain. Additional areas of concern for trauma patients are

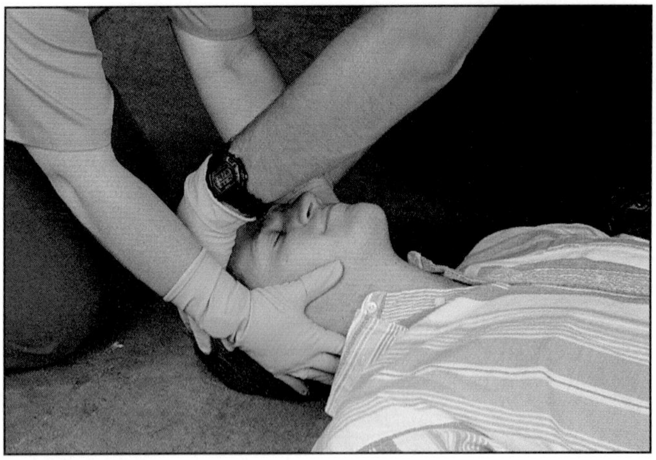

Figure 10-10

While maintaining in-line stabilization, feel along the skull and face for deformities.

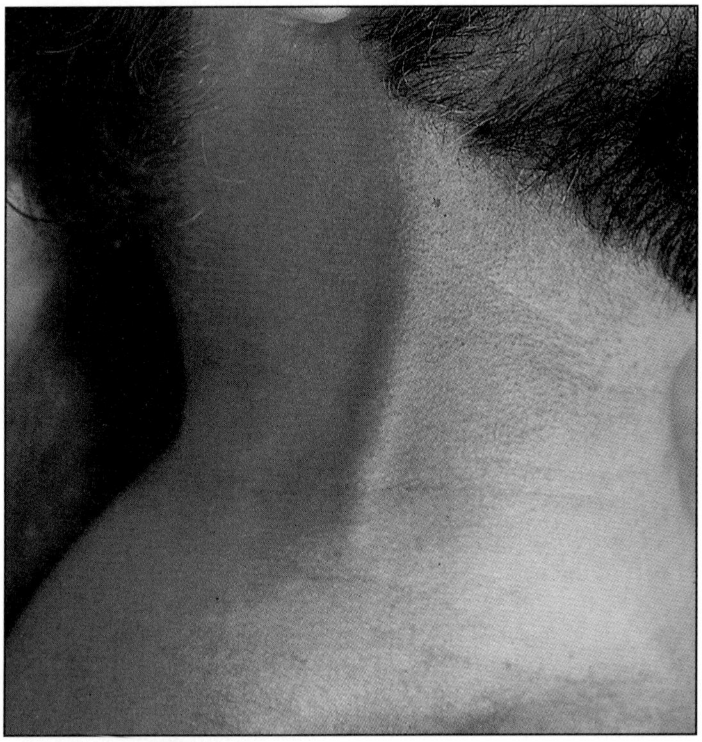

Figure 10-11

Distended jugular veins in an upright patient indicate a backup of blood in the venous system.

the pelvis, back, and thighs. Injuries to these areas of the body can result in paralysis or significant blood loss.

As you perform the physical examination, use the letters DCAP-BTLS to remember what to check for in each area of the body. The letters stand for:

Deformities (abnormal position or shape)
Contusions (bruising)
Abrasions (scrapes)
Punctures (penetrating objects)
Burns
Tenderness (sensitivity to touch)
Lacerations (cuts)
Swelling

While all of these items are appropriate for a trauma patient, only tenderness and swelling are commonly assessed for medical patients.

Begin by examining the patient's head and neck. In trauma patients, make sure that someone is maintaining in-line stabilization of the head and neck. Look and feel quickly along the skull and face for obvious deformities such as protrusions or depressions (Figure 10-10). Check for bleeding from the head, nose, or ears. A nosebleed could be caused by trauma or a medical condition such as hypertension.

Examine the neck, looking and feeling for abnormalities. In addition to the DCAP-BTLS items, assess the jugular veins. If the patient is seated, the jugular veins are often not visible. If the patient is lying down, the veins are somewhat distended. Flat jugular veins in a patient who is lying down could indicate blood loss. **Jugular vein distention** (JVD) in an upright patient indicates a backup of blood in the venous system, a possible sign of heart failure (Figure 10-11). Check to see that the trachea is also in the center of the neck and not deviating to one side, which could indicate a significant chest injury.

If you suspect that the patient may have suffered trauma to the head or spine, apply a cervical collar to minimize movement. When you complete the physical examination and have a backboard available, log-roll the patient onto one side and examine the back before placing the patient on the board (Figure 10-12). If the patient has head injuries and is unconscious, consider this patient a high priority and transport immediately.

Examine the chest by looking for obvious problems, such as contusions, abrasions, or punctures that could indicate lung injury. Palpate the sternum and ribs and auscultate breath sounds. The presence of pain during breathing could mean a fractured rib or a medical problem such as pneumonia. **Paradoxical movement** or **crepitus** could indicate multiple rib fractures and a more serious condition, flail chest. Paradoxical movement often occurs when multiple consecutive ribs are broken in more than one place. This causes movement of one part of the chest wall in opposition to the rest of the chest during breathing. Crepitus is the sound and feel of broken bones grinding against one another or air under the skin (subcutaneous emphysema).

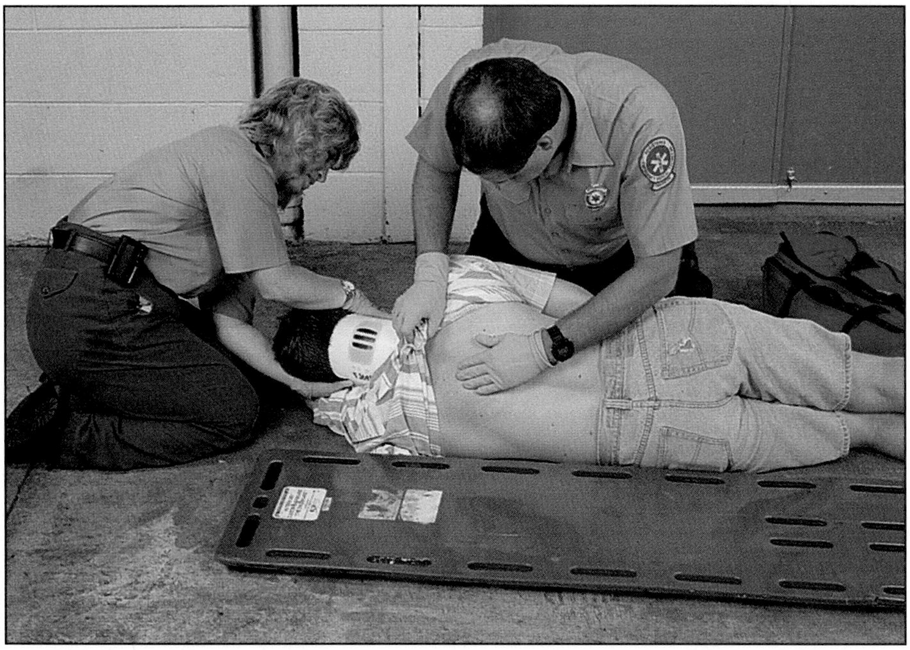

Figure 10-12

Before placing the patient on the backboard, perform a log-roll and examine the back for abnormalities.

Auscultate the patient's breath sounds. Listen to the lungs on each side of the chest by placing a stethoscope on the upper anterior and then the lower lateral chest (see Figure 10-4). Breath sounds should be present and equal bilaterally. The absence of breath sounds on one side of the chest could indicate a significant lung injury, such as a **pneumothorax.** Wheezing and crackles are likely signs of medical problems such as asthma or pulmonary edema. Also listen to the back, if possible.

Examination of the abdomen involves checking the four quadrants for discoloration, pain, tenderness, guarding, distension, and rigidity. While looking at the abdomen, place your hands on each of the quadrants and apply gentle pressure to the abdomen (Figure 10-13). Note whether the abdomen is rigid or if the patient reports pain in any of the quadrants. A rigid abdomen could signify internal bleeding. A distended abdomen may be a sign of air in the stomach, as is sometimes seen in crying children. Some patients will attempt to protect areas of the body that are painful. This is known as guarding and can also indicate a significant problem in the abdomen.

Unlike the chest, which is protected by the ribs, the vital organs of the abdomen lack bony protection. Only the upper two quadrants of the abdomen, which contain the liver, stomach, and spleen, are provided some protection by the lower ribs. Organs in the abdomen can

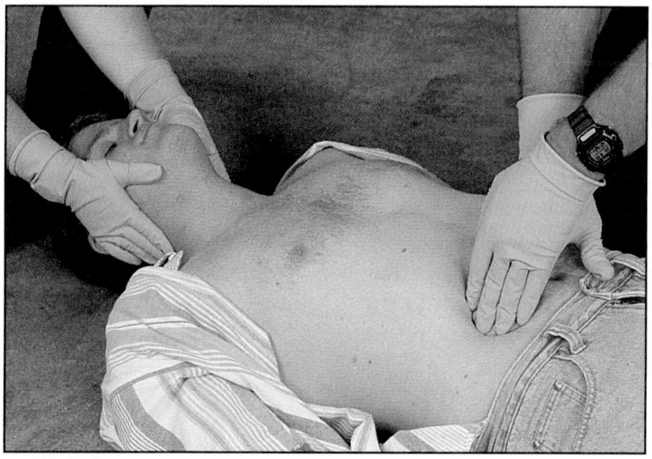

Figure 10-13

Examine all four quadrants by looking and applying gentle pressure. Note any pain, rigidity, or guarding.

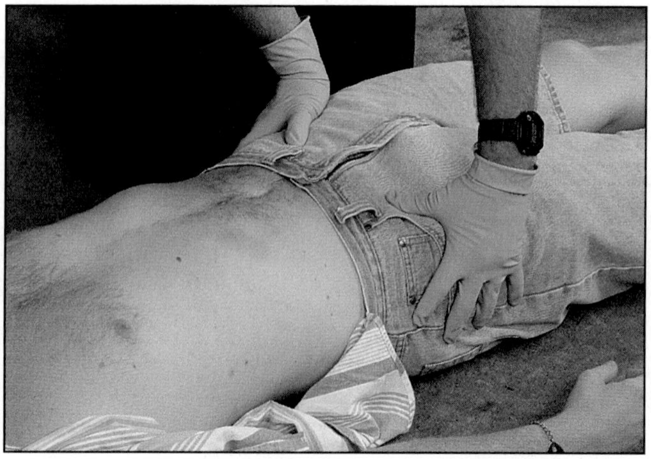

Figure 10-14

Determine the stability of the pelvis by pressing first downward, then inward, on the iliac crests.

therefore easily be injured. Some organs, such as the liver and spleen, tend to bleed profusely when injured. With internal injuries, your rapid assessment will only be able to identify the possible organs involved. Fortunately, this examination is often enough to locate a potentially life-threatening condition and identify the need for rapid transport, even when the exact injury is uncertain.

Move from the abdomen to assess the pelvis. Again, consider the mechanism of any injury, the patient's age, and the overall condition. Elderly patients can suffer significant hip and pelvic injuries from what otherwise might seem to be minor falls. A pelvic fracture can result in significant blood loss or a ruptured bladder. It requires pelvic stabilization and rapid transport.

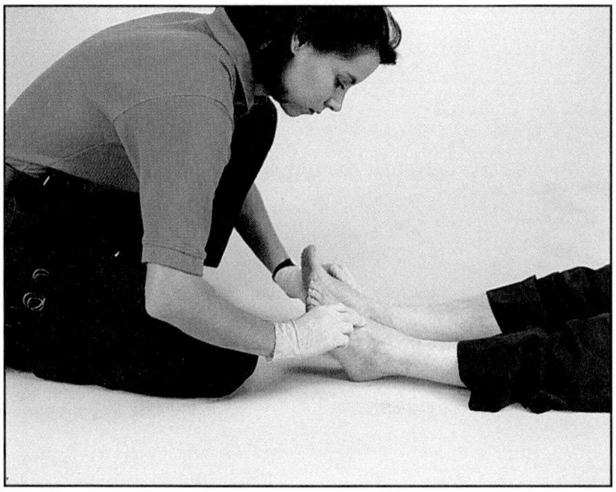

Figure 10-15

Assessing the dorsal pedis pulse.

Examine the pelvis by placing your hands at the **iliac crests.** To determine the stability of the pelvis, press downward to flex the pelvis and then inward to compress the pelvis (Figure 10-14). This procedure is only done on patients who do not initially complain of pain in the pelvic area. If the procedure produces pain, stop immediately and assume a pelvic injury.

Finally, check the patient's extremities, beginning with the legs. In addition to the usual check for deformity, crepitus, and tenderness, look for appropriate movement, sensation, and circulation. Ask a conscious patient to wiggle the fingers and toes. Touch different areas of the hands and feet, and ask if the patient can feel where you are touching. This helps indicate that the patient has appropriate sensation. An unconscious patient will not be able to respond to a verbal request for movement and feeling but may still respond to stimuli. For example, an unconscious patient may withdraw or extend a limb in response to pain. This tells you that the patient has both sensation and motor response.

To check circulation in the extremities, locate one of the pulse sites in the feet. There are two commonly checked sites, the dorsalis pedis pulse on the top of the foot (Figure 10-15), and the posterior tibial pulse on the medial side of the ankle (Figure 10-16). The absence of **distal pulses** may indicate poor circulation caused by shock or heart failure. Edema of the ankles and feet may also indicate a significant heart problem. Once you have finished checking the legs and feet, examine the arms and hands in the same manner as you did the legs and feet. Check circulation by feeling the radial pulse at the wrist (Figure 10-17).

While trauma patients with multiple injuries or a significant mechanism of injury should receive this rapid physical examination, not all trauma patients need it. A patient with an isolated injury, such as an injured hand or

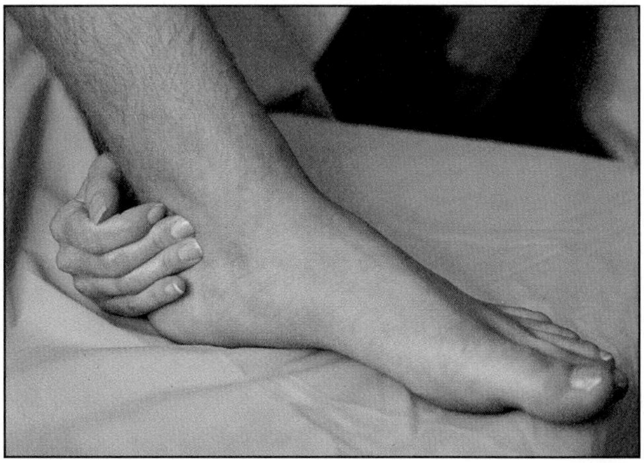

Figure 10-16

Assessing the posterior tibial pulse on the medial side of the ankle.

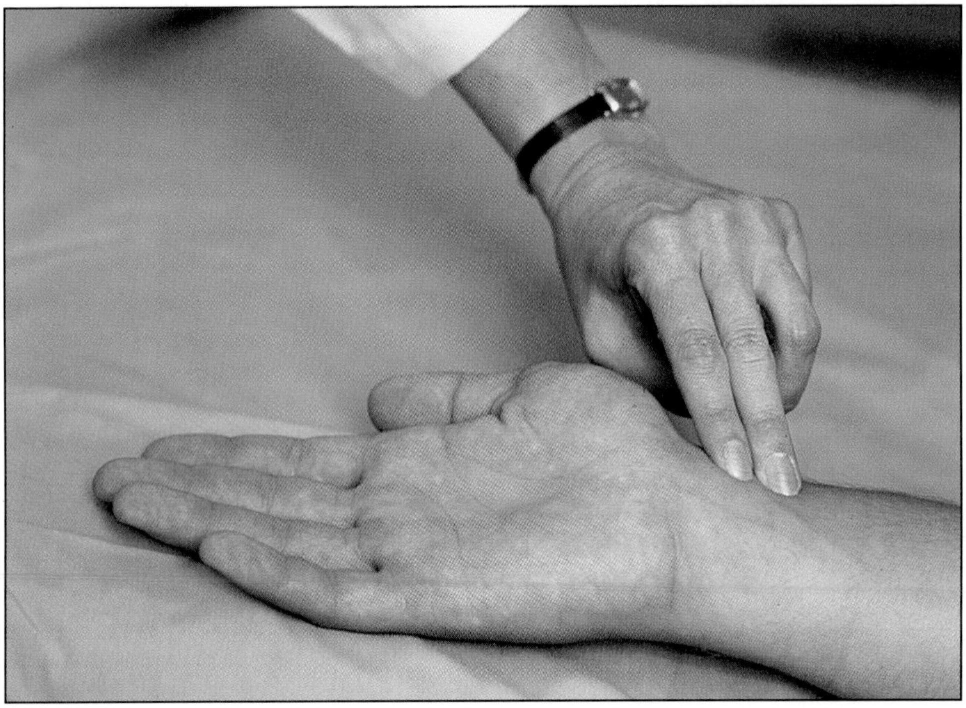

Figure 10-17
Extremity circulation also can be checked by assessing the radial pulse at the wrist.

foot, will normally require only a focused examination on that part of the body. However, you should still do an initial assessment and gather pertinent information through the focused history. Be alert for mechanism of injury or other signs that could indicate additional injuries.

While the physical examination helps you identify external problems such as wounds, it is not as certain to reveal the exact nature of internal problems. When examining a patient with a medical problem, the past and present medical histories may help. The following examples demonstrate how this information can be used in conjunction with a focused physical examination.

You are dispatched to a 35-year-old male complaining of abdominal pain. As you arrive, his screaming makes it obvious that he is conscious, his airway is clear, he is breathing, and he has a pulse. His chief complaint is pain in his left side and back that is constant and excruciating. He describes the events leading up to this problem, including a recent marathon run, inadequate fluid replacement, and the inability to urinate without discomfort. He denies suffering any form of injury.

As you palpate the abdomen, you note that the patient is guarding his abdomen. You find the abdomen to be somewhat rigid, and the patient complains of pain confined to the left side and radiating around to the back. His vital signs include a rapid pulse and rapid respirations without any problem exchanging air. He also states that he had kidney stones about 2 years ago and that the pain was in the same area and felt the same. Based on this information, it is likely that he is having a recurrence of the same problem.

At other times, although a patient may not have similar past problems to relate, the information you gather will still be adequate to provide the proper care. Consider the following example:

You respond to a call for a 75-year-old female complaining of shortness of breath. When you arrive, the patient is seated in a chair. She is alert and oriented, but states that she feels lightheaded. Her chief complaints are substernal chest pain and difficulty breathing. She states that the pain is constant and does not vary during breathing. She describes it as a dull pain that has been there for about a day and has been getting worse over the last hour. Her breath sounds indicate that she has crackles, and her jugular veins are distended. She denies having any medical problems or allergies and is not taking any medications. You take her vital signs and find an abnormally slow and irregular pulse; rapid, labored respirations; lower-than-normal blood pressure; and pale, diaphoretic skin. You examine her ankles and find some edema.

You conclude that the patient's problem is likely cardiac in origin and decide to treat this patient ac-

cording to your protocols for chest pain and difficulty breathing. This includes helping the patient achieve a position of comfort, administering high-concentration oxygen and assisting ventilations, requesting ALS personnel, and preparing the patient for transport without delay.

When a patient is unconscious, the medical history may not be readily available. Consider the scenario presented at the beginning of the chapter as you read the conclusion below. In this case, the physical examination provided a clue as to what the problem was. This clue did help, but it would not have affected the treatment that you provided.

IT'S YOUR CALL
CONCLUSION

You were dispatched to an unconscious patient and arrived to find a woman motionless on the floor. The only information provided by a bystander is that the woman collapsed and was lowered to the floor, where she appeared to have a seizure.

You have completed your initial assessment, which showed the patient's condition to be unstable. You summon ALS personnel and begin the focused history and physical examination. Unable to get any additional verbal information from the patient or bystanders, you focus on the physical examination, assessing vital signs and doing a rapid physical assessment from head to toe.

You note a medical identification bracelet indicating the patient is a diabetic. You complete your assessment and do not find any abnormalities. You follow your protocols for treating an unconscious patient, which include proper positioning and immobilization of the patient, airway management, summoning ALS personnel, and preparing for transport without delay.

After applying a cervical collar and securing the patient to a backboard, you place the patient on a wheeled stretcher and move her to the ALS unit that has pulled up in front of the building. You relay your information to the paramedic and get on board to assist with some ALS procedures. After the paramedic starts an intravenous line and administers a glucose solution, the patient responds. The patient was experiencing a diabetic emergency involving a low blood-sugar level.

The Detailed Physical Examination

Once the focused history and physical examination have been completed, initial care has been provided, and the patient has been moved to the ambulance, you may need to complete a **detailed physical examination.** The detailed physical examination is done in the same systematic manner as the focused history and physical examination, but more slowly and with greater attention to detail. This reassessment should routinely be accomplished in a few minutes.

Once again, inspect the body from head to toe, moving from the head to the neck, chest, abdomen, pelvis, and extremities. It will not be possible to check the patient's back if he or she has already been immobilized on a backboard (this should have been done before placing the patient on the backboard). It will also not be necessary to conduct this detailed physical examination in all situations. A patient with breathing difficulty caused by asthma does not require palpation of the head, abdomen, pelvis, or extremities. A reassessment of the airway, neck, and chest are all that would be needed in such a case.

While positioned alongside the patient, look for obvious injuries, bruising, bleeding, or abnormal skin temperature or moisture. Also note facial expression. Feel for soft spots, indentations, bone instability, and impaled objects. Listen for respiratory abnormalities. Ask questions to learn how the patient is feeling generally and whether the patient feels any pain as you touch specific areas of the body. Record any abnormal findings. Palpate the body to discover any hidden problems, such as undetected injuries or painful areas. Keep in mind that a painful injury in one area of the body may override the patient's feeling of any pain in a different area. Use your sense of smell to detect characteristic odors such as alcohol.

When reassessing the head, pay particular attention to soft spots or indentations on the surface. Be alert for sharp bony fragments, shards of glass, or other foreign objects. These objects may cause injuries to become more extensive if they are accidentally pressed. They may also tear through your gloves, destroying the disease barrier and possibly injuring you. Indentations in the skull and changes in mental status are indications that a serious brain injury may be present. Check the patient's face around the eyes, nose, maxilla, and mandible. Observe the patient for the presence of raccoon eyes, caused by blood seeping into the tissue around both eyes and giving the face a mask-like appearance (Figure 10-18). This possible sign of a basilar skull fracture does not usually appear right away. If it is present immediately, it more likely indicates direct trauma to the face. Feel the entire facial bone structure beginning at the bridge of the nose and extending laterally to the ears.

Feel the bones surrounding the eyes and the forehead for any deformity or instability. Looking at each eye individually, note whether the eyes are working together. Look at the pupils to see that they are round, the same size, and react to light. The eyes should be able to work in conjunction with each other, looking up, down, left, and right. Sluggish pupil responses can reflect a lack of oxygen or the use of depressants.

Note any discoloration of the face, such as pallor or cyanosis, beginning to develop. This could indicate a lack of oxygen in the tissues. Look at the nose and ears for signs of bleeding or cerebrospinal fluid (CSF). When fluid containing CSF leaks onto a gauze dressing, the CSF may separate from other fluid and make a double ring on the gauze. This is commonly known as the "halo effect." Generally, you will not need to specifically test leaking fluid for this, but note it if it is present. Look behind the ears for signs of bruising, called *Battle's sign,* another indication of skull fracture that will not appear until several hours after the injury (Figure 10-19).

Check the mouth for tongue lacerations and make sure there are no broken teeth or other foreign bodies. Have suction ready because swallowed blood can cause vomiting. Make note of any odors on the patient's breath. Alcohol and the fruity smell of a diabetic are two common and important odors you may detect. For dark-skinned individuals, the inside of the lips is also a good place to assess skin color.

When reexamining the neck, check for swelling, bruising, lacerations, and JVD. If the patient has a cervi-

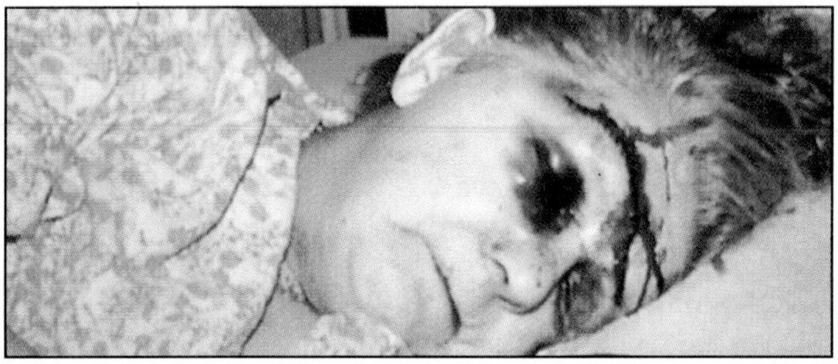

Figure 10-18

Raccoon eyes usually do not appear immediately. If this mask-like appearance is immediately present, it indicates direct trauma to the face or skull.

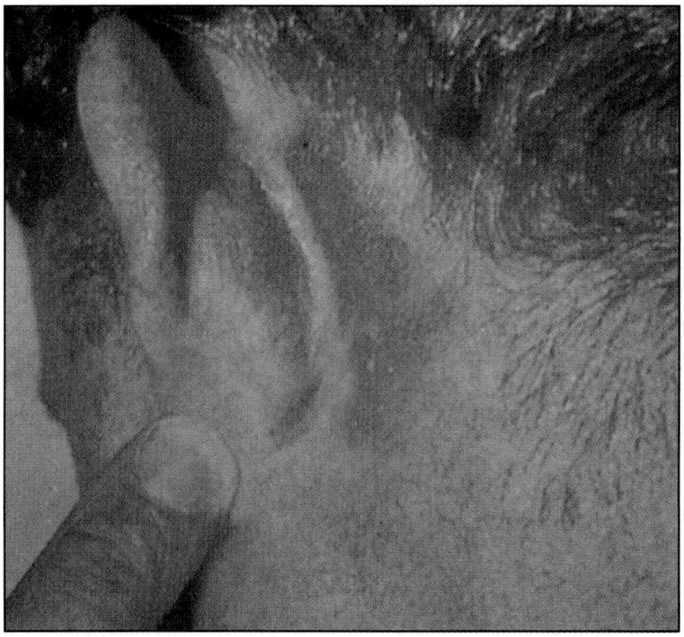

Figure 10-19

Bruising behind the ears is called Battle's sign and does not usually appear for several hours after the injury.

cal collar in place, assessment of the neck will be limited to the anterior portion. This is why it is important to check the neck during the initial examination, before applying the collar. Feel the neck for *subcutaneous emphysema,* which will feel like air bubbles just under the skin. Subcutaneous emphysema develops when air from the lungs or from a tear in the trachea leaks into the tissues of the upper chest and neck; when these areas are palpated, the tissue will crackle under the finger tips. The patient will take on a bloated appearance. The anterior portion of the neck also needs to be rechecked for tracheal deviation. Ask the patient if there is any neck pain or any tightness, numbness, tingling, or burning in the shoulders, down the arms, or down into the legs.

Reconfirm that the trauma patient has been properly placed in a cervical collar and secured to the backboard. If the collar is occluding the airway or creating difficulty breathing, ensure that it is the proper size and has been applied correctly.

Examine the chest for signs of bruising, swelling, paradoxical movement, use of accessory muscles while breathing, and open chest wounds. Bruising that may not have been evident initially can appear later. Feel the entire chest: the length of the clavicles, the sternum, and the rib cage, including as much of the posterior ribs as can be reached safely. Feel for signs of tenderness, deformities, crepitus, and subcutaneous emphysema. Check the chest for symmetry. Look for scars that could indicate previous surgery.

Auscultate breath sounds and compare them to what you heard initially. A medical patient who has been placed supine may now develop fluid in the lungs that you did not hear earlier, or a patient with chest trauma could gradually lose lung sounds on one side. These sounds are not easy to hear in a moving ambulance.

Feel all four quadrants of the abdomen, noting any rigidity, tenderness, or guarding. The normal abdomen feels soft. A patient who is guarding or who has a rigid or pulsating abdomen could have a serious condition, and you should expedite the transport.

Reexamine the pelvic bones for deformity or instability. For patients who are not complaining of pain, push gently down on the anterior portions of the iliac crests, then gently push both sides toward the midline. If this causes pain at any point or if you detect instability, do not continue. Deformity and tenderness of the pelvis could indicate a fracture. If the force was great enough to fracture the pelvis, it could easily have been great enough to cause major structural and vascular injuries, such as a ruptured bladder.

Evaluate the genital region for injury and to determine if the patient has lost bladder or bowel control. Incontinence can result from coma, seizure, stroke, or brain or spinal injury.

When rechecking the extremities, observe for signs of bruising, bleeding, open wounds, deformities, swelling, loss of motor function and sensation, and abnormal pulses or skin condition. Look and feel the entire length and girth of each extremity. Compare one extremity to the other, looking for any abnormalities. In patients complaining of chest pain or difficulty breathing, check the ankles for signs of peripheral edema, which may indicate congestive heart failure. Ask if the patient is able to feel where you are touching; this is done to confirm sensory perception. To test motor function, ask the patient to wiggle the fingers and toes and squeeze or push against your hand. Reevaluate capillary refill in the fingers or toes.

Examine the back if the patient is not yet immobilized on a backboard. Check the flank regions toward the sides of the patient's back if you have not already done so during the abdominal exam. Palpate the small of the back. Poor circulation can cause edema in the lumbar region.

As you document any new findings, compare them with previous examination results to identify changes in the patient's condition. This could indicate a trend toward either improvement or deterioration and may require further action.

Ongoing Assessment

Ongoing assessment enables you to identify subtle changes, either good or bad. A patient who was initially alert and oriented could begin to show signs of decreased consciousness related to head trauma, inadequate oxygenation, stroke, **hypoglycemia,** or a number of other conditions. Significant changes in vital signs would also be considered abnormal. The ongoing assessment is performed while you are en route to the hospital. The patient should be reevaluated every 15 minutes if stable, and every 5 minutes if unstable.

A stable patient is one who has a simple, specific injury, such as a hand laceration or injured ankle, and who has normal vital signs. A patient whose only complaint is nausea or vomiting may also be considered stable, as would a patient with generalized illness, such as the flu. Such a patient is considered stable if vital signs are unchanging and normal for the patient's condition and age group.

Unstable patients include any trauma or medical patients with a significant mechanism of injury or nature of illness. These patients may be unstable upon your arrival or may become unstable later. Even if the patient's vital signs are within normal limits, the patient should be reevaluated frequently based on the mechanism of the injury or illness. Other patients likely to be unstable are those complaining of difficulty breathing, chest or abdominal pain, or those with altered consciousness.

The ongoing assessment will usually be conducted in the ambulance. Occasionally this will not be true if you are attending a patient while awaiting an ALS crew or if a multiple casualty incident (MCI) is in progress. Though not all patients receive a complete physical assessment as

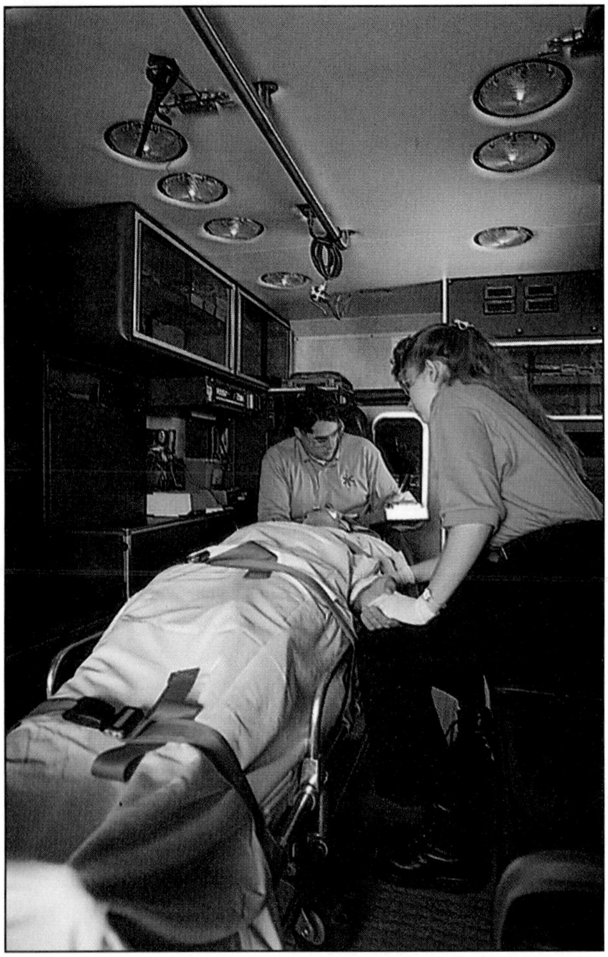

Figure 10-20

Perform an ongoing assessment during transport, taking vital sign measurements and checking the patient's condition every few minutes.

part of the focused history and physical examination, all patients do receive an ongoing assessment.

The ongoing assessment requires you to repeat some assessment steps already done. Be sure to:

- Repeat the initial assessment of consciousness, airway, breathing, and circulation.
- Recheck historical information to see if new information is offered.
- Measure and record all vital signs.
- Repeat the physical examination, focusing on the patient's chief complaint.
- Reevaluate the treatment provided so far.

Reevaluating the treatment you have provided will help ensure that it has been effective. Among the interventions that deserve particular attention are:

- The adequacy of supplemental oxygen
- Ongoing control of bleeding
- Effectiveness of immobilization
- Attention to the patient's comfort

The length of the transport will determine how often the patient needs to be reevaluated. The last assessment should occur a few minutes before arrival at the hospital. You will have the latest information for hospital staff and will be ready to comment on any trends noticed since the initial assessment. This will also leave time to prepare the patient and any equipment for movement into the hospital (Figure 10-20).

SUMMARY

The focused history and examination is a rapid, systematic plan for evaluating every patient, regardless of the problem. If a patient's complaint is confined to a particular area of the body, then the physical examination will focus on that area. The length of time it takes to complete the focused history and examination varies depending on the number of EMTs available, but it is usually completed in only a few minutes.

The focused history gathers information such as previous medical history (SAMPLE) and history of the present event. It also includes questions about any pain that is present (OPQRST). The physical assessment involves recording vital signs and conducting a head-to-toe check of the patient.

A more detailed physical examination can be done as you begin transporting the patient. This involves reassessing the items already checked but more slowly and in greater detail. Once the detailed physical examination is complete, you will continue to assess the patient periodically. This ongoing assessment indicates whether treatment has been successful and identifies trends in the patient's condition.

Section 5

Airway Management

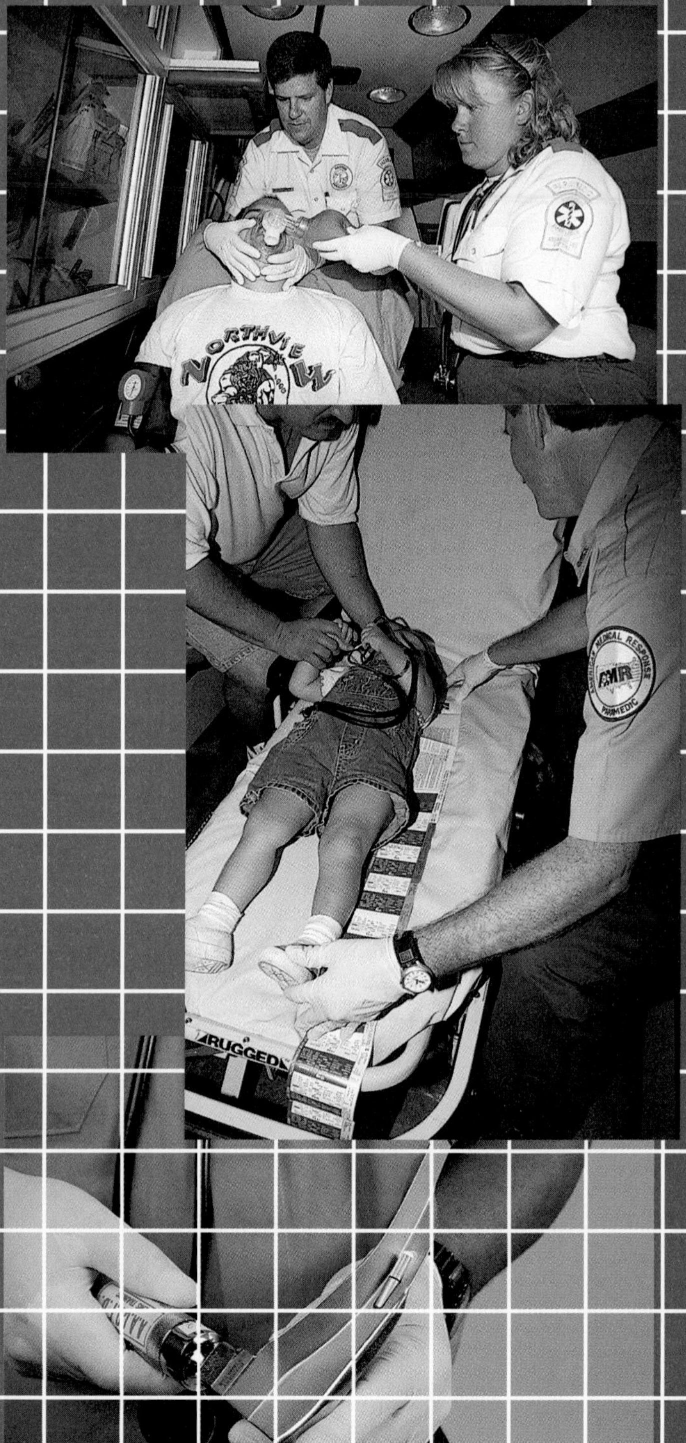

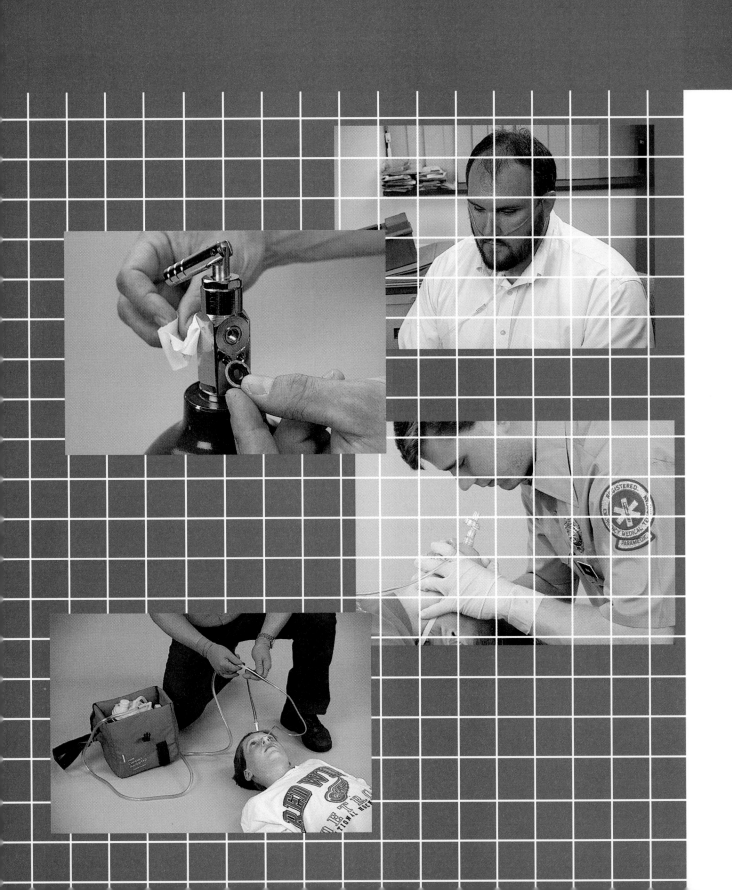

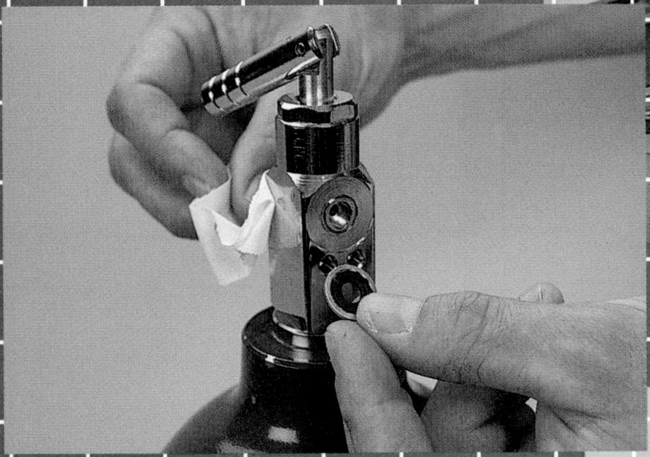

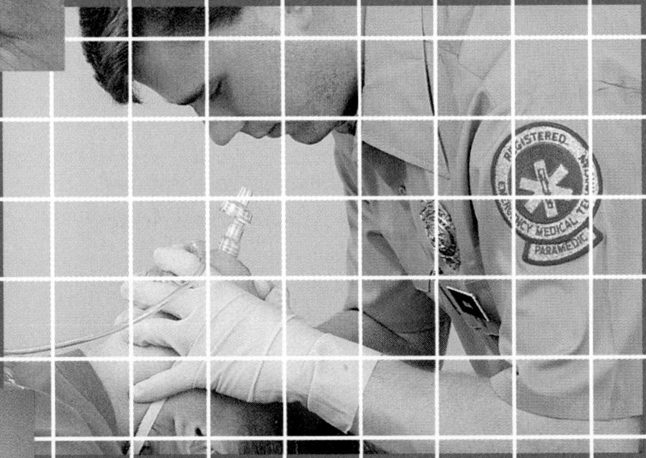
REGISTERED
PARAMEDIC

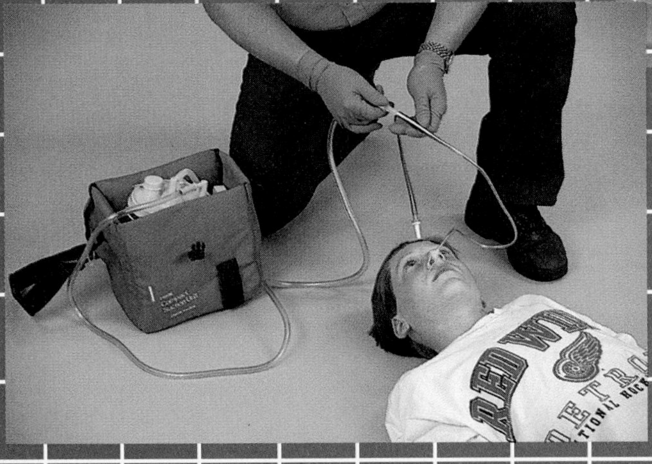

Chapter 11

Basic Airway Management

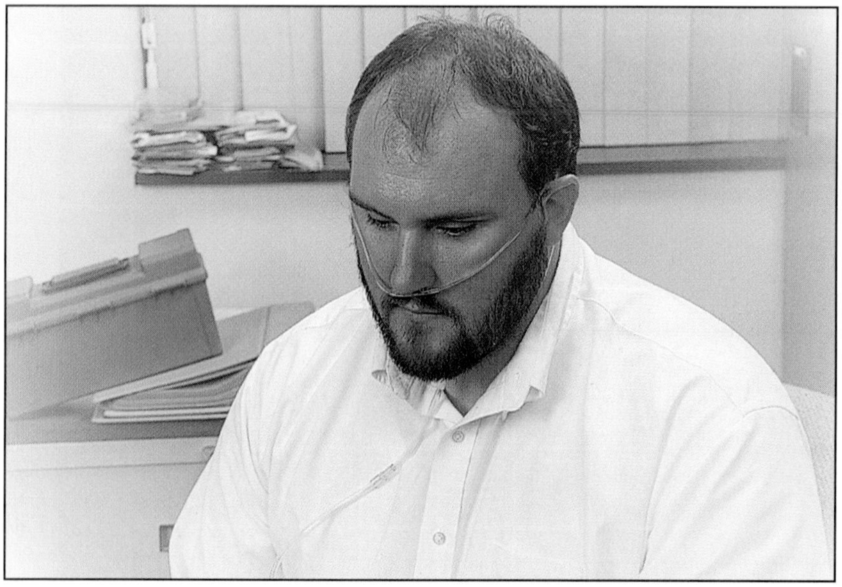

Knowledge Objectives

As an EMT-Basic, you should be able to:

OBJECTIVES

1. Identify the major structures of the respiratory system.
2. Describe how the respiratory system works with other systems in the body.
3. List the signs of adequate and inadequate breathing.
4. List the steps to take when treating a patient with respiratory distress.
5. Describe the steps for relieving airway obstructions in conscious adult, child, and infant patients.
6. Describe the steps for relieving airway obstructions in unconscious adult, child, and infant patients.
7. Describe how to identify a nonbreathing patient.
8. Describe how to open an airway using the head-tilt–chin-lift and modified jaw-thrust techniques.
9. Describe the various techniques for ventilating a nonbreathing patient with one rescuer and with two, including:
   - Mouth-to-mask
   - Bag-valve-mask ventilation
   - Flow-restricted, oxygen-powered ventilation devices
10. Describe the signs of adequate artificial ventilation.
11. Explain how you would provide artificial ventilation to a patient with a laryngectomy.
12. Describe the equipment and techniques used to suction a patient.
13. Describe when it would be appropriate to use a suction device.
14. Describe when to use oropharyngeal and nasopharyngeal airways and how to insert them properly.
15. Define the components of an oxygen delivery system.
16. Describe the procedures used to set up an oxygen system and administer oxygen.
17. Describe when to use a nasal cannula and a nonrebreather mask, and list the oxygen flow requirements for each.

OBJECTIVES

Skill Objectives

As an EMT-Basic, you should be able to:

1. **Demonstrate how to relieve airway obstructions in conscious adult, child, and infant patients.**
2. **Demonstrate how to relieve airway obstructions in unconscious adult, child, and infant patients.**
3. **Demonstrate how to open an airway using the head-tilt–chin-lift and modified jaw-thrust techniques.**
4. **Demonstrate how to perform artificial ventilation using mouth-to-mask breathing with a pocket-size mask and one-way valve.**
5. **Demonstrate how to perform artificial ventilation with one rescuer and with two, using a resuscitation mask, bag-valve-mask, and a flow-restricted, oxygen-powered delivery device.**
6. **Demonstrate how to ventilate a patient who has a stoma.**
7. **Demonstrate the techniques used to suction an airway.**
8. **Demonstrate how to insert oropharyngeal and nasopharyngeal airways.**
9. **Demonstrate how to set up an oxygen cylinder and regulator for the delivery of oxygen.**
10. **Demonstrate how to use oxygen delivery devices.**

Attitude Objectives

As an EMT-Basic, you should be able to:

1. **Defend the idea that artificial ventilation and airway-management skills take priority over most other basic life-support skills.**
2. **Describe your feelings about performing artificial ventilation on a nonbreathing patient.**
3. **Defend the rationale for providing adequate oxygenation by giving high concentrations to patients who in the past have received only low concentrations.**
4. **Act as a role model for others in regard to the use of basic airway adjuncts.**

KEY TERMS

1. **Airway:** The structures of the respiratory system through which air passes.
2. **Alveoli:** Microscopic air sacs in the lungs where gas exchange occurs.
3. **Artificial Ventilation:** The process of ventilating a nonbreathing or inadequately breathing patient; can be done with mouth-to-mask breathing or breathing adjuncts such as a bag-valve-mask device.
4. **Aspiration:** The inhalation of foreign matter into the trachea and lungs; a life-threatening problem that EMTs must anticipate and try to prevent.
5. **Bag-Valve-Mask:** A device that can be attached to supplemental oxygen and used for artificial ventilation; consists of a self-inflating bag, a one-way valve, and a face mask.
6. **Dyspnea:** Shortness of breath; difficulty breathing.
7. **Gag Reflex:** A protective mechanism designed to protect the airway from aspiration; occurs when the back of the throat is stimulated.
8. **Head-Tilt–Chin-Lift:** A technique used to open a patient's airway by tilting the head back and lifting the chin forward.
9. **Hypoxia:** Inadequate oxygenation; can refer to the cellular level, a particular organ, or the entire body.
10. **Laryngectomy:** A surgical procedure in which the larynx is removed.
11. **Modified Jaw-Thrust:** A technique used to open the airway of a patient with suspected spinal injury; the head remains in a neutral position while the jaw is lifted forward.
12. **Nasal Cannula:** A flexible tube used to administer oxygen through the nostrils of a breathing patient.
13. **Nasopharyngeal Airway:** A flexible, rubber, tubelike device inserted into one nostril and the nasopharynx to prevent the tongue from obstructing the airway.
14. **Nonrebreather Mask:** A mask that covers the mouth and nose and is used to administer oxygen to a breathing patient.
15. **Oropharyngeal Airway:** A curved plastic tube inserted into the mouth and oropharynx of a patient without a gag reflex; prevents the tongue from obstructing the airway.
16. **Oxygenation:** The process of bringing oxygen into the body and delivering it to the tissues.
17. **Regulator:** A device attached to an oxygen cylinder that reduces the pressure within the cylinder to an amount that can be safely administered to a patient.
18. **Respiratory Arrest:** Cessation of breathing.
19. **Respiratory Distress:** Difficult or inadequate breathing.
20. **Stoma:** A surgical opening in the neck; the primary (or only) breathing opening for a person whose larynx has been removed.
21. **Stridor:** An abnormal, high-pitched breath sound caused by an obstruction in the upper airway.
22. **Suctioning:** The use of manual or mechanical devices to draw vomitus and secretions, such as saliva and blood, from a patient's mouth and throat.
23. **Ventilation:** The movement of air into and out of the lungs.
24. **Wheezing:** A musical breathing noise caused by air flowing through narrowed airway passages in the lungs (the lower airways); commonly associated with asthma.

IT'S YOUR CALL

You are dispatched to the home of a 66-year-old man complaining of difficulty breathing. Upon arrival, you find your patient sitting on the couch, leaning forward, and in obvious distress. His chief complaints are shortness of breath and tightness in his chest. You notice that the patient is already on oxygen. The patient's wife tells you that her husband has a history of emphysema and has been on oxygen for the last year.

As you assess the patient, you notice that his breathing is faster than normal, at 32 breaths per minute, and is labored and noisy. His heart rate is 120 beats per minute, and his blood pressure is 160/90. His skin is cyanotic and moist. His lung sounds include crackles (rales) on both sides. You notice that the patient's oxygen is being delivered through a nasal cannula at 4 liters per minute (lpm). His wife tells you that the oxygen is usually set at 2 lpm. He raised it when he began having trouble breathing hours ago, but it has not helped. The patient tells you that the chest pain feels like pressure in the middle of his chest. It began about 40 minutes ago and has not gone away. He says he does not have any heart problems. Besides emphysema, he has been hospitalized for pneumonia and has been a smoker for 25 years.

Based on this assessment, you believe that the patient is having a significant breathing problem, which might also be related to a heart problem. You remove the patient's nasal cannula and place him on a nonrebreather mask at 15 lpm. Several minutes later, after the patient is placed in the ambulance, you notice that there is no change in his respiratory status. You then begin to assist his breathing with a bag-valve-mask connected to oxygen at a flow rate of 15 lpm. However, the patient's wife reports that his physician told him never to use more than 4 lpm of oxygen. Are your actions appropriate, or should you follow the advice given to the patient by his physician?

As an EMT-Basic, prompt recognition and management skills for airway and breathing emergencies are essential. Whether you are dealing with a trauma or a medical emergency, ensuring that your patient has an open airway and is breathing adequately is the first priority in patient care. An understanding of how the respiratory system works and the ability to recognize when a patient is having difficulty breathing will help you provide the best possible care.

Airway adjuncts are available to help care for a patient with breathing difficulty. These include devices designed to clear a patient's airway of debris, keep an unconscious patient's airway open, and deliver oxygen. These devices help oxygenate and ventilate the patient adequately. This chapter will help you learn how to provide care in a wide variety of breathing emergencies, from a patient who is having mild distress to one who is not breathing at all. Whether the patient is an adult, child, or infant, proper airway and breathing care are essential parts of the EMT's job.

Reviewing the Body Systems

To function properly the human body needs oxygen. Without it the body is not able to carry out any of its vital functions. While the respiratory system is primarily responsible for getting oxygen into the body and removing carbon dioxide, it must rely on other systems to circulate the oxygen and regulate its use. These include the circulatory, musculoskeletal, and nervous systems.

The Respiratory System

Every human activity is fueled by oxygen; without it the body cannot create or use energy. The **respiratory system** is made up of the lungs and a series of **airways** that conduct air into the lungs during inhalation and remove waste products in used air during exhalation. Air enters the body through the mouth and nose, then passes into the oral and nasal cavities, through the pharynx and vocal cords, and down the windpipe, known as the *trachea* (Figure 11-1). The **trachea** is located in front of the esophagus and divides into two tubes, the bronchi, which lead to the lungs. These bronchi break into even smaller tubes, called *bronchioles,* which further divide into grapelike clusters of air sacs in the lungs, called **alveoli** (Figure 11-2), where the gas exchange takes place. It is here that the blood picks up oxygen and releases carbon dioxide. The cell membranes in the alveoli are very thin to allow for this exchange of oxygen and carbon dioxide.

Interrelationship of Body Systems

While the respiratory system is responsible for providing oxygen, the circulatory system carries oxygenated blood to the tissues. In the lungs, red blood cells pick up the oxygen in the alveoli. As the heart pumps, the oxygenated blood is distributed throughout the body. As it exits the heart through the aorta, the coronary arteries deliver some of that oxygenated blood to the heart itself. Other arteries deliver the blood to the various organs. There,

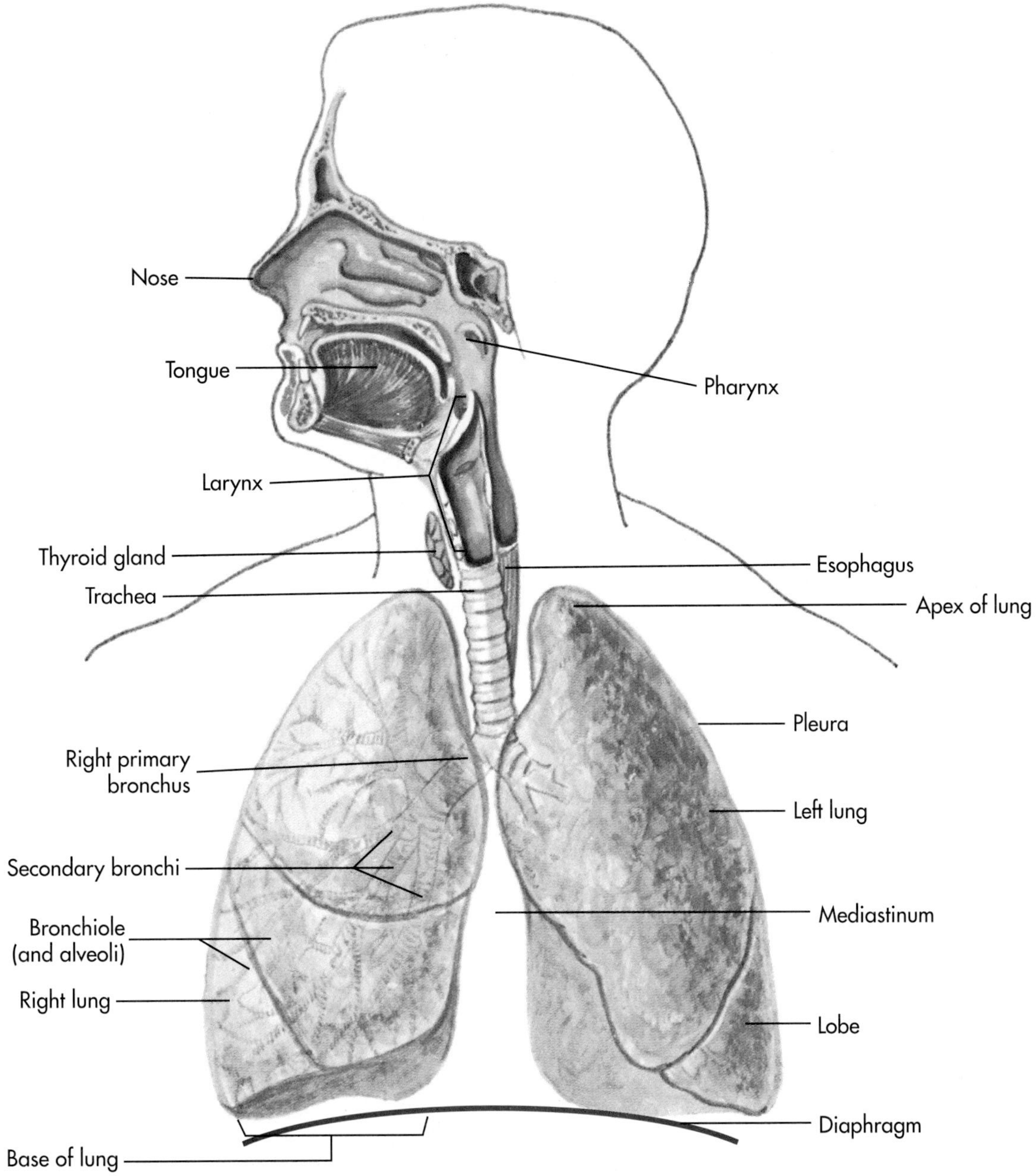

Figure 11-1

Basic structures of the respiratory system.

cells pick up the oxygen and release carbon dioxide and other waste products back into the blood. This deoxygenated blood returns to the heart and is pumped back into the lungs. There the blood picks up fresh oxygen and releases carbon dioxide, which is breathed out of the body. The cycle continues.

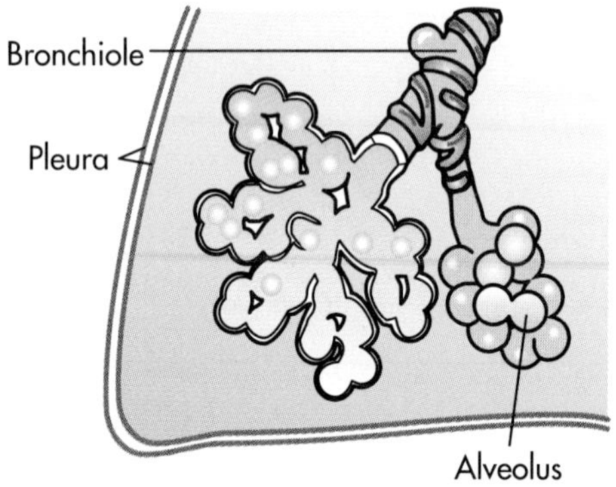

Figure 11-2

Blood picks up oxygen and releases carbon dioxide in the alveoli.

For the respiratory system to function properly, there must be adequate expansion and contraction of the lungs. The lungs have no muscular tissue and cannot move air by themselves. The musculoskeletal system makes this happen. Structures such as the rib cage, the diaphragm, and the intercostal muscles cause the movement of air in and out of the body. The diaphragm is a specialized muscle that separates the thoracic and abdominal cavities. During inhalation, the diaphragm and intercostal muscles contract, increasing the thoracic area, decreasing the pressure inside the chest, and pulling air into the lungs. During exhalation, the diaphragm and intercostal muscles relax, which causes the thoracic cavity to decrease, the pressure inside to increase, and air to be forced out of the lungs (Figure 11-3).

Another important system that works with the respiratory system is the nervous system. The brain sends signals to the respiratory and musculoskeletal systems when there is a need for increased ventilation. The nervous system also helps regulate the depth of breaths and the size of blood vessels. This allows for changes in the amount of blood that goes through the lungs and through vessels in other tissues as the demand for oxygen changes in various parts of the body. When oxygen is low or carbon dioxide is high, the nervous system stimulates the respiratory system to breathe faster.

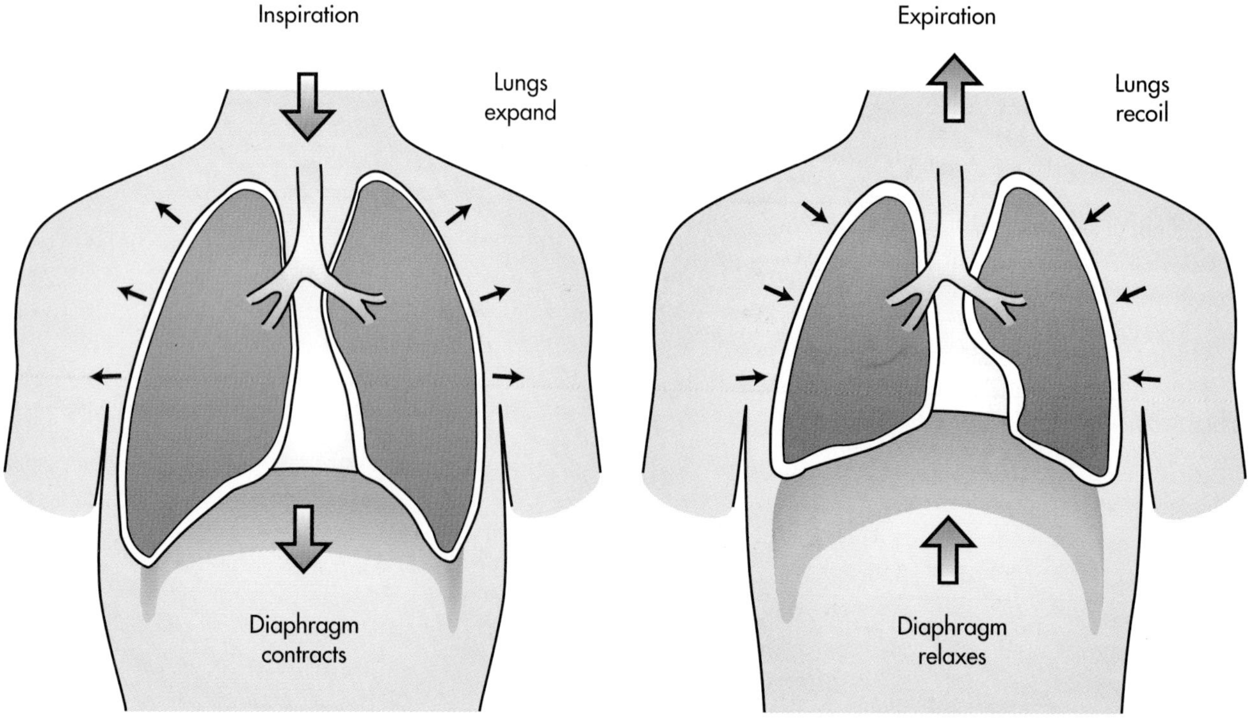

Figure 11-3

The diaphragm and intercostal muscles control the movement of air in and out of the body.

The Patient With Breathing Difficulty

One of the most common emergencies that an EMT-Basic will deal with is difficulty breathing or shortness of breath **(dyspnea).** This condition can be caused by a variety of medical and traumatic problems. Regardless of the cause, it is important to address the situation quickly. To recognize a patient with breathing difficulty, you must be familiar with the characteristics of normal breathing, including rate, rhythm, quality, and depth.

Rate: The number of times a person breathes in a minute is the respiratory rate. The normal rate for an adult is 12 to 20 times per minute. However, this may vary slightly depending on age, physical condition, and size. People in excellent physical condition may have a normal rate of 10 breaths per minute. Children and infants breathe more quickly than adults. A child's normal respiratory rate is 15 to 30 breaths per minute, and an infant's is 25 to 50 breaths per minute. Breathing rates in children and infants also vary with age, sex, size, and physical condition.

Rhythm: In a normal rhythm, the time between breaths and the length of each breath will be constant. The chest will also rise and fall smoothly and symmetrically.

Quality: A person who is breathing normally will have clear and equal lung sounds from side to side (bilaterally), will have adequate and equal chest expansion, and will breathe with minimal effort. An important abnormal sign can be seen in patients with spinal cord injury at the cervical level; these patients may show exaggerated abdominal movement with breathing. The cord injury interrupts nervous control of chest muscles, leaving movement of the diaphragm as the only way to breathe.

Depth: The depth of breathing, also referred to as **tidal volume,** indicates the amount of air entering the airways with each breath. The average adult has a tidal volume of 500 to 800 ml. Of this, only about 350 ml makes it all the way to the alveoli. The remaining air fills the air passages, also called the *dead air space.* Air in these passages is not available for oxygen and carbon dioxide exchange in the alveoli. When a person is breathing adequately, the depth of breathing will be constant and normal.

Breathing varies from person to person. Observing people breathing normally helps one learn to recognize abnormal breathing. It is also important to know when breathing changes are normal. For example, it is normal for a person who just ran a mile to breathe faster and more deeply than a person at rest. This person may even have an irregular breathing pattern and gasp for air. It is not normal for a person relaxing in the living room to have fast, irregular, or shallow breathing, or to be struggling to breathe.

Recognizing Respiratory Distress

Consider all the characteristics of breathing when determining the extent of a patient's **respiratory distress,** which can have the following signs:

- Rapid or slow breathing rate. A person who is laboring to breathe, or who has a respiratory rate of less than 8 or more than 24 times per minute, may be in respiratory distress. Although the normal range is 12 to 20 breaths per minute, rates outside of 8 and 24 may be normal in some populations (e.g., athletes or infants, as noted earlier). Use common sense to consider the possible causes, and observe other clinical signs.
- Irregular breathing rhythm. The patient may be breathing very fast, then slow, then fast again.
- Shallow or deep breathing.
- Abnormal or absent breath sounds. A patient with an upper airway obstruction may make a high-pitched sound **(stridor)** when attempting to breathe. Narrowing (constriction) of the lower airways can result in a **wheezing** sound, often most prominent during exhalation. Extreme lower airway constriction can make it impossible to hear any breath sounds at all.
- Inadequate or unequal chest expansion. The patient may avoid taking deep breaths, or you may only see one side of the chest rise. This may result from trauma or from a partial or complete obstruction of a bronchus.
- Inability to speak in full sentences. A patient who can speak only short phrases or one to two words at a time is in significant distress.
- Increased breathing effort. *Retractions* are the inward motions of *accessory muscles*—including the muscles above the clavicles, between the ribs, or below the rib cage—during inhalation to aid in breathing. Retractions are most commonly seen in children and infants as they increase the force of muscle contractions to draw in more air.
- Nasal flaring in children and infants. When the openings of the nostrils move in and out with breathing, the child is working hard to draw in air.
- "Seesaw" breathing. An infant's chest falls as the abdomen rises, followed by chest rise as the abdomen falls.
- Grunting (audible, forceful breathing noises). This is another common sign of respiratory distress in children.
- Agonal respirations. These are occasional gasps for air, often seen just before breathing stops.
- Pale or blue (cyanotic) skin color. This indicates a lack of oxygen in the bloodstream. (Visible cyanosis requires good peripheral circulation. A patient in shock with constricted peripheral vessels may simply look pale, even if the patient is **hypoxic** and the blood is bluish.)
- Position of patient. A seated position usually allows patient to breathe more easily.

A patient with signs of breathing difficulty needs immediate treatment. If not recognized or managed properly, a

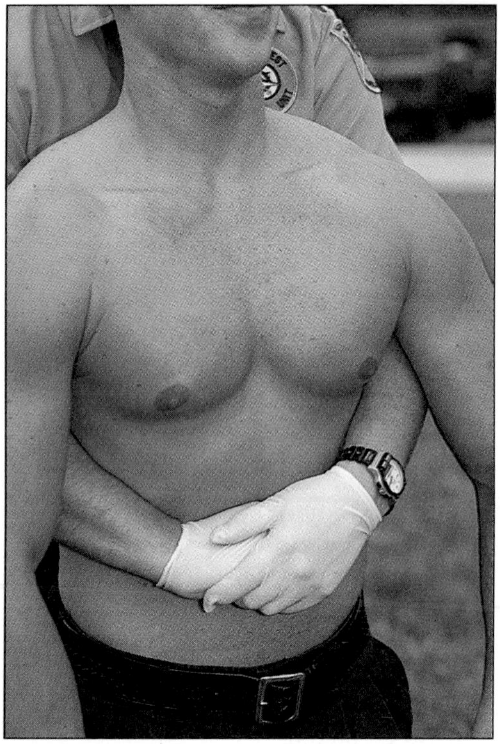

Figure 11-4

Correct hand placement for performing the Heimlich maneuver in a conscious adult patient.

A

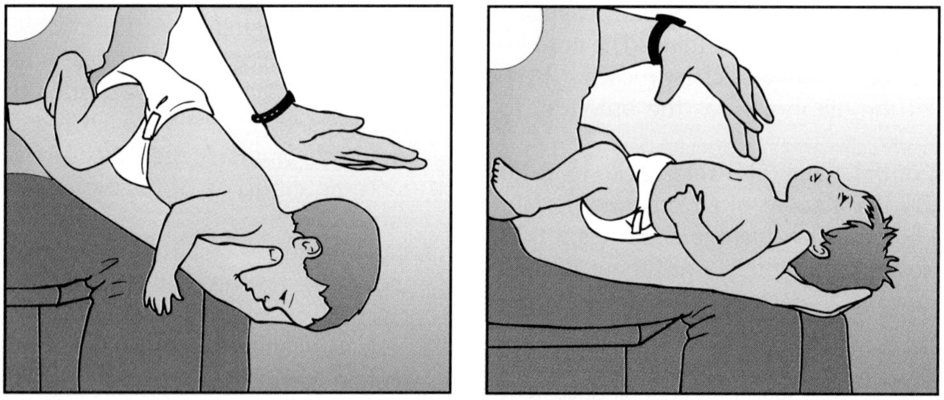

B

Figure 11-5

Correct body placement for treating an infant with an airway obstruction.

patient in respiratory distress may stop breathing altogether, a condition known as **respiratory arrest,** discussed on p. 247.

Caring for Patients in Respiratory Distress

There are three primary objectives in caring for a patient in respiratory distress:

1. Ensuring that the patient's airway is open (clear of obstructions).
2. Assisting breathing if the patient's breathing efforts are not effective on their own.
3. Providing supplemental oxygen to meet the needs of the body.

By meeting these three objectives, you will provide the initial care needed by your patient, regardless of the cause of the respiratory emergency.

Relieving Airway Obstruction in a Conscious Patient

The most common cause of an airway obstruction is a foreign body, such as a piece of food, that gets lodged in the airway. Conscious patients often display a universal sign that they are choking. This is the characteristic grasping at the throat. A patient who cannot cough, breathe, or speak is choking and has a complete airway obstruction. You must intervene immediately by using abdominal thrusts, commonly referred to as the *Heimlich maneuver,* to try to relieve the obstruction. Follow these steps:

1. Determine that the patient cannot breathe, cough, or speak.
2. Stand behind the patient and wrap your arms around the patient's waist.
3. Make a fist with one hand. Place the thumb side of your fist right above the patient's navel and well below the rib cage. Grasp that fist with your other hand (Figure 11-4).
4. Deliver forceful inward and upward thrusts. Each thrust should be a separate attempt to relieve the obstruction. Deliver sets of five thrusts until the object is expelled or the patient loses consciousness.

Do not attempt abdominal thrusts if the patient is able to cough forcefully. In that case, the patient has only a partial airway obstruction. Coughing is the body's natural attempt to clear the airway. Encourage the patient to continue to cough while you transport to the hospital. Sometimes the patient will report being able to feel the object stuck in the throat. If the patient can talk, the airway is clear enough to breathe and move adequate air for the moment. Give supplemental oxygen, monitor breathing closely during transport, and be ready to intervene if the airway becomes completely obstructed.

You should not attempt abdominal thrusts if your patient is in the late stages of pregnancy or is markedly obese.[1] Instead, stand behind the patient and wrap your arms around the patient's chest, placing your fist directly on the middle portion of the sternum. Perform chest thrusts instead of abdominal thrusts until the obstruction is removed.

Choking is a common emergency in children and infants because they are quick to put objects in their mouths. If a choking child is 1 to 8 years old, use the same technique described for an adult. You may have to position yourself on one knee to be at the correct level with the patient, and you will also need to use less force with the thrusts. Ensure that the patient is breathing adequately after relieving the obstruction.

An infant (less than 1 year old) with an obstruction will not be able to cry, cough, or breathe, and will usually become cyanotic quickly. Because of the anatomic and physiologic differences in infants, your care for an airway obstruction must be different. Follow these steps:

1. Place the infant along your arm face down, supporting the head and neck. Rest your arm on your thigh (Figure 11-5, *A*).
2. Using the heel of your hand, deliver up to five back blows between the infant's shoulder blades.
3. Support the back of the infant's head. Turn the infant over onto your other arm and rest that arm on your thigh (Figure 11-5, *B*). Imagine a line between the infant's nipples. Place your middle and index finger on the sternum, one finger-width below this line. Deliver up to five chest thrusts, pressing straight down onto the chest.
4. Continue this sequence of back blows and chest thrusts until the object is removed. If you dislodge the object and can see it in the patient's mouth, you may have to use a finger to sweep the object from the mouth. This technique is discussed in detail in the next section. When abdominal thrusts, back blows, or chest thrusts have removed an obstruction, transport the patient to the hospital for evaluation.

Relieving Airway Obstruction in an Unconscious Patient

You may also encounter an unconscious patient who has stopped breathing as a result of an airway obstruction. If the patient is not breathing, attempt to ventilate. With an airway obstruction, the air will not go in even after you have repositioned the airway. You must clear the airway before your ventilations will be effective.

Follow these steps:

1. Reposition the patient's head using the **head-tilt–chin-lift** or **modified jaw-thrust** technique (see p. 247) and attempt again to ventilate. If breaths do not go in, assume that the person has an obstructed airway.
2. Straddle the patient's legs and place the heel of one of your hands just above the patient's navel. Place your other hand on top of the first.

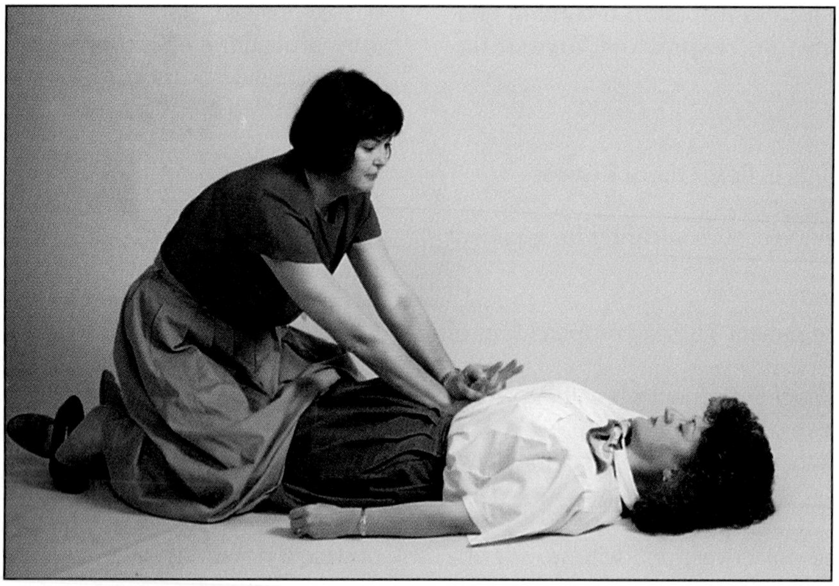

Figure 11-6

After positioning the patient's head, deliver up to five abdominal thrusts to dislodge the object.

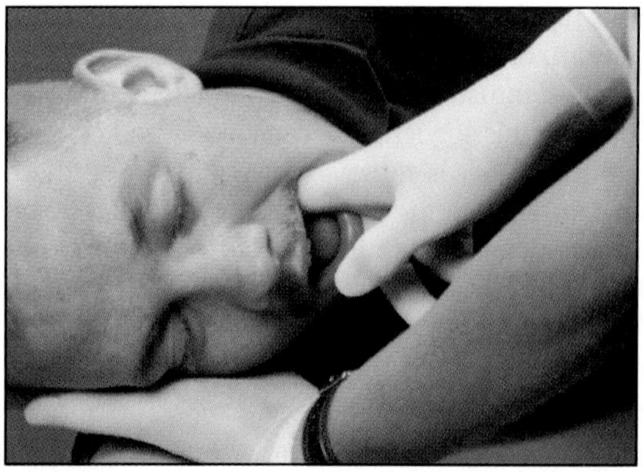

Figure 11-7

Perform a finger sweep on an unconscious patient to remove a visible object.

3. Deliver up to five abdominal thrusts to dislodge the object (Figure 11-6).
4. Grasp the patient's lower jaw and tongue with your thumb and index finger and lift the jaw upward.
5. Look in the patient's mouth and perform a finger sweep to remove any visible object (Figure 11-7).
6. Position the patient's head and attempt to ventilate. If your breaths still do not go in, repeat these steps.

These steps are the same for children, with two exceptions: do a finger sweep only if the object is clearly visible, and do not press as forcefully on a child's abdomen.

The steps are different if you are caring for an unconscious infant with an obstructed airway. However, they are very similar to the care you learned earlier for a conscious infant with an obstructed airway:

1. Place the infant along your arm face down, supporting the head and neck. Rest your arm on your thigh.
2. Using the heel of your hand, deliver up to five back blows between the infant's shoulder blades.
3. Support the infant's head and turn him or her over onto your other arm. Rest that arm on your thigh. Use two fingers to deliver up to five chest thrusts.
4. Place the infant on a firm surface such as a table. Look inside the infant's mouth. If you see an object, attempt to remove it using a finger sweep.
5. Open the infant's airway and attempt to give two breaths. If breaths do not go in, reposition the head and try to ventilate.
6. If breaths still do not go in, continue the sequence of back blows, chest thrusts, finger sweeps (if the object is visible), and ventilation attempts until the object is removed. Once breaths go in, check the patient's pulse and breathing and provide care as necessary.

The Nonbreathing Patient

If not managed early, a patient in respiratory distress may proceed to respiratory arrest. The brain can only last for

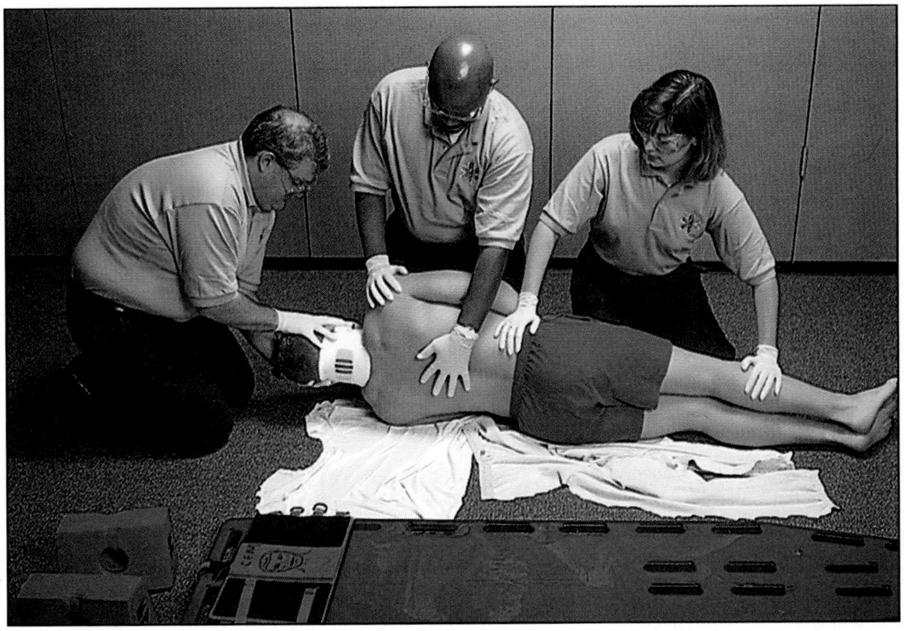

Figure 11-8
Log-roll the patient face up, watching, listening, and feeling for air movement.

a few minutes without oxygen before permanent damage begins to occur. It is important to recognize a person in respiratory arrest right away and begin to ventilate before the condition deteriorates further. As with respiratory distress, you do not need to know the cause to take the proper action.

Recognizing Respiratory Arrest

To determine whether a patient is breathing, *look* for the rise and fall of the chest, *listen* for air exchange, and *feel* for air coming out of the patient's mouth or nose. This can often be done without moving the patient. If the patient is supine, checking for breathing is easy. If not, you may need to log-roll the patient onto the back and ensure an open airway before checking. A patient that has suffered trauma, particularly to the head or spine, should be moved carefully. With a second EMT stabilizing the patient's head and neck, the two of you should log-roll the patient face up (Figure 11-8). Be sure the airway is open. If you do not see any movement of the chest, hear air exchange, or feel any air escaping, then the patient has stopped breathing and is in respiratory arrest.

Opening the Airway

The tongue is the most common cause of an airway obstruction in an unconscious patient. The tongue is attached to the muscles of the lower jaw. In an unconscious, supine patient, the tongue may drop back and block the airway when the jaw muscles relax. Another important cause of obstruction, especially in children, is upper airway swelling. Chapter 26 discusses childhood diseases that cause airway swelling.

There are two common techniques to relieve obstruction caused by the tongue. The head-tilt–chin-lift is used in nontraumatic cases, and the modified jaw-thrust is used when you suspect head or spinal injury.

Head-Tilt–Chin-Lift Technique

The most common way to open the airway of a nontrauma patient is the head-tilt–chin-lift technique. Place one hand on the patient's forehead and the other under the bony part of the front of the chin (mandible). Lift the chin and tilt the head back (Figure 11-9). This will help lift the tongue away from the back of the throat and open the airway. When lifting the chin, be careful not to push on the soft tissue under the chin, closing the mouth. You may have to pull the lower lip down with your thumb to keep the mouth open.

Modified Jaw-Thrust Technique

When treating a patient with a suspected neck or back injury, open the airway using the modified jaw-thrust technique. Kneeling at the top of the patient's head, place your fingers at the angle of the jaw just below the patient's ears. Lift the jaw forward with both hands, minimizing any head and neck movement. This will displace the jaw and move it forward, lifting the tongue out of the way (Figure 11-10) while allowing you to prevent the head and

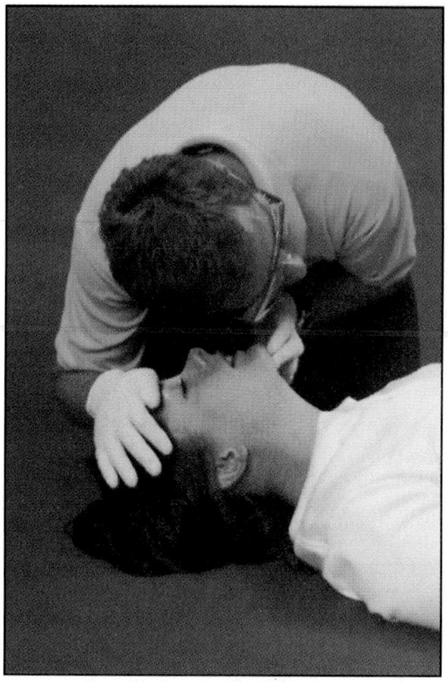

Figure 11-9

The head-tilt–chin-lift technique can be used on nontrauma patients to open the airway.

neck from moving. If the patient's lips close, use your thumb to pull down on the lower lip. The modified jaw-thrust technique should also be used to open the airway in an unconscious patient when the nature of the problem is unknown (you should suspect possible spinal injury in that situation).

Once you have opened the airway, you will have to maintain the opening. It may close quickly if you let go. Watch also that nothing new appears to obstruct the airway, such as vomit or blood. Have one rescuer monitor the airway constantly. Adjuncts that are available to help open and maintain an airway are discussed on p. 257.

Ventilating the Nonbreathing Patient

Oxygenation refers to supplying a sufficient concentration of oxygen in the air entering the lungs. **Ventilation** is the actual process of moving air in and out of the lungs. Imagine that you place an oxygen mask over the face of a nonbreathing patient. The device is delivering oxygen, but the oxygen cannot reach the lungs. Supplemental ventilation will be necessary to ensure adequate oxygenation to the body.

Once you have opened the airway and determined that the patient is not breathing or is breathing inadequately, you will need to provide some form of **artificial ventilation.** What method you use depends on the situation and the equipment available. Whether you use mouth-to-mask breathing or a ventilation device such as a bag-valve mask, it is important that your patient is ventilated quickly and effectively.

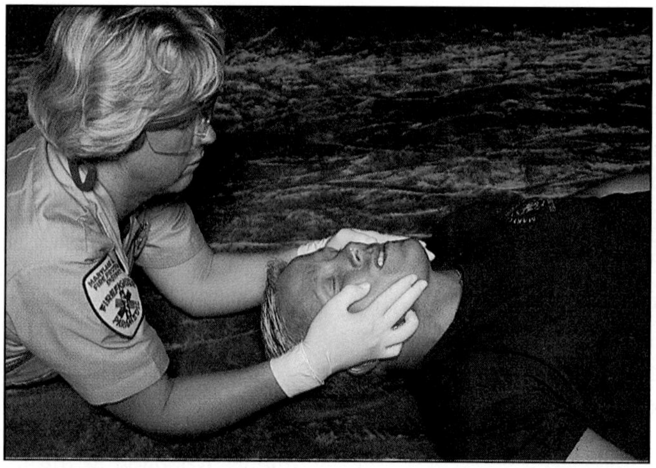

Figure 11-10

The jaw-thrust technique displaces the patient's jaw forward, lifting the tongue out of the way. This technique should be used on any patient with a suspected spinal injury in whom the airway must be opened.

Mouth-to-Mask Ventilation

Mouth-to-mask ventilation replaces the older mouth-to-mouth technique. Mouth-to-mouth ventilation involved breathing directly into a patient's mouth. The method was developed in 1959 and proved effective at oxygenating patients.[3] However, because of the potential for disease transmission, mouth-to-mouth ventilation is no longer considered appropriate for routine use by rescuers. It may be required in unusual situations in which you know the patient and have no other equipment immediately available. Whenever doing mouth-to-mouth ventilations, however, you should use some type of barrier device. While not a complete protection from secretions, the barrier device will provide some protection from disease transmission.

Effective mouth-to-mask ventilation using a resuscitation mask with a one-way valve provides an adequate barrier against disease transmission. Ventilations with a mouth-to-mask technique allow the rescuer to determine the ease of ventilating the patient and how deep to provide the ventilations.

Resuscitation masks come in a variety of styles, but they all have the same general features. They are made of pliable, transparent plastic, with an inflatable cuff that allows for a tight seal on the patient's face (Figure 11-11). These masks have a standard 15-mm coupling and are often supplied with an attached one-way valve. The valve prevents the patient's exhaled air and any body fluids from coming in contact with the rescuer. Most masks also now have a filter that further reduces the risk of disease transmission. Try to use a mask with both a valve and a filter.

Many resuscitation masks also have an oxygen inlet. As with mouth-to-mouth breathing, using the resuscitation mask without oxygen delivers only about 16% oxygen to the patient (the amount of oxygen in exhaled air). With oxygen attached to the mask, the amount of oxygen delivered to the patient may reach 50% to 55%.

To use a resuscitation mask, follow these steps:

1. Kneel at the patient's head and assemble the mask, attaching the one-way valve.
2. Place the mask on the patient's face, with the bottom edge of the mask on the patient's chin and the top above the bridge of the nose.
3. Open the airway. Place your thumbs on the sides of the mask and press down. Grasp the lower jaw with your fingers and lift the jaw while tilting the head back (Figure 11-12).
4. Breathe into the one-way valve until you see the chest rise. Give one breath every 5 seconds for adults, and one breath every 3 seconds for children and infants.
5. If you suspect a neck or back injury, use the modified jaw-thrust technique to maintain neutral alignment and stabilization of the head and neck while ventilating.

If oxygen is available, connect it to the resuscitation mask and run it at a rate of 15 lpm.

Simultaneously maintaining the mask seal and keeping the airway open can be difficult to master. If you are having trouble, have another rescuer help. One of you can maintain the airway while the other attends to the mask seal and provides ventilations.

Bag-Valve-Mask Ventilation

The **bag-valve-mask** device, commonly called a *BVM*, is another device to provide artificial ventilation. As the

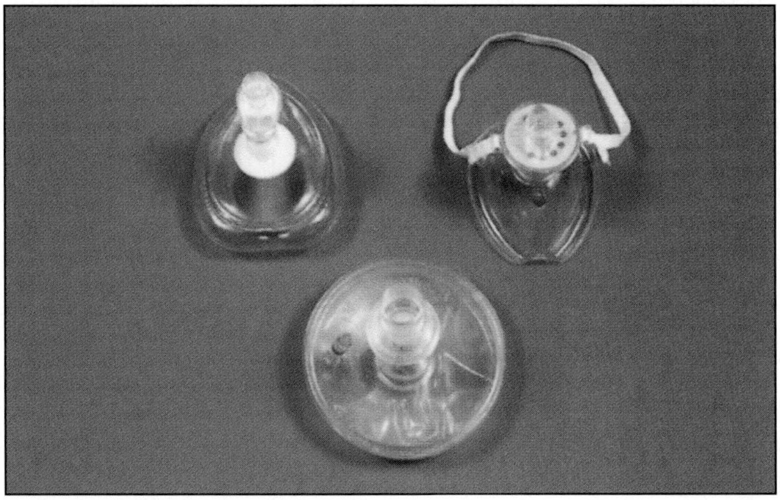

Figure 11-11

Resuscitation masks.

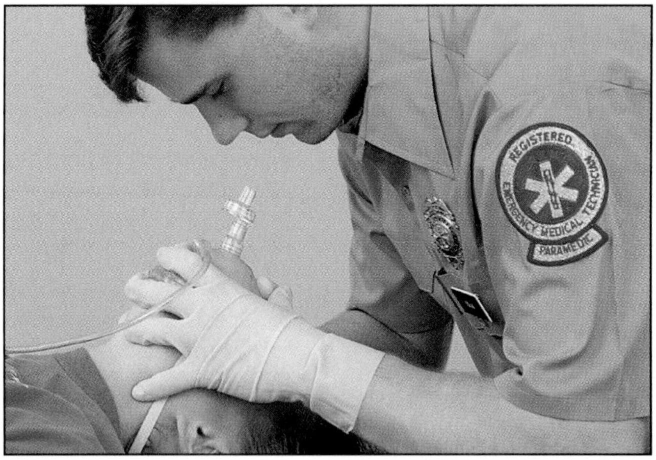

Figure 11-12

Correct finger and thumb positioning to seal the mask and lift the patient's lower jaw.

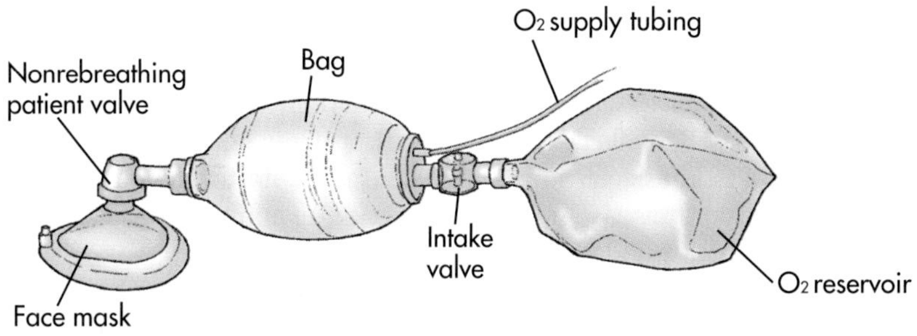

Figure 11-13

Most bag-valve-masks will accept a reservoir bag, an oxygen supply tube, or both.

name suggests, the device consists of a self-inflating bag, a one-way valve, and a face mask. It also makes it possible to give supplemental oxygen when ventilating a patient. Most BVM devices will accept a reservoir in the form of a bag or a length of tubing that attaches to the end of the bag (Figure 11-13). Without oxygen, the BVM delivers about 21% oxygen (atmospheric air). If oxygen tubing is attached to the BVM and a reservoir attachment is used, the delivered percentage of oxygen can be as high as 95%.

The BVM is the most widely used ventilation device among EMS providers. The device prevents direct contact of the rescuers with potentially infectious body substances. It also gives a sense of when increasing resistance in the airways makes ventilation more difficult. However, studies have shown that EMTs have difficulty maintaining good mask seal and delivering proper ventilation volumes when "bagging" by themselves. Keeping the patient's airway open, maintaining a tight mask seal, and squeezing the bag adequately may require more than two hands. It is best to have two properly trained EMTs use the BVM whenever possible. One EMT can open the airway and hold the mask in place while the second squeezes the bag. It is important that you be aware of the common deficiencies in the one-person technique. You may find it is easier and more effective to use the mouth-to-mask method when you have to ventilate a patient without assistance.

The average adult BVM holds about 1600 ml of air. Though there are various styles of BVMs, they should all have the following characteristics:

- Self-refilling bag that can be easily cleaned and sterilized or is disposable
- Nonjamming one-way exhalation valve to prevent rebreathing of exhaled air
- Standard 15-mm or 22-mm fittings
- Oxygen inlet, preferably with a reservoir to deliver high oxygen concentrations

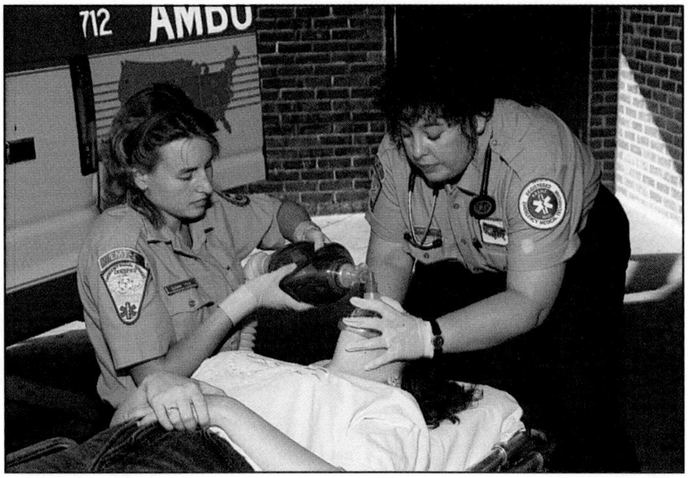

Figure 11-14

When two rescuers are using a bag-valve-mask on a patient, a rescuer opens the airway and maintains the mask seal while the other rescuer controls the bag.

- Clear, soft plastic mask capable of creating a tight seal against the patient's face
- Adult, child, and infant sizes
- Construction with materials that perform well in various environmental conditions and temperature extremes

Some BVMs are manufactured with a special valve, called a *pop-off valve,* designed to prevent over-inflation of the patient's lungs. However, these valves have been shown to prevent adequate ventilation in some situations, including patients with poor lung compliance and those receiving cardiopulmonary resuscitation (CPR).[2] In these situations, the pressure needed to ventilate adequately may exceed the pop-off limits; and you will have to disable the pop-off valve. When this occurs, watch the patient's respiratory status very closely. Higher ventilation pressures increase the chance of causing a pneumothorax.

When using a BVM with two rescuers, follow these steps:

1. One EMT kneels at the top of the patient's head, while the second kneels at the side of the head.
2. The EMT at the side inserts an **oropharyngeal airway** (see p. 257), if available and tolerated by the patient, to help keep the airway open.
3. The EMT at the top assembles the BVM and places the mask on the face. Using both hands, this EMT applies firm pressure on the mask and opens the airway using the head-tilt–chin-lift method (nontrauma patients) or the modified jaw-thrust technique.
4. The other EMT uses both hands to squeeze the bag smoothly until the patient's chest rises. Do not continue to force oxygen in after the chest starts to rise. Give one breath every 5 seconds, allowing the bag to refill between ventilations (Figure 11-14).

If you use the BVM by yourself:

1. Position yourself at the top of the patient's head and assemble the equipment.
2. Position the mask on the patient's face.
3. Using one hand, wrap your index finger and thumb around the dome of the mask and grasp the patient's jaw using your other fingers (Figure 11-15).
4. Press down on the mask to form a seal on the face as you tilt the head back and lift the jaw.
5. Use your other hand to squeeze the bag firmly until the chest rises.

The one-rescuer technique is difficult to master and should be practiced regularly on a manikin. This method should not be used for a patient with a suspected neck or back injury. It is more difficult for a single rescuer to open and maintain an airway and ventilate a patient using the modified jaw-thrust technique.

Ventilation of children and infants requires the same technique but with the appropriate-size bag and face mask. It is usually not necessary to tilt the child's head back as far as an adult's to open the airway. In fact, tilting too far back may kink the airway and obstruct it. Because children and infants normally breathe more frequently than adults, they should be ventilated more frequently, at the rate of one breath every 3 seconds.

Flow-Restricted, Oxygen-Powered Delivery Devices
Another common device used to ventilate nonbreathing patients is the *flow-restricted, oxygen-powered delivery*

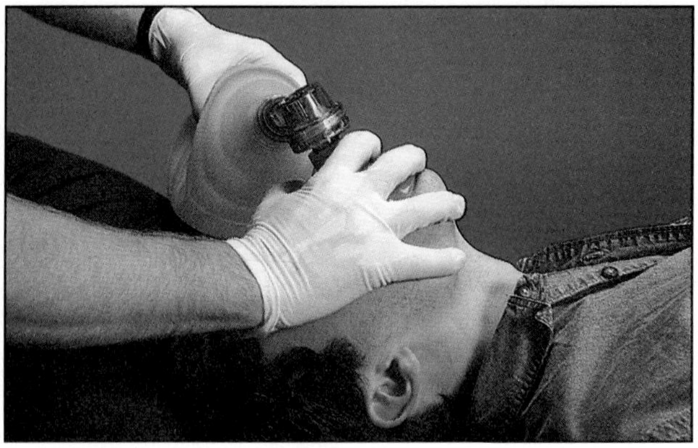

Figure 11-15

Correct hand positioning for a single rescuer using a bag-valve-mask.

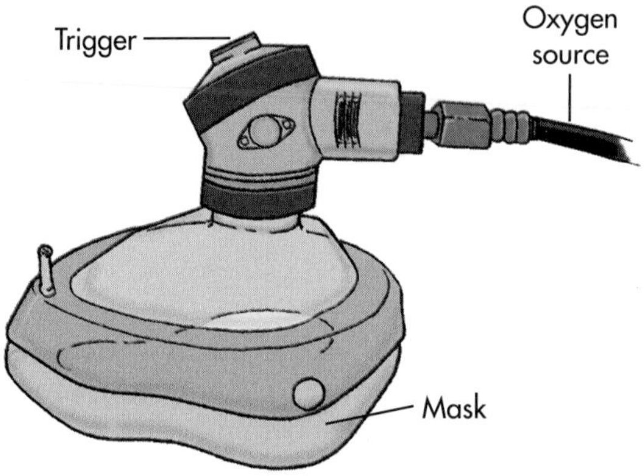

Figure 11-16

Demand valve device.

device. This device, also known as a *positive-pressure ventilator* or *demand valve,* allows delivery of 100% oxygen by depressing a button on the valve (Figure 11-16). It has a flow restricter that limits oxygen delivery to a maximum rate of 40 lpm. It also has a pressure-relief valve that opens when pressure exceeds a certain level, usually 60 cm of water. This adapter reduces the risk of injuring the lungs by overinflating them.

Because of the pressures this device will deliver, you must be very careful with its use. For this reason, it is not to be used at all for children or infants. As soon as the patient's chest starts to rise, release the valve and stop forcing oxygen into the lungs. In most situations, use of other methods, such as mouth-to-mask and the BVM device, are safer and more appropriate and are preferable to the use of a demand valve.

To use a flow-restricted, oxygen-powered ventilator use the following steps:

1. Position yourself at the top of the patient's head and place the face mask as you would a BVM.
2. While holding the mask in place, gently squeeze the trigger to allow air to flow into the patient's lungs (Figure 11-17).
3. Watch for the chest to begin to rise. Stop the ventilation as soon as you see the chest rise. Deliver one ventilation every 5 seconds.

The predecessor to this device was known as a demand valve because it delivered a greater amount of oxygen on demand as the patient breathed. A patient with difficulty breathing could simply inhale and activate the valve, allowing 100% oxygen to flow. This was commonly used by firefighters suffering smoke inhalation. While this worked well on breathing patients, the greater pressure was not appropriate for the nonbreathing patient because it tended to cause air to enter the stomach, resulting in gastric distention. This is why manufacturers placed a restricting valve on the device. To overcome the problem, some manufacturers now make a flow-restricted, oxygen-powered delivery device that has a switch to allow the device to be used as a ventilation device for both breathing and nonbreathing patients (Figure 11-18).

Special Situations

There are some situations in which you will have to modify the way you ventilate a patient. One such situation is a patient with a laryngectomy.

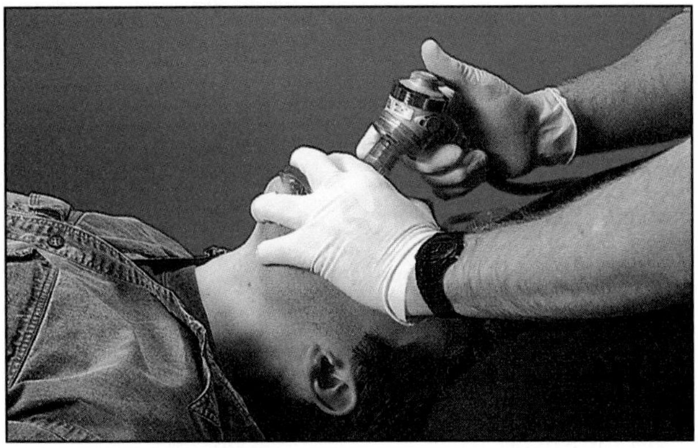

Figure 11-17

Stop the ventilation as soon as the patient's chest begins to rise.

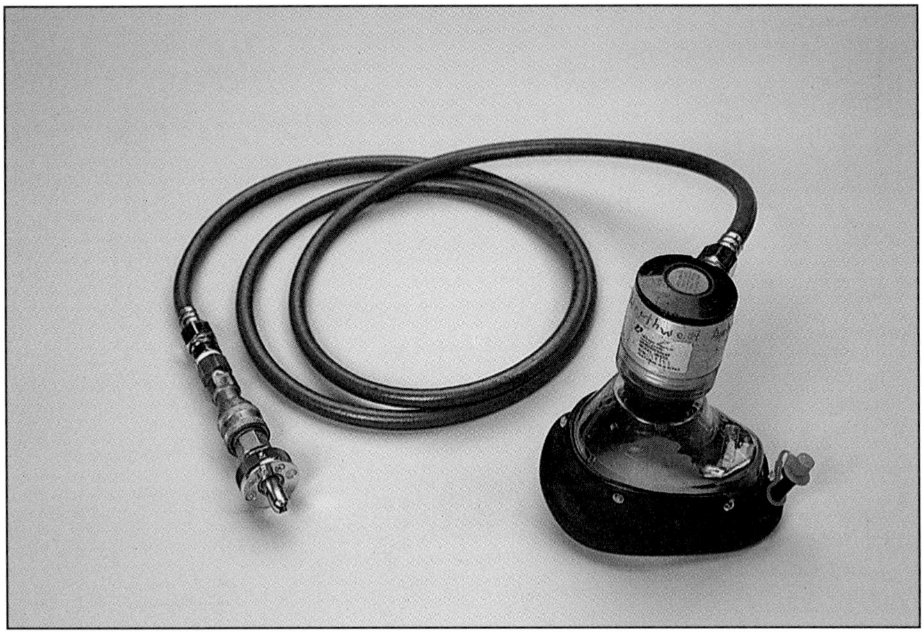

Figure 11-18

Flow-restricted, oxygen-powered delivery device.

Laryngectomies. A **laryngectomy** is a surgical procedure that removes part or all of the voice box (larynx). A laryngectomy patient will usually not breathe through the mouth or nose. Instead, there is an opening in the front of the neck, called a **stoma** (Figure 11-19). When checking to see if a person is breathing, it is important to check the patient's neck for a stoma. In these patients, you may see a rise and fall of the chest but not feel any air exchange at the mouth or nose.

When ventilating through a stoma, the ventilation device is placed directly over the stoma. To maintain a good seal, apply pressure to the ventilation device and mold it around the patient's neck. If you are using an inflatable mask, you have to change the volume of air in the cuff to get a better seal. If the patient's chest does not rise, check to see if air is escaping through the mouth and nose. Some stoma patients are partial neck breathers; they breathe through the neck, but still have an open air passage to the pharynx. In this case, you will need to seal the mouth and nose as you ventilate through the stoma.

Tracheostomies. In some situations, the patient may have a tracheostomy tube in place in the stoma (Figure 11-20). Attach the bag-valve device directly to that tube and ventilate the patient without the mask.

Ventilation Assessment

If you note that a patient's chest does not rise when you attempt to ventilate, make sure that you have an open airway. Reposition the head and attempt to ventilate again. If you are unable to deliver adequate ventilations, switch to another ventilating device. If you determine that there is an obstruction, attempt to remove the obstruction manually (see p. 245) or with equipment (see p. 257).

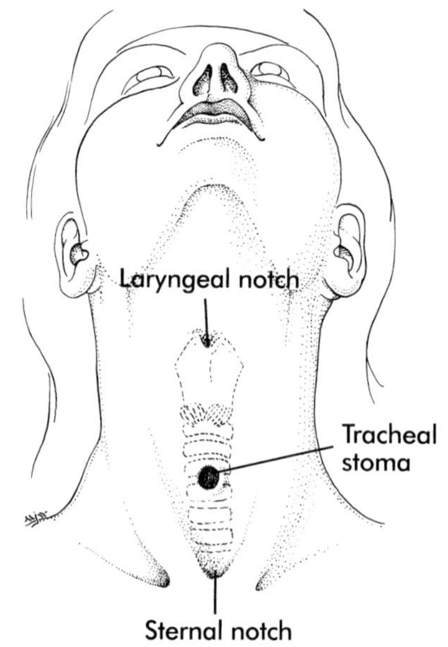

Figure 11-19

Stoma.

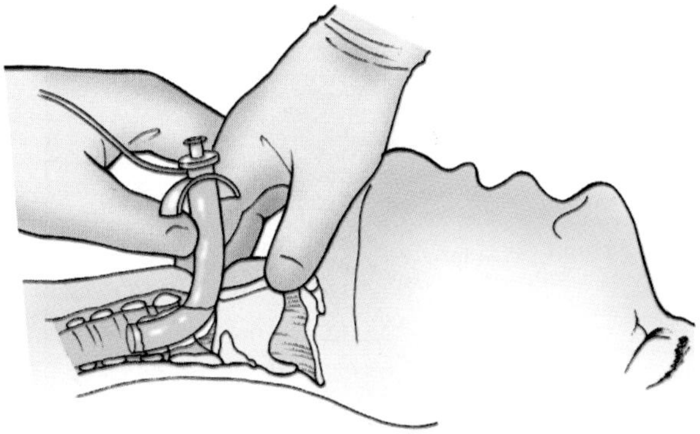

Figure 11-20

If the patient has a tracheostomy tube in place in the stoma, ventilate the patient directly through the tube.

Basic Airway and Breathing Adjuncts

There are several tools or adjuncts to help manage airway and breathing emergencies. These include suction devices, oropharyngeal and nasopharyngeal airways, and oxygen. Keep the following points in mind regarding the use of these adjuncts:

- Make sure that these adjuncts are easily accessible and functioning properly. However, never withhold or delay care if they are not readily available.
- Make sure you understand the proper use of any adjuncts that you carry.
- Keep these tools clean and disinfected; replace if necessary.

Suctioning

After checking the patient's level of consciousness (LOC), the next step is to check the airway. There may be vomitus or other materials in the mouth obstructing or blocking the airway. Fluids such as blood and saliva can also drain into the patient's airway and be aspirated.

Aspiration is the inhalation of foreign material, such as vomitus, into the lungs. **Suctioning** is the use of manual or mechanical devices to remove vomitus or other secretions from the mouth and throat. Good airway care requires that suction equipment be within easy reach and ready for action at all times. This is especially true when the patient has airway problems or is not conscious enough to protect the airway.

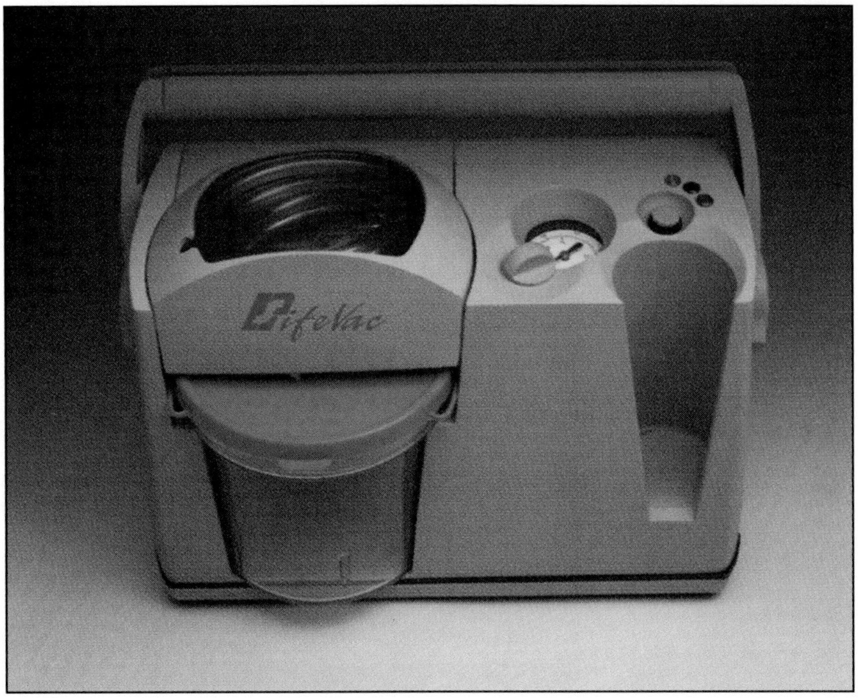

Figure 11-21
Mechanical suction device.

Suction Devices

A *suction device* is used to clear the mouth of vomitus, blood, or other liquid and food particles obstructing the airway. There are two types of suction devices available: manual and mechanical. Both types can be portable, but mechanical suction devices can also be mounted as fixed units in ambulances (Figure 11-21).

These devices should be powerful enough to provide vacuum pressure of more than 300 mm Hg when the tube is clamped. Mechanical devices are powered by a vacuum system from the vehicle's engine or by an electric pump. Manual devices require the operator to squeeze or pump a handle to create suction. Both kinds have collection bottles, often lined with a plastic bag, making it easy to dispose of suctioned fluids or to carry fluids to the emergency department for evaluation. Wide-diameter tubing connects the suction unit to the suction catheter.

Portable suction units can be taken with you to the patient. Many of these units are battery powered and are kept charged in the vehicle (Figure 11-22). These suction units should also be able to generate a vacuum of 300 mm Hg when the tube is clamped. The biggest disadvantage of portable electric units is the need for constant charging.

The simpler portable suction devices are manually operated, hand-held units. Unlike battery operated portables, these units do not require an external energy source. The operator creates vacuum pressure by squeezing a handle. These devices are much lighter and easier to carry than electric units and have proved reliable in the field.

Another hand-held, manual suction device is a bulb syringe, the preferred device for suctioning infants. It is frequently used to suction the nose and mouth of newborns and infants up to approximately 4 months of age. Because newborns and young infants breathe primarily through their noses, it is particularly important to keep their nasal passages clear.

Tips and Catheters

EMTs usually carry a variety of catheters and suction tips with their suction units (Figure 11-23). The most common tip is the rigid suction tip, which is also referred to as a *tonsil tip* or *Yankauer tip.* This type of tip can be operated with one hand, leaving the other hand free to open the patient's mouth. Rigid tips have a fairly wide-diameter opening that allows rapid suctioning of liquids and small particles.

The soft or French catheter is usually used only for fluid removal. Because of the small diameter of the tube, it can easily become clogged. However, it is good for nasal suctioning and for suctioning through an endotracheal tube (see Chapter 12). Because it is flexible, the soft catheter is somewhat harder to control than the rigid catheter.

With the exception of hand-held, manual suction devices, the tips and catheters on other devices have a hole in the side to allow the EMT to control suctioning by covering the hole with a thumb or finger (Figure 11-24). With the hole covered, a vacuum is created and suctioning is possible. When the hole is uncovered, the vacuum is broken and the tip will not suction.

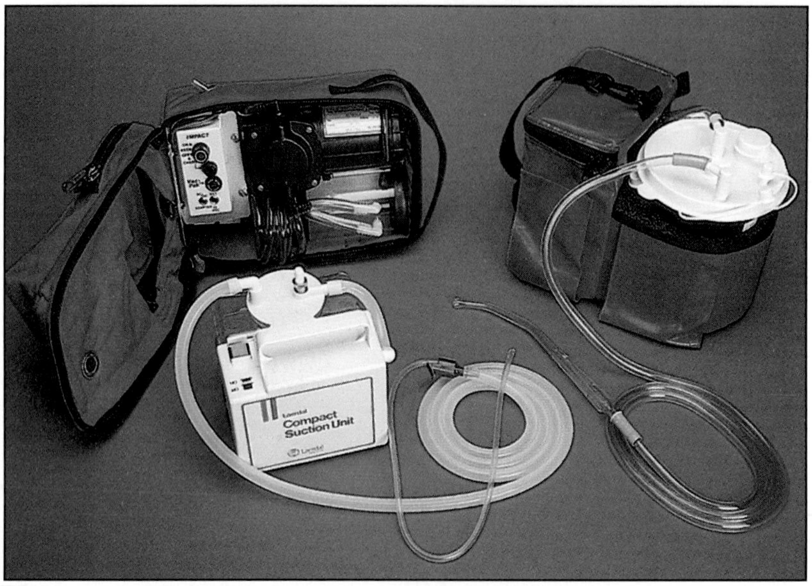

Figure 11-22

Portable electric suction units.

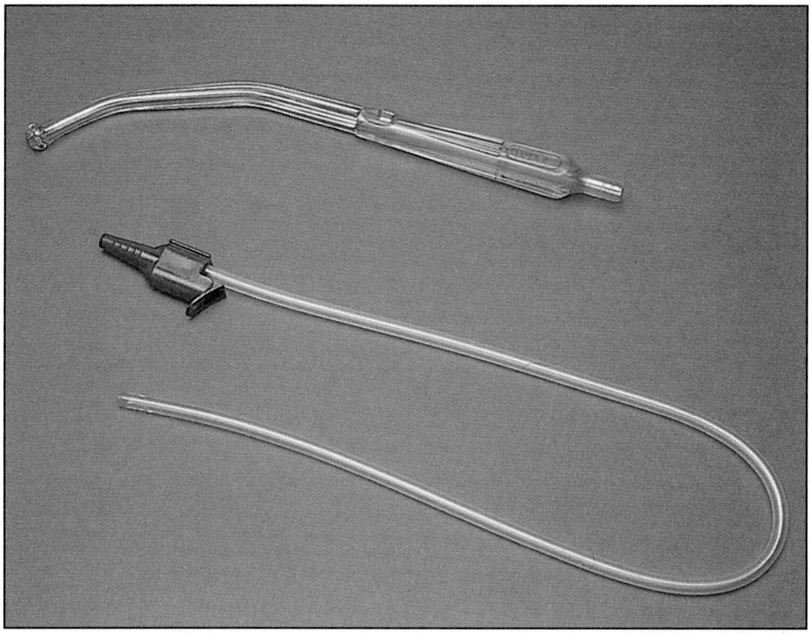

Figure 11-23

Rigid (wide-diameter) and soft (small-diameter) catheters.

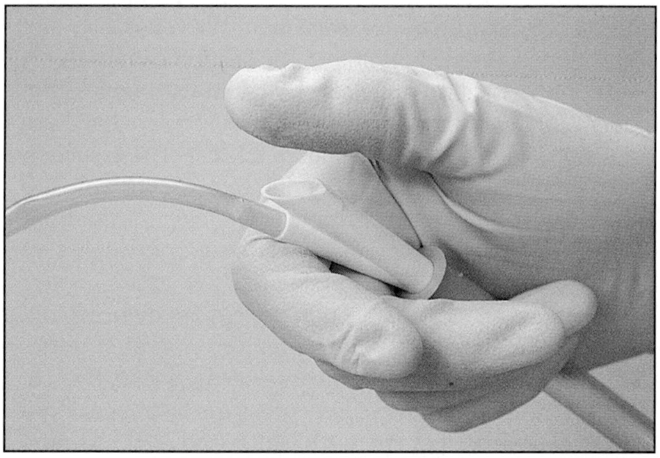

Figure 11-24

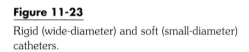

The tips and catheters on many suction devices have a hole in the side to allow control of the suctioning.

Suctioning Techniques

Make sure that you know how to operate your suction equipment. It is also important to understand how to provide suction without damaging the airway. Be prepared to suction if you hear a gurgling sound or see vomitus or fluids. You will only suction the oropharynx, not deeper areas. To avoid going too deep into the throat, measure the catheter or tip from the corner of the patient's mouth to the earlobe (Figure 11-25). Mark this distance on the device with your fingers to prevent inserting it too far. With a hand-held device, suction only as deep as you can see.

When you are using a mechanical suction device to clear a patient's airway, follow these steps:

1. Take precautions against body substances by wearing gloves and a face shield or goggles.
2. Turn on the unit and check that it is working by placing your thumb over the end of the tubing and feeling for suction.
3. Select and attach a catheter.
4. Measure the catheter to determine how far it can safely be inserted into the patient's mouth.
5. Turn the patient's head to the side. (If you suspect spinal injury, log-roll the patient onto the side.) Insert the catheter into the mouth. Do not cover the opening in the catheter until you are ready to begin withdrawing it.
6. Cover the opening and begin to suction as you withdraw the catheter. Do not suction the patient for more than 15 seconds at a time.

Because debris may get caught in the tip or tubing, have sterile water or saline readily available to flush the catheter. After removing the suction tip or catheter from the patient, place it in the sterile water and allow it to suction water to clean the tube. Remember that suctioning fluid from the airway also suctions oxygen from the airway and lungs. After suctioning, ventilate the patient immediately with supplemental oxygen.

Maintaining an Open Airway

Once you have opened and cleared the airway, you must ensure that the airway remains open. A conscious patient will usually be able to do this without any problem. However, if the patient is unconscious, you may have to help maintain the airway. This can be accomplished by using either an oropharyngeal or nasopharyngeal airway.

Oropharyngeal (Oral) Airways

The tongue is the most common cause of anatomic obstruction in an unconscious patient. The oropharyngeal airway is an airway adjunct designed to keep the tongue from blocking the upper airway. It is also used to keep the patient's mouth open to allow for easier suctioning and to prevent mouth clenching that could close the airway. The biggest drawback of the oropharyngeal airway is that it can only be used on patients who do not have a **gag reflex,** which is a protective reflex that causes a patient to gag when the back of the throat is stimulated. Attempting to insert an oropharyngeal airway into a patient with a gag reflex may cause the patient to vomit, which could actually worsen the airway situation.

The oropharyngeal airway should be used routinely when ventilating a patient with a BVM device. It is also helpful to have in place when suctioning an unconscious patient. Oropharyngeal airways come in sizes to fit patients from neonates to large adults (Figure 11-26). Using an oropharyngeal airway that is too small or too large

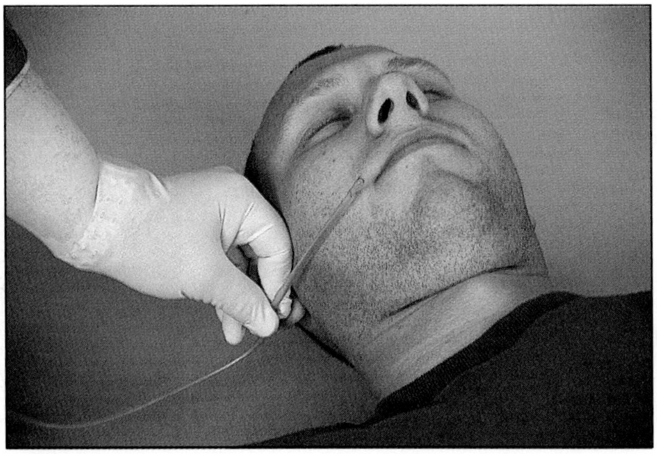

Figure 11-25

Avoid suctioning deeper than the oropharynx by measuring the catheter tip from the patient's mouth to his or her earlobe.

may further compromise the patient's airway. To find the proper size, measure as you would a suction catheter, from the corner of the mouth to the earlobe. The oropharyngeal airway is designed to displace the tongue away from the back of the throat and allow for the clear passage of air. However, inserting the airway improperly can push the tongue back and block the back of the throat.

Follow these steps when inserting an oropharyngeal airway:

1. Take standard precautions against disease transmission.
2. Determine the proper airway size (Figure 11-27).
3. Open the patient's mouth by lifting the jaw and tongue.
4. Insert the airway upside down, with the tip toward the roof of the mouth (Figure 11-28). It is also acceptable to insert the airway sideways, with the tip pointing toward one of the cheeks. Either way, the goal is to avoid pushing the tongue back into the throat.
5. Slide the airway along the roof of the mouth until it is nearly all the way in, then rotate it 180 degrees so that the flange (upper end) comes to rest against the patient's lips (Figure 11-29). (If the airway is initially inserted sideways, it will only need to be rotated 90 de-

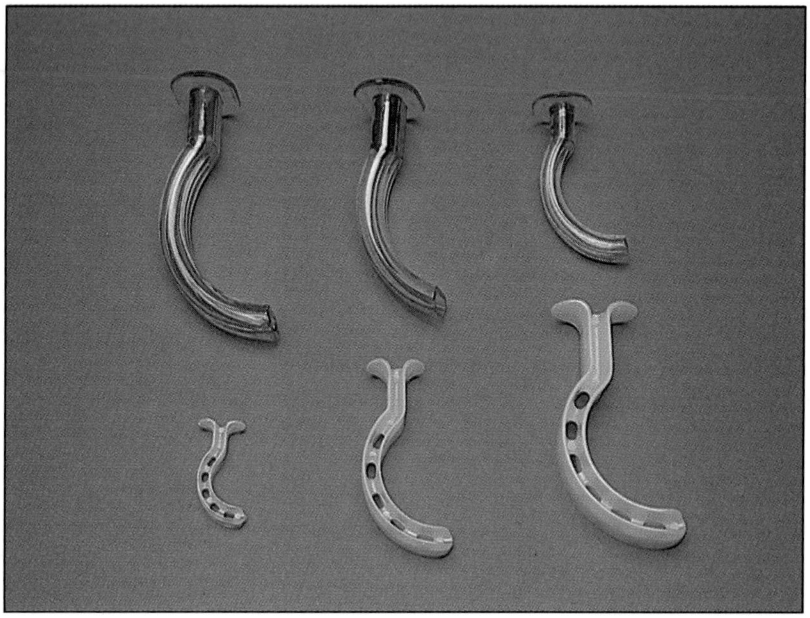

Figure 11-26

Oropharyngeal airways.

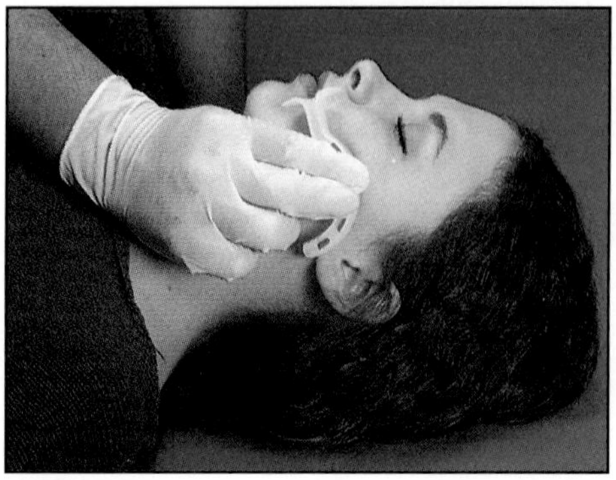

Figure 11-27

The oropharyngeal airway should measure from the patient's earlobe to the corner of the mouth.

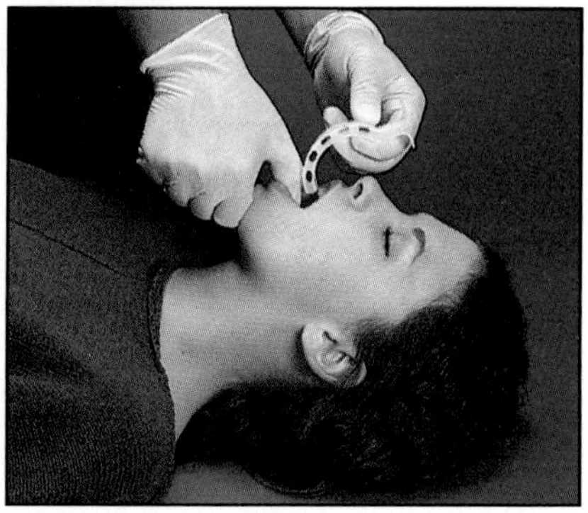

Figure 11-28

Avoid pushing the tongue back into the throat by inserting the airway upside down or sideways.

grees.) Do not attempt to force an airway into place. Remove it if the patient begins to gag.

6. Continue to monitor the airway. The oropharyngeal airway is not foolproof. You may still need to maintain a manual airway maneuver such as a modified jaw-thrust.

Another technique for inserting the airway is to hold the tongue down with a tongue depressor and insert the airway right side up. This technique is recommended for children and infants (Figure 11-30).

Nasopharyngeal (Nasal) Airways

The **nasopharyngeal airway** is an alternative to the oral airway. The nasal airway has an advantage over the oropharyngeal airway in that it is less likely to stimulate a gag reflex and therefore can be used on conscious patients. The nasopharyngeal airway is inserted in the nose and slides down the back of the nasopharynx into the hypopharynx (lower throat), bypassing the major area of the gag reflex.

The nasopharyngeal airway is also the adjunct of choice for patients with severe mouth injuries, and for

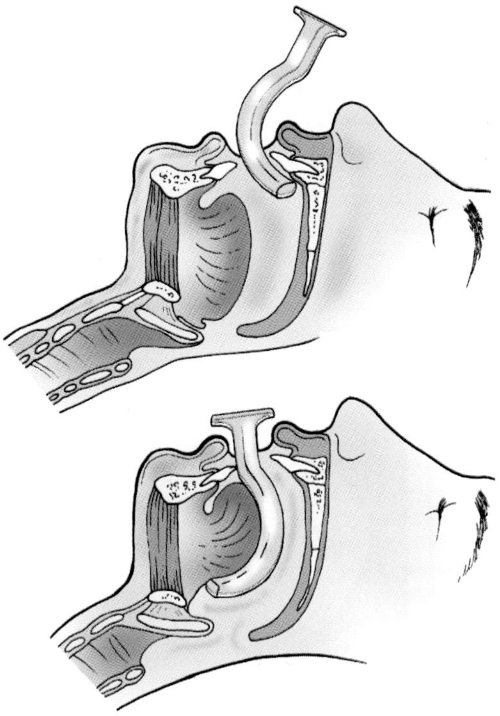

Figure 11-29

Rotate the airway when it is nearly all the way in.

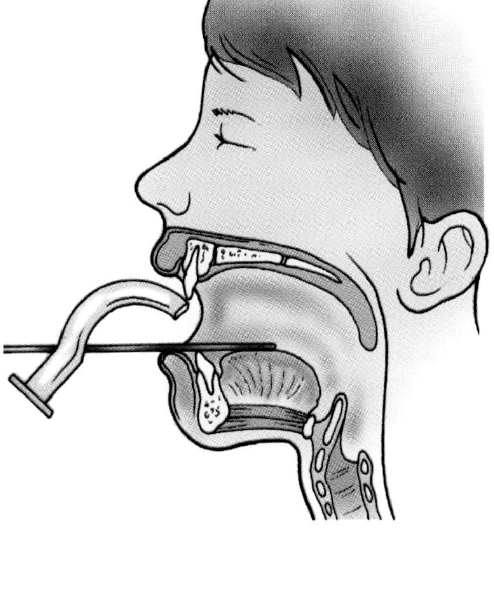

Figure 11-30

For children, it is recommended that the airway be inserted right side up while holding the tongue down with a tongue depressor.

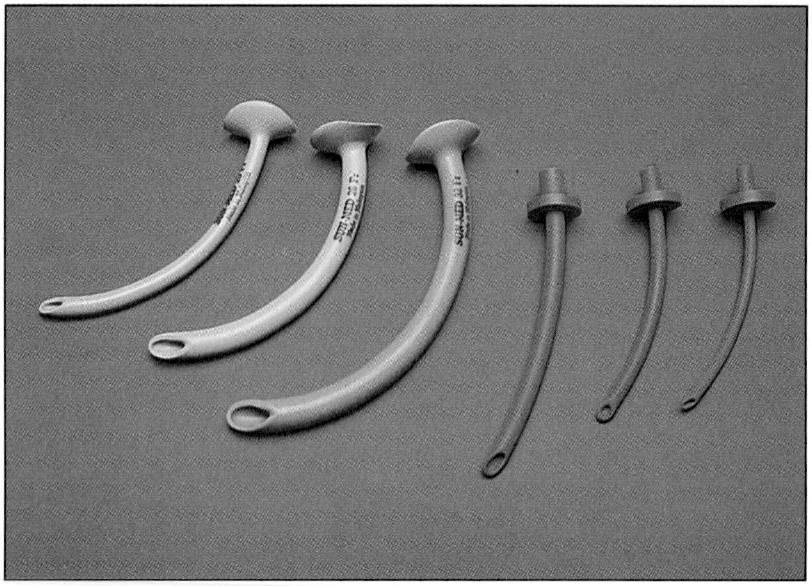

Figure 11-31

Nasal airways.

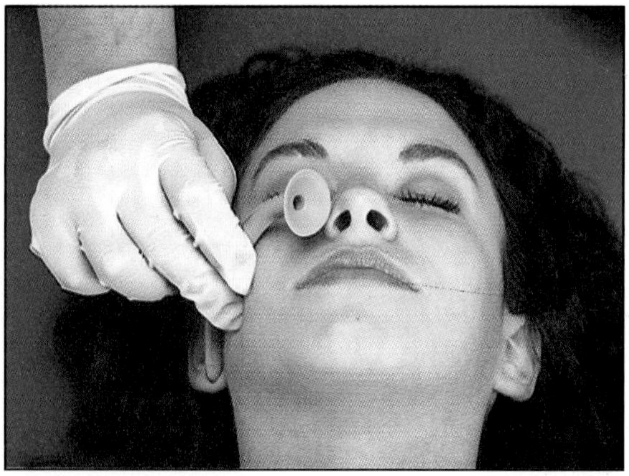

Figure 11-32

The nasal airway is measured from the earlobe to the nostril.

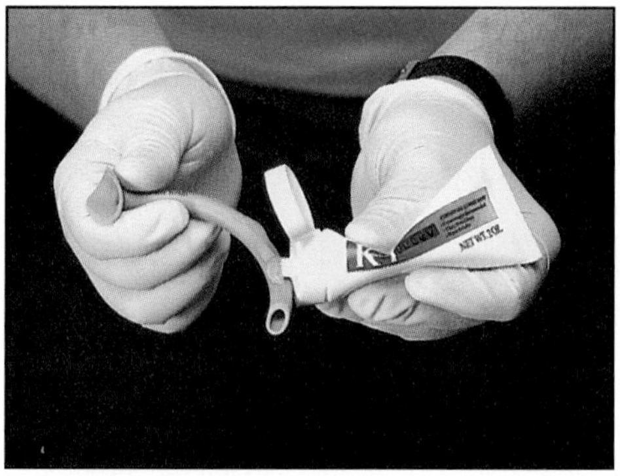

Figure 11-33

Lubricate the airway before insertion.

problems that prevent opening the mouth, such as seizures. The nasal airway comes in various sizes and diameters (Figure 11-31). To select the proper size, measure the distance from the nostril to the earlobe. Also consider the diameter of the airway by looking at the size of the patient's nostrils and choosing a tube slightly smaller than the visible opening.

To insert a nasopharyngeal airway, follow these steps:

1. Determine the proper airway size (Figure 11-32).
2. Lubricate the airway with a water-soluble lubricant (Figure 11-33).
3. Position the patient's head in a neutral position and place gentle pressure on the tip of the nose. This method of positioning will help open the nostrils enough for insertion.
4. Insert the airway into the nostril, with the bevel facing the nasal septum. The natural curve of the airway makes it work most easily in the right nostril (Figure 11-34).
5. Slide the airway into the nose until the flange rests against the nostril (Figure 11-35, *A* and *B*). If you feel resistance during insertion, do not force it. Remove the airway and try the other nostril.

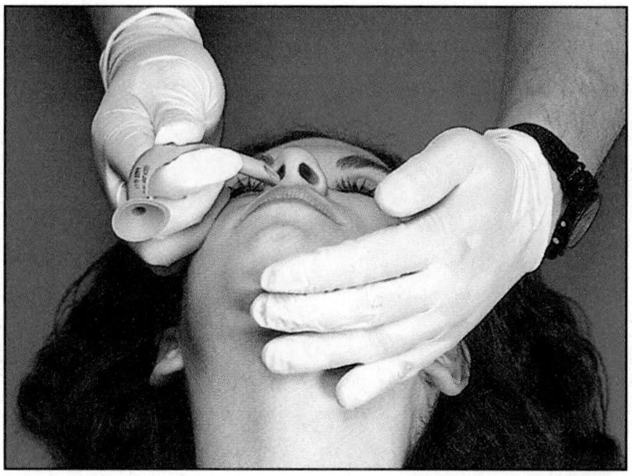

Figure 11-34

The bevel of the airway should face the nasal septum as the airway is being inserted.

Nasopharyngeal airways are contraindicated in patients that may have a basilar skull fracture, nose fracture, or deviated septum.

Oxygen Administration

Any seriously ill or injured patient will generally need supplemental oxygen. There is no reason why oxygen should ever be withheld from a patient in a prehospital setting. The following discussion covers the types of oxygen equipment most commonly used in EMS systems. Familiarize yourself with the specific oxygen delivery devices that you will use.

Oxygen Cylinders

Oxygen is a pressurized gas that comes in various sizes of cylinders made of aluminum or stainless steel. Full cylinders are usually filled with 2,000 to 2,200 pounds per square inch (psi) of pressure. The smallest, a D size, is commonly used as a portable cylinder. The medium size is an E cylinder. The large M cylinder supplies the onboard oxygen system in most ambulances (Table 11-1).

All oxygen cylinders must have the following information on the cylinder:

- United States Pharmacopeia (USP) labeling (Figure 11-36) (Oxygen cylinders are green, a color code established by the USP, with a yellow label.)
- Interstate Commerce Commission (ICC) specification number and date of manufacture
- Service pressure
- Name and identification mark of manufacturer
- Date that the cylinder was last hydrostatically tested (This is testing done to ensure that the cylinder is free of defects, such as corrosion, and will withstand the pressure. Cylinders should be hydrostatically tested every 5 years.)

TABLE 11-1 Capacity of Oxygen Cylinders

Cylinder size	Capacity	Use
D	350 liters	Small; portable system
E	625 liters	Medium; portable system
M	3,000 liters	Large; ambulance system
H	6,900 liters	Largest; hospital system

An additional safety system for pressurized gases is the use of gas-specific **regulators.** Oxygen regulators will only fit on oxygen cylinders.

While handling oxygen is safe for the most part, you should handle the equipment with care. The following guidelines will help ensure safe handling of oxygen equipment:

- Handle cylinders gently because their contents are under pressure.
- Cylinders should be stored lying down rather than standing up to prevent the cylinder from falling and damaging the valve-gauge assembly, which could turn the cylinder into a dangerous projectile.
- Do not allow smoking around oxygen equipment or while oxygen is in use. Oxygen promotes combustion (speeds burning).
- Do not use grease, oil, or adhesives (tape) around oxygen cylinders or regulators.
- Ensure that all cylinders in use are within dates for hydrostatic testing.

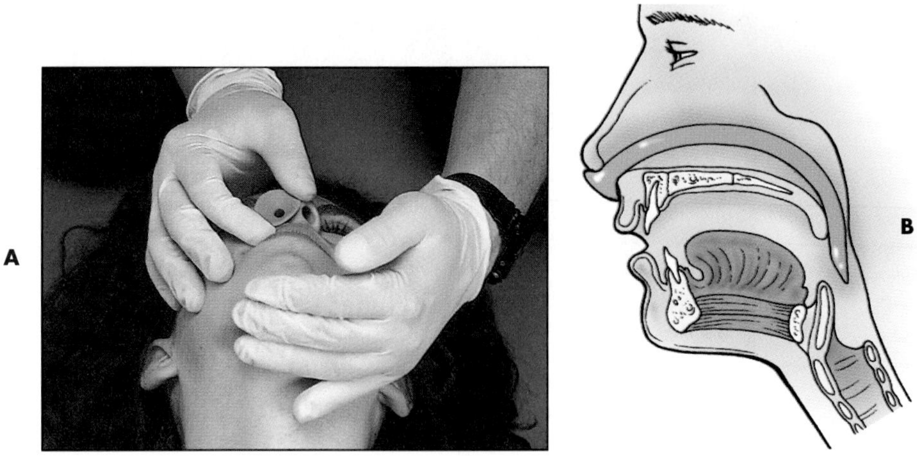

Figure 11-35

A, Slide the airway in the nose until the flange rests against the nostril. **B,** Proper positioning of the nasal airway.

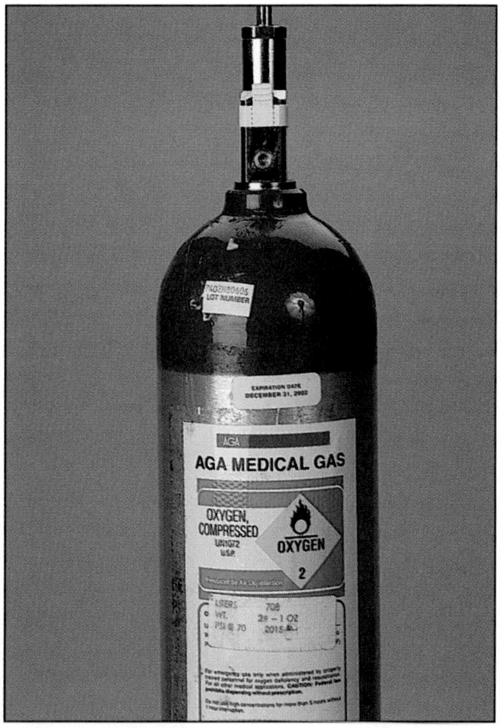

Figure 11-36

A green oxygen cylinder with a yellow label.

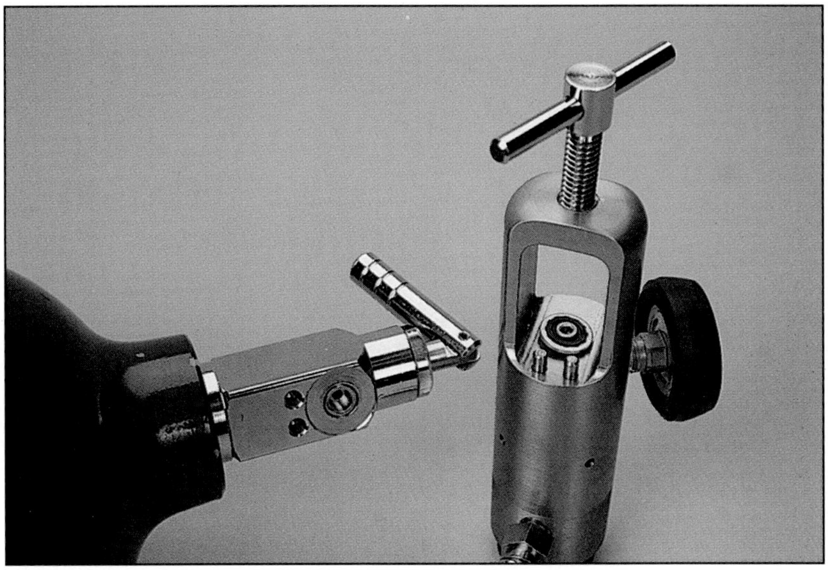

Figure 11-37
Pin-index safety system.

Pressure Regulators
Supplemental oxygen is a compressed gas. A full cylinder is under a pressure of approximately 2,000 psi. This pressure is far too high for patient use and therefore needs to be reduced before patient administration. This is done with a pressure regulator. The pressure regulators for smaller tanks (D and E) are yoke-type regulators. They use a pin-index safety system to ensure that only an oxygen tank can be attached to them (Figure 11-37). Larger tanks use a threaded-valve assembly that is part of a diameter-index safety system.

Once a pressure regulator is attached to the cylinder, the oxygen pressure is dropped to about 40 to 70 psi. In this range, the gas can be delivered safely. A flow meter determines how fast the regulator delivers the oxygen to the patient, within a range of 1 to 25 lpm.

Flow Meters
Most flow meters used in prehospital settings are attached to a pressure regulator (Figure 11-38). Types of flow meters include the Bourdon gauge, pressure-compensated, and constant-flow meters.

Bourdon Gauge. The Bourdon gauge flow meter is commonly used on portable oxygen cylinders. It is calibrated to indicate lpm and is part of the regulator. Usually you will see two gauges side by side. One gauge will indicate the amount of oxygen left in the tank; the other gauge will indicate the lpm. Unlike other regulators, the Bourdon gauge is not gravity dependent and can be placed in any position. It uses a clocklike dial that indicates the liter flow.

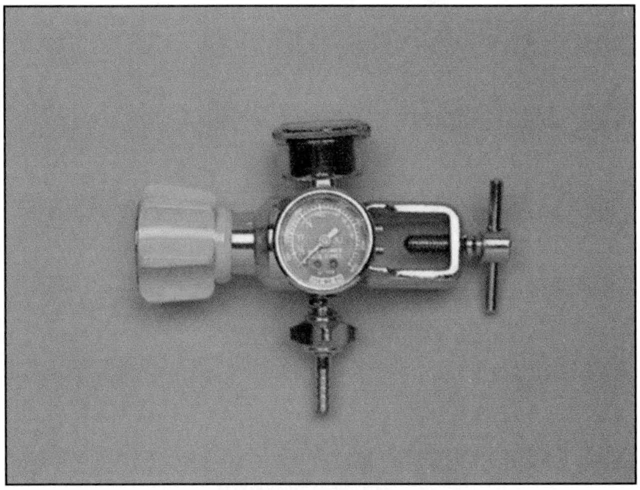

Figure 11-38
Flow meter.

Pressure-compensated Flow Meters. The biggest difference between a pressure-compensated flow meter and other types is that it is gravity-dependent. It shows the flow rate with a ball float that moves up and down inside a calibrated glass tube. The advantage of this device is that it will show a drop in flow rate if there is an obstruction, such as a kink in the tubing. In other types of flow meters, such an obstruction may go unnoticed. Pressure-compensated meters are most often found on fixed oxygen delivery systems in ambulances, but do not work well on portable oxygen tanks.

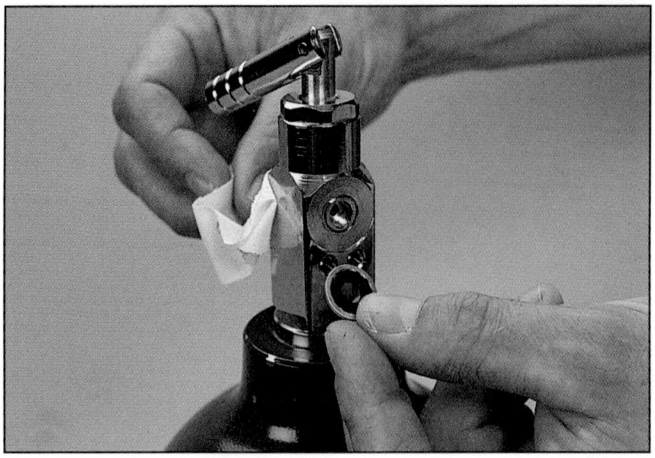

Figure 11-39

Remove the protective seal.

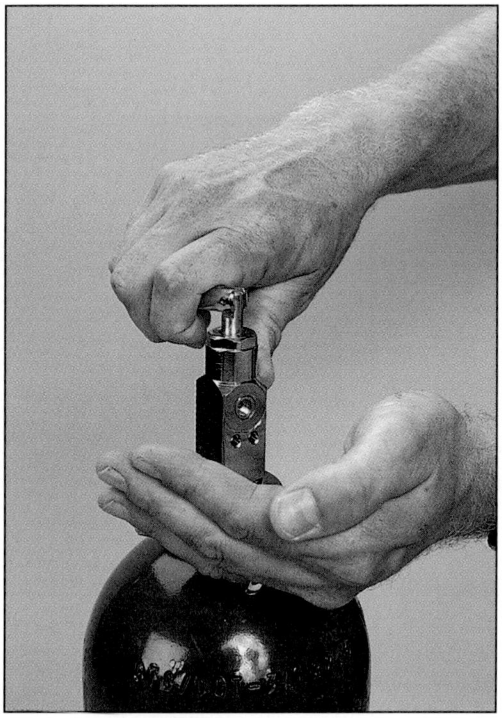

Figure 11-40

Remove any dirt from the valve.

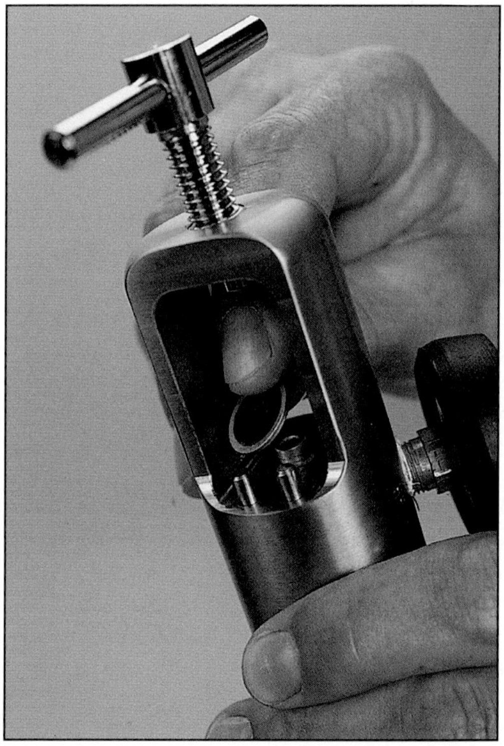

Figure 11-41

Check for a working washer on the regulator's inlet port.

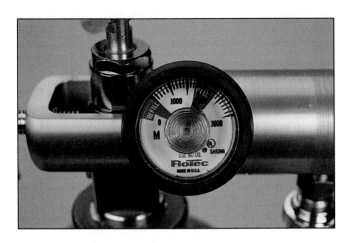

Figure 11-42

Check how much oxygen is available.

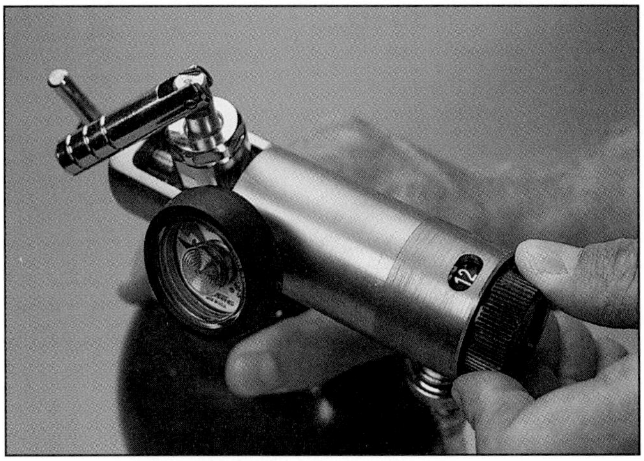

Figure 11-43

Turn the knob to the desired flow rate.

Constant-flow Meters. The newest type of flow meter, usually seen on portable oxygen systems, is the constant-dial flow meter, also called a constant-flow selector valve. This flow meter does not have a gauge. It is calibrated so that you can adjust the liter flow in stepped increments, from 2 to 25 lpm.

Regardless of the type of pressure regulator and flow meter, steps for connecting the regulator to the oxygen cylinder are the same:

1. Ensure that the cylinder contains oxygen.
2. Remove the protective seal from around the cylinder valve and save the washer (Figure 11-39).
3. Briefly open and close the valve to remove any dirt from the tank opening (Figure 11-40).
4. Check to see that a washer is on the regulator's inlet port. If not, attach the one provided with the cylinder (Figure 11-41). (Washers eventually compress to the point that they will not maintain a good seal. If reusing a washer, double check for leaks by ensuring that the gauge does not gradually fall.)
5. Attach the regulator to the cylinder and tighten the screw.
6. Open the valve to ensure that there are no leaks; check how much oxygen is available. The pressure regulator will indicate the psi in the cylinder (Figure 11-42).
7. Attach an oxygen delivery device to the flow meter, turn the knob to the desired flow rate (Figure 11-43), and place the oxygen delivery device on the patient (Figure 11-44).

To disconnect the oxygen system, reverse the process. Make sure to bleed (discharge) pressure from the cylinder before removing the flow meter. Do this by opening the flow meter after you have closed the valve on the cylinder. This will release pressure from the system. The needle on

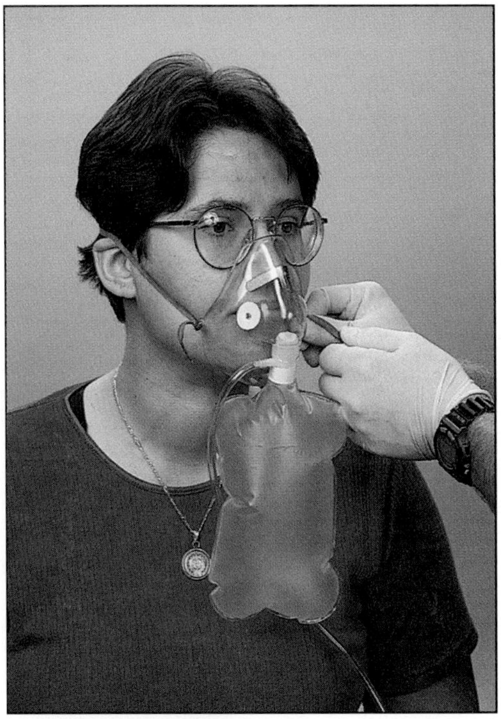

Figure 11-44

Place the delivery device on the patient.

the pressure regulator should drop to zero, and you will not feel or hear any more gas moving. At this point, it is safe to remove the regulator from the tank.

Free-Flow Oxygen Delivery Devices

With the previously discussed positive-pressure devices used to ventilate a nonbreathing patient, the operator provides the force to get the oxygen into the patient by blowing into a mask, squeezing a bag, or depressing a button to force oxygen from an oxygen cylinder. But what if your patient is breathing but not receiving an adequate oxygen concentration? A number of free-flow devices deliver extra oxygen to a patient who is already moving adequate volumes of air. Free-flow oxygen should always be humidified to prevent unnecessary drying of the airways. Two oxygen devices are in common prehospital use: the nonrebreather mask and the nasal cannula.

Nonrebreather Mask. The **nonrebreather mask** is the usual choice for delivering high-concentration oxygen to a breathing patient (Figure 11-45). It can deliver up to 90% oxygen when the flow rate is set at 15 lpm. This device has an oxygen reservoir bag attached to a mask that covers the mouth and nose. The mask has one-way valves on each side, which allow exhaled air to escape so that the patient does not rebreathe it. Oxygen fills the bag during exhalation; inhalation draws the oxygen from the bag into the mask.

A nonrebreather mask should be used for any patient with signs of shock, cardiac problems, or severe respiratory distress. To use the nonrebreather mask, connect the attached tubing to the flow meter and adjust the flow to 10 to 15 lpm. Place your finger over the port between the reservoir bag and the mask to allow the bag to fill before applying the mask. Once the bag is inflated, place the mask over the patient's face and adjust the straps on either side. The bag should deflate to about one-third full when the patient inhales, then fill up during exhalation. If the bag deflates completely during inhalation, increase the oxygen flow rate. The patient may have difficulty getting a full breath otherwise.

In the past, there has been controversy about giving high-concentration oxygen to patients with a history of chronic obstructed pulmonary disease (COPD), such as emphysema. EMTs were advised to avoid high concentrations for fear that these patients might stop breathing. However, this is no longer considered a significant problem. All patients should receive high-concentration oxygen through a nonrebreather mask if they need it. More information about the treatment of COPD patient appears in Chapter 14.

Some patients become anxious or apprehensive when a mask is placed over their face. To reduce this problem in a child, hold the mask slightly away from the child's face. Have a parent or other adult guardian hold the mask if possible. Some children feel more comfort-

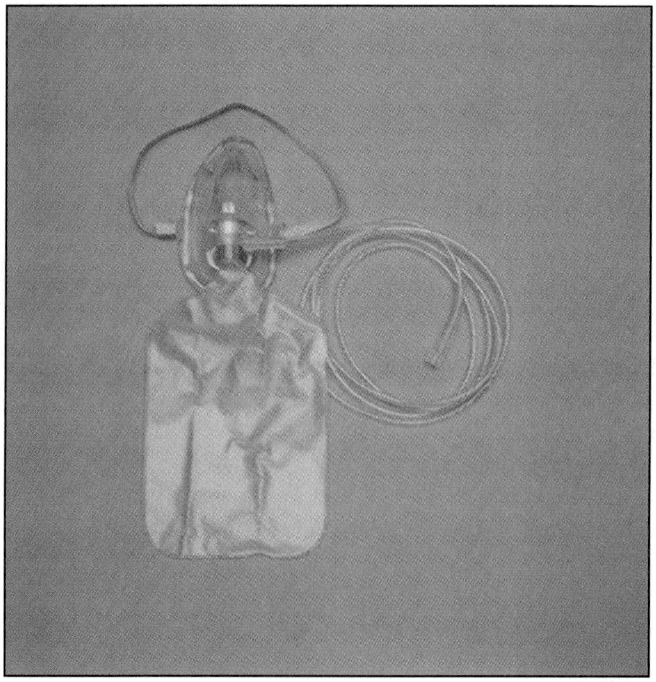

Figure 11-45

Nonrebreather mask.

able if they can hold the mask themselves. If you encounter a child or adult patient who is still uncomfortable with a mask covering the face, you may have to use a nasal cannula.

Nasal Cannula. A **nasal cannula** delivers oxygen through two prongs that are placed in the patient's nostrils. The tubing is wrapped behind the patient's ears and secured under the chin (Figure 11-46). A nasal cannula is used at a flow rate of 2 to 6 lpm. The device can provide only low-concentration oxygen in the range of 28% to 44%. At 2 lpm, a nasal cannula delivers 28% oxygen. The oxygen percentage increases by 4% for each additional lpm added. A nasal cannula should never be used to deliver oxygen at a flow greater than 6 lpm. Even at that rate, a patient may feel an uncomfortable jet of air rushing through the nose. Over time, this moving air can dry the nasal passages, especially if the oxygen is not humidified.

There are two situations in which you may decide to give low-concentration oxygen through a nasal cannula. One is a patient who cannot tolerate a mask. The second is a patient who is already on home oxygen. You may simply be continuing this low-concentration oxygen therapy or be treating a nonemergent condition.

A nasal cannula does not work well if the patient breathes only through the mouth. The oxygen from a nasal cannula is going into the nose. Unless inhalation is primarily through the nose, there will be less force to draw the oxygen into the body. (Mouth breathing will draw in some but not all oxygen provided by a nasal cannula.) For a patient who is not in immediate distress, some rescuers start with a nasal cannula immediately and then switch to a nonrebreather mask after assessing the patient. This allows the patient to speak without having to do so through a mask.

Other Masks. Although the nonrebreather mask and the nasal cannula are the two devices used primarily in emergency care, there are other types of oxygen delivery masks used in hospitals and other health care settings. The Venturi mask (Figure 11-47) is commonly used on patients being treated with oxygen for a long period of time who need specific oxygen concentrations, such as patients with COPD. These masks allow adjustment of the delivered oxygen to a desired concentration between 24% and 40%, using flow rates of 4 to 8 lpm.

Other masks include the simple face mask and partial nonrebreather mask. These masks deliver a medium concentration of oxygen (50% to 60%) at a flow rate of approximately 10 lpm. The simple face mask is commonly used by athletes at sporting events. The partial nonrebreather mask is similar to the nonrebreather mask except that it only has one exhalation valve. This allows a certain amount of exhaled air to be rebreathed. You will probably not carry these masks, but you may see them on patients that transport from one medical facility to another. If you are transporting a patient with a mask that you are not familiar with, make sure to ask a staff member for information before you begin transport.

If a resuscitation mask has an oxygen inlet, it can also be used on patients that are having difficulty breathing. However, it will not deliver the high oxygen concentrations needed in major hypoxic emergencies. The nonrebreather mask is the first choice in these situations. If you do use a resuscitation mask for free-flow oxygen administration, keeping the one-way valve attached to the mask will reduce the amount of oxygen that escapes. If the patient stops breathing, you can then begin ventilating immediately.

Bag-Valve-Mask. BVMs are commonly used to ventilate nonbreathing patients (see p. 249); however, they can also be used to assist ventilations in a person with difficulty

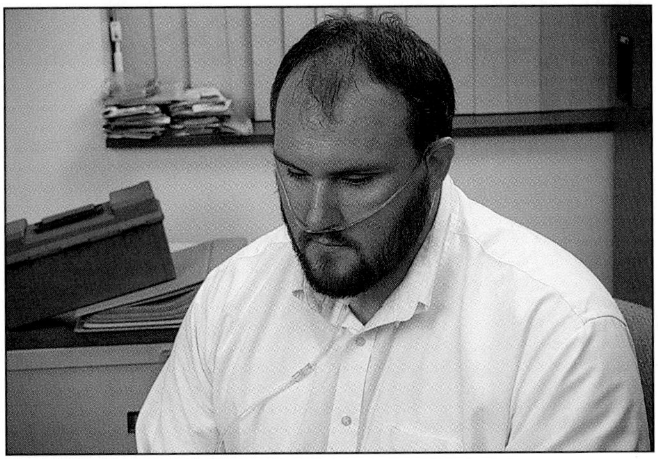

Figure 11-46
Nasal cannula.

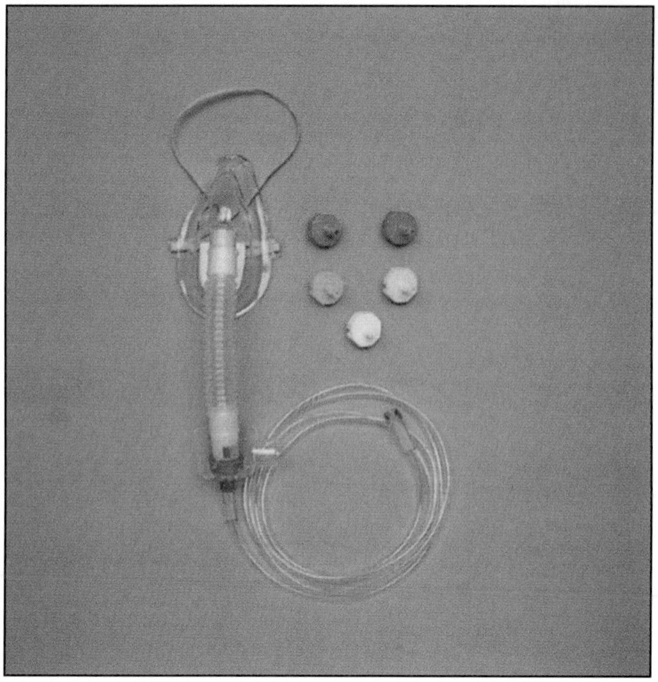

Figure 11-47

Venturi mask.

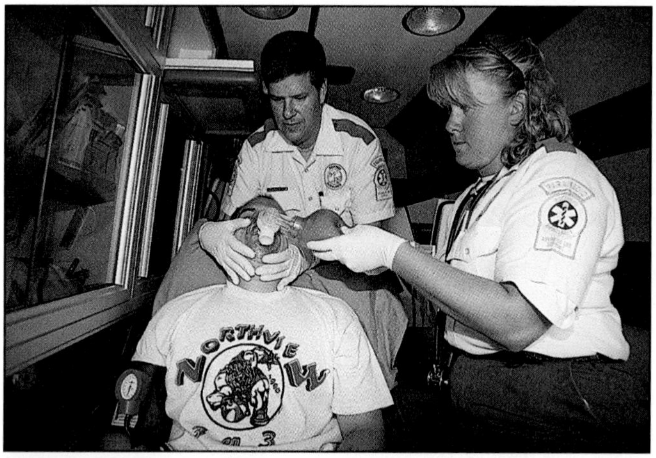

Figure 11-48

A patient with difficulty breathing can also be assisted with a bag-valve-mask.

breathing. A patient having difficulty breathing whose respiratory rate is less than 8 or more than 24 per minute may benefit from assisted ventilations. (Though 12 to 20 is the normal range for respiratory rate, patients can usually vary slightly from the normal range before ventilation is needed. Remember also to check clinical signs in addition to respiratory rate in assessing the need to assist ventilations.) Connect the BVM to an oxygen source and allow the reservoir to fill. Assist by squeezing the bag in rhythm with the patient's own inhalations (Figure 11-48).

Flow-Restricted, Oxygen-Powered Delivery Devices
In addition to its use on nonbreathing patients, the flow-restricted, oxygen-powered delivery device may be useful in assisting a patient that is having difficulty breathing. However, this device is limited in the amount of air that it can deliver to a breathing patient. Some patients will not be able to get enough oxygen from the device because of its valve that restricts a flow rate over 40 lpm.

IT'S YOUR CALL
CONCLUSION

Your patient has difficulty breathing, with a rate of 32 breaths per minute and crackles evident when auscultating lung sounds. His cyanotic color indicates that he is hypoxic. This patient is in serious respiratory distress and needs high-concentration oxygen. Because he is laboring to breathe, your patient is likely breathing through his mouth; therefore the nasal cannula will not be effective. Also, because he has fluid in the lungs, his ability to absorb oxygen is decreasing. The oxygen mask has not improved his respiratory status. You decide that assisting ventilations with a BVM device is the best way to improve oxygenation. You connect it to supplemental oxygen at a flow rate of 15 liters per minute as you begin to ventilate the patient.

SUMMARY

The respiratory system is responsible for taking in oxygen and eliminating carbon dioxide from the body. For this to occur effectively, the respiratory, circulatory, musculoskeletal, and nervous systems work together to regulate the amount of oxygen and carbon dioxide in the body. If problems occur with any of these body systems, the result could be a breathing emergency such as respiratory distress or respiratory arrest.

One common type of breathing emergency is choking. Both conscious and unconscious choking patients receive sequences of maneuvers to relieve the obstruction, followed by airway checks. The sequences differ depending on patient age and condition. There are several adjuncts available to help keep the patient's airway clear and assist breathing. Manual and mechanical suction devices can be used to clear the patient's mouth of obstructions such as vomitus and other fluids. With the airway clear of foreign objects, you can use oropharyngeal or nasopharyngeal airways to keep the tongue from occluding the airway in an unconscious patient.

Once you are certain that the airway is clear and adequately maintained, administer supplemental oxygen to the patient. If the conscious patient is experiencing severe respiratory distress, evidenced by labored or noisy respirations, abnormal respiratory rate, or other clinical signs, assist ventilations with an appropriate positive-pressure device, in rhythm with the patient's inhalations.

REFERENCES

1. **American Heart Association:** Emergency Cardiac Care Committee and Subcommittees: Guidelines for cardiopulmonary resuscitation and emergency cardiac care. II. Adult basic life support, *J Am Med Assoc* 268:2184, 1992.
2. **Elam JO, Greene DG:** Mission accomplished: successful mouth-to-mouth resuscitation, *Anesth Analg* 40:578, 1961.
3. **American Heart Association:** Emergency Cardiac Care Committee and Subcommittees: Guidelines for cardiopulmonary resuscitation and emergency cardiac care. V. Pediatric basic life support, *J Am Med Assoc* 268:2251, 1992.

Chapter

Advanced Airway Management

12

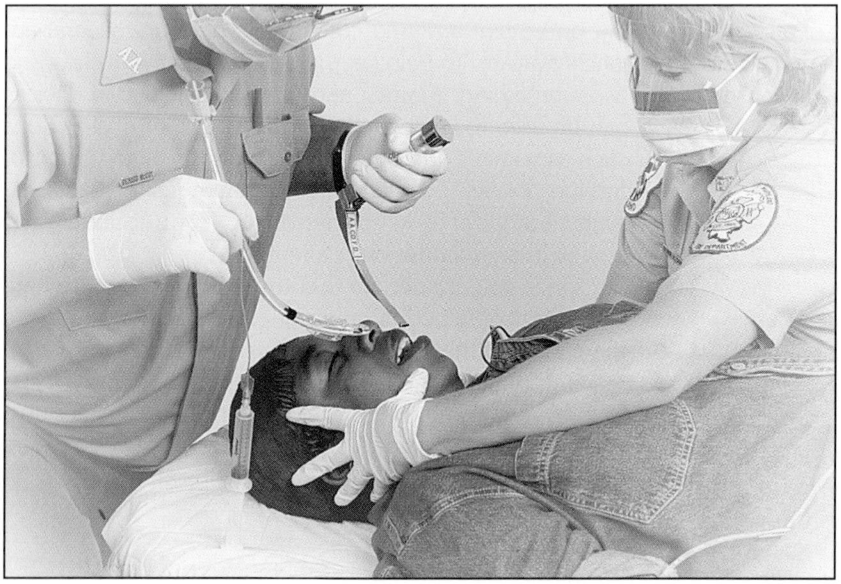

Knowledge Objectives

As an EMT-Basic, you should be able to:

OBJECTIVES

1. Describe when advanced airway-management techniques are indicated.
2. Describe the anatomic structures of the airway that are important in advanced airway management.
3. Discuss the differences in airway anatomy between adult and pediatric patients.
4. List the equipment required for orotracheal intubation.
5. Describe how to select an appropriate-size endotracheal tube for an adult, child, or infant.
6. Explain the reasons for using a stylet while placing an endotracheal tube, and describe how to use a stylet properly.
7. Describe how to perform orotracheal intubation.
8. Describe how to perform the Sellick maneuver (cricoid pressure) during orotracheal intubation.
9. Describe how to confirm endotracheal tube placement.
10. Explain the consequences of an unrecognized esophageal intubation.
11. Describe the use of carbon dioxide detection devices to confirm and maintain proper endotracheal tube placement.
12. Describe how to secure an endotracheal tube.
13. List complications associated with orotracheal intubation.
14. Explain the anatomic and physiologic differences between adult and pediatric patients relative to orotracheal intubation.
15. Discuss the differences among other advanced devices available to help maintain an airway.
16. Describe the technique for performing tracheal suction.
17. Explain the importance of sterile technique in both endotracheal intubation and tracheal suction.
18. Describe the indications, contraindications, and techniques for the placement of nasogastric tubes in pediatric patients.
19. Explain how to manage the airway of a laryngectomee properly.

OBJECTIVES

Skill Objectives

As an EMT-Basic, you should be able to:

1. **Demonstrate how to perform the Sellick maneuver.**
2. **Demonstrate orotracheal intubation for an adult, child, and infant patient, using sterile technique.**
3. **Demonstrate how to confirm proper endotracheal tube placement.**
4. **Demonstrate how to ventilate a patient properly with an endotracheal tube in place.**
5. **Demonstrate tracheal suction using sterile technique.**
6. **Demonstrate the use of alternative devices to maintain an airway.**

Attitude Objectives

As an EMT-Basic, you should be able to:

1. **Describe your feelings about performing invasive, advanced airway-management procedures.**
2. **Explain the value of performing advanced airway-management procedures.**
3. **Discuss your professional responsibility in maintaining skill competency in endotracheal intubation.**

KEY TERMS

1. **Aspiration:** The inhalation of blood, vomitus, or other foreign matter into the trachea and lungs.
2. **Carina:** The point at which the trachea divides into the two mainstem bronchi.
3. **Cricoid Cartilage:** The cartilage ring just inferior to the larynx.
4. **Endotracheal Intubation:** The process of inserting an endotracheal tube into a patient's trachea to maintain an open airway and provide effective oxygenation and ventilation.
5. **Epigastrium:** Area of the abdominal surface directly anterior to the stomach and just inferior to the xiphoid process.
6. **Epiglottis:** A leaf-shaped structure that prevents food and fluid from entering the trachea.
7. **Esophagus:** The tube leading from the pharynx to the stomach.
8. **Gastric Distention:** Inflation of the stomach with air, often caused by the use of too much force or volume during emergency ventilation; can make ventilations less effective or cause vomiting.
9. **Glottis:** The opening between the vocal cords, leading to the trachea.
10. **Laryngoscope:** An instrument that allows one to see the vocal cords directly before inserting an endotracheal tube during orotracheal intubation.
11. **Mainstem Bronchi:** The two main airway branches that lead from the trachea to the lungs.
12. **Nasogastric Tube:** A tube passed through the nose and esophagus into the stomach to relieve the pressure that causes gastric distention.
13. **Orotracheal Intubation:** The primary type of endotracheal intubation in which the tube is passed through the mouth into the trachea.
14. **Sellick Maneuver:** Pressure applied to the cricoid cartilage to prevent passive aspiration and assist in visualizing the vocal cords; also called *cricoid pressure.*
15. **Stylet:** A semiflexible device placed in an endotracheal tube to help hold the tube's shape and assist during endotracheal intubation.
16. **Thyroid Cartilage:** Cartilage covering most of the larynx; the Adam's apple.
17. **Vallecula:** A space between the base of the tongue and the epiglottis into which the tip of a curved laryngoscope blade is inserted during endotracheal intubation.
18. **Vocal Cords:** The two folds of tissue at the entrance to the larynx that vibrate and produce sounds as air passes between them.

IT'S YOUR CALL

You are dispatched on a report of an unconscious man in the street. A paramedic unit from a neighboring jurisdiction has been dispatched to provide mutual aid but is several minutes behind you. Upon arrival, you see a man lying on the ground. As you approach the patient, bystanders tell you that he was placing groceries in his vehicle when he suddenly clutched his chest and collapsed. Your initial survey shows that he is breathless and without a pulse. You initiate cardiopulmonary resuscitation (CPR) as your partner hooks up the automated external defibrillator (AED) to check the patient's heart rhythm. After administering three shocks without success, you contact medical control to get approval to intubate the patient.

As you are making the request, your partner prepares the intubation equipment while bystanders continue CPR. What size laryngoscope blade and endotracheal tube should you use? Because the patient is now vomiting, what will you do to visualize the vocal cords for correct placement of the tube?

As you learned in earlier chapters, one of your primary responsibilities is to ensure that your patient has a patent airway. As an EMT-Basic you have learned basic techniques to manage the airway, including opening the airway and using oral and nasal airways to prevent the tongue from occluding the airway. You have learned to use a pocket mask or bag-valve-mask (BVM) to deliver oxygen to a nonbreathing patient. However, with the addition of new equipment and techniques and permission from medical direction, you will be even better equipped to manage difficult airway problems.

This chapter examines these other devices and skills, particularly the endotracheal tube and its insertion. You will also learn when it is appropriate to use these skills and the complications that can occur if they are used incorrectly. (Note: Endotracheal intubation is an optional skill in the EMT-Basic curriculum. Approval to use it in a particular EMS system depends on local regulations and policy in the system and medical direction judgments regarding training resources and skills maintenance.)

Using Advanced Airway Adjuncts

The use of advanced airway adjuncts enables you to provide and protect a patent airway. Basic airway procedures, such as a jaw thrust and placement of an oropharyngeal airway, help maintain the airway in an open position. However, these procedures do not prevent the potential entry of blood or vomitus into the trachea or lungs. **Endotracheal intubation,** with the tube cuff inflated in the correct location in the trachea, provides partial, direct protection against **aspiration.** The endotracheal tube also allows ventilation directly into the lungs.

Other adjunctive devices block the **esophagus** and prevent **gastric distention** by keeping air from entering the stomach and forcing air toward the trachea and lungs; however, these other airway adjuncts are less direct and effective at preventing aspiration. They use inflatable cuffs placed outside of the trachea but inside the esophagus and pharynx. Fluid can still enter the trachea, especially when there is bleeding in the airway. Even with an endotracheal tube, fluid leakage past the tracheal cuff is possible, but aspiration of large amounts is much less likely.

Earlier chapters presented the basic function and structures of the respiratory system. To use advanced airway adjuncts properly, it is important to become even more familiar with the anatomic features that serve as landmarks during intubation (Figure 12-1).

To get to the lungs, air must pass through the pharynx (throat) to a point where the openings of the trachea and esophagus meet. The **epiglottis,** a leaflike structure just superior to the trachea, opens during inhalation and exhalation to allow air movement into and out of the trachea, but closes over the trachea during swallowing to prevent food and fluid entry. Between the epiglottis and the base of the tongue is a space known as the **vallecula.** Just beneath the epiglottis is the **larynx,** which contains the **vocal cords.** The **glottis** is the opening between the vocal cords, which leads to the trachea. The larynx is supported by the semicircular **thyroid cartilage.** The lower portion of the larynx is surrounded by the full ring of the **cricoid cartilage,** which prevents the trachea from collapsing during forceful air movement. The cricoid cartilage is the only area of the trachea completely surrounded by cartilage. The trachea bifurcates, or divides, into two **mainstem bronchi** at the **carina.** The left mainstem bronchus leaves the trachea at a sharper angle than does the right mainstem bronchus. Consequently, objects such as aspirated food or misplaced endotracheal tubes pass more easily into the right side. The mainstem bronchi subdivide further into smaller air passages known as **bronchioles** until they reach the **alveoli,** where gas exchange takes place.

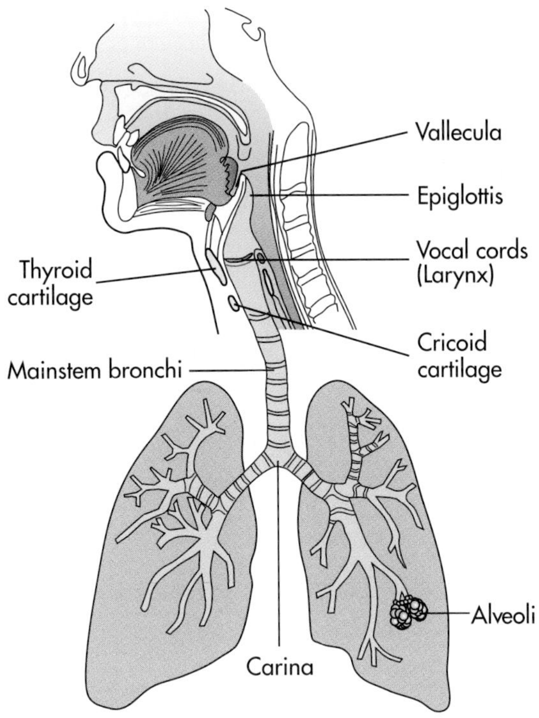

Figure 12-1
Anatomic landmarks.

Endotracheal Intubation

Endotracheal intubation is the most effective way to maintain an open airway, prevent aspiration, and deliver adequate oxygenation and ventilation. Passing an endotracheal tube into a patient's trachea allows oxygen delivery directly into the patient's lungs. **Orotracheal intubation,** in which the endotracheal tube is passed through the mouth into the trachea, is the most common method of endotracheal intubation. Inserting the tube through the nose and into the trachea is called **nasotracheal intubation** (Figure 12-2). This technique is more difficult and limited than the orotracheal method. It is usually performed "blind" (the vocal cords are not visible) and is generally not used in nonbreathing patients because the procedure relies on listening for breath sounds. For these reasons, it is a skill reserved for paramedics and physicians, or in some systems, for physicians only.

Once you learn to perform orotracheal intubation, ongoing practice is a particularly important part of skill maintenance for endotracheal intubation. When possible, practicing with anesthesia personnel in an operating room is ideal. However, frequent review and practice with a manikin, under direction of a qualified instructor, is also very valuable. Because this is such a critical skill, some EMS systems require personnel to demonstrate adequate performance on a regular basis, as often as every 3 to 6 months.

Indications and Complications

As an EMT-Basic, you may be trained in orotracheal intubation of apneic patients. This will allow you to control the airway, reduce the risk of aspiration, deliver better oxygenation and ventilation, and suction the airways below the larynx. You should be thoroughly familiar with local protocols regarding orotracheal intubation.

There are two basic indications for performing EMT-Basic endotracheal intubation:

- Inability to oxygenate and ventilate the apneic patient
- Concerns that a patient who is unresponsive to painful stimuli, has no gag reflex, or otherwise shows indications of inability to protect the airway, may aspirate blood or vomitus

While orotracheal intubation will greatly benefit the patient, it is an invasive skill requiring placement of an object inside the body. Complications can occur, especially if you perform the skill incorrectly:

- Prolonged intubation attempts can lead to hypoxia. This is the primary reason why there is a time limit on intubation attempts.
- Stimulation of the airway during intubation can slow the heart rate significantly. This normally resolves quickly, but it is another reason for a time limit during intubation attempts. It is important that you closely monitor the patient's pulse during the intubation procedure.

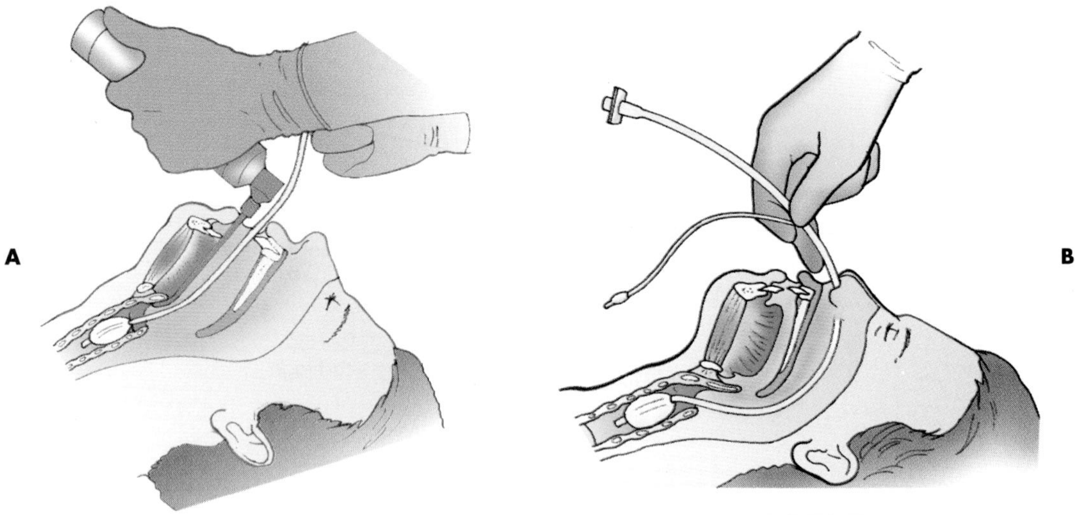

Figure 12-2
A comparison of orotracheal **(A)** and nasotracheal **(B)** intubation.

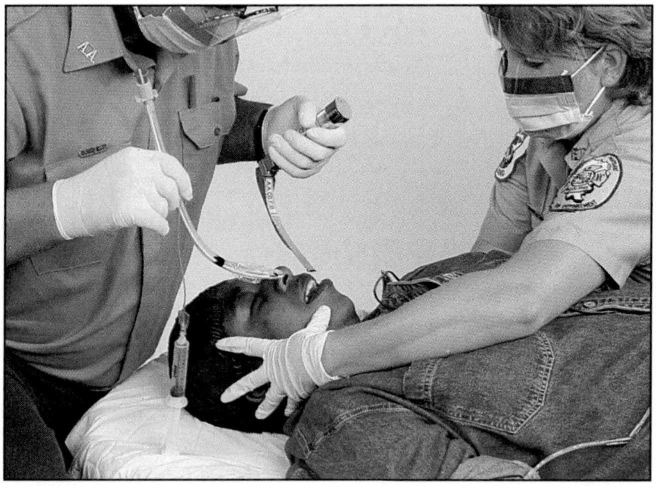

Figure 12-3
BSI precautions for intubation include the use of gloves, a mask, and goggles.

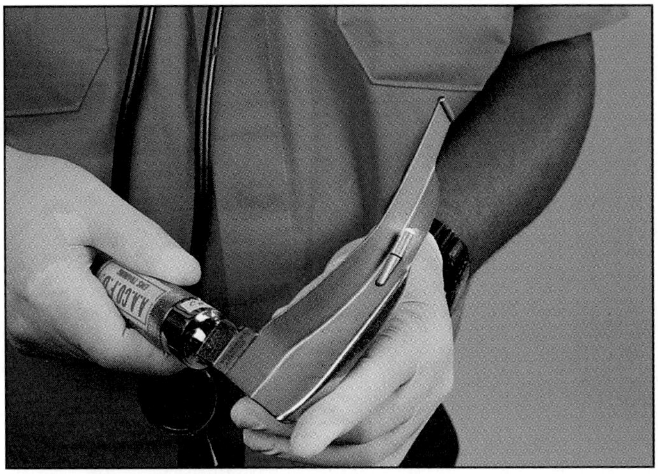

Figure 12-4
A laryngoscope with a Macintosh blade.

- When performed improperly, intubation can cause trauma to the lips, teeth, tongue, gums and airway structures such as the trachea, vocal cords, and bronchi.
- Placing the tube into the right mainstem bronchus can lead to inadequate oxygenation and collapse of lung tissue in the left lung.
- Placing the tube into the esophagus instead of the trachea will result in inadequate oxygenation and anoxia, gastric distention, and vomiting. When unrecognized, the anoxia can quickly cause cardiac arrest.
- Vomiting may occur if the patient regains consciousness.
- Upon gaining consciousness, a patient may attempt to remove the endotracheal tube, causing injury to the larynx and airways.
- The procedure can increase intracranial pressure, which may be particularly dangerous in patients with head injuries (see Chapter 25). This makes it important to place the tube as quickly and as smoothly as possible in head injury and stroke patients.

Preparing Equipment

Orotracheal intubation requires special equipment. Because you are entering a patient's body, infectious disease hazards are a concern. Proper body substance isolation (BSI) precautions, including the use of gloves, a mask, and goggles, must be observed when intubating a patient (Figure 12-3).

Placing a tube into the trachea also creates an infection concern for the patient. Endotracheal intubation is ideally performed as a sterile technique. It may be more realistic to consider it clean rather than sterile in some field settings; however, procedures should remain as close to sterile as possible. The endotracheal tube is sterile in its container; you should attempt to keep it sterile at least until it is time for placement into the trachea.

Laryngoscope. The device used to visualize the vocal cords and allow placement of the endotracheal tube into the trachea is the **laryngoscope** (Figure 12-4). Its handle contains batteries and a locking bar. Its other part is a blade, which snaps into place on the locking bar and has a small light on the tip. The two most common types of blades are curved Macintosh blades and straight Miller blades.

Laryngoscope blades come in a variety of sizes, ranging from 0 to 4 (Figure 12-5). The larger the number, the larger the blade. Most adult patients require a size 3 or 4 blade; pediatric patients need smaller blades. The decision between straight and curved blades is a personal preference that develops over time as one gains skill in intubating. However, a small straight blade should be used for all children under 8 years of age. The proportionally larger size of the epiglottis and the relatively superior location of the vocal cords in small children creates a sharp angle between the mouth and the cords that can make visualization difficult. The straight blade is the most effective in moving the tongue and elevating the epiglottis to reduce that angle.

To assemble the laryngoscope, insert the locking bar of the handle into the notch at the end of the blade until it clicks. Then lift upward, which locks the blade in place and activates the light (Figure 12-6). Check that the light is bright and screwed tightly to the blade. A loose light that falls into the airway is a serious, although preventable, complication.

Endotracheal Tubes. Like laryngoscope blades, endotracheal tubes come in various sizes. The size refers to the internal diameter of the tube. The average tube used in an adult male patient is 8.0 to 8.5 mm in diameter; sizes 7.0 to 8.0 are commonly used in adult females. As a general rule, a 7.5 tube will fit most adults. The size of endo-

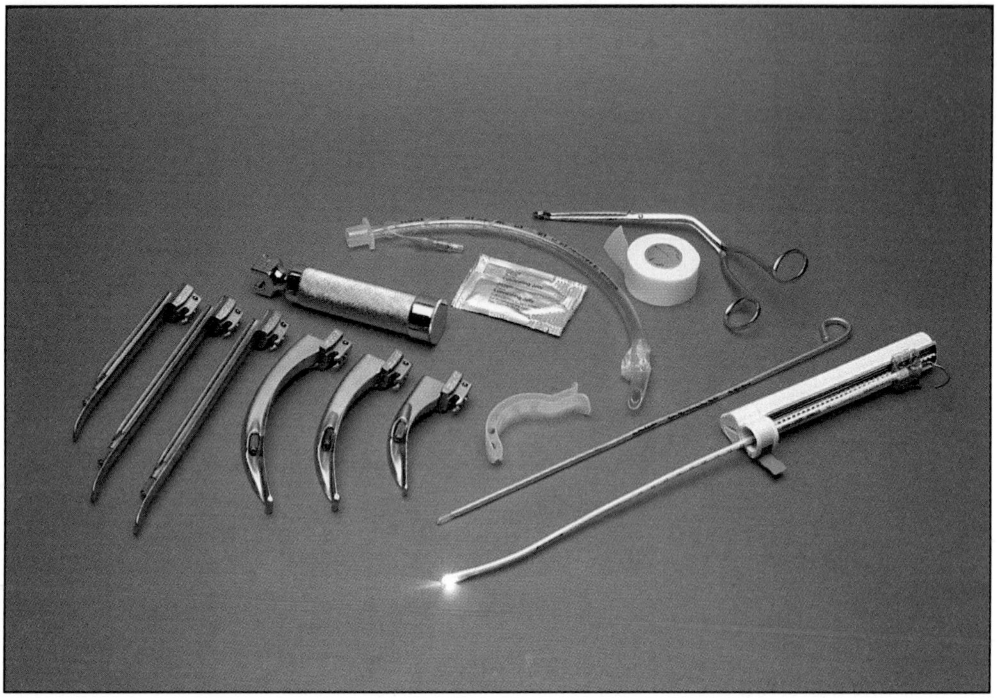

Figure 12-5

Endotracheal equipment, including several sizes of straight and curved laryngoscope blades, Magill forceps, and a lighted stylet.

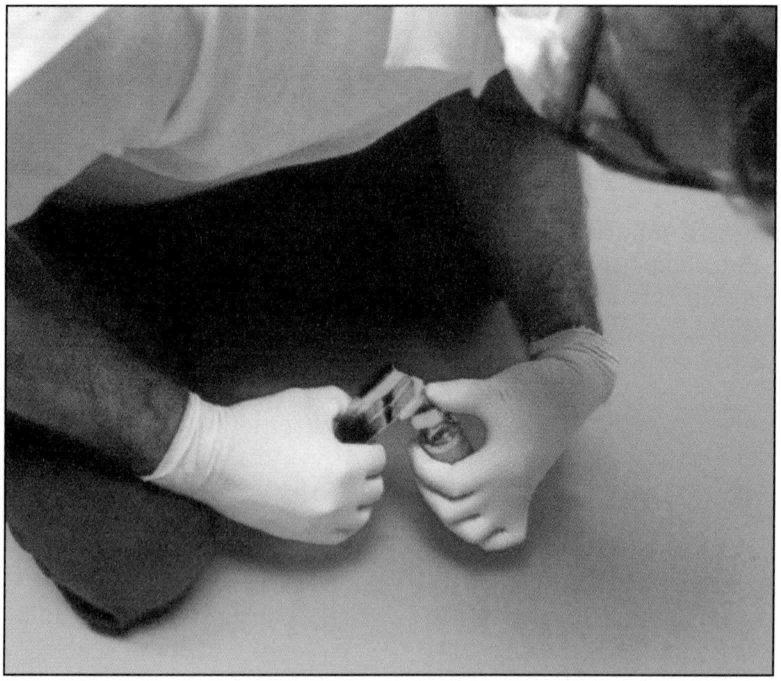

Figure 12-6

Lift to lock the blade in place.

tracheal tubes used for children will be discussed later in the chapter (see p. 286).

The top of the tube has a 15-mm adapter for attaching a bag-valve device to the tube for ventilating the patient. A tiny inflation tube runs along the main tube. At the top of the inflation tube is the inflation valve, and just below it is the pilot balloon (Figure 12-7). The inflation valve accepts a 10-ml syringe for inflating the cuff at the distal end of the endotracheal tube. The pilot balloon inflates at the same time, verifying that the cuff is inflated.

Correctly placed in the trachea, the cuff at the end of the endotracheal tube prevents air from leaking back out of the lungs during inspiration. It also helps protect against aspiration of foreign matter into the lungs (Figure 12-8). Because the narrowest portion of the adult airway is at the vocal cords, the balloon is needed to protect the larger airway just below the cords. Endotracheal tubes for infants and children do not have cuffs; their small tracheas are more sensitive to the pressure caused by inflation; and the narrowing of the trachea at the cricoid ring (the narrowest portion of the pediatric airway) helps make a natural seal below the larynx.

The small side hole at the distal end of the tube, opposite the bevel (angled cut), is called the *Murphy eye.* It provides a backup for air passage in case an obstruction blocks the end of the tube. Adult endotracheal tubes are commonly 33 cm in length. On an average adult, the front teeth are about 20 cm from the sternal notch and 25 cm from the carina. Because the tip of the tube should come to rest between these two levels, a depth of 22 to 23 cm is usually appropriate in adults (Figure 12-9). The markings on the side of the tube can be used as reference points to verify that the tube remains at the proper depth once it has been placed. This is not an absolute indicator; clinical signs, particularly breath sounds, still demand regular monitoring. However, tube markings can be useful during the intervals between auscultations.

Accessories. A **stylet** is a semiflexible wire that is inserted into the endotracheal tube to provide shape and partial rigidity for easier insertion. Use of a stylet should be a routine method to stabilize the tube and guide it quickly into place. The stylet becomes even more important in warm weather when tubes soften and are more difficult to control.

The tip of the stylet should never be inserted past the Murphy eye; doing so may allow the stylet's tip to lacerate the airway as the tube is advanced into the airway. The tube and stylet should be formed into a hockey-stick shape to help pass the tip through the vocal cords. Applying a water-soluble lubricant to the distal end of the endotracheal tube also eases insertion.

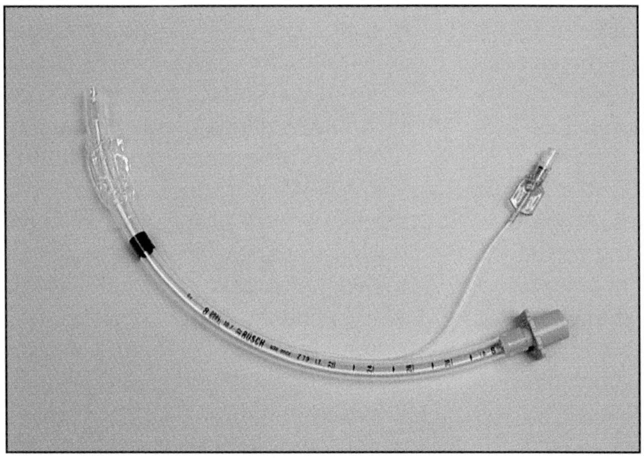

Figure 12-7

Endotracheal tube.

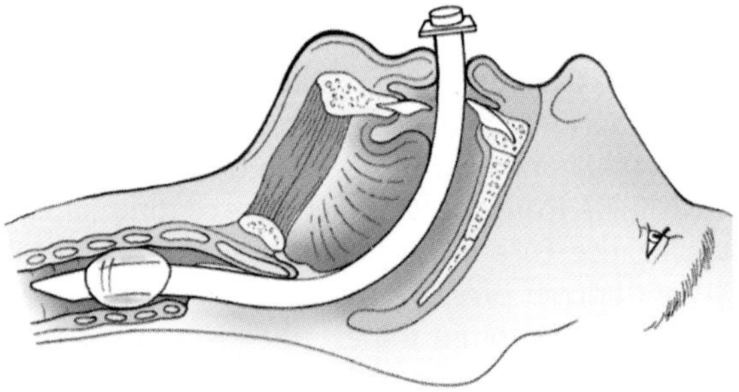

Figure 12-8

A correctly placed endotracheal tube prevents air leakage and helps protect the patient from aspiration.

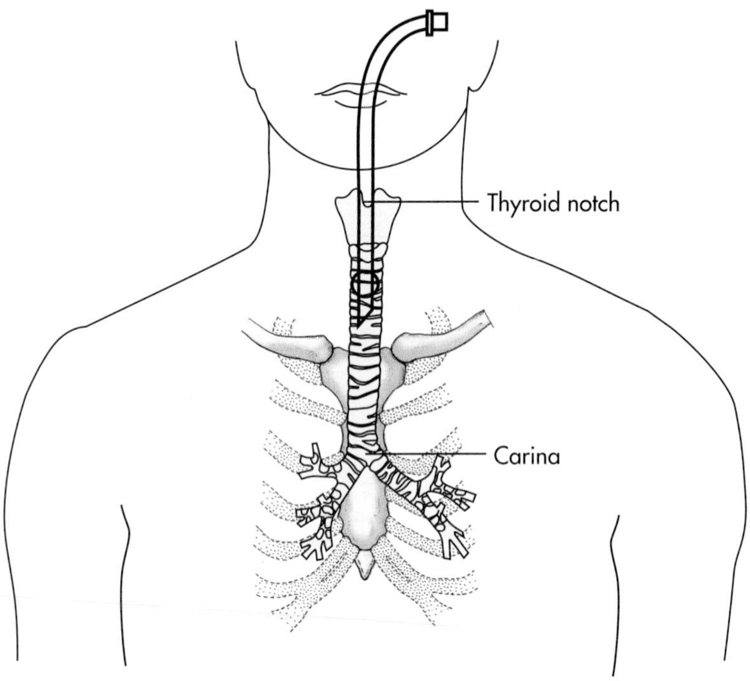

Figure 12-9

Correct depth for the endotracheal tube.

A 10-ml syringe is attached to the inflation valve to inflate the cuff. Before insertion, the cuff should be inflated briefly to test for leaks. This can be done with the endotracheal tube left in the sterile wrapper; the end can be opened for access to the inflation valve and to place the stylet. When the cuff is inflated, the pilot balloon also inflates (Figure 12-10).

Tape, umbilical tie, or a special tube holder can be used to secure the endotracheal tube in place. An oropharyngeal airway is also sometimes inserted to prevent the patient from biting down on the tube and potentially occluding it (Figure 12-11). Some commercial tube holders have built-in bite blocks.

Before intubation, suction equipment should be prepared in case the patient vomits. A large-bore tip will speed the process of clearing the airway of any fluid. After intubation, a flexible French catheter can be used for endotracheal suctioning through the endotracheal tube.

A stethoscope is needed to confirm the proper placement of the endotracheal tube. A carbon dioxide detector can also help assess tube placement.

Intubation Techniques

Endotracheal intubation requires organization and a division of duties. While one EMT performs the intubation, a second attends to ventilating, assisting with equipment, and perhaps performing the **Sellick maneuver.** Preparation includes attention to sterile technique as much as possible, as well as to the steps of the procedure.

Sellick Maneuver. Gastric distention, regurgitation, and aspiration are common problems that occur during ventilation of a patient with an unprotected airway. The Sellick maneuver, also called *cricoid pressure,* is a helpful technique to prevent all three of these problems. It is performed by applying gentle pressure on the cricoid cartilage (Figure 12-12). This pushes the cricoid ring into the esophagus, which lies directly posterior, and closes the esophagus. The maneuver also pushes the vocal cords back, thereby reducing the angle between the mouth and the cords and making visualization and tube insertion easier.

To find the correct position, feel for the cricoid membrane. It is located in the depression just below the Adam's apple (thyroid cartilage). The prominence just below this membrane is the cricoid ring. This cartilage, which completely encircles the trachea, is the correct place to apply the Sellick maneuver. Grasp the sides of the cricoid ring using your thumb and index finger; and apply gentle, firm pressure from anterior to posterior. If you are performing this maneuver on a child or infant, be careful that you do not apply too much force. The pediatric trachea is softer than an adult's, and excessive pressure can cause tracheal obstruction.

This maneuver can be useful in blocking some of the flow of fluids from the stomach, preventing aspiration. However, use care if the patient is forcefully vomiting; persistent cricoid pressure held against a forceful emesis can damage or rupture the esophagus. Cricoid pressure should *not* be used if the patient is actively vomiting.

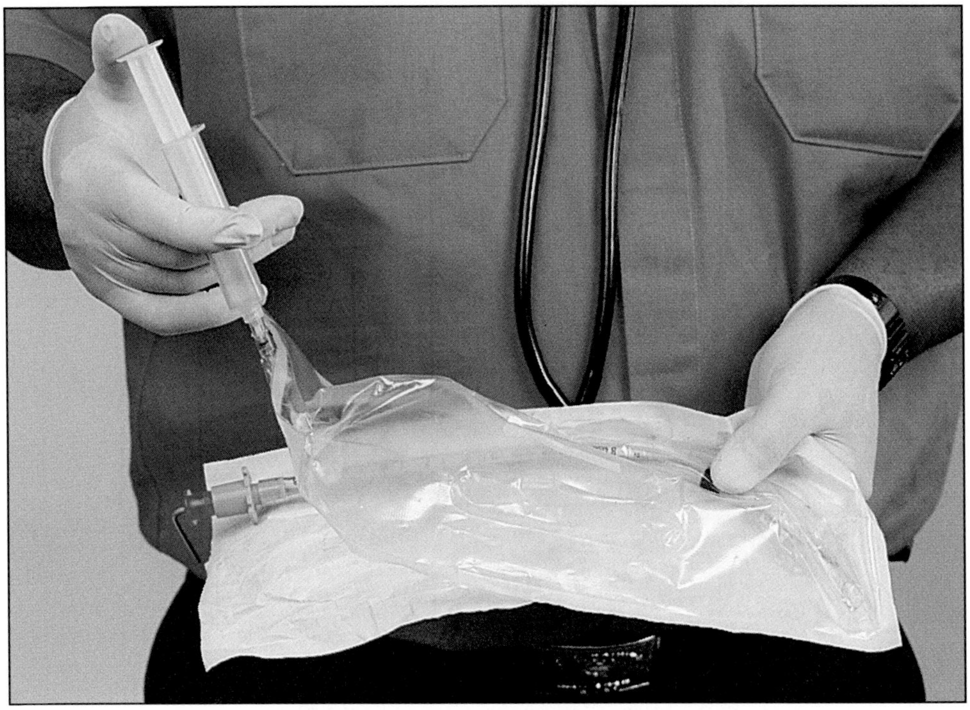

Figure 12-10

Inflate the cuff before insertion to test for leaks.

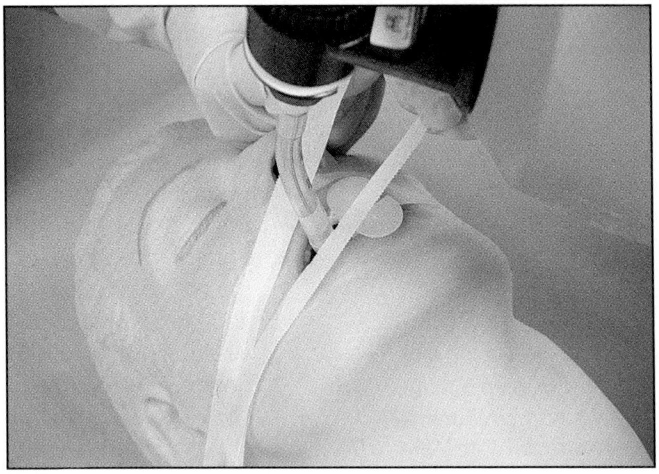

Figure 12-11

An orotracheal airway can be used to prevent a patient from biting down on the endotracheal tube and occluding it.

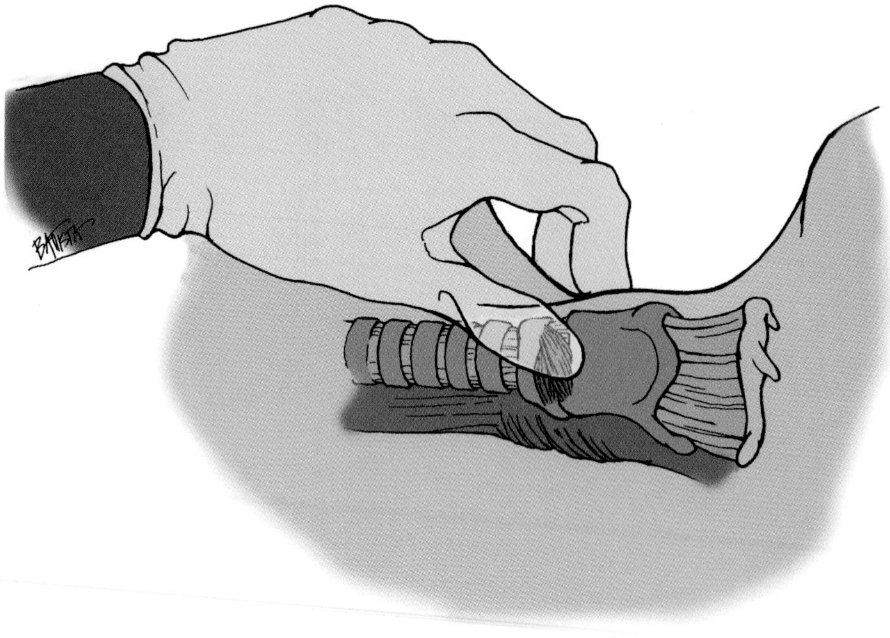

Figure 12-12

The Sellick maneuver is performed by applying pressure on the cricoid ring to compress the esophagus.

IT'S YOUR CALL CONTINUED

In the opening scenario, an adult male was found in cardiac arrest and in need of advanced airway management. You have decided to perform orotracheal intubation. The proper size endotracheal tube for this patient is 8.0 to 8.5 mm. After suctioning the patient, your partner uses the Sellick maneuver to minimize aspiration and help you visualize the vocal cords. You pass the endotracheal tube through the glottis and begin to ventilate the patient as your partner checks for lung sounds. They are present only on the right side, and you hear gurgling sounds there as you ventilate. Should you secure the tube in place and continue to ventilate? Are there additional measures you could take to get bilateral lung sounds and reduce the gurgling? What can you do to confirm that the tube is in the correct position?

Endotracheal Tube Insertion. Placing an endotracheal tube requires recognition of certain anatomic landmarks and coordination of several activities. Follow these steps:

1. Ensure that the patient has an open airway and is being ventilated adequately. In a medical patient, tilt the head back and lift the chin; it is sometimes helpful to place a towel under the patient's head as well. This is referred to as the *sniffing position* and aids visualization of the vocal cords. However, if you suspect trauma, maintain the head in a neutral position. Have another EMT hyperventilate the patient with a BVM at a rate of one breath approximately every 2½ seconds.
2. Select the proper equipment, assemble it, and test it. Check to see that the laryngoscope works properly and the light is bright and secure. While handling the endotracheal tube, try to keep it sterile until inserting it into the trachea. Check the tube to ensure that the cuff inflates and holds air. Insert the stylet and lubricate the tube.
3. Take BSI precautions.
4. Position yourself at the top of the patient's head. Have your partner stop ventilating. Your partner can perform the Sellick maneuver at this point, if needed. Holding the laryngoscope with your left hand, insert the blade into the right side of the patient's mouth. Move the tongue with a sweeping motion from right to left (Figure 12-13). Gently guide the blade into the throat until you are able to visualize the epiglottis and the vocal cords. If you are using a curved blade, place

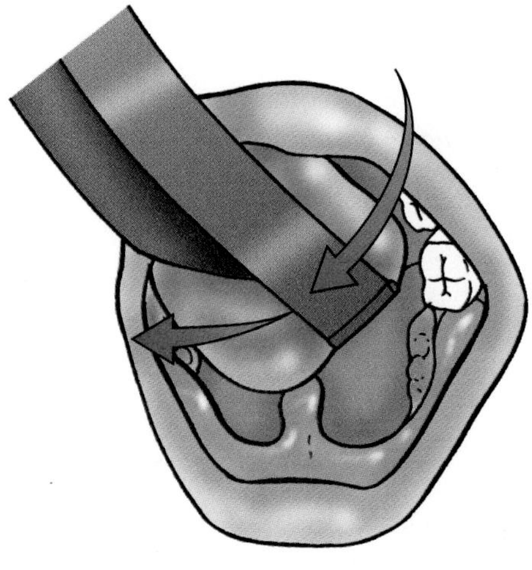

Figure 12-13

Inserting the blade in the right side of the patient's mouth, use a sweeping motion to move the tongue.

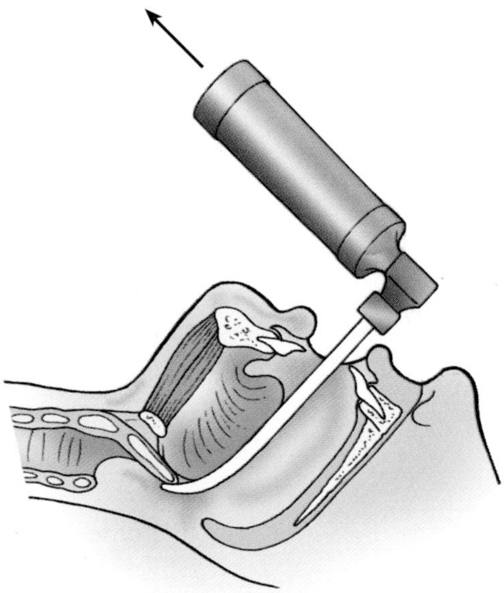

Figure 12-14

Lift the laryngoscope up and away.

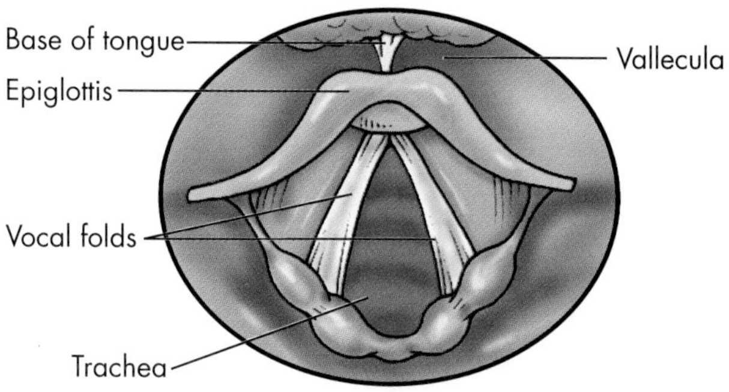

Figure 12-15

Vocal cords.

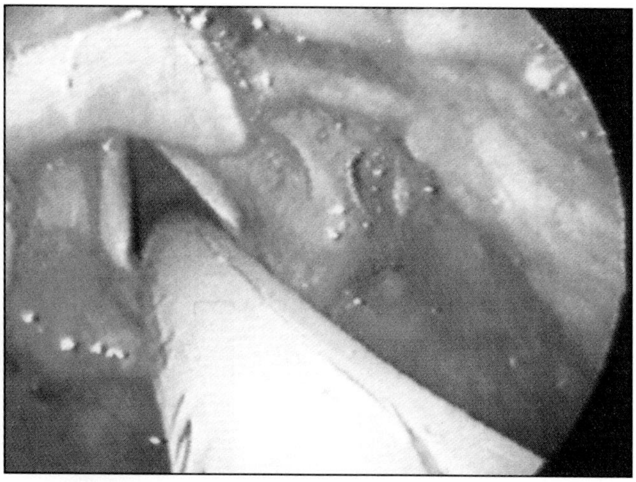

Figure 12-16

Pass the endotracheal tube through the vocal cords.

the tip of the blade into the vallecula and lift anteriorly. If you are using a straight blade, advance the blade tip past the epiglottis and lift anteriorly, trapping the epiglottis above the blade.

5. Lift the laryngoscope up and away from the patient to visualize the glottic opening (Figure 12-14). Do not pull back on the laryngoscope; this uses the teeth as a fulcrum and may damage the teeth.
6. Visualize the vocal cords (Figure 12-15).
7. From the right side of the mouth, insert the endotracheal tube until the cuff passes completely through the vocal cords (Figure 12-16). If you are intubating a child, the tube will not have a cuff. Instead, look for the black ring marker at the distal end and insert the tube so that this point just passes the cords.
8. Remove the laryngoscope and stylet. Note the number marking on the tube at the level of the lips. The tube should be kept at this level.
9. If the endotracheal tube has a cuff, inflate it with 8 to 10 ml of air to maintain a good seal. Also check firmness of the pilot balloon to confirm that the cuff is inflated and holding air.
10. While holding the tube firmly in place, attach a bag-valve device and ventilate. Look for a symmetrical rise and fall of the chest. Auscultate for the presence of breath sounds on both sides of the chest, both ante-

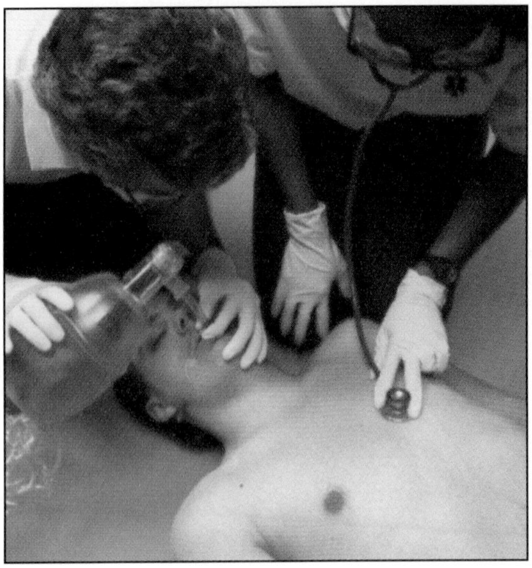

Figure 12-17

While ventilating, auscultate for breath sounds on both sides of the chest, using both anterior and posterior auscultation sites and over the epigastrium.

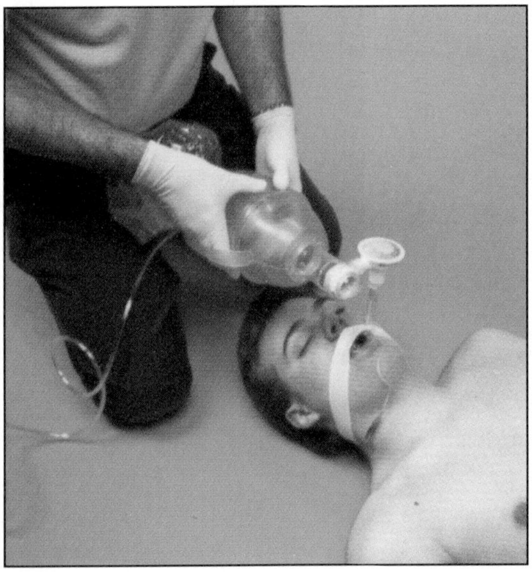

Figure 12-18

Once the placement has been confirmed, secure the tube and continue ventilations.

riorly and laterally (Figure 12-17); listen to confirm the absence of air sounds over the **epigastrium.** If your protocols allow, attach an end-tidal carbon dioxide detector (see p. 283) to verify and monitor placement of the tube (Figure 12-18).

11. Once you confirm tube placement, secure the tube and continue to ventilate. Reconfirm proper chest rise, presence of bilateral lung sounds, and absence of air sounds at the epigastrium.

Note that steps 4 through 9 should not take more than 15 to 30 seconds to complete. If you have difficulty locating landmarks and correctly placing the tube, withdraw the tube and laryngoscope and hyperventilate the patient with a BVM before the next attempt at placement. Some EMTs find it useful to hold their own breath while placing a tube. One's own air hunger is a good reminder to stop and ventilate before the patient becomes hypoxic.

Carbon Dioxide Detection. Carbon dioxide detection equipment can help you monitor tube placement (technically this is called *end-tidal carbon dioxide detection*). When ventilation is adequate and the patient has adequate cardiac output, each exhalation will expel carbon dioxide. This will be detected by the device and will confirm presence of the endotracheal tube in the lungs. A cardiac arrest patient will not produce carbon dioxide without CPR. Even with CPR, there may not be enough of the gas exhaled to make a carbon dioxide detector work correctly. Using carbon dioxide detection in cardiac arrest patients is therefore controversial.

The colorimetric type of carbon dioxide detector, which is most often used in prehospital care, is attached at the end of the endotracheal tube between the tube and the bag-valve device. (Electronic carbon dioxide detectors are more commonly seen in hospitals.) The color of the detector should change with elevated carbon dioxide levels when the tube is in the trachea. There is no color change when the tube is in the esophagus because there is no significant carbon dioxide expelled. An appropriate color change indicates that the tube is in the trachea.

Colorimetric carbon dioxide detectors will not work properly when wet. Also, low-perfusion states make them unreliable. A patient in shock or cardiac arrest may not produce any color change, even when the tube is in the proper position. Do not assume that shock or cardiac arrest is the problem. Use the laryngoscope and direct visualization of the vocal cords to reconfirm tube placement if there is no color change. The following is a memory aid to help with the colors and their meanings:

- *Y*ellow = *Y*es (Tube is in place.)
- *T*an = *T*hink about it (Tube may not be properly placed.)
- *P*urple = *P*roblem (Tube is not in the trachea.)

Esophageal Detection Device. Another method of confirming endotracheal placement of the tube is with an esophageal detection device. This device has an endotracheal tube adapter attached to a large syringe. Once the endotracheal tube has been placed, the syringe is attached to the tube and aspiration is performed. If the tube is in the trachea, air will be freely aspirated by the syringe; if the tube is in the esophagus, when aspiration is attempted, the esophagus will collapse around the end of the endotracheal tube and the syringe will not be able to aspirate air. Although these devices seem fairly reliable, there is some controversy about their effectiveness.

Both the end-tidal carbon dioxide detector and the esophageal detection device should be viewed as an adjunct to help confirm endotracheal tube placement. If there is any question, visualize the vocal cords to confirm the tube's position.

Endotracheal Suctioning. You may sometimes hear gurgling sounds and feel resistance as you ventilate a patient. First, check tube placement; these signs could indicate a tube in the esophagus. Then consider the possibility that fluid in the trachea or bronchi is obstructing the exchange of air through the endotracheal tube. Some EMS systems will allow EMT-Basics to directly suction the trachea through the endotracheal tube.

In this situation, you should hyperventilate the patient and select a flexible, French catheter for suctioning through the endotracheal tube. Using sterile gloves, insert the catheter into the tube and advance it 25 cm, which should be approximately at the level of the carina. Cover the hole in the catheter with your thumb or finger to begin suctioning. Withdraw the catheter, using a twisting motion to ensure that the tip does not stick to an airway wall. Use sterile technique to keep the suction catheter sterile during this process. Because suctioning pulls oxygen out of the airways and lungs, it should be limited to 10 seconds.

IT'S YOUR CALL
CONCLUSION

After your intubation attempt, the patient only had lung sounds on the right side; and gurgling was heard during ventilation. It is possible that you passed the endotracheal tube too deeply, intubating the right mainstem bronchus. By deflating the cuff and withdrawing the tube slightly, you are likely to position it better and achieve bilateral breath sounds. If you hear no sounds when auscultating directly over the stomach, the gurgling sounds you hear when ventilating could mean that the patient has aspirated foreign matter, such as vomitus. By advancing a soft suction catheter through the endotracheal tube, you can apply suction and try to clear the tube.

Alternative Advanced Devices for Airway Management

Endotracheal intubation is considered the most effective form of airway management. However, the technique is a demanding one. The time and practice needed to learn and maintain the skill make it impractical for some EMS services.

For years, EMS researchers have sought a device for airway management that would approach the effectiveness of the endotracheal tube but would be simpler to learn and use. The first generation of devices included the esophageal obturator airway (EOA) and the esophageal gastric tube airway (EGTA). Both featured a long tube designed for easy insertion into the esophagus, with a large inflation cuff at the distal end to block regurgitation of stomach contents and prevent air from entering the stomach.

Unfortunately, this first wave of esophageal tubes depended on a good seal with a face mask for effective ventilation. They offered improved protection against aspira-

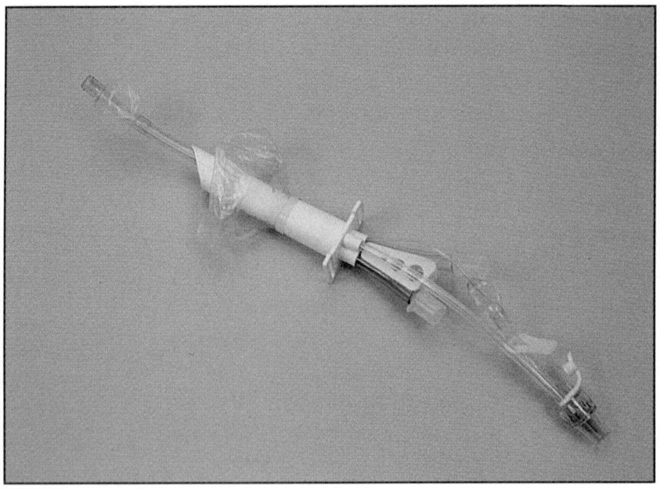

Figure 12-19
A pharyngeotracheal lumen airway.

tion of vomitus, but not against blood in the airway; and all too often their use was associated with inadequate oxygenation and ventilation. There also were periodic instances in which the tube came to rest in the trachea, completely preventing ventilation until it was removed.

Further development led to a second generation of easier-to-use tubes. Both of the examples discussed below solve the mask-seal problem with the addition of a pharyngeal balloon that prevents air from escaping through the mouth and nose during inhalation with a bag-valve device. Because the tube is placed blindly, both are also designed to work effectively, whether the tube enters the esophagus or the trachea. These devices are referred to as esophageal-tracheal double-lumen airway (ETDLA) devices.

Pharyngeotracheal Lumen Airway

The Pharyngeotracheal Lumen Airway, commonly called the *PtL airway,* is a double-lumen tube with two cuffs (Figure 12-19). Because it does not require visualization of the vocal cords or additional equipment such as a laryngoscope, it is easier to use than the endotracheal tube.

The device is blindly placed; you do not need to see the vocal cords for placement. The shorter tube of the PtL rests in the oropharynx, and the longer tube passes into either the esophagus or the trachea. Because it is a blind insertion, you will initially be uncertain about where the tube is positioned. A large balloon at the end of the short tube seals the oropharynx when inflated, eliminating the need for a face mask. A cuff at the end of the longer tube secures it in place and prevents any leak, regardless of whether the tube has entered the trachea or the esophagus.

A stylet inside the tube aids insertion of the tube. The tube is designed either to block or allow airflow, depending on its location. If the tube is placed in the esophagus, which occurs most frequently, the cuff at the end blocks the esophagus. Air is delivered through the short tube into the pharynx. Because the esophagus and the oropharynx are both blocked, air can only go into the trachea. If the tube is in the trachea and you ventilate through the short tube, the lungs will not rise and no lung sounds will be present. Remove the stylet and attach the bag-valve device to the other lumen and air will go directly into the trachea. In this case, the distal cuff secures the tube in the trachea.

Esophageal Tracheal Combitube

The Esophageal Tracheal Combitube (ETC) is also a double-lumen tube with two inflatable cuffs. It is similar to the PtL, but its structure is simpler and it offers some possible advantages. The pharyngeal balloon is designed to position and adjust itself, and the lack of a stylet simplifies the process (Figure 12-20). The ETC has also shown very good oxygen-administration capability. As with the PtL, it is blindly placed and the tubes are ventilated to determine the location of the distal end of the device.

There are many similarities in the use of the PtL and ETC airways, including the need to hyperventilate the patient in advance, check the cuffs, lubricate the distal end of the device, place the patient's head in a neutral position, inflate two different cuffs after insertion, check breath sounds to determine whether the long tube has entered the trachea or the esophagus, and ventilate through the appropriate port depending on the location of the tube. As with the endotracheal tube, these airways are for use in unresponsive patients with no gag reflex. They may be especially useful when you cannot see the vocal cords or when patient position or possible neck injury makes endotracheal intubation impractical.

Once placed, all advanced airway devices should be left in place if possible. If the patient regains consciousness and the airway must be removed, follow these steps:

1. Have suction ready. The patient is likely to vomit after removal of the airway.
2. Turn the patient to the side.

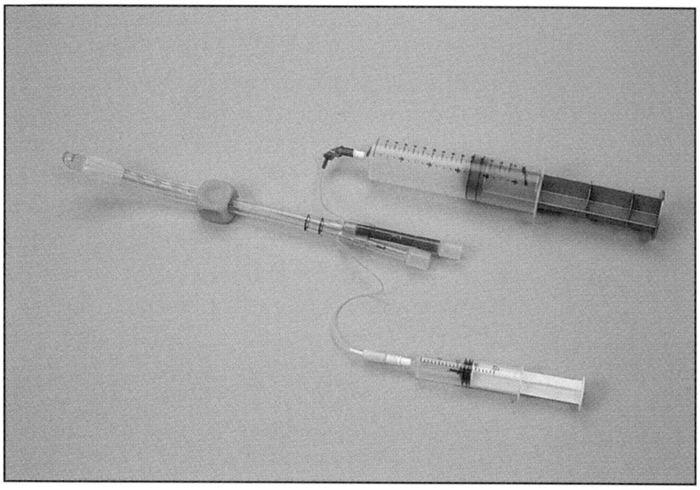

Figure 12-20

An esophageal tracheal Combitube.

AUTOMATIC VENTILATION

Using a BVM to manually ventilate a patient has drawbacks. One is that, as you tire, the ventilation rate and tidal volume can become inconsistent. Another is the difficulty in providing adequate ventilation while the patient is being moved. To overcome these problems, some EMS systems are using devices known as automatic transport ventilators (ATVs) (Figure 12-21). Although they have been in use in Europe for many years, they have just begun to gain popularity in the United States.

ATVs are compact devices with adjustable settings for the ventilation rate and tidal volume. They connect to an oxygen cylinder and are capable of delivering 100% oxygen at rates and tidal volumes appropriate for the full range of patients over 5 years of age. They can be used either through an endotracheal tube or a ventilation mask and have built-in alarms to alert you in the event of ventilation problems.

It is important to monitor the patient and the device as it functions. Using it with a ventilation mask requires constant attention to mask seal. It can also cause gastric distention, which creates resistance to effective ventilation and may lead to vomiting. To prevent distention, keep the ventilator adjusted to the lowest volume that will produce good chest rise.

Despite the possible drawbacks, an ATV can provide a measure of freedom to concentrate on patient movement and other aspects of care. It can effectively ventilate the patient during movement up or down stairs, over rough terrain, or for prolonged periods of time.

Follow local medical direction protocols for the use of ATVs if they are available.

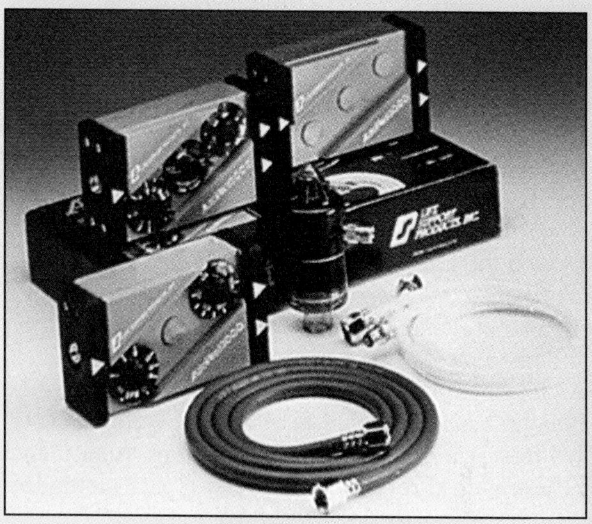

Figure 12-21

Automatic transport ventilators.

3. Deflate the cuff.
4. Remove the airway.
5. Suction the airway if necessary.
6. Ensure that the patient remains well ventilated and oxygenated after the tube is removed.

Special Considerations

When you perform advanced airway skills, there will be instances that require modification of the standard techniques. This is especially true when dealing with pediatric patients and patients with special conditions, such as laryngectomies.

Pediatrics

Pediatric emergencies tend to cause extra anxiety in EMS personnel. When managing the airway of an infant or child, remember that they are not just small adults. Their bodies are anatomically and physiologically different and need to be treated differently.

Anatomic and Physiologic Differences

The head of a child is proportionally larger than an adult's, and the tongue is proportionally larger and more anterior than an adult's tongue. A child's epiglottis is also larger and more anterior and superior and extends farther into the pharynx.

A child's larynx is located more anterior and superior than an adults, at the level of cervical vertebrae 3 to 4. This makes it difficult to create a clear visual plane from the mouth through the pharynx to the glottis for orotracheal intubation in children. The higher position of the larynx also increases the temptation to hyperextend the neck to improve the view of the cords. However, hyperextension may kink and close off the trachea. A child's epiglottic folds, which are larger and more elastic than an adult's, also may interfere with visualization of the vocal cords.[1] For these reasons, the best way to manage a child's airway is in a neutral sniffing position. Because the smaller and more delicate tissue in a child's airway can be more easily damaged than an adult's, intubation requires a gentle approach and should be performed by the most experienced rescuer present (Figure 12-22).

A child's trachea is more flexible than an adult's and may collapse easily. Its diameter is only a fraction of that of an adult trachea. For this reason, endotracheal tubes for children younger than 8 do not have cuffs. The cricoid ring, which is the narrowest part of the airway in this age group, will help provide a seal around the tube; however, this is not likely to be as effective as an inflated cuff. Intubated children are at greater risk of aspiration than intubated adults. Also, more care is required to ensure that the tube is not dislodged. If applying cricoid pressure during intubation, remember that the cricoid cartilage is not as strong as an adult's; it can be obstructed or damaged if too much force is applied.

Because a child's airway changes significantly between birth and adolescence, the equipment used for advanced airway management must also be different. This is most noticeable in the sizes and types of endotracheal tubes, laryngoscope blades, and suction catheters (Table 12-1). Because it is not always possible to know a child's age or weight, a measuring tape has been devised that estimates weight based on a length (height) measurement and suggests equipment sizes accordingly. Known as the *Broselow tape,* this device is used in many EMS systems

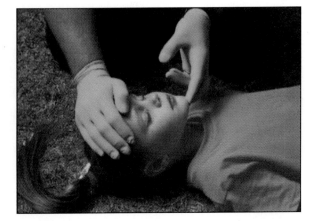

Figure 12-22

The neutral sniffing position should be used for managing a child's airway.

TABLE 12-1 Equipment Used for Pediatric Orotracheal Intubation

Age	Endotracheal tube size (mm)	Laryngoscope blade size	Suction catheter size
Newborn	2.5-3.0	#0-#1 straight	6 French
6 months	3.5	#1 straight	8 French
18 months	4.0	#1 straight	8 French
3 years	4.5	#2 straight	8 French
5 years	5.0	#2 straight	10 French
6 years	5.5	#2 straight	10 French
8 years	6.0	#2 straight or curved	10 French
12 years	6.5	#3 straight or curved	10 French

Modified from EMT-*Paramedic National Standard Curriculum:* Washington, DC, 1985, U.S. Department of Transportation, U.S. Government Printing Office.

for quick selection of the proper equipment for pediatric intubation and for dosages in medication administration (Figure 12-23). If you do not have a chart or tape to guide you in choosing endotracheal tube size, select a tube that is approximately the diameter of the child's little finger or nostril.

Nasogastric Tubes

Gastric distention is a common problem among children. It can be relieved by inserting a **nasogastric tube,** a procedure available to EMT-Basics in some systems. The procedure involves inserting a tube through the nose and pharynx into the stomach (Figure 12-24). The most common use of the nasogastric tube relative to airway management is to remove air from the stomach. This improves ventilation because a distended stomach obstructs normal movement of the diaphragm during inspiration. Relieving gastric distention also reduces the risk of vomiting and aspiration.

A nasogastric tube should not be used when there is major facial, head, or spinal trauma. In these situations, orogastric techniques are used. When inserting a nasogastric tube, be aware of the possible complications, including vomiting and inadvertent tracheal intubation.

To insert a nasogastric tube you will need the following equipment:

- Appropriate-size nasogastric tube:

Newborn/infant	8 French
Toddler/preschool	10 French
School-age	12 French
Adolescent	14-16 French

- 20-ml syringe
- Water-soluble lubricant
- Emesis basin
- Tape
- Stethoscope
- Suction unit and catheters

Follow these steps when inserting a nasogastric tube:

1. Assemble and check the equipment.
2. Measure for proper tube size. Measure the tube from the tip of the patient's nose, around the ear, and to a point 1 or 2 inches below the xiphoid process (Figure 12-25).
3. Lubricate the distal end of the tube with a water-soluble lubricant.
4. Place the patient in a supine position.

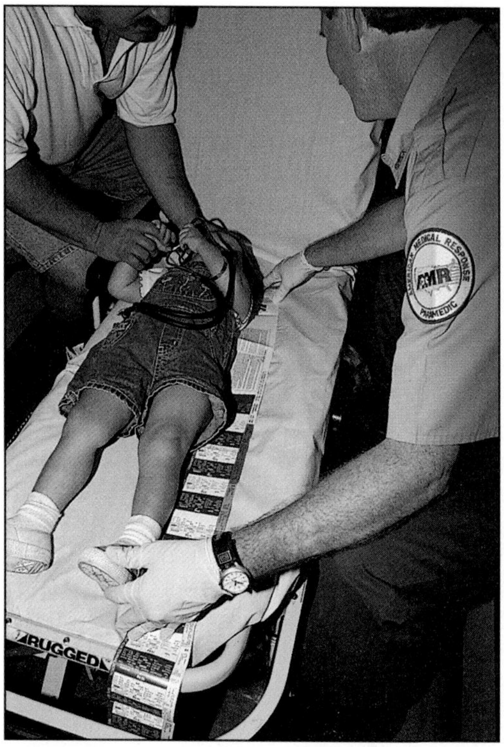

Figure 12-23

Measuring a pediatric patient against a Broselow tape can provide some important information about the sizes and types of equipment that are appropriate.

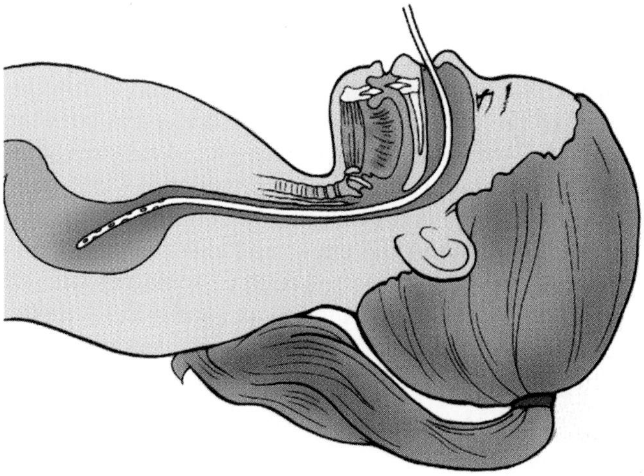

Figure 12-24

Proper placement of the nasogastric tube in a pediatric patient's stomach.

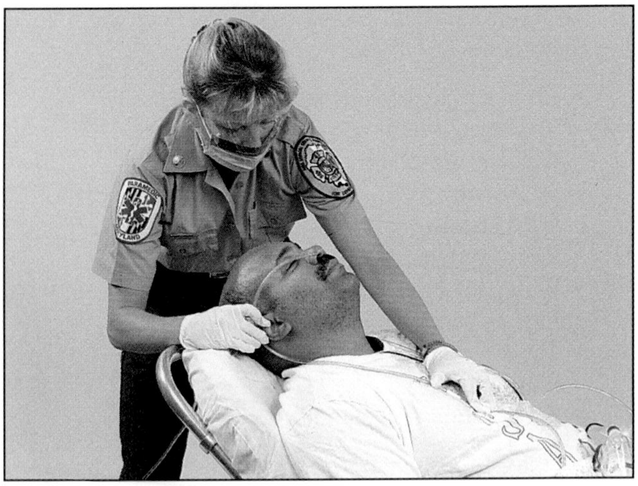

Figure 12-25

Physical landmarks to measure nasogastric tube length.

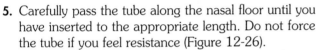

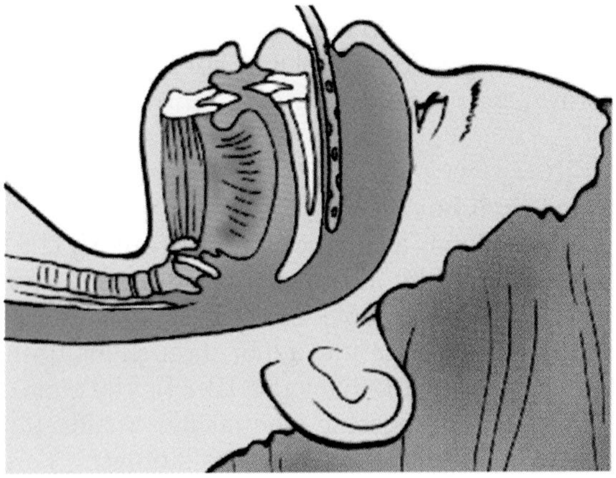

Figure 12-26

Pass the tube along the nasal floor.

5. Carefully pass the tube along the nasal floor until you have inserted to the appropriate length. Do not force the tube if you feel resistance (Figure 12-26).
6. Check placement of the tube either by using the syringe to withdraw stomach contents, or by listening for gurgling sounds over the stomach while injecting 10 to 20 ml of air into the tube.
7. Attach the tube to a suction device to reduce stomach distention (Figure 12-27). Irrigate the tube with saline or sterile water if it becomes clogged.
8. Tape the tube in place.

Laryngectomees

You may treat a patient, called a **laryngectomee,** whose larynx has been removed surgically. Laryngectomees are also referred to as *neck breathers* because they breathe through an opening in the front of the neck known as a **stoma.** A complete neck breather has had a total removal of the voice box; there is no connection between the upper and lower airways. This person only breathes through a stoma. A partial neck breather may still have part of the voice box in place and continues to have a connection between the upper and lower airways. This person primarily breathes through a stoma but will still have slight air exchange at the mouth and nose. A metal, plastic, or silicone tracheostomy tube is usually in place in the stoma.

When performing an initial assessment, it is important to check for a stoma. If one is present, you will need to adapt the way you manage the airway. Check for breathing by feeling for air exchange at the stoma. If the patient is not breathing, deliver oxygen and ventilations through the stoma. The head can be kept in a neutral position because the tongue will not cause an obstruction.

To ventilate a patient who does not have a tube in the stoma, use a bag-valve device with an infant-size mask to make a tight seal around the stoma. If the patient has a tracheal tube in place, the bag-valve device will attach directly to the tube. When ventilating, check for chest rise. If there is none, feel for air coming out of the mouth and nose. If you feel air escaping, you will need to seal the mouth and nose to ventilate effectively. If there is difficulty with a tracheal tube already in place, suction is usually all that is needed. If suction does not clear the stoma tube, deflate its cuff, remove it, and replace it with an endotracheal tube.

To deliver oxygen to a laryngectomee who is breathing spontaneously, place an oxygen mask over the stoma. A pediatric nonrebreather mask works well for administering high oxygen concentrations. There are oxygen masks specifically made for neck breathers, but they are not commonly carried on ambulances.

Intubating a laryngectomee requires several adjustments to the standard technique. First, you will probably not need the laryngoscope because you will usually not be entering the mouth and visualizing the vocal cords. (Some

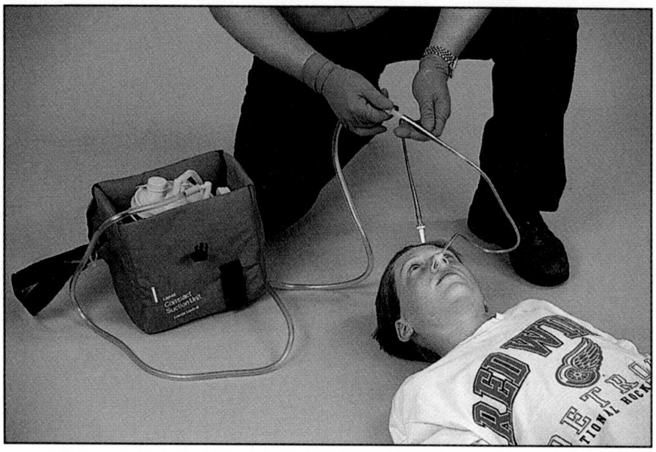

Figure 12-27
Attach the tube to a suction device.

laryngectomees can be intubated orally, but this is not the first technique to try.) Second, you must consider the size of the stoma—which varies from patient to patient—and choose a tube that will fit through that opening. Extend the patient's head and insert the endotracheal tube directly through the stoma until the cuff has disappeared about 2 cm into the neck. Inflate the cuff, check breath sounds, and secure the tube to the patient's neck.

SUMMARY

Several advanced techniques are available to help the EMT-Basic manage airways. Endotracheal intubation is the most effective method. Orotracheal intubation allows direct access to the patient's lower airway without the danger of tongue obstruction and greatly reduces the risk of aspirating foreign matter. Other devices are also available to help secure an airway. The PtL and ETC allow for either esophageal or tracheal intubation without direct visualization of the vocal cords and can provide good ventilation either way. Though these devices have shown their effectiveness in airway maintenance, some controversy still exists about their use. Local protocols are the final word.

Anatomic and physiologic differences in the airways of infants and children mean that their airways require somewhat different management. Structures that are proportionally larger and are located more superior than in adults create special challenges. Nasogastric tube placement can be helpful in dealing with specific situations common to pediatric patients, such as gastric distention.

Laryngectomees are another special population. Neck-breathing patients require a number of adaptations in ventilating, intubating, and administering oxygen through a stoma.

Though you have learned several advanced airway-management techniques, it is important to remember the basic airway-management skills that you already know (see Chapter 11). Advanced techniques will not be successful unless preceded and supported by good basic skills.

REFERENCES

1. **Eichelberger M et al:** *Pediatric emergencies,* Englewood Cliffs, NJ, 1992, Brady.

SUGGESTED READINGS

1. **International Association of Laryngectomies:** *Rescue breathing of laryngectomees and other neck breathers,* Atlanta, 1995, American Cancer Society.

Section 6
Medical Emergencies

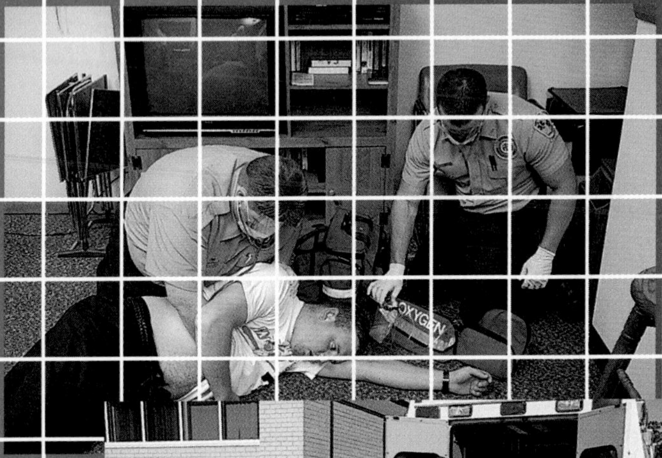

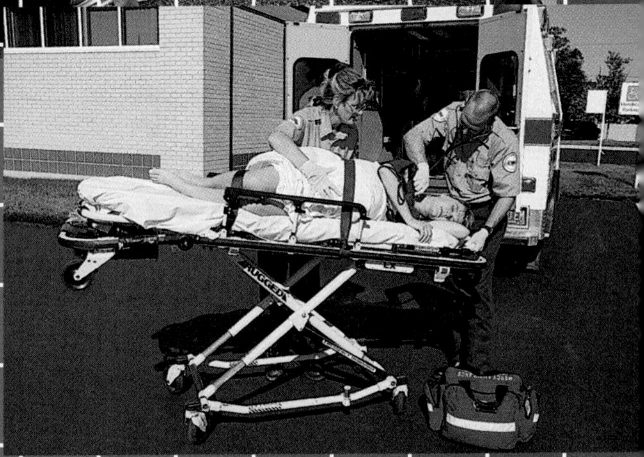

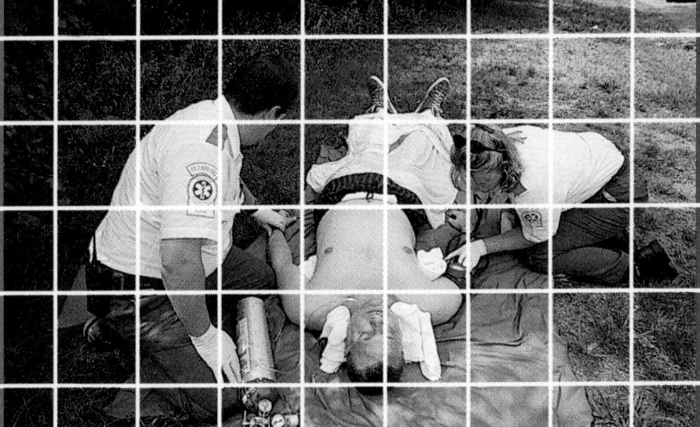

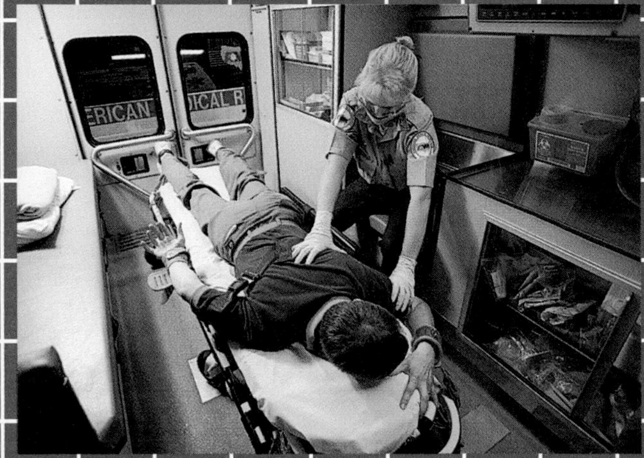

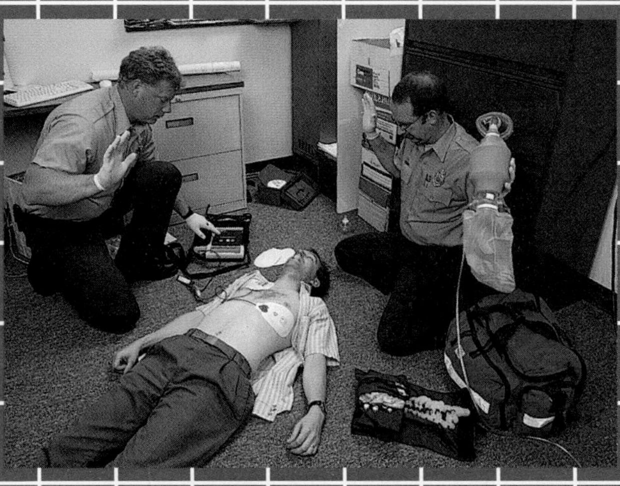

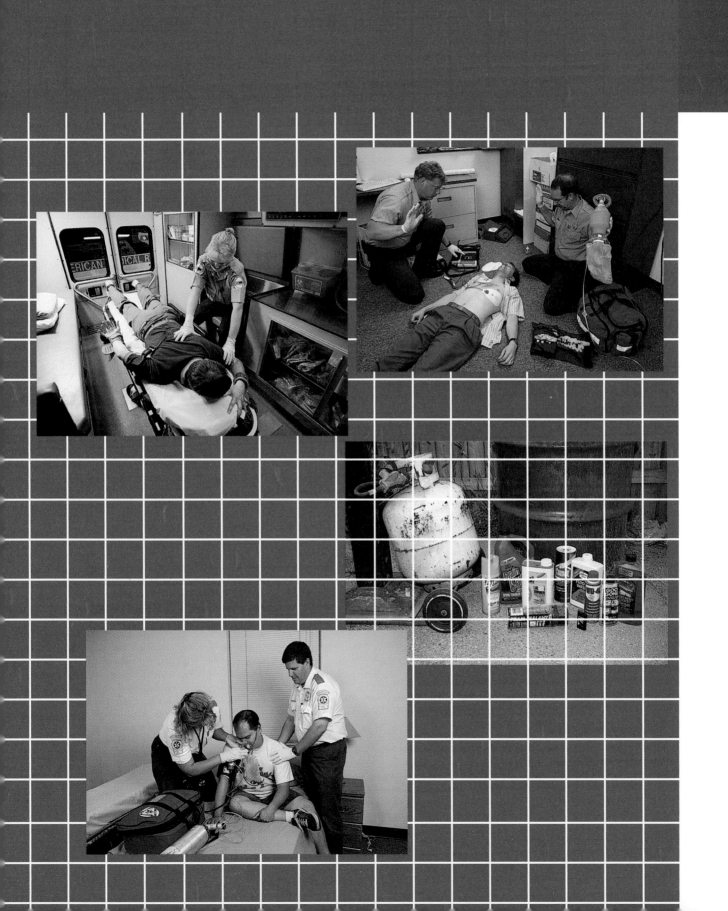
WD-40

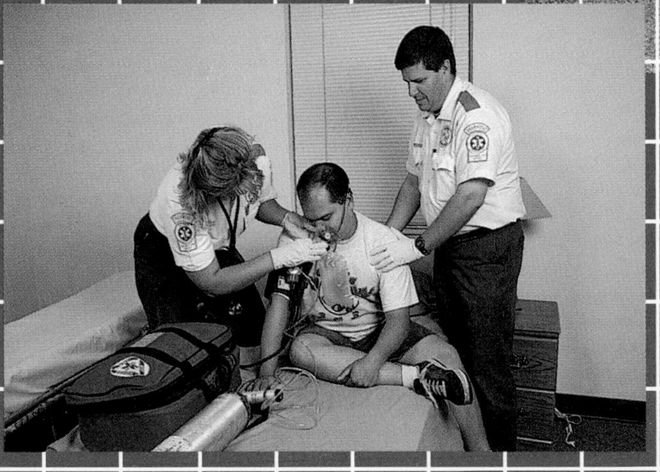

Chapter

Understanding Medications

13

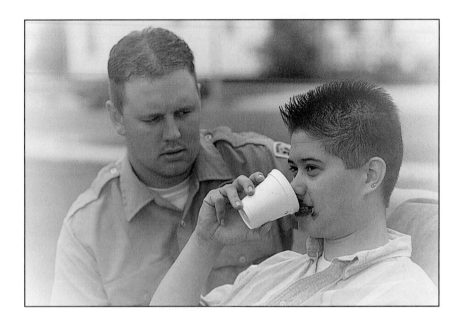

Knowledge Objectives

As an EMT-Basic, you should be able to:

OBJECTIVES

1. Differentiate between the generic and trade names of the medications that you are qualified to administer.
2. Describe the physical forms in which medications are available.
3. Differentiate between a medication's actions and its side effects.
4. Describe the routes of medication administration that you will commonly use and their potential advantages.
5. Discuss items that you need to document after the administration of a medication.
6. Identify the medications commonly carried on a basic life support (BLS) ambulance.
7. Identify the prescribed medications that you may assist patients in self-administering.
8. Describe the medical conditions under which you may administer the following medications:
   - Activated charcoal
   - Oral glucose
   - Oxygen
   - Bronchodilator inhalers
   - Nitroglycerin
   - Epinephrine

OBJECTIVES

Skill Objectives

As an EMT-Basic, you should be able to:

1. **Demonstrate how to assist a patient with self-administration of the following prescribed medications:**
   - **Bronchodilator inhalers**
   - **Nitroglycerin**
   - **Epinephrine auto-injector**
2. **Demonstrate how to administer the following medications:**
   - **Oxygen**
   - **Activated charcoal**
   - **Oral glucose**
   - **Bronchodilator inhalers**
   - **Nitroglycerin**
   - **Epinephrine auto-injector**
3. **Read the labels and inspect the following medications to determine the forms in which they are supplied, their expiration dates, and the appropriate routes for their administration:**
   - **Oral glucose**
   - **Activated charcoal**
   - **Bronchodilator inhalers**
   - **Nitroglycerin**
   - **Epinephrine auto-injector**

Attitude Objective

As an EMT-Basic, you should be able to:

1. **Discuss your personal feelings, attitudes, and beliefs about administering medications.**

KEY TERMS

1. **Activated Charcoal:** A medication that is taken orally for the management of certain ingested poisonous substances; charcoal adsorbs (sticks to) the substance and prevents its absorption by the digestive system.
2. **Bronchodilator Inhalers:** A group of medications for the treatment of certain respiratory emergencies; administered through inhalation; called *bronchodilators* because they dilate bronchial passages.
3. **Contraindication:** Situation in which a medication should not be used because it may harm the patient.
4. **Dose:** The correct amount of medication to administer.
5. **Drug:** A chemical substance that alters the body's function when introduced into the body.
6. **Epinephrine:** A medication commonly used to relieve the signs and symptoms of a severe allergic reaction; constricts blood vessels, dilates bronchial passages, and helps block histamine response.
7. **Generic Name:** A medication's noncommercial name; often an abbreviated version of the chemical name (see also: *trade name*).
8. **Indication:** A situation in which a specific medication should be given because of its potential ability to improve a condition; the condition for which a drug is prescribed.
9. **Medication:** A drug used in patient care to treat or prevent a specific disease or condition.
10. **Mechanism of Action:** The manner in which a medication works in the body; also simply called its *action*.
11. **Nitroglycerin:** A medication taken sublingually to reduce chest pain of cardiac origin.
12. **Oral Glucose:** An oral sugar medication administered for the treatment of altered consciousness that may result from low blood sugar during a diabetic emergency.
13. **Route:** The way in which a medication enters the body; oral, sublingual, intramuscular, and inhalation are examples.
14. **Side Effect:** Any action other than the desired action that a medication causes.
15. **Sublingual:** Administered under the tongue.
16. **Trade Name:** The commercial brand name under which a manufacturer of a medication markets the product (see also: *generic name*).

IT'S YOUR CALL

Your crew has been reviewing new protocols for administering medications to patients when you are dispatched to an unconscious person. Because your agency does not have an advanced life-support (ALS) provider available today, one has been dispatched from a neighboring county to assist with the call. However, it will likely be 15 minutes before this provider can reach the patient.

When you arrive at the scene, you find a woman in her mid-50s seated on a sofa and attended by a family member. An initial assessment reveals that she is conscious but disoriented. Her pulse and breathing are rapid, and her skin is cool and moist. Family tells you that she has not suffered any trauma. After performing a focused history and physical examination, you determine that the patient's chief complaints are a headache and dizziness. The patient states that her headache has been present for several hours, and her pain is about a 4 on a scale of 1 to 10. The SAMPLE (see Chapter 10) questions reveal that the patient has a history of diabetes for which she is taking insulin. You learn that the patient has been taking her insulin appropriately but has had the flu for the last 24 hours and has not been eating or drinking properly.

In addition to standard BLS skills, what can you do for this patient? Is there any medication that could help her? If so, how would it work, how much should you administer, how would you administer it, and are there any precautions you should follow?

You will frequently encounter patients who are taking prescribed medications, as well as those who have failed to take their medications properly. There are a variety of reasons why patients do not use a medication as prescribed. They may be hesitant to take it because they are uncertain about exactly how to administer it or even whether they should administer it. Some patients will not take their medication simply because they do not want to or do not realize its importance. Possibly, a patient may just be too weak to self-administer medication without help; these patients can benefit from your assistance in administering their prescribed medications. In some cases, you may have medications in your ambulance that a patient needs but does not have.

This chapter provides the basic information about medications that you will be qualified to administer. To administer medications properly, you must follow guidelines established for their safe use. These guidelines include an understanding of the following:

- How a medication works
- The conditions under which a medication should and should not be administered (indications and contraindications, respectively)
- The common side effects of a particular medication
- How much of a particular medication to administer
- How to administer the medication
- The local medical direction protocols for the administration of the medication

Understanding Medications

Pharmacology is the study of drugs and how they affect the body. **Drugs** are chemical substances that alter the body's function in some way when introduced into the body. **Medications** are specific drugs that are used in patient care to treat or prevent a specific disease or condition. Although the terms *drug* and *medication* are sometimes used interchangeably, your patients may think of a drug as an illegal or abused substance. The term *medication* will be used in this chapter to refer to substances that you can administer to a patient.

Sources of Medications

Medications are derived from five sources: plants, animals and humans, minerals, microorganisms, and man-made or synthetic materials (chemical substances produced in a laboratory). A well-known pain medication, morphine, is derived from opium, which comes from a plant. Codeine is another pain medicine that is a synthetic derivative of morphine. Medications such as insulin and epinephrine were originally extracted from animal organs, but recent genetic engineering has enabled pharmaceutical companies to develop synthetic versions of these medications. Iron is derived from a mineral source. The most well-known antibiotic, penicillin, is produced from a microorganism. A commonly used sedative, Valium, is an example of a synthetic medication. The majority of emergency medications are produced synthetically.

Medication Names

Medications can be identified by three different names:

- Chemical name: This name represents the exact chemical structure of a medication.
- Generic name: A **generic name** is a medication's most frequently used name, often a shortened version

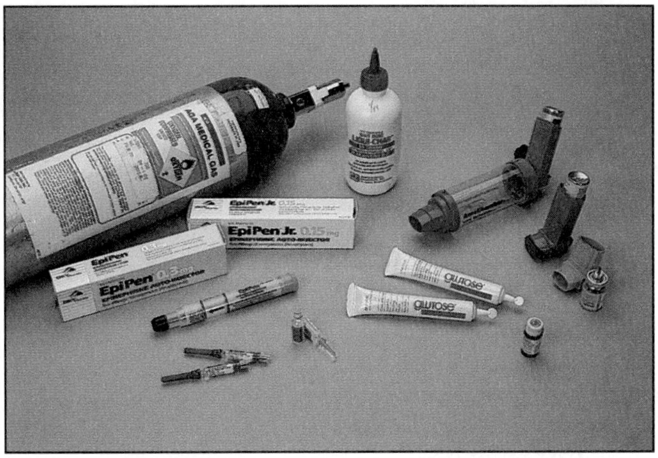

Figure 13-1

Various medications an EMT-Basic can administer.

of the chemical name. It is also the name listed in the *United States Pharmacopeia* (USP), a document that defines the quality standards of medications in use in the United States. Generic names are not capitalized.
- Trade (brand) name: A **trade name** is the name given to a medication by the company manufacturing it. This name is protected by trademark laws and is always capitalized.

Generic and trade names are those that you will most frequently encounter when administering medications, reading labels on a patient's prescribed medications, or asking a patient about current medications being used. Because more than one company may produce a medication, it can have several trade names but only one generic name. For example, consider albuterol, a common respiratory medication used to dilate the bronchial tubes:

- Chemical name: alpha1[(tert-butyl-amino)methyl]-4-hydroxy-m-xylene-alpha-alpha'-diol
- Generic name: albuterol
- Trade names: Proventil, by the Schering Corporation; Ventolin, by Allen and Hanburys

Medication Forms

Medications come in a variety of forms. The three most common forms are solids, liquids, and gases (Figure 13-1). Solid medications are most often administered orally. These include capsules, tablets, and fine powders that are diluted for ingestion. They also include gel-type medications, such as **oral glucose.**

Common liquid medications include:

- Syrups: Medications suspended in water and sugar, like most cough preparations.
- Elixirs: Medications containing alcohol, often with flavoring added, such as Nyquil.
- Suspensions: Medications in which fine powders are distributed throughout a liquid. Suspensions tend to separate after sitting for a short time and need to be shaken before administration. Examples of suspensions include activated charcoal and the antibiotic amoxicillin.
- Solutions: Medications dissolved in a solvent, such as water. This type of liquid medication is used for injection, inhalation, and oral ingestion and is the most common type of liquid medication used in prehospital settings.
- Pastes or gels: Medications supplied in tubes for oral administration, such as oral glucose, or in the form of skin patches. The latter type includes nitroglycerin patches, which may have to be removed from the chest before applying defibrillator patches. It is difficult to classify pastes or gels as either solids or liquids because they are partially both.

The most common medication administered in gas form is oxygen.

How Medications Work

It is helpful to understand how medications work in general, as well as the specific actions of the medications you can administer. This is important because medications affect the body in different ways, both positive and negative. How a medication works on the body is called its **mechanism of action.** Every medication has a specific mechanism of action. What a medication does in the body is referred to as its *effect.* Some medications also have undesired **side effects.** For example, the effect of **activated charcoal** is a reduction in the level of a poison that can be absorbed by the digestive system. Its mechanism is to adsorb the poison to itself. Nausea is a possible side effect of activated charcoal.

Actions (Primary Effects)

When a medication is administered, it works on certain areas of the body, such as blood vessels, lung tissue, muscles, or the nervous system. Medications are absorbed into the bloodstream after being administered. For example, **epinephrine** is injected into the thigh muscle and absorbed into the blood vessels in the muscle. Medication can also be absorbed through tissues in the mouth (**nitroglycerin,** oral glucose) or lungs **(bronchodilator inhalers).** Most tablets are absorbed into the bloodstream from the digestive tract.

Some of the medications you will administer stimulate internal functions, while others depress them. The particular actions of the medications that EMTs can administer are discussed later in this chapter.

Side Effects

As previously mentioned, most medications do have some undesirable side effects. A side effect is any action that a medication causes other than the desired action. For example, nitroglycerin is used to relieve chest discomfort that may be associated with a heart problem. However, it can cause a headache and reduce blood pressure. Some medications can cause nausea and vomiting. Even oxygen has side effects, such as drying out mucous membranes and causing headache or nose bleed. You should know the likely side effects of the medications you administer and explain them to your patients.

Administering Medications

An understanding of medications includes the various ways in which they can be administered, the situations in which they should and should not be given, and the proper doses to be administered.

Routes

Medications can be administered by several **routes;** some get the medication into the bloodstream faster than others. A medication that is inhaled into the lungs starts to work faster than one that is ingested and has to be absorbed through the digestive tract. Oral medications are usually the slowest to be absorbed and take effect. Medications administered intravenously (IV) cause their effect most rapidly. Some medications are administered under the skin (subcutaneously); there is fairly rapid absorption by this route, but not as fast as IV administration. Some medications are absorbed topically through the skin, such as creams and ointments, but this generally results in comparatively slow absorption into the bloodstream. Finally, medication can be administered rectally as either a liquid or suppository. This route has a slightly faster onset than the oral route. While ALS providers can potentially administer some medications via all these routes, you will be limited to administering medications through only four routes: oral, **sublingual** (under the tongue), inhalation, and intramuscular injection. Table 13-1 provides an overview of these routes.

Inhalation requires the patient to inhale medication into the lungs. It is among the fastest of the four routes of medication administration that EMTs can use because there are a lot of blood vessels (capillaries) in the lungs to

COMMON MEDICATIONS

Did you ever wonder how many different prescribed medications there are in the United States or how these medications are recognized? What about the most commonly prescribed medications? The USP is a nongovernmental agency that works in conjunction with the Food and Drug Administration (FDA), a governmental agency, to list medications that have met the FDA's quality standards. The USP provides information on approximately 4000 medications.

Some of the more commonly prescribed groups of medications in the United States are listed below:

- Antibiotics: Medications used to fight infection
- Anticonvulsants: Medications used to treat seizure disorders
- Antidysrhythmics: Medications used for heart conditions
- Antihypertensives: Medications used to control high blood pressure
- Antiinflammatories: Medications used to reduce swelling and inflammation
- Antipyretics: Medications used to treat fever
- Analgesics: Medications used to relieve pain
- Bronchodilators: Medications used to relax the bronchial passages
- Hypoglycemics: Medications used to promote the normal use of sugar in body tissues

Some medications have more than one action. Aspirin, for instance, has analgesic, antiinflammatory, and antipyretic actions.

Because it is not possible to memorize all of the medications that you will encounter in the field, it is a good idea to invest in a simple reference guide. These pocket guides provide information on several hundred of the most frequently used medications.

absorb the medication. The onset of action is normally less than 3 minutes. Inhaled medications are fine mists found in bronchodilator inhalers and in gases, such as oxygen (Figure 13-2).

Sublingual administration involves placing medication under the patient's tongue. If the medication is in tablet form, it will dissolve and be absorbed by the capillaries under the tongue. If a spray is used sublingually, absorption is slightly faster because the medication is already dissolved. Medications administered sublingually work rapidly, often within 3 minutes. Nitroglycerin is the medication that EMTs can administer sublingually (Figure 13-3).

The intramuscular route involves injecting liquid medication into a large muscle where it is absorbed by the capillaries in the muscle. This route is slower than the two routes previously described. The onset of action usually begins in 3 to 5 minutes. You will use intramuscular injection when you assist a patient with the administration of a prescribed epinephrine auto-injector (Figure 13-4). Intramuscular injections are the easiest form of injection to administer.

The oral route is convenient and safe but slow in comparison to other routes. Oral medications that require digestion often need 30 minutes or longer before they begin to take effect. Another drawback to oral administration is that the patient must be alert and able to swallow. Activated charcoal is one medication that EMTs administer by the oral route (Figure 13-5). This medication works much more quickly than other oral medications because it does not need to be digested or absorbed. Another medication that is placed in the mouth, although not swallowed, is oral glucose. It is absorbed through the mucosal lining of the cheeks and gums, making it speedier than substances requiring intestinal absorption. This medication can also be given sublingually.

Faster routes are generally preferred so that the pa-

TABLE 13-1 Medication Routes

Route	Definition	Approximate rate of absorption	Advantages/disadvantages
Inhalation*	Inhaling medication in an aerosol or gas form	Rapid	Used only in conscious patients
Subcutaneous	Injecting medication into the subcutaneous skin layer; above the muscle	Slow	Absorption varies
Intramuscular*	Injecting medication into the muscle	Moderate	Greater tissue blood flow beneath the subcutaneous skin layer; allows for faster absorption
Intravenous	Injecting directly into a vein	Rapid	Direct access ensures delivery of medication into the bloodstream and quick onset of action
Oral*	Placing medication in the mouth, between cheek and gum Ingesting the medication	Moderate Usually slow	Used only in conscious patients Used only in conscious patients
Sublingual*	Placing or spraying the medication under the tongue	Rapid	Used only in conscious patients

*Indicates route of administration that can be used by EMTs.

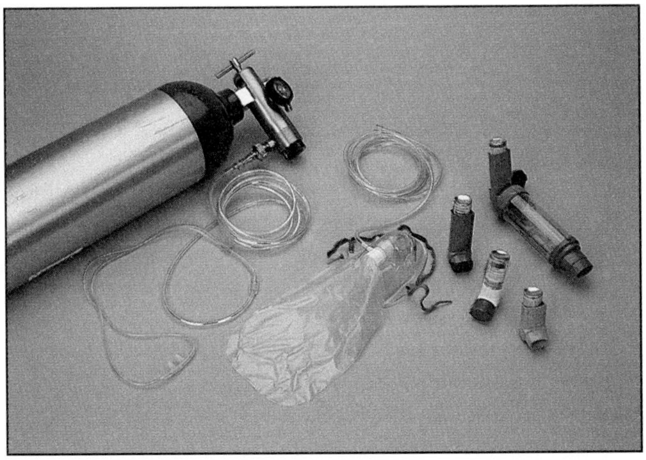

Figure 13-2
Inhalation medications, including bronchial inhalers and oxygen.

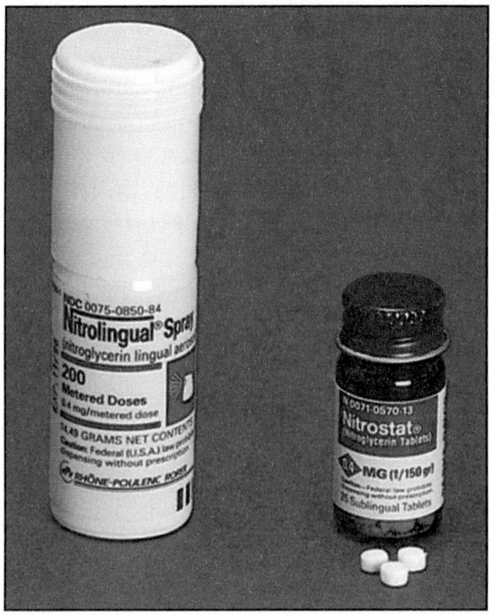

Figure 13-3

Nitroglycerin comes in a spray and a pill form.

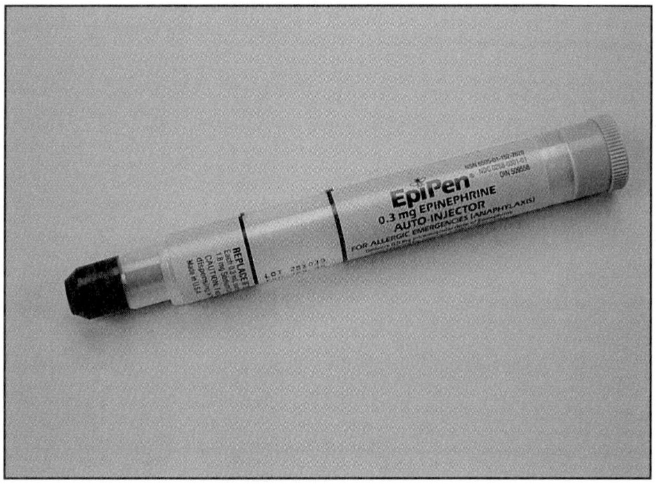

Figure 13-4

Epinephrine auto-injector.

tient will feel the effects of medication sooner. If the proper medication is given in the proper amount, the effect on the patient will likely be positive. However, if the wrong medication or an improper amount is given, fast onset may only increase the risk to the patient.

Indications and Contraindications

Most of the medications that EMTs can administer have certain **indications** for their use and **contraindications** that prohibit their use. These should be outlined in local protocols. The indication is the intended use of the medication—the reason that you are giving it. For example, a patient with a history of allergic reactions to bee stings may have a prescribed epinephrine auto-injector. This medication is indicated when the patient has been stung and is experiencing certain signs and symptoms of a severe allergic reaction.

Contraindications are conditions in which a medication should not be used because it may be dangerous to the patient. Contraindications include problems that could occur if incompatible medications are already being used by the patient. Some medications are contraindicated in

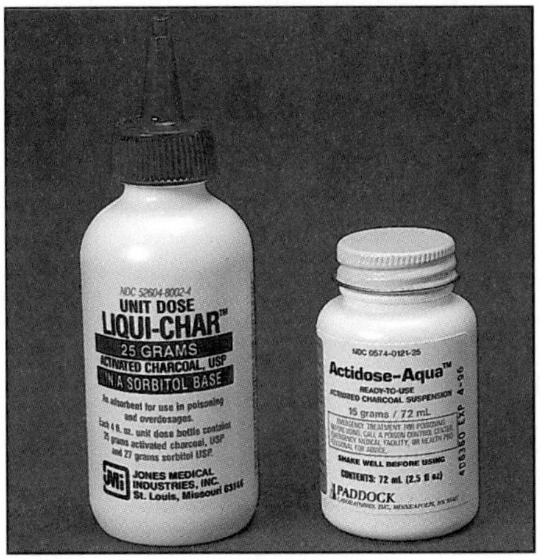

Figure 13-5

Activated charcoal must be thoroughly mixed before administration.

children. Other contraindications involve the patient's vital signs before administration of the medication. For example, a patient with a blood pressure below 90 systolic could be harmed by administering nitroglycerin because it may further reduce blood pressure.

Dosage

All medications have a prescribed **dose,** the amount that should be administered in a specific situation to produce the desired effect. While some medications have standard dosages, others vary according to the patient's age or weight. The doses of the medications that EMTs can administer are simple to remember and usually do not require calculations. Table 13-2 lists the correct doses of medications you will be using.

Preparation

Before administering any medication, ensure that the patient's condition fits your protocols for medication administration. This includes review of the patient's vital signs and chief complaint, a thorough assessment of the patient's condition, medications the patient may presently be taking, present medical conditions, and allergies to medications. Much of this information is gathered during the SAMPLE history.

Begin by examining the medication container. Make sure that it is the appropriate medication. Look for the expiration date; do not administer medication that has expired. Next, look at the clarity of the medication itself; it should not be discolored or crystallized (Figure 13-6).

Whether you are planning to assist a patient with the administration of a prescribed medication or administer a medication carried on the ambulance, the guidelines for medication administration can be summarized with the rule of the "Five Rights":

> *Give the right* medication, *in the right* dose, *by the right* route, *to the right* patient, *for the right* condition.

Rechecking is the other key to correct medication administration. Check these five elements before, during, and after administering the medication to the patient.

If you are preparing to assist a patient with the administration of a prescribed medication, make sure the patient's name is on the container. If the medication is kept in a pill container with other medications, ensure that the patient is certain of which medication to take. Contact the supervising medical direction physician to discuss any problems or issues that are not clearly outlined in protocols. If the medication is not in the proper container and you cannot verify the name on the label, notify your online physician. In this case, you may not be able to assist the patient with the administration of this medication.

Medical Direction

Protocols are general standards for patient care. Local protocols for EMTs are likely to address two general types of medical activity:

1. Assessment and treatment procedures that require direct, online permission from medical direction

TABLE 13-2 Common Medications That You Will Administer

Medication	Trade name	Indication	Form	Dosage	Route	Action
Glucose	Glutose 15 Insta-Glucose	Diminished consciousness; known diabetic emergency	Paste or gel	1 tube (15 gm)	Oral	Supplies glucose to cells
Activated charcoal	Actidose Liqui-Char SuperChar InstaChar	Ingested poisons	Liquid or powder	Adult: 25-50 gm Pediatric: 12-25 gm	Oral	Binds with the poison to prevent its absorption
Oxygen		Any unconscious patient or any medical- or trauma-related incident in which a patient could benefit from increased oxygen concentration	Gas	10-15 lpm	Inhaled	Enables body cells to function properly with oxygen
Bronchodilator Inhalers:		Respiratory difficulty from bronchioconstriction	Fine powder/vaporized aerosol	1-2 sprays	Inhaled	Opens breathing passages and improves air exchange
Albuterol	Proventil Ventolin					
Metaproterenol sulfate	Alupent Metaprel					
Isoetharine	Bronkosol Bronkometer					
Nitroglycerin	NitroStat NitroSpray	Chest pain from suspected cardiac causes	Sublingual tablet or spray	1 tablet or spray every 3-5 minutes to maximum of 3 doses	Sublingual	Dilates blood vessels to improve oxygen supply to the heart
Epinephrine	Adrenalin EpiPen	Severe allergic reaction	Injection via auto-injector	Adult: 0.3 mg Pediatric: 0.15 mg	Intramuscular	Counteracts the allergic reaction to improve blood pressure and breathing

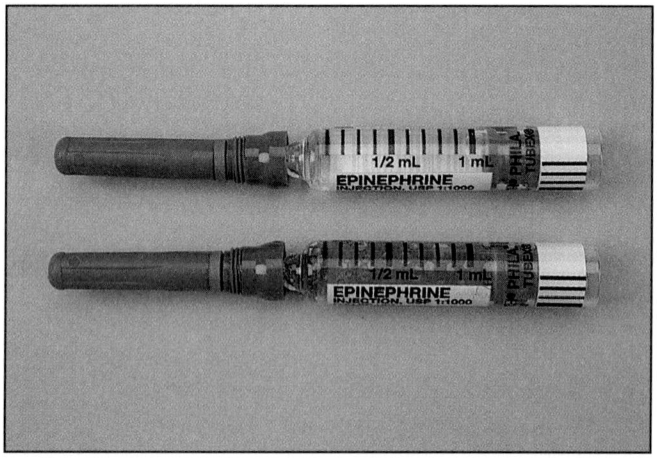

Figure 13-6

After checking the expiration date, always check for color and clarity. The medication in the lower syringe has become discolored.

2. Procedures that the EMT is authorized to do without calling for permission first (in the form of written standing orders)

Some services may rarely authorize EMTs to administer medications beyond the six discussed in this chapter. This will usually be done only under direct, online physician supervision.

Your protocol may require contact with the online physician to discuss the patient's condition before administering any medication. Begin by identifying yourself. Provide a concise report of the patient's condition, including vital signs. If you think the patient's condition fits your protocol for medication administration, ask for permission to administer the medication. Whenever you are given an order authorizing you to administer a medication, repeat the order back to the physician to verify that you have understood it correctly. This is both a professional courtesy and an excellent way to document the order. It may sound something like this:

> *I copy an order at 18:20 to administer 25 g of activated charcoal orally and initiate transport to your facility. I will contact you en route if there is any change in the patient's condition.*

Monitoring the Patient

Once you have given the medication, monitor the patient closely to see if the medication is working. Reassess the patient's vital signs and overall condition and compare these findings with the initial findings. Determine whether the patient is experiencing the proper effects or any side effects. You should be able to see some positive changes in the patient's condition. For example, a patient who was having difficulty breathing should be breathing easier after the administration of a bronchodilator inhaler. While the patient's breathing rate and quality may not return to a normal range, there should be improvement over time. Similarly, a diabetic patient who has undereaten or overexercised and is feeling lightheaded should improve in response to glucose administration.

Sometimes it may be necessary to give an additional dose of the medication. This often occurs when nitroglycerin is given to relieve chest pain of cardiac origin. If the pain is only partially relieved and the patient's vital signs allow it, your protocols may call for a repeat dose.

Documentation

Documentation of medication administration is very important. The written patient-care report must show that the patient's condition fits your protocols to administer the medication. Document this by recording a complete set of vital signs, the patient's chief complaint, SAMPLE history findings, and pertinent results of the focused history and physical examination, including the patient's description of any pain. Record the name, time, dose, and route of the medication. Note the patient's response to the medication by reassessing vital signs and repeating the SAMPLE questions. Also, when completing your patient-care report, be sure to document the time and the name of the physician who gave you the order. Adequate documentation is very important if you have to explain the case and your actions later. Remember the saying, "If it's not written down, it didn't happen."

If you ever discover that you have mistakenly administered the wrong medication or given the correct substance improperly (e.g., wrong dose), report the situation immediately to your medical direction physician. The physician will determine if anything further needs to be done to correct the situation and will advise you of other things to monitor. The exact sequence of events must also be clearly documented on the patient-care report.

Medications That EMTs Can Deliver

There are six different medications that EMTs may be able to administer in the field. These fall under two general classifications: (1) medications carried on the BLS ambulance, and (2) medications that the patient has had prescribed by a personal physician. All of these medications can only be administered to patients who fit criteria established in your local protocols. Before administering these medications, you will need to be operating under standing orders or must directly contact your medical direction physician. For example, many protocols include a standing order to administer oxygen to any patient with signs of a condition that could deprive vital organs of essential oxygen. These signs include difficulty breathing, chest pain, altered consciousness, or blood loss. Other protocols require EMTs to contact the physician directly before administering a medication carried in the ambulance or assisting a patient with the self-administration of a prescribed medication.

Medications Carried on an Ambulance

Three medications that you may carry on the ambulance are oxygen, oral glucose, and activated charcoal. The following sections describe their actions, indications and contraindications, dosages, and side effects (see Table 13-2).

Oxygen

Oxygen is the most common medication that EMTs use. You will provide supplemental oxygen to any patient who is having difficulty breathing or whose condition otherwise indicates the need for it, such as any serious medical or trauma condition. It should be administered to any unconscious patient or patient with an altered mental status. Oxygen can be delivered through a variety of devices that provide different concentrations of oxygen (see Chapter 11). If it is delivered for a prolonged period, it tends to dry out mucous membranes, which can result in nosebleeds and headaches. This is unlikely to occur during short intervals of field care, however.

Other than these few side effects, the only major considerations with oxygen are to use caution around open flames and avoid dropping the cylinder and damaging the regulator. Oxygen administration often does not require advance contact with online medical direction. Standing orders should clearly state how much oxygen to deliver in specific situations.

Activated Charcoal

Activated charcoal is used to treat patients who have ingested certain poisons. It is effective against poisons that have been swallowed because it binds the poison and prevents its absorption by the digestive system. The poison and the charcoal are then excreted from the body together. Activated charcoal is most often supplied in suspension form, although it also comes as a powder that must be diluted. Activated charcoal is the generic name of the medication. It is available under numerous trade names.

Activated charcoal is indicated for a patient who is conscious and able to swallow, has an intact gag reflex, and has the signs, symptoms, and history of an ingestion poisoning. Contraindications include an altered level of consciousness (LOC) or the suspicion that the patient may become unconscious, the presence of vomiting, an inability to swallow, or ingestion of a corrosive, caustic, or petroleum product.

Unlike other oral medications that must be absorbed by the digestive tract before they begin to work, the onset of action of activated charcoal is immediate because it binds with the poison in the stomach. Activated charcoal

A

B

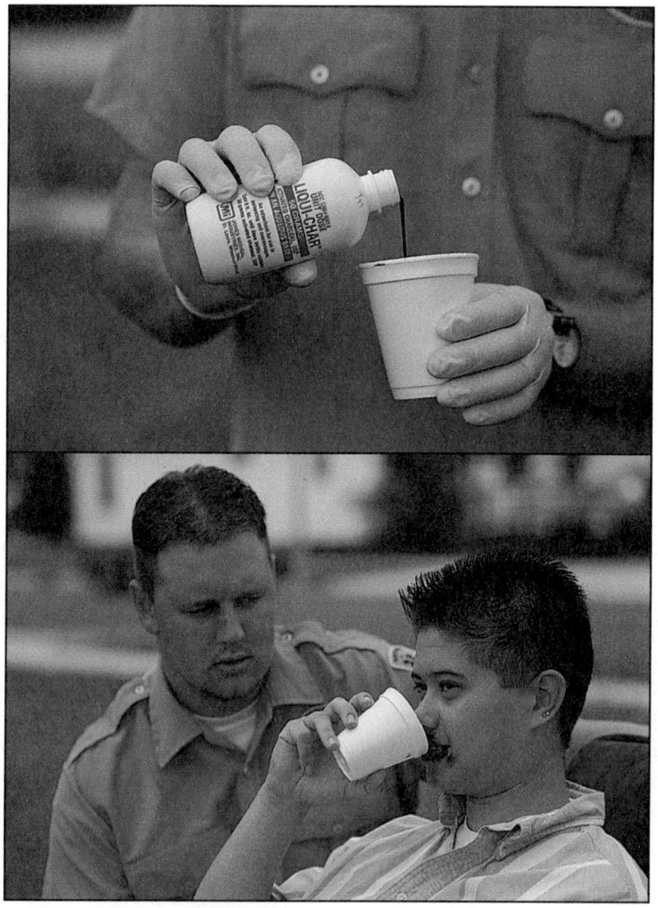

Figure 13-7

A, When administering activated charcoal, pour the correct dose into a cup immediately after mixing. **B,** The patient should drink the medication quickly, before it has settled. If the patient is hesitant, using a lid and straw may help.

is supplied in plastic bottles containing 15 to 25 g of the medication suspended in water. A typical dose of activated charcoal is 1 g/kg of patient's body weight for both adults and children. The normal amount given to an adult is 25 to 50 g. This means that you may need to administer more than one bottle to an adult. For children, this dose is usually cut in half. Although 50 g is the typical maximum dose, you may receive orders for a larger dose based on the patient's weight.

Before administering activated charcoal, consult with your online physician. If you are advised to administer the medication, shake the container thoroughly. Activated charcoal looks much like mud, and patients may be hesitant to drink it (Figure 13-7). It sometimes helps to place it in a covered container and have the patient drink it through a straw or sipper lid. It may also help to have patients close their eyes or hold their noses as they drink it. It is important that the medication be ingested quickly or it will begin to settle and need to be shaken again. Side effects include nausea, vomiting, constipation, and black stools. If the patient vomits after the administration of the activated charcoal, repeat the dose once if local protocol allows it or if ordered by medical direction.

Oral Glucose

Oral glucose is a form of sugar that can be taken by mouth. It is used for diabetic emergencies in which the patient's blood sugar level is too low. Many patients have a home glucose-testing device to measure their blood sugar level. This may provide additional information but should not change your approach to patient care based on history and examination findings. The medication comes as a gel that is easily absorbed when placed in the mouth along the inside of the cheek. Because it does not have to be swallowed, the onset of action is rapid. It increases a diabetic's LOC by rapidly increasing the blood sugar level. Like other medications, oral glucose is marketed under several trade names, including Insta-Glucose, Glutose, and Glutose 15 (Figure 13-8).

Oral glucose is indicated for any awake but disoriented patient with a known history of diabetes. The medication is generally contraindicated for a patient who is unable to swallow, such as an unresponsive patient. However, some systems allow glucose paste to be administered carefully under the tongue or between the gum and cheek of an unresponsive patient. This requires placing the patient in the lateral recumbent position (on the side) to promote drainage of secretions away from the airway. It also commits the EMT to close, constant airway monitoring. Although this procedure is allowed for some EMTs and other trained health care professionals, it should not be recommended to family members or bystanders.

Oral glucose is supplied in tubes that contain 15 to 25 g of medication. The normal dose for a child or adult is one tube. Local protocol may allow you to administer it by standing order under certain conditions or may require you to contact the online physician for permission. Oral glucose can be placed under the tongue or between the cheek and gum by squeezing small amounts on a tongue depressor and using it to apply the paste (Figure 13-9). There are no side effects associated with the administration of oral glucose.

The Patient's Prescribed Medications

You will sometimes care for patients who have a medication of their own for a specific medical condition but who need your assistance administering it. There are three medications that you can help a patient self-administer: bronchodilator inhalers, nitroglycerin, and epinephrine. Local protocol should indicate whether you have indirect,

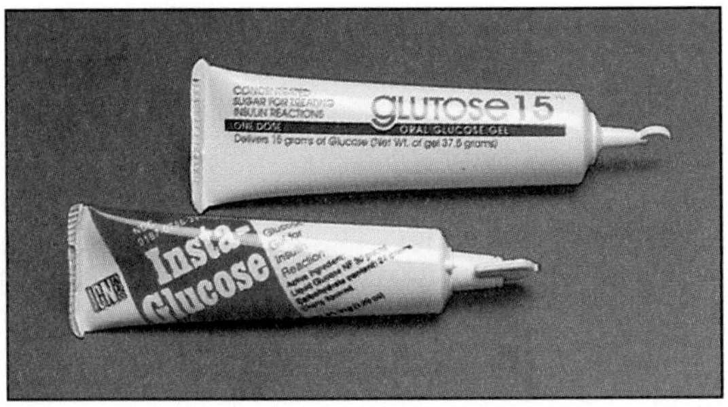

Figure 13-8

Oral glucose products.

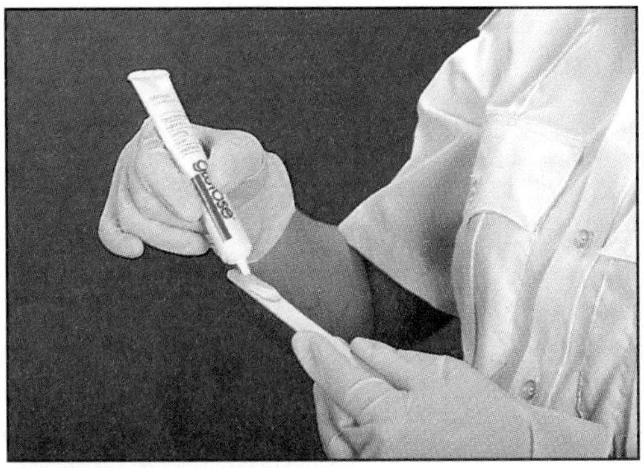

Figure 13-9

Oral glucose can be applied to a tongue depressor so it can be more easily placed between the cheek and gum.

IT'S YOUR CALL
CONCLUSION

Your patient is a diabetic who has been unable to maintain proper nutrition. You suspect she is suffering from a diabetic condition in which she has too much insulin and not enough sugar. You quickly contact your online physician and discuss the patient's situation. You advise that the patient is conscious enough to eat and drink and that you would like to administer one tube of oral glucose. The physician is aware of the lengthy response time of the ALS provider and approves your request to administer the medication. The patient's condition improves in minutes as an ALS provider arrives. The patient remains awake and is transported to the hospital for further evaluation. After the call, you note under "Treatment" in your patient-care report: "25 g oral glucose given on Dr. Hanson's order at 18:20 hrs. Patient responded quickly with return to normal consciousness."

offline approval (through written standing orders) to help a patient with these medications, or if you need direct permission from the online physician. Patients may also have other medications that they request assistance in administering. Because you are not trained to administer other medications, you can only honor this request after contacting the online physician.

Bronchodilator Inhalers

Some patients use bronchodilator inhalers for breathing problems such as asthma, emphysema, and chronic bronchitis (Chapter 14 presents specifics about these diseases). A bronchodilator inhaler is a device that delivers a premeasured amount of medication for inhalation into the lungs, where it dilates bronchial tubes and makes it easier for the patient to breathe. There are three common generic medications used in bronchodilator inhalers: albuterol, metaproterenol sulfate, and isoetharine. Albuterol is packaged under two commonly known trade names: Proventil and Ventolin. Metaproterenol sulfate's trade name is Alupent, and isoetharine's is Bronkosol (see Table 13-2 on p. 300).

Bronchodilator inhalers are indicated for patients who have been diagnosed by a physician as having a medical condition that can be improved by the use of bronchodilators, have a prescribed inhaler, and exhibit signs and symptoms of respiratory distress. Contraindications include patients who are not experiencing difficulty breathing, are unable to help with use of the device themselves, have an inhaler that has not been prescribed for them, or have already taken the prescribed maximum dose before your arrival.

Bronchodilator inhalers deliver a premeasured amount of medication, referred to as a *metered dose,* with each spray. The normal dose for adults and children is usually two sprays. Because patients with difficulty breathing can be anxious and excited, they do not always use their inhaler properly. For this reason, it can be very helpful for an EMT to coach a patient through the administration steps. To assist a patient with self-administration of a bronchodilator inhaler, follow these steps:

1. Determine that the patient's condition fits your protocol for administering the medication.
2. Verify the name of the medication, that the medication belongs to the patient, and that the medication has not expired.
3. Contact your online physician to gain approval, if required by protocol.
4. Shake the inhaler several times.
5. Have the patient exhale forcefully.
6. Have the patient close his or her lips around the canister opening. Some patients use a device known as a *spacer* attached to the inhaler. The spacer acts as a reservoir for the medication, allowing more complete inhalation of the spray once it has been released from the canister (Figure 13-10).
7. Have the patient squeeze the inhaler to activate the spray, inhale deeply as they squeeze, and hold the inhalation breath as long as possible before exhaling.
8. The sequence listed above may be repeated for a second inhalation, depending on prescription and protocol.

Side effects associated with the use of bronchodilator inhalers include increased heart rate, tremors, and nervousness.

Nitroglycerin

Some patients with heart disease use a prescribed medication called *nitroglycerin.* Nitroglycerin is a **vasodilator,** which means that it dilates blood vessels. By dilating the coronary arteries, nitroglycerin increases blood flow and oxygen to the heart muscle. Because it also dilates blood vessels in the periphery, resistance to blood flow drops, the heart does not have to work as hard, and the demand for oxygen is reduced. Both of these effects can help reduce chest pain.

Nitroglycerin is manufactured in several forms and under several trade names. The forms of nitroglycerin include pill, spray, ointment, and patch. You will only be administering nitroglycerin by pill or spray. Common trade names for nitroglycerin in these forms include Nitrostat and Nitrolingual Spray.

Nitroglycerin is indicated for patients experiencing chest pain that is likely to be of cardiac origin. You are allowed to administer nitroglycerin to your patients only when the following four conditions are met:

1. The patient must show signs and symptoms of chest pain of cardiac origin, such as crushing chest pain, shortness of breath, and sweating.
2. The patient must have physician-prescribed nitroglycerin in the form of a pill or spray.
3. The patient must have a systolic blood pressure greater than 90 to 100 mm Hg (the specific level will be determined by your local protocol).
4. You must have approval, either standing orders or by direct permission from the online physician.

Nitroglycerin is contraindicated in patients who do not have their own prescribed medication. It is also contraindicated when a patient has a systolic blood pressure below 90 to 100 mm Hg, a diminished LOC or head injury, or has already taken the maximum prescribed dose before your arrival.

Whether you are administering nitroglycerin in the form of a pill or a spray, one dose of the medication is administered sublingually; give one pill or one spray under the tongue (Figure 13-11, *A* and *B*). Vital signs should be repeated within 3 minutes after the administration of nitroglycerin. Observe the patient's response and report to medical direction. If the pain is still not relieved, you may

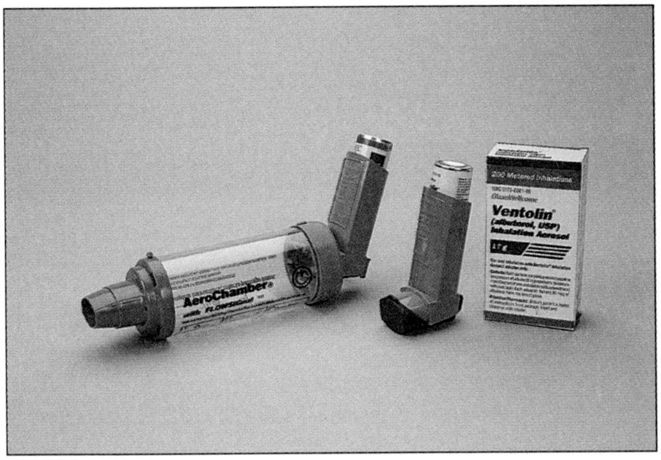

Figure 13-10

Bronchial inhaler with and without a spacer.

A

B

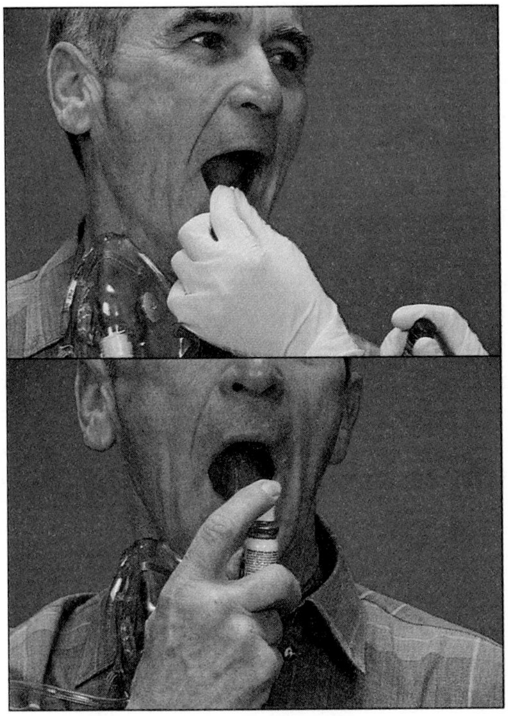

Figure 13-11

A, Use gloves when administering nitroglycerin tablets. The medication can be absorbed through the mucous membrane under the tongue. **B,** Nitroglycerin spray should be applied sublingually.

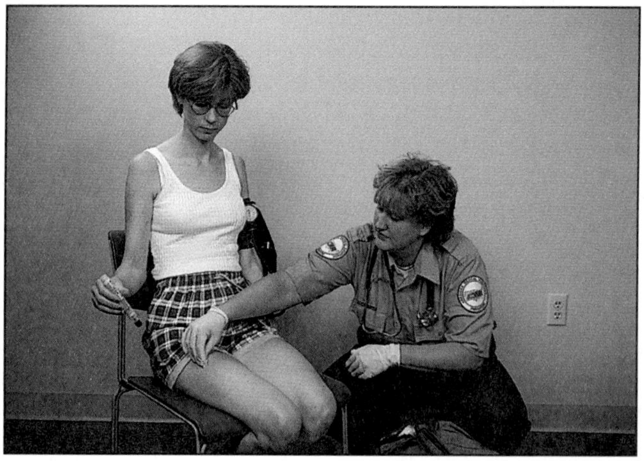

Figure 13-12

Move clothing away from the injection site, cleaning the site if possible.

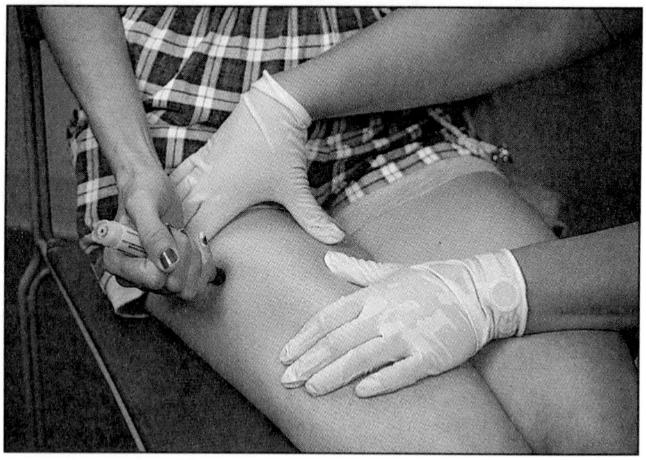

Figure 13-13

The auto-injector should be perpendicular to the leg.

receive orders to administer additional nitroglycerin every 3 to 5 minutes for up to three total doses.

To administer nitroglycerin, follow these steps:

1. Check the label; confirm that the medication belongs to the patient and has not expired.
2. Ask the patient how many doses have already been taken.
3. Check under the patient's tongue to see if there is a pill already there.
4. Contact the online physician for approval, if required.
5. Place the patient in a comfortable, seated position. Consider a semireclining position to minimize possible effects of a drop in blood pressure.
6. Administer one pill or spray under the patient's tongue.
7. Prepare the patient for transport.
8. Check the patient's vital signs within 3 minutes. If the systolic blood pressure drops below 90 to 100 mm Hg after administration, place the patient in Trendelenburg's position and contact medical direction. If the pain has not been relieved and systolic blood pressure remains above 90 to 100 mm Hg, administer another dose if allowed by standing orders or approved by medical direction.

Side effects that could occur after administering nitroglycerin include a drop in blood pressure and pulse (pulse may also increase), headache, and a burning or tingling sensation under the tongue.

Epinephrine Auto-injector

Epinephrine, sometimes supplied under the trade name Adrenalin, is commonly used to relieve the signs and symptoms of a severe allergic reaction. When given, it does three important things:

1. Constricts blood vessels, causing blood pressure to rise. A patient experiencing a severe allergic reaction usually has low blood pressure from dilated blood vessels.
2. Dilates bronchial passages. A patient with an allergic reaction also often has significant difficulty breathing because of bronchial constriction.
3. Acts to decrease the actions of *histamine,* which is a powerful blood vessel dilator that is released as part of an allergic reaction.

The epinephrine you administer will be packaged in a sealed plastic auto-injector. It has a premeasured dose of 0.3 mg for an adult or 0.15 mg for a child. It may appear under the trade name EpiPen (see Figure 13-4 on p. 298). It is indicated for a patient who is experiencing a severe allergic reaction, including respiratory distress and shock. There are no absolute contraindications to the use of epinephrine in this life-threatening setting. However, some protocols do restrict its use in older patients, particularly those with cardiac conditions.

To administer epinephrine with an auto-injector, follow these steps:

1. Determine that the patient's signs and symptoms meet your protocol for the administration of epinephrine for a severe allergic reaction.
2. Check the label to confirm that the medication belongs to the patient and has not expired. If the liquid is visible, ensure that it is not discolored or crystallized.
3. Get approval from the online physician to administer the medication, if required.
4. Remove the safety cap from the medication.
5. Remove clothing from the patient's thigh, which will be used as the injection site. If this is not possible, the injection can be administered through clothing as thick as jeans.
6. Locate the injection site on the lateral portion of the thigh, midway between the waist and knee (Figure 13-12).
7. Clean the skin if possible.
8. Place the tip of the auto-injector perpendicular to the leg (at a 90-degree angle) and push firmly to inject the medication. The device will trigger itself when pressed against the skin (Figure 13-13).
9. Hold the auto-injector in this position for 10 seconds to allow all of the medication to be injected.
10. Immediately deposit the used auto-injector in a biohazard container, taking care to avoid an accidental needlestick injury. Your training in the use of auto-injectors should include standard precautions for needle handling.
11. Record the time of administration.
12. Monitor the patient's vital signs for indications of improvement. If the patient's condition does not improve in a few minutes and the patient has an additional injector, contact medical direction to discuss administering a second dose.

The side effects of epinephrine include increased heart rate, pale skin, dizziness, headache, nausea, and vomiting. In severe cases, or when too much epinephrine is given, it can cause dangerously fast heart rates or cardiac arrest.

SUMMARY

As an EMT-Basic, you will be qualified to administer six medications to patients who are either taking their own prescribed medications or are in need of medications carried on the BLS ambulance.

Before administering any medication, be certain that your patient fits the protocol for its administration. This involves completing the initial patient assessment and the focused history and physical examination. When required, contact the online physician to discuss the patient's condition and request an order to administer a medication. Remember the rule of Five Rights when administering any medication: give the right *medication,* in the right *dose,* by the right *route,* to the right *patient,* for the right *condition.* Record your findings, the order for the medication, the amount and route administered, and your reassessment of the patient's condition.

This chapter has provided the basic information about the medications that EMTs can administer. It has presented guidelines that have been established for the safe use of these medications. These guidelines include understanding how the medications work, the indications and contraindications for administration, dosages, the most common side effects, and the routes and methods of administration. You will have the opportunity to review these medications in the chapters that follow on medical emergencies.

REFERENCES

1. **LeSage P, Derr P, Tardiff J:** *EMS field guide,* ed 9, Lake Oswego, Ore, 1993, InforMed.
2. **Madigan KG:** *Prehospital emergency drugs pocket reference,* St Louis, 1990, Mosby.
3. **McHenry L, Salerno E:** *Mosby's pharmacology in nursing,* ed 18, St Louis, 1992, Mosby.
4. **Ray O, Ksir C:** *Drugs, society, and human behavior,* ed 5, St Louis, 1993, Mosby.

Chapter 14
Respiratory Emergencies

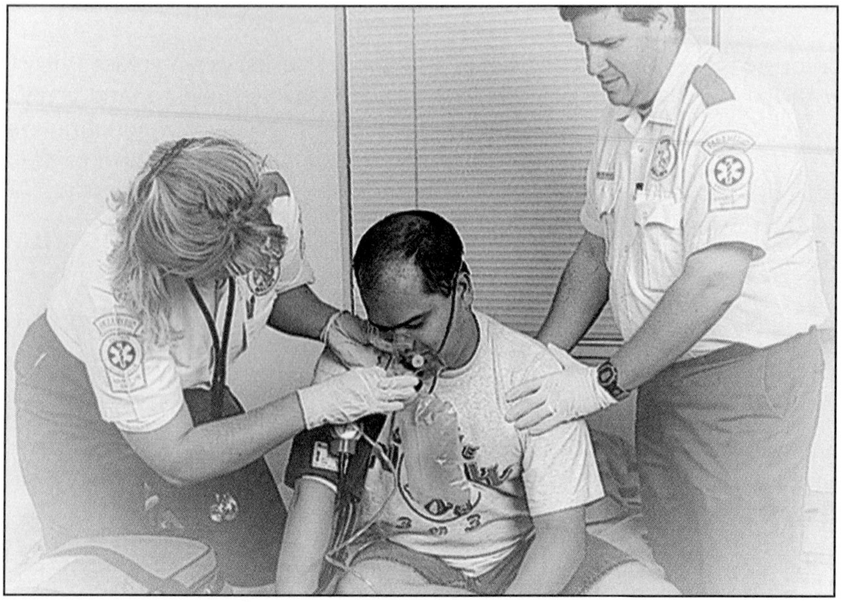

Knowledge Objectives

As an EMT-Basic, you should be able to:

OBJECTIVES

1. Identify and describe the structure and function of the respiratory system.
2. Explain how to recognize pediatric and adult patients with difficulty breathing.
3. Describe how to treat pediatric and adult patients with difficulty breathing.
4. Explain the relationship between airway management and the treatment of a patient with difficulty breathing.
5. List signs of respiratory distress that are common in pediatric patients and may appear earlier than in adult patients.
6. Differentiate between adequate and inadequate air oxygenation.
7. State three generic and trade names for bronchial inhalers.
8. Identify the medication dosage, route, actions, indications, contraindications, and procedures for administration of common bronchial inhalers.
9. Explain treatment for infants, children, and adults with breathing difficulty.
10. Distinguish between upper and lower airway obstruction recognition and treatment in infants, children, and adults.
11. Identify the signs and symptoms of the following conditions:
    - Asthma
    - Chronic bronchitis
    - Croup
    - Emphysema
    - Epiglottitis
    - Hyperventilation
    - Pneumonia
    - Pulmonary embolism

OBJECTIVES

Skill Objectives

As an EMT-Basic, you should be able to:

1. **Demonstrate how to provide general care for a patient in respiratory distress.**
2. **Demonstrate how to perform rescue breathing for a patient in respiratory arrest.**
3. **Demonstrate the steps for assisting a patient with the administration of a bronchial inhaler.**

Attitude Objectives

As an EMT-Basic, you should be able to:

1. **Understand the importance of contacting your medical direction physician for advice about treating a patient with difficulty breathing.**
2. **Defend the treatment steps for various respiratory emergencies.**

KEY TERMS

1. **Aerosol:** A fine mist of liquid droplets; particularly, a mist of liquid medication produced by an inhaler.
2. **Asthma:** A condition that results in excessive mucus production, inflammation, and narrowing of the bronchiolar air passages.
3. **Auscultation:** Evaluation by listening, usually through a stethoscope.
4. **Bronchiodilator Inhaler:** A device used to administer inhaled, aerosolized medication that dilates bronchial tubes, reducing the effects of respiratory distress in patients with asthma, chronic bronchitis, and emphysema.
5. **Chronic Bronchitis:** A form of chronic obstructive pulmonary disease that causes an increase in mucus production, primarily in the bronchioles; limits adequate ventilation and gas exchange.
6. **Chronic Obstructive Pulmonary Disease (COPD):** A chronic condition in which air is trapped behind obstructions, including secretions, in the bronchioles; emphysema and chronic bronchitis are two forms of COPD.
7. **Croup:** A respiratory infection that causes inflammation and swelling of the laryngeal lining and narrowing of the trachea below the vocal cords; usually seen in younger children.
8. **Dyspnea:** Difficulty breathing; shortness of breath.
9. **Emphysema:** A form of COPD that results in the destruction of the alveoli and the bronchioles; occurs more commonly in adults than in children.
10. **Epiglottitis:** A severe infection causing swelling of the epiglottis that can lead to complete airway obstruction.
11. **Hypoxia:** Inadequate oxygenation of tissues; can be localized or systemic (body wide).
12. **Pleuritic Chest Pain:** Chest pain associated with breathing movement or other motion; usually caused by an injury or infection of the pleural membranes or chest wall.
13. **Pneumonia:** An infection that results in the accumulation of fluid, bacteria, and inflammatory cells between the alveoli and the capillaries.
14. **Pulmonary Embolism:** The blockage of a pulmonary artery by foreign matter, such as a blood clot, fat, tumor tissue, or air.
15. **Pulse Oximeter:** An electronic device that uses colored-light technology to measure the percentage of blood hemoglobin that is saturated with oxygen.
16. **Respiration:** The exchange of gases, either between the body and the environment or between the cells and the blood.
17. **Respiratory Arrest:** Cessation of breathing; apnea.
18. **Respiratory Distress:** Difficult or inadequate breathing.
19. **Ventilation:** The movement of air between the lungs and the environment.
20. **Wheezing:** A musical breathing noise caused by air flowing through narrowed passages in the lower airways; commonly associated with asthma.

IT'S YOUR CALL

It has been a hot and humid spring day. Despite the heat, humidity, and high pollen count, you have not had any patients with breathing problems . . . until now. You are dispatched at 15:40 for "difficulty breathing."

You arrive at a tennis court and locate your patient, a 13-year-old male who is sitting upright on the court. Initial observation reveals a thin patient who is conscious, struggling to breathe, diaphoretic, and mildly cyanotic. Obtaining an accurate history is difficult because he is only able to speak in short phrases. You learn that he has **asthma.** A friend states that he was becoming short of breath while they played a match and that he used his **bronchial inhaler** twice without relief. You check the inhaler and find that it is empty. Another friend has gone to the patient's nearby home in the hope of bringing back another inhaler.

How should you assess this patient?

Respiratory emergencies are among the most common emergencies that EMTs encounter. They range from problems such as mild shortness of breath and short choking spells to life-threatening conditions caused by infection, disease, trauma, blood clots, mucus obstructions, and bronchiolar constriction. As an EMT-Basic, one of your primary responsibilities is to identify patients experiencing breathing problems and take immediate steps to help. This may involve administering oxygen, relieving an airway obstruction, assisting a patient with the administration of medication, inserting a device to help establish an airway, and assisting with **ventilations.**

This chapter begins with a brief review of the structure of the respiratory system. It identifies inadequate breathing, explores some causes of breathing emergencies, and concludes with the steps for treating these conditions.

Reviewing Respiratory Anatomy and Function

The respiratory system is divided into the upper and lower airways (Figure 14-1). The upper airway warms, filters, and humidifies air as it flows in from the environment. The upper airway begins with the oral and nasal cavities and extends to the larynx. The larynx is the portion of the upper airway that joins the pharynx to the trachea and houses the vocal cords. Both the larynx and trachea are protected by the epiglottis, a leaf-shaped, soft-tissue structure that prevents food and fluid from entering the trachea during swallowing.

The lower airway begins with the trachea, just beneath the larynx, and extends to the microscopic air sacs in the lungs, the alveoli. Air passes through the vocal cords and enters the trachea, which divides into the two main bronchi that lead to the lungs. The bronchi divide into secondary bronchi, which further divide into bronchioles. The bronchioles end in the alveoli, where oxygen enters the blood from the air sacs and carbon dioxide leaves the blood to be exhaled (Figure 14-2). Oxygenated blood returns to the heart through the pulmonary veins and is pumped into arteries for distribution to all parts of the body. Oxygen is delivered to the cells of the body by the capillaries. Because capillaries are very thin, oxygen and carbon dioxide pass easily between the capillaries and blood cells. As the cells take in oxygen, they release carbon dioxide back into the blood. Deoxygenated blood returns to the heart through the veins and is pumped to the lungs. There, carbon dioxide is released and the cycle begins again.

Respiration is controlled by the central nervous system. Chemical sensors in the brain detect changes in oxygen and carbon dioxide levels in the blood. When oxygen levels fall or carbon dioxide increases, these sensors detect those changes and cause stimulation of the respiratory mechanism, leading to faster, deeper breathing in an attempt to increase the oxygen or decrease the carbon dioxide. Of these two respiratory drive mechanisms, carbon-dioxide sensing is more sensitive to changes in blood concentrations.

The nerve impulses responsible for controlling respiratory muscles originate in the part of the brain stem known as the *medulla.* The intercostal nerves originate in the thoracic region of the spine and cause movement of the intercostal muscles between the ribs. The phrenic nerve, which exits the spinal cord in the cervical spine region, causes the diaphragm to contract and move down. Because of the location of the phrenic nerve, cervical spine injuries may damage it, causing paralysis of the diaphragm, which can significantly affect a patient's respiratory status.

The process of respiration occurs as a result of pressure changes in the thoracic cavity that make the lungs expand and contract. During inspiration, the diaphragm contracts (lowers and flattens) and the intercostal muscles contract, expanding the chest wall. The contraction of the diaphragm and intercostal muscles increases the size of the thoracic cavity. The increase in volume decreases the pressure inside the chest relative to air pressure outside the body. The higher external pressure causes air to flow

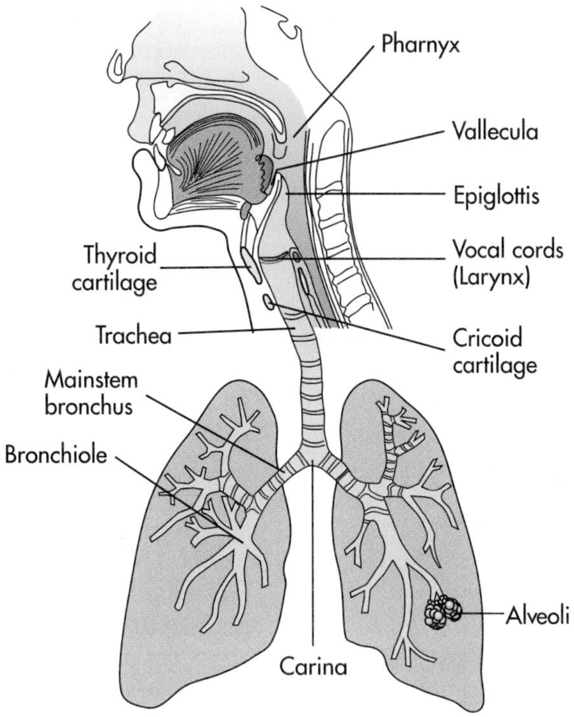

Figure 14-1

Upper and lower airways.

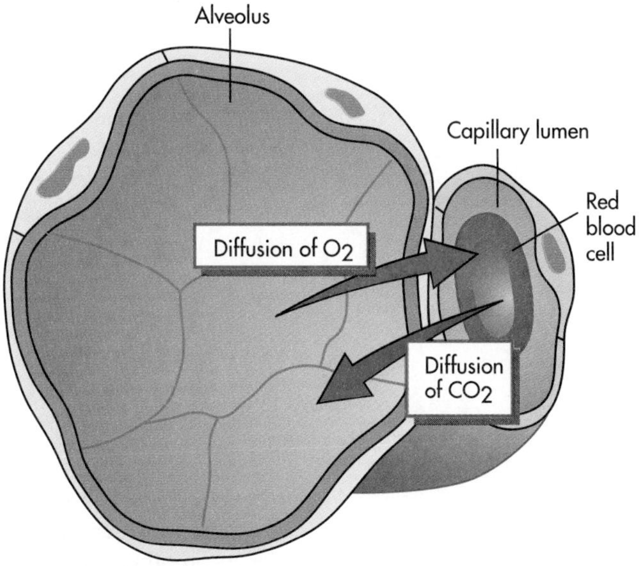

Figure 14-2

Gas exchange at the cellular level.

into the lungs. During exhalation, the intercostal muscles and the diaphragm relax, thereby reducing lung volume, increasing pressure in the lungs, and forcing air out.

Pediatric and adult airways differ in a number of ways. In general, the respiratory system of a child is smaller and more flexible than an adult's. A child's tongue is also larger in proportion to the airway than that of an adult. The chest wall is less developed, so a child relies more on the diaphragm to breathe. These differences result in a greater susceptibility to distress when something goes wrong with the child's respiratory system. Common problems include foreign-body airway obstruction and respiratory infections that cause swelling of the tissue around the larynx and trachea. The pediatric airway is discussed in detail in Chapter 26.

Assessing Breathing Difficulty

Breathing should be an effortless, involuntary task. Any condition that interferes with the proper exchange of oxygen and carbon dioxide can lead to inadequate breathing.

BOX 14-1 Recognizing Respiratory Distress

Use your senses of sight, sound, and touch to identify a patient who is in respiratory distress. As you conduct the assessment, remember to look, listen, and feel.

Look for:

- Restlessness, agitation, confusion
- Patient posturing in an erect, seated position
- Diminished consciousness
- Abdominal breathing
- Abnormal breathing rate and rhythm
- Pale, cyanotic, or flushed skin
- Use of accessory muscles, including intercostal muscle retractions

Listen for:

- A patient complaining of shortness of breath or pain during respirations
- A patient unable to speak or only able to speak a word or short phrase at a time
- Noisy respirations
- Coughing
- Unequal or diminished breath sounds
- Abnormal breathing rate and rhythm

Feel for:

- Abnormal chest movement
- Abnormal pulse (The heart rate tends to increase when a person is struggling to breathe. In children, it decreases after prolonged **hypoxia,** just before **respiratory** arrest.)

It is important to determine the adequacy of every patient's breathing early in the assessment process. Rapid identification of a breathing problem can lead to early corrective action and a positive patient outcome (Box 14-1).

Adequate Breathing

Adequate breathing can be determined by noting the patient's breathing rate, rhythm, and quality. The average, healthy adult breathes at a rate of 12 to 20 times a minute, exchanging approximately 500 ml (one pint) of air with every breath. The depth and pattern should be regular.

The patient should not appear to be in any distress when breathing and should be able to speak without shortness of breath or a need to limit speech to short phrases. Normal speaking may cause some irregularity in breathing. Breathing should be quiet, not noisy. Respiration depth should be normal, not shallow or deep. The chest rise should be symmetrical, with adequate expansion upon visual examination and palpation.

When **auscultated,** breaths sounds should be equal bilaterally. Check this with stethoscope placements on the chest corresponding to the upper and lower lobes on both the right and left sides. Remember that the lower placement locations are lateral rather than anterior. When possible, also check the four corresponding locations on the back (see Figure 10-4, p. 221).

Inadequate Breathing

There are a number of conditions that can result in inadequate breathing, including injury, illness, stress, anxiety, and excitement. Inadequate breathing is usually identified by abnormal signs involving one or more of the following:

- Breathing rate
- Breathing rhythm
- Breathing quality
- Chest expansion
- Breath sounds

The breathing rate may be too fast or too slow. Rhythm may be irregular, meaning that the timing and length of breaths are not constant. Quality may reflect a labored effort to breathe, characterized by nasal flaring and the use of accessory muscles that cause retraction of the intercostal muscles or of the neck muscles or supraclavicular areas. Respiration depth may be shallow or deep. Chest expansion may be unequal or inadequate (Figure 14-3). **Auscultation** can reveal diminished, unequal, or absent breath sounds.

Besides these specific signs, a patient may also complain of shortness of breath or **dyspnea.** The phrase *one- to two-word dyspnea* is often used to describe a patient with difficulty breathing who can speak only a word or two at a time.

While conducting the focused history, ask pertinent questions about the present problem. Try to get the patient to describe the breathing difficulty clearly. Quote the patient's own words in the narrative portion of the patient-care report. Use the acronym OPQRST (see Chapter 10) to determine:

- *O*nset of breathing difficulty
- Whether anything *P*rovoked the onset
- *Q*uality of the distress
- Whether any pain *R*adiates to another body location
- How *S*evere the distress is, on a scale of 1 to 10
- The *T*ime at which the distress was first noted

A patient experiencing inadequate breathing is in **respiratory distress,** the most common type of breathing emergency. If not corrected, this condition could deteriorate to **respiratory arrest** and death. The presence of agonal respirations is an ominous sign that occurs just before respiratory arrest. These respirations are characterized by sporadic, irregular, and infrequent gasping for air. Respiratory failure is the inability of the respiratory and cardiovascular systems to maintain an appropriate transfer of oxygen and carbon dioxide in the lungs. This could be caused by either a lack of oxygen or a problem with gas exchange. Injuries and diseases such as asthma, **emphysema,** lung cancer, **pneumonia,** and tuberculosis can result in respiratory failure.

Inadequate oxygenation of the tissues, called hypoxia, is the end result of airway and breathing problems. In addition to the classic signs of **hypoxia** (cyanosis, respiratory distress), its effect on the brain often influences the way a patient presents. Along with other possible causes of altered mentation, hypoxia should always be considered in patients who are confused, irritable, agitated, or even combative.

The visible, clinical signs outlined above are the primary indicators for recognizing hypoxia. Some EMTs will also be able to use electronic technology in the form of a **pulse oximeter.** When available, this tool can confirm the clinical signs of hypoxia or give an early warning before they appear.

Children and infants breathe at faster rates than adults. Normal respiratory rates are 15 to 30 breaths per minute for a child and 25 to 50 for an infant. As a sign of respiratory distress in children, muscle retractions are more common than in adults and usually appear earlier. Nasal flaring is also a frequent sign. In infants, grunting often accompanies the extra breathing effort in respiratory distress.

Oxygen and ventilation therapies for children are

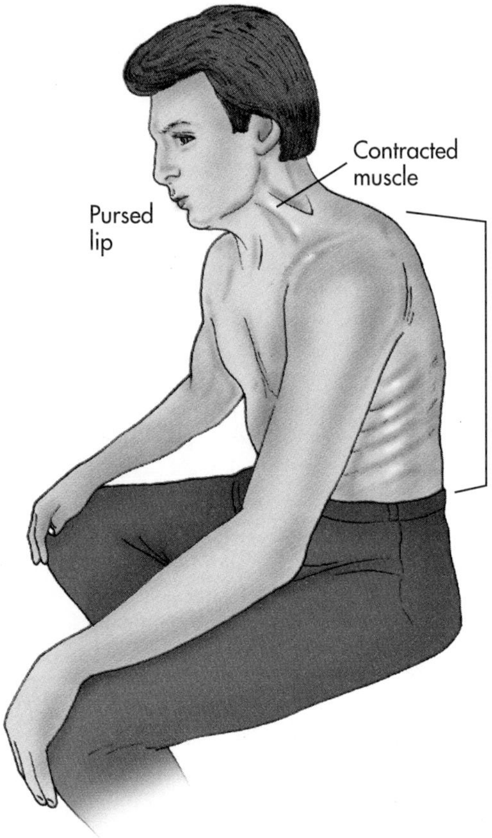

Figure 14-3

Pursed lips and use of accessory muscles reflect a labored effort to breathe.

PULSE OXIMETRY: MEASURING ARTERIAL BLOOD OXYGENATION

The fact that blood changes color from red to blue as the oxygen content increases makes skin appearance a good clinical sign of oxygenation; pink skin suggests good oxygenation, blue (cyanotic) skin suggests poor oxygenation. The pulse oximeter is an electronic device that measures the percentage of oxygen saturation in arterial blood. Saturation is the extent to which oxygen is attached (bound) to available **hemoglobin.**

Almost all oxygen transported in the blood is bound to hemoglobin, although a small fraction travels free, or dissolved, in the blood. Each hemoglobin molecule has four attachment sites for oxygen molecules. A fully saturated hemoglobin molecule, carrying oxygen at all four sites, has a bright red color, the color of normal arterial blood. Fully desaturated hemoglobin (no oxygen attached) is dark blue, the color that causes cyanosis. Venous blood, usually partially saturated, is an in-between color: dark brownish red.

The pulse oximeter shines a red and then a blue light in rapid sequence through an area of tissue, such as a fingertip. It then collects and analyzes the light that reaches the far side of the tissue. Using physical laws of light reflection and absorption, the oximeter's circuitry decides how much of the blood is red, blue, or in between. It then displays a number indicating arterial oxygenation saturation: the percentage of available hemoglobin sites that are carrying oxygen. Oxygen in arterial blood is the true measure of what is available to the tissues.

How do you interpret these readings? In healthy patients who are breathing normally, expect a saturation above 95%. A reading of 90% to 95% indicates a potential developing problem, but not yet an immediate threat to the patient. Below 90%, most patients are hypoxic.

Patients with **chronic obstructive pulmonary disease (COPD)** can be the exception. They sometimes maintain normal saturations as low as 80%. COPD patients below 80% should be considered hypoxic, and they may be in danger at higher levels. Watch clinical signs. (Your training and local protocols should address interpretation of saturation readings in COPD patients in more detail.)

To ensure that the oximeter works correctly, the operator must keep several things in mind. Most important is the machine's pulse signal. Every oximeter has an indicator that shows whether it can detect changes in blood flow with each heart contraction. For an accurate saturation reading, the pulse indicated on the oximeter should be the same as the patient's measured pulse.

Patients in shock or those with hypothermia may have peripheral pulses too weak to allow measurement with an oximeter. Cardiac arrest is the extreme example. Cardiopulmonary resuscitation (CPR) will probably not generate a good pulse signal. Most oximeters provide an audible beep tone to confirm pulse signal without the need to watch the machine's display panel. Leaving this tone turned on may also occasionally give you an early signal of decreasing perfusion.

To ensure appropriate measurements, make sure that the finger clamp closes snugly on the patient's finger. A very loose fit can allow external light to reach the sensor, thereby causing inaccurate measurements.

Other cautions apply to all medical equipment, especially electronic ones. The operator must:

- Value clinical signs above all else.
- Understand the equipment and its limitations.
- Apply common sense to the readings and compare them thoughtfully to the clinical situation.

A number of medical conditions can make oximeter readings inaccurate or make them misleading when they are accurate. Consider these examples:

1. Bleeding and anemia: Both reduce the total amount of hemoglobin in the blood. The hemoglobin present could be well saturated, but there may not be enough of it to deliver sufficient oxygen to the tissues.
2. Carbon monoxide poisoning: Like oxygen, carbon monoxide binds to hemoglobin and turns it red. However, it does not nourish the tissues, so the oximeter generates a falsely elevated measurement. If you suspect carbon monoxide, turn off the oximeter and focus on aggressive, high-concentration oxygen therapy.
3. Other poisons that produce alterations in hemoglobin: A number of other toxic substances bind to hemoglobin and change its color. These poisons reduce oxygen-carrying capacity and produce incorrect oximeter readings. These poisons include:
   - Nitrate compounds (Amyl nitrate is sometimes used as a drug of abuse.)
   - Cyanide
   - Sulfur-containing compounds

   The last two substances are seen most commonly in smoke-inhalation situations.
4. Hypoventilation: A patient breathing inadequately may maintain a good saturation, especially if you give supplemental oxygen. However, carbon dioxide can build up to a level that threatens to disrupt tissue function and threaten organs. Good saturation does not guarantee adequate ventilation.
5. Sickle-cell anemia: Use clinical findings—especially pain complaints—to assess oxygenation, and concentrate on treatment.
6. Other problems: Other situations that may negatively affect oximetry readings include excessive hand motion, jaundiced skin, metal-flake or other unusually opaque nail polishes, and electronic interference (radios, malfunctioning fluorescent lights, or other electronic devices). Your training and the oximeter's operating manual should address these issues more thoroughly.

Using electronic equipment in patient care poses new challenges. If you let it, it can remove you from direct observation of your patient's condition and from direct personal contact with your patient. Here are some final reminders:

1. If the saturation reading is low, act immediately to improve oxygenation.
2. If the reading is high, make sure it is not falsely high. Consider the problems listed above before you agree with the machine.
3. Continue to monitor clinical signs.
4. Keep talking to your patient. Do not let the machine become too important.

generally similar to those for adults. The differences lie principally in sizes and volumes, both of the patient's anatomy and of the equipment the EMT uses. Chapter 26 discusses pediatric breathing issues more fully.

Assessing Specific Respiratory Conditions

Some breathing problems can result from problems in other body systems, such as the circulatory system. When a heart attack occurs, the patient may be struggling to keep up with the increased oxygen demand on the heart. Congestive heart failure (CHF) can be a primary cause of respiratory distress as blood backs up behind the failing heart and causes fluid to build up in the lungs. Other respiratory problems can result from injury or drug toxicity. However, many breathing problems are associated with specific medical conditions that directly affect the respiratory system (Box 14-2).

Table 14-1 presents a comparison chart of signs and symptoms of the various respiratory conditions frequently seen by EMT-Basics. Some of the most common and most serious include:

- COPD (emphysema and chronic bronchitis)
- Asthma
- Respiratory infections (pneumonia, croup, and epiglottitis)
- Pulmonary embolism
- Hyperventilation

BOX 14-2 Conditions Resulting in Respiratory Distress

Medical Conditions

Airway obstruction
Altered mental status
Anaphylaxis
Asthma
Chronic bronchitis
Croup
Drug overdose
Emphysema
Epiglottitis
Heart conditions
Pneumonia
Poisoning
Pulmonary embolism

Injuries

Brain injuries
Burns to the face, neck, and airway
Cervical spine injury
Drowning
Electrocution
Fractured larynx or trachea
Pneumothorax
Rib fractures

Chronic Obstructive Pulmonary Disease

COPD is the fourth leading cause of death in the United States.[1] It is a condition in which air is trapped behind secretions or other obstructions in the bronchioles. This ir-

TABLE 14-1 Differentiating Conditions that Cause Respiratory Distress

Condition	Possible cause	Signs, symptoms	Lung sounds
Asthma	Allergy, stress, infection, exercise	History, nonproductive cough	Wheezing or diminished
COPD	Smoking, smoke exposure	History, productive cough	Often diminished, possible wheezes or coarse crackles (rhonchi)
Pneumonia	Infection	Fever, pleuritic chest pain	Diminished or absent, possible wheezes, crackles, or coarse crackles
Congestive heart failure (CHF)	Heart failure, pulmonary hypertension	Ankle edema, dyspnea on exertion	Crackles, possible wheezes
Croup	Viral infection, laryngeal or tracheal edema	Recent illness and fever, barking cough, younger patient (3 months-3 years)	Upper-airway stridor
Epiglottitis	Bacterial infection, epiglottal edema	Sudden onset, fever, sore throat, no cough, drooling, older child (3-7 years)	Upper-airway stridor
Pulmonary embolus	Venous clot that travels to pulmonary arteries	History, inactivity, rapid breathing and pulse	Normal or diminished in affected area

reversible and deteriorating condition encompasses several different diseases; emphysema and **chronic bronchitis** are the two most common ones. The chronic form of asthma is sometimes also considered to be a COPD, especially in older patients. These diseases are characterized by irreversible airway obstruction and air trapping that compromises the ability of the lungs to exchange oxygen and carbon dioxide. As a result, carbon dioxide is retained and hypoxia develops.

Emphysema is a degenerative disease that begins with the destruction of the alveoli and bronchioles. As the condition worsens, the number of capillaries in the lungs decreases, causing an increased resistance to pulmonary blood flow. This may lead to pulmonary hypertension, right-sided heart failure, and death.

The typical emphysema patient is an older, thin male with a significant history of cigarette smoking. Assessment often reveals a patient who complains of shortness of breath and tightness in the chest. The patient's skin may appear to be flushed. For this reason, the patient is sometimes referred to as a "pink puffer." The chest will appear to be barrel shaped, the result of gradual but continuous air trapping in the lungs. This occurs because the lungs can no longer relax completely. Breath sounds are usually diminished, and **wheezing** and coarse crackles (rhonchi) may be present. The patient breathes with the assistance of well-developed accessory muscles. The lips appear to be pursed, a maneuver that helps maintain pressure in the alveoli.

Chronic bronchitis is another type of COPD. It results from an increase in mucus production, primarily in the bronchioles, that limits adequate ventilation and gas exchange. Chronic bronchitis is associated with prolonged cigarette smoking and exposure to cigarette smoke. Like emphysema, pulmonary hypertension may also develop, leading to right-sided heart failure. The disease is progressive and can be fatal. A patient with chronic bronchitis often appears to be overweight and cyanotic, with a history of frequent respiratory infections and considerable production of sputum. Because of their weight and cyanosis, these patients are sometimes called "blue bloaters."

Asthma

Asthma is a common respiratory condition affecting patients of all ages. Although a chronic condition, in many cases asthma affects a patient only at certain times. An asthma attack can be triggered by infection, stress, exercise, or exposure to allergens. Exercise-induced asthma commonly afflicts both children and adults. Asthma results in excessive mucus production and inflammation and narrowing of the bronchioles (Figure 14-4). As the disease progresses, it can become a life-threatening emergency; some cases of acute asthma are fatal.

Initially, an asthma patient breathes normally upon inhalation as bronchioles open adequately, but wheezing occurs during exhalation through the obstructed air passages. As the asthma attack progresses, the patient may also wheeze during inhalation. In some cases, the wheezing can be so prominent that it can be heard without a stethoscope. In severe cases, wheezing and other breath sounds cease entirely as airways close too tightly to allow significant airflow. Besides the characteristic wheezing, asthma patients will likely be tired from rapid breathing and may have a persistent cough. The cough is often nonproductive (no sputum is produced).

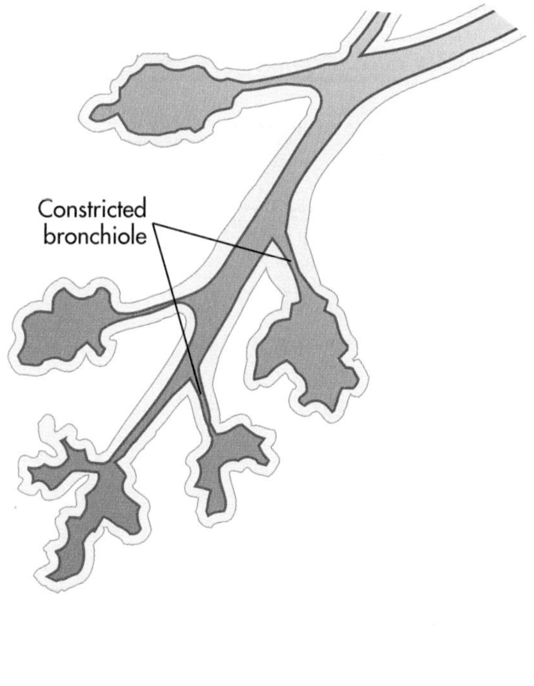

Figure 14-4

Excessive mucus production and inflammation and narrowing of the bronchioles obstructs the asthma patient's airways.

Respiratory Infections

Respiratory infections vary from the common cold that everyone contracts occasionally to more serious conditions such as pneumonia. These infections most often affect children and the elderly. A common cold can cause swelling of the mucous membranes and draining of the sinuses. These effects rarely result in inadequate breathing for adults, but they can be more severe for children because of their narrower airways. Acute respiratory infections are the most common illnesses among children. This is especially true during fall and winter months when the influenza and respiratory syncytial viruses (RSV) are most common. Respiratory infections can also easily affect the elderly and other adults with compromised respiratory status.

Croup and **epiglottitis** are the most common serious respiratory infections among children. These are viral (croup) and bacterial (epiglottitis) infections that result in occlusion of the airway in the area of the epiglottis and larynx. These conditions can result in inadequate oxygenation because of an inability to ventilate properly through the narrowed airways.

Epiglottitis is the more severe of the two infections because the swelling of the epiglottis may be so severe and rapid that it can cause sudden, complete airway obstruction. A patient with epiglottitis often looks very ill, has a high fever and sore throat, and may be drooling because of an inability to swallow. The patient is often sitting up and forward in an attempt to keep the airway open (Figure 14-5).

Although airway obstruction is a serious problem in epiglottitis, it should not discourage the EMT about the possibility of effective treatment. In fact, the airway is rarely occluded completely. The patient is more likely threatened by inadequate breathing and by fatigue from the extra effort of breathing against the obstruction. Generally, allow the patient to sit in the position of most comfort; do not force the patient to lie down. Provide supplemental oxygen by whatever route the patient will tolerate. If the patient has a change in mental status or is unable to breathe unassisted, gently assisting ventilations with bag-valve or mouth-to-mask techniques and supplemental oxygen will nearly always force enough air past the obstruction to maintain minimal oxygenation until further medical care can be obtained. Advanced medical care must be obtained immediately in these situations. Fortunately, with recent immunization programs, epiglottitis occurs much less frequently than in the past.

Croup causes inflammation and swelling of the lining of the larynx and trachea just below the vocal cords. Because this is normally the narrowest point in a child's airway, any swelling can cause some degree of obstruction. The patient often presents with a high-pitched, bark-like cough, an indication of a serious airway problem.

Both croup and epiglottitis present problems related to anatomic airway obstruction, but inability to move adequate air is not the direct threat to the child. The more immediate danger is fatigue. As the child tires from the extra work of breathing through narrowed passages, respiratory effort will begin to decrease and will eventually

RSV . . . WHAT'S IT MEAN TO ME?

Acute respiratory infections are common illnesses among children of all ages. You will likely encounter a larger number of these patients during fall and winter months, when more people stay indoors. Confined indoor air flow increases the chance of disease transmission by airborne infections. One such infection that is present in epidemic proportion during the winter is respiratory syncytial virus, commonly called *RSV.* This highly contagious virus is transmitted by direct and indirect contact with respiratory secretions. Sneezing commonly spreads the disease. Infection occurs when the virus contacts mucous membranes of the upper airway, primarily the nose.

Once the virus enters the body, RSV enters cells in the respiratory tract and matures in about a week, at which time the signs and symptoms begin to appear. Among the most significant symptoms are increased secretions in the airway, sore throat, cough, and low-grade fever. If the disease progresses, the lower airway becomes affected, causing an increase in respiratory rate, the use of accessory muscles, intercostal retractions, nasal flaring, and decreased food and fluid intake. These signs and symptoms can seem similar to pneumonia; RSV is believed to be the cause of nearly half of all cases of pneumonia in young children. Children between 6 weeks and 2 years of age are especially susceptible to the lower-airway complications associated with RSV.

Treatment of advanced stages of RSV includes oxygen therapy, bronchiodilator medications, and fluid replacement. Children with severe disease may have to be hospitalized. The virus is not as severe in adults, but you should still take precautions. Once infected, you also may be able to infect others for as long as 1 month. Keep yourself protected and your equipment clean to help prevent the spread of this disease.

Halpern JS: Respiratory syncytial virus (RSV): a common health problem, *J Emerg Nurs* 18:61, 1992.

Hoekelman RA et al: *Primary pediatric care,* ed 2, St Louis, 1992, Mosby.

Wald E: Respiratory syncytial virus and viral pneumonia. In Blummer J, editor: *A practical guide to pediatric intensive care,* St Louis, 1990, Mosby.

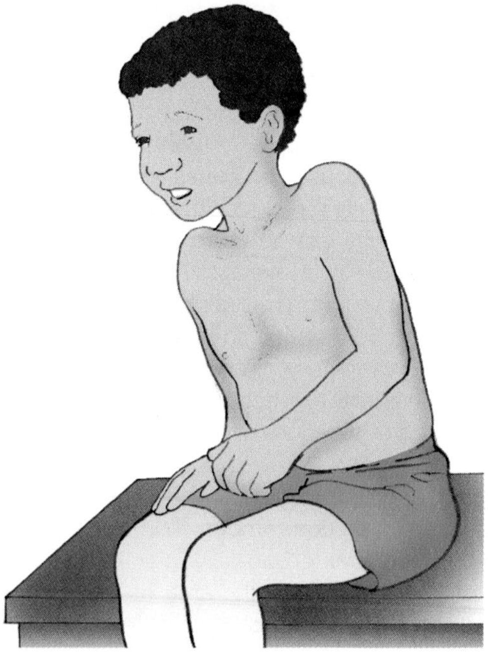

Figure 14-5

Signs of epiglottitis include a high fever, sore throat, drooling, and an upright, forward-leaning posture.

cease. The EMT who recognizes early signs and intervenes with ventilatory support and supplemental oxygen can therefore make a big difference in patient outcome. Additional information on the cause and management of croup and epiglottitis is presented in Chapter 26.

Pneumonia is the sixth leading cause of death in the United States.[1] It afflicts patients of all ages but is especially common in the young, the elderly, and those with HIV. Either a bacteria or a virus can infect a part or all of a lung. The infection results in inflammation and fluid accumulation between the alveoli and the capillaries (Figure 14-6), thereby reducing the ability to exchange carbon dioxide and oxygen efficiently.

A patient with pneumonia often complains of flulike symptoms such as general weakness, fever, and chills. There may also be shortness of breath and chest tightness. Auscultation of breath sounds may reveal wheezes, crackles (rales), or coarse crackles (rhonchi) or sounds may simply be diminished. There is often a deep cough, frequently producing yellow-green sputum.

Trauma

Although they are not medical conditions, injuries can also have a direct effect on the adequacy of breathing. Chest trauma (rib fractures, flail chest, pneumothorax, hemothorax) can affect the respiratory system in two ways. One is interference with normal chest movement during breathing. Pain upon chest motion and disruption of the chest's normal single-unit structure can make the mechanical part of moving air less effective. The other potential effect of chest trauma is interference with gas exchange in the alveoli. This can be caused by reduction in the alveolar surface area available for gas exchange (pneumothorax, hemothorax) or by direct interference with gas exchange (bleeding in or into the lungs).

Injuries to other parts of the body can also influence the adequacy of breathing. Head injuries can affect respiratory drive, which is controlled by the medulla in the brain stem. Spinal cord damage in the cervical spine can interrupt the flow of nerve impulses from the medulla to the respiratory muscles, especially the diaphragm. Injury to the upper airway can cause airway obstruction or bleeding into the airway.

Pulmonary Embolism

A **pulmonary embolism** is the blockage of a pulmonary artery by foreign matter such as fat, air, tumor tissue, or a blood clot. Pulmonary embolism is often associated with prolonged inactivity during fracture immobilization, lengthy travel, recovery from surgery, or blood clotting problems. Some medications, such as birth control pills, predispose patients to blood clots and pulmonary emboli.

A blood clot may form in the large veins of the lower extremities and move through the circulatory system to the right side of the heart, where it is pumped to the lungs through a pulmonary artery. The clot lodges in that artery or in a smaller arterial branch and blocks blood flow to the area of the lung supplied by the occluded vessel (Figure 14-7).

Assessment usually reveals a patient complaining of a sudden onset of unexplained severe dyspnea. There may also be **pleuritic chest pain.** Breathing and heart rate are typically rapid. History may reveal recent hospitalization, prolonged immobilization, or the fact that the patient has stopped using blood thinning medications. Lung sounds may be normal or diminished in the affected area.

Hyperventilation

Hyperventilation is rapid breathing, usually defined as a rate greater than 20 breaths per minute. It can occur in

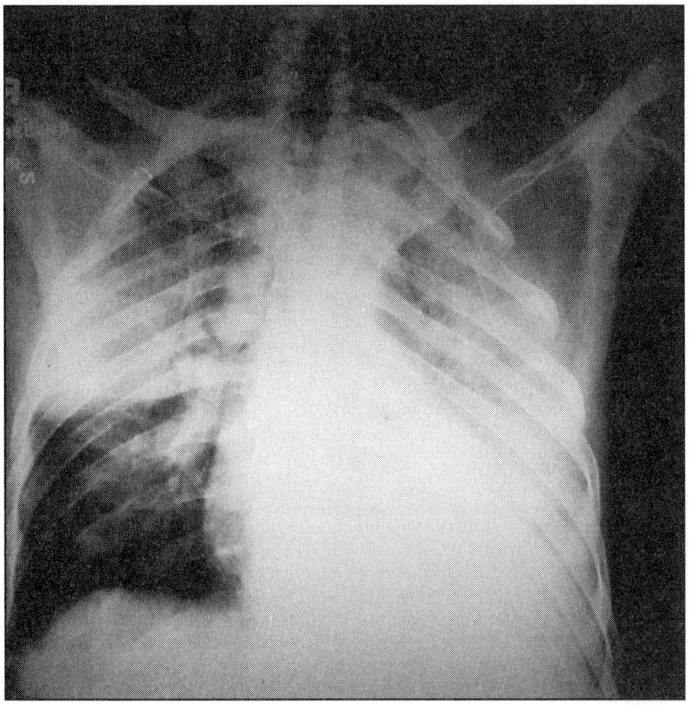

Figure 14-6

This severe case demonstrates replacement of air by fluid in the whiter areas of the radiograph.

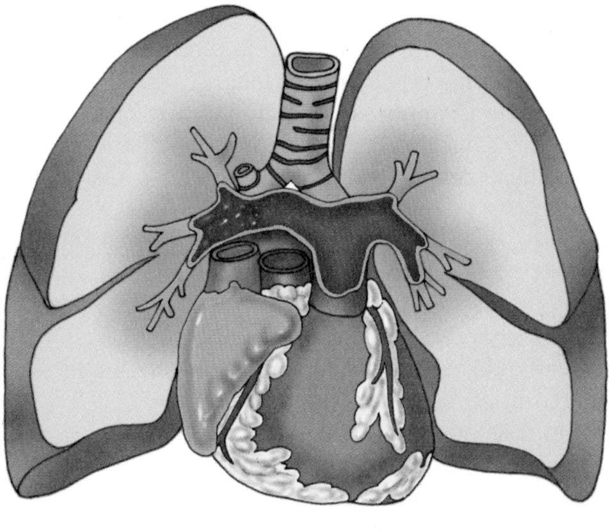

Figure 14-7

A pulmonary embolism occurs when foreign matter, such as a blood clot, lodges in an artery or smaller arterial branch, blocking blood flow.

a patient who has suffered an acute injury or illness, simply because of the anxiety created by the incident. On the other hand, the rapid respirations may be an indicator of the body's increasing need for oxygen because of a serious medical problem.

Hyperventilation is sometimes associated with an isolated emotional event or a buildup of nervous tension. The patient often states, "I can't catch my breath." The rapid breathing causes excess elimination of carbon dioxide and can lead to chest pain, extremity numbness or tingling, or numbness of the tongue or around the mouth. This type of hyperventilation can often be resolved with reassurance and a conscious effort by the patient to control breathing. However, hyperventilation always calls for thorough consideration of the possibility of a serious, underlying medical or trauma problem.

Caring for Breathing Emergencies

The breathing characteristics that you assess will help identify the extent of a patient's respiratory distress and the care you need to provide. An adult patient who is seated upright, cyanotic, diaphoretic, struggling to breathe, and has a respiratory rate of 36 is experiencing

IT'S YOUR CALL
CONTINUED

Your patient has a history of asthma and now is having trouble breathing. Further assessment includes inspection and palpation of the chest and auscultation of lung sounds. The patient has wheezes in all lung fields. Intercostal retractions indicate that he is using accessory muscles during inspiration. Respiratory rate, which had been 36 breaths per minute and labored, is now slow and shallow. He seems to be getting weaker and may be ready to collapse.

As you prepare to provide care, the patient's friend returns with another bronchial inhaler. How will you treat this patient?

BOX 14-3 Treating Respiratory Distress

When caring for a patient experiencing a respiratory emergency:

1. Place the patient in a comfortable position.
2. Ensure that the patient's airway is open and clear of obstructions.
3. Provide supplemental oxygen.
4. Assist ventilations if the patient is unable to breathe effectively.
5. Request ALS assistance according to local protocols.
6. Contact your medical direction physician.
7. Assist the patient with prescribed medications, when appropriate.
8. Transport to a receiving facility without undue delay.

significant respiratory distress. This patient needs ventilatory assistance and may have prescribed medication that you can help administer. On the other hand, a patient who is able to talk in complete sentences, is comfortable in a reclined position, and is not cyanotic or diaphoretic likely has no more than mild respiratory distress and may need only oxygen. The aggressiveness of care will be based on your assessment of the patient's degree of distress. Box 14-3 provides an approach to caring for a patient in respiratory distress regardless of its cause.

Comfortable Position

Most patients experiencing respiratory emergencies prefer to be seated upright because it is easier for them to breathe in that position. You may respond to a respiratory emergency and find a patient lying supine in bed and struggling to breathe. If the patient is able to sit up or can be supported in an upright position, that may lessen the respiratory distress (Figure 14-8). Many patients will have found the most comfortable position for them before you arrive. Ask about comfort level before moving the patient into another position.

Airway Adequacy

Anyone who is able to talk clearly or cry loudly has a clear airway. If the patient is unable to do this, consider the possibility of an airway obstruction. If the airway is obviously obstructed by food or fluid in the mouth, remove the obstruction. Use a gloved hand and suction to remove any obvious loose debris. However, if you suspect an anatomic obstruction caused by swelling from croup or epiglottitis, do not probe the mouth or throat. This could worsen the condition.

Avoid using a suction catheter in the mouth of someone with epiglottitis. This could increase swelling or cause laryngospasm and thus worsen the airway obstruction. Continue to ventilate and provide supplemental oxygen. It will usually be possible to force adequate air past the obstruction until further care can be obtained.

In cases of foreign-body airway obstruction, perform airway-clearing procedures as taught in basic CPR certification (see Chapter 11). Pediatric airway procedures are generally similar to those for adults, but there are important differences. Chapter 26 discusses the pediatric airway.

Oxygenation and Ventilation

Earlier chapters discussed administering oxygen. As a general rule, do not withhold oxygen from a patient with any form of respiratory distress; a patient will only benefit from its administration. Most of your patients should receive oxygen through a nonrebreather mask at a rate of 15 liters per minute (lpm) (Figure 14-9). Patients experiencing only mild distress or those unable to tolerate a mask can receive oxygen through a nasal cannula at approximately 2 to 4 lpm. A young child often does not tolerate a mask covering the face. If it appears that the child will fight the mask, have a parent or other helper hold the mask near the patient's face.

Oxygen administration by itself will not always be adequate. Patients having difficulty moving air, breathing less than 8 or more than 24 times per minute, or breathing too shallowly need breathing assistance with a bag-valve-mask (BVM) or mouth-to-mask technique. Local training and protocols should define when to assist ventilations and administer oxygen, what type of administration device to use, and how much oxygen to provide.

If your patient is unconscious and not breathing, maintain an open airway with the head-tilt–chin-lift or the

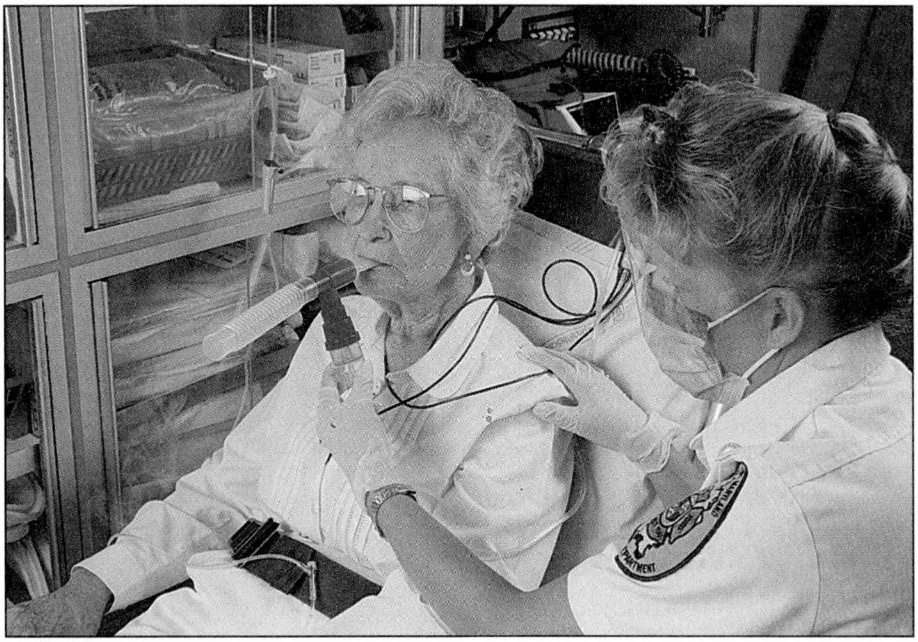

Figure 14-8

Helping a patient into a seated upright position may make it easier for him or her to breathe.

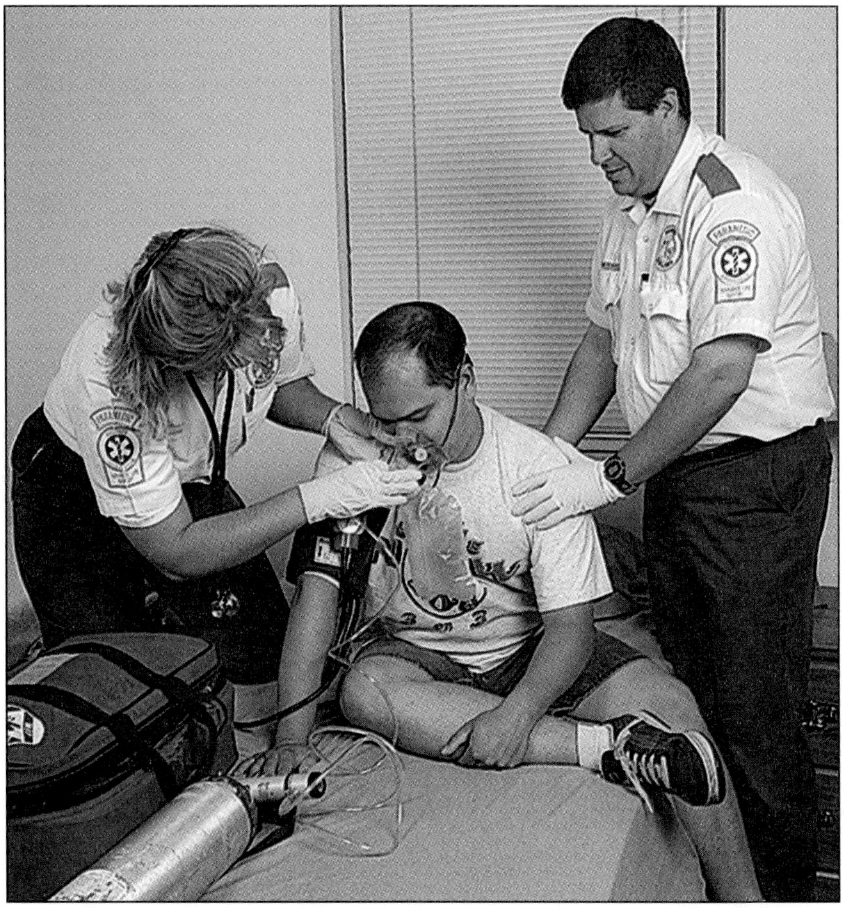

Figure 14-9

It may be necessary to assist some patients with a nonrebreather mask.

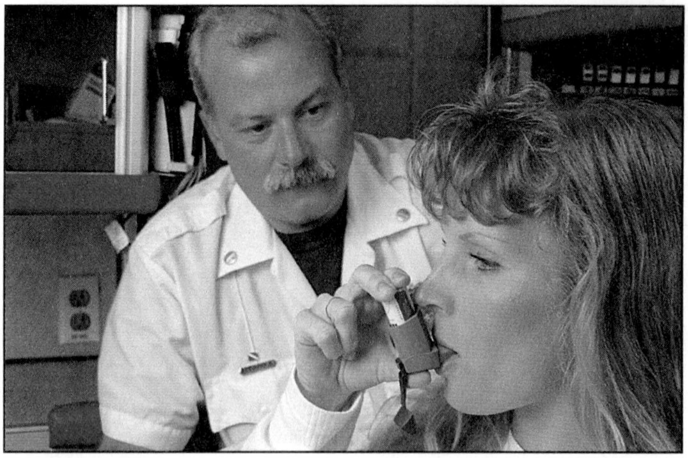

Figure 14-10

Have the patient press the inhaler, inhale slowly and deeply, and hold his or her breath as long as possible before exhaling.

modified jaw thrust. Place an oropharyngeal or nasopharyngeal airway in the patient's mouth or nose to keep the tongue from blocking the airway. Using a BVM or mouth-to-mask breather, ventilate the patient at a rate and depth that approximates normal breathing. This will be one breath every 5 seconds for an adult (12 per minute) and one breath every 3 seconds for a child or infant (20 per minute).

Assisting With Inhalers

Some patients use prescribed bronchial inhalers for specific medical conditions including asthma, emphysema, and chronic bronchitis. A bronchial inhaler is a device used to administer **aerosolized** medication that dilates bronchial tubes, providing better ventilation. A patient with a prescribed inhaler is usually familiar with its use. However, a patient who is anxious or weak may need your assistance to administer the medication (see Chapter 13).

A bronchial inhaler delivers a premeasured amount of medication, referred to as a *metered dose,* with each spray. The normal dose for adults and children is one to two sprays. Albuterol, metaproterenol, and isoetharine are among the most common medications used in bronchial inhalers. Consider the use of an inhaler when:

- The patient's condition meets local protocols for administering a bronchial inhaler during respiratory distress.
- The patient possesses an inhaler prescribed in the patient's name.
- Your medical direction physician approves the procedure.

Avoid assisting with the administration of bronchial inhalers when:

- The patient has someone else's inhaler.
- The patient has taken the maximum prescribed dose or demonstrates side effects such as rapid heart rate, nervousness, or tremors.

IT'S YOUR CALL
CONCLUSION

Given the patient's history of asthma, his belief that this is an asthma attack, and the signs and symptoms revealed in your initial and focused assessments, it is likely that he is suffering an asthma attack. This patient should be treated aggressively by:

- Maintaining/placing him in a comfortable position
- Administering high-concentration oxygen (15 lpm)
- Assisting ventilations with a BVM
- Assisting with the administration of his bronchial inhaler after confirming that it is appropriate in this situation
- Contacting your medical direction physician to approve treatment and offer any additional treatment
- Requesting ALS assistance, if available
- Transporting the patient to the nearest hospital without delay

- The patient is unable to at least assist in using the device.
- Your medical direction physician denies permission.

When helping the patient with inhaler administration, begin by shaking the container. Have the patient exhale forcefully and make a lip seal around the canister opening. If the patient uses a spacer, attach it to the inhaler. A spacer is a reservoir chamber that holds the medication and allows the patient to inhale as much of the delivered dose as possible. Have the patient press the inhaler to activate the spray, inhale deeply, and hold the breath as long as possible before exhaling (Figure 14-10). Resume oxygen therapy. Record the medication name, the time it was administered, and the dose. Reassess the patient and note any change. The medication should quickly provide relief. If the patient's condition does not improve, repeat the dose if your medical direction physician approves it.

SUMMARY

Air should proceed unimpeded through the mouth and nose, pass through the larynx, enter the trachea and main bronchi, and finally arrive in the alveoli for the exchange of oxygen and carbon dioxide with the blood. However, respiratory conditions resulting from disease, injury, infection, and obstruction can disrupt this coordinated activity. Rapid recognition of a patient experiencing inadequate breathing will lead to early treatment. There are many signs of inadequate breathing, but the typical signs are abnormalities in respiratory rate, rhythm, and quality.

A thorough assessment of the patient's respiratory status includes a focused history and physical examination. Obtaining the patient's pertinent medical history will not only help identify the potential cause of the problem but may also reveal a way to resolve it.

The first step in caring for a patient with a breathing emergency is to ensure that the airway is clear. Then administer oxygen and assist ventilations if necessary. If the patient's condition warrants the use of a bronchial inhaler, contact your medical direction physician for approval to assist the patient with the medication.

REFERENCES

1. **National Safety Council:** *Accident facts,* 1995 edition, Itasca, Ill, 1995, National Safety Council.

SUGGESTED READINGS

1. **Angus GE:** *Case studies in prehospital care: adult respiratory emergencies,* St. Louis, 1994, Mosby.
2. **Halpern JS:** Respiratory syncytial virus (RSV): a common health problem, *J Emerg Nurs* 18:61, 1992.
3. **Hoekelman RA et al:** *Primary pediatric care,* ed 2, St. Louis, 1992, Mosby.

Chapter 15
Cardiovascular Emergencies

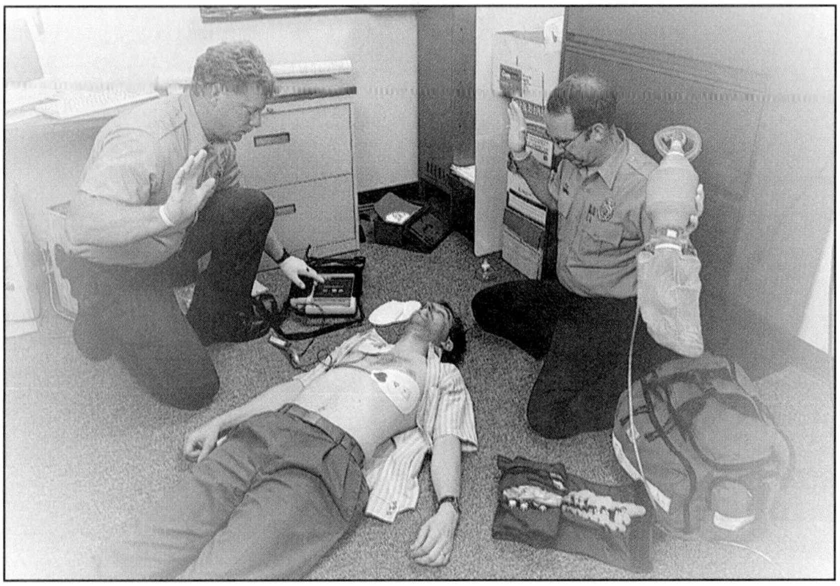

Knowledge Objectives

As an EMT-Basic, you should be able to:

OBJECTIVES

1. Describe the structure and function of the cardiovascular system.
2. Discuss circulatory compromise.
3. Discuss the relationship between angina pectoris and acute myocardial infarction.
4. Describe the process of assessing a patient with chest pain or discomfort.
5. Describe the signs and symptoms of circulatory compromise.
6. Describe how to provide care for a patient experiencing chest pain or discomfort.
7. Describe the mechanism of action, indications, contraindications, side effects, and dosage for nitroglycerin.
8. Explain the circumstances in which it is appropriate to interrupt cardiopulmonary resuscitation (CPR).
9. Explain the need for early defibrillation.
10. List the indications and contraindications for automated defibrillation.
11. List the steps for operating an automated external defibrillator (AED).
12. State the reasons for ensuring that a patient is pulseless and apneic before using an AED.
13. Explain the importance of rapid advanced cardiac life support (ACLS) intervention in patients experiencing chest pain or discomfort or in cardiac arrest.

Skill Objectives

As an EMT-Basic, you should be able to:

OBJECTIVES

1. **Demonstrate how to assess a patient with chest pain or discomfort.**
2. **Demonstrate how to care for a patient with chest pain or discomfort.**
3. **Demonstrate how to check, operate, and maintain an automated external defibrillator.**
4. **Demonstrate how to assess and document a patient's response to the use of an automated external defibrillator.**
5. **Demonstrate how to assist a patient with the administration of nitroglycerin.**
6. **Demonstrate how to complete a prehospital care report for a patient with cardiac emergencies.**

Attitude Objectives

As an EMT-Basic, you should be able to:

1. **Value the importance of early defibrillation for patients in cardiac arrest.**
2. **Serve as a positive role model for other EMS personnel in regard to the assessment and management of a patient with circulatory compromise.**

KEY TERMS

1. **Acute Myocardial Infarction (AMI):** Death of an area of heart muscle; commonly called a *heart attack*.
2. **Angina Pectoris:** Chest pain associated with a cardiac emergency. The pain is caused by inadequate blood supply to the heart muscle.
3. **Asystole:** The absence of electrical activity in the heart; electrical flat line.
4. **Automated External Defibrillator (AED):** An automated device used to recognize lethal dysrhythmias and to defibrillate (shock) a patient's heart. (See *defibrillation.*)
5. **Cardiogenic Shock:** Shock (hypoperfusion) caused by failure of the heart's mechanical (pumping) function.
6. **Circulatory System:** The organs and structures that transport oxygen and other nutrients in the blood to all parts of the body.
7. **Congestive Heart Failure (CHF):** The backup of venous blood returning to the heart when the heart fails to pump as much as it receives; raises venous pressure, which can force fluid into the lungs and other tissues, such as the legs. (See *pulmonary edema.*)
8. **Defibrillation:** The process of delivering an electric shock to the heart in an effort to restore normal electrical and mechanical activity.
9. **Dysrhythmia:** Abnormal electrical rhythm in the heart.
10. **Ischemia:** Lack of oxygen in an area of tissue.
11. **Myocardium:** A thick layer of muscle cells that makes up the majority of the heart wall.
12. **Nitroglycerin:** Cardiac medication used to dilate blood vessels and relieve chest pain.
13. **Pulmonary Edema:** The collection of fluid in the lungs, often caused by rising venous pressure in CHF.
14. **Stroke Volume:** The amount of blood ejected from each of the ventricles with each contraction of the heart.
15. **Ventricular Fibrillation:** A state of disorganized electrical activity in the heart that results in quivering of the heart chambers and loss of effective pumping activity; can sometimes be corrected by defibrillation.
16. **Ventricular Tachycardia:** A rapid contraction of the ventricles; often does not allow the heart chambers to fill completely with blood; can sometimes be corrected by defibrillation.

IT'S YOUR CALL

Dispatched for "chest pain," you arrive to find a female in her mid-70s who is in obvious distress. She has difficulty breathing and severe chest pain that radiates to the shoulder and jaw. She states that she has a history of cardiac problems for which she takes numerous medications including **nitroglycerin.** She also reports that the chest pain came on suddenly, approximately 45 minutes before your arrival, and has become progressively worse.

You take the patient's vital signs and note the following:

Level of consciousness (LOC):	Alert and oriented
Pulse:	100, weak, and irregular
Respiration:	28 and labored; lung sounds are clear and equal bilaterally
Blood pressure:	110/72
Skin:	Moist, pale

A paramedic unit is on the way but will not arrive for about 8 minutes. How are you going to provide care for this patient until the paramedics arrive? What additional information do you need?

Cardiovascular disease affects more than 5,000,000 people annually in the United States and results in more than 600,000 deaths. More than 350,000 of those deaths occur suddenly without any warning signs or symptoms, most of them outside of a hospital.

When a cardiac emergency occurs, circulation can be compromised. Based on observation of the signs and symptoms, you will be able to recognize patients whose problems may be cardiac in nature. These patients need rapid intervention to minimize heart damage and, in some cases, to restore normal cardiac activity.

In this chapter, you will learn how to provide the appropriate initial care for a patient with a cardiac emergency even before the exact cause or degree of the problem is certain. You will review the anatomy and function of the circulatory system and learn about cardiac conditions that could compromise it. You will also learn how to recognize and treat cardiac emergencies. Treatment always begins with basic life support that includes placing the patient in a position of comfort and administering oxygen. In some situations, you will be able to further help the patient by assisting with the administration of medication. If the patient is unconscious, not breathing, and pulseless, you will perform cardiopulmonary resuscitation (CPR). You may apply a device known as an automated external defibrillator (AED), if it is available, in an effort to correct a problem with heart rhythm.

Reviewing Circulatory Anatomy and Function

The **circulatory system** distributes oxygen and other nutrients to all parts of the body and removes waste products such as carbon dioxide. This process occurs when the heart pumps blood through the network of blood vessels. A detailed description of this process appears in Chapter 8. The discussion here reviews the most important elements.

Blood and Blood Vessels

The larger blood vessels, arteries and veins, carry blood throughout the body. Arteries normally carry oxygenated blood away from the heart, while veins return deoxygenated blood to the heart.

Blood leaves the heart through the aorta, off of which branch arteries. As arteries move further away from the heart, they branch into small arterioles and then into even smaller capillaries. Oxygen and other nutrients are transferred to body tissue across the thin capillary walls. Capillaries join together to form venules, which lead to the larger veins. The superior vena cava returns deoxygenated blood to the heart from the upper body, as the inferior vena cava does from the lower body. Both empty into the right atrium (Figure 15-1).

From the right atrium, blood passes through the tricuspid valve into the right ventricle. Blood leaves that ventricle through the pulmonic valve and travels through the pulmonary arteries into the lungs. Oxygenated blood returns to the heart through the pulmonary veins. The lungs are the only place where deoxygenated blood travels in arteries and oxygenated blood travels in veins.

From the lungs, this oxygenated blood enters the left atrium and then passes through the mitral (bicuspid) valve and into the left ventricle. Blood leaves the left ventricle through the aortic valve and enters the aorta for distribution to the body. As the blood leaves the heart, some of it enters the coronary arteries that supply nutrients to the **myocardium** muscle of the heart. Deoxygenated blood

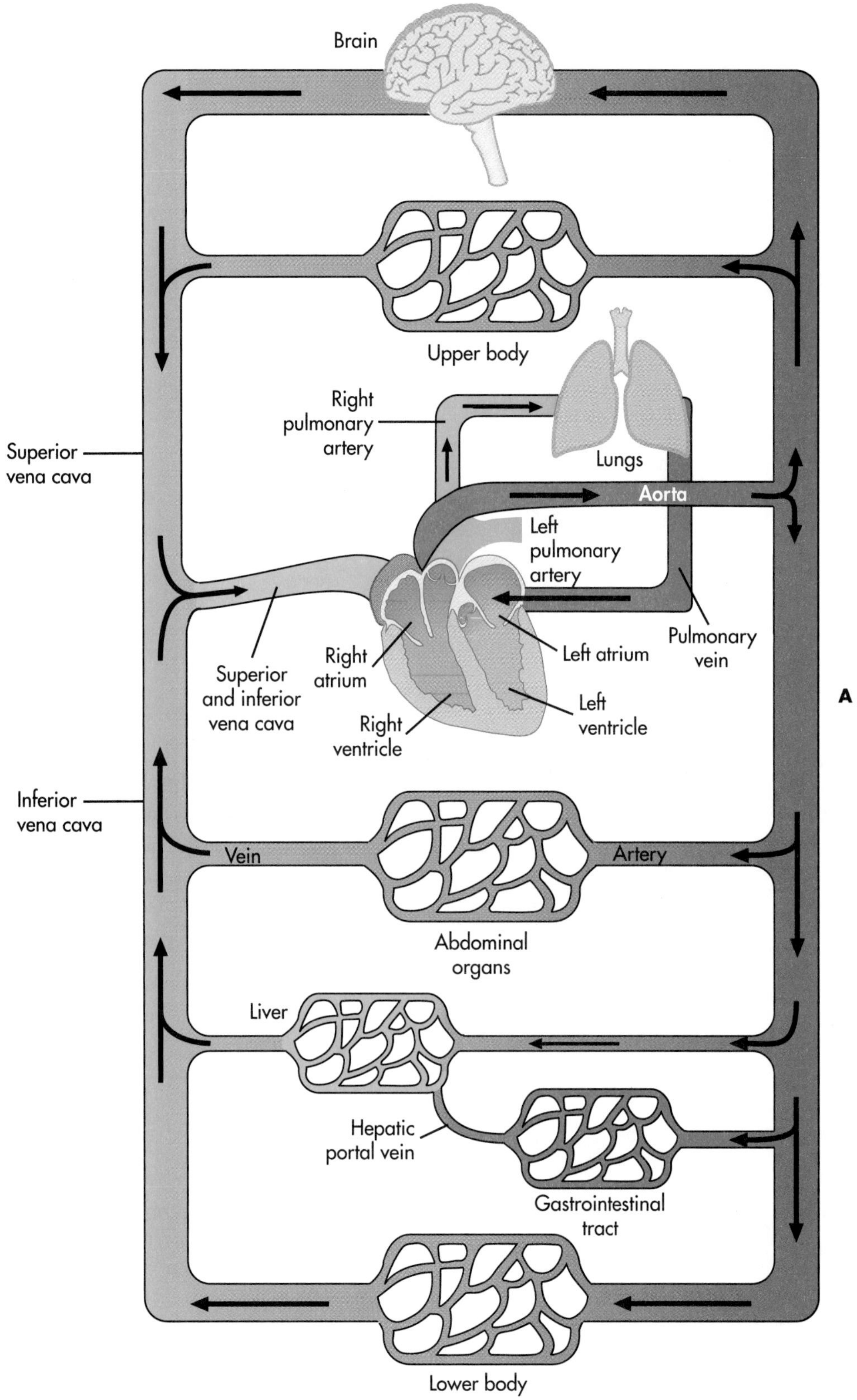

Figure 15-1

A, Blood circulates through a closed system of arteries and veins.

Continued

B

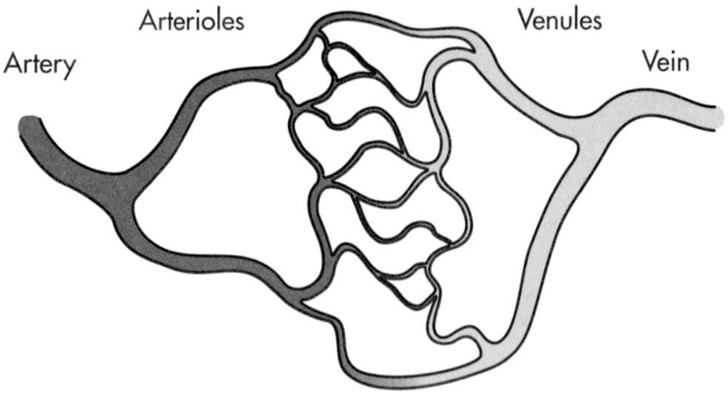

Figure 15-1, cont'd

B, Microcirculation.

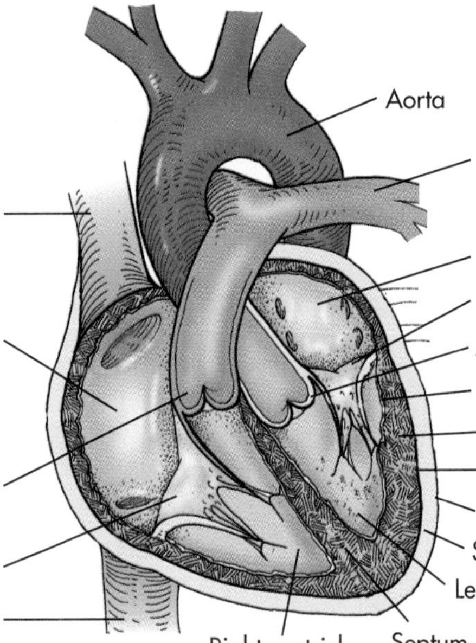

Figure 15-2

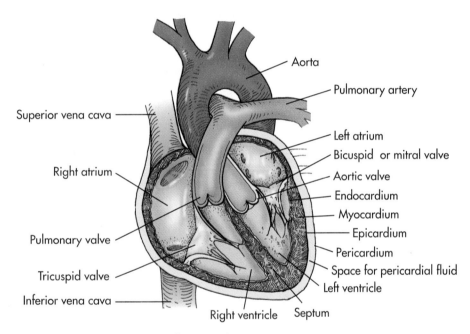

Basic anatomy of the heart.

leaves the heart through the coronary veins, which drain into the right atrium.

The Heart as a Pump

The heart is a muscular organ about the size of a fist, with four chambers and several layers of tissue. The outermost protective layer around the heart is the pericardium. Just under the pericardium is the epicardium, the outermost layer of the heart muscle itself. A small amount of pericardial fluid is present between the pericardium and epicardium. This reduces friction as the heart moves inside the pericardial sac.

Continuing inward, the myocardium is the thick muscle mass responsible for the forceful contractions that eject blood from the heart. The left side is much thicker than the right because it has to force blood throughout the body. The myocardium is the layer most commonly affected during serious heart attacks. The innermost tissue layer, lining the chambers of the heart, is the endocardium (Figure 15-2).

The heart's pumping action results from the coordinated efforts of the atria and ventricles as they contract and relax. The right and left atria contract at the same time, filling the ventricles with blood. The two ventricles also contract at the same time, ejecting blood into the pulmonary arteries and the aorta.

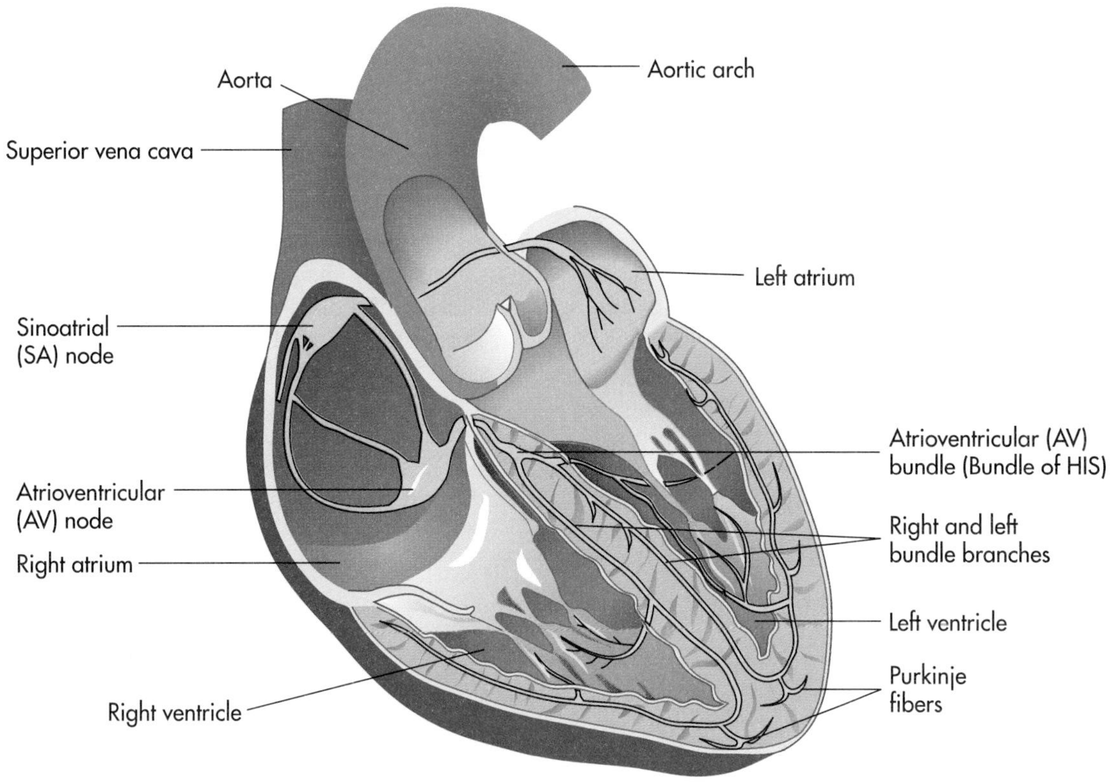

Figure 15-3

Conduction system of the heart, showing the cardiac pacemaker cells.

The amount of blood ejected from each of the ventricles during contractions is referred to as the **stroke volume.** Because the left ventricle is more muscular than the other chambers, it ejects blood more forcefully. In both ventricles, the amount of blood pumped and the strength of pumping depend on how much blood returns through the veins. Think of the heart as a giant rubber band. Increased blood return stretches the muscle fibers further, and they contract with more force.

When the heart works harder, as it does during physical exertion, the demand for oxygen and blood flow increases. A healthy heart will be able to meet this demand. The coronary arteries dilate to supply more blood to the heart muscle itself, and the heart rate increases. However, if heart disease causes a blockage in the coronary arteries, blood flow may not meet the demands on the heart. This blockage is commonly called atherosclerosis. The patient may experience chest pain when the heart needs more blood than the coronary arteries can deliver.

Electrical Activity of the Heart

The heart's ability to circulate blood depends on its electrical system (also called the *conduction system*). The electrical system's proper function is crucial to effective pumping. Specialized cardiac cells have unique electrical properties that allow for the rapid generation, transmission, and reception of electrical impulses. When one cell is excited, others nearby are also excited in a manner that ensures coordinated muscle contraction and good blood flow. The heart's unique ability to generate its own electrical impulses, independent of commands from the brain, is called automaticity.

You can think of the conduction system as a pathway of cells through which electrical impulses travel (Figure 15-3). These impulses originate at special points called *pacemaker cells,* which are cells with the property of automaticity that spontaneously produce electrical impulses and feed them into the network. Healthy pacemakers operate rhythmically. The pacemaker that usually controls heart rate and rhythm (the sinoatrial [SA] node) fires naturally at a rate of 60 to 100 times per minute, the normal heart rate at rest. The conduction system also has backup pacemakers in case the normal mechanism fails. The backups usually fire at slower rates.

A heart monitor allows a trained technician to analyze electrical activity in the conduction system. The electrocardiogram (ECG; also often called *EKG*) is a tracing on paper or on an electronic screen that illustrates electrical activity during the heart's working and relaxing phases. Electrical disturbances in the heart produce abnormal cardiac rhythms called **dysrhythmias.** Illness, injury, lack of oxygen, and numerous kinds of chemical imbalances can cause these disturbances.

The most common lethal dysrhythmia is **ventricular fibrillation.** It is present in approximately two thirds of all adult patients who suffer cardiac arrest. Ventricular fibrillation is a state of completely disorganized electrical activity that makes the heart chambers quiver (fibrillate). The quivering will not make the chambers contract, so the heart does not pump blood or produce a pulse. This dysrhythmia appears as a chaotic, irregular waveform on the ECG (Figure 15-4).

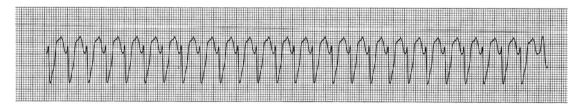

Ventricular tachycardia is another life-threatening dysrhythmia. The term *tachycardia* means rapid heart rate. Ventricular tachycardia is a rapid contraction of the ventricles. Because the rate is so fast, the heart chambers are unable to fill completely and usually cannot generate adequate cardiac output. Occasionally, the heart is temporarily able to compensate for the rapid rate. There may be a pulse, and blood pressure can even be adequate; however, this is unusual, and the compensation will not continue indefinitely. At some point the pulse is likely to disappear. Ventricular tachycardia is characterized by rapid, regular, wide spikes on the ECG (Figure 15-5). It usually occurs in the presence of myocardial **ischemia** or significant heart disease.

If these lethal ventricular rhythms are not corrected quickly, they will deteriorate into a less correctable dysrhythmia called **asystole.** Asystole is the absence of any electrical activity. It appears as a flat-line ECG (Figure 15-6). This is considered a terminal rhythm, indicating a dead heart that is unlikely to be resuscitated. Because

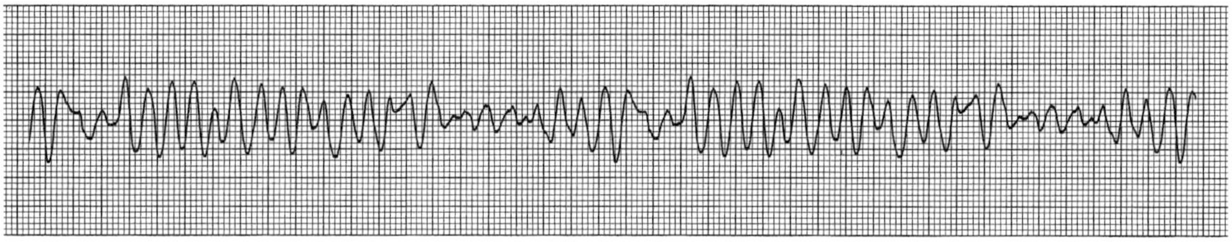

Figure 15-4

Ventricular fibrillation.

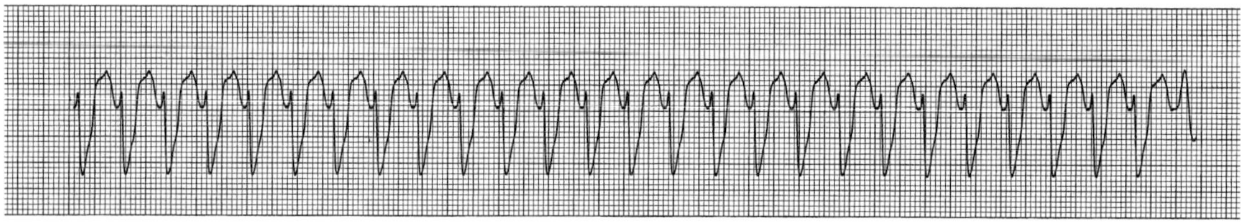

Figure 15-5

Ventricular tachycardia.

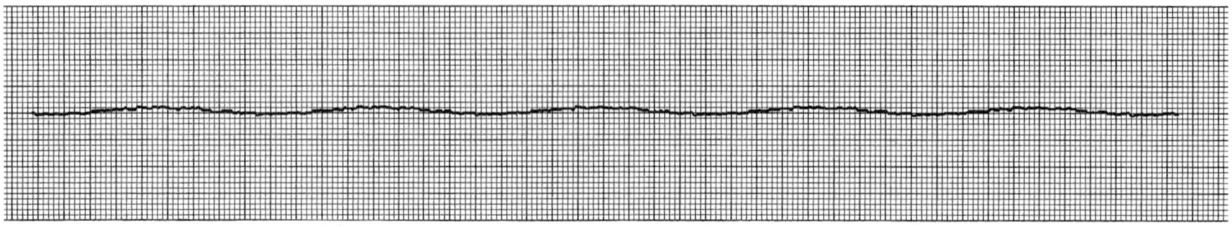

Figure 15-6

Asystole.

there is no electrical activity, no blood is pumped from the heart and the patient will always be pulseless.

Although you are not expected to identify dysrhythmias in the field, it is important to know that the common causes of cardiac arrest are ventricular rhythms, which can sometimes be corrected with prompt delivery of an electrical shock **(defibrillation).** Defibrillation will be discussed on p. 337.

It is equally important to understand that the ECG only measures the heart's electrical activity, not its mechanical (pumping) function. There may be electrical activity on a monitor, but you must assess clinical signs to ensure that perfusion is adequate. Clinical signs include level of consciousness (LOC), pulse, blood pressure, and skin signs. When caring for a patient who may be having a serious heart problem, assess these signs every few minutes.

Understanding Compromised Circulation

Several conditions can compromise circulation. A significant problem occurs when there is inadequate oxygenated blood circulating throughout the body. This could result from the heart's failure to pump effectively, from inadequate blood volume, or from a blockage that impairs blood flow. Any condition associated with the insufficient delivery of oxygen and nutrients necessary for normal tissue and cellular function is known as *shock* (hypoperfusion). Chapter 22 discusses the different types of shock in detail.

Specific Cardiovascular Conditions

Among patients with cardiovascular disease, compromised circulation may result from atherosclerosis, a blockage in a coronary artery supplying the heart with oxygenated blood (Figure 15-7). It could also be caused by dysrhythmias, inadequate blood volume, or failure of either of the ventricles to pump adequately.

Angina Pectoris

If the heart is deprived of oxygen for more than a few seconds, the patient will usually complain of chest pain. The specific character of the pain varies with the patient. It is often described as a crushing or squeezing substernal pain, like a heavy weight being placed on the chest. It may radiate into the back, shoulder, arm, or jaw. Exertion, excitement, stress, and anxiety can increase cardiac oxygen demand and cause pain if the vessels cannot meet that demand. In addition to vessel blockage, vessels may also spasm (contract) and cause decreased blood flow; however, spasms occur less frequently than blockages.

In either case, the condition producing the pain is **angina pectoris,** commonly called *angina.* It usually indicates the presence of cardiovascular disease. When the patient ceases activity or reduces stress, the pain often subsides. Nitroglycerin is a medication used to alleviate the pain by dilating blood vessels and increasing the flow of oxygenated blood to the heart muscle. You will review the use of nitroglycerin later in this chapter.

Acute Myocardial Infarction

If a coronary artery becomes blocked to the point of compromising blood flow to a particular area of the heart, the tissue in that area can die. Heart muscle death is called **acute myocardial infarction (AMI),** or more commonly, a *heart attack* (Figure 15-8). In most cases, the damage is to the left ventricle. Because it is the largest and thickest chamber, it requires the most oxygen. Damage to this area can cause pain, cardiac dysrhythmias, and impaired pumping activity. The pain associated with AMI is often severe and is not relieved by rest.

For some patients, blood circulation to the heart is impaired to the point that the heart is unable to pump

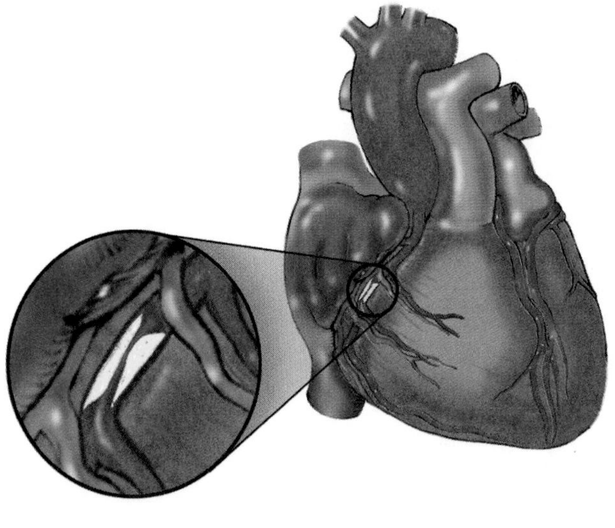

Figure 15-7

Blockage in a coronary artery can cause compromised circulation and damage myocardial tissue.

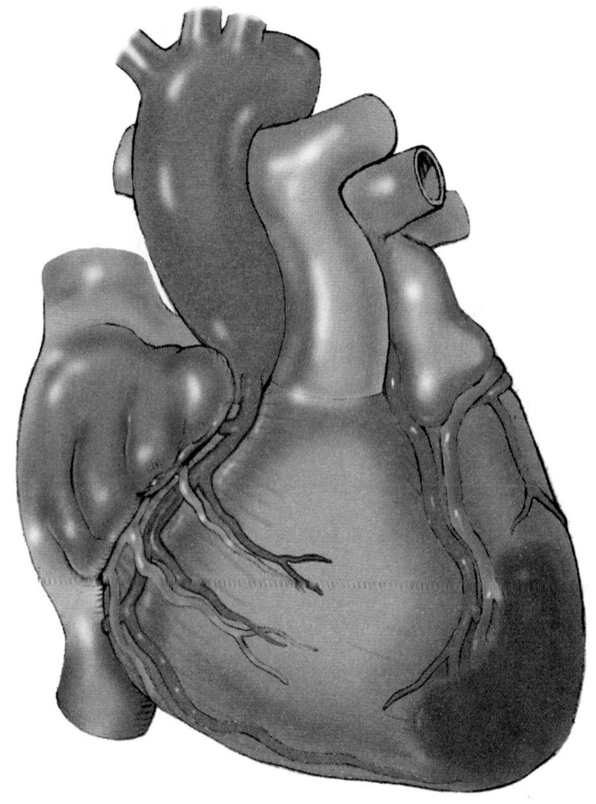

Figure 15-8

Acute myocardial infarction (heart attack) occurs when the heart muscle tissue dies due to compromised blood flow.

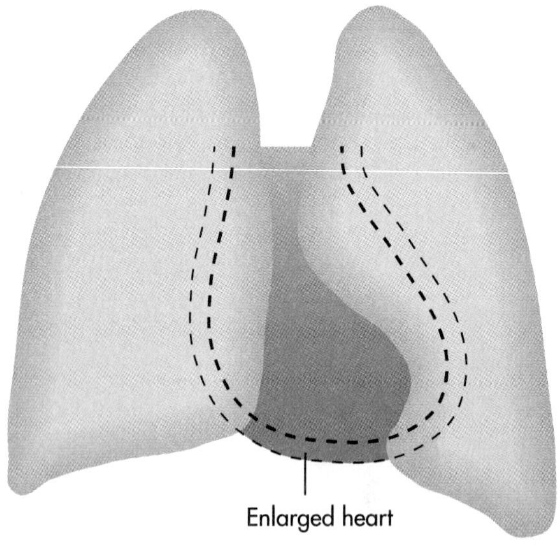

Figure 15-9

In cases of congestive heart failure, the heart muscle becomes enlarged and lung capacity is impaired.

enough blood to deliver adequate circulating blood volume to the body. This serious condition is known as **cardiogenic shock.**

Congestive Heart Failure (CHF)

The heart attempts to deal with disease that threatens circulation in several ways. It does this by beating faster, increasing the force of contractions, and increasing the size of the left ventricle to pump more blood. If these adjustments are ineffective, **congestive heart failure (CHF)** can develop. CHF gets its name from the backup of blood, usually in the pulmonary veins, as the left ventricle fails to pump as much blood as it is receiving.

As the blood accumulates in the pulmonary veins, the pressure in the pulmonary capillaries increases to a point where fluid passes through the walls of the capillaries and into the alveoli (Figure 15-9). This is the condition called **pulmonary edema.** With increased fluid buildup, the lungs become less able to exchange gases and the patient feels short of breath. Auscultation of breath sounds may reveal crackles or wheezing. A patient with CHF is usually unable to lie down because this increases breathing difficulty by spreading fluid over a greater area inside the lungs. CHF patients often also have peripheral edema, particularly in the ankles, because of the backup of pressure in the venous system.

Recognizing Compromised Circulation

When circulation is compromised, the body tries to preserve blood flow to vital organs such as the heart and brain. It does this by increasing the heart rate and the force of contractions and by redistributing blood flow from noncritical organs (the skin, skeletal muscles, and abdominal organs) to more vital ones. These are temporary measures to maintain adequate blood flow to the important organs of the body. Because there is less blood flowing to peripheral areas, the skin becomes pale, cool, and moist. If blood flow to the brain is impaired, the patient's LOC is altered.

Over time, the force of contractions and the amount of blood circulated decrease. Blood pressure drops, and perfusion of vital organs becomes inadequate. **Perfusion** is the circulation of blood to the tissues, delivering nutrients and removing wastes. At this stage, circulation is significantly compromised. As the heart becomes ischemic, a variety of other signs and symptoms emerge:

- Chest pain or discomfort, often described as a squeezing or crushing sensation that may radiate to the arms, back, neck, or jaw
- Weakness
- Difficulty breathing
- Sweating
- Dysrhythmias (as indicated by a pulse that is irregular or very rapid or slow)
- Abnormal vital signs (LOC, pulse, respiration, skin signs, blood pressure)

Patient Assessment

As with other situations, start with the initial assessment to check for and correct any immediately life-threatening problems such as absent pulse or breathing. Once this check is complete, conduct the focused history and physical examination of the medical patient. This entails gathering important past and present medical history, establishing baseline vital signs, and doing a rapid physical assessment. During transport, you may have time to do a more detailed physical examination.

As you assess a patient with compromised circulation, you are likely to find variations in normal vital-sign measurements, including:

- LOC: If the heart fails to provide sufficient oxygenated blood flow to the brain, the result will be an altered LOC. The patient may feel faint or light-headed, become confused or combative, or lose consciousness.
- Pulse: Check both central (carotid) and peripheral (radial) pulses. The absence of a radial pulse while the carotid pulse is present indicates impaired circulation. The pulse could also be irregular, slow, rapid, or weak. Identify pulse rate in one of the following three standard categories:

  Slow (bradycardia): less than 60 beats per minute
  Normal: 60 to 100 beats per minute
  Fast (tachycardia): more than 100 beats per minute

- Respiration: It is common for a patient who is having a heart problem to experience some change in respiration. As the demand for oxygen increases, the patient will begin to breathe faster. Some patients may gasp for air. If the lungs are filling with fluid, as with CHF, there may be rapid, deep gasping. If the pain is severe or breathing worsens the pain, breathing may become shallow.
- Skin: Skin color, temperature, and moisture can also indicate compromised circulation. Pale or cyanotic skin indicates poor perfusion. The patient may also be sweating because of a sympathetic nervous system response.
- Blood pressure: When combined with assessment of pulse, skin signs, and LOC, blood pressure can help confirm suspected circulation problems. However, dropping blood pressure is a late sign of compromised circulation. It may still appear to be high or normal if the patient has a history of hypertension (high blood pressure). History of what is normal for a particular patient is therefore an important part of a blood pressure assessment.

Several other signs and symptoms should alert you to the potential for a serious cardiac emergency. The most important symptom is chest pain or discomfort. If the patient is complaining of pain or discomfort, try to qualify it using the OPQRST format (see Chapter 9):

Onset: What were you doing when the pain began?
Provokes: Is there anything you can think of that might have caused the pain or that makes it worse?
Quality: Can you describe the pain (sharp, dull, throbbing)?
Radiation: Does the pain spread anywhere else in your body, such as the arm or jaw?
Severity: How bad is the pain on a scale of 1 to 10, with 10 being the worst you have ever experienced?
Time: When did the pain first begin? Has it changed since it started?

Caring For a Patient With Compromised Circulation

Timely intervention may dramatically change the outcome for a patient with compromised circulation. If the initiation of proper treatment is delayed until the patient arrives at the emergency department, permanent damage may already have occurred. You should call for advanced life support (ALS) personnel, if they are available, as soon as you recognize that the patient is experiencing circulatory compromise, including chest pain. If you are able to begin transporting the patient before ALS personnel arrive, coordinate a location where they can meet you on the way. If ALS is not available, begin transport to the hospital as soon as possible.

Caring for a patient with cardiac problems always begins with basic life support measures and then continues to more advanced care. The steps include:

- Controlling blood loss
- Positioning the patient properly and maintaining body heat
- Administering oxygen
- Relieving pain
- Circulating blood mechanically (CPR)
- Correcting dysrhythmias

Controlling Blood Loss

Control any external bleeding by applying direct pressure to the site of a wound or to a nearby pressure point. Other methods of hemorrhage control are discussed in Chapter 22.

Positioning and Body Warmth

As soon as possible, the patient should be placed on a stretcher in a position that is comfortable and that helps improve circulation; the patient should not be allowed to walk any distance, particularly to the ambulance. The preferred position is often supine or semi-Fowler (Figure 15-10). Once positioned, the patient should be kept warm to decrease energy needs.

Oxygenation

Oxygen is indicated for any patient with a circulatory problem. As the heart works harder, the demand for oxygen increases. Besides satisfying myocardial oxygen demand, supplemental oxygen can help meet the increased oxygen needs in other organs and tissues. Administer the highest concentration of oxygen possible. This usually

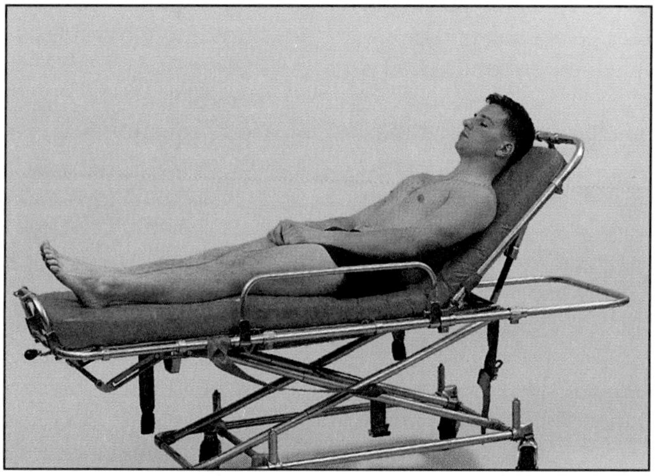

Figure 15-10

The semi-Fowler's position may be comfortable for patients with compromised circulation.

means 15 liters per minute (lpm) through a nonrebreather mask. If the patient is experiencing significant difficulty breathing, as evidenced by respiratory rate and quality, assist breathing with positive-pressure ventilation. This can be done with a bag-valve-mask (BVM) and oxygen reservoir.

Relieving Pain

Nitroglycerin is a medication commonly used to relieve cardiac chest pain. By relaxing the smooth muscle in blood vessel walls, it causes the coronary vessels to dilate, increasing the blood flow and oxygen to the heart muscle. This action may produce some relief from the ischemic pain.

If local protocols allow (Box 15-1), you can assist a patient in the administration of prescribed nitroglycerin. Check the name of the medication, the patient's name, and the expiration date. Also check blood pressure. Systolic pressure should be above 100 mm Hg or the level indicated in your protocol. If required by local protocol, contact your medical direction physician for approval to assist with the medication.

BOX 15-1 Sample Nitroglycerin Protocol

Assist the patient with nitroglycerin administration if:

- Patient reports symptoms of chest pain similar to previous angina episodes.
- Nitroglycerin is prescribed in the patient's name.
- Nitroglycerin is within expiration date.
- Systolic blood pressure is greater than 100 mm Hg.
- Medical direction physician approves the request.

The medication, either a nitroglycerin tablet or a metered-dose spray, is placed in the patient's mouth. A tablet is placed sublingually (under the tongue), while the spray can be given sublingually or on the cheek lining (Figure 15-11, *A* and *B*). Some patients wear a nitroglycerin patch on the chest; this is not something an EMT assists with.

Nitroglycerin usually begins to work within a few minutes. Protocols normally call for the administration of a dose every 5 minutes to a maximum of three doses, as long as the pain continues and the patient's systolic blood pressure remains above 100 mm Hg. When the nitroglycerin is still potent, patients often report a headache and a tingling or burning sensation in the mouth. Because blood pressure may drop after administering nitroglycerin, place the patient in a seated or semi-Fowler position before giving the medication.

Reevaluate the patient's vital signs every few minutes after the administration of nitroglycerin. Document the time that the medication is administered and the response (i.e., whether the medication reduced the pain and whether vital signs changed). If the pain is not relieved after three doses, the patient should be assumed to have a more serious cardiac emergency, such as an AMI.

It is possible that the pain is not from a cardiac emergency. Sometimes chest pain associated with respiratory problems can mimic the pain of a heart attack. However, this often cannot be determined until after evaluation at the hospital. For your treatment, assume that the cause is cardiac.

Maintaining Circulation

If the patient's condition deteriorates to the point of unconsciousness, apnea, and pulselessness, you must circulate blood for the patient. This is done by performing CPR. Even under the best of circumstances, CPR only generates about one third the normal blood flow. How-

A

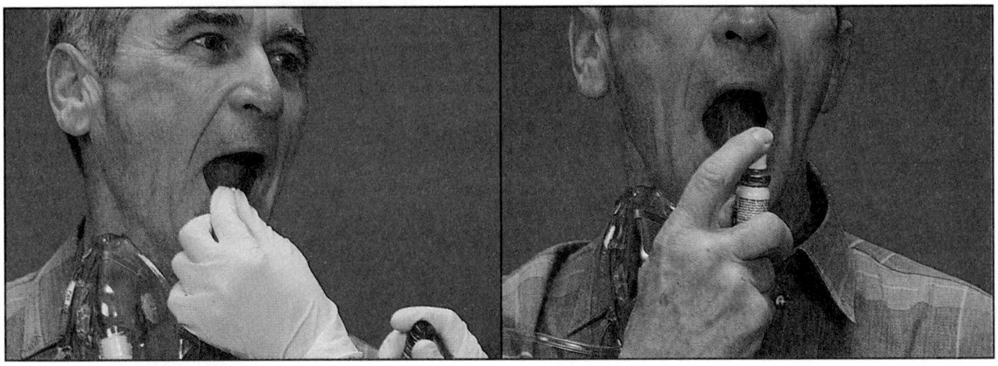

B

Figure 15-11

A, Administering nitroglycerin tablets. **B,** Administering nitroglycerin spray.

IT'S YOUR CALL
CONTINUED

From your patient's medical history and description of pain, you believe she has a cardiac problem. Additional information that you need includes whether the patient took her nitroglycerin before your arrival. If so, how many doses did she take, and was the medication current or expired? If the patient placed the pill under her tongue, check to see if it has dissolved and ask if she experienced any of the normal side effects such as tingling or headache.

The care you provide until the ALS unit arrives includes administering oxygen at 15 lpm through a nonrebreather mask, helping the patient into a comfortable position, and contacting medical direction for approval to assist the patient with nitroglycerin, if allowed by local protocol. If ALS assistance is not available, begin transporting the patient to the hospital as soon as possible.

As you are on the radio discussing the patient's condition with hospital staff, the patient suddenly gasps for breath and loses consciousness. Your partner's attempt to arouse the patient is unsuccessful. Breathing and pulse are assessed and both are found to be absent. Faced with this sudden change in the patient's condition, how will you provide care?

ever, done properly and started early, CPR can provide the patient a chance for survival. CPR can help keep the heart fibrillating longer, increasing the chance that a defibrillator can be used to correct the dysrhythmia and return the heart to a perfusing rhythm. Usually, CPR by itself will not restore normal cardiac activity.

Whether you are performing one- or two-person CPR, the object is to provide the patient with oxygen and compress the chest to circulate oxygenated blood to the heart and brain. What follows is a brief overview of CPR procedures. An approved CPR-certification course teaches the details and the techniques of CPR procedures.

Open the airway and check breathing. After determining the absence of breathing, provide two slow ventilations. Check the carotid artery for a pulse. If the pulse is absent, prepare to perform CPR. To perform CPR effectively, expose the patient's chest. The correct position for your hands on an adult patient is over the lower half of the sternum. Place two fingers on the xiphoid process at the lower end of the sternum. Place the heel of your other hand on the sternum, just above the two fingers. Apply pressure to the sternum with the heel of your hand. Remove your fingers from the xiphoid process and place this hand on top of the hand already on the sternum (Figure 15-12). This position minimizes the risk of injuring internal organs by breaking ribs or the xiphoid process.

Kneel close to the patient's side with your hands on the chest. Straighten your arms at the elbows so that they are directly over the sternum. Press straight down. Compress the chest of an adult 1 to 1½ inches and allow your hands to return to the original position. Do this 15 times before giving two breaths if performing one-person CPR or five times before one breath if performing two-person

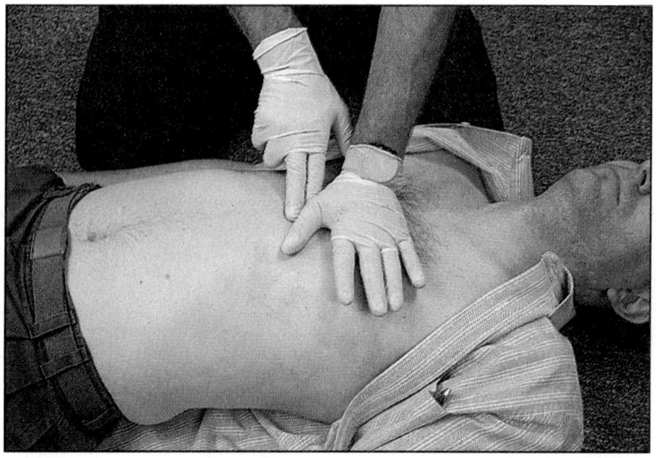

Figure 15-12

To find the correct hand placement for adult CPR, place two fingers over the xiphoid process. Place the heel of the other hand just above those two fingers.

CPR. For a child or infant, you do not need to compress the chest as deeply as you do for an adult. Also, you will only use the heel of one hand for a child (Figure 15-13, *A*), or two to three fingers for an infant (Figure 15-13, *B*). Table 15-1 provides a comparison of hand placement, depth of compression, and compression and ventilation ratios for adults, children, and infants.

Once you start CPR, you should continue as long as the patient is in cardiac arrest or until:

- You become exhausted and can no longer continue.
- Another rescuer takes over CPR.
- The patient regains a pulse.
- A defibrillator is applied to the patient.
- ALS personnel ask you to stop CPR during a procedure.
- In some EMS systems, after CPR and defibrillation have been unsuccessful, your medical direction physician may instruct you to stop resuscitation.

Correcting Dysrhythmias

While CPR provides a mechanical means of circulating small amounts of blood, it does not correct the underlying

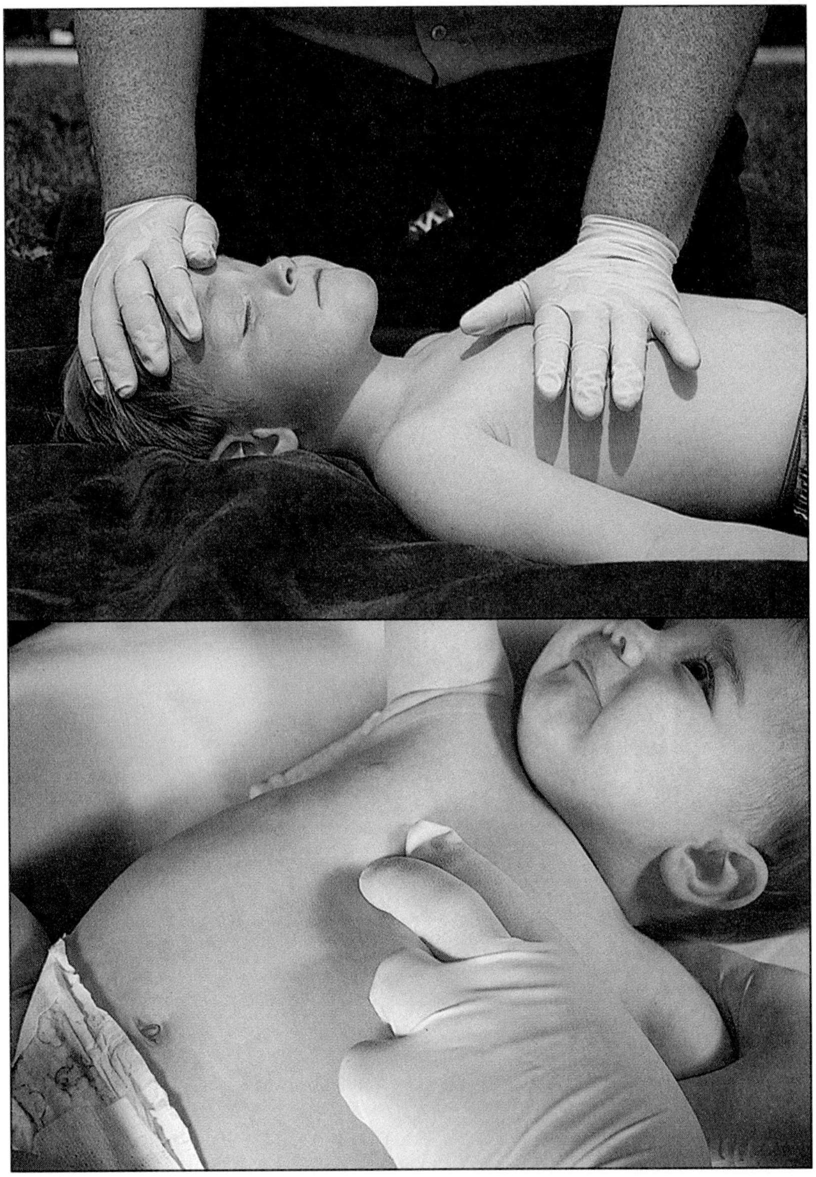

Figure 15-13

A, Only use the heel of one hand when doing chest compressions on a child. **B,** Two or three fingers should be used for infant chest compressions.

TABLE 15-1 CPR for Adults, Children, and Infants

Action	Adult (over age 8)	Child (1-8 yrs)	Infant (birth-1 yr)
Assess responsiveness	Tap and shout.	Tap and shout.	Tap and shout.
Airway	Tilt head and lift chin.	Tilt head back (not as far as adult's) and lift chin.	Tilt head back (not as far as child's) and lift chin.
Breathing	Look, listen, and feel for breathing. Pinch nose and cover mouth. Give two slow breaths (about 1.5 sec each).	Look, listen, and feel for breathing. Pinch nose and cover mouth. Give two slow breaths (about 1.5 sec each).	Look, listen, and feel for breathing. Cover mouth and nose. Give two slow breaths (about 1.5 sec each).
Circulation	Check carotid pulse. Use two hands to compress chest 15 times. Compress 1½-2 in; 80-100 compressions per min.	Check carotid pulse. Use one hand to compress chest 15 times. Compress 1-1½ in; 80-100 compressions per min.	Check brachial pulse. Use two fingers to compress chest five times. Compress ½-1 in; at least 100 compressions per min.
Cycles	15 compressions and two breaths; if two-rescuer CPR, five compressions and one breath.	Five compressions and one breath.	Five compressions and one breath.

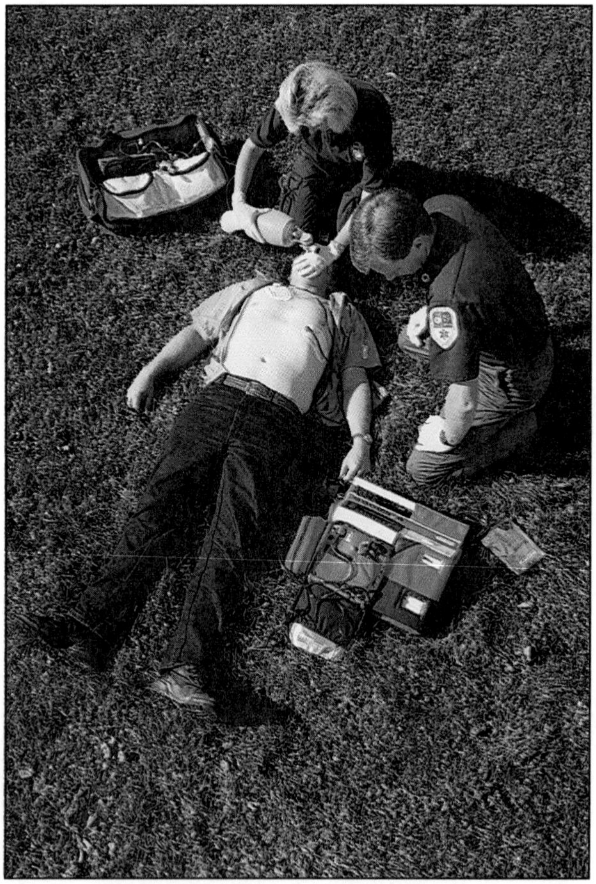

Figure 15-14

An automated external defibrillator.

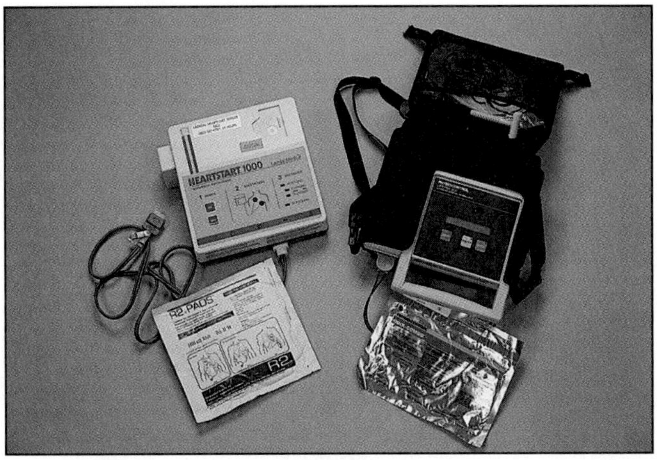

Figure 15-15

Different models of AEDs.

dysrhythmia that may be causing the problem. To correct these electrical rhythm disturbances, the patient needs early defibrillation. Research has proved defibrillation to be the element that can make the greatest difference in the survival of cardiac arrest patients. Defibrillation is the delivery of an electric shock to the heart in an attempt to stop the ineffective electrical activity of the heart and restore normal pumping function. The development of automated defibrillators has enabled EMTs, first responders, and lay people to bring this life-saving treatment to patients more rapidly (Figure 15-14).

Automated External Defibrillation

Learning to interpret ECGs and use a manual defibrillator is time consuming and expensive. To enable more people to deliver defibrillation in cardiac arrests, **Automated External Defibrillations (AEDs)** were created (Figure 15-15). AEDs interpret a patient's heart rhythm and deliver a defibrillation shock automatically, if appropriate. While some machines display a tracing of the patient's rhythm on a screen, you will not need to interpret that tracing. The device will analyze the rhythm with internal computer circuitry. Your job, once the device has been applied, is to follow the instructions provided by the AED.

An AED is a combination of a monitor that analyzes cardiac rhythm and a defibrillator that can deliver a shock. AEDs are designed to identify two rhythms that can be corrected by defibrillation: ventricular fibrillation and ventricular tachycardia. Two adhesive electrodes are placed on the patient's chest and connected to the device with cables. The electrical activity from the patient's heart is picked up by the electrodes and transmitted through the cables for analysis by the computer. If a shockable rhythm is present, the machine develops an electrical charge for the defibrillation shock. While charging, the AED initiates a warning for bystanders to stand clear and then administers a shock at a predetermined energy level.

Some devices are fully automated, meaning that once the machine is attached to the patient and turned on, it will do everything: analyze the rhythm, charge the defibrillator, and deliver the shock. Other AEDs are semiautomatic, meaning that the operator will follow commands provided by the machine such as pressing a button to analyze the rhythm, charge the machine, or administer a shock. All types of AEDs are capable of automatically recognizing a dysrhythmia that requires a shock.

Operating the AED. All AEDs require you to perform the same basic steps:

1. Confirm cardiac arrest (absence of consciousness, breathing, and pulse) (Figure 15-16).
2. Attach the device to the patient with electrodes (patches) and cables (Figure 15-17).
3. Turn on the AED.
4. Stop all movement or touching of the patient and stand clear (Figure 15-18). Also, be sure the patient is not wet or in water.
5. Allow the AED to analyze the rhythm (Figure 15-19).
6. Deliver a shock if required.

Once you confirm cardiac arrest, one rescuer should remove clothing from the patient's chest and begin CPR while another attaches the electrode pads and turns on the AED. If the AED has been applied before cardiac arrest occurs, proceed immediately with AED use rather than beginning CPR. Some machines contain a recording device to record sounds from the event. Provide a brief status report including:

- Your identity ("EMT Jacobs with ambulance 4-2")
- Assessment findings ("Male in his mid-60s found in cardiac arrest; bystander CPR was in progress.")
- Any significant event (electrocution, drowning, other trauma)

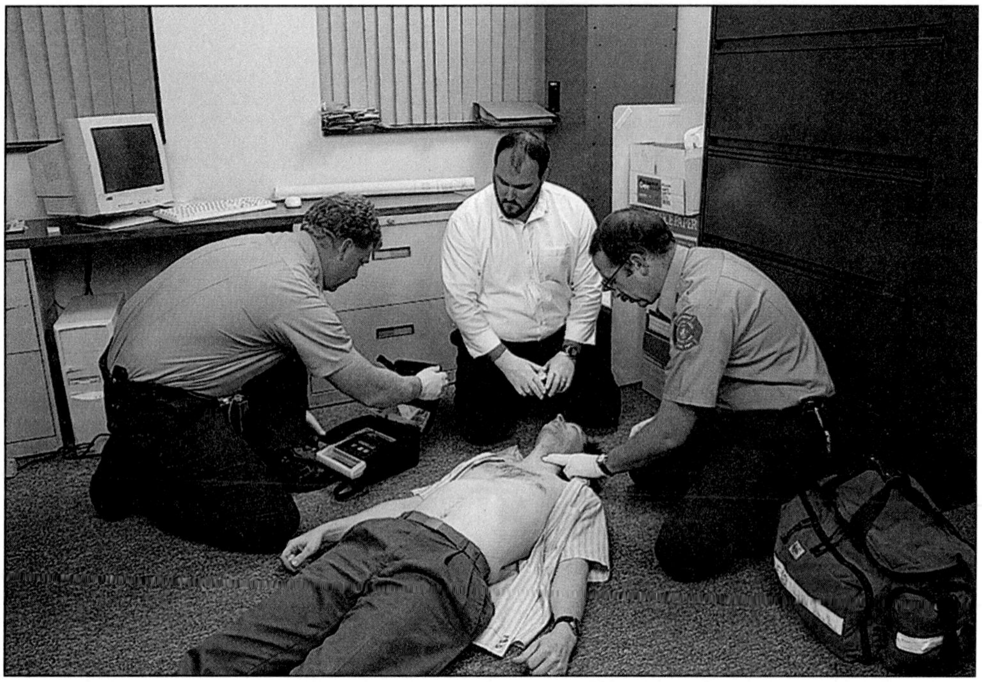

Figure 15-16

To confirm cardiac arrest, check for absence of consciousness, breathing, and pulse.

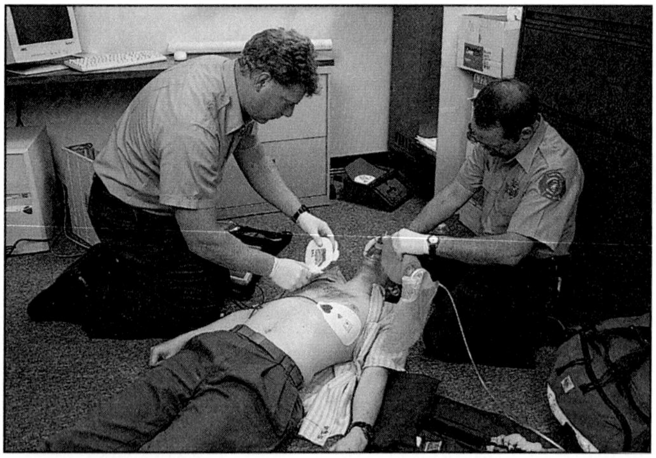

Figure 15-17

Attach the AED patches to the patient in the correct positions.

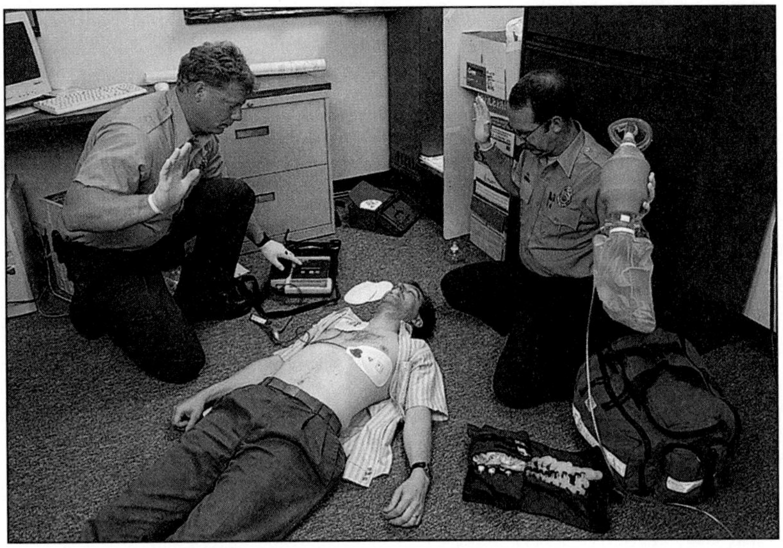

Figure 15-18
After turning the AED on, stand clear of the patient.

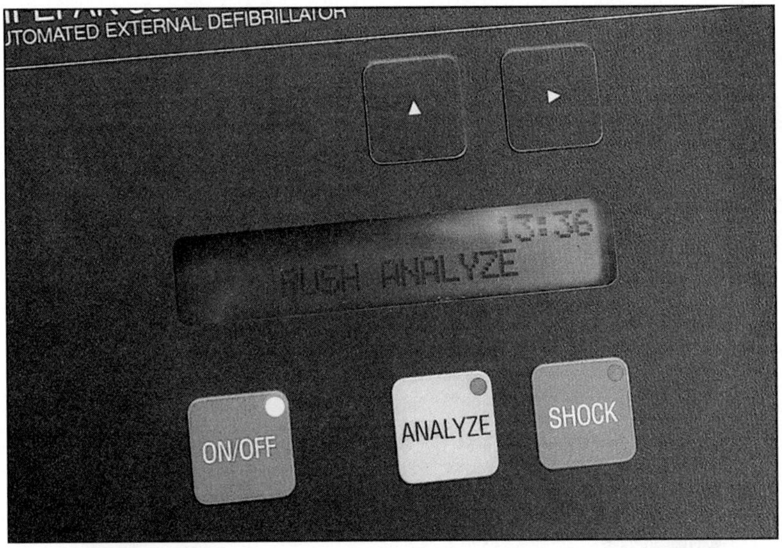

Figure 15-19
Follow the instructions on the AED to analyze the patient's rhythm and shock if required.

AEDs also record the heart's electrical activity, either onto a cassette tape or an electronic module, for later analysis and review in training.

The electrodes are adhesive patches about the size of a hand. They have a special gel on the underside that provides good contact with the patient's skin for accurate detection of electrical impulses and delivery of the shock (Figure 15-20). Remove the electrodes from their package and attach them to the two color-coded cables. Peel away the protective backing from the electrodes, stop CPR, and attach the electrodes to the patient's chest in the positions indicated for defibrillation. If the chest is moist, wipe it dry with a towel before applying the electrodes.

Stop CPR so that you can apply the electrodes efficiently. Place one electrode on the upper right side of the patient's chest and the other on the lower left chest (Figure 15-21). If you are uncertain about placement of patches or cables, there is usually a diagram on the package.

Stop all movement of the patient, stand clear, and check that no one else is in contact with the patient. This is necessary so that the AED can accurately analyze the patient's heart rhythm. If the AED detects a shockable rhythm, it will either charge and advise you of the need to push a button to defibrillate (semiautomatic units) or it will charge and deliver the shock itself (fully automatic units). Some semiautomatic devices also require pushing a button to charge the unit. The EMT operating the device advises everyone to stand clear. After the shock, the rhythm will be reanalyzed. If the dysrhythmia has still not been corrected, additional shocks will be needed. The energy level delivered by the AED is preset and will depend on the type of shock waveform delivered. Most AEDs currently marketed will deliver successive energy levels, typically of 200, 300, and 360 joules. Recently, AED devices with an alternative shock waveform (biphasic) have been developed; these devices require lower levels of energy for the shock.

Local protocols have been developed to reflect American Heart Association (AHA) guidelines for the use of

BOX 15-2 AED Protocol

1. Confirm cardiac arrest (absence of consciousness, breathing, and pulses).
2. Perform CPR until the AED can be attached.
3. Analyze rhythm.
4. Verify that no one is touching the patient and state "all clear."
5. Defibrillate with energy levels preprogrammed in the unit up to three times if advised by the AED.
6. Confirm that the patient is still in cardiac arrest (absence of consciousness, breathing, and pulses).
7. Perform 1 minute of CPR.
8. Repeat Steps 3 and 4.
9. Confirm that the patient is still in cardiac arrest (absence of consciousness, breathing, and pulses).
10. Perform 1 minute of CPR.
11. Repeat Steps 3 and 4.
12. If the patient remains in cardiac arrest, continue CPR and advise medical direction, who may advise you to transport if the hospital is near or if no ALS providers are available. You may also be advised to administer additional shocks at the scene until the dysrhythmia is resolved or the "no shock" advisory is given.

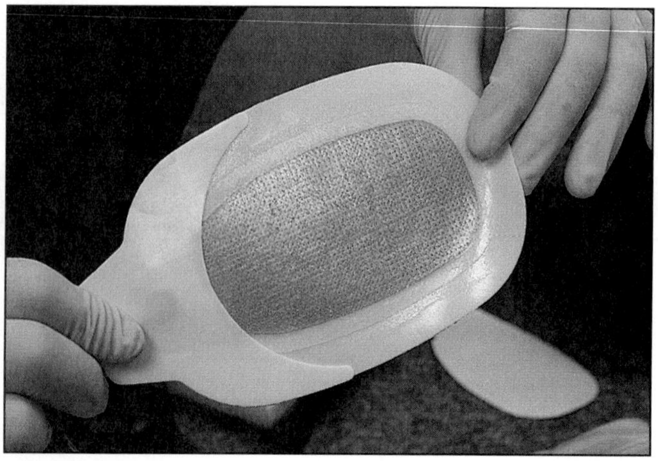

Figure 15-20

Gel on the underside of AED patches helps to provide good contact with the patient's skin.

AEDs. Box 15-2 provides a sample protocol, consistent with AHA guidelines. This protocol calls for shocks to be given in sets of three until a pulse returns, a nonshockable rhythm is detected by the AED, or ALS personnel arrive and take over.

Any time the AED advises that a shock is not necessary, check the patient's pulse. If the pulse is still absent, begin CPR for 1 minute and reanalyze the rhythm with the AED. The patient may be in cardiac arrest with a dysrhythmia that is not correctable with defibrillation. If the pulse has returned, continue to manage the patient's airway and breathing and transport immediately.

As noted above, the AED you use will probably record the patient's cardiac rhythm either on a cassette tape or with an electronic module, providing a summary of the heart rhythm immediately before and after defibrillation. A copy of the summary, along with the cassette tape or memory module, should be reviewed as part of the EMS system's routine quality-improvement process. A copy of the code summary may also be included as part of the patient's medical record.

Precautions. You should be aware of several precautions when operating an AED:

- Do not attempt to defibrillate a patient who has a pulse.
- Do not defibrillate until everyone around the patient is clear of the patient (not touching the patient). Otherwise, the shock could be transmitted through the patient to the other person.
- Do not defibrillate a patient younger than 12 years old or less than 90 pounds. These patients generally require less electrical current than preprogrammed AEDs deliver.
- Do not defibrillate a patient lying in water or other fluid.
- Remove any nitroglycerin patches from the patient's chest before defibrillating. The patches could spark from the electric shock.

Special Situations

- If you are alone with a patient in cardiac arrest and have a defibrillator, apply it as soon as possible.
- Withhold CPR whenever you can immediately apply the AED.
- A hypothermic patient is not likely to respond well to defibrillation until rewarmed. In this situation, most protocols call for administering some or all of the first three shocks. If the shocks are unsuccessful, perform CPR and rewarm the patient before delivering any additional shocks.

Maintenance. An AED requires regular maintenance to ensure that it continues to function properly. Your EMS system should have a maintenance checklist to be completed daily for each AED. The list should include the following instructions:

- Verify that the device is clean.
- Check that the cables are in good condition.

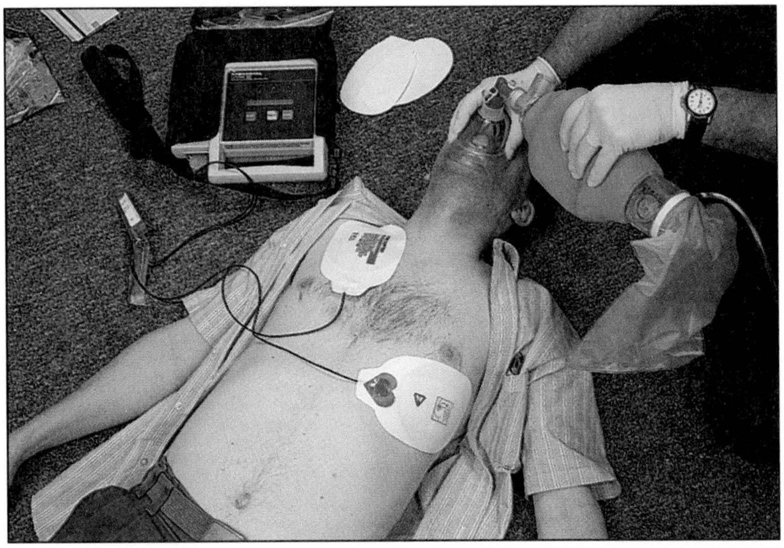

Figure 15-21

Place one electrode on the upper right side of the patient's chest and the other electrode on the patient's lower left chest. There is often a diagram on the electrode package.

- Check for needed supplies such as electrodes, a spare battery, a cassette tape or electronic module, a towel, and a razor for chest hair.
- Replace the battery on a periodic basis as specified by the manufacturer.
- Check to see that the AED powers up appropriately and that all indicator lights and prompts work properly. Many systems have a simulator that tests the device's ability to analyze rhythm, charge the defibrillator, and deliver a shock.

You must also maintain your AED skills. This requires periodic review and testing. EMS systems have different requirements regarding the length of time between competency assessments. Some require it quarterly; others assess skills every 6 months or every year. It is also a good idea to review actual events recorded by the AED and discuss them with a physician or higher-level EMS provider.

IT'S YOUR CALL
CONCLUSION

The absence of consciousness, breathing, and pulse confirms that your patient is now in cardiac arrest. Your crew begins two-person CPR. You quickly notify dispatchers of the situation, who will tell the paramedic unit that is on the way. You place the AED electrodes, connect the cables, and stop CPR to allow the device to analyze cardiac rhythm. The AED advises of the need to defibrillate the patient. You have your crew stand clear before administering the shock. Additional analyses and shocks are needed. After the third shock, the patient's pulse returns. You continue to assist ventilations. The paramedic unit arrives and the medics begin advanced care to stabilize the patient. A few minutes later you are on the way to the receiving hospital.

SUMMARY

Cardiac emergencies are among the most challenging problems you will encounter in the out-of-hospital setting. They range from patients who are having brief periods of angina to those who are in cardiac arrest and need defibrillation. Your ability to quickly assess and manage a patient with a cardiac problem may make a significant difference in the patient's outcome.

Compromised circulation can produce shock (hypoperfusion), which results in marked changes in the patient's vital signs and may cause symptoms such as chest pain. A thorough assessment includes information about the patient's pertinent medical history and any pain or discomfort they may be experiencing. Responsive patients with a cardiac history and prescribed nitroglycerin may benefit from its administration.

If the patient's circulatory compromise is so severe that cardiac arrest occurs, begin CPR until you can apply an AED. You must be familiar with the AED your local system uses, and you must refresh your training periodically. By keeping these skills current, you can continue to provide the most effective care for patients with compromised circulation.

SUGGESTED READINGS

1. **American Heart Association:** *1996 Handbook of emergency cardiac care for healthcare providers,* St Louis, 1996, Mosby.
2. **Paradis NA, Halperin HR, Nowak RM:** *Cardiac arrest: the science and practice of resuscitation medicine,* Baltimore, 1996, Williams & Wilkins.
3. **Awoke S, Mouton CP, Parrott M:** Outcomes of skilled cardiopulmonary resuscitation in a long-term care facility: futile therapy? *J Am Geriatr Soc* 40:593, 1992.
4. **Becker LB et al:** CPR Chicago: outcome of CPR in a large metropolitan area—where are the survivors? *Ann Emerg Med* 20:355, 1991.
5. **Gray WA, Capone RJ, Most AS:** Unsuccessful emergency medical resuscitation: are continued efforts in the emergency department justified? *N Engl J Med* 325:1393, 1991.
6. **Halperin HR, Weisfeldt ML:** New approaches to CPR: four hands, a plunger, or a vest, *J Am Med Assoc* 21:2940, 1992.
7. **Cohen TJ et al:** Active compression-decompression: a new method of cardiopulmonary resuscitation, *J Am Med Assoc* 21:2916, 1992.

Chapter 16

Altered Consciousness

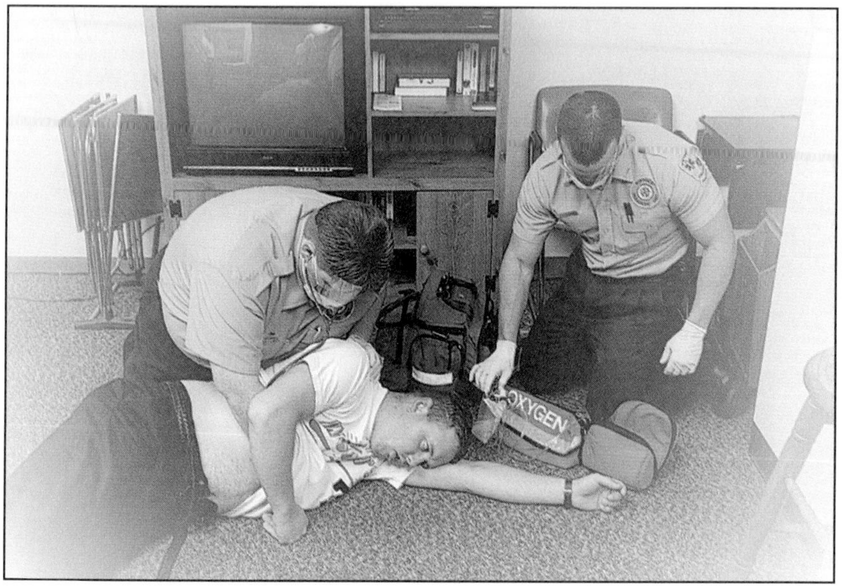

Knowledge Objectives

As an EMT-Basic, you should be able to:

OBJECTIVES

1. Describe how to recognize a patient with an altered level of consciousness (LOC).
2. Describe the general care to provide for any patient with an altered LOC.
3. Discuss the relationship between airway management and a patient with an altered LOC.
4. List possible causes of an altered LOC.
5. Explain what is meant by a "syncopal episode."
6. Discuss the implications of an altered LOC in a diabetic patient.
7. Recognize the signs and symptoms of a diabetic emergency.
8. Differentiate hypoglycemia from hyperglycemia.
9. Explain how knowing that a patient has a history of diabetes will affect the care you provide if the patient has an altered LOC.
10. State the generic and trade names, medication form, action, indications and contraindications, dose, and administration procedures for oral glucose.
11. Describe how to provide care for a seizing patient.
12. Describe what occurs when a patient suffers a stroke.
13. Describe how to provide care for a patient who may be having a stroke.
14. Evaluate the need for advanced life support (ALS) assistance or physician medical direction when caring for a patient with an altered LOC.

OBJECTIVES

Skill Objectives

As an EMT-Basic, you should be able to:

1. **Demonstrate how to provide care for a patient who has had a syncopal episode.**
2. **Demonstrate how to provide care for a patient with an altered LOC who also has a history of diabetes.**
3. **Demonstrate how to administer oral glucose.**
4. **Demonstrate how to assess and document a patient's response to the administration of oral glucose.**
5. **Demonstrate how to complete a patient-care report for a patient having a diabetic emergency.**
6. **Demonstrate how to provide care for a patient having a seizure.**
7. **Demonstrate how to provide care for a patient having a stroke.**

Attitude Objectives

As an EMT-Basic, you should be able to:

1. **Express your feelings about the importance of administering oral glucose.**
2. **Defend the need to adhere strictly to the indications for the administration of oral glucose.**
3. **Advocate the need for summoning ALS personnel or contacting physician medical direction to ensure adequate care for a diabetic patient.**
4. **Serve as a role model for others when assessing and caring for a patient with an altered LOC.**
5. **Value the need to maintain privacy for a seizure patient.**

KEY TERMS

1. **Altered Level of Consciousness:** A condition in which a patient is not appropriately oriented to elements such as person, place, time, or recent events; an abnormal state of mind.
2. **Diabetes Mellitus:** A disease associated with inadequate insulin production; commonly called *diabetes* or *sugar diabetes*.
3. **Epilepsy:** A chronic nervous system disorder with characteristic seizure patterns; the type and duration of seizures varies.
4. **Glucose:** A simple form of sugar found in foods and produced by the digestion of carbohydrates; serves as the body's primary source of energy.
5. **Hyperglycemia:** A condition in which there is too much glucose in the blood.
6. **Hypoglycemia:** A condition in which there is too little glucose in the blood.
7. **Insulin:** A hormone produced by the pancreas that enables the body to use glucose for energy; also manufactured commercially for use by diabetic patients.
8. **Insulin-dependent Diabetic:** A diabetic patient who requires insulin injections for proper sugar metabolism.
9. **Oral Glucose:** A form of sugar administered orally.
10. **Seizure:** A disorder of the electrical activity in the brain that causes sudden changes in level of consciousness (LOC) or behavior and sometimes causes uncontrolled muscle movement.
11. **Stroke:** A disruption of blood flow to the brain caused by an occluded or ruptured artery; also called a *cerebrovascular accident (CVA)*.
12. **Syncope:** A sudden, temporary loss of consciousness; a fainting episode.

IT'S YOUR CALL

You are dispatched at 7:30 am for an illness in a 45-year-old female. You arrive at the home of the patient's neighbor who called 9-1-1 for her. The neighbor states that the patient walked nearly a half mile through deep snow to get to this house because her phone was not working and she was afraid to drive in the snow.

You are led to the kitchen, where you find the patient seated in a chair, resting her head in her arms on the table. Her chief complaint is dizziness. She states that she has had flulike symptoms for the past 12 hours, including weakness, nausea, and vomiting, and has not been able to eat adequately. Further assessment reveals that she is an **insulin-dependent diabetic.** When asked if she knows what day and time it is, the patient responds inappropriately, indicating an altered mental status.

What other questions are pertinent, given this patient's history? What do you believe her problem is? How would you provide care for this patient?

Medical and trauma emergencies can lead to an altered mental status or decreased level of consciousness (LOC). Medical emergencies can occur suddenly or develop over a period of days. The most common cause of altered consciousness is a momentary reduction in blood flow to the brain, causing fainting. This can be caused by any condition causing hypoxia, including respiratory problems. Some causes of altered mental status, including respiratory problems, head trauma, and poisoning, are discussed in other chapters. This chapter specifically considers additional causes such as **syncope,** diabetic emergencies, **seizures,** and **strokes.** Finally, you should also consider the possibility of a central nervous system (CNS) infection or a systemic body infection in patients with a fever and altered mental status.

For a patient experiencing sudden altered consciousness, without any prior history of a similar event, the care you provide will be general in nature. This care includes:

- Positioning the patient properly and maintaining the airway
- Providing adequate oxygenation and ventilation
- Maintaining normal body temperature
- Summoning advanced life support (ALS) personnel, if available
- Contacting your medical direction physician for medical direction

For a patient with a known medical condition such as diabetes, care may be more specific, including administration of an **oral glucose** medication. This chapter explores several of the most common causes of altered consciousness and describes both general and specific care for these conditions.

Recognizing Altered Consciousness

Normal consciousness implies that patients are alert and oriented to who they are (person), where they are (place), the day and approximate time (time), and what has just happened (recent events). Patients who are not alert and aware of the situation and surroundings are considered to have an **altered level of consciousness;** this can also be called *altered mental status.*

An altered LOC can vary from slight confusion to complete unresponsiveness. As you question a patient during the focused history, you will be able to form a general impression of LOC. The patient may respond to questions but seem confused or have difficulty remembering or answering the questions. Some patients will respond only to loud sounds or painful stimuli or will not respond at all. As you gather more information, such as vital-sign measurements, you may find that the patient has a low blood pressure or an abnormal heart or respiration rate. These signs may be either the cause or the result of the altered LOC.

General Care for Altered Consciousness

There are general steps to take that will help the patient, regardless of the exact cause of the patient's condition. You have learned about each of these in previous chapters. If your patient is unconscious:

1. Place the patient in a supine position; for a nontrauma patient, use the recovery position.
2. Protect the cervical spine if there is any possibility of spinal injury.
3. Maintain an open airway.
4. Provide oxygenation and ventilation.
5. Check the carotid pulse. Perform cardiopulmonary resuscitation (CPR) if the pulse is absent.
6. Summon ALS personnel or notify your medical direction physician, if appropriate.
7. Immobilize the patient on a backboard if trauma is suspected.
8. Transport without delay.

A patient who has altered mental status or is complaining of dizziness or faintness should not be left standing or seated. Help the patient into a safe and comfortable position. This may be a supine position, perhaps on your stretcher with the side rails raised and straps secured, to prevent injury. If trauma is not a consideration, use the recovery position to protect the airway. There are times when a horizontal position would not be appropriate; difficulty breathing is likely to be worsened by supine positioning. In this case, place a nontrauma patient in a seated or semireclining position.

Ensure that the patient's airway is clear and administer oxygen through a nonrebreather mask at 15 liters per minute (lpm). Gather pertinent medical history and take a complete set of vital-sign measurements. Maintain the patient's body temperature. If the patient feels cool, apply blankets and circulate warm air to raise the temperature. If the patient is hot from exertion, remove excess clothing and blankets in an attempt to cool the patient. You will learn more about warming and cooling patients in Chapter 19.

When appropriate, summon ALS personnel or notify your medical direction physician. If the patient has a specific medical condition, such as diabetes, discussing the patient's condition with the online physician may result in orders for additional care.

Specific Conditions Resulting in Altered Consciousness

This section will discuss the causes, signs, and symptoms of four common medical conditions that lead to altered consciousness:

- Syncope
- Diabetic emergencies
- Seizures
- Strokes

Many conditions discussed in other chapters can also alter a patient's mental status. These include poisoning and overdose, head trauma, hypoxia, systemic infection, and localized CNS infection. When treating a patient with altered mental status of unknown cause, you will have to consider all of these possibilities. However, the basic treatment described above will be appropriate in all cases.

Syncope

Syncope is a sudden, temporary loss of consciousness, often called a *fainting episode.* It is often preceded by a feeling of dizziness or light-headedness. One of the most common medical conditions leading to altered consciousness, syncope is caused by a temporary reduction of blood flow to the brain. This frequently occurs when blood pools in the abdominal organs and the legs as a result of gravity or of dilation in the peripheral vessels. When a patient who has been lying supine gets up suddenly, the circulatory system must overcome gravity and pump blood to the brain. Sometimes this does not occur quickly enough, and the person feels dizzy or light-headed. When the brain is deprived of blood flow, for whatever reason, it is also deprived of oxygen. This can cause a momentary loss of higher brain function, and the patient may collapse and lose consciousness.

Other causes of syncope include overexertion, heart disease that leads to reduced cardiac output or rhythm problems, and emotional shock, such as the sight of blood. Heart disease is a particularly important consideration in elderly patients who experience syncope. In pregnancy, the increasing demands of the fetus may deprive the mother of nutrients and lead to syncope.

Recognizing Syncope

By definition, syncope is a brief loss of consciousness. EMTs will usually arrive to find a patient who has already at least partially regained consciousness and normal orientation. The patient who has not started to come around should be suspected of having a more serious problem. The dizziness or light-headedness before a syncopal episode may last for seconds or minutes before the loss of consciousness. With some cardiac rhythm problems, the loss of consciousness occurs abruptly without any preliminary symptoms. Signs of hypoperfusion will often be present after the episode, including pale, cool, moist skin, and altered pulse and respiratory rates. The patient may complain of nausea and numbness and tingling in the extremities. Some syncope patients present with a slow heart rate rather than the fast rate you would expect as a compensation for the hypoperfusion. You may hear other caregivers call this a *vasovagal episode.*

Treating Syncope

Syncopal episodes usually resolve themselves without assistance. When a patient moves from an upright to a horizontal position, the body no longer has to work as hard to pump blood against gravity, and the temporary reduction in blood flow to the brain is corrected. This often leads to the return of consciousness within a short time, usually about 1 or 2 minutes. However, a person who falls after fainting can have serious injuries to the head or other areas. In caring for a patient who fell during a syncopal episode, assume that there could be head or spine injury and treat them accordingly.

Further care for a syncope patient should include loosening any restrictive clothing, administering oxygen, and elevating the legs above the level of the heart to increase circulation to the vital organs. For a patient without any mechanism of head or spine injury or any likelihood of cardiac problems, this can be done by lifting the legs about 12 inches (Figure 16-1). When you are concerned about head or spine injury, place the patient on a long

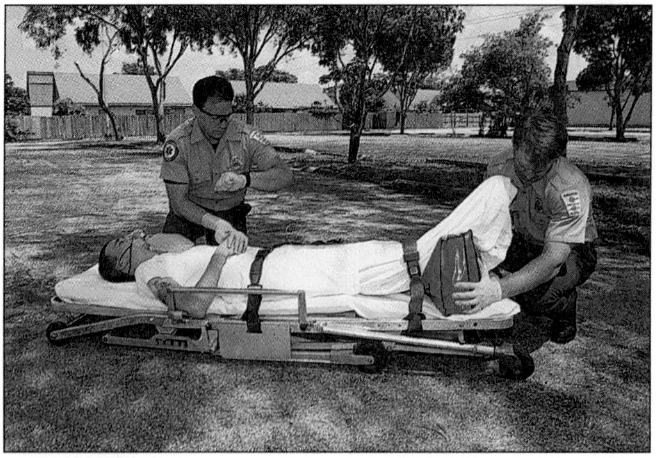

Figure 16-1

This variation of the shock position can be used on patients who are not suspected of having head or spinal injuries.

backboard and elevate the foot end of the board (Figure 16-2) (see Chapter 25). Repeating vital-sign measurements every few minutes will help track the patient's progress.

Often a patient will feel better and want to get up. This should only be allowed if vital-sign measurements are within normal limits and there is no trauma that movement would worsen. Proceed cautiously. Have the patient move slowly to a seated position. Repeat vital-sign measurements to see that there is no significant change, such as a rise in pulse rate of more than 10 per minute or a drop in blood pressure of more than 10 mm Hg. (Pulse usually changes before blood pressure does.) If the patient insists on standing, assist with the process and repeat vital-sign measurements.

Syncope is caused by some underlying condition. For this reason, it is always advisable to summon ALS personnel, talk with your medical director, and try to transport the patient to a hospital for further evaluation to determine the cause.

Diabetic Emergencies

Body cells need sugar as an energy source in order to function properly. **Glucose,** a simple form of sugar found in foods and produced by the digestion of carbohydrates, serves as the body's primary energy source. The food that a person consumes on a daily basis is converted into glucose and is absorbed into the blood. However, glucose cannot pass freely from the blood into the cells. It needs **insulin,** a hormone produced by the pancreas, to act as an "escort" (Figure 16-3).

When both insulin and glucose are present, the body can use glucose effectively as a source of energy. Without sufficient insulin, the cells are surrounded by glucose but cannot use it. Without adequate glucose, the body will not have enough sugar to satisfy the body's demands and the patient will lose consciousness. Brain cells may die if deprived of glucose for a prolonged period of time.

Diabetes mellitus, more commonly called *diabetes* or *sugar diabetes,* is a disease in which the pancreas does not produce sufficient insulin. There are two primary types of diabetes:

- Type I, or insulin-dependent diabetes (juvenile-onset diabetes).
- Type II, or non–insulin-dependent diabetes (adult-onset diabetes).

In insulin-dependent diabetes, the pancreas either does not produce enough insulin or it produces none at all. This type of diabetes often develops during childhood and results in the need to take supplemental insulin in the form of an injection (Figure 16-4). Insulin cannot be taken by mouth because the gastrointestinal tract will not absorb it.

Non–insulin-dependent diabetes, on the other hand, tends to occur later in life. It has been associated with obesity. As in Type I diabetes, decreased insulin production is the problem. However, in this case, the diabetes may be controlled through dietary restrictions, exercise, and smoking cessation and does not require the use of insulin. Some non–insulin-dependent diabetics must take oral medications to control the diabetes. These medications stimulate the cells in the pancreas to produce more insulin.

A diabetic patient can suffer from two common diabetic emergencies. These emergencies affect the insulin-dependent diabetic more often because these patients are more prone to severe fluctuations in blood glucose levels:

Hypoglycemia: A condition of too little sugar in the blood

Hyperglycemia: A condition of too much sugar in the blood

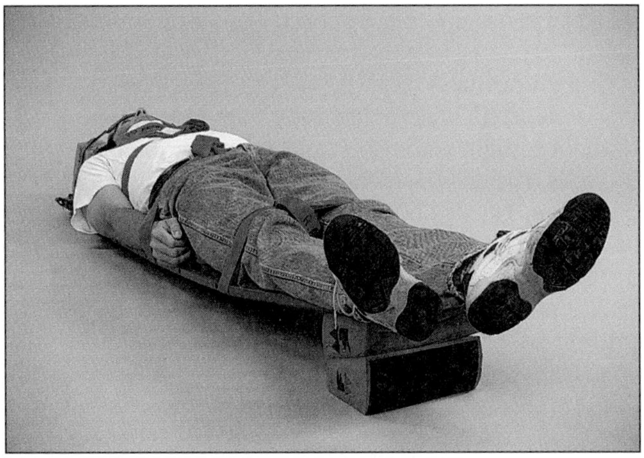

Figure 16-2

If head or spinal injuries are a possibility, the patient may be placed on a long backboard with feet elevated.

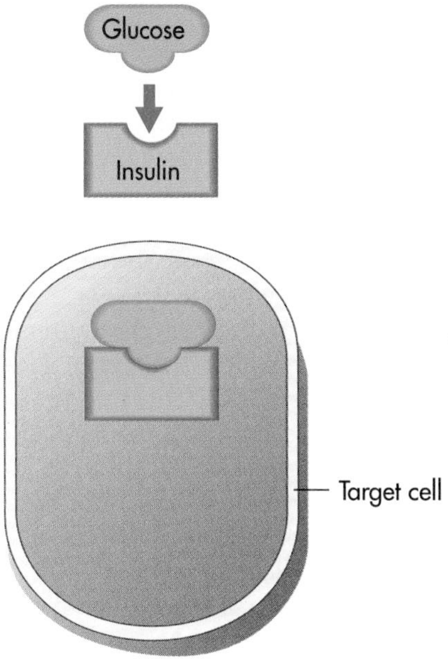

Figure 16-3

Insulin is needed to carry glucose through the cellular membranes and into cells.

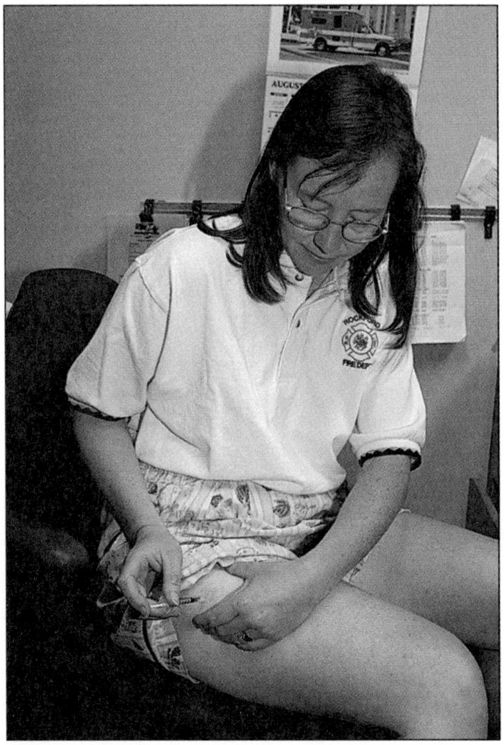

Figure 16-4

A patient with insulin-dependent diabetes will need to take supplemental insulin in the form of an injection.

Hypoglycemia

Hypoglycemia is the more common of the two emergencies. It can affect both insulin-dependent and non–insulin-dependent patients and can actually be more worrisome in the latter; it is more difficult to correct and may reappear after the initial correction because of the long duration of action of the medications these patients take.

A diabetic who has adequate insulin but fails to eat properly will not have sufficient sugar in the blood. The body draws what energy it can from any remaining glucose and from other sources in the tissues. However, this will only satisfy the body for a short period of time. As the blood sugar levels continue to drop, there is not enough glucose for the brain to function properly. If left untreated, this can lead to unconsciousness, seizure, and death. If corrected early, the patient's condition will improve dramatically in a few minutes.

Hypoglycemia can occur when the patient:

- Takes too much insulin or oral medication.
- Fails to eat adequately.
- Overexerts either physically or emotionally, causing sugar to be used faster than normal.
- Has an illness that makes it impossible to keep food and fluid in the stomach for normal digestion. (Illness also stresses the body, changing its need for and ability to use glucose; this can lead to either hypoglycemia or hyperglycemia.)

Following are important points that should be part of your questioning of a diabetic patient or family members.

- Does the patient take medication to control diabetes? What medication?
- Has the patient taken insulin or other diabetic medication today?
- Did the patient take the proper dose?
- Did the patient eat a normal meal, and when was the last meal?
- Has the patient been very active physically or under emotional stress?
- Has the patient been ill?

Look for medications, either pills or injectable solutions. Insulin has to be kept cold, so check the patient's refrigerator.

Hyperglycemia

Hyperglycemia is an abnormally high blood sugar level. Without insulin to transport glucose from the blood into the cells, the cells become starved for energy. However, over time, glucose builds up in the blood, finally spilling over into the urine. This leads to increased urine production and dehydration and makes the patient thirsty. As the process continues, the body begins to use fat and protein as primary energy sources. These metabolic changes produce large amounts of ketone, a type of acid; this is a serious complication called *diabetic ketoacidosis*. If not corrected, it can cause serious changes that lead to coma. Unlike the simpler problem of hypoglycemia, which you can correct by giving glucose, hyperglycemia requires insulin and other treatments that EMTs are not trained to administer. In hyperglycemia, a patient often has:

- Forgotten to take the required insulin.
- Eaten too much, causing an abundance of glucose to be present.
- Developed an infection that disrupts the normal glucose-insulin balance.
- Developed symptoms gradually over hours or days.

Recognizing Diabetic Emergencies

Ask the patient to describe any symptoms while you look for signs. The common signs and symptoms of diabetic emergencies include:

- Altered mental status
- Rapid pulse

BOX 16-1 Hypoglycemia and Hyperglycemia Comparison

Hypoglycemia	Hyperglycemia
Causes	Causes
Too much insulin (or oral medication)	Too little insulin
Too little food	Too much food
Overexertion	Infection
Illness	
Signs and Symptoms	Signs and Symptoms
Rapid onset	Gradual onset
Altered consciousness	Altered consciousness
Rapid pulse	Rapid pulse
Rapid respirations	Rapid and deep respirations
Cool, pale, moist skin	Warm, flushed, dry skin
	Fruity odor on breath (like alcohol)

- Rapid and deep respirations
- Weakness
- Sweating
- Abnormally warm and dry or cool and moist skin
- General ill feeling that may include nausea and headache
- In extreme cases, seizures

Box 16-1 provides a detailed comparison of the typical indicators of hypoglycemia and hyperglycemia. These conditions can sometimes present very similarly; the signs and symptoms may overlap. Do not assume that you are certain which one is present.

Treating Diabetic Emergencies

In addition to the general care that you provide for altered mental status, a diabetic patient may benefit from the administration of **oral glucose,** which is a form of sugar that can be taken by mouth and is helpful when the patient's blood sugar level is too low. The medication is supplied as a gel that is readily absorbed when placed in the mouth. Because it does not have to pass through the digestive system, its onset of action is rapid.

Oral glucose is indicated for any awake but disoriented patient with a known history of diabetes. It is generally contraindicated in a patient who is unable to swallow, such as an unresponsive patient. However, your protocols may allow you to roll the patient on the side to prevent aspiration and place the oral glucose under the patient's tongue or inside the cheek. There are no side effects associated with the administration of oral glucose. It is marketed under several trade names, including Insta-Glucose, Glutose, and Glucose 15. It is supplied in tubes that contain approximately 15 to 25 g of medication. The normal dose is one tube.

Follow local protocols for the administration of oral glucose. You will either be contacting your online physician or following standing orders that allow you to give the medication under certain conditions. Oral glucose should be placed between the patient's cheek and gum or under the tongue. This can be done by repeatedly placing small amounts on a tongue depressor and inserting it in the patient's mouth or simply by squirting it under the tongue (Figure 16-5, *A* and *B*). When the patient's LOC is reduced, place the patient in the recovery position and monitor the airway closely. This position will let saliva and extra medication drain out of the mouth rather than into the airway. After administration of the glucose, continue to reassess the patient's condition every 5 minutes to determine if the glucose has had a positive effect.

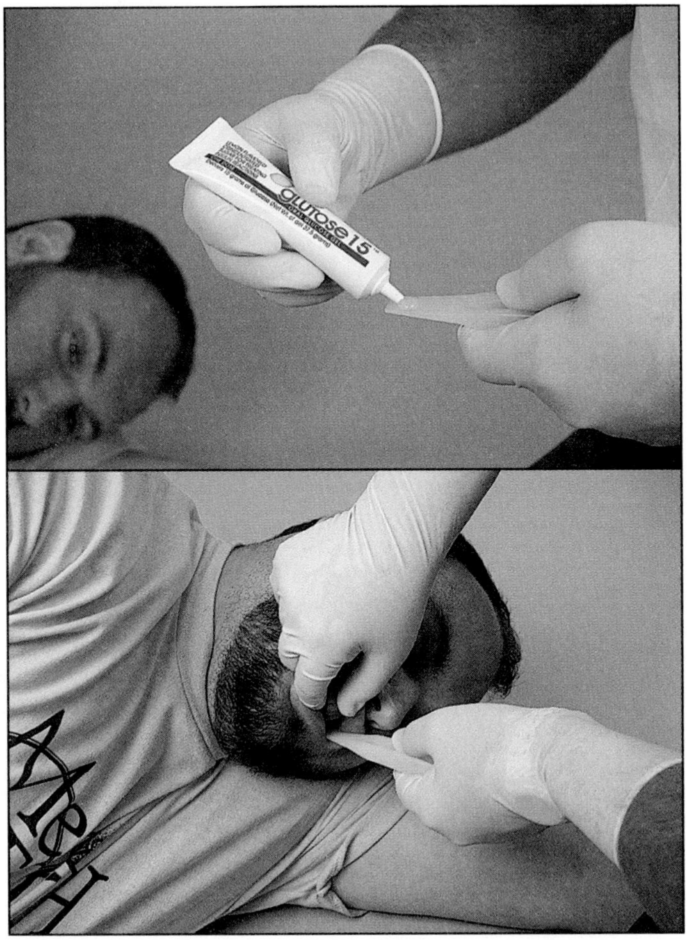

A

B

Figure 16-5

A, Glucose can be placed on a tongue depressor. **B,** If the patient is able to swallow, but the level of consciousness is reduced, local protocols may allow the patient to be placed in recovery position for glucose administration.

IT'S YOUR CALL
CONCLUSION

Your patient is an insulin-dependent diabetic who is complaining of dizziness. Her flulike symptoms of the last 12 hours have limited her food intake, and she had a strenuous walk through the snow to her neighbor's house.

You attempt to find out if she took her insulin today. She replies that she took it this morning. Reviewing the pertinent information, you now know that she took her insulin, has not been eating adequately, has vomited in the last 12 hours, and has overexerted herself this morning. Taking vital signs, you note that her skin is moist and cool, and respirations and pulse are rapid. As you assess her, she starts to become more confused.

The patient's history and vital signs suggest that she is having a diabetic emergency, most likely hypoglycemia. The care that you should provide includes positioning her on her side, giving oxygen, maintaining normal temperature, and following protocols for administering oral glucose.

Seizures

Seizures, also called ***convulsions,*** are another cause of altered consciousness. When the normal functions of the brain are disrupted by disease, including diabetes, fever, infection, and injury, the electrical activity of the brain can become irregular, resulting in a random discharge of electrical impulses (Figure 16-6). A seizure is a disruption in the brain's electrical activity that causes sudden changes in a person's LOC, behavior, and muscle movement. Although hypoxia, hypoglycemia, and infections of the CNS can cause seizures, in many cases the exact cause of seizures cannot be determined. They can be chronic or acute. Chronic seizure activity may be caused by **epilepsy.** Epilepsy can usually be controlled with medication.

Recognizing Seizures

Seizures can range from mild to severe. In a mild state, a person experiencing a seizure can look like someone who is daydreaming. The patient simply exhibits a blank look, staring off into space. In the most severe state, seizures can involve uncontrolled muscular movement of the entire body, called *tonic-clonic* activity. In some cases, the patient has an **aura,** a sensation of light, smell, color, or warmth that precedes the onset of a seizure. During the seizure, the patient may lose bladder or bowel control. Seizures can last for a few seconds or several minutes. The longer the seizure, the greater the likelihood of complications. Some seizures can last for a prolonged time or stop and start again without a period of consciousness in between. This is called **status epilepticus,** a condition

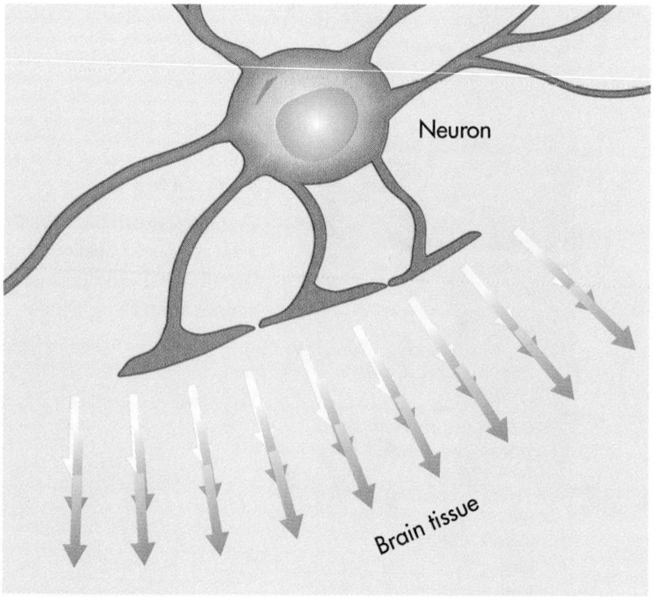

Figure 16-6

A seizure is caused by excessive firing of neurons in the brain.

that can result in permanent neurologic damage, respiratory failure, and death. Seizures caused by fever are called *febrile seizures.* This is especially common among children. Febrile seizures are discussed in Chapter 26.

After a tonic-clonic seizure, a patient usually enters a postictal state, which is a period of rest, like a deep sleep. The patient is usually responsive only to painful stimuli, or may be unresponsive. During this state, the brain is recovering from the large discharge of electrical impulses, and the body from the muscle contractions. Like the seizure, the postictal state varies in duration, but is normally 5 to 30 minutes. During this time, the muscles are completely relaxed. A patient emerging from this state may be confused, agitated, and even combative. Fatigue, muscle soreness, and headache are also common after seizures.

Treating Seizures

Most seizures are self-limited and are not life threatening, despite how frightening they are for bystanders and the patient. Basic guidelines to follow when caring for a seizure patient, regardless of the type of seizure, include:

- Protecting the patient from harm: This means placing the patient on the floor and moving away objects that could cause injury if struck during muscle contractions (Figure 16-7).
- Positioning the patient in the recovery position (Figure 16-8): The patient may breathe inadequately or be apneic during the seizures and could have saliva or even vomit in the mouth. The jaw may also be clenched shut, denying you access to the airway. Positioning the patient on the side, if possible, promotes drainage during the seizure and postictal period. Do not place any objects in the patient's mouth. Be ready with suction.
- Loosening any restrictive clothing: This could include things such as a necktie and the top button of a shirt.
- Providing psychologic support: A patient coming out of a seizure and postictal period may be frightened and embarrassed. It may help to ask bystanders to leave the area. Try to calm and reassure the patient.
- Summoning ALS personnel: Generally, seizures are not life threatening unless the seizure activity is prolonged, as in status epilepticus. If the patient is still seizing when you arrive, assume status epilepticus; this is likely to be either an additional seizure or a very long initial one. Providing oxygen is the primary concern during a prolonged seizure. There is usually some breathing, so holding a nonrebreather mask near the face will help prevent what could otherwise be very dangerous hypoxia.

SEIZURE ACTIVITY

Each year more than 300,000 Americans discover that they have a seizure disorder. Of these, 120,000 are younger than 18 years old. In the past, the terms *seizure* and *epilepsy* were used interchangeably, but there is a significant difference between them. An isolated seizure is a sign of an underlying problem, such as hypoglycemia or fever, that, once corrected, will no longer cause seizures. Epilepsy is a condition in which the cause of recurrent seizures may be unknown and is often irreversible, although the seizures themselves may be controllable. In almost two thirds of epilepsy cases, a specific cause cannot be identified. In the remaining cases, the cause can be traced to factors such as infection, head injury, or lack of oxygen before or during birth. Once a person is diagnosed with epilepsy, treatment generally involves suppressing the electrical activity with medications because the underlying cause often cannot be treated.

Seizures can be classified as either partial or generalized. Generalized seizures are further divided into:

- Tonic-clonic: This is also commonly called a *grand mal seizure,* after the French terms for *big* and *bad.* This type of seizure may or may not be preceded by an aura before the patient collapses into a state of uncontrolled muscle movement. The tonic phase is a period of rigidity that lasts for approximately the first 30 seconds. This is followed immediately by the clonic phase in which violent convulsions occur, usually for less than 2 minutes.
- Absence: Also called *petit mal,* this is brief seizure—usually less than 10 seconds—that lacks the obvious signs of a tonic-clonic seizure and can easily go unnoticed. The patient often exhibits a blank stare and lacks any significant motor activity. Children can have many absence seizures a day, causing teachers to think that they are daydreaming in class.

Partial seizures are said to be either simple or complex. A simple partial seizure involves tingling, rigidity, and spasm of a particular part of the body, such as an arm. In some cases, this can progress to a generalized tonic-clonic seizure. A complex partial seizure is characterized by abnormal behavior such as confusion, pacing, staring (similar to an absence seizure), or an intoxicated appearance.

Seizures are generally not life threatening unless the seizure activity is prolonged, as in status epilepticus. Whether the patient has epilepsy or an isolated seizure, you will provide the same care. Protect the patient from injury, manage the airway, and request ALS assistance.

Cox C: Seizures and epilepsy: understanding the differences, *Emerg* 26:32, 1994.

Hoekerman R et al: *Primary pediatric care,* St Louis, 1992, Mosby.

Moshe S et al: *The Parke-Davis manual on epilepsy,* Morris Plains, NJ, 1993, KSF Group.

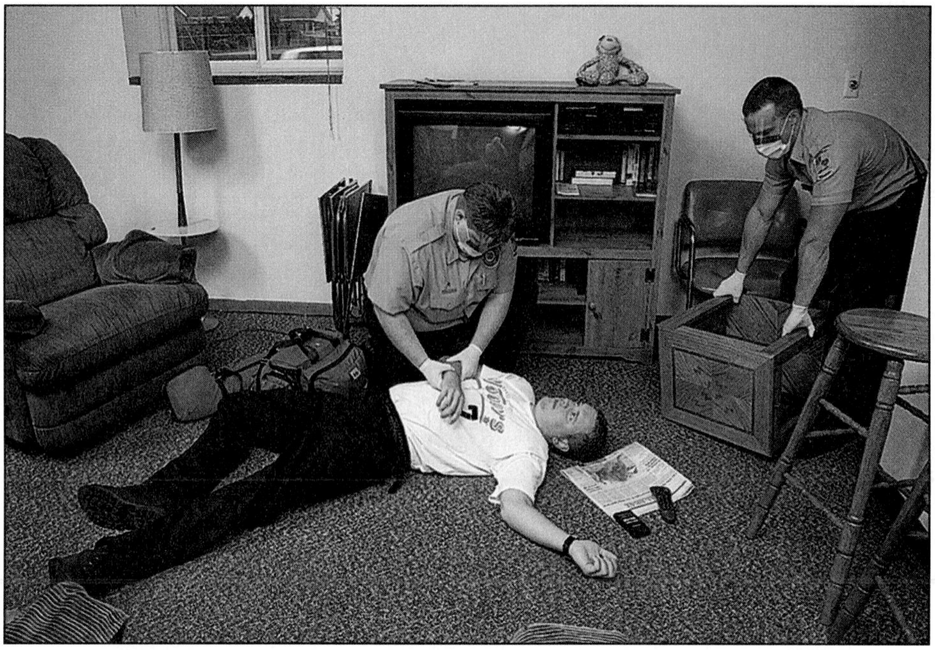

Figure 16-7

Place the patient on the floor and move objects away that could cause injury.

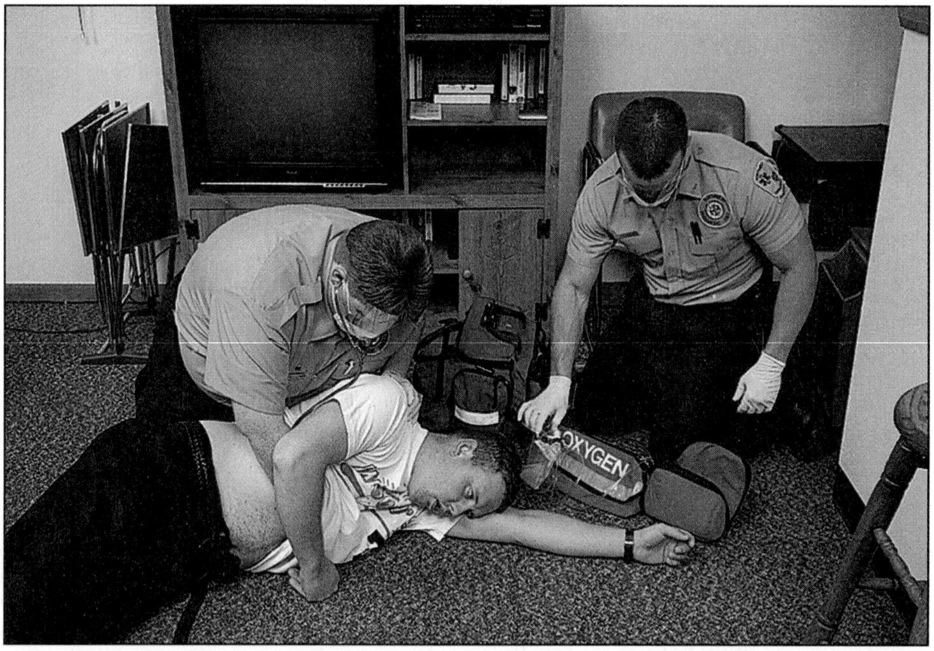

Figure 16-8

If possible, place the patient in recovery position and loosen any restrictive clothing.

After reorienting, the patient may refuse to go to the hospital. Try to explain to the patient that a seizure is a serious condition that needs evaluation by a physician. Also, injuries may have occurred during the seizure. If the patient continues to refuse, contact your medical direction physician to discuss the situation.

Stroke

Stroke is another possible cause of altered consciousness. Also called *cerebrovascular accident (CVA),* it is the third leading cause of death, claiming the lives of more than 150,000 Americans each year.[1,2] Many strokes result in permanent mental or physical disability.

A stroke is the loss of brain function resulting from the disruption of blood flow to the brain; the disruption in blood flow is usually caused by an occluded artery or bleeding from a ruptured or leaking artery in the brain. Both of these prevent adequate oxygen from reaching an area of the brain. The symptoms seen depend on the area of the brain affected.

Most often, a blockage occurs as a result of a blood clot, called a thrombus or embolus. High blood pressure or a weak spot in an artery wall **(aneurysm)** can cause an artery to leak or rupture. Head injury or a tumor can also compress an artery in the brain and cause a stroke, although this is less common. Sometimes a patient will experience a temporary or transient episode similar to a stroke, but that resolves spontaneously. This is called a *transient ischemic attack (TIA),* and usually lasts for only a few minutes or hours.

In the past, it was felt that very little could be done to improve the outcomes for stroke patients. However, hospitals today can provide treatment that improves outcomes for at least some of these patients. The National Stroke Association refers to stroke as a "brain attack" to emphasize the importance of early recognition and treatment.

Recognizing a Stroke

Altered LOC, sudden behavior changes, headache, impaired speech, visual changes, and numbness or weakness of the face, arm, and leg on one side of the body are among the common signs of stroke. In addition, the patient's pupils may be unequal, and vision may be distorted.

Treating a Stroke

Caring for a stroke patient involves considering the possibility of a stroke early on and providing supportive care designed to minimize the damage to brain tissue. As with other conditions leading to an altered LOC, begin by managing the airway. The stroke patient may have difficulty swallowing, and fluid or vomitus may need to be suctioned from the airway. Administer oxygen through a nonrebreather mask at 15 lpm. Attempt to calm and reassure the patient, and keep all comments friendly and professional. Although these patients may be unable to respond, they can often understand what is being said. Summon ALS personnel and prepare to transport the patient. If the patient is conscious and the airway can be adequately managed, the patient can be transported in a reclined position. If the patient is unconscious or you are unable to guard the airway, place the patient in the recovery position on the side of the body that has been affected.

Some stroke patients will survive the initial event but continue to worsen over the next few hours, even though the damage has already occurred. There are new medications that can be given in the hospital to some stroke patients that limit the amount of permanent damage done to the brain and thus the disability caused by the stroke. Therefore, the patient should be transported to the hospital as quickly as possible. EMS public education programs should educate the community about the signs and symptoms of strokes so patients will seek medical attention early in the process.

SUMMARY

Altered consciousness can occur for a variety of reasons, most notably diabetic emergencies, syncope, seizure, and stroke. You can provide general care to any patient experiencing altered consciousness, regardless of the exact cause. This care includes proper positioning of the patient so that you can ensure an open airway; providing oxygenation and, if necessary, ventilation; summoning ALS personnel or notifying your medical direction physician; transporting the patient without delay; and acting in a calm and reassuring manner. The care that you provide is supportive, designed to help prevent the condition from becoming worse.

Diabetic emergencies are usually the result of illness, overexertion, or failure to properly eat or take medication. Care for a diabetic patient is the same as for any other patient with altered mental status, with the exception of administering oral glucose according to local protocols.

When caring for seizures, remember that most seizures are not life threatening unless the seizure activity is prolonged, as in status epilepticus. Whether the patient has epilepsy or an isolated seizure, you will provide the same care. Protect the patient from injury, manage the airway, request ALS assistance, and reassure the patient.

Stroke care is generally supportive, with particular emphasis on airway maintenance, oxygen therapy, and immediate transport to the hospital for further evaluation and treatment.

REFERENCES

1. **American Heart Association:** *Heart and stroke facts,* Dallas, 1993, American Heart Association.
2. **National Safety Council:** *Accident facts,* Itasca, Ill, 1995, National Safety Council.

SUGGESTED READINGS

1. **Cox C:** Seizures and epilepsy: understanding the differences, *Emerg* 26:32, 1994.

Chapter

Poisoning

17

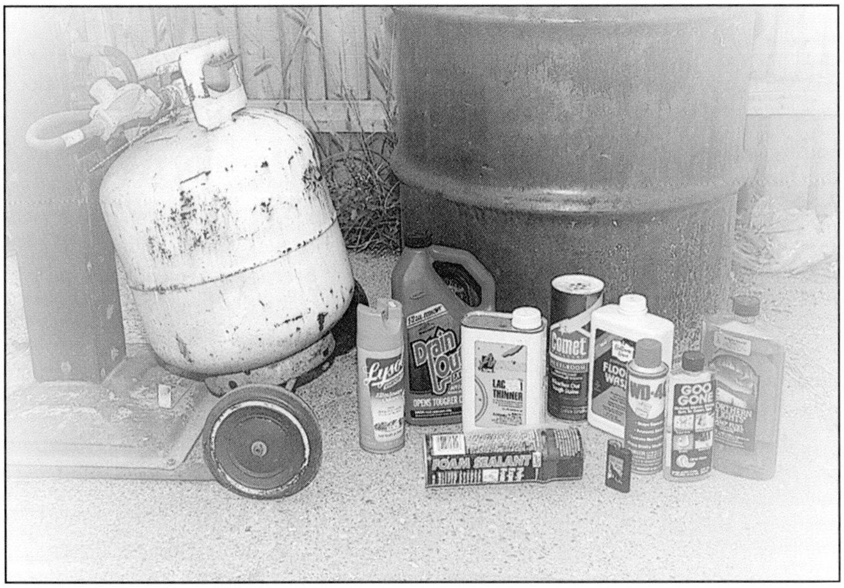

OBJECTIVES

Knowledge Objectives

As an EMT-Basic, you should be able to:

1. Identify the various ways that poisons enter the body.
2. Recognize signs and symptoms associated with poisoning.
3. Describe how to care for a patient with a suspected poisoning.
4. Discuss the care that should be provided for a patient with a suspected drug overdose.
5. Discuss the importance of airway management in a poisoned patient.
6. Identify the generic and trade names, indications, contraindications, medication form, dose, administration, actions, and side effects of activated charcoal.
7. Recognize the need for medical direction in caring for a patient with poisoning or drug overdose.

Skill Objectives

As an EMT-Basic, you should be able to:

1. Demonstrate how to care for a patient with suspected poisoning or drug overdose.
2. Demonstrate how to administer activated charcoal.
3. Demonstrate how to assess and document patient response (positive, negative, or no response) to the administration of activated charcoal.
4. Demonstrate proper disposal of activated charcoal after administration.
5. Demonstrate how to complete a prehospital care report for patients with a poisoning emergency.

Attitude Objectives

As an EMT-Basic, you should be able to:

OBJECTIVES

1. **Describe the feelings you may experience when dealing with a patient who has tried to commit suicide.**
2. **Discuss how your feelings about an overdose patient may affect the care you provide.**

KEY TERMS

1. **Absorbed Poison:** A toxic substance that enters the body through the skin, eyes, or mucous membranes.
2. **Activated Charcoal:** A medication taken orally for the management of certain poisonous ingestions; binds with the poison to prevent it from being absorbed in the digestive tract.
3. **Antivenin:** A commercially produced substance that counteracts the effect of animal or insect venom.
4. **Emesis:** Vomiting.
5. **Ingested Poison:** A toxic substance that enters the body through the mouth and is absorbed into the digestive tract.
6. **Inhaled Poison:** A toxic substance that enters the body through the lungs during inhalation.
7. **Injected Poison:** A toxic substance that enters the body through a puncture in the skin.
8. **Overdose:** Administration of a toxic quantity of a medication or other substance that is not harmful in smaller amounts. Some refer to *overdose* as intentional and *poisoning* as accidental.
9. **Poison:** Any substance that produces adverse effects when it enters the body through absorption, ingestion, inhalation, or injection; also called a *toxin*.
10. **Toxin:** A poison.

IT'S YOUR CALL

You have just completed checking your unit when you are dispatched for a poisoning. The address is in a new housing development that is popular with young married couples. Information is sketchy. The dispatcher states that a 5-year-old girl has ingested something in the bathroom.

When you arrive, you find the child and her mother crying. The cabinet over the bathroom sink is open. It contains toiletries and medications. With difficulty, your partner takes the patient's vital signs while you try to talk to her and her mother to find out what happened. The mother points to several open containers of over-the-counter medications, including Tylenol. They were in the child's hands when she discovered her sitting on the edge of the sink. The containers still have pills in them, but the mother does not know how many chewable Tylenol pills were in the bottle before this happened. In addition, the child took several of her mother's birth control pills and other medications, such as cough drops. The child's vital signs are normal.

Your dispatcher advises that there are no ALS providers available. How should you proceed? What resources can the hospital staff provide for you? What additional patient assessment should be performed? What medication is available to help this patient? How would you determine if you should administer it? How would you administer it? How does it work?

It is estimated that 1 to 2 million poisonings occur every year in the United States. More than 90% of them take place in the home. Children under age 5 account for most unintentional poisonings. Adults account for almost all intentional poisonings. While street drugs such as cocaine and heroin capture the headlines, abuse and misuse of prescription drugs is a greater problem.

According to the National Safety Council, approximately 9000 people died in 1994 from poisonings. Approximately 8000 of those deaths came as a result of poisoning from liquids and solids, such as drugs, medicines, mushrooms, and shellfish. Another 700 victims died from poisoning by gases and vapors, usually carbon monoxide produced by motor vehicles and cooking and heating equipment, and smoke inhalation from fires. The other deaths were caused by foods and other substances.[1]

As an EMT-Basic, you will encounter calls involving both intentional **overdoses** and unintentional poisonings. Your scene assessment will involve detective work when the situation involves young children or uncooperative or unconscious patients. This chapter provides the information you will need to understand how poisons enter the body, how to recognize poisoning, and how to care for patients who have ingested, inhaled, injected, or absorbed poison.

How Poisons Enter the Body

Any substance that produces adverse effects when it enters the body is a **poison,** also called a **toxin.** Terminology relating to poisonings can sometimes be confusing. Generally, *poisoning* refers to accidental exposure to a toxin and *overdose* refers to intentional exposure to a toxin. For purposes of this chapter, the term *poisoning* will be used to refer to both.

There are four principal methods or routes of poisoning:

- Ingestion
- Inhalation
- Injection
- Absorption

Ingestion

An **ingested poison** enters the body through the mouth and is absorbed in the digestive tract. About 80% of all poisonings are by ingestion. Types of ingested poisons include drugs, plants, alcohol, and household products (Figure 17-1). Many substances that are not poisonous when taken in small amounts, such as normal doses of medications, can be poisonous in larger quantities. Drugs account for most cases of ingested poisonings. These include over-the-counter medications, including pills such as aspirin and acetaminophen (Tylenol) and liquids such as NyQuil and cough preparations. Other liquids and solids, such as cleaning products and insecticides, represent about one third of all ingested poisonings. Among children, plants are also a common source of poisoning. Because children are curious, they like to touch and often bite the leaves of bushes and plants. Alcohol is also a common cause of poisoning by ingestion, especially among teenagers and college students.

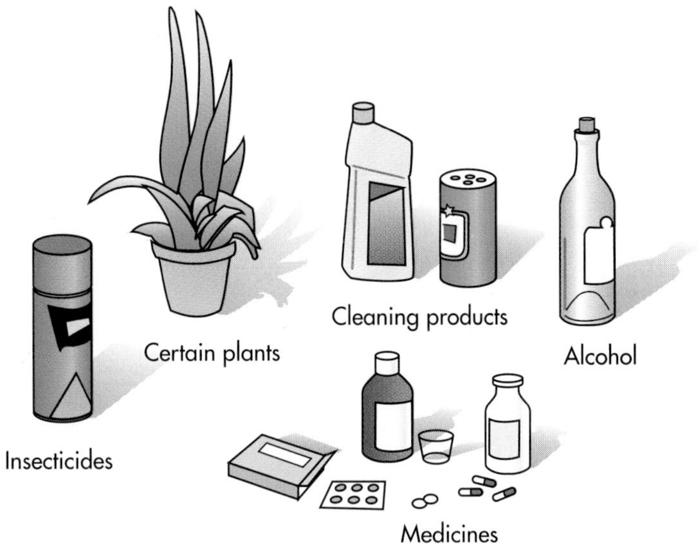

Figure 17-1

Many ingested poisons are common household items.

Contaminated food can be a source of ingested poison. Foods left out too long or prepared in an improper or unclean manner can cause food poisoning. This presents as an upset stomach, sometimes with vomiting and diarrhea (acute gastroenteritis). Food poisoning can be fatal, especially among young children, if it leads to severe dehydration.

Food poisoning can also be caused by various types of bacteria, such as ***Salmonellae, Staphylococci,*** and ***Clostridium*** species. Proper cooking and cleanliness usually kills salmonellae. Staphylococci produce toxins when contaminated food is kept at a warm temperature that encourages bacterial growth. Spores of ***Clostridium*** organisms can grow in food and produce a toxin that can cause **botulism,** a potentially fatal condition caused by eating improperly canned food.

Poisonous plants, fruits, berries, or nuts eaten by inexperienced collectors can also cause poisonings. Some of these substances can result in death.

Inhalation

An **inhaled poison** is a toxic substance taken into the lungs during inhalation. Smoke inhalation is one type of inhalation poisoning, usually caused by **carbon monoxide** (Figure 17-2). This was a common problem among firefighters before the use of self-contained breathing apparatuses (SCBA). It remains a frequent problem among fire victims, who more often die as a result of smoke inhalation than heat injury. Other sources of inhalation poisoning include natural gas, fumes from drugs such as crack cocaine, carbon monoxide from car motors and other sources of combustion, gas from chlorine used at swimming pools, and fumes from household products such as paints, thinners, and glues. Some people, mostly young teenagers, inhale fumes from glue, paint, butane lighters, and aerosol containers. Such inhalant abuse, often called "sniffing" or "huffing," causes severe damage to the brain and other vital organs. It can also be immediately fatal when it causes heart dysrhythmias and cardiac arrest.

The odors of some inhaled poisons, such as chlorine and smoke, are obvious. Some fumes irritate the airway. Others, such as carbon monoxide, are less obvious. Carbon monoxide is invisible, odorless, and tasteless. Hemoglobin, the oxygen-carrying component of red blood cells, has a strong affinity for carbon monoxide. It binds approximately 250 times more readily to carbon monoxide than it does to oxygen, causing displacement of oxygen from hemoglobin and leading to hypoxic tissue damage.

When you suspect carbon monoxide poisoning, your own safety is always the first priority. Do not enter or remain in an area that may contain carbon monoxide unless you are equipped with an SCBA.

Injection

An **injected poison** enters the body when the skin is punctured. Injection methods include hypodermic syringes and the bites and stings of spiders, ticks, insects,

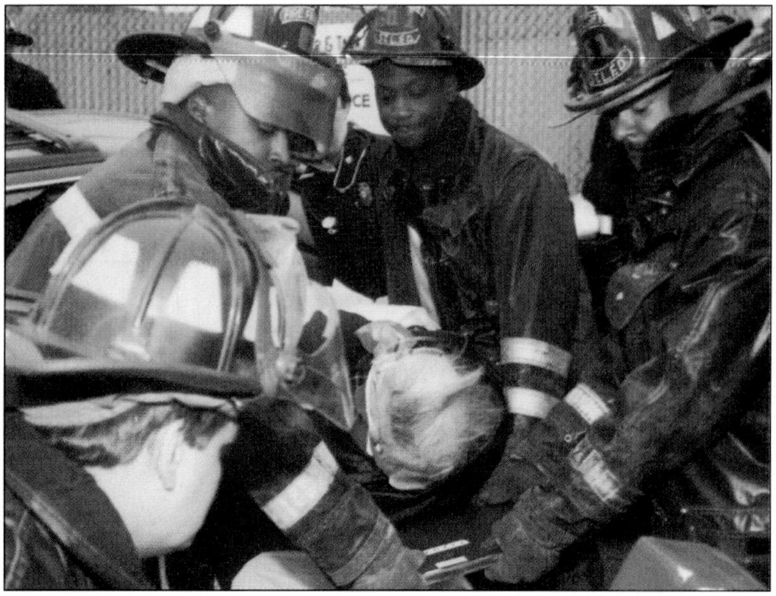

Figure 17-2

Smoke inhalation is a frequent problem among fire victims and firefighters.

animals, people, snakes, and marine life (Figure 17-3). When dealing with bites and stings, remember that the attacking creature could still be present and could attack the rescuer. It can sometimes be difficult to determine exactly what was responsible for a bite or sting, especially if the creature fled.

In cases of narcotics and drug injections, the victim or companions may try to hide illegal drugs and needles and may provide inadequate or inaccurate histories. Be particularly careful when examining and moving a patient with a possible injection overdose. An uncapped needle in a pocket creates the risk of a contaminated needle-stick injury for a responder (see Chapter 3).

Absorption

An **absorbed poison** enters the body by contact with the skin, eyes, or other membranes of the body. Absorbed poisonings often involve home and commercial compounds such as pesticides, acids, petroleum products, and other liquids (Figure 17-4). Powdered cocaine is an

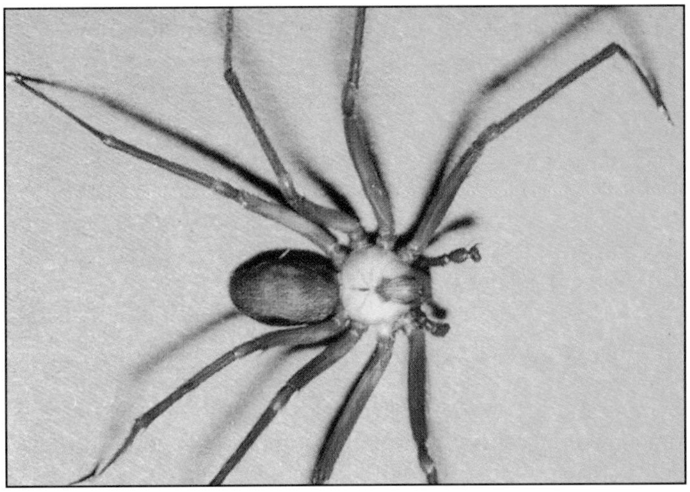

Figure 17-3

Injected poisons can come from brown recluse spider bites.

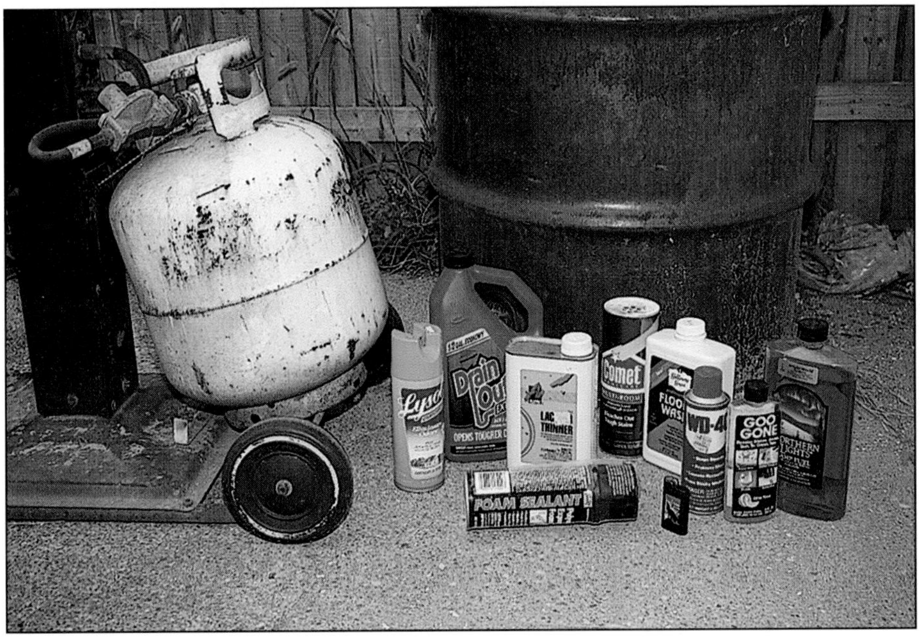

Figure 17-4

A variety of common household substances can also be absorbed poisons.

example of an intentional poisoning by absorption through the mucous membranes in the nose and mouth.

Recognizing Poisoning

In cases of suspected poisonings, scene safety is critical. Whatever substance poisoned the patient may harm you. Be wary and protect yourself. Approach the scene and survey it with caution. Look for flames and smoke. Be watchful for signs of what the toxic substance might be. Be aware of unusual smells. Open medication containers, an overturned house plant, scattered pills, a spilled liquor bottle, drug equipment, or the remains of food and drink may provide clues to the source of the poisoning (Figure 17-5).

Critical Questions

If the patient is responsive or bystanders can provide information, try to get answers to a few critical questions:

- What type of poisoning occurred?

Begin by determining how the poisoning occurred. Look around the scene and ask the patient or bystanders what happened. In situations involving poisoning of small children, consider the possibility of abuse or neglect.

- What specific substance was involved?

Sometimes you will be able to learn the exact substance that caused the poisoning. In other cases, such as a bite or sting, the exact poison will not be as easy to determine.

- How much poison was involved?

When poisoning involves ingestion of drugs, such as prescription or over-the-counter medications, you may be able to determine how much was taken by looking at the prescription or medication bottle. This will tell you how many pills were in the container when the prescription was filled. By looking at the prescription date, considering how many pills may have been taken previously, and counting the pills still in the container, you can sometimes estimate the number of pills that were ingested.

- When did the poisoning occur?

Try to learn how long it has been since the poisoning occurred. This can be important in treatment decisions.

- What has happened since the poisoning?

Determine if the patient feels ill, has vomited, has taken any home remedies, or has contacted a physician or poison control center for advice.

- How much does the patient weigh?

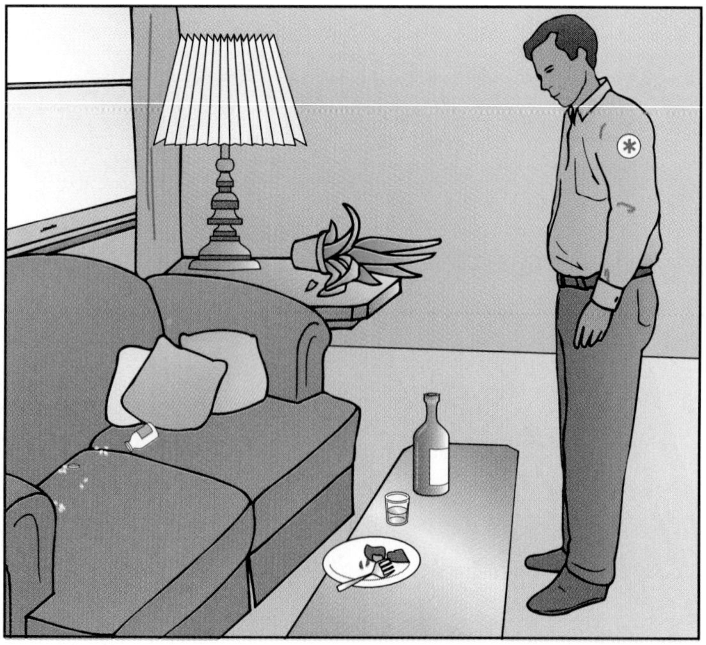

Figure 17-5

Examine the scene carefully for clues about the source of poisoning.

The effects of a poison can depend on the body weight of the patient. Small amounts of poison are more likely to produce toxic effects in children and in small adults.

If the patient is unresponsive or uncooperative, question bystanders or family members. Observe the scene and consider the patient's signs and symptoms for clues to what might have caused the poisoning.

Common Signs and Symptoms

There are many different general signs and symptoms associated with poisoning, including:

- Nausea or vomiting
- Difficulty breathing
- Diarrhea
- Excessive salivation
- Burns in or around the mouth
- Peculiar breath odor
- Abdominal pain
- Skin irritation, redness, itching, or burns
- Constriction or dilation of the pupils
- Altered level of consciousness (LOC)
- Headache
- Seizures

Caring for the Poisoned Patient

Although care depends somewhat on the form of poisoning, there are common elements of care. All patients should be positioned to protect the airway. An unconscious patient may vomit, so position the patient on the side whenever possible. Administer oxygen to any patient experiencing difficulty breathing or altered consciousness. Try to keep the patient calm. Repeat vital signs frequently, particularly if the patient's condition is unstable.

Ingested Poisons

Ingestion is the most common kind of poisoning that EMTs encounter. Try to determine what type of poison was ingested, how much was taken, how long ago it was taken, and the patient's approximate age and weight. Follow your local protocols and contact your medical direction physician or a poison control center.

If the patient is unresponsive, open the airway. If the airway is obstructed by vomitus, pills, or other foreign substances, use suction to clear it. Insert an oral or nasal pharyngeal airway, administer oxygen, and begin ventilation, if necessary. Monitor vital signs. Because poisoned patients can deteriorate quickly, they require frequent reassessment. Most ingested poison incidents are caused by drugs. Some drugs such as sedatives, opiates, and barbiturates depress the central nervous system (CNS), causing respiratory depression.

Activated Charcoal

Activated charcoal counteracts ingested poisons by binding with them and preventing absorption in the digestive tract. Some activated charcoal products also contain sorbitol, a sugar that acts as a laxative to speed elimination from the body. Activated charcoal is produced in both powder and premixed liquid forms. When dry, it must be mixed with water to make a drinkable liquid. This

SYRUP OF IPECAC

Syrup of ipecac, long the standard treatment for many ingested poisonings, is a powerful medication made from the extract of a shrub found in Latin America. Ipecac is classified as an emetic, which means that it causes vomiting. When ingested, it acts as a local irritant in the gastrointestinal tract and stimulates vomiting receptors in the brain. These actions cause vomiting in nearly all of the patients to whom it is administered, usually within 15 to 20 minutes and often without warning. Because the patient must drink this medication and then is likely to vomit, the patient must be conscious and alert. Make sure an emesis basin is handy.

Ipecac is available over the counter, but most protocols allow it to be administered only under direction of medical authority, such as a physician or poison control center. Usual doses are as follows:

Adults: 30 ml, followed by approximately two glasses of water

Children: 15 ml, followed by approximately one glass of water

Infants: 5 to 10 ml, followed by approximately one-half glass of water

Use of ipecac is no longer commonplace. Studies have shown that it is no more effective than activated charcoal in preventing absorption of a poison. There are also instances in which vomiting is not desired. Ipecac should not be given to patients:

- Who are unable to swallow.
- Who are unconscious.
- Who are less than 6 months old.
- Who have heart problems or are pregnant.
- Who have ingested corrosive substances such as alkalis and acids, or petroleum products such as gasoline, lighter fluid, and paint thinner.

IT'S YOUR CALL
CONCLUSION

Your patient is a young child who may have ingested Tylenol and several other medications. Her mother is uncertain how many pills the child has taken.

With the mother's help, you complete your scene assessment by calculating approximately how many pills were in the containers, and counting how many are now left. Your assessment of the child's mouth reveals purple coloring on her tongue and teeth, consistent with the color of the chewable medication.

Because there are no ALS providers to assist and you have an extended transport time, you decide to transport the patient without delay and contact the emergency department en route. You advise the hospital staff that the patient may have ingested nearly an entire bottle of Tylenol and an unknown quantity of other medication approximately 30 minutes ago. The hospital advises you to administer 20 g of activated charcoal. You place it in a covered container and are able to persuade the child to drink it. You continue to observe the patient during transport; her condition does not change.

powder form is messy and hard to mix under emergency conditions; it is seldom used in the field.

Premixed activated charcoal is often supplied in 25- or 50-g doses in plastic bottles (see Figure 13-5). The usual dosage for both adults and children is 1 g per kilogram of body weight. This means adults typically receive between 50 to 100 g of activated charcoal, while children receive half as much, usually 12.5 to 25 g. However, exact dosage and procedures vary; follow local protocols.

Shake the bottle thoroughly before administering it. Convince the patient to drink it all at once, before the charcoal and water separate again. Activated charcoal is not very attractive to consume. Placing it in a drinking cup with a lid and straw, so that the patient (especially a child) will not see the murky liquid, sometimes helps.

A possible side effect of activated charcoal is vomiting, so have suction and an **emesis** basin at hand. Activated charcoal is contraindicated in patients who are unable to swallow, such as unresponsive patients or those having seizures, because the patient cannot protect the airway. It is also contraindicated for anyone suspected of having ingested an acid or alkali. It is not effective with these substances, and may cause additional problems if it makes the patient vomit.

Inhaled Poisons

Your initial concern with inhaled poisons is your own safety. An inhaled poison may still be in the air around the victim and could harm you and other rescuers. A patient who has suffered an inhalation poisoning needs to be removed from the area as soon as possible. If you cannot enter the area safely, summon specialized personnel with the proper rescue equipment.

Some poisons, such as carbon monoxide, are invisible, tasteless, and odorless. Carbon monoxide is produced by incomplete combustion of natural gas, propane, kerosene, coal, oil, and wood—often when these substances are used for heating and cooking. Other inhaled poisons include chemicals, paint vapors, ammonia, and other products that have been used in areas without proper ventilation.

Patients who have been poisoned through inhalation may experience the following:

- Flulike symptoms
- Headache
- Weakness
- Drowsiness
- Difficulty breathing
- Hoarseness, coughing, gagging
- Altered consciousness
- Conspicuous breath odor
- Stained clothing
- Staggering gait
- Cardiac dysrhythmias

Providing proper patient care begins by removing your patient from the source of the poison. Ensure that the patient has an open airway. Administer oxygen to all of these patients and be ready to use suction to clear the airway.

Oxygen is needed to help reverse the effects of inhaled poisons, especially carbon monoxide. In a conscious patient, it can take up to 5 hours breathing normal air to reduce the amount of carbon monoxide in the blood by one half. Administration of 100% oxygen lowers this time to about 90 minutes. Some patients may be treated with hyperbaric oxygen to reduce the carbon monoxide level more rapidly. Hyperbaric oxygen also may decrease the likelihood of permanent neurologic problems associated with carbon monoxide intoxication. Many people describe "cherry red skin" as a classic sign of carbon monoxide poisoning. Although this does occur, it usually is seen in fatal cases and therefore is not a reliable sign to look for in most patients.

Monitor your patient carefully and transfer without delay to a hospital emergency department for evaluation, even if the patient looks fine. If you can safely do so, bring labels, containers, and bottles with you to the emergency department. This will help physicians identify the inhaled poison.

Injected Poisons

Injected poisons are those that enter the body through a skin puncture. They often occur from natural causes, such as bites and stings from bees, spiders, marine life, scorpions, snakes, animals, and even humans (infections). But

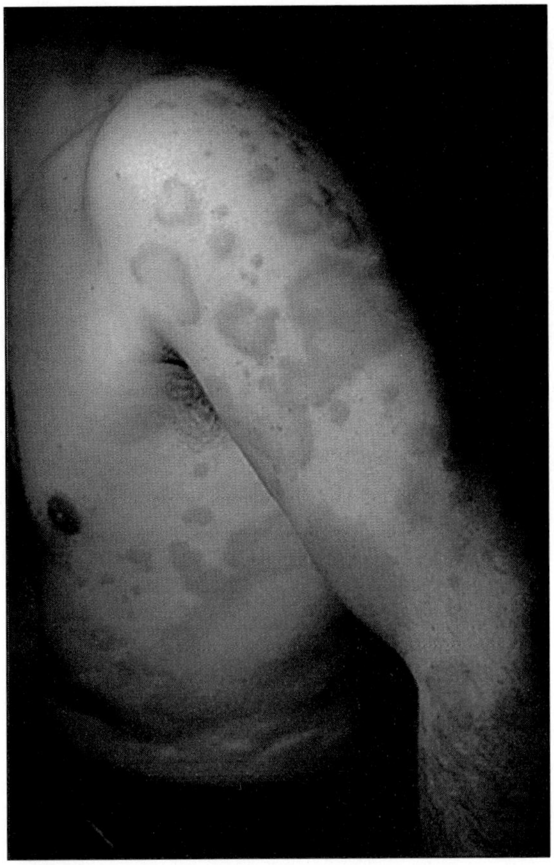

Figure 17-6
For an allergic patient, a wasp sting can cause a severe reaction.

they can also occur as a result of a drug overdose, such as heroin or cocaine.

Bites and Stings

Bees, Wasps, and Hornets. For most people, a sting from a bee, wasp, or hornet is a minor irritation with localized swelling and itching (Figure 17-6). However, for a severely allergic person, one sting can quickly become life threatening. Even nonallergic persons can die if stung enough times.

Bees can only sting once. When a bee injects venom through its barbed stinger, the stinger and part of the bee's abdomen remain in the victim while the bee flies away and dies, enabling the sting organ to continue injecting venom for several more minutes. Hornets and wasps have unbarbed stingers and can sting repeatedly.

Signs and symptoms of insect stings include pain, swelling, redness, burning, and itching (Figure 17-7). Sometimes, a welt forms at the injury site; this is a raised, red elevation of the skin with a whitish center. If a stinger is present, do not squeeze or pluck it to remove it. Instead, you may be able to gently scrape the sac away using a tongue blade or the edge of a credit card. Clean the wound and apply an antiseptic. Applying cold packs may reduce pain and swelling.

In some cases, reaction to insect stings and bites will be more pronounced. Severe allergic reaction, or anaphylaxis, can be life threatening (see Chapter 18).

Signs that a patient is having a mild or moderate allergic reaction to a sting include:

- Flushed skin
- Hives (urticaria) (Figure 17-8)
- Itching
- Swelling and numbness of the lips and tongue
- Cramps
- Diarrhea

Signs of a severe reaction can include any of those listed above, plus:

- Cyanosis
- Difficulty breathing, with or without wheezing
- Altered consciousness as a result of oxygen deprivation
- Signs of shock

About 5% of the population is allergic to insect stings, and about 200 deaths from insect stings are reported annually. Two thirds of those who die from severe allergic reaction do so within an hour after being stung.[2] These

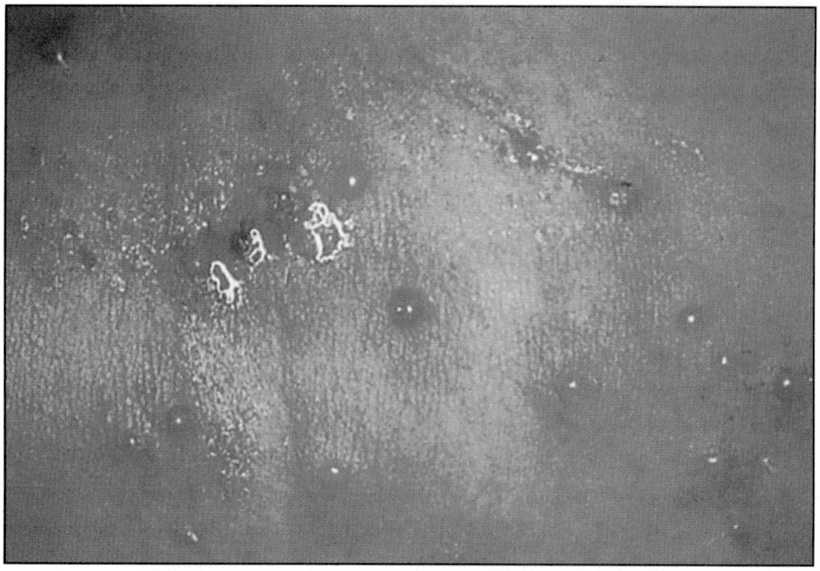

Figure 17-7

Signs of an insect sting include redness, pain, and welts.

Figure 17-8

Hives can be recognized as red, edematous patches usually surrounded by a faint, white halo.

patients need advanced medical care. Maintain an open airway and administer high-flow oxygen. If available, summon ALS personnel if you suspect an allergic reaction. Transport these patients immediately to the hospital. If the patient has epinephrine in an autoinjector, you can assist with the administration of the medication (see Chapters 13 and 18 for additional information).

Snakebites. Approximately 40,000 to 50,000 people are bitten by snakes every year. About 8000 of these bites involve poisonous snakes, although only about 12 incidents each year are fatal.[2] Of approximately 150 species of snakes that live wild in the United States, only four are poisonous:

- Rattlesnake (Figure 17-9, *A*)
- Copperhead (Figure 17-9, *B*)
- Cottonmouth, also called *water moccasin* (Figure 17-9, *C*)
- Coral snake (Figure 17-9, *D*)

The rattlesnake is the most common poisonous snake in the United States. Along with the copperhead and water moccasin, it belongs to a group of snakes called pit vipers. The name comes from the heat-sensitive pits between

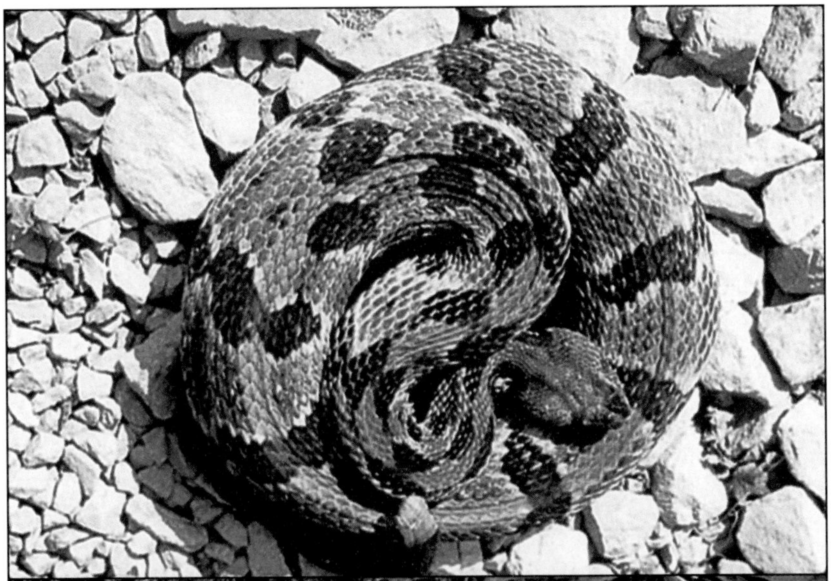

A

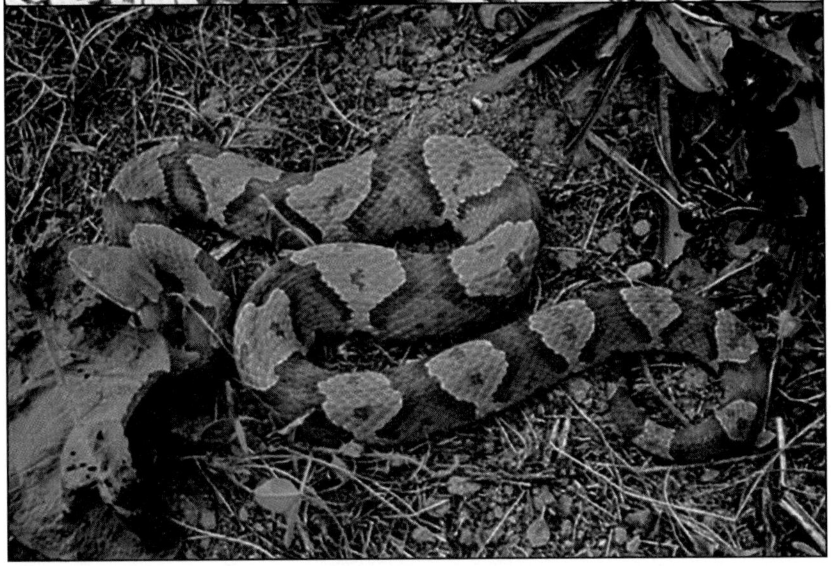

B

Figure 17-9

A, The timber rattlesnake is widely spread throughout the eastern United States. **B,** Copperheads may be the leading cause of snakebites in the United States, but fatalities from their bites are very rare. *Continued*

C

D

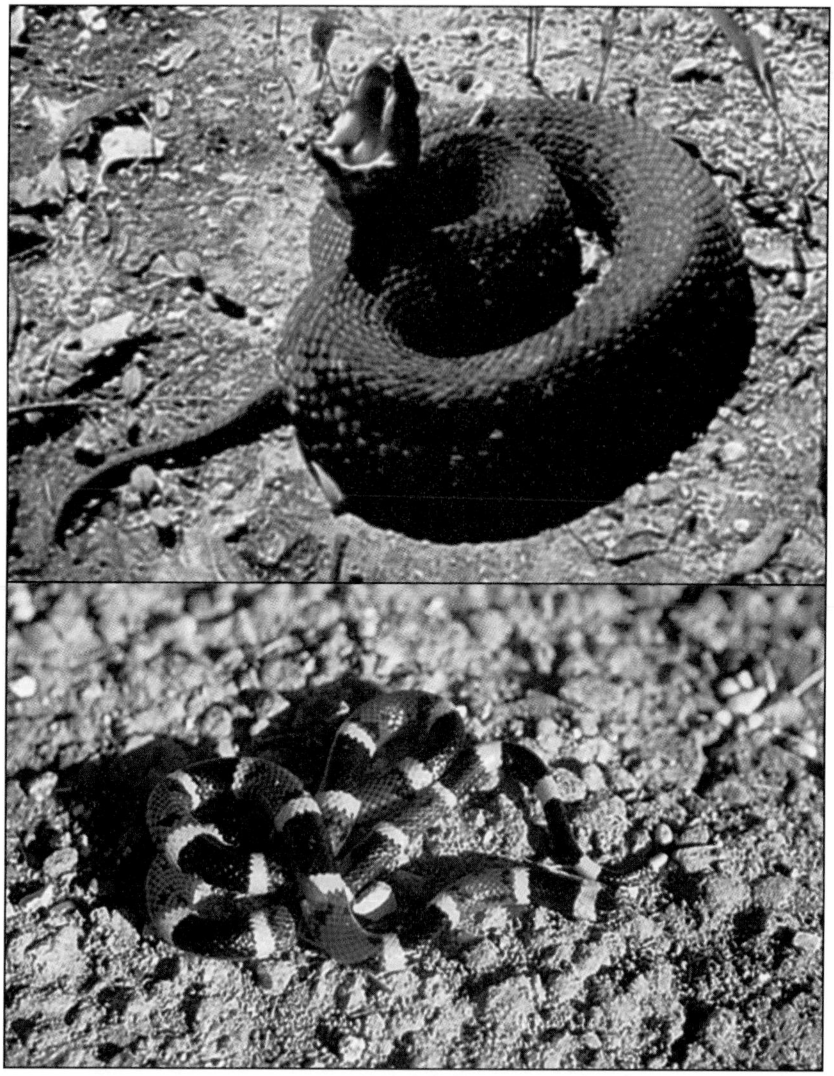

Figure 17-9, cont'd

C, The cottonmouth is a semiaquatic pit viper. **D,** The North American coral snake is the northernmost living coral snake.

their eyes and nostrils. These pits help locate warm-blooded prey to kill and eat. Pit vipers are also recognizable by their triangular, flat heads that are wider than their necks. They have two large, hollow fangs through which they inject venom.

The most poisonous snake in the United States is the coral snake. This is an extremely shy snake that lives primarily in Florida and southwestern states. It injects a potent neurotoxin (poison affecting the nervous system) through small teeth with a chewing action. Coral snakes are much smaller than pit vipers and are quite colorful. They have red, yellow, and black bands around their bodies. A number of harmless snakes have a similar coloring. To differentiate between the coral snake and a harmless imitator, consider the color bands. The red and yellow bands of the coral snake are next to each other and encircle the snake's body. This is not true of other snakes. Remember this old rhyme: "Red on yellow, kills a fellow. Red on black, venom will lack."

Most snakes, poisonous or nonpoisonous, are timid. They avoid humans and will readily attempt to flee. People are usually bitten because they deliberately corner and provoke a snake or accidentally surprise or injure a snake by stepping on it. Even when poisonous snakes bite, about a quarter of the time they do not inject any venom.

Most patients are able to tell you that they were bitten by a snake. The most common signs and symptoms of snake bites include (Figure 17-10):

- Two small puncture wounds about ½ inch apart
- Discoloration at the site of the bite
- Burning pain around the bite
- Swelling
- Nausea, sweating, vomiting, and weakness in severe cases

Caring for a patient with a snake bite begins with efforts to calm the patient. Keeping the victim's heart rate as slow as possible helps prevent absorption of the poison.

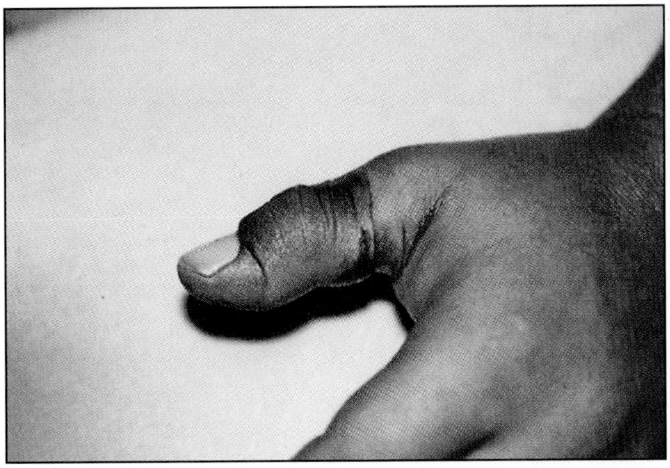

Figure 17-10

This patient was bitten by a rattlesnake on the thumb. Careful examination reveals both puncture wounds as well as the typical discoloration and swelling around the bite.

Some people have an almost disabling fear of snakes and will need reassurance. Remember that snakebites are rarely poisonous and almost never fatal.

Cleanse the area to remove any surface poison. Immobilize any bitten extremity, and try to keep it below the level of the heart if possible. Minimizing movement helps slow the absorption and distribution of the poison. Give oxygen as needed. Maintain normal body temperature. If extended patient care and transport time are an issue, local protocol may call for the application of a constricting band around an extremity to help slow the flow of the poison. This constricting band partially restricts venous blood flow. When applied, you should still be able to slide one to two fingers under the band. This is not the same as a tourniquet, which is applied more tightly to stop blood flow entirely. Track the progression of swelling with pen marks on the skin, noting the time the mark was made. Call poison control, if allowed by local protocol.

There are also several things that you should *not* do when caring for a snake bite.

- Do not apply cold packs or ice.
- Do not apply a tourniquet.
- Do not cut into the wound or attempt to suck out the venom.
- Do not apply any form of electric shock.

These do little good and may cause harm. In all but the most remote locations, a hospital emergency department is usually close enough that effective treatment can be given after transport. Provide the staff with as much information as possible about the kind of snake involved. Hospital treatment may include the administration of a snake **antivenin,** which is a fluid that counteracts the injected toxin.

Animal and Human Bites. Dogs account for most animal bites, and most of the patients are small children (Figure 17-11). Dog bites should be treated by a physician because they can become seriously infected. A tetanus shot and antibiotics are often needed. Some dog bites require stitches. Dog bites generally must be reported to public health authorities. Bites from both domestic and wild animals pose the threat of rabies, as well as soft-tissue injuries and infection.

Rabies is caused by a virus transmitted through the saliva of wild animals such as skunks, raccoons, bats, and foxes, and domestic animals such as cattle, cats, dogs, sheep, and pigs. Vaccination programs have reduced the incidence of rabies from domestic animals, but it can still occur. Not every animal that has rabies can transmit it. If transmitted, this viral infection affects the nervous system. The infection can be treated effectively with a vaccine if it is given soon enough, but is nearly always fatal if left untreated.

Unusual animal behavior could point to rabies. For example, a normally nocturnal animal like a raccoon should not be moving about openly in daylight. A fox should flee when approached; rabid animals are usually aggressive. Do not attempt to handle any strange dog or wild animal. Summon animal control personnel to capture the animal.

Your initial care for animal bites involves maintaining your own safety and, when appropriate, removing the patient from the presence of the animal. Reassure the patient. Control any bleeding, apply sterile dressings over the wound site, and transport the patient to a hospital.

Human bites also come under the category of poisoning by injection. The human mouth contains much more infectious bacteria than most animals. It does not require a deliberate bite to cause serious injury. Striking

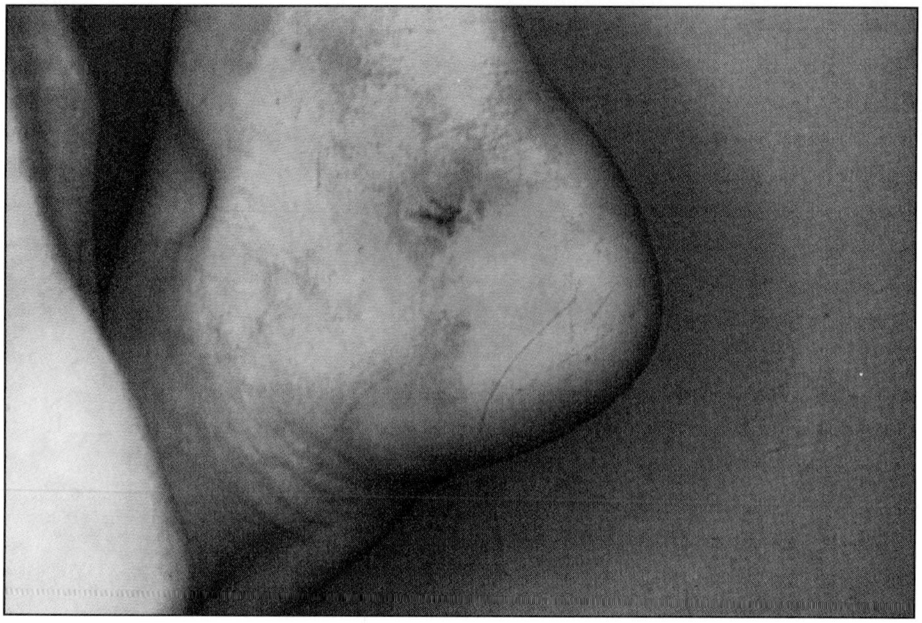

Figure 17-11

Dog bites can cause puncture wounds such as this one and should be treated by a physician because of the possibility of infection.

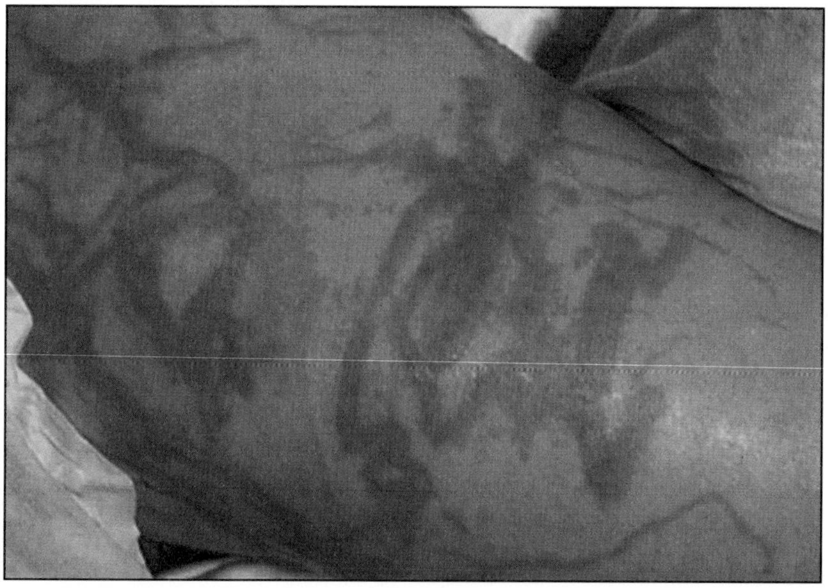

Figure 17-12

The intense necrosis of these stings is typical of a severe box-jellyfish sting.

someone in the mouth during a domestic dispute could cause a hand laceration from striking a tooth. This wound should be treated in the same manner as an animal bite. The patient will likely receive a tetanus shot and antibiotics at the hospital. EMS personnel bitten by a patient should clean and dress the wound and report it to supervisors and hospital personnel immediately after the response is concluded. It may require follow up for possible infectious exposure (see Chapter 3).

Marine Life. Stings from marine animals such as jellyfish, sting rays, sea urchins, and sea anemones occur in coastal areas that attract large numbers of swimmers. Stings from the tentacles of jellyfish, Portuguese men-of-war, and anemones can cause redness, welts, and serious allergic reactions (Figure 17-12).

To provide care for jellyfish and Portuguese man-of-war stings, remove any tentacles, if present, without stinging yourself; use a tongue blade, not your bare hands. Clean the wound with isopropyl (rubbing) alcohol.

Sting rays and sea urchins cause puncture wounds when swimmers step on their barbs. The feet and lower legs are usually involved. The pain can be intense. The poisons are heat sensitive, so treatment is simple and effective. Soak the affected limbs in hot water and transport to the hospital. It normally takes about 30 to 60 minutes for the heat to destroy the poison. The patient may still require a tetanus shot and care for potential infection.

Scorpions. Scorpions look like small crayfish or lobsters and have stingers at the end of their upraised tails. They live in dry regions of the southwestern United States. Only a few species are considered to be fatally poisonous, such as the Arizona scorpion (Figure 17-13). They normally hide during the day under rocks and logs, and they avoid humans.

A sting from a scorpion causes pain and burning around the sting site. Children are usually affected most severely by poisonous scorpions. Some patients experience difficulty breathing, muscle spasms, and even paralysis. Management of a scorpion sting involves cleaning the site with isopropyl (rubbing) alcohol, or soap and water. Apply a cold pack and transport the patient to the hospital. Monitor the patient's vital signs and administer oxygen if the patient begins to show signs of respiratory difficulty.

Ticks. While most tick bites are harmless, a few are associated with the spread of serious disease, such as Rocky Mountain spotted fever (RMSF). This disease can cause paralysis or even death. Cases of RMSF have been reported in nearly all states, as well as Canada and Mexico. Typically, a patient has sudden onset of high fever, chills, headache, rash, abdominal pain, nausea, and vomiting. In later stages, RMSF can cause respiratory and cardiac failure. Effective treatment requires early administration of antibiotics.

More recently, attention has focused on ticks because of the spread of **Lyme disease,** which has been reported in 40 states. This disease gets its name from the Connecticut town in which it was first discovered. Not all ticks carry Lyme disease. The type of tick responsible for Lyme

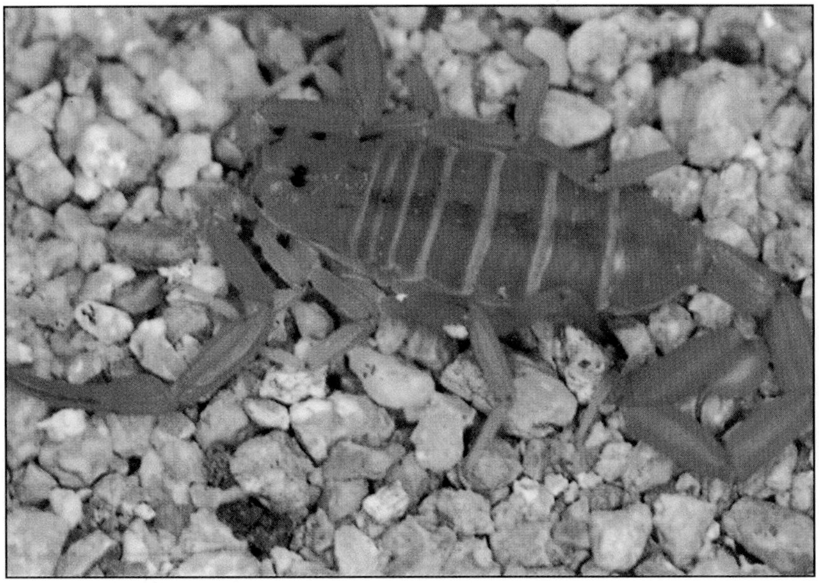

Figure 17-13

The Arizona scorpion is one of the few species considered fatally poisonous.

disease is the deer tick, which usually attaches itself to deer and small rodents. Deer ticks are much smaller than common wood or dog ticks. They can be as small as the head of a pin and are found in wooded and grassy areas and on beaches. They will attach themselves to any warm-blooded animal, including humans.

The first symptoms of Lyme disease appear approximately 3 days after a tick bite. A red rash develops and spreads (Figure 17-14). Days later, painful swelling begins in the joints, especially the knees. If not treated, Lyme disease can cause memory loss, arthritis, and vision and hearing problems. Antibiotics are effective in treating Lyme disease.

Most people do not realize they have been bitten by a tick; the bite is often painless. It may be noticed only after it has become engorged with blood and swells as large as ¼ inch in diameter.

When caring for a tick bite, use tweezers to pull the tick off slowly. If you do not have tweezers, wear gloves to protect your fingers and grasp the tick as close to the bite site as possible. Do not twist, or you will leave part of the tick inside. Once the tick is removed, wash the area thoroughly. If you are not transporting the patient, advise the patient to see a physician about the tick bite. Early treatment for infection is most effective.

Practices once thought to be effective for the treatment of tick bites have proved useless. Some cause more harm by triggering a release of additional infectious material.

- Do not apply fingernail polish, petroleum jelly, or alcohol to the tick.
- Do not try to prick it with a pin.
- Do not apply a hot match or cigarette to the tick; this is likely to burn the patient.

Spiders. Spiders are widespread in the United States. Out of sight, in dark and remote corners, they present little threat to humans. Spider bites usually occur on hands and arms as people reach into the areas where spiders live, such as wood piles, closets, basements, attics, and garages.

While many spiders bite, only the black widow is likely to cause significant systemic reactions. These can even be fatal. The black widow appears glossy black to dark brown, measuring about 1 to 1½ inches long, with legs extended. The female has a red-orange or yellow hourglass marking on her abdomen (Figure 17-15). The male does not have this marking and is not poisonous.

Black widow venom is neurotoxic and more deadly than rattlesnake venom. The first sensations after a black widow spider bite are pain and redness at the site. Other complaints include cramping of large muscles, dizziness, headache, chills, nausea, vomiting, and abdominal cramping. Victims can also experience tightness in the chest and trouble breathing. About 5% of victims of black widow spider bites die from asphyxiation caused by respiratory paralysis. Most patients improve after 48 hours.

Treatment for a black widow spider bite includes applying cold packs at the bite site. Maintain the airway and provide oxygen at the first sign of breathing difficulty. Keep the victim calm and transport to the emergency department. Antivenin is available to treat black widow bites.

The brown recluse spider is smaller than the black widow spider and dark brown to light yellow in color.

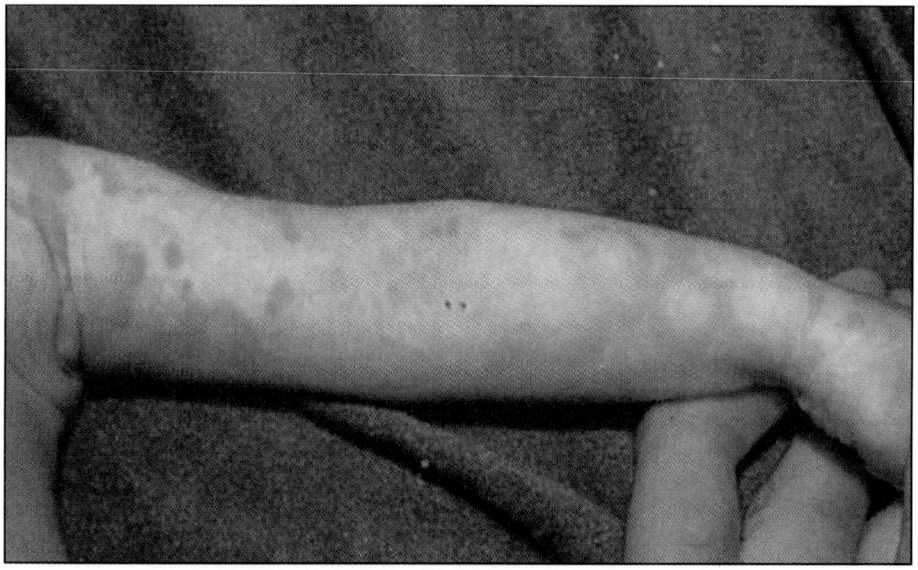

Figure 17-14

The first sign of Lyme disease is a rash such as this, which can develop within 3 days after the initial bite.

This spider has a characteristic dark violin-shaped mark on its back (Figure 17-16). While the bite of the black widow attacks the nervous system, the brown recluse spider's bite causes local tissue damage that often produces a draining sore. The initial bite may not even be noticed by the victim. About 2 to 8 hours later, pain begins, accompanied by blisters, bleeding, and swelling. There may also be nausea, chills, and fever. There is no specific antivenin for the treatment of brown recluse spider bites. Clean the area with isopropyl alcohol. Apply cold packs to reduce pain and swelling, and transport the patient to a hospital.

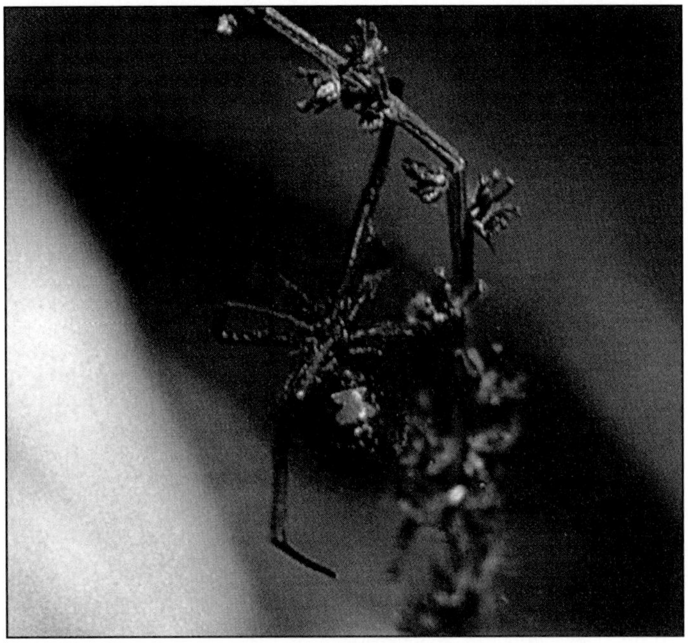

Figure 17-15

Black widow venom is more deadly than that of a rattlesnake.

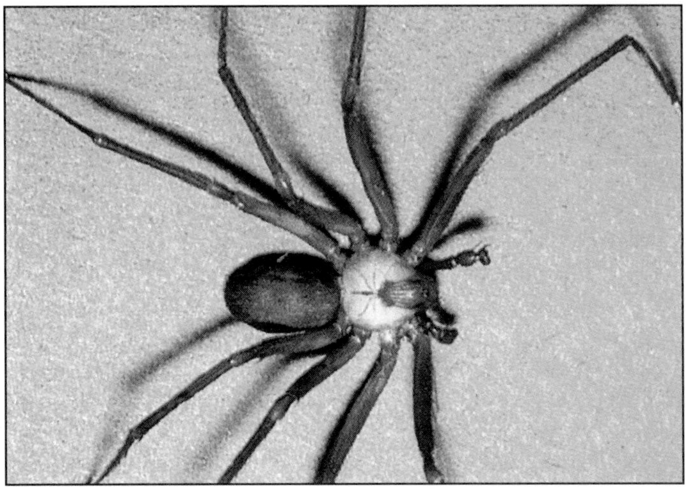

Figure 17-16

The brown recluse is smaller and lighter in color than the black widow and bears a violin-shaped mark on its back.

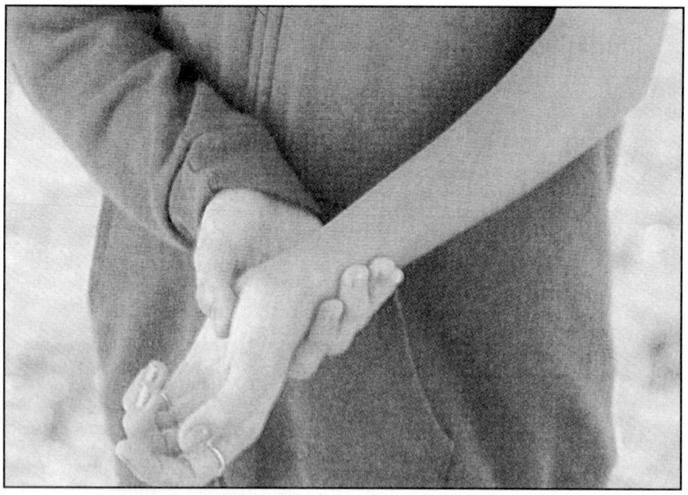

Figure 17-17

Absorbed poisons can cause irritation and burns.

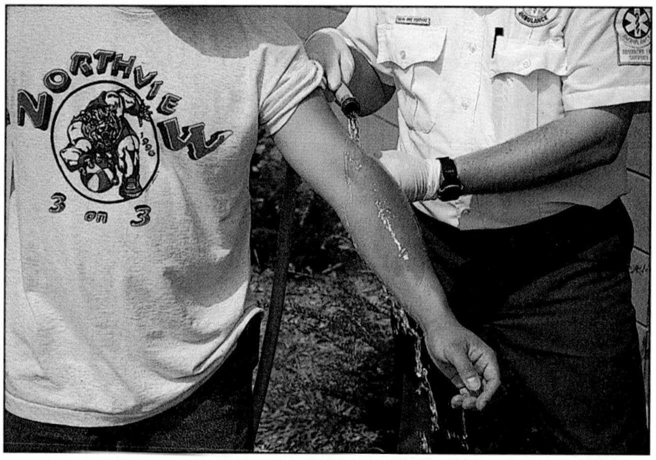

Figure 17-18

Apply water in a way that prevents further contamination.

Absorbed Poisons

Poisonous substances can also enter the body by absorption through the skin. Common absorbed poisons include dry and wet chemicals, such as industrial chemicals and insecticides. Corrosive substances such as acids, alkalis, and petroleum products can damage skin, eyes, and mucous membranes upon contact. This often results in irritation and burns (Figure 17-17).

To care for contact with toxic liquids, flush the affected areas with large amounts of water for at least 20 minutes and transport the patient to a hospital. Summon ALS personnel, particularly if the poison has affected the airway. Dry chemicals, such as lime, should be brushed off before flushing. Even though water activates some dry chemicals, continuous running water can flush away the substance before it causes harm. Protect yourself from contamination while flushing, and apply water in a way that protects the patient's unaffected areas from contamination (Figure 17-18). As with other poisoning, contact your medical direction physician as soon as possible with the name of the absorbed poison.

Although not absorbed into the skin, plant toxins such as poison ivy, poison sumac, and poison oak cause contact irritation in millions of people every year (Figure 17-19, *A* and *B*). The sap and juice of these plants can cause an allergic reaction that involves a burning or itch-

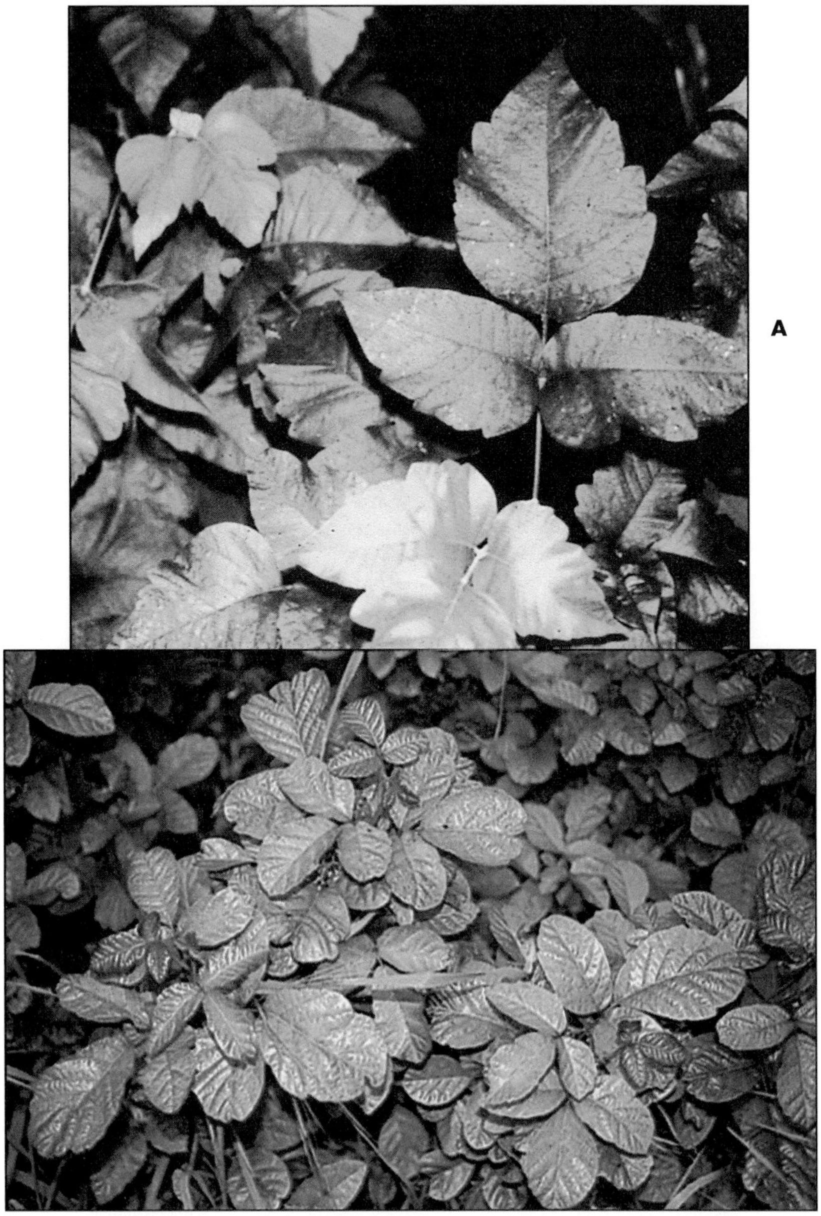

Figure 17-19
A, Poison ivy. **B,** Poison oak.

ing sensation. Swelling and blisters form, and in severe cases, can cause additional skin infections.

The immediate treatment for skin contact with a poisonous plant is to wash the affected area with soap and water within 30 to 60 minutes after exposure; however, many victims are not aware they have touched poisonous plants until 1 or 2 days later, when the signs and symptoms appear. If you respond to a call for a patient that has weeping and oozing wounds indicative of poisonous plants, transport the patient to the hospital for treatment. Home treatments such as Calamine lotion or baking soda soaks and compresses can help, but prescribed medicine may be necessary to reduce the swelling. Remind the patient to wash any exposed clothing before wearing it again.

Substance Misuse and Abuse

Substance misuse and abuse occur among people of all ages and at all levels of society. **Substance misuse** refers to the use of a substance for unintended purposes or for appropriate purposes but at an improper dose. **Substance abuse** refers to the deliberate, excessive use of a substance without regard for the health consequences, generally with the intention of causing some mental effect or physical sensation. When the amount of the substance causes harm, it is commonly referred to as a **drug overdose.** This can be either intentional or unintentional; although the term usually refers to intentional misuse. Overdose is commonly associated with the use of

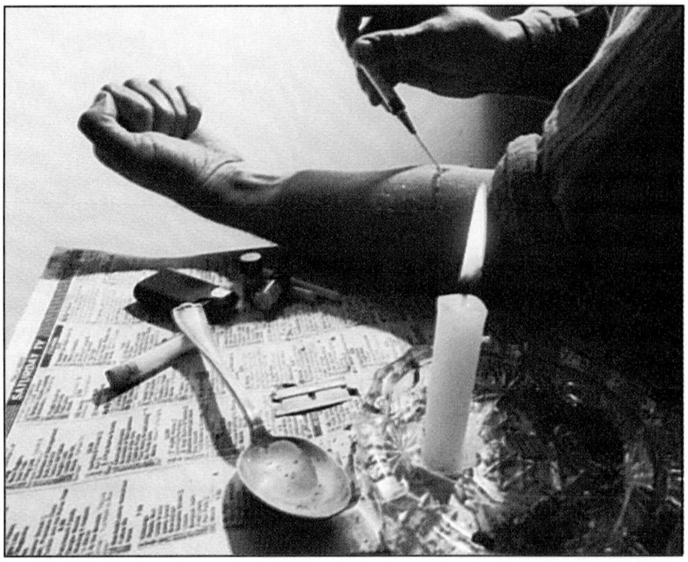

Figure 17-20

Intravenous heroin.

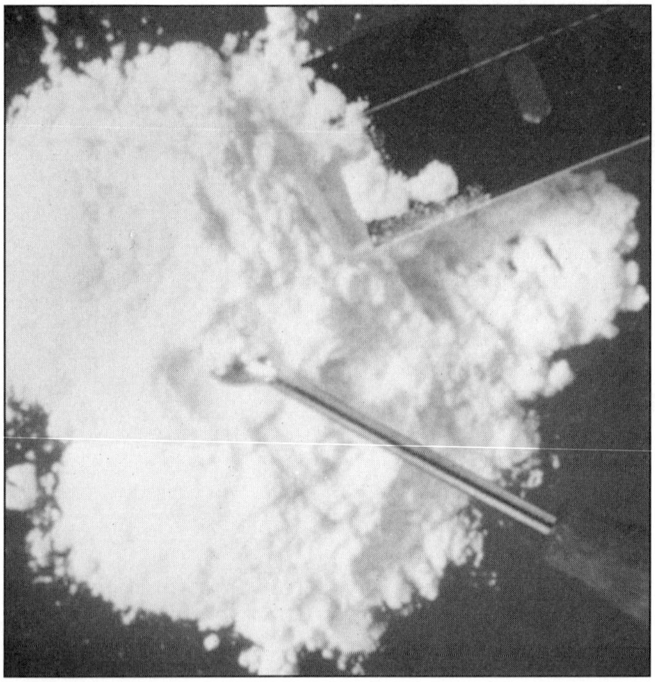

Figure 17-21

Cocaine in powdered form can be either inhaled or mixed with other drugs and injected.

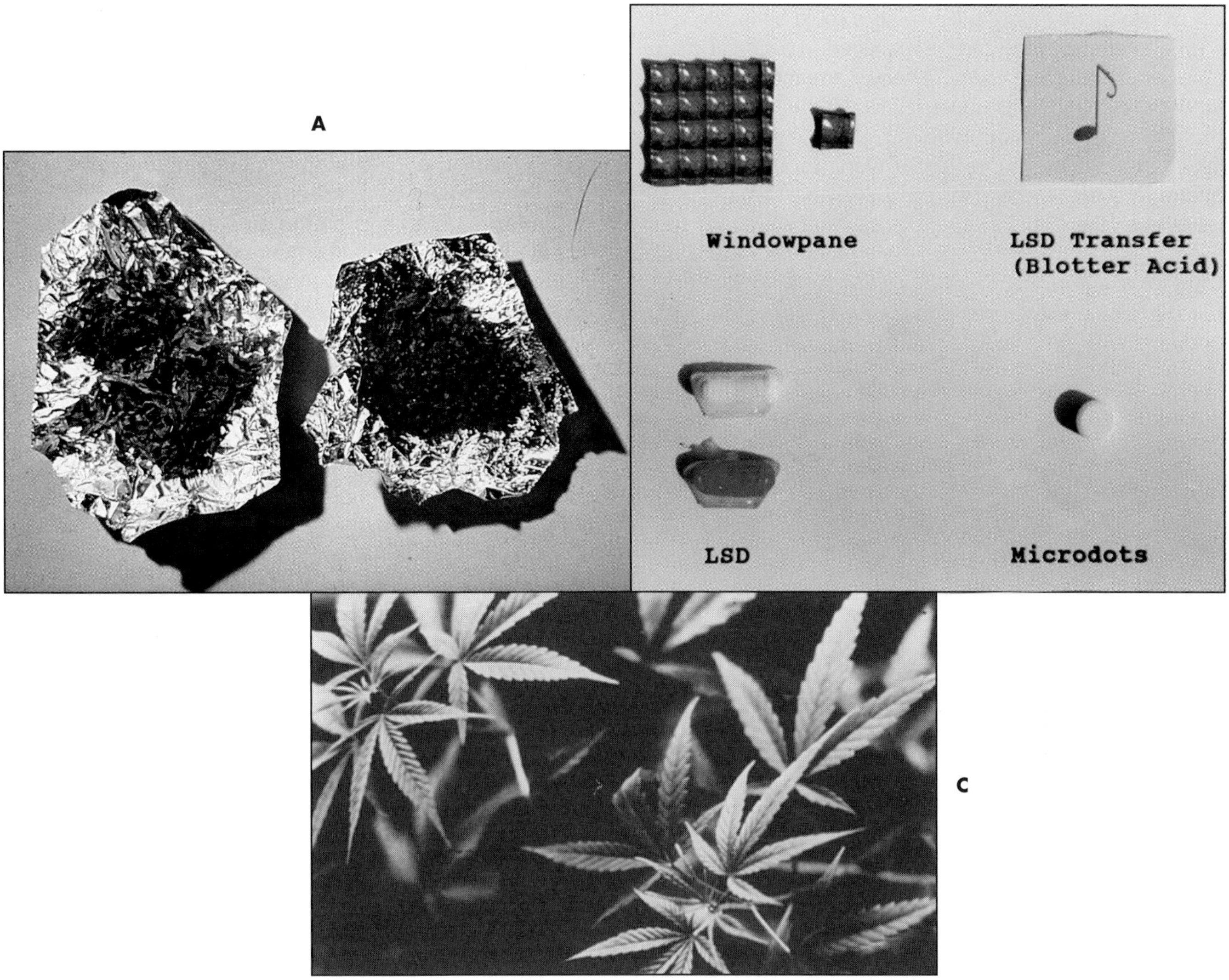

Figure 17-22

A, PCP is found naturally occurring on plants. **B,** LSD in some of its more common forms. **C,** Marijuana is derived from the cannabis plant.

illegal substances such as heroin, cocaine, and lysergic acid diethylamide (LSD). However, overdoses of legal substances such as alcohol, prescription medications, over-the-counter medications, and vitamins are also possible.

Narcotic substances such as heroin are common causes of drug overdose (Figure 17-20). Narcotics depress the CNS, causing altered consciousness, respiratory depression, and constricted pupils. Because illegal activity may be involved with use of these drugs, you may have difficulty getting cooperation from victims and bystanders. Other CNS depressants include barbiturates, benzodiazepines, and alcohol, the most widely abused depressant.

Other drugs resulting in overdose include stimulants such as amphetamine and methamphetamine. The most publicized and potent stimulant is cocaine. Whether injected, snorted (inhaled nasally), or smoked, cocaine poses a serious threat because of its addictive properties and its effect on heart rate and rhythm (Figure 17-21).

There are also substances that produce delusions and alter perception of time and space. Known as *hallucinogens,* they change mood, sensation, thought, and self-awareness. The most widely abused hallucinogens are marijuana, LSD, phencyclidine (PCP), and psilocybin mushrooms (Figure 17-22, *A, B,* and *C*).

While many different substances could be involved in a drug overdose, they can be managed in a similar manner. Ensure that the scene is secure; maintain an open airway if the patient is unconscious. Use suction to clear the airway if necessary. Provide high-concentration oxygen and ventilate the patient if respirations are inadequate. Request ALS assistance, if available. Try to determine from the victim and witnesses what substance was used, when it was used, and how much was involved. Care for any significant conditions that have resulted from the use of the substances and for any injuries that have occurred.

SUMMARY

This chapter covered basic information about poisonings and guidelines for treating poisoning victims. Remember to maintain an open airway, administer oxygen, and ventilate the patient as needed. Because vomiting is common, be ready to suction the airway. Try to collect the poison and take it with you or carefully document what it is. Transport the patient to the nearest hospital. If appropriate, you may receive an order to administer activated charcoal to manage ingested poisoning. Some poisons will result in severe allergic reactions.

REFERENCES

1. **National Safety Council:** *Accident facts,* Itasca, Ill, 1995 edition, National Safety Council.
2. **Auerbach PS, Geehr EC:** *Wilderness medicine: management of wilderness and environmental emergencies,* ed 3, St Louis, 1995, Mosby.

Chapter 18

Allergic Reactions

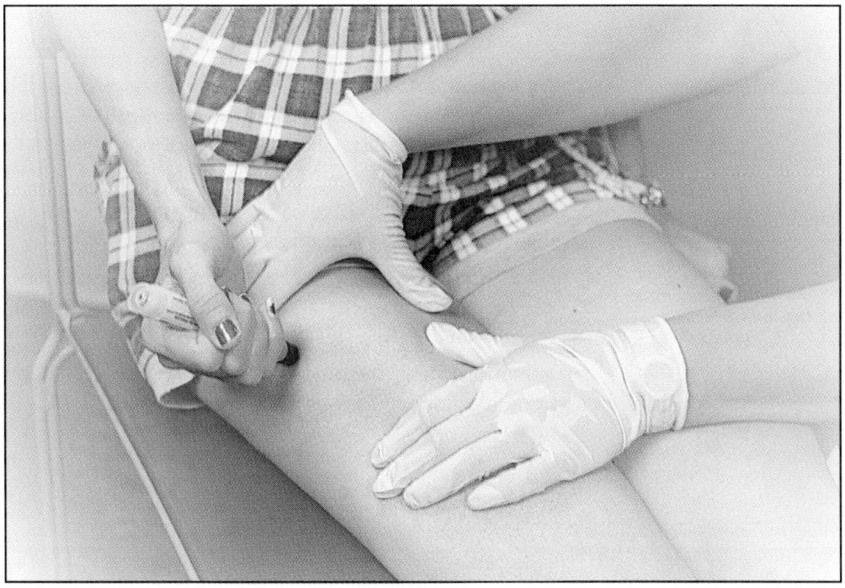

OBJECTIVES

Knowledge Objectives

As an EMT-Basic, you should be able to:

1. Recognize an allergic reaction.
2. Describe the mechanism of an allergic reaction and how it can affect the airway.
3. Describe how to manage the airway in allergic reactions.
4. Describe the general emergency care for a patient with an allergic reaction.
5. Identify the generic and trade names, medication form, dosage, route, action, indications, and contraindications for the epinephrine autoinjector.
6. Identify signs indicating an allergic reaction that requires immediate medical care, including administration of epinephrine.
7. Explain when it is important to contact medical direction about a patient with an allergic reaction.

Skill Objectives

As an EMT-Basic, you should be able to:

1. Demonstrate how to provide emergency medical care for a patient experiencing an allergic reaction.
2. Demonstrate how to use an epinephrine autoinjector, including how to assess and document patient response to the injection and how to properly dispose of the equipment.
3. Demonstrate how to complete a prehospital care report for patients with allergic emergencies.

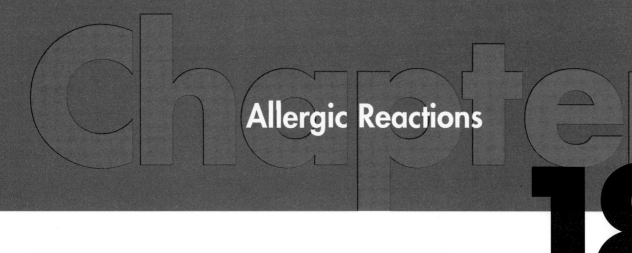

Attitude Objectives

As an EMT-Basic, you should be able to:

OBJECTIVES

1. **Describe what a patient may be feeling who develops trouble breathing after a bee sting.**
2. **Discuss how you might feel as a rescuer the first time you help a patient with an epinephrine autoinjector.**

KEY TERMS

1. **Allergen:** A foreign substance that produces an allergic reaction.
2. **Allergic Reaction:** An immune response to contact with an allergen.
3. **Anaphylaxis:** A severe, potentially life-threatening, allergic reaction.
4. **Autoinjector:** A sealed, plastic-encased syringe that automatically injects medication when pressed against the injection site.
5. **Edema:** Swelling produced by fluid (plasma) seeping from capillaries into surrounding tissues.
6. **Epinephrine:** A medication commonly used to relieve the signs and symptoms of a severe allergic reaction. It constricts blood vessels, dilates bronchial passages, and helps block the histamine response.
7. **Histamine:** A chemical released by the immune system in response to exposure to an allergen.
8. **Hives (Urticaria):** A type of rash produced by an allergic reaction; characterized by itching and swollen areas of skin.
9. **Immune System:** The organ system that protects the body from infection and invasion by foreign substances.

IT'S YOUR CALL

You are working on a summer day when your ambulance is dispatched to a local park for an unspecified illness. At the scene, you find a 19-year-old female who works as a counselor for a local day camp. She and her kindergarten campers have been having a picnic. Now she feels ill and is seated on a park bench while other counselors take charge of her group. The counselor says she feels ill because she was stung by a bee.

In your initial assessment, you see some blotching around the patient's face, neck, and arms. You also notice a red, swollen area on her left forearm where she says the bee stung her. She is sweating although she is sitting in the shade. Her pulse and breathing have become faster since your arrival. You also detect slight wheezing when auscultating her lung sounds. You determine that the patient has a history of **allergic reactions** to bee stings.

An allergic reaction can be a medical emergency requiring advanced life support (ALS) intervention. You notify dispatch of the need for ALS personnel, but the nearest medic unit is just clearing the hospital approximately 15 minutes away. What basic life support treatment should you provide? What medication will help the patient? How does it work? How is it administered? What precautions should be taken?

The **immune system** functions to protect the body from infection and from invasion by foreign substances. It consists of the lymphatic system, the spleen, and a number of components in the blood.

An allergic reaction is an immune response to contact with a foreign substance. In some cases, a patient can develop a severe and potentially life-threatening allergic reaction—**anaphylaxis**—caused by an exaggerated immune response. Patients with severe allergic reactions often have prescribed medication to carry with them, such as **epinephrine** in an **autoinjector.** Even though patients carry such medication, they are sometimes uncomfortable administering it themselves or are uncertain whether to do so. They may also be too weak or disoriented to administer it. These patients can benefit from your assistance administering the medication.

This chapter provides basic information about allergic reactions, including their possible causes and their signs and symptoms. You also will learn about emergency medical care for allergic reactions with emphasis on airway management. Finally, this chapter provides information about epinephrine: how it works, its side effects, the conditions under which it should and should not be given, and how to use an autoinjector to administer it.

The Allergic Response

Substances that cause allergic reactions are called **allergens.** For most people, these substances are harmless. However, for some, insect bites and stings and common substances such as shellfish, peanuts, medications, milk, and even dust, can cause allergic reactions. About 5% of the population is allergic to the venom of bees, hornets, and wasps. Allergic reactions are often caused by substances from one of the following four groups (Figure 18-1). (The examples listed are among the most common; however, many other specific substances in these categories can be allergens.)

- Food (shellfish, peanuts, milk)
- Plants (pollen or other plant materials)
- Medications (especially penicillin and other antibiotics)
- Insect bites and stings (honey bee, yellow jacket, wasp, hornet)

The rate at which allergic reactions develop varies widely based on the type of allergen, the route of contact with the allergen, and the type of reactions the patient has previously experienced. Generally, stings or allergens from injection develop fairly quickly; those ingested may take longer. Patients with prior severe reactions tend to react quickly.

Anaphylaxis is a severe, potentially life-threatening reaction to an allergen. Anaphylaxis can develop very quickly. Most related deaths are caused by an inability to breathe and a decrease in blood pressure.

Histamine, a powerful blood vessel dilator, is one of several chemicals released during the immune response. This physiologic protection system works well when the reaction is localized. However, it can cause a medical emergency if these substances provoke a generalized, sys-

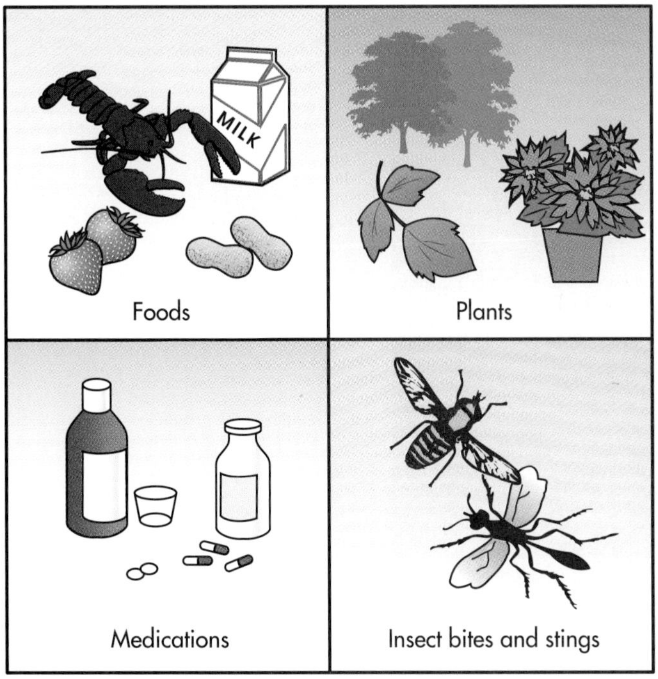

Figure 18-1

Allergens are often common substances that are harmless for most people.

temic reaction. A response that dilates blood vessels throughout the body can quickly lower blood pressure and cause shock.

Histamine and the other allergic responder chemicals have important effects beyond dilating vessels. They produce **edema** by making capillaries "leaky," and they trigger smooth-muscle constriction in the lungs (bronchoconstriction). This allergic response actually cannot take place during a first exposure to an allergen. The first contact sensitizes the body to recognize the substance as an allergen. An allergic reaction, either mild or severe, can then occur when the patient is reexposed to the same allergen.

Some people who experience severe allergic reactions are treated with repeated, small doses of the allergen (allergy shots) to desensitize themselves to the allergen so that they will not develop such severe reactions. Those with severe reactions should also be careful to avoid possible exposure. For example, those allergic to insects should always wear long pants and shoes when outdoors, avoid areas where insects typically are found (e.g., gardens, flower beds), and avoid cosmetics and perfumes, which often attract insects.

Recognizing Allergic Reactions

Allergens, usually protein substances, stimulate the immune system to produce an allergic response. The reaction is usually mild. Inhaled allergens can produce a runny nose, sneezing, watery eyes, and headache. With insect bites and stings, the normal reaction is often only localized pain and swelling; however, this is not always the case. The signs and symptoms of a severe reaction can present quickly. The skin is almost always a good early warning indicator of allergic reactions. It becomes flushed as the blood vessels dilate, and the redness may progress to a rash called **hives (urticaria)** (Figure 18-2). The patient may also complain of itching and burning of the skin. Edema, swelling produced by fluid (plasma) seeping from capillaries into surrounding tissues, is often present. This can be seen in several areas, especially around the face, neck, tongue, hands, and feet (Figure 18-3).

Fluid leaking into throat tissues can cause edema that constricts the airway. A patient may experience difficulty breathing and complain of tightness in the throat. A hoarse voice or stridorous breathing sounds may indicate that the patient's upper airway is swelling and in danger.

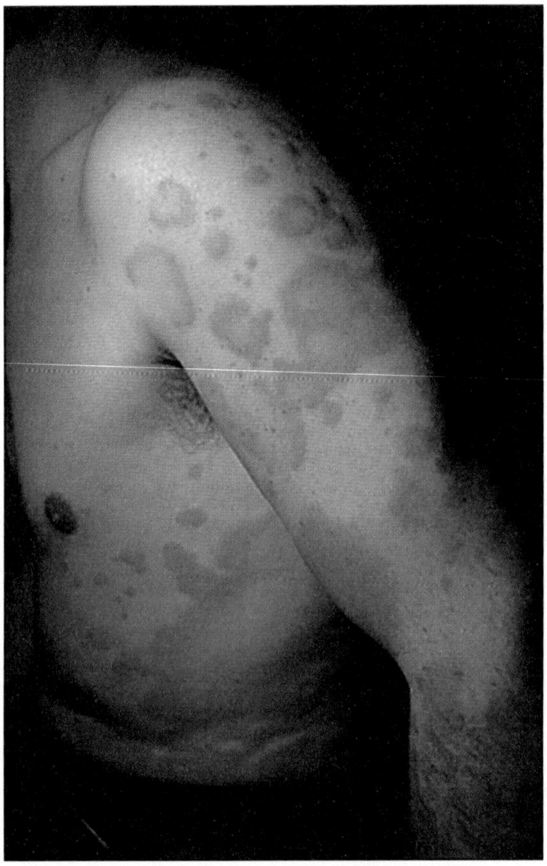

Figure 18-2

Hives are one of the quick presentations of an allergic reaction.

Signs and symptoms of an allergic reaction include:

- Coughing and sneezing; itching, watery eyes
- Stridor: a high-pitched or crowing sound caused by upper-airway swelling
- Wheezing: musical or whistling sounds produced by lower-airway spasm (constriction) or obstruction
- Respiratory distress: rapid, labored breathing
- Nausea, vomiting, or diarrhea
- Cyanosis in the lips, mucous membranes, or nail beds
- Confusion, dizziness, or unconsciousness caused by inadequate perfusion
- A rapid, weak pulse as the body tries to compensate for decreased perfusion
- A sense of fear brought on by the combination of symptoms, especially difficulty breathing
- Sweating, a part of the sympathetic response to decreased perfusion

Caring for Allergic Reactions

Severe allergic reactions can become life threatening within minutes. You must be able to recognize the signs and symptoms of a severe allergic reaction, or anaphylaxis, and act quickly to correct the problem. If ALS providers are not already en route, have them dispatched immediately; the patient may benefit from intravenous (IV) fluid therapy that ALS personnel can provide. If an ALS unit is not available or will be delayed, transport the patient promptly.

Gather pertinent information from the patient or bystanders, such as the allergen the patient may have been exposed to and the method of exposure. Determine how the patient's reaction has progressed. Ask if the patient has had a previous allergic reaction to this or other allergens. Also try to learn whether the patient has prescribed epinephrine for self-administration. Complete the remaining components of the SAMPLE history (see Chapter 9).

Mild reactions create minor skin reddening, itching, and other signs that do not include swelling, widespread hives, difficulty breathing, or signs of perfusion compromise. These patients do not require specific emergency care, but some may need transport for further evaluation and monitoring. Transport is especially important if there is any sign that a mild reaction is spreading or worsening. Make the patient comfortable, monitor respiratory status and level of consciousness (LOC), and frequently reassess vital signs. These patients may benefit from oxygen administration. It is important to understand that, because patients having an allergic reaction can deteriorate rapidly, they must be monitored closely.

In more severe reactions, place the patient in a comfortable position. If the patient is conscious and having difficulty breathing, this position is usually seated upright. If the patient's LOC is deteriorating, place the patient in the recovery position or Trendelenburg's position. Keep the airway clear. Administer high-flow oxygen through a nonrebreather mask. Be ready to assist breathing with a bag-valve-mask (BVM) if it becomes labored, too fast, or too slow. Calm the patient as much as possible and reassess vital signs continually. If the patient has epinephrine, prepare to administer it.

Administering Epinephrine

Follow local protocols for administration of epinephrine. Some EMS systems require online medical direction before administering the medication; others authorize the administration of epinephrine by standing order. Epi-

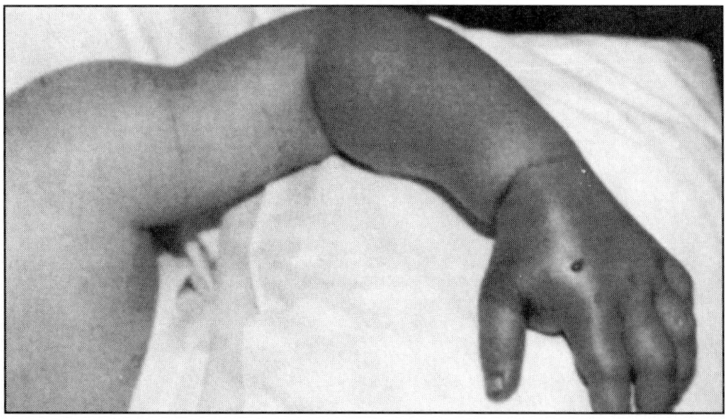

Figure 18-3

Edema can readily be seen around the hands.

nephrine is widely used to relieve the signs and symptoms of a severe allergic reaction.

Epinephrine constricts blood vessels, which raises blood pressure and improves LOC. It also dilates bronchial passages that have been constricted by histamine and the other chemicals released during the allergic response.

The epinephrine that patients carry with them may be packaged in a sealed plastic autoinjector. It contains a premeasured dose of 0.3 mg for adults or 0.15 mg if prescribed for children. Epinephrine is indicated for severe allergic reactions that include respiratory distress or shock. The side effects of epinephrine include increased heart rate, pallor, dizziness, headache, nausea and vomiting, and excitability or anxiousness.

In a life-threatening situation, there are no conditions that absolutely prohibit the use of epinephrine. However, some cautions do apply. Patients older than 40 years may develop cardiac ischemia (oxygen deficiency) that can cause chest pain and lead to heart muscle damage (myocardial infarction) after being given epinephrine. Epinephrine can also cause dangerous heart rhythms in this group. Older patients with a history of heart or coronary vessel disease such as angina, high blood pressure, or heart attacks, are at even greater risk. These situations should be discussed with the online physician before administering epinephrine.

Some patients carry allergy kits with epinephrine in a container other than an autoinjector. The kits may also include different medications, including antihistamines. These medications, like diphenhydramine hydrochloride (Benadryl) are designed to directly counteract the effects of histamine release. These alternate delivery systems and medications are not covered in the standard EMT-Basic scope of care. EMTs will not normally be able to assist in their administration.

To administer epinephrine with an autoinjector:

1. Confirm that the patient's signs and symptoms meet your protocol for administering epinephrine for a severe allergic reaction.
2. Check that the medication belongs to the patient and has not expired (see Figure 13-6).
3. Get approval from your online physician or follow off-line standing orders to administer the medication.
4. Remove clothing from the thigh. If this is not possible, the medication can be administered through clothing as thick as denim.
5. Locate the injection site on the lateral portion of the thigh, midway between the waist and knee.
6. Remove the protective cap to activate the device.
7. Place the tip of the autoinjector at a 90-degree angle (perpendicular) to the leg and push firmly (Figure 18-4).
8. Hold the autoinjector in this position for 10 seconds to ensure that all of the medication is injected.
9. Deposit the used autoinjector in a biohazard container.
10. Record the time of the administration and monitor the patient's vital signs for indications of improvement. If the patient's condition does not improve in a few minutes and the patient has an additional injector, contact the online physician to discuss administering an additional dose.

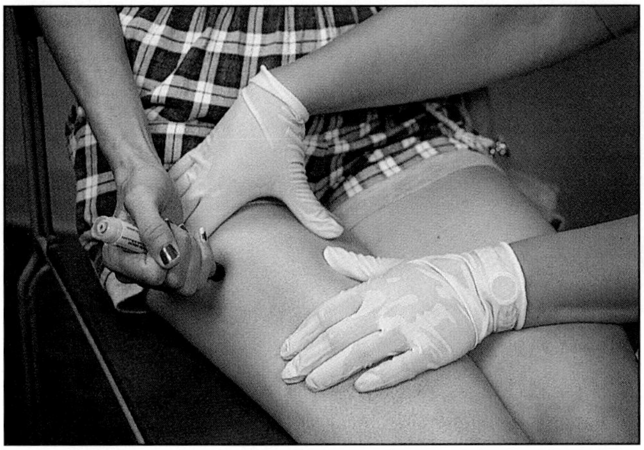

Figure 18-4

The autoinjector device will automatically administer the medication when it is pressed firmly.

IT'S YOUR CALL
CONCLUSION

Your patient has been stung by a bee and has signs and symptoms indicating an allergic reaction that is becoming more severe. The patient reaches into her backpack and produces an epinephrine autoinjector. You place the patient on high-flow oxygen as your partner inspects the injector to ensure that the medication is hers and has not expired. You contact your online physician for authorization to administer the medication. After receiving approval, you follow instructions for use of the autoinjector. After giving the medication, you transport the patient without delay. You reassess the patient's vital signs en route. By the time you pull up next to the ALS unit at a prearranged meeting point, her blood pressure has begun to rise, her breathing is improving, and she states that she is feeling somewhat better.

SUMMARY

This chapter explained how to recognize the signs and symptoms of mild and severe (anaphylactic) allergic reactions. The most significant signs—edema, shock, and difficulty breathing—can be life threatening. It also presented information on how to care for patients suffering from allergic reactions. Care for anaphylaxis involves patient positioning, airway and breathing management, requesting ALS personnel, the possible use of epinephrine, and rapid transport to a hospital.

As an EMT-Basic, you will be able to administer epinephrine to patients who carry autoinjectors with them. Before administering this medication, be certain that your patient fits the protocol for epinephrine administration. An initial patient assessment and physical examination must be completed quickly. Contact your online physician to discuss the patient's condition and request an order to administer epinephrine. Follow the proper steps for injection, then monitor the patient closely and document response to the medication.

Chapter 19

Environmental Emergencies

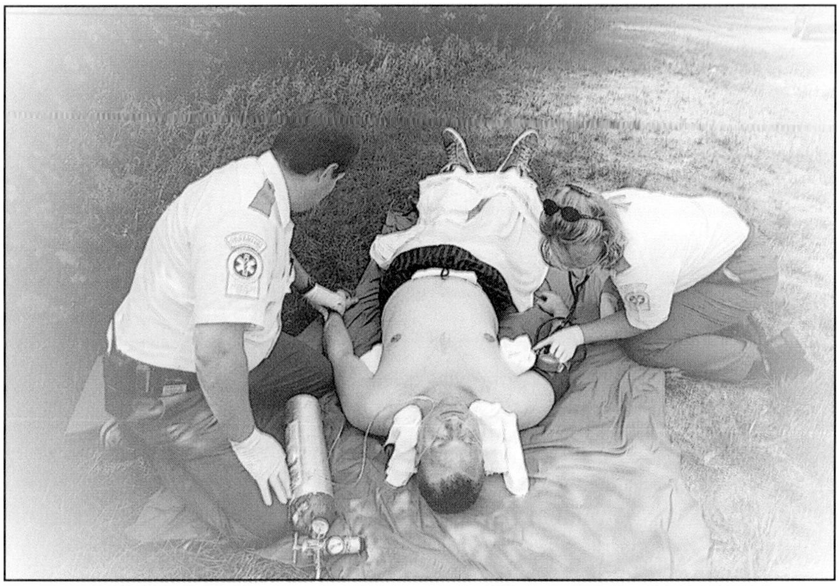

Knowledge Objectives

As an EMT-Basic, you should be able to:

OBJECTIVES

1. Name and describe the methods by which the body retains and loses heat.
2. List the signs and symptoms of cold exposure.
3. Differentiate the signs and symptoms of hypothermia and frostbite.
4. Describe the general steps of care for a patient with a cold-related emergency.
5. Describe the specific steps of care for hypothermia and frostbite.
6. List the signs and symptoms of heat exposure.
7. Describe the difference between heat cramps, heat exhaustion, and heat stroke.
8. Describe how to provide care for a patient with a heat-related emergency.
9. Recognize the signs and symptoms of water-related emergencies.
10. Explain the difference between drowning and near-drowning.
11. Describe the complications associated with near-drowning.
12. Describe how to provide care for a patient who has experienced a near-drowning.
13. Describe how to provide care for a patient who has experienced barotrauma.
14. Describe the signs and symptoms of high-altitude illness.
15. Describe how to provide care for a patient who has experienced high-altitude illness.
16. Explain how to provide general care for bites and stings.

OBJECTIVES

Skill Objectives

As an EMT-Basic, you should be able to:

1. **Demonstrate how to assess a patient who has suffered a heat-, cold-, water-, or altitude-related emergency.**
2. **Demonstrate how to provide care for a patient with a heat-, cold-, water-, or altitude-related emergency.**
3. **Demonstrate how to complete a patient-care report for a patient with a heat-, cold-, water-, or altitude-related emergency.**

Attitude Objectives

As an EMT-Basic, you should be able to:

1. **Defend the need to take spinal precautions when caring for a near-drowning victim.**
2. **Advocate the need for summoning advanced life support (ALS) personnel or contacting physician medical direction to discuss the care of a patient who has suffered an environmental emergency.**
3. **Serve as a role model for others when assessing and caring for a patient with an environmental emergency.**

KEY TERMS

1. **Ambient Temperature:** The environmental temperature to which the body is exposed; the surrounding air or water temperature.
2. **Barotrauma:** Tissue damage that results when a person is exposed to increased environmental pressure; commonly associated with scuba diving injuries.
3. **Conduction:** The direct transfer of heat from a warmer object to a colder object or fluid.
4. **Convection:** The transfer of heat from the body to colder moving air or water vapor.
5. **Decompression Sickness:** An illness that occurs when nitrogen bubbles expand in the tissues in which they have dissolved; usually caused by ascending too rapidly during scuba diving; also called the *bends*.
6. **Drowning:** Death resulting from submersion in fluid, most commonly water.
7. **Evaporation:** The process in which a liquid changes to a gas; also involves transfer of heat and can thus be a mechanism of heat loss.
8. **Frostbite:** A cold-related emergency in which body tissues freeze.
9. **High-altitude Illness:** Illness associated with insufficient oxygen from decreased atmospheric pressure at high altitude.
10. **Hyperthermia:** A condition in which the body retains more heat than it loses, causing body temperature to rise above normal levels.
11. **Hypothermia:** A condition in which the body loses more heat than it retains, causing body temperature to fall below normal levels.
12. **Near-drowning:** A submersion incident in which the patient survives.
13. **Radiation:** The transfer of heat from a warm surface to the cooler environment.

IT'S YOUR CALL

It is noon on a hot, humid summer day—the last day of a grueling, 3-day ultratriathalon event. Day 1 involved a 3-mile swim at a nearby lake. Day 2 featured a 100-mile bike ride over rolling hills. Today, the event is a 26-mile run. Many participants had muscle cramps during the first 2 days, and yesterday there were several bike crashes. Heat may play a factor today; hot temperatures and high humidity are forecasted.

You and your partner are positioned at the 19-mile mark. It is about here that runners sometimes begin to have problems. Most have passed your point already, leaving only a few behind in the rising temperatures. Several runners passing by complain that there were no drinks at the previous station. You advise that the next station is about a mile ahead. A female runner approaches, staggers momentarily, then regains her footing. Her pace is slow. You approach her and ask how she is feeling, noticing that her skin appears very flushed. She refuses any assistance, pushes on at a quicker pace, and is soon out of sight.

A few minutes later, you are dispatched to assist a "runner down" at the 20.5-mile mark. As you and your partner arrive in the ambulance, you see the same woman, lying at the side of the roadway and not moving. Runners and bystanders state that she staggered and collapsed to her knees. Another runner assisted her to the ground, where she failed to respond to his questions.

How are you going to assess and provide care for this patient? What signs and symptoms might you look for? What is this patient's most likely problem?

The environment can sometimes be a hostile setting. Sport, recreation, and work activities can lead to environmental emergencies, whether indoors or outdoors. These emergencies are often related to heat, cold, water, and altitude. They can also involve bites and stings of insects and animals (see Chapter 17). During your assessment, you are likely to uncover clues that point to a particular problem. Once you consider the mechanism of injury or nature of illness and evaluate the patient's signs and symptoms, you will be able to provide appropriate care. In general, care involves rewarming a patient who is cold, cooling a patient who is hot, and immobilizing and resuscitating a patient who has suffered a serious water-related emergency.

Regulating Body Temperature

Normal body temperature is 98.6° F (37° C). The body must maintain this temperature fairly closely to function properly. While slight changes in body temperature can be normal, significant variations cause life-threatening changes in the body. Among these changes is the failure of the sweat mechanism to function properly when the body is exposed to extreme heat for a prolonged period; core temperature can rise to the point that it causes unconsciousness and death. Loss of body temperature can also lead to major problems.

The body should respond quickly to changes in **ambient temperature,** the surrounding environmental temperature, in order to maintain a normal internal temperature. The body tries to regulate internal temperature by balancing heat loss with heat production. Heat can be generated through metabolism (converting food to energy) and through muscle contraction. If body temperature is warmer than ambient temperature, heat is lost to the environment. If the body is unable to continue to manufacture and retain adequate heat, body temperature drops. The body conserves heat by constricting blood vessels near the skin. This shunts warm blood to the body core, limiting the amount of heat escaping through the skin. If this fails to control heat loss, rapid contraction of the muscles, or shivering, increases heat production.

The body loses heat in four major ways (Figure 19-1):

- **Conduction:** The direct transfer of heat from a warmer object to a colder one, such as the loss of body heat from the skin when lying on cold ground or when submerged in cold water.
- **Convection:** The transfer of heat from the body to cooler moving air or water vapor. This commonly occurs when an individual is exposed to cold wind and takes place more quickly when the air is very humid.
- **Evaporation:** The transfer of heat that occurs when liquid turns to gas. The common example is sweating. As sweat evaporates, it takes heat away from the body.
- **Radiation:** The transfer of heat from a warm surface to a cooler environment. This occurs when body temperature is warmer than the surfaces of objects around it (e.g., skin to cooler air). Clothing and blankets can help reduce heat loss through radiation.

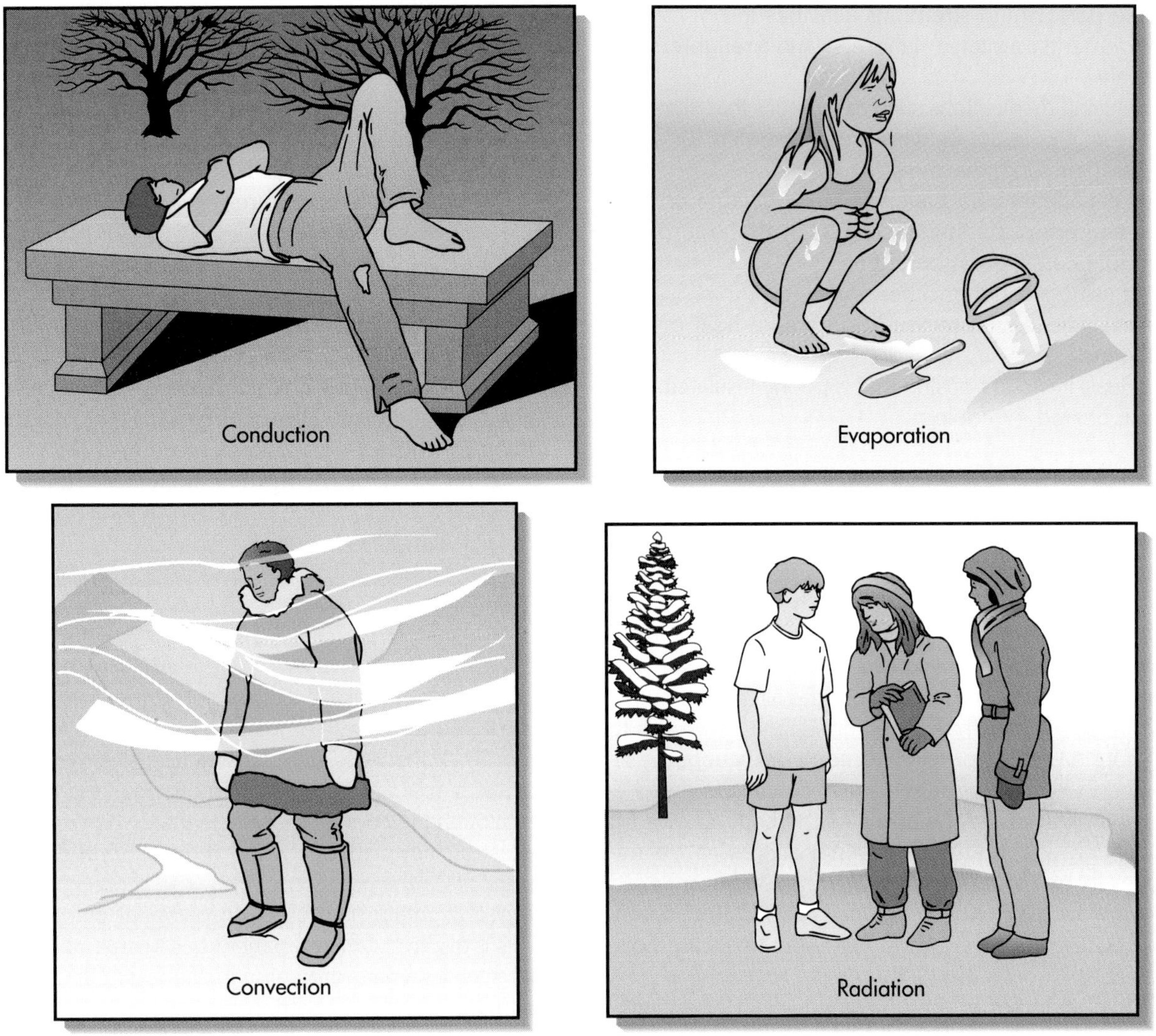

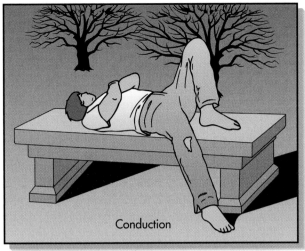

Figure 19-1

The body can lose heat through direct transfer to an object or fluid (conduction), through transfer to moving air or vapor (convection), through evaporation of fluids, and through radiation to the environment.

Respiration combines two of these mechanisms, evaporation and convection, in a hidden form of heat loss. The rate and depth of respirations determine how much heat is lost in the form of exhaled warm air and water vapor.

If the environment is warmer than the body, the body absorbs this heat and must find a way to remove what it does not need. It does so by dilating blood vessels near the surface of the skin, allowing more blood to come to the surface and radiate heat away. Sweating adds evaporative heat loss.

Other elements such as fluid intake and the type and amount of clothing a person wears also help regulate body temperature. Blood circulates heat that is produced in the core throughout the body, including the skin, where heat can be given off.

Predisposing Factors for Heat and Cold Emergencies

Those at increased risk for heat or cold emergencies include:

- Young and elderly individuals. A child's body is not capable of adequately regulating heat and cold. Children have a relatively large surface area to body mass, making it easy to experience temperature changes. They have less body fat, and their smaller muscle mass does not allow for efficient shivering. In the elderly, disease and aging lead to poor circulation.
- Individuals with preexisting health problems that cause poor circulation, such as cardiovascular disease and diabetes.

- People performing strenuous activities in hot or cold environments; athletes, laborers, and firefighters are examples.
- Those using medications such as diuretics that eliminate fluid from the body, or who are dehydrated for other reasons (vomiting, diarrhea).
- Trauma patients who have lost blood volume or have been injured in the spinal cord or in the area of the brain that controls temperature.
- Those using alcohol or other drugs.
- Patients who have previously suffered a heat or cold emergency.
- Individuals living in housing that is poorly insulated, ventilated, heated, or cooled.

The three external factors that have the greatest effect on heat loss or gain are ambient air temperature, wind, and humidity (moisture in the air). Wind and humidity can enhance the effects of ambient air temperature, making them seem hotter or colder. When exposed to wind, the body loses heat at a more rapid rate through convection. Humidity refers to the moisture content in the air; the greater the humidity, the more moist the air. A hot, humid day often feels hotter than a hot, dry day. It also tends to cause more breathing problems among the young, the elderly, and those with certain medical conditions. In addition, as humidity rises, the ability of the body to give off heat through evaporation (sweating) decreases. At humidity levels of 75%, evaporation drops significantly. At levels approaching 90% humidity, evaporation nearly ceases because the air is almost fully saturated with moisture already.

Wind-chill factor is the combined effect of air temperature and wind and plays an important role in cold-related emergencies. Humidity and air temperature combine to produce a heat index. Weather forecasters often refer to these two terms when discussing what the temperature really feels like. This can provide individuals with a better idea of how serious the environmental conditions really are.

General Assessment

When assessing a scene, look for a mechanism that may have caused the problem. For example, if you find a person lying on the roadway on a cold evening, consider whether the person collapsed as a result of a cold-related emergency. Even if the collapse was caused by some other condition, cold may now be part of the problem. Question the patient or bystanders to determine the degree that the environment played a factor in the condition. Consider these factors:

- The source of heat or cold
- The length of exposure to heat or cold
- Whether the exposure resulted in altered consciousness that contributed to further injury if the patient collapsed or failed to respond properly
- The patient's pertinent medical history, if known
- Whether the problem is localized, affecting a specific body part, or generalized, affecting the entire body
- The patient's temperature

Cold-Related Emergencies

There are two types of cold-related emergencies: generalized and localized. **Hypothermia** is a generalized condition in which the body loses more heat than it retains, resulting in a below-normal body-core temperature. **Frostbite** is a localized condition in which body tissues in particular areas freeze.

Hypothermia

Contrary to popular belief, hypothermia is more likely to occur with moderate ambient temperatures between 40° and 50° F than it is with extremely cold temperatures because people are more likely to overlook the need for extra clothing in cool temperatures than when it is very cold. Moist air coupled with wind reduces temperature even more. If clothing becomes wet, the protective layers designed to retain heat begin to pull heat out of the body. This is also true when a patient has been immersed in water, such as a near-drowning incident. Hunters and fishermen are prone to hypothermia, especially if weather conditions change suddenly, catching them unprepared and far from shelter. Always suspect the possibility of hypothermia in these situations.

Recognizing Hypothermia

As body temperature drops, the patient will pass through various stages of hypothermia, from mild to severe. In the mildest stage of hypothermia, core temperature is approximately 94° to 97° F. The most noticeable sign is shivering. These rapid muscle contractions are an attempt to generate more heat. As hypothermia progresses and body temperature drops to 86° to 94° F, shivering may still be present but the patient will experience loss of sensation, difficulty speaking, altered consciousness (usually confusion and dizziness), and muscle rigidity. In the most severe stage of hypothermia, core temperature is below 86° F. In this stage, shivering is usually absent and the patient is responsive only to pain, if responsive at all. Respirations and pulse become slow and irregular.

Because blood flow to the extremities is diminished when the body cools, checking the skin peripherally will reveal cool skin. To get a better indicator of the presence of hypothermia, check the abdomen. If the abdomen is cool, the patient is probably hypothermic. Altered con-

TABLE 19-1 Stages of Hypothermia

Vital signs	Mild hypothermia 94°-97° F	Moderate hypothermia 86°-94° F	Severe hypothermia <86° F
Level of consciousness	Usually normal	Alert but disoriented	Responsive to painful stimuli only, or unresponsive
Respirations	Rapid	Slowing	Slow, shallow, or absent
Pulse	Rapid	Slowing	Slow, irregular, barely palpable
Blood pressure	Normal	Falling	Low or absent
Skin	Normal or flushed	Pale, cool	Pale or cyanotic, cool
Pupils	Normal (reactive)	Sluggish	Dilated, slow to respond

sciousness and decreased motor function are among the most significant signs that hypothermia is serious. When a patient is in the late, severe stage of hypothermia, pulses may be barely palpable or undetectable. Check carefully for pulses in the carotid and femoral arteries; you may need to palpate for 30 seconds or longer. Table 19-1 illustrates how vital signs change as hypothermia progresses.

Caring for Hypothermia

The care you provide for a hypothermic patient will vary depending on the patient's level of consciousness (LOC). The common element of care is that all hypothermic patients need to be rewarmed. There are two general methods: passive and active rewarming. Active rewarming, in turn, can be done in two ways: internally and externally.

Passive rewarming, the most basic method, can be thought of as self-rewarming. In this situation, you simply move the patient from the cold environment to a warmer one, such as an ambulance with the heat turned up. Remove cold, wet clothing, and cover the patient in warm, dry material. The patient generates enough heat to rewarm the body naturally.

Active rewarming, on the other hand, requires you to add heat to the patient's body. Active external rewarming, which is more effective than passive rewarming, is done by applying heat packs or other heat sources to the outside of the patient's body. Active internal rewarming, the most aggressive method and the most effective for severe hypothermia, can be accomplished with warmed, humidified oxygen. ALS personnel may follow this with warmed intravenous fluids, and hospital personnel may flush the stomach with warm fluid or use a cardiac bypass machine to warm the blood directly.

There are several general steps to follow when treating a hypothermic patient, regardless of the stage.

- Maintain an open airway.
- Rewarm the patient. Begin by preventing further heat loss. Remove the patient from the cold environment, remove any wet clothing, and wrap the patient in warm blankets. Turn up the heat in the ambulance.
- Administer high-flow oxygen, preferably warmed and humidified (Figure 19-2).
- Handle the patient gently; rough handling can cause life-threatening cardiac rhythm problems.
- If your protocols allow, attempt to measure body temperature with an oral or rectal thermometer.
- Summon advanced life support (ALS) personnel or contact your medical direction physician.
- Transport the patient to a hospital for evaluation.

You can also begin active external rewarming. Wrap chemical heat packs in towels and place them at the patient's armpits, groin, and neck. Monitor the patient closely because active external rewarming could cause cardiac rhythm disturbances by returning cold peripheral blood to the core.

If the patient is without signs of life, assess the pulse for at least 30 seconds. Because of impaired circulation, the pulse may be very hard to find in a severely hypothermic patient. If there is no pulse, begin cardiopulmonary resuscitation (CPR). Apply patches for the automated external defibrillator (AED). If the AED identifies a shockable rhythm, the patient can be defibrillated up to three times. Follow local protocols for the use of the AED in hypothermia patients. These may require you to contact medical direction for further treatment orders.

Frostbite

Frostbite is a localized condition in which specific body tissues freeze. Water lies in and around body cells. When the water freezes, it causes swelling and ice crystal formation, both of which can damage cells. The severity of frostbite is based on the depth of tissue destruction. In the most severe cases, gangrene (local tissue death) can lead to the loss of the affected body part (Figure 19-3).

Temperature, including wind chill, and exposure time are the two environmental factors that most influence the severity of frostbite. Smoking is another predisposing factor for frostbite. Smoking causes peripheral blood vessels to constrict, and the reduced blood flow lowers heat and

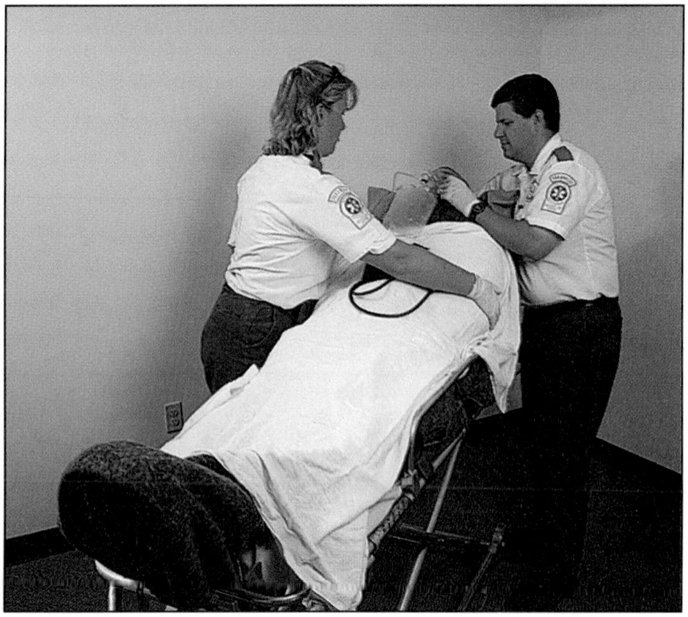

Figure 19-2

In caring for a hypothermic patient, maintain the airway and administer oxygen while performing rewarming measures.

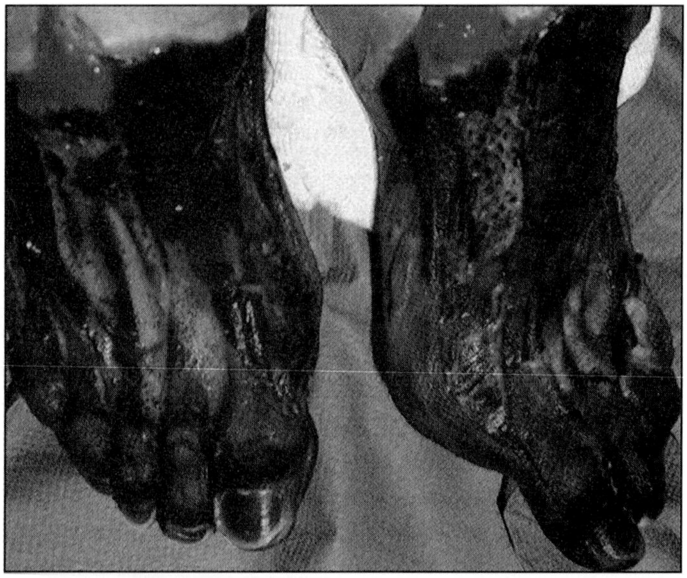

Figure 19-3

Necrosis of tissue 1 week after a severe, local, deep, cold injury.

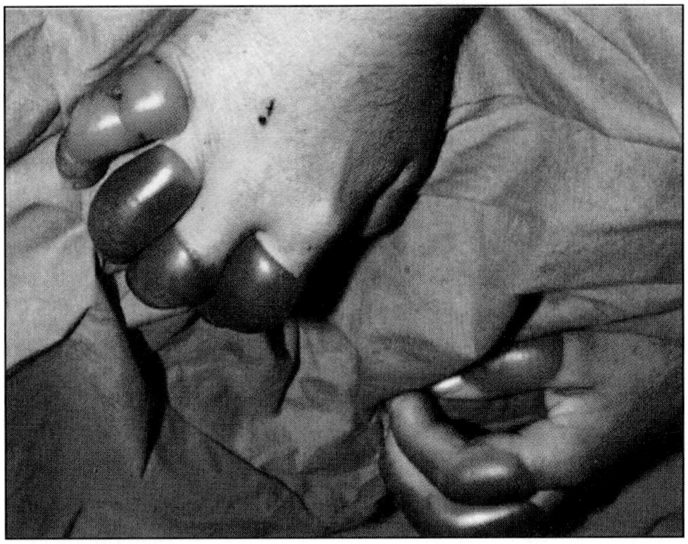

Figure 19-4

The waxy look and blisters here are common indications of a frostbite cold injury.

oxygen delivery to peripheral tissues. The most common body areas affected by frostbite are the fingers, toes, ears, nose, and face. There are several reasons for this:

1. Blood vessels in these areas are very close to the skin surface and are among the first to constrict and deprive the tissue of blood flow, which is being shunted to the core to maintain temperature there.
2. These areas are supplied by smaller-diameter vessels (capillaries), as compared with other areas with larger veins and arteries.
3. These areas are farthest from the central circulation.

Recognizing Frostbite

Superficial damage to tissue may occur at an early stage. This is commonly called *frostnip* and is characterized by pale skin; the patient will experience a tingling or loss of sensation in the affected area. As the extent of damage increases, deeper tissue destruction occurs. This makes the skin firm or "waxy," with swelling and blistering (Figure 19-4). The patient loses sensation in the affected part, making movement difficult or painful. When the area is completely frozen, it will be firm, numb, and white or gray. If the tissue has begun to thaw, the skin could appear discolored, with a combination of pale, red, cyanotic, and purple areas.

Caring for Frostbite

Frostbitten tissue needs to be rewarmed. However, this is best accomplished in a hospital setting. Your role in the care of frostbite should be to avoid further damage to the affected area. Remove the patient from the source of the cold. This includes removing cold, wet clothing. Because swelling is likely, also remove any jewelry. Cover the injured area with sterile, dry dressings and bandage loosely. If the fingers or toes are affected, place dressings between them before bandaging (Figure 19-5). If an extremity is affected, immobilize it. Administer oxygen. Do not rub the area, break blisters, or apply heat to the affected part. Do not allow the patient to walk if the feet are involved.

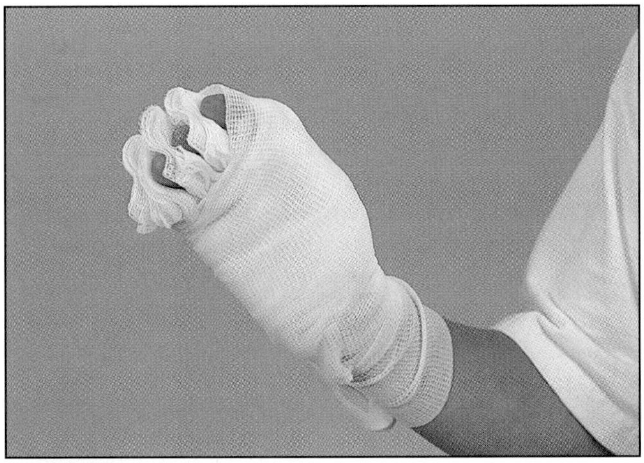

Figure 19-5

Cover the injured tissue with dry, sterile dressings. Also place dressings between fingers and toes if they are affected.

In situations involving extended transport time, you may seek medical direction and be instructed to begin rewarming. In this case, the affected part must not be allowed to refreeze during transport. Refreezing greatly increases tissue damage.

To rewarm, immerse the affected body part in warm water (102° to 104° F). Maintain this temperature by adding more warm water as the water begins to cool from contact with the cold tissue. Handle frostbitten tissue very gently; it is sensitive and easily damaged. Once the skin is soft and color and sensation have returned, gently dry, bandage, and immobilize the area.

Heat-Related Emergencies

The opposite of hypothermia is **hyperthermia,** in which the body retains more heat than it loses and body temperature rises above normal. Any time the body is unable to cool itself properly, signs and symptoms of heat illness will appear.

Recognizing Heat-Related Emergencies

As hyperthermia progresses, the patient may experience the following signs and symptoms:

- Muscle cramps: Often one of the first signs of hyperthermia, these are painful muscle spasms, usually in the legs. They can also occur in other body areas, such as the abdomen. Heat cramps result from a loss of fluid and salt during heavy sweating. Heat cramps often occur before normal body temperature has risen much above normal.
- Weakness or exhaustion: If fluid and salt loss are more severe, the patient can experience generalized weakness and exhaustion. This condition is commonly called *heat exhaustion* and may progress to hypovolemic shock.
- Changes in skin color, temperature, and moisture: The skin may look pale or flushed, feel cool or hot, or be moist or dry. An altered LOC and hot, flushed, dry skin may indicate that the sweat mechanism is not functioning properly. This can quickly become a life-threatening problem called *heat stroke.*
- Altered LOC: This can vary from disorientation to unresponsiveness.
- Rapid pulse and respirations.
- Nausea and vomiting.
- Abdominal cramps.

Caring for Heat-Related Emergencies

If you think a patient is suffering from hyperthermia:

- Remove the patient from the source of heat. This means moving the patient to a cool environment, such as an air-conditioned ambulance. Cool areas out of direct sunlight will also help if an ambulance is not immediately available.
- Remove any excessive or restrictive clothing.
- Fan the patient to promote cooling.
- Administer oxygen.
- If the patient is conscious, position in the shock position. If unconscious or vomiting, position the patient on the left side.

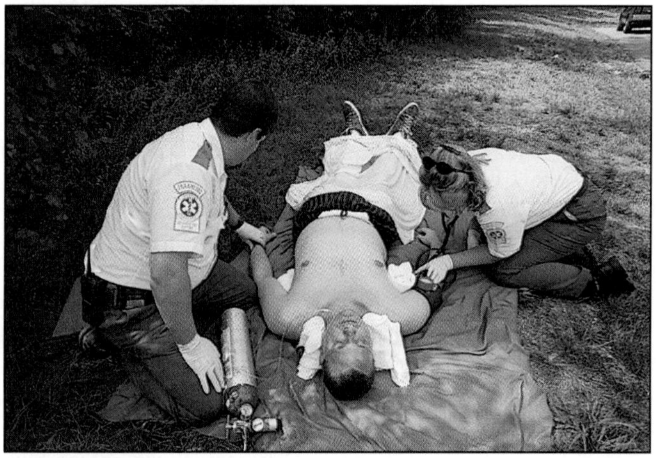

Figure 19-6

If it is necessary to cool the patient rapidly, apply moist towels or sheets and place cool packs wrapped in towels at the armpits, groin, and neck.

- If the patient is conscious and oriented and is not nauseated or vomiting, give cool water to drink.

If the patient has hot skin and an altered LOC, cool the patient rapidly. In addition to the steps discussed above, apply cool, moist sheets or towels over the patient's body and place cool packs wrapped in towels at the armpits, groin, and neck (Figure 19-6). Transport immediately and contact medical direction on the way.

Water-Related Emergencies

Water is a source of recreation for millions of Americans each year. Unfortunately it is also a source of death and disability to thousands. Drowning and near-drowning are the two most frequent water-related emergencies that you will encounter. Scuba diving also results in injuries and death as a result of pressure problems underwater.

IT'S YOUR CALL
CONCLUSION

The female runner that you spoke with minutes earlier has collapsed. You and your partner arrive to find her lying motionless on the ground.

You begin with an initial assessment of LOC, adequacy of the airway, breathing, and pulse. Recognizing that the patient is responsive only to painful stimuli and that she has a rapid pulse and respirations, you instruct your partner to apply oxygen at 15 liters per minute (lpm) with a nonrebreather mask. You rule out trauma as a problem and focus on the patient's skin, which feels hot and relatively dry despite her physical activity. You suspect that the patient is suffering from a serious heat-related emergency that requires rapid cooling.

You place the patient on your stretcher and move her to the ambulance, where you have already turned on the air conditioning. Once inside, your partner manages the patient's airway, while you remove clothing, take the patient's temperature, and begin to cool the patient with moist towels and cool packs. You notify dispatch of your situation, request an ALS unit to meet you en route, and advise the hospital. A paramedic who joins you on the way to the hospital applies a cardiac monitor and starts two intravenous lines to provide fluid. You note that the patient's temperature has begun to drop, and you continue to monitor vital signs and manage the airway. As you arrive at the hospital, the patient's condition is improving.

Drowning and Near-Drowning

Drowning is fatal submersion in fluid, most commonly water. **Near-drowning** is a submersion incident that the patient survives. Approximately 4000 Americans die each year from drowning, and nearly twice that many suffer near-drowning incidents that require hospitalization. About 30,000 are injured seriously enough to require treatment in a hospital emergency department.[1,2,3] Children under age 2 and teenagers from 15 to 19 are the most frequent victims. The three most common factors involved in drowning and near-drowning are lack of supervision, high-risk behavior, and the use of drugs, including alcohol.

Caring for Near-Drowning

Managing submersion victims always requires consideration of the possibility of associated trauma to the head and spine. Any patient found unconscious around water should be suspected of having a possible head or spine injury. If the mechanism of injury clearly indicates the potential for head and spine injury (such as a person injured when diving in shallow water), it is extremely important to manage the airway and spine appropriately from the start. This is true even of victims who have been removed from the water by lifeguards or bystanders before your arrival.

You will occasionally be on the scene before the patient is removed from the water and will participate in a search and rescue effort. In this case, remember the need to put personal safety of the rescuers first. Water rescue is a specialized activity. The rule is: rescue from shore or from very shallow water unless you have the special training and equipment required to work in deeper water.

Removing the patient from the water is a team effort. Begin by positioning the patient face up in the water. If there is any chance of spinal injury, support the head and spine. There are several methods that can be used to position and immobilize the patient. This is one of the simplest:

1. Hold the head in line with the body.
2. Rotate the patient toward you into a face-up position while supporting the head, neck, and back (Figure 19-7, *A*).
3. Have your partner submerge a backboard and raise it under the patient (Figure 19-7, *B*).
4. Control the patient's head while your partner and other rescuers support the board, secure the patient, and move to safety (Figure 19-7, *C*).

If the patient's airway is clear and breathing is adequate, apply a cervical collar and secure the remainder of the straps while still in the water (Figure 19-8). Depending on conditions, this may require more help. If the victim is unresponsive, pulseless, or in respiratory distress or arrest, appropriate care can only be accomplished on land. If adequate personnel are available to assist, remove the patient from the water immediately and begin care. Proper care requires managing the airway while stabilizing the

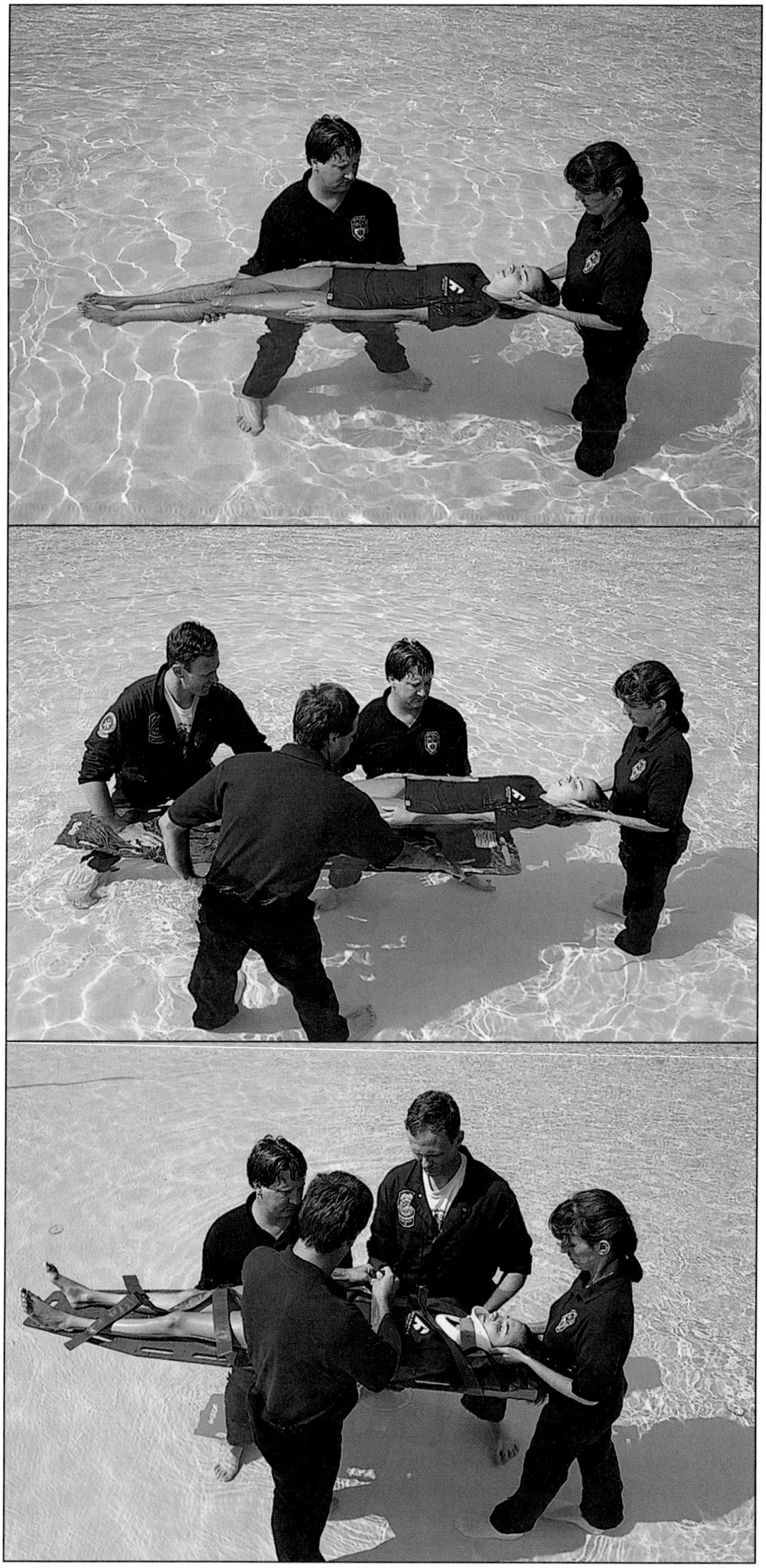

A

B

C

Figure 19-7

A, Rotate the patient while supporting the head, neck, and back. **B,** While maintaining stabilization, submerge a backboard and raise it under the patient. **C,** Secure the patient and move to safety. A cervical collar should be applied.

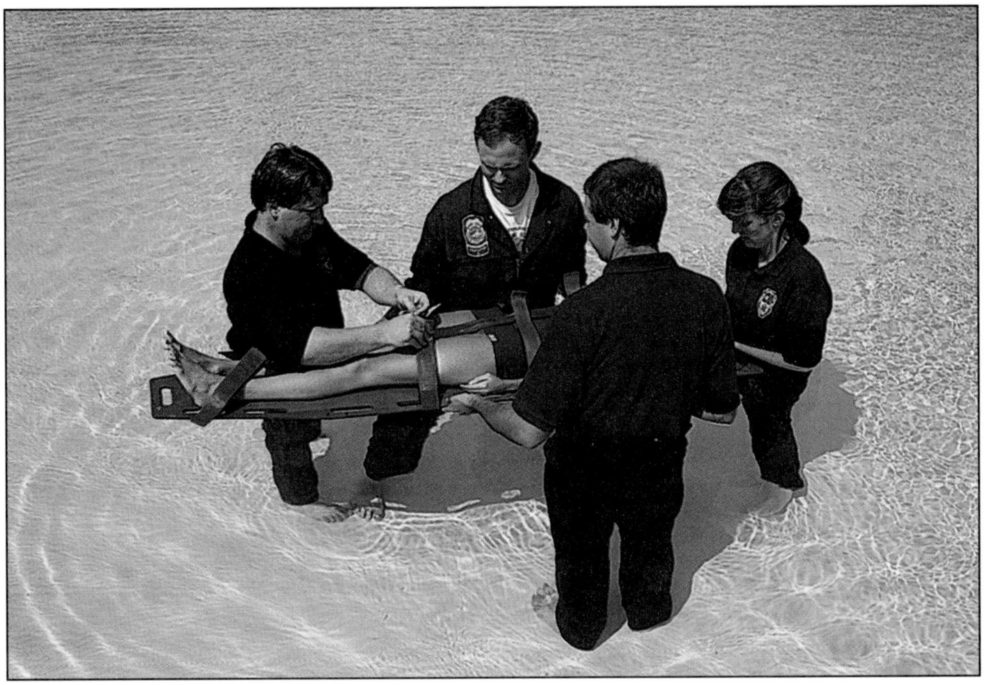

Figure 19-8
Secure all straps before moving the patient.

cervical spine and preventing hypothermia. This generally means that rescuers should not take the time to use all of the usual straps. Maintaining inline stabilization, get the patient out of the water as quickly as possible.

Once removed from the water, the patient's airway may need to be suctioned, and oxygen and ventilation provided. If the patient is pulseless, start CPR and apply an AED. If you are unable to ventilate properly, the airway may be obstructed. Attempt to relieve the obstruction by turning the head to the side (unless you suspect cervical trauma) and giving five abdominal thrusts (adult or child) or back blows and chest thrusts (infant). Endotracheal intubation is also indicated if the victim is unresponsive and in respiratory or cardiac arrest. Perform endotracheal intubation only if your protocols allow and you have been properly trained.

Scuba Diving Emergencies

The sport of scuba diving continues to grow rapidly. There are more than 3 million divers in the United States, and each year approximately 200,000 more are trained. Most scuba diving emergencies occur during underwater descent or ascent. These emergencies fall into a category of injuries known as either **barotrauma** or **decompression sickness.**

Barotrauma is tissue damage to the ears, sinuses, and other tissues that occurs from exposure to increased environmental pressure. Barotrauma during descent results from the compression of gas within enclosed spaces, such as the inner or middle ears. As the diver descends, outside pressure increases. The eustachian tube connects the nasopharynx and the inner ear and allows air pressure in the inner ear to equalize with pressure outside the body. If this tube is blocked or a diver fails to equalize pressures in the tube by exhaling during descent, severe pressure can be exerted on the ears. Besides pain, symptoms include dizziness and ringing in the ears and, in severe cases, the pressure can rupture the eardrum. These pressure changes can also affect facial sinuses if sinus congestion prevents pressure equalization.

Any air trapped in enclosed body spaces will expand as external pressure decreases during ascent. This most commonly occurs when a diver ascends rapidly while holding his or her breath after running out of air or panicking for some other reason. This can result in serious injury to the lungs. If expanding air is not exhaled, the alveoli may rupture. This can force air bubbles into the circulatory system, where they may obstruct blood flow. An air embolism resulting from rapid ascent can obstruct the pulmonary vessels and can also affect the brain and spinal cord. If air enters the pleural space, it could cause a pneumothorax.

Decompression sickness, commonly called the *bends,* involves nitrogen bubbles in the veins. The diver breathes nitrogen as part of the air mixture in the scuba tank. Higher pressures at depth make this nitrogen dissolve in the blood. As the diver ascends and pressure drops, the dissolved nitrogen expands and forms bubbles in small blood vessels and the surrounding tissue. As with air embolism, these bubbles can expand and obstruct blood flow. The patient often complains of severe extremity, chest, or abdominal pain. Additional signs and symptoms include numbness, nausea, headache, dyspnea, and loss of consciousness. The problem may appear rapidly, but not be serious enough to make the diver seek immediate attention. However, most patients with decompression sickness seek treatment within 12 hours of the onset of symptoms.

Caring for Scuba Diving Emergencies

Barotrauma during ascent is the most likely reason that you would be summoned for a scuba diving emergency. (Problems during descent usually involve the sinuses and ears and tend to be less severe.) Air embolism and decompression sickness are both caused by the same mechanism: gas expansion during a too-rapid ascent. The definitive care for these problems is recompression in a specialized chamber. This restores the patient to the pressure experienced underwater, then allows for gradual decompression that will ease the signs and symptoms. You should be familiar with the location of the nearest recompression chamber.

General care for barotrauma injuries that occur during ascent includes:

- Gathering pertinent information on the dives, such as the time under water, depth of the dive, amount of air used, whether a specialized gas mixture was used, and whether there was more than one dive in the same day.
- Protecting against hypothermia.
- Assessing lung sounds.
- Providing oxygen at 15 lpm through a nonrebreather mask. If necessary, place the patient in a supine position and assist ventilations. If there is significant concern for air embolism, the patient should be placed in Trendelenburg's position on the left side. This helps prevent air bubbles from entering the brain and coronary arteries.
- Summoning ALS personnel and contacting your medical direction physician.
- Transporting the patient without delay; this may be to a facility with a recompression chamber.

High-Altitude Emergencies

High-altitude illness is caused by insufficient oxygen that is the result of decreased atmospheric pressure at high altitude. Individuals most often affected by high-altitude emergencies are mountain climbers and hot-air balloonists. As a person is rapidly exposed to the reduced atmospheric pressure of high altitude, several serious conditions can occur.

- Acute mountain sickness
- High-altitude pulmonary edema (HAPE)
- High-altitude cerebral edema (HACE)

These conditions usually begin 24 hours after exposure to high altitude, often at 8000 feet or higher. The signs of acute mountain sickness are often the first to occur and include symptoms such as light-headedness, shortness of breath, headache, nausea and vomiting, and weakness. This can progress to a loss of muscle coordination and altered consciousness, such as confusion, disorientation, and impaired judgment. These more severe signs can indicate HACE, which can progress to blurred vision and unconsciousness. As the condition worsens, fluid can build up in the lungs and cause respiratory distress (HAPE). HACE and HAPE require immediate descent and rapid transport for emergency care. General care for less severe cases of acute mountain sickness includes oxygenation, ventilation, and descent to a lower altitude, where conditions often improve rapidly. These patients should still be transported for further evaluation and treatment.

Reviewing Bites and Stings

As you learned in Chapters 17 and 18, bites and stings are forms of injected and contact poisons that can range from mild local reaction and pain to systemic effects if the patient has an allergic reaction. Whether the bite or sting is from an insect, spider, snake, scorpion, tick, or marine animal, you should be able to assess the patient and provide appropriate care. In most cases the patient will be able to tell you what happened and possibly even exactly what type of animal is involved. During your assessment, look for signs such as a stinger embedded in the skin, bite marks, and local redness and swelling.

Use these guidelines to provide care for a patient who has been bitten or stung:

- Ensure your own safety.
- Maintain airway, breathing, and circulation.
- If a stinger is imbedded in the skin, scrape it away with the edge of a rigid item, such as a credit card or piece of cardboard.
- Clean the area.
- Remove any jewelry in case of swelling.
- Position an affected extremity lower than the heart to limit absorption of the venom.
- Follow local protocols in regard to any additional specialized care for snakebite or marine life.
- Summon ALS personnel or contact your medical direction physician if signs of an allergic reaction develop.

SUMMARY

While the signs and symptoms of environmental emergencies vary, your care has one common element: remove the patient from the source of the problem. If heat is the problem, move the patient to cool surroundings and lower the body temperature. If the patient is cold, move the patient to a warm area and begin rewarming. In the water, remove the patient to dry ground and manage the airway, breathing, and circulation problems that are likely to be present if the patient has been deprived of oxygen. If problems occur at high altitude, descend.

Some early signs and symptoms warn of more serious potential conditions. Heat cramps are often an early indicator of a heat-related emergency. If the patient ceases strenuous activity in a hot environment at that time, the problem often resolves itself. The same can be said for cold-related emergencies. Early signs such as shivering and tingling or numbness in the extremities are often indicators that the body is suffering either a generalized or localized cold-related emergency. Ignoring these early signs will cause the conditions to worsen. The care you provide for temperature-related emergencies is based on the severity of the condition.

Manage water-related emergencies such as near-drowning by maintaining the airway and cervical spine stabilization. Provide care assuming that a head or spinal injury has occurred. Administer oxygen, and ventilate if needed. If the patient is pulseless, begin CPR.

Care for scuba diving emergencies also includes providing oxygen and ventilation. Position the patient for comfort, and transport the patient to the nearest hospital or to a recompression chamber for definitive care.

High-altitude illnesses occur when people ascend too rapidly to adapt to the reduced oxygen supply at higher altitudes. The patient should be treated during descent to a lower altitude and then transported for further care.

REFERENCES

1. **Association of Trial Lawyers of America and Johns Hopkins Injury Prevention Center:** *Good sports: preventing recreational injuries,* Baltimore, 1992.
2. **National Safety Council:** *Accident facts,* Itasca, Ill, 1995, National Safety Council.
3. **Wintemute GJ:** Childhood drowning and near-drowning in the United States, *Am J Dis Child* 44:633, 1990.

SUGGESTED READINGS

1. **Auerbach PS, Geehr EC:** *Management of wilderness and environmental emergencies,* ed 2, St Louis, 1989, Mosby.
2. **Clarke JR:** The perils of puddles, pails, and pools: preparing for pediatric submersions, *J Emerg Med Serv* 17:38, 1992.

Chapter 20

Behavioral Emergencies

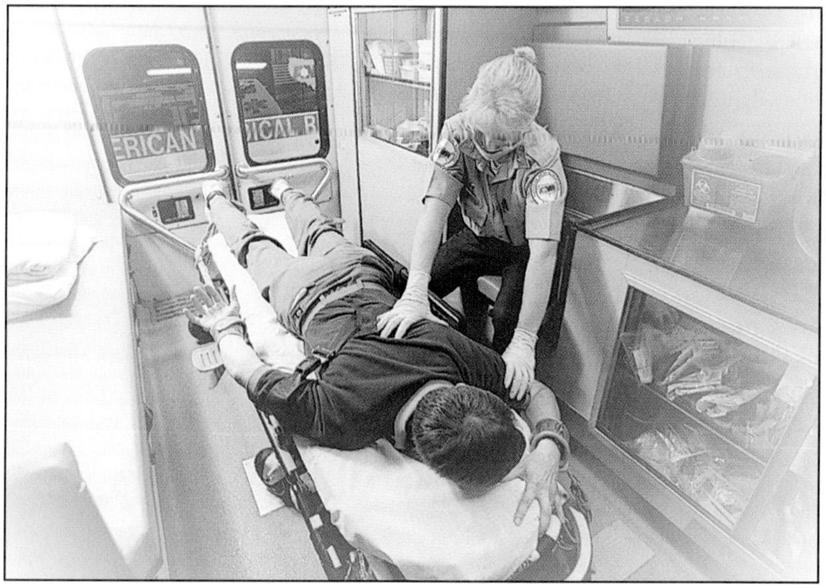

Knowledge Objectives

OBJECTIVES

As an EMT-Basic, you should be able to:

1. Define a behavioral emergency.
2. Discuss the general factors that may cause alterations in behavior.
3. Describe alterations in behavior that could indicate a behavioral emergency.
4. Discuss the behavioral characteristics that indicate a risk of violence.
5. Discuss the factors and behavioral characteristics that indicate a risk of suicide.
6. Describe how to assess a patient with a behavioral emergency.
7. Describe how effective communication techniques can help calm a patient having a behavioral emergency.
8. Discuss the legal and ethical considerations associated with the management of behavioral emergencies.

Skill Objectives

As an EMT-Basic, you should be able to:

1. Demonstrate how to assess and care for a patient having a behavioral emergency.
2. Demonstrate safe restraint of a patient having a behavioral emergency.
3. Demonstrate how to complete a patient-care report for a patient experiencing a behavioral emergency.

Attitude Objectives

As an EMT-Basic, you should be able to:

OBJECTIVES

1. **Value the importance of modifying your own behavior when dealing with a patient who is having a behavioral emergency.**
2. **Serve as a role model for other EMS providers when assessing and caring for a patient who is having a behavioral emergency.**

KEY TERMS

1. **Behavior:** How a person acts, including mental and physical activities.
2. **Behavioral Emergency:** A situation in which a patient exhibits abnormal behavior that places the patient or others in danger.
3. **Depression:** An emotional state in which there are extreme feelings of sadness, dejection, lack of worth, and emptiness.
4. **Mania:** A state in which a patient is severely agitated, often marked by rapid speech or constant physical activity such as pacing.
5. **Paranoia:** Irrational fear that others intend to harm or kill one.
6. **Psychosis:** A severe mental disorder that involves a distorted sense of reality; may include hallucinations (false impressions of the senses) or delusions (imaginary ideas or beliefs).
7. **Reasonable Force:** The minimal force necessary to keep a patient from injuring self, rescuers, or bystanders.
8. **Schizophrenia:** A form of mental illness in which a patient loses touch with reality and is no longer able to think or act normally (rationally).
9. **Suicide:** The act of taking one's own life.

IT'S YOUR CALL

You are dispatched to a **suicide** attempt. It appears that an adult female has tried to end her life by ingesting a large quantity of pills. Deciding that she did not want to die after all, the patient called 9-1-1 only minutes after taking the pills. Dispatch advises you that police should be arriving in 4 to 5 minutes. This is the second time that you have responded to this patient for an attempted suicide in the past 6 months. Dispatch also advises that this patient is considered a danger to herself and others. Based on this information, you decide to stage your ambulance several blocks from the scene and await police arrival.

After their arrival, you are notified that the scene is secure and you can enter. You encounter a large, agitated woman in her mid-30s who states that she took approximately 20 antidepressants and about 20 more assorted pills from the medicine cabinet, including aspirin, antibiotics, and sedatives. The patient begins to cry and now repeatedly refuses treatment, stating that no one understands what she is going through. She says she hears voices telling her to kill herself, these voices are becoming more vocal, and she is unable to sleep. She requests to be left alone to die. She suddenly stops speaking to you in mid-sentence and begins to talk aloud to herself.

How would you describe this patient's level of consciousness (LOC)? Is she experiencing a behavioral emergency? How would you continue to assess and care for this patient? Does it matter that this patient is refusing treatment?

This kind of situation can pose unique management problems. **Behavior** refers to mental and physical actions that are noticeable by others. A **behavioral emergency** is a situation in which a patient exhibits abnormal behavior that places the patient or others in danger. Such is the case with patients who become violent, attempt to take their own lives, or believe that people are out to harm them. This chapter examines the most common behavioral emergencies and describes how to assess and care for a patient who is experiencing one.

Causes of Behavioral Emergencies

Injury, physical or mental illness, and extreme stress are the most common causes of behavioral emergencies. Any condition that results in impaired oxygen flow or glucose supply to the brain can also lead to a significant behavior change. A normally calm person who is deprived of oxygen can suddenly become upset, confused, or even violent. Physical illness as a result of substance abuse, diabetic emergencies, environmental emergencies, and neurologic conditions associated with aging can all lead to behavior changes. Finally, head trauma can cause behavioral problems such as combativeness.

Mental illness can also be a source of behavioral emergencies. The exact cause of mental illness is often not known. The behavior can be bizarre. Among the possible behaviors are manic and depressed states. **Mania** is a state in which a patient is speaking rapidly and pacing and may be severely agitated. **Depression** is an emotional state in which there are extreme feelings of sadness, dejection, lack of worth, and emptiness.

Schizophrenia is another form of mental illness. It encompasses a large group of mental disorders in which a patient loses touch with reality and is no longer able to think or act normally. It can be mild and treated with medications or serious enough to require hospitalization. **Psychosis** is a form of mental illness in which a person holds false or mistaken beliefs (delusions) or sees or hears things that are not present (hallucinations).

Emotional crisis can lead to extreme stress, which affects people differently. An emotional incident and the way a patient copes or fails to cope with the stress can lead to moods and behaviors and can present as uncontrollable crying, denial, anger, frustration, or depression.

It is felt that many of these mental illnesses are caused or contributed to by chemical (hormonal) abnormalities in the brain.

Recognizing Behavioral Emergencies

There are many signs and symptoms that indicate a possible behavioral emergency. The four most common are as follows:

- Violent behavior toward self or others
- Loss of touch with reality (hallucination and delusion)
- Threatening or attempting suicide
- Frustration, anger, and depression associated with emotional crises

Violent Behavior

Violence can take many forms, from verbal abuse to punching, kicking, biting, and using weapons. Violent behavior is common with behavioral emergencies. A violent situation may erupt as a result of a seemingly trivial discussion. While the violence may not be directed toward you, you could easily become an indirect victim caught in the middle of an altercation. On the other hand, some violent acts are targeted only at individuals in uniform or in positions of authority.

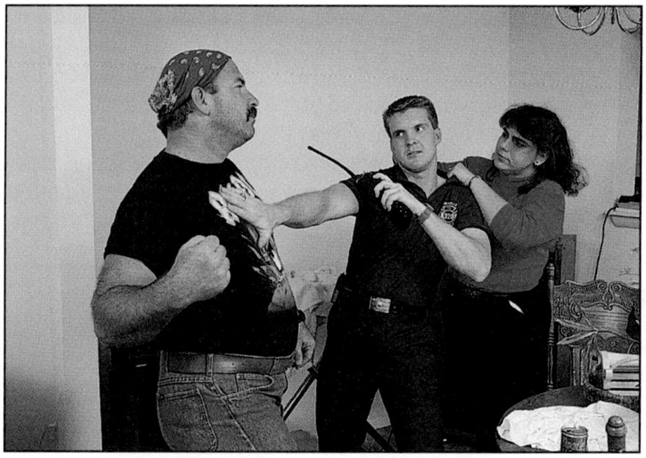

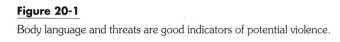

Figure 20-1

Body language and threats are good indicators of potential violence.

A patient's body language, comments, and overall demeanor are the best indicators of potential violence. Threatening comments and posture provide good clues to the patient's intentions (Figure 20-1). When a patient assumes a physical position of readiness to fight, take the body language seriously and approach very cautiously. Comments provided by family members about past violence should also make you approach with care.

Psychologic Disorders

Mental illness can cause a patient to lose touch with reality. A patient's behavior is often characterized by irrational thinking and actions, including visual or auditory hallucinations. A psychotic patient can experience a significant variation in mood over a short period of time. The patient may initially appear willing to cooperate with your assessment, but then become withdrawn and uncooperative or suddenly violent. This unpredictability can pose a threat to the patient, rescuers, and others. Some patients may experience **paranoia,** the belief that others want to harm or kill them. Because patients experience different psychoses, there is no one typical kind of behavior. A schizophrenic patient may show signs such as confusion, fear, depression, withdrawal into fantasy, or failure to communicate.

Suicide Risk

Suicide is the act of taking one's own life. Any situation in which a person has tried suicide but not succeeded is called a suicide attempt.

Suicide is a national health problem. More than 30,000 deaths each year are attributed to suicide, and 500,000 more individuals make unsuccessful attempts. On average, there is a suicide attempt every 90 minutes in the United States. While more suicide attempts are made by females, males are more successful at suicide. The most common method of attempting suicide is drug overdose. However, firearms account for more than 50% of all successful suicides.[1,2,3]

Several factors seem to play a role in a patient's decision to attempt suicide. These include:

- Failure to achieve success in personal or business affairs
- Serious personal illness, physical or emotional
- Alcoholism or drug dependence
- Serious illness or death of a loved one
- A failing relationship
- Chronic depression, which may not be linked to current situations in life

If family members or friends are present, ask them if they have witnessed any recent behavior changes. Any patient who has discussed or attempted suicide in the past is at risk. This is particularly true if the individual has discussed a definite plan for the suicide attempt.

Emotional Crisis

Emotional crisis can affect people in different ways. A patient who has recently experienced an emotional shock or loss, such as the death of a loved one, may experience extreme and unfamiliar emotions. There is often a common and visible pattern in these emotions, called the *stages of grieving*. People tend to grieve in this pattern for any loss; this can include the loss of a job or an important possession, as well as a death. The stages are as follows:

- Denial
- Anger
- Bargaining
- Depression
- Acceptance

Patients in emotional crisis may follow this sequence, but people react differently. They may experience these emotions in a different order, skip one or more entirely, or remain in one stage for a long time. An EMT should recognize that these feelings are a coping mechanism that helps shield the patient from the shock of the crisis and the difficulty of dealing with it. In general, if these emotions pose no threat to the patient or others, they are normal. These emotions may be expressed in the form of frustration, withdrawal, or aggressive verbal or physical behavior. Protect yourself and others if necessary, but remember not to take negative comments or actions personally.

It is also possible that the grief reaction will be delayed. You may learn by history that the patient experienced a loss or emotional crisis some time ago. This delayed stress reaction often occurs on anniversaries of the event and occasionally helps explain unusual mood changes or more extreme behavioral problems. Again, this can be a normal part of emotional reaction and healing.

It is important for EMTs to understand that they themselves may experience some of these feelings as a result of tragic or stressful events experienced on the job (e.g., several persons killed in a serious motor vehicle collision). Critical incident stress management programs can help EMS personnel work through these issues (see Chapter 3).

Assessing and Caring for Behavioral Emergencies

Your personal safety should always be a concern when dealing with a patient experiencing a behavioral emergency. Size up the scene and gather information as part of your assessment. This information should include pertinent medical history (including psychiatric or emotional problems), medications, alcohol or other drug use, and

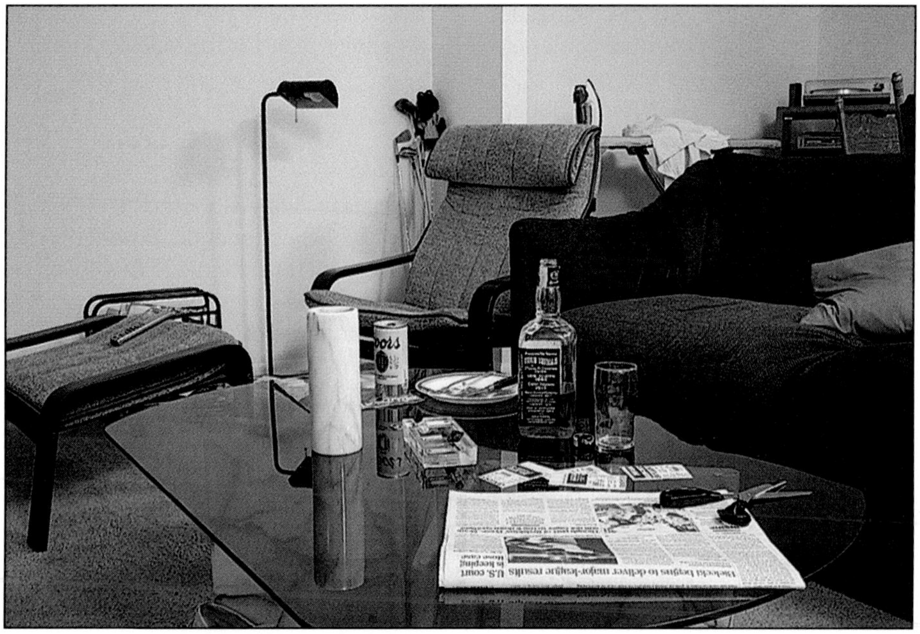

Figure 20-2

Common items can become weapons if a violent situation erupts.

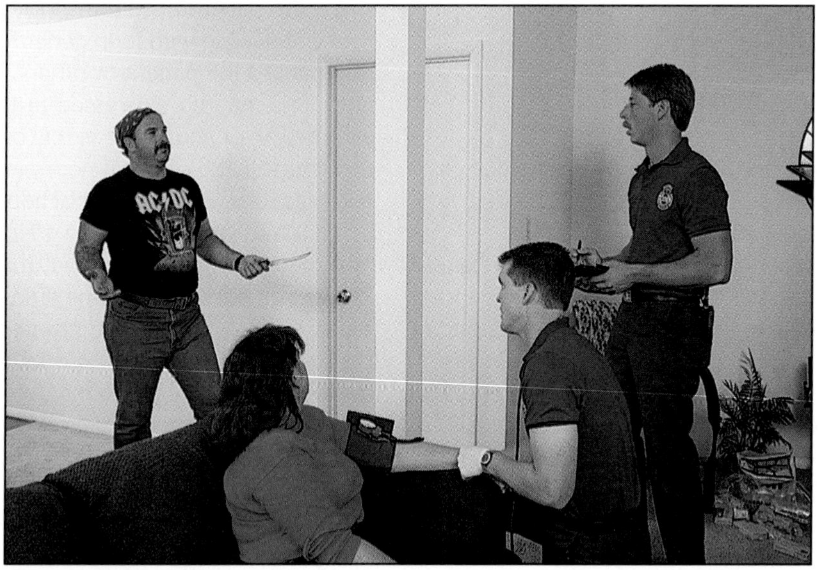

Figure 20-3

Be certain a path to the exit remains open when dealing with a potentially violent situation.

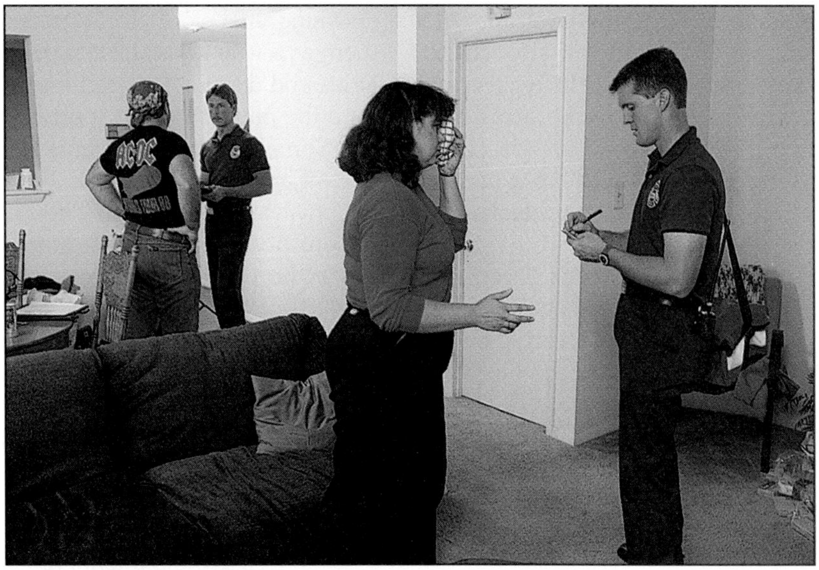

Figure 20-4
The EMT's nonverbal and verbal communication should be quiet and nonthreatening.

any recent life events that may have triggered the problem. Provide appropriate care as you proceed through your assessment. This includes protecting the patient, yourself, and bystanders from injury. Occasionally, this requires the use of restraints.

Scene Safety

Before you assess a patient, consider scene hazards. Do not enter a dangerous situation until it can be corrected. This sometimes means waiting until law enforcement personnel arrive to help control a situation. When it is safe to enter, remain cautious as you approach the patient. The scene may not be as safe as it appears. The patient may be carrying weapons or have them nearby (Figure 20-2). Always be prepared for safety threats. Know where the nearest exit is, and do not allow the patient to get between you and the exit (Figure 20-3).

Recognizing signs of a potentially violent situation is an important first step in avoiding violent confrontation.

- Threats or shouting
- Knowledge of previous violent behavior by the patient
- A patient who is carrying weapons or who has them within reach
- Body language, including clenched fists or a fighting stance
- Possible alcohol intoxication or other drug use

Approach the patient cautiously, looking for items that could be used as weapons. Keep your portable radio with you; it is your immediate method to call for help. Keep your eyes on the patient and do not turn your back. Stay between the patient and the exit. In some situations you will have additional personnel that can stand near the exit and observe from a distance. If there is a problem, the exit can be kept clear for a rapid retreat. Extra help may also be needed to apply restraints and prevent injury to the patient and others. You and your partner should communicate verbally and nonverbally so that each understands the situation and plan of response.

Regardless of the reason for violent behavior, there are steps that you can take to help calm it. Talk with the patient in a quiet, nonthreatening manner. Assume a relaxed body position, facing the patient with your arms at your sides (Figure 20-4). This allows you to move freely if you need to. Standing in a rigid position with your arms crossed is often seen as threatening by patients. If you are unable to retreat from the immediate area and must try to control a violent patient, again try to assume a nonthreatening posture and speak in a normal tone of voice. If this does not work, you may have to defend yourself. Use only the force necessary to subdue the patient or to retreat to a safe area.

Effective Communication

Behavioral emergencies can pose unique communication problems. Establishing good rapport is critical. Effective communication can help calm a patient and will usually make assessment and care easier. Try to minimize causing problems when communicating with a patient. Your words and body language can be misinterpreted. Body position can send positive or negative messages. Get in front of the patient and stand at the same level. Maintaining eye contact shows that you are attentive to what the patient has to say. Some patients will try to avoid eye contact; do not force it. Avoid crossing your arms or standing sideways because this suggests an impersonal, disinterested, or threatening position. Maintain a comfortable distance from the patient, and do not make any quick or sudden moves.

Speak slowly, clearly, and in simple terms. Use the patient's name whenever possible. This shows respect. Rephrase patient statements so that the patient knows you are listening and that you care. Acknowledge the patient's feelings.

Discuss issues honestly. Do not falsely reassure the patient, but explain that everything possible will be done to help. Do not "play along" or make statements to support a patient's delusions. Always act in a calm, compassionate, and professional manner.

Patient History and Physical Examination

Begin by making eye contact with the patient. Introduce yourself and learn the patient's name. Ask about the chief complaint. A patient who did not summon EMS personnel may be confused by the new people present. Ask if the patient knows why you are there. Begin with simple questions. Encourage the patient to talk by using open-ended questions that ask for more than a yes or no response.

Observe the patient's general appearance and behavior as you talk. Determine the consciousness and activity level. Is the patient active or subdued? How is the speech? Explain what you would like to do, including checking vital signs. If the patient has any injuries, use them as a way to establish rapport. Begin care for the injuries and discuss the need for further medical care. Prepare the patient for transport, if possible.

Some patients may refuse to go to the hospital. Be patient and continue to talk. Over time, you may be able to convince the patient that you can be trusted. When the patient needs further care and you are not able to persuade the patient after repeated attempts, contact your medical direction physician to discuss the options. You may need to ask police officers to place the patient in protective custody. However, state laws vary widely in this regard, as do policies and procedures of specific law enforcement agencies. You need to know local laws and policy in advance of these situations.

Patient Protection

A patient with a behavioral emergency needs to be evaluated by professionals trained to handle this type of problem. It is your job to see that the patient gets to a hospital without injury to self, rescuers, or others. Try to transport the patient in a comfortable position. Unfortunately, this will not be possible in all situations. If the patient is or may become violent, you should restrain the patient. This is for the patient's and your personal safety during transport.

Using Restraints

Consider using restraints as a means of patient protection in very limited circumstances. As discussed in Chapter 2, restraining a person without justification can give rise to a

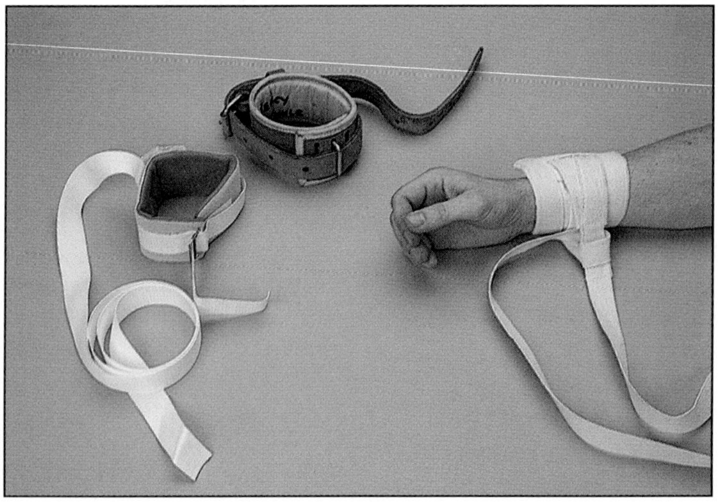

Figure 20-5

Common restraints:

claim of assault and battery. Restraints should only be used when behavior indicates danger to the patient or to those providing care. Place a patient in restraints only if the measures discussed above are clearly inadequate. When deciding whether or not to restrain a patient, consider the relative size of the patient, the availability of others to assist in applying restraints, the type of behavior known or expected, and the likely consequences of both using and not using restraints. Be sure to document your reasoning for the decision in the patient-care report.

If restraints are needed, decide how to position the patient and apply the restraints. Work with others to restrain the patient before leaving the scene. Applying restraints can be much more difficult during transport, and the ambulance is a dangerously confined space for violence.

Use **reasonable force** when applying restraints. This is the minimal force necessary to prevent injury and to get the job done. Avoid overly aggressive behavior. Use soft, wide, leather or cloth restraints (Figure 20-5). Position the patient in a manner that will minimize any injury and maintain an open airway. The best position for this is often the left lateral recumbent position, with the patient on the side. This position protects the patient's airway and respiratory status; however, it is difficult to restrain a violent patient in this position. Therefore the prone or supine positions are effective for a violent patient (Figure 20-6, *A*).

Applying restraints requires several rescuers who have been adequately trained in the equipment and techniques used by your agency. Law enforcement personnel should be present to help and to witness the process when possible. Ideally, there should be enough helpers to assign one person to each extremity. It is also useful to assign one person to the patient's head. This person can control the head and help calm the patient by talking and remaining fully visible. All four extremities should be placed in restraints; sometimes restraints are also needed for the torso. Once the patient has been re-

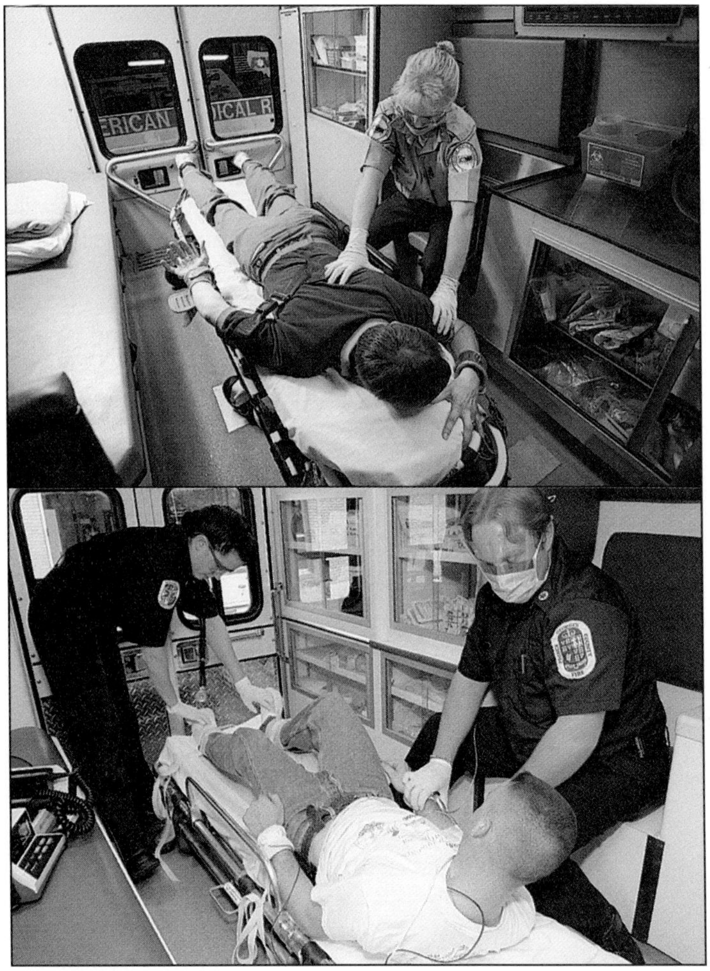

A

B

Figure 20-6

A, The prone position may be best for minimizing injury and maintaining an airway. **B,** The patient should be continuously monitored while in restraints.

strained, monitor continually to ensure that breathing is adequate and circulation to the extremities is not impaired (Figure 20-6, *B*). Appropriately restraining patients requires special training and practice.

Legal and Ethical Considerations

Dealing with behavioral emergencies involves three significant legal and ethical issues (see Chapter 2):

- Consent
- Reasonable force
- Documentation

Consent

Consent is the verbal or written acceptance of medical treatment. In a nonemergency situation, a patient has the right to decide whether to accept or refuse treatment. In a life-threatening emergency, other legal principles such as implied consent may apply. The patient gives **informed consent** to the care that is going to be given after being told of the nature of the situation, the treatment to be provided, the potential risks of treatment (if any exist), and the possible results of refusing care. The patient must be mentally competent to give an informed consent or informed refusal of care.

Before providing care or honoring the patient's refusal, assess the patient's ability to give an informed consent or refusal. Ask questions to determine if the patient is alert, oriented, and able to hear and understand what you are saying. These factors will help you confirm the patient's ability to think rationally. A patient who refuses treatment and wants to die as a result of ingesting a toxic substance, for example, is not considered to be thinking rationally. In this situation, you will have to consider other legal alternatives.

In many behavioral emergencies, the patient's competence to consent or refuse is questionable. You may have to apply restraints and transport involuntarily. The law in most states allows this, in limited circumstances, regardless of the patient's desire. There must be documentable facts, not speculation or unfounded fear, that the patient is dangerous to self or others. The patient can often be held involuntarily for evaluation by a physician. You are usually free from legal risk when you act in good faith by transporting a patient having a behavioral emergency involuntarily to the hospital for evaluation.

Local law enforcement personnel can help guide your actions. They may be able to place the patient in protective custody, although willingness to do this varies widely. If possible, talk with your medical direction physician in cases that seem to call for involuntary transport.

Reasonable Force

You must limit the force you use to that which is reasonable for the particular situation. A claim of battery may arise if you use inappropriate force when restraining a patient. Intentional and unjustifiable detention against a patient's will can also lead to a claim of false imprisonment. This can only be claimed if the patient understands the circumstances. If the patient is unaware of the surroundings and unable to provide informed consent or refusal, transport for evaluation is justified.

Documentation

It is important to accurately document events regarding your assessment and care during a behavioral emergency. Proper documentation will provide support for your actions if they are challenged at a later date. Essential elements for your documentation include the following:

- Physical signs and symptoms of the patient and a description of the scene.
- Description of the patient's behavior, including mental status.
- Statements made by the patient that help support your position. If you determine that the patient is not thinking rationally, use the patient's exact words.
- Any care provided—including the use of restraints, the method of restraint used, the type of restraints used—and assessment done before and after the restraints were applied (breathing, circulation).
- Instructions or direction from your medical direction physician.
- Law enforcement intervention.
- Witness statements and signatures.

IT'S YOUR CALL
CONCLUSION

You have been called to assist a woman who has overdosed on medication in an attempt to kill herself. The patient told you that she hears voices and is now talking to herself.

In assessing LOC, you would describe her as conscious but disoriented. Her suicide attempt, the report of hearing voices, and her current disorientation indicate that she is unable to respond rationally. You recheck the scene to ensure that the patient does not have any weapons in her possession or nearby that she could use to harm herself or others. You gather history by asking questions about the medications she took and you encourage her to discuss her problem. You express concern for the patient's condition as you take a set of vital signs. Because of the nature of the overdose, you summon advanced life support (ALS) personnel.

You believe that this patient's problem is a serious behavioral emergency because she appears to be a threat to herself and she needs medical care. After repeated, unsuccessful attempts to obtain the patient's permission to transport, you discuss the situation with your medical direction physician. The physician directs you to request the assistance of the police officers in persuading her to consent to transport. She again refuses, and the officers place her under protective custody for transport to a hospital for medical and mental health evaluation. She becomes combative, and you are forced to restrain her. You request an officer to accompany you and the patient during transport.

SUMMARY

When you are responding to a patient with a behavioral emergency, begin by assessing the scene for dangers. If the situation is unsafe, do not approach the patient until law-enforcement personnel have secured the scene. Approach cautiously, without making any rapid movements. Talk to the patient in a normal tone of voice and try to learn the patient's problem. Provide care for any injuries.

As you assess the patient, determine the LOC and mental status. Talk with any relatives or bystanders who may be able to provide additional insight into the patient's behavior. If you note behavior that is threatening or violent, try to calm the patient. If this does not work, you may have to use reasonable force to restrain the patient for safe transport to a receiving facility. Document the situation carefully to support your conclusions and actions.

REFERENCES

1. **Koop CE, Lundberg GD:** Violence in America, *J Am Med Assoc* 6:3075, 1992.
2. **National Safety Council:** *Accident facts,* Itasca, Ill, 1995, National Safety Council.
3. **Pallikkattayil L, Flood M:** Adolescent suicide: prevention, intervention, and post intervention, *Nurs Clin N Am* 9:623, 1991.

SUGGESTED READINGS

1. **Dernocoeur KM:** *Streetsense: communication, safety, and control*, ed 3, Redmond, Wash, 1996, Laing Research Services, Laing Communications, Inc.
2. **Meade DM, Lynch BA, Fuller R:** Adolescent suicide, *J Emerg Med Serv* 24:27, 1995.
3. **Nordberg M:** Call weighting, *J Emerg Med Serv* 24:23, 1995.

Chapter 21

Obstetrics and Gynecology

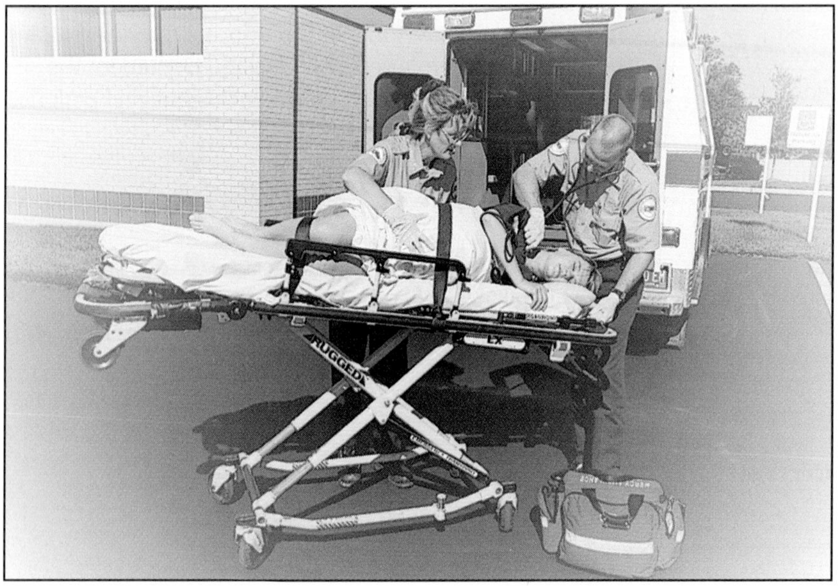

Knowledge Objectives

As an EMT-Basic, you should be able to:

OBJECTIVES

1. Identify the structures of the internal and external female genitalia.
2. List and describe complications associated with pregnancy.
3. Identify and explain the use of the contents of an obstetric kit.
4. List signs suggesting that delivery is imminent.
5. Explain the difference between the care you would provide during a normal delivery and the care you would give to a patient with pregnancy complications.
6. Identify the steps you would take to prepare for delivery.
7. Establish the relationship between body substance isolation practices and childbirth.
8. Describe the steps you would take to assist in the delivery of an infant.
9. Describe how to provide care for an infant during childbirth, once the head emerges.
10. Describe how and when to cut the umbilical cord.
11. Describe how to deliver the placenta.
12. Describe how to provide routine care for a newborn.
13. Describe when and how to resuscitate a neonate, including any special equipment that might be required.
14. Describe the procedures for the following abnormal deliveries: breech birth, prolapsed cord, and limb presentation.
15. Describe how to provide care for the birth of multiple infants.
16. Describe the special considerations associated with meconium in the amniotic fluid.
17. Describe the special considerations associated with delivery of a premature infant.
18. Describe the care to provide for a patient with a gynecologic emergency, including excessive vaginal bleeding.
19. Discuss the need to summon advanced life support (ALS) personnel for a patient experiencing an obstetric or gynecologic emergency.

OBJECTIVES

Skill Objectives

As an EMT-Basic, you should be able to:

1. **Demonstrate how to assist in the normal delivery of an infant.**
2. **Demonstrate how to provide care for a neonate once the head emerges during childbirth.**
3. **Demonstrate how to provide general care for a newborn.**
4. **Demonstrate how to resuscitate a neonate.**
5. **Demonstrate how to cut an umbilical cord.**
6. **Demonstrate how to deliver a placenta.**
7. **Demonstrate how to provide care for a mother following childbirth.**
8. **Demonstrate how to provide care for the following abnormal deliveries: breech birth, prolapsed cord, and limb presentation.**
9. **Demonstrate how to provide care for a patient with excessive vaginal bleeding.**
10. **Demonstrate how to complete a prehospital care report for patients with obstetric or gynecologic emergencies.**

Attitude Objectives

As an EMT-Basic, you should be able to:

1. **Discuss the importance of maintaining a patient's modesty and privacy during assessment and care of an obstetric or gynecologic emergency.**
2. **Serve as a role model for other EMS personnel when assessing and caring for a patient with an obstetric or gynecologic emergency.**

KEY TERMS

1. **Abortion:** Delivery of an embryo or fetus before it is able to live on its own, usually in the first trimester of pregnancy; spontaneous abortion is often called *miscarriage.*
2. **Amniotic Sac:** A thin membrane surrounding the fetus, containing up to 2 L of amniotic fluid that helps cushion and protect the developing fetus.
3. **Cervix:** The lower, necklike portion of the uterus.
4. **Contraction:** A rhythmic tightening of the muscles in the uterus, often indicating labor.
5. **Delivery:** The process in which the baby is expelled from the uterus.
6. **Embryo:** The developing baby inside the uterus during the first 2 months of pregnancy.
7. **Fetus:** The developing baby inside the uterus during the third and following months of pregnancy.
8. **Gynecology:** The branch of medicine dealing with women's health care.
9. **Labor:** The process of childbirth; proceeds from the beginning of contractions, through delivery of the newborn, to delivery of the placenta.
10. **Menstruation:** The periodic discharge of blood, mucus, and tissue from the lining of the uterus; associated with normal function of the uterus and ovaries.
11. **Miscarriage:** Another term for spontaneous abortion.
12. **Neonate:** A newborn baby.
13. **Obstetrics:** The branch of medicine dealing with pregnancy and childbirth.
14. **Ovulation:** The release of an egg (ovum) from one of the ovaries; occurs approximately 14 days after the beginning of the previous menstrual cycle.
15. **Placenta:** The structure that develops during pregnancy and attaches to the wall of the uterus; it serves to deliver oxygen and other nutrients from the mother to the fetus and to receive carbon dioxide and other wastes back from the fetus.
16. **Trimester:** One of the three approximately 13-week intervals in a normal pregnancy.
17. **Umbilical Cord:** The supply line between the fetus and placenta through which nourishment of the fetus and removal of fetal wastes take place.
18. **Uterus:** The hollow, muscular organ within which the fetus develops; the womb.

IT'S YOUR CALL

Your unit is dispatched to a woman believed to be in active **labor.** En route, you are advised by dispatch that a neighbor will meet you. You arrive to find a woman lying on the living room floor, in obvious pain. You notice bloody fluid on the floor. You learn that she is 28 years old and that this is her third pregnancy; however, she has had only one other child. The patient states that she is having strong, frequent, long contractions and feels like she needs to move her bowels. Faced with this situation, how do you proceed to assess and care for this patient? What additional questions would you ask? What physical examination steps should you perform? How would you provide care for this patient and, if necessary, for the newborn?

Obstetric and gynecologic emergencies are rare but require immediate attention when they do occur. **Obstetrics** is the branch of medicine dealing with pregnancy and childbirth. **Gynecology** is the area of medicine concerning health care specific to women.

When faced with a situation requiring you to assist with the delivery of a baby, you can take some comfort in knowing that less than 10% of births have any complications. Childbirth is a natural process that you can assist by following a few simple steps. Things become slightly more complicated once the baby is born because you then have two patients for whom to provide care. This requires you to work well with a partner, sharing the care for both patients. If you are alone and assisting with a delivery, you will find it a challenge. However, by following the basic steps, you will be able to provide the appropriate care for both patients.

This chapter covers the steps in assisting in childbirth and providing care for both mother and infant during the process. It also reviews the anatomy of female reproductive system and discusses some of the complications that can occur during pregnancy and childbirth. Gynecologic problems related to injury or infection of female reproductive organs are also discussed.

A

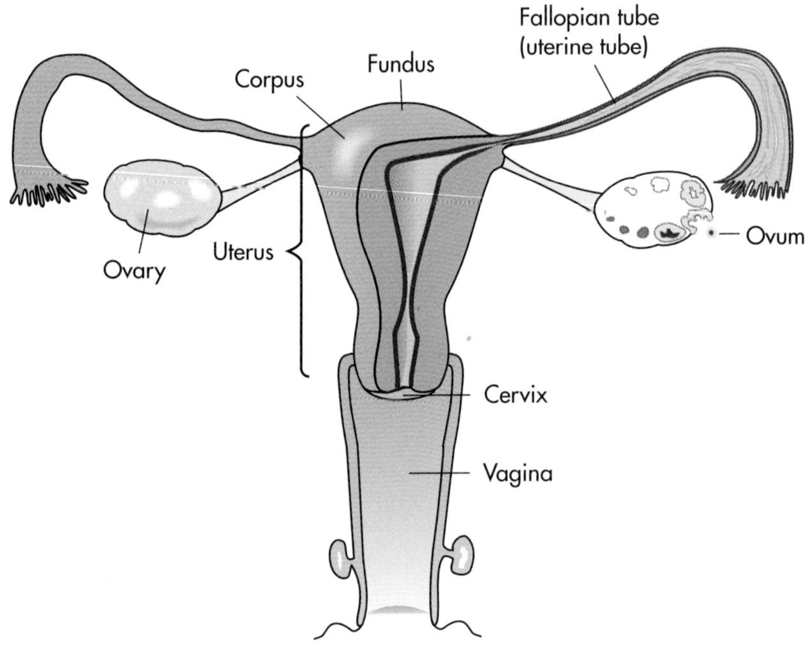

Figure 21-1

A, Internal female genitalia.

Anatomy and Physiology of the Female Reproductive System

The female reproductive system includes the internal and external genitalia (Figure 21-1). The periodic discharge of blood, mucous, and tissue in a nonpregnant female, known as **menstruation,** is a normal function of the **uterus** and ovaries. A new menstrual cycle begins about every 28 days and lasts 4 to 6 days. Menstruation begins with the onset of puberty and ends at menopause, often when a woman is in her forties.

Approximately 14 days after the beginning of the previous menstrual cycle, ovulation occurs. **Ovulation** is the release of an egg (ovum) from one of the two ovaries. As the egg passes through the fallopian tube, it may be fertilized if sperm is present. If fertilization does not occur, the egg passes with blood and other tissue from the uterus as part of the menstrual period.

Pregnancy

If fertilization does occur, it marks the beginning of pregnancy. The ovum changes after the first week into an **embryo,** the term for the new organism as it implants in the uterus (womb) and undergoes the first 2 months of growth and development (Figure 21-2). The uterus is a muscular organ capable of expanding as the **fetus** grows and contracting and expelling the fetus during childbirth. *Fetus* is the term for the developing infant after the second month of pregnancy. The fetus is surrounded in the uterus by the **amniotic sac,** a thin, dual-layered membrane that contains up to 2 L of amniotic fluid. This fluid-filled sac provides some cushion and protection for the fetus during development. As the process of childbirth begins, the amniotic sac ruptures, releasing the fluid. This is commonly referred to as the "water breaking."

The fetus receives nourishment through the **placenta,** a structure that develops during pregnancy. Attached to the wall of the uterus, it is the transfer point between the mother's circulation and that of the fetus. The **umbilical cord** connects the placenta and fetus. Oxygen and other nutrients pass through the cord from the placenta to the fetus. Carbon dioxide and other wastes pass in the other direction. The fetus depends completely on maternal circulation. Any factor that lowers maternal blood pressure (bleeding, dehydration) or depletes nutrient levels in maternal blood (hypoxia, hypoglycemia) also threatens the fetus.

The fetus continues to develop for approximately 40 weeks. This interval consists of three **trimesters** of approximately 13 weeks each (Table 21-1). To meet the demands of the growing fetus, several changes occur in the mother. Two of the most significant are increases in blood volume and heart rate. These changes permit adequate blood flow to allow for exchange of nutrients and waste products between mother and baby. As childbirth nears, the **cervix**—the lower, necklike portion of the uterus—begins to dilate and become thinner. This enables the fetus to pass through the birth canal. A mucus plug that fills the cervix during pregnancy becomes dislodged and is expelled. This plug usually contains mucus and fluid that is streaked with blood. Its expulsion indicates widening of the cervix and a shift of fetal weight down into the pelvis. Both of these are signs that labor is likely to begin soon. As the muscles of the uterus contract, the fetus is

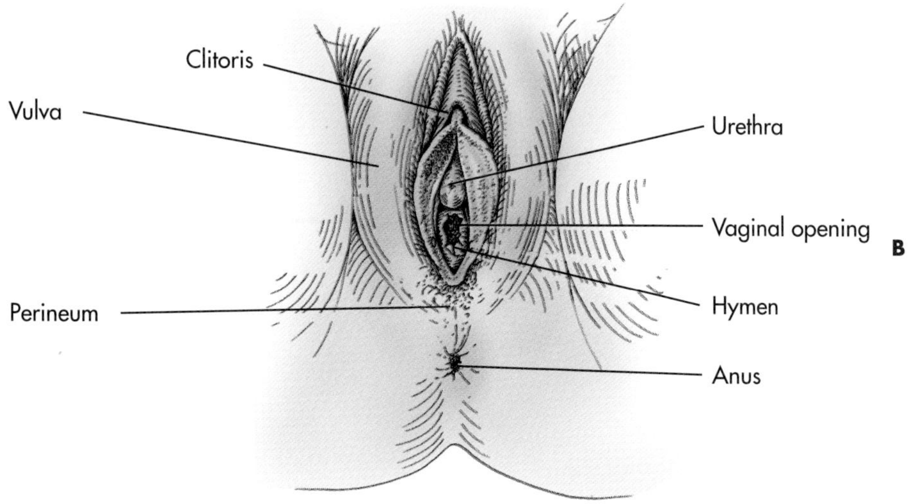

Figure 21-1, cont'd

B, External female genitalia.

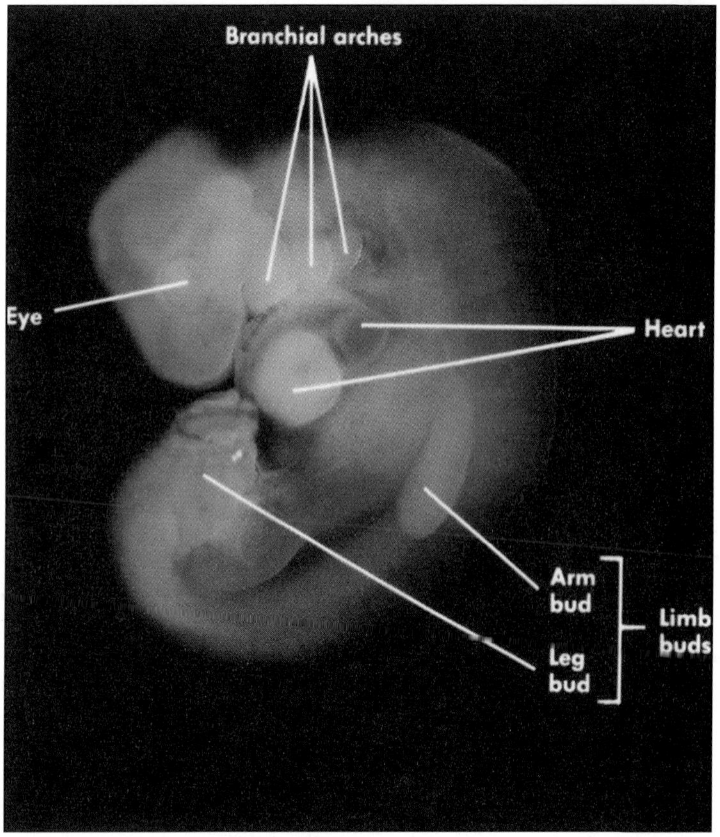

Figure 21-2
Human embryo at 35 days.

TABLE 21-1 Trimesters of Fetal Growth

Within first trimester (first 13 weeks)	Within second trimester (about 13 to 28 weeks)	Within third trimester (about 28 to 40 weeks)
• Foundations of body systems are formed.	• Heart beat is present.	• Fetus is viable if born early (eighth month).
• Arms and legs begin to develop.	• Kidneys secrete urine.	• Skin is pink and becomes smoother.
• Brain begins to develop.	• Fetal movements are felt by mother.	• Eyelids open.
• Placenta is complete.	• Eyebrows and fingernails develop.	• Vigorous movement occurs.
• Gender differentiation begins.	• Gender differentiation complete.	• Bones of the skull are nearly together at the sutures.
• Eyes, ears, and nose appear.		

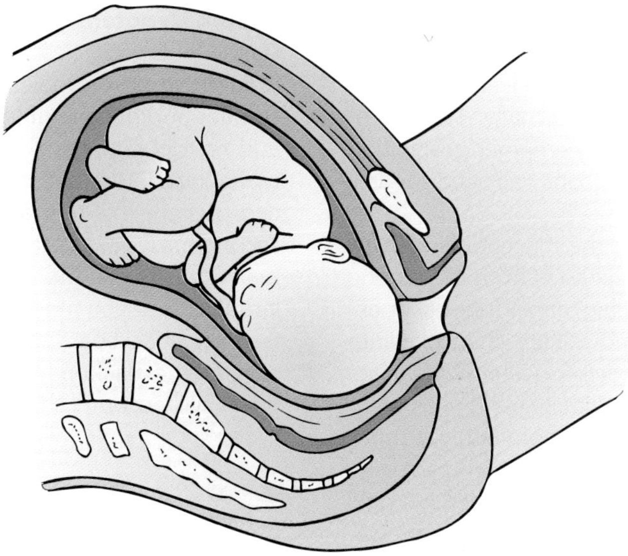

Figure 21-3

The fetus in position for normal delivery.

forced downward into the birth canal and through the opening of the vagina during delivery (Figure 21-3).

During pregnancy, the mother's vital signs may not be as helpful during patient assessment as they are in a nonpregnant woman. The patient's blood volume increases, but production of red blood cells does not keep up. This means that the oxygen-carrying capacity of the blood is decreased even when blood pressure is normal. A slight tachycardia is normal, so this is not as helpful as usual as an early sign of shock. Additionally, the blood pressure may remain normal when there is fluid loss. Finally, pregnant patients are often slightly tachypneic (having rapid breathing). In a pregnant patient, pay more attention to history, especially abdominal pain, and other signs (e.g., diaphoresis, normal blood pressure with increased pulse) that may indicate early blood loss.

Complications of Pregnancy

Most pregnancies proceed without complication. However, occasionally trauma or a medical condition can cause complications. The most likely signs and symptoms of complications are abdominal pain and vaginal discharge or bleeding.

Medical Conditions

Several specific medical conditions can cause pregnancy complications:

- Ectopic pregnancy
- Placenta previa
- Abruptio placentae
- Miscarriage (abortion)
- Preeclampsia and eclampsia
- Supine hypotension

Because the signs, symptoms, and care for many of these conditions are similar, it will usually not be necessary for you to differentiate them. All are serious and require care by a physician. Your responsibility is to recognize the problem and provide basic care. To do this, you will position the patient correctly, administer oxygen, provide basic shock treatment to help counteract internal bleeding, summon advanced life support (ALS) personnel, transport the patient to the nearest hospital, and contact medical direction for any additional orders.

Ectopic Pregnancy

Ectopic pregnancy is a condition in which the ovum develops outside of the uterus, usually in a fallopian tube. It occurs in about 1 of every 200 pregnancies and is most commonly identified in the first trimester. The primary concern is that, as an ectopic pregnancy grows, it will rupture the tube and cause serious, potentially life-threatening, bleeding. As the ectopic pregnancy begins to cause problems, the mother complains of severe abdominal pain that may radiate to the back. Vaginal bleeding is often present, but may be minimal or absent. Heavy internal bleeding is possible, and the mother may be in shock. Surgery is the definitive care for this patient.

Problems with the Placenta

In **placenta previa,** the placenta implants in the lower portion of the uterus, covering the opening of the cervix.

It occurs in approximately 1 of every 300 deliveries. The placenta can hemorrhage, and there may be bright red vaginal bleeding, generally without significant pain. Major bleeding can also be concealed internally. The loss of blood can lead to fetal hypoxia. This emergency situation requires hospital care because the baby will need surgical **delivery** (cesarean section).

Another condition involving the placenta is **abruptio placentae.** The placenta separates from the uterine wall, resulting in significant bleeding, either internal or external. Abruptio placentae is more likely than placenta previa to cause pain, and it may develop after physical activity or trauma. It occurs in approximately 2% of all pregnancies and, like placenta previa, is commonly a third-trimester problem. If the bleeding is retained internally, the mother's lower abdomen will become tender and rigid and she may show signs of shock. Like placenta previa, abruptio placentae requires immediate delivery by cesarean section.

Miscarriage (Abortion)

An **abortion** occurs when a fetus delivers too early, before it is able to live on its own. When it is spontaneous, this condition usually occurs during the first trimester and is often called a **miscarriage.** It can also be caused deliberately, either in a health care setting or in an attempt by the patient to self-abort the pregnancy. By definition, abortion results in loss of the fetus. During a miscarriage, the mother will often experience severe abdominal cramping, vaginal bleeding, and discharge of clots and tissue. As with other conditions involving abdominal pain and vaginal bleeding, position the patient for comfort, administer oxygen, control bleeding, summon ALS personnel if available, and transport to a hospital.

It is important to understand that not all abdominal pain and bleeding during early pregnancy indicate a miscarriage. These signs can occur normally during early pregnancy; however, these patients should be evaluated by a physician to ensure that no other conditions are present.

Preeclampsia and Eclampsia

Preeclampsia is a serious condition that occurs in about 6% of all pregnancies. The signs and symptoms are different from the other conditions that have been discussed. Preeclampsia is a condition of high blood pressure that occurs in the third trimester. The mother often complains of headache and fluid retention and has excessive weight gain. As the condition worsens, it can lead to seizures **(eclampsia),** which can be life threatening to both mother and fetus. This patient needs advanced medical care as soon as possible. Transport the patient on her left side. This helps reduce any pressure from the weight and position of the fetus on the inferior vena cava that may be restricting the mother's circulation. Administer oxygen and avoid stimuli that could trigger seizures, such as bright lights, siren noise, and rough handling or transport.

Supine Hypotension

As the fetus grows, especially during the third trimester, its weight can pose problems for the mother's circulation. If she lies supine, the uterus can compress the vena cava and restrict venous blood return to the heart. This can make the mother hypotensive and the fetus hypoxic. You can prevent this by transporting any patient in the late second trimester or later in a left-lateral position. This will make gravity pull the weight of the uterus away from the large veins. If you must immobilize a pregnant trauma patient on a backboard, prop a rolled blanket under the right side of the backboard; even a moderate angle of the board will accomplish the same thing.

Trauma

Any injury involving a pregnant patient requires consideration of the chance of injury to the fetus as well. Patient assessment follows normal trauma evaluation steps with the addition of history and examination factors related to possible fetal injury. Was there direct impact to the abdomen? (This includes impact against restraint belts in a vehicle.) Is there abdominal pain? Does the abdomen show bruising or other signs of direct trauma? Is there vaginal bleeding or any sign of possible internal bleeding?

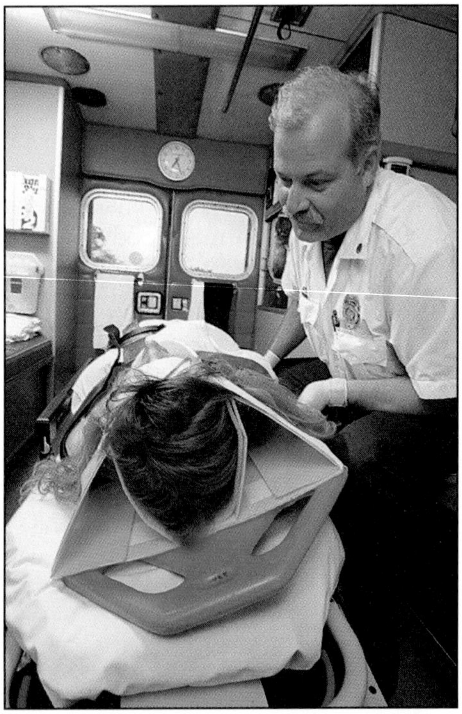

Figure 21-4

Transport the patient with her right side raised 30 degrees to reduce pressure from the uterus on the inferior vena cava.

When a pregnant patient has experienced trauma, administer oxygen through a nonrebreather mask. Transport the patient on her left side, if possible, to avoid pressure from the uterus on the inferior vena cava. If the patient has suffered a head or spine injury, secure her to a backboard and raise the right side of the board by placing blankets or pillows underneath it (Figure 21-4).

If the mother suffers cardiac arrest as a result of trauma, follow local protocols for patients in cardiac arrest. These include performing cardiopulmonary resuscitation (CPR), possibly intubating the patient, summoning ALS personnel, and transporting the patient to a hospital without delay. Once at the hospital, the fetus may be saved through emergent delivery by cesarean section.

Childbirth

The process of childbirth is often defined as stressful, exhausting, exciting, painful, and even frightening. Fortunately, childbirth is a natural process that usually proceeds without complication. Your role in childbirth is to assist the mother with the delivery of the newborn infant and then provide care for both mother and child.

Labor is the process of childbirth, beginning with the first rhythmic **contractions** of the uterus. As contractions continue, they dilate the cervix (enlarge its opening), allowing the fetus to move from the uterus into the vagina (birth canal). Delivery is the actual expulsion of the fetus from the uterus, through the vagina. This labor and delivery process usually takes about 14 hours for first-time mothers. The process is often much quicker for subsequent deliveries.

Stages of Labor

There are three distinct stages of labor:

- Stage 1: Onset of contractions and dilation of the cervix
- Stage 2: Delivery of the baby
- Stage 3: Delivery of the placenta

The first stage of labor is one in which the mother's body prepares to give birth. It begins with the onset of uterine contractions and is completed when the cervix is fully dilated. Beginning gently, contractions gradually become more intense. They begin at intervals approximately 10 to 15 minutes apart. As time passes, they last longer and become more intense and frequent. This first stage of labor lasts several hours and is substantially longer than the remaining two stages.

The second stage of labor begins when the cervix is fully dilated and ends when the infant is actually delivered. When the infant's head begins to emerge from the vagina, called *crowning,* it is time to prepare for immediate delivery (Figure 21-5).

The third stage of labor begins immediately after the delivery of the infant and ends with the expulsion of the placenta. About 15 to 30 minutes after the delivery of the infant, the placenta disengages from the uterine wall and exits the birth canal.

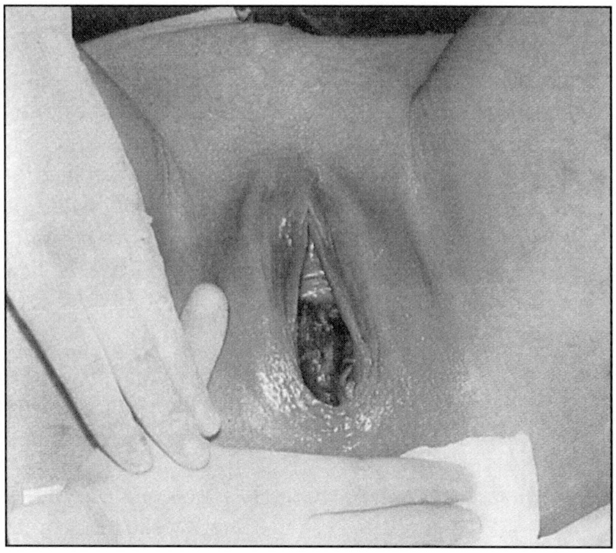

Figure 21-5

During crowning, the labia are stretched to form a ring around the infant's head.

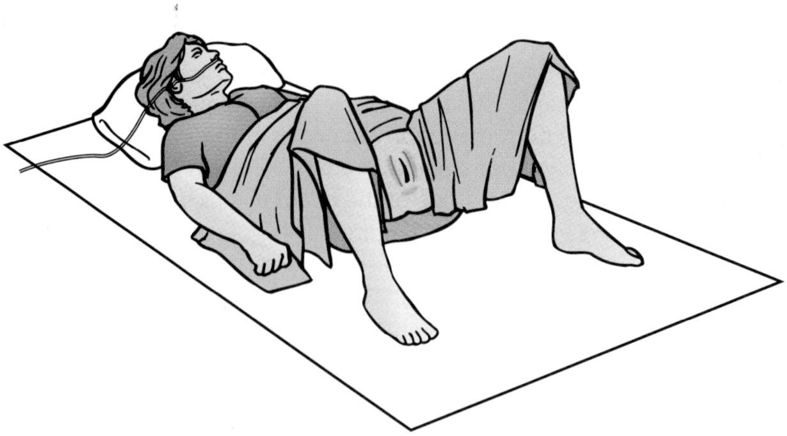

Figure 21-6
When positioning the patient, use clean sheets to create a warm, clean area for the delivery.

Assessing Labor

When you respond to an obstetric call, first verify that the patient is in labor (having regular contractions). If so, consider whether you have enough time to transport the patient to the hospital. It is preferable to transport an expectant mother whenever possible. However, if you feel there are only a few minutes before delivery, prepare for delivery at the scene.

To determine how far along the labor is, conduct a physical examination and ask these key questions:

- Is this the first pregnancy? Labor is usually longer in the first pregnancy.
- When is the baby due? This helps determine if the fetus is full-term or premature. Labor may proceed more quickly with significant prematurity.
- When did the contractions begin, and what are they like now? As labor progresses, the contractions occur more frequently and last longer. Time the length of a contraction from beginning to end. Contractions occurring only 2 to 3 minutes apart and lasting 1 minute or longer indicate that delivery will occur shortly.
- Has the amniotic sac broken? Labor will usually proceed quickly after the sac ruptures, especially in patients who have previously delivered babies.
- Is there a feeling of vaginal pressure or the need to push or have a bowel movement? As the fetus moves through the birth canal, it exerts pressure on the bladder and rectum. This feeling indicates that delivery is near.
- Is crowning present? Appearance of the top of the infant's head indicates the beginning of delivery.

Assisting With Normal Delivery

Once you decide that an expectant mother is going to give birth, quickly prepare the patient, area, equipment, and supplies. Begin by following body substance isolation (BSI) practices. Because of the likelihood of splashing body fluids, BSI practices should include the use of gloves, gown, goggles, and mask. Position the patient on her back, with her legs bent and knees drawn up and apart. Administer oxygen even if the delivery appears to be progressing normally. Create a clean area for delivery by placing clean sheets, blankets, or towels under the patient's buttocks and across her legs (Figure 21-6). Place hot packs in a folded blanket to warm it for the infant. Locate and open the obstetric kit. It will contain sheets for draping the mother and items for clearing the newborn's airway. Also included are items for clamping and cutting the umbilical cord and for keeping the baby warm. A list of the contents in a typical disposable obstetric kit appears in Box 21-1.

BOX 21-1 Contents of an Obstetric Kit

- Bulb syringe for suctioning the newborn's mouth and nose
- Clamps, umbilical tape, and scissors/scalpel for tying and cutting the umbilical cord
- Several pairs of sterile gloves
- Sterile gauze pads for cleaning and drying the newborn
- Sheets for draping the mother
- Blanket for warming the baby
- Sanitary napkins for absorbing blood
- Plastic bag for the placenta

Position yourself between the patient's legs. As crowning occurs, follow these steps to deliver the infant:

1. Place one of your hands on the bony part of the infant's skull and apply light pressure (Figure 21-7, *A*). This will ensure that the head emerges slowly, to prevent an "explosive delivery" (rapid, forceful expulsion) that could injure the mother or infant. Do not apply pressure to the soft areas of the infant's head **(fontanelles).**

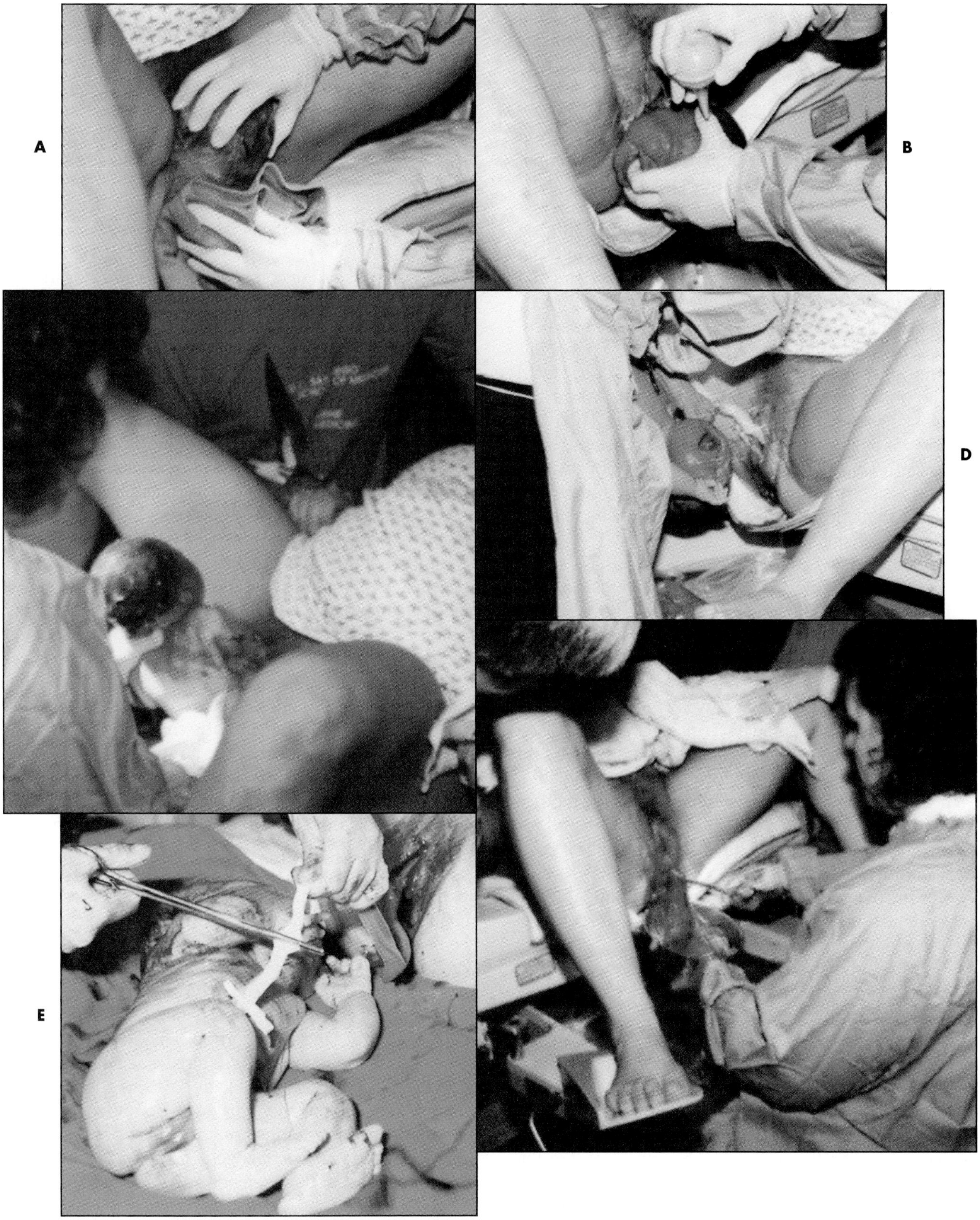

Figure 21-7

A, Apply light pressure to the bony parts of the infant's head. **B,** After the infant's head has emerged, use a bulb syringe to suction the nose and mouth. **C,** Grasp the infant's arm near the shoulder and support the body as it delivers. **D,** Wrap the infant in a warmed blanket, being careful to keep the infant and the mother at the same level. **E,** Cut the cord between the two clamps. **F,** The placenta will deliver on its own. Do not pull on the umbilical cord.

2. Usually the baby will be born with the head facing down (toward the mother's buttocks). Once the infant's head has emerged, support it and allow it to turn to the side, which it usually does naturally during delivery. If the amniotic sac is still intact, rupture and remove it from the infant's face. If the umbilical cord is wrapped around the infant's neck, gently slip it over the occiput of the head to remove it. If this is not possible, immediately clamp and cut the cord (see step #8).
3. Using the bulb syringe, suction the mouth and nose (Figure 21-7, *B*). Squeeze the bulb, insert it into the cavity, and release it. Withdraw the bulb syringe and squeeze the contents onto a towel or into a basin. (Note: Although some sources recommend a particular order for suctioning, it does not make a major difference whether you suction the mouth or nose first.)
4. The upper shoulder usually delivers first. Lower the infant's head to help ease the shoulder out. Then support the infant with both hands and guide the body upward. This will allow the lower shoulder to emerge. Grasp the arm firmly near the shoulder; the remainder of the body will deliver quickly and will be slippery to handle (Figure 21-7, *C*).
5. Place the infant between the mother's legs and repeat suctioning to remove any further secretions. Dry the infant's body. This stimulus should be all that is necessary to make the infant cry and begin breathing. If this is not enough, try flicking the soles of the feet and briskly rubbing the infant's back.
6. Discard the wet items that have been used to dry the baby. Wrap the infant in a warmed blanket and place the infant on its side to help promote drainage and keep the airway clear. Be sure to cover the infant's head. Keep the infant at the same level as the mother to avoid circulatory compromise caused by blood returning to the placenta through the umbilical cord (Figure 21-7, *D*).
7. Record the time of birth and complete an APGAR score at 1- and 5-minute intervals. (APGAR scoring is discussed on pp. 425-426.)
8. Feel the umbilical cord for pulsations. Once they cease, clamp or tie the cord. Place one clamp about 4 inches from the infant, and the second clamp four inches beyond the first clamp. Make sure they are securely fastened. Cut the cord between the two clamps (Figure 21-7, *E*). After the cord is cut, the baby can be given to the mother.
9. Reevaluate both the infant and the mother. If you are not already on the way to the hospital, prepare for immediate transport.
10. As the placenta prepares to deliver, the mother will again feel strong contractions. The placenta will emerge on its own; do not pull on the umbilical cord. Wrap the placenta in a towel and place it in a plastic bag (Figure 21-7, *F*). Hospital personnel will need to examine it for completeness.
11. Once the placenta has delivered, clean the mother and place a sterile pad over the vaginal opening. Have the mother lower her legs and place them together. The mother will be very tired; you may have to help her lower her legs.
12. Begin uterine massage and follow other guidelines discussed later in this chapter (p. 427).

Complications During Delivery

Most deliveries are uncomplicated. However, for the few that are complicated, the care that you provide can be critical to the infant's survival. This section reviews seven complications that can occur during delivery.

Meconium

Meconium is material that collects in the intestines of a fetus, forming the first stool of a newborn. It is a thick, sticky, green or black substance. If meconium is present in the amniotic fluid, it means that the infant has already had a bowel movement. This often occurs because the fetus has experienced some distress before delivery. Possible aspiration of meconium into the lungs is a major concern because it can lead to fetal distress after birth. It causes blockage of the airway, failure of the lungs to expand, and other respiratory problems, such as pneumonia. If meconium is present at delivery, suction the newborn repeatedly to clear the airway. In this situation, you should definitely suction the infant's mouth before the nose. Allow oxygen to blow by the infant's mouth and nose and closely assess respiratory effort. If the infant is in respiratory distress, assist ventilations with a bag-valve-mask (BVM). The patient should be transported quickly to the hospital; notify the hospital of the situation while en route.

Breech Presentation

In a breech birth, the fetus' buttocks or legs present first (Figure 21-8). Surgical intervention (cesarean section) may be needed for delivery. Because this is not possible in the prehospital environment, other options must be considered. Field delivery is difficult and risky. The safest choice may simply be to position the patient in a manner that delays delivery, and transport quickly. Place the patient on her left side with legs and hips elevated (left-lateral Trendelenburg's position) (Figure 21-9, *A*). In this position, gravity will pull the fetus away from the cervix. Another effective position is the knee-chest position. Place the patient on hands and knees, then have her lower her head and chest to the stretcher or floor (Figure 21-9, *B*). Though useful in stationary environments, knee-chest position is difficult to maintain safely in a moving ambulance.

The other option is to deliver the infant. As the baby emerges, support the body with both hands. The infant will deliver without difficulty up to the shoulders. At this point, you will need to manipulate the shoulders gently,

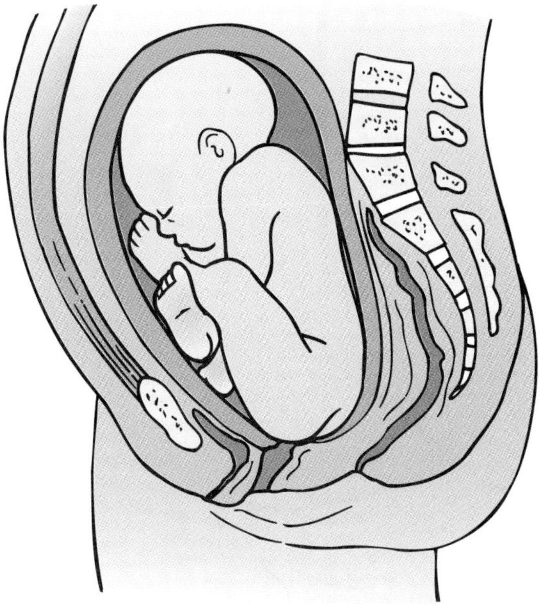

Figure 21-8

Position of the fetus in a breech birth.

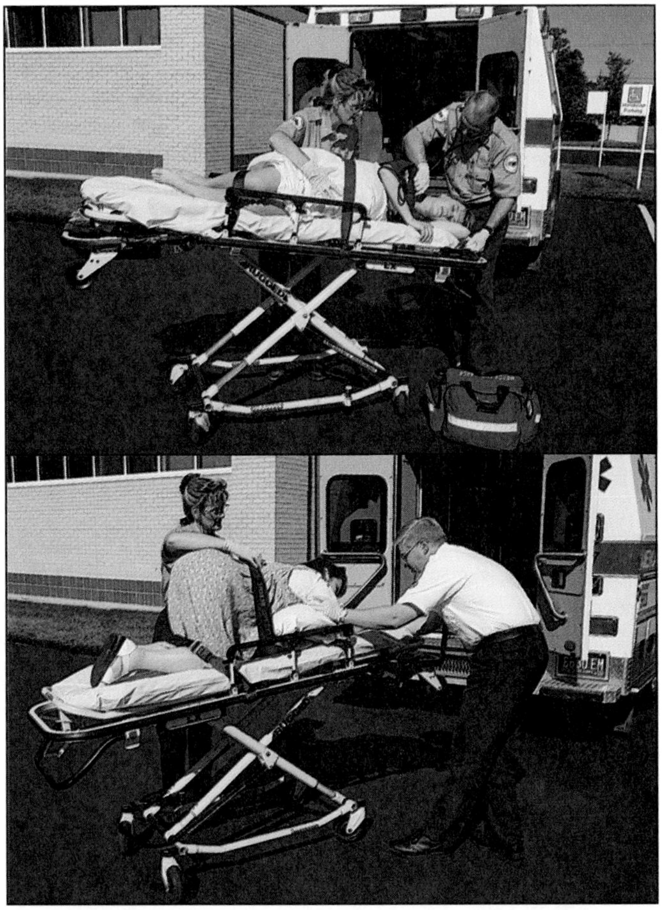

A

B

Figure 21-9

A, The left-lateral Trendelenburg's position may help delay a breech birth. **B,** The knee-chest position may also be useful in delaying a breech birth but can be difficult to maintain in a moving ambulance.

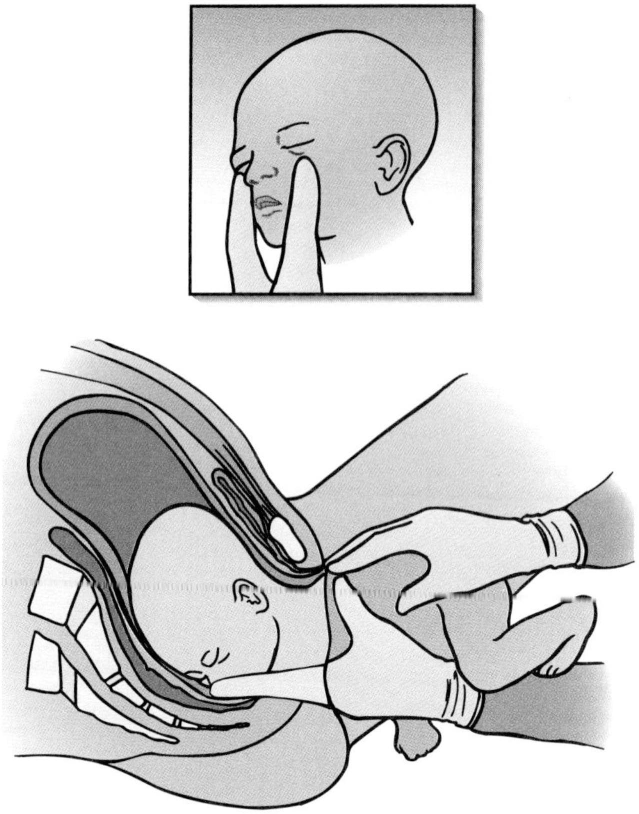

Figure 21-10

Push the vaginal wall gently away from the infant's face. This will allow the infant to breathe and may enable the head to deliver.

one at a time, to allow them to deliver. Lower the body to deliver the upper shoulder, then raise the body to deliver the lower one. Once this occurs, the head may emerge without difficulty. Never pull on the infant's legs or trunk in an effort to force delivery of the head.

If the head does not deliver immediately, you must provide care to prevent suffocation of the infant. With its face against the birth canal, the baby will be unable to breathe. The cord may also be compressed by the infant's head, restricting oxygenated blood flow. Wearing sterile gloves, insert two fingers into the vagina so that they are on each side of the infant's nose. Push the vaginal wall away from the infant's face to allow the head to deliver (Figure 21-10). If this does not enable the head to deliver, maintain the position as a means of airway support during transport.

Limb Presentation

Although rare, a limb presentation represents a significant medical emergency because the infant cannot be delivered in this position. If you notice a limb presenting through the vagina when you check for crowning, position the mother to lessen pressure on the umbilical cord. Use left-lateral Trendelenburg's or the knee-chest position, as described above. Transport immediately.

Prolapsed Cord

Occasionally, a portion of the umbilical cord will protrude from the vagina before the infant presents; this is called a *prolapsed cord.* As in a breech birth, the infant's head can compress the umbilical cord against the wall of the birth canal, compromising blood flow to the infant. To resolve this problem, you must reduce the pressure on the umbilical cord, similar to the way in which it is done for a limb presentation. Begin by placing the mother in left-lateral Trendelenburg's or the knee-chest position. Gently insert several fingers (using a sterile glove) into the vagina, only far enough to push the infant's head away from the umbilical cord (Figure 21-11). Do not attempt to replace the cord. Cover any exposed portion of the cord with moist, sterile dressing. Transport rapidly and maintain this position.

Disproportion

On rare occasions, the infant's head will not fit through the mother's pelvis. This can be caused by a small pelvis, a large fetus, or fetal abnormalities. The condition is seen most frequently in mothers giving birth for the first time. You will only be able to recognize this condition after it becomes obvious that the infant's head is not progressing through the birth canal and vagina. Even though the

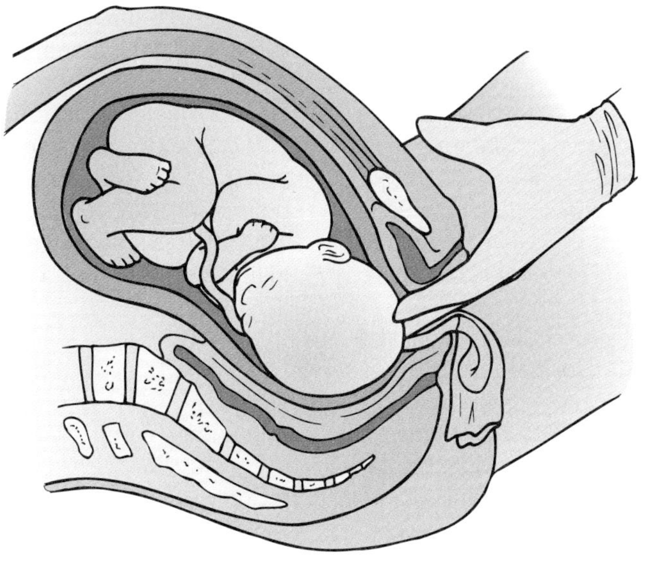

Figure 21-11

When a portion of the umbilical cord delivers before the infant, gently insert fingers into the vagina to push the infant's head away from the cord.

mother is experiencing frequent, prolonged contractions, no progress is made toward a full delivery.

With proper prenatal care, the mother may know that her physician suspects a **disproportion** problem. If so, transport the patient immediately. A cesarean section will likely be necessary to avoid rupture of the uterus, a life-threatening event.

Premature Birth

An infant is considered premature if delivered earlier than 7 months (28 weeks) after conception or at a weight of less than 5.5 pounds. Premature infants are prone to complications because their body systems have not had time to develop fully. They often do not have the necessary body fat to help insulate against hypothermia. Premature infants also more frequently require resuscitation. Pay special attention to maintaining body heat. Shivering can use up the premature baby's limited stores of oxygen and blood sugar very quickly. Administer oxygen and assist ventilations or provide CPR as needed. Transport immediately.

Multiple Births

Multiple births, such as twins, often result in premature deliveries. Even when not premature, low birth weight of multiple fetuses makes problems more likely. Call for extra help to care for multiple patients, when possible. It is estimated that twins are born in about one out of every 90 births, and triplets in one out of every 8000 births.

A mother who has received good prenatal care is likely to know that she is carrying multiple fetuses. In this case, you know in advance that you need additional equipment, supplies, and personnel. Normally, multiple births occur before the delivery of the placenta. Each infant could be attached to a separate placenta, or they may all be attached to the same one. Deliver and care for additional infants in the same manner as you do for the first. Remember that prematurity and small size raise the priority level for maintaining body heat and monitoring respiratory status.

Caring for a Newborn

Once the infant has been delivered, you must assess and evaluate its status as well as provide routine and emergency care.

Assessment

Assessing the newborn should be a continuous process. It begins with a brief, initial assessment of respirations, heart rate, and skin color. Assessment then continues with APGAR scoring at 1 minute and 5 minutes after birth. The APGAR scoring system (Table 21-2) uses the following components:

- **A**ppearance: This refers to skin color. Determine if it is blue, pale, or pink. Does this color extend to the entire body or only specific areas? It is normal for peripheral areas to be cyanotic initially, but the torso should be pink.

- **P**ulse: The infant's pulse should be greater than 100 beats per minute. A slower rate may indicate compromised circulation and a distressed infant.
- **G**rimace: Grimace refers to response to stimulus. Determine this by flicking the soles of the infant's feet. This should generate motion and crying.
- **A**ctivity: This reflects the amount of movement (muscle tone) that the infant exhibits. It may involve limited movement, such as flexion of the extremities, or active movement of the limbs.
- **R**espiration: A newborn infant's respirations should be normal in both rate and effort. (Normal rate is 40 to 60 breaths per minute, but color and respiratory effort are both more important than rate.) Forceful crying indicates an open airway and adequate breathing. Insufficient oxygenation can result in labored respirations, which will affect other elements of the APGAR score. Infants should begin breathing within 30 seconds after delivery. If this does not occur, the infant will need further stimulation and may need ventilatory support.

TABLE 21-2 APGAR Scoring for Newborn Evaluation

Sign	0 points	1 point	2 points
Appearance	Body blue, pale	Body pink, extremities blue	Body pink
Pulse	Absent	<100 bpm	>100 bpm
Grimace	No response to stimulus	Some motion, weak cry	Vigorous motion, strong cry
Activity	Limp	Some flexion of extremities	Active movement
Respiration rate and effort	Absent	Slow, irregular, or labored	Normal

Do not delay resuscitation or transport to record an APGAR score. This scoring can be completed during transport. Once your assessment is complete, total the points on the APGAR scale. A good initial score is 7 to 10. Scores less than 6 after initial stimulation and oxygen indicate distress that requires more active resuscitation.

Routine Care

The routine care for a newborn includes:

- Supporting the infant. Because newborns are slippery, use both hands to support the head and torso. Work close to the surface of the bed, stretcher, or floor.
- Clearing the airway by suctioning the mouth and nose.
- Clamping and cutting the umbilical cord.
- Quickly cleaning, drying, and warming the infant. Preventing shivering reduces oxygen needs and helps conserve the infant's blood sugar.
- Positioning the infant to maintain a clear airway.
- Using tactile stimulation to verify adequate response.

The Distressed Newborn

Fortunately, less than 10% of all deliveries require resuscitation. Most newborns respond to drying, warming, positioning, suction, and tactile stimulation. If this does not adequately stimulate the newborn, begin providing emergency care.

If respirations are slow, shallow, labored, or absent or the pulse is less than 100 beats per minute, assist ven-

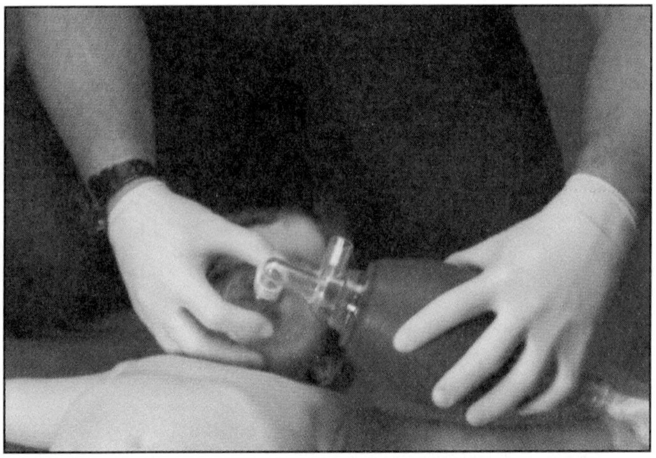

Figure 21-12

Use a BVM attached to oxygen to assist ventilation on a newborn.

tilations. This should be at a rate of 60 per minute, with a neonatal BVM attached to oxygen (Figure 21-12).

If the newborn's pulse is less than 60 beats per minute, or less than 80 beats per minute and not responding to ventilation efforts, begin chest compressions. Reassess the infant after 1 minute and every few minutes thereafter. If the infant responds appropriately to these resuscitative efforts (pulse greater than 100 and respirations normal), cease resuscitation and administer oxygen by holding a face mask or the end of the oxygen tubing near the infant's face. Oxygen should also be administered any time the infant continues to show signs of cyanosis. If you recognize the need for resuscitation, you should also recognize the need for additional help and rapid transport. Summon ALS personnel and contact the medical direction physician to discuss additional care.

Newborn resuscitation is a specialized process, and you need special equipment to do it. Be sure in advance that your ventilation kit includes neonatal sizes of items such as ventilation bags and masks, suction catheters, and bulb syringes. Your ambulance should be stocked with enough blankets and other warming gear to care for two **neonates.**

Caring for the Mother

While one provider cares for the infant, another should attend to the mother. After placental delivery, clean the mother and begin uterine massage to speed uterine contraction and help control bleeding. Using both hands, gently knead the lower abdomen (Figure 21-13). Once the newborn has been assessed and cared for, allow the mother to begin to nurse the infant. This also stimulates the uterus to contract and slow bleeding. If the infant will

IT'S YOUR CALL
CONCLUSION

Your 28-year-old female patient is preparing to give birth to her second child. You learned from the initial history that this is her third pregnancy, but she only has one child. Additional questioning reveals that she lost a child because of a miscarriage about 1 year ago. Other questions should include whether she has had prenatal care, whether the infant is due now (full term), and whether her water has broken. You should also check to see if the infant is crowning. Because the patient said that she feels the need to move her bowels, it is likely that birth is near.

The baby is crowning, and you prepare the patient for immediate delivery. You position the mother, prepare your supplies and equipment, and begin to administer oxygen. Positioning yourself between the patient's legs, you apply light pressure to the infant's head and assist with delivery. You clear the airway after the head presents. After delivery, you dry and wrap the baby to maintain warmth, and use a position that will keep the airway clear and prevent backflow of blood to the placenta. After the cord stops pulsating, you clamp and cut the umbilical cord, record APGAR scores, and place the baby at the mother's breast. Your partner has tended to the mother while you cared for the neonate. After a normal, uncomplicated delivery, you are ready to transport your two patients to the hospital.

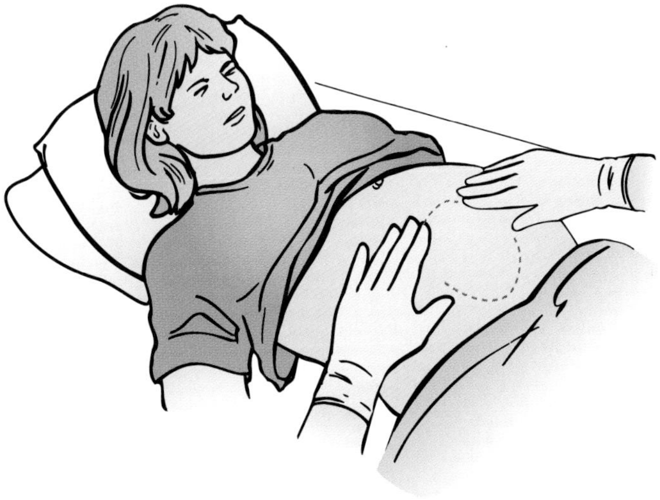

Figure 21-13

Kneading the lower abdomen with both hands can speed uterine contractions and help control bleeding after delivery.

not nurse, have the mother massage her nipples. Place sanitary pads over the vagina and have the mother lower and place her legs together. If the mother shows signs of shock, continue to administer oxygen, maintain normal body temperature, massage the uterus, and transport immediately. Contact the receiving hospital to discuss the patient's status.

Gynecologic Emergencies

Gynecologic emergencies can affect women who are pregnant as well as those who are not. Abdominal pain and vaginal bleeding are the two most frequent complaints associated with gynecologic emergencies. The pain and blood loss can be the result of trauma, infection, or sexual assault. The general care for these conditions is similar to the care for a pregnant patient.

Infection

Pelvic inflammatory disease (PID) affects about 1 million women annually. It is associated with a bacterial infection. The pathogen enters the body through the vagina and ascends to other organs, including the cervix, uterus, fallopian tubes, and ovaries. This infection can result in septic shock and infertility. A woman with PID often complains of lower abdominal pain, fever, and vaginal discharge. The patient usually experiences the onset of these signs and symptoms within approximately 1 week of her menstrual period. This patient should be cared for in the same manner as any other female patient experiencing nontraumatic abdominal pain. Place her on oxygen and transport to the hospital for evaluation by a physician.

Trauma

Injury to the external genitalia can result from mechanisms such as childbirth, sexual assault, and direct trauma to the **perineum** (straddle injuries). Treat as you would for any soft-tissue injury. If bleeding is present, control it with pressure. If the area is bruised and swollen, cold can be applied to reduce the pain and swelling. Apply an ice pack by wrapping it in a thin covering before applying it. This will minimize any damage to the tissue that could occur from direct contact with cold. Treat penetrating injury with direct pressure to control any bleeding. Assess carefully to determine the possibility of internal bleeding and organ damage.

Care for any additional signs or symptoms that you notice. Injuries to the genitalia should be evaluated by a physician. Monitor the patient's condition for signs of improvement or deterioration while en route to the hospital. Injuries of this type can be embarrassing and emotional. Act professionally and attempt to maintain the patient's privacy.

Sexual Assault

Sexual assault can have devastating consequences for the victim and family members. Though males can be sexually assaulted, females are much more frequent victims. Care for injuries associated with sexual assault as you would for any other injury. Only examine the external genitalia if external bleeding is present. The emotional support you can provide is of equal importance to your medical care:

- Limit physical examination to what is necessary to maintain the patient in a stable condition. Conduct the necessary examination in a private manner that protects the patient's modesty. Whenever possible, have an EMT of the same gender conduct the examination. If this is not possible, try to locate a police officer or family member of the same gender that can assist.
- Avoid being judgmental. The patient needs your reassurance. Remain calm and professional while questioning, examining, and providing care for the patient.
- Use a gentle manner. Explain what you are doing. Ask permission, and gain the patient's cooperation.
- Protect crime scene evidence. Discourage the patient from cleaning wounds, bathing, or urinating because this may destroy evidence essential to solving the crime. Preserve clothing and weapons for the same reason.
- Transport patients with life-threatening emergencies immediately.
- Document what the patient tells you about the incident and what you observe.

SUMMARY

Pregnancy usually proceeds without complication, but there are problems that can complicate pregnancy and delivery. These include problems associated with the location of the ovum, the location or separation of the placenta, early expulsion of the fetus, and preeclampsia. All of these situations are serious and require advanced care by a physician. Your responsibility is to recognize the problem and provide basic care while transporting the patient for further evaluation.

As childbirth begins, your role will be to assist with the delivery of the infant. The stages of labor usually progress gradually in first-time mothers, but may proceed quite quickly in later pregnancies. As you assess the mother, ask key questions to learn about her history and determine whether she is in active labor and about to give birth.

After delivery you will have two patients to care for. Tend to the mother after ensuring that the baby is dry and warm and in stable condition. After placental delivery, take measures to enhance uterine contraction and slow post-delivery bleeding.

Gynecologic emergencies arise from infection, trauma, and sexual assault. The care for infection and trauma is usually routine, but sexual assault requires special sensitivity to the patient's emotional needs. Privacy, gentle care, and a nonjudgmental attitude are all important. Friends and family members may also need emotional support.

Section 7

Trauma Emergencies

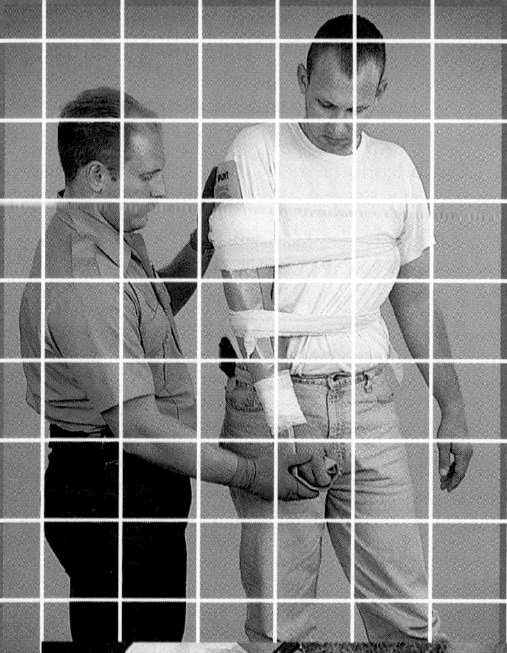

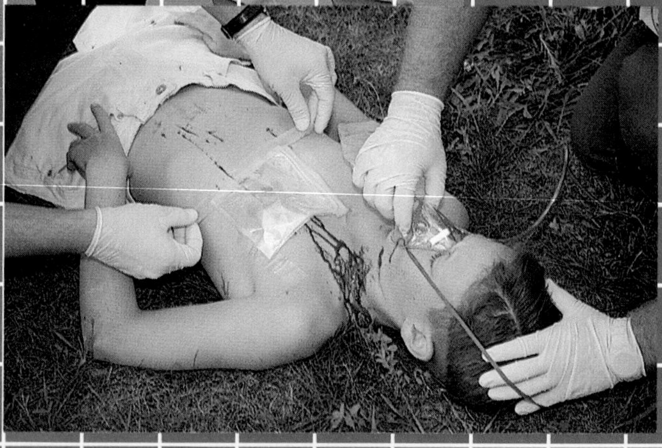

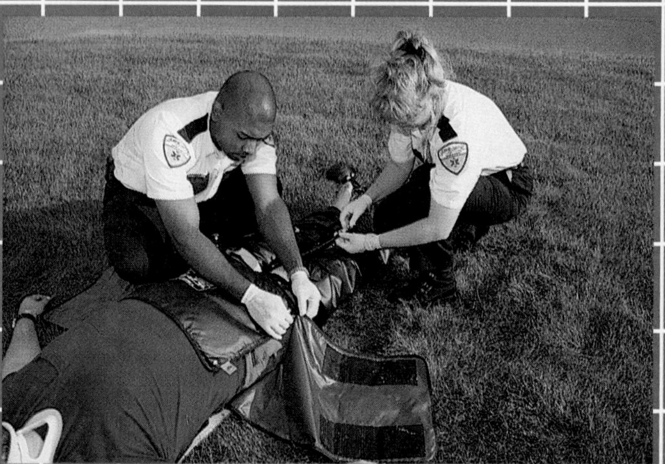

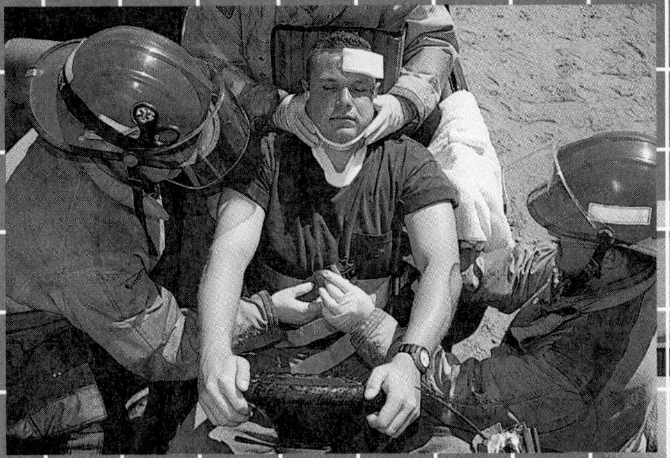

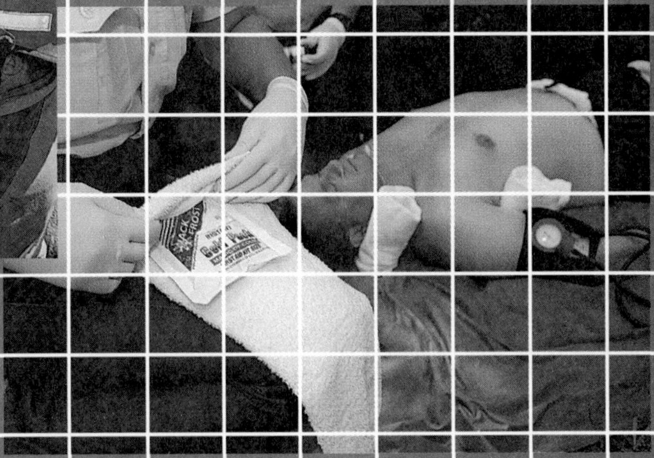

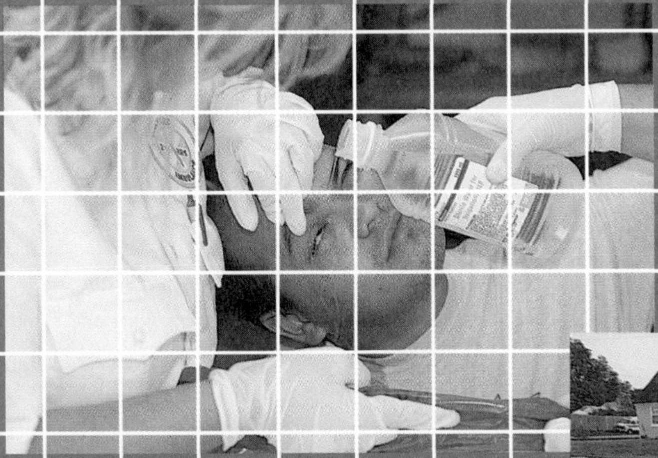

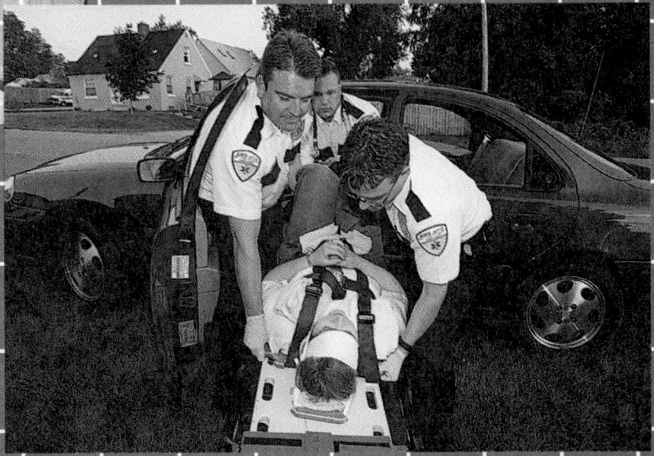

Chapter 22
Bleeding and Shock

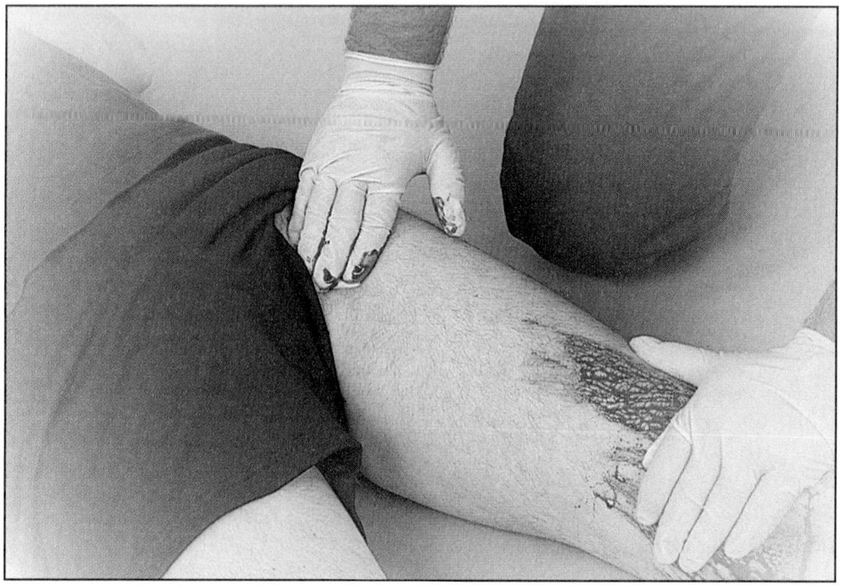

Knowledge Objectives

As an EMT-Basic, you should be able to:

OBJECTIVES

1. List the major components of the circulatory system.
2. Describe the function of the circulatory system in perfusing the tissues.
3. Explain the differences between arterial, venous, and capillary bleeding.
4. Describe the importance of airway management in a trauma patient.
5. Describe the importance of body substance isolation (BSI) when dealing with external bleeding.
6. Identify the methods of controlling external bleeding.
7. Describe how to apply a pressure bandage.
8. Describe the effects of an improperly applied bandage or tourniquet.
9. List the signs and symptoms of internal bleeding.
10. Describe the care for a patient with the signs and symptoms of internal bleeding.
11. Describe the relationship between mechanism of injury and internal bleeding.
12. Differentiate between compensated and uncompensated shock (hypoperfusion).
13. Identify the signs and symptoms of shock.
14. Describe the steps in providing care to a patient with the signs and symptoms of shock.
15. Describe the indications for the use of the pneumatic antishock garment (PASG).

OBJECTIVES

Skill Objectives

As an EMT-Basic, you should be able to:

1. **Demonstrate the use of direct pressure, elevation, pressure bandage, and pressure points to control external bleeding.**
2. **Demonstrate care of a patient with the signs and symptoms of internal bleeding.**
3. **Demonstrate care of a patient with the signs and symptoms of shock.**
4. **Demonstrate the use of the PASG.**
5. **Demonstrate how to complete a patient-care report for a patient with bleeding or shock.**

Attitude Objective

As an EMT-Basic, you should be able to:

1. **Defend the rationale for rapid transport of trauma patients.**
2. **Serve as a role model for other EMS personnel regarding the care of a patient who is bleeding or in shock.**

KEY TERMS

1. **Direct Pressure:** The first step in controlling external bleeding, by using the hand (with appropriate protective barriers) to apply pressure directly to the wound.
2. **Hemorrhage:** The loss of blood internally or externally.
3. **Hypoperfusion:** Inadequate blood flow through the tissues, which results in inadequate delivery of oxygen and nutrients to the cells and inadequate removal of waste products; also known as *shock*.
4. **Perfusion:** The circulation of blood to all organs of the body, carrying oxygen and other nutrients to the cells and removing waste products.
5. **Pneumatic Antishock Garment (PASG):** Inflatable garment used as a pressure splint to stabilize pelvic or lower-extremity fractures; may assist in the treatment of shock. Also called *MAST* (military antishock trousers) or *MAST pants*.
6. **Pressure Bandage:** A bandage applied to control external bleeding.
7. **Shock:** See *hypoperfusion*.

IT'S YOUR CALL

You are dispatched to a vehicle collision on a freeway. Upon arrival, you find two badly damaged cars. The driver of one car is walking around and denies any problem. The driver of the other is still inside the car. As you approach that patient, you notice that the car has severe damage to the front end and a crack in the windshield. The patient is sitting in the car and appears to be dazed. It does not appear that he was wearing restraint belts, and there is damage to the steering wheel. He is complaining of a headache, chest pain, and pain in his abdomen. As your partner begins inline spinal stabilization, you request a paramedic unit to assist. You are advised by dispatch that the medic unit is returning from a hospital at the other end of town and is at least 10 minutes away.

As your partner maintains C-spine immobilization, you check your patient's airway and breathing and put him on oxygen. He is breathing fast, about 30 breaths per minute, and his pulse is 100. He remembers his name, but not the day, where he is, or what happened. His blood pressure is 130/80. Lung sounds are diminished on one side.

Fire department personnel help you package the patient, who is now breathing about 38 times per minute and has a weak, rapid pulse of 120 and a tender, rigid abdomen. You reassess the patient's ventilations as your partner starts the ambulance toward the nearest hospital. Was your decision to "load and go" with your patient appropriate, or should you have waited for the paramedic unit?

As an EMT-Basic, you will deal with many types of trauma patients. Caring for them requires you to manage airway and breathing emergencies and any other life-threatening conditions before treating minor injuries such as minor bleeding and isolated extremity fractures. Trauma patients bring a unique challenge to assessment and care. The potential for hidden internal injuries is great, and these injuries can cause patients to deteriorate rapidly. Your goal is rapid assessment, treatment of life-threatening injuries, and transport to a hospital that can provide prompt definitive care. Serious trauma patients often require surgery.

Reviewing the Circulatory System

In understanding trauma and injuries affecting the circulatory system, it is important to remember that system's major structures. You may wish to review Chapter 8, Understanding the Human Body, for more detail.

The main function of the circulatory, or cardiovascular, system is to provide oxygen and nutrients to the tissues. It consists of three major components: the heart (pump), blood vessels (piping), and blood (fluid) (Figure 22-1).

- The heart: The heart is the pump that pushes blood through the body. With every contraction, the right side of the heart collects deoxygenated blood from the body and pumps it to the lungs. The left side of the heart receives oxygenated blood back from the lungs and pumps it to the rest of the tissues.
- Blood vessels: The blood vessels are the tubes through which blood flows. The three types of blood vessels are arteries, veins, and capillaries. Arteries carry blood away from the heart. Veins carry blood back to the heart. Capillaries are a network of blood vessels that connect arteries with veins. It is in the capillaries that oxygen, carbon dioxide, nutrients, and wastes are exchanged between the tissues and the blood.
- Blood: Blood is the fluid that is pushed through the vessels. Blood provides oxygen to all of the organs, helps fight infections, and forms clots to help stop bleeding. The average adult has about 5 L of blood.

The circulatory system plays such an important role in the body that its condition needs to be monitored constantly. Many of the vital signs measured during patient assessment are indicators of circulatory system function.

Perfusion

When **perfusion** is adequate, blood reaches all parts of the body and passes through all of the organs. This allows for delivery of oxygen and other nutrients to the cells and removal of carbon dioxide and other waste products. Injury to any of the components of the circulatory system may result in inadequate perfusion.

A failure to provide adequate circulation to the tissues is known as **hypoperfusion,** commonly called **shock.** Without good perfusion, the body's organs will not function properly. This can lead to death if not corrected. Shock has many possible causes. Regardless of the cause, the immediate problem is that the tissues are not receiving enough oxygen. Your job is to improve oxygenation. Shock is discussed in detail later in this chapter.

Sources of Bleeding

The term **hemorrhage** describes the loss of blood, either internally or externally. The amount and type of bleeding that occurs depend on the type of blood vessel that has been injured. Recognizing the type of bleeding will help you decide the type and extent of care necessary.

Arterial Bleeding

As the heart contracts, blood is forced through the arteries under pressure. The walls of the arteries expand and contract as the blood wave passes. When an artery is severed, bright red, well-oxygenated blood spurts out every time the heart contracts. This pressure wave makes it harder to control arterial bleeding. Bleeding from a large artery is life threatening because large amounts of blood can be lost quickly. As the patient's blood pressure drops, the amount of bleeding decreases because the pressure behind it decreases.

Venous Bleeding

Bleeding from veins is dark red or maroon in color. This is because venous blood lacks the high concentration of oxygen found in arterial blood. The blood in the veins is returning to the heart and is under less pressure. Venous bleeding therefore flows steadily, rather than in spurts. Bleeding from veins can also be profuse, but because of the reduced pressure, is usually easier to control than arterial bleeding.

Capillary Bleeding

Capillary bleeding is the most common type of bleeding from minor wounds. Bleeding from capillaries oozes because of their small size. However, it may appear that there is more major blood loss when large numbers of capillaries bleed at the same time. This is often seen in cuts to the face, which is very vascular. Because capillar-

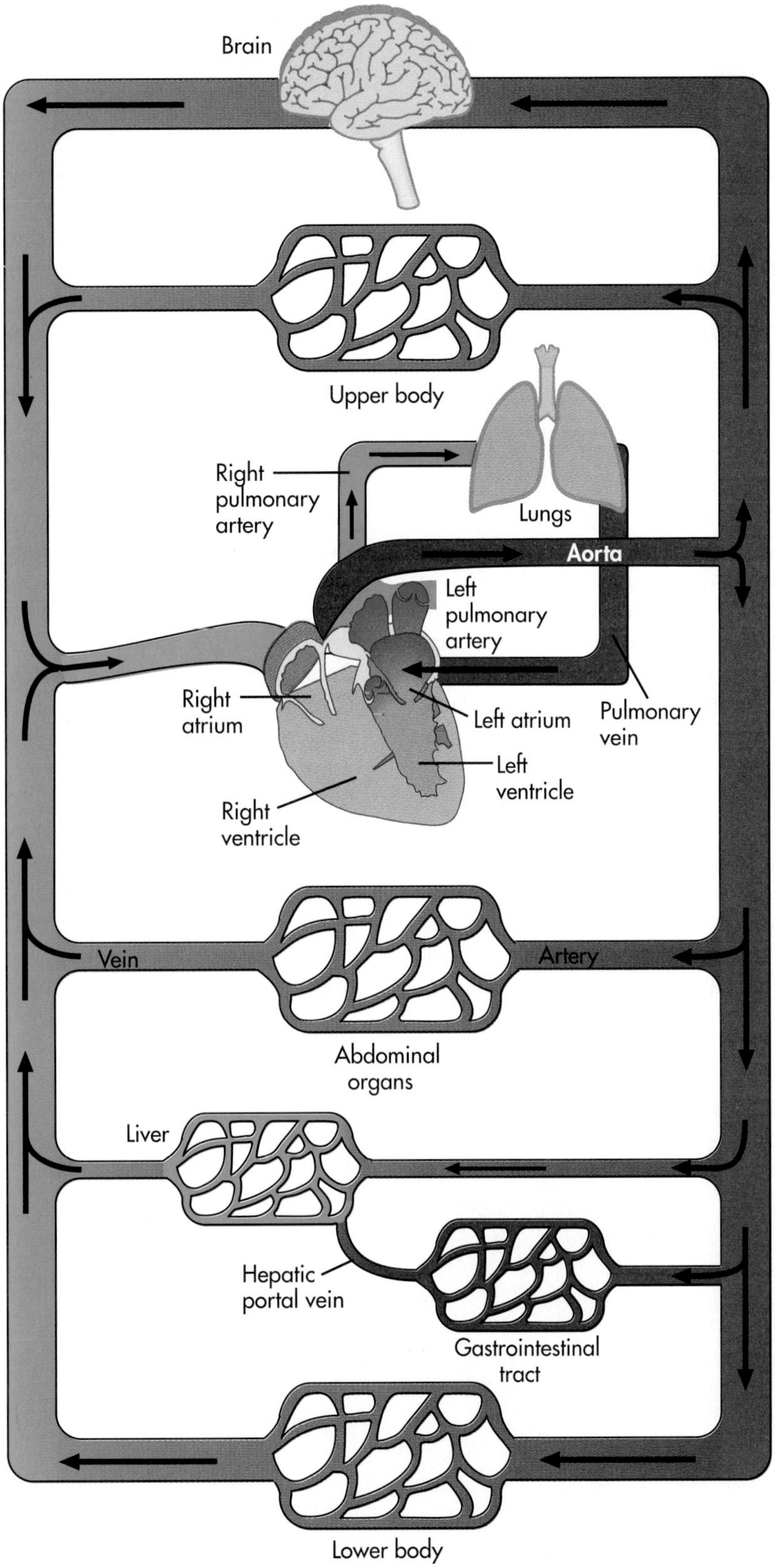

Figure 22-1

The heart, vessels, and blood make up the circulatory system.

ies connect arteries to veins, the color of capillary blood is neither as bright as arterial blood nor as dark as venous blood. Capillary bleeding is the easiest type to control because of the small size of the vessels and the low pressures involved.

External Bleeding

External bleeding results from any type of injury that penetrates the skin and severs blood vessels. If not cared for promptly, heavy external bleeding can cause shock.

Severity

The average adult has approximately 5 to 6 L of blood, compared with 3 L for a child and just under 1 L for an infant. The sudden loss of 1 L of blood in an adult patient, ½ L in a child, or 100 to 200 ml in an infant is considered serious. The severity of blood loss is reflected in the patient's signs and symptoms. As blood loss increases, perfusion decreases. A patient exhibiting signs and symptoms of shock has sustained severe blood loss.

Managing External Bleeding

Controlling bleeding is important in all trauma situations. Once airway and breathing have been addressed, check circulation. This means checking for a pulse and any severe bleeding that may affect the patient's condition. Minor bleeding can be cared for after treating more serious injuries.

Bleeding may initially appear to be serious. However, upon closer examination, the patient may have other more serious conditions requiring your immediate attention. Do not let appearance be the only factor in determining patient condition. Maintain a systematic approach to the assessment. This may be easier if you assign a helper to control bleeding while you continue the assessment.

The body has a natural response system, known as *clotting,* to stop bleeding. However, a serious injury resulting in massive blood loss or persistent bleeding may prevent effective clotting from occurring promptly. For this reason, you must generally act quickly to control any type of bleeding. Most external bleeding can be controlled simply by applying firm pressure to the wound. Because external bleeding provides a means for transmission of disease, first take the proper precautions to minimize exposure to the patient's blood or other body fluids.

Body Substance Isolation Practices

Chapter 3 discussed body substance isolation (BSI), or universal precautions, which are measures taken to minimize the risk of disease transmission. When caring for a bleeding patient, it is important for the EMT to wear gloves and other appropriate personal protective equipment to create a barrier against the patient's blood. If bleeding is profuse, goggles, a face shield, and even a gown may be needed to avoid splattering blood. If you are directly exposed, follow local protocols for informing appropriate personnel and arranging for follow-up.

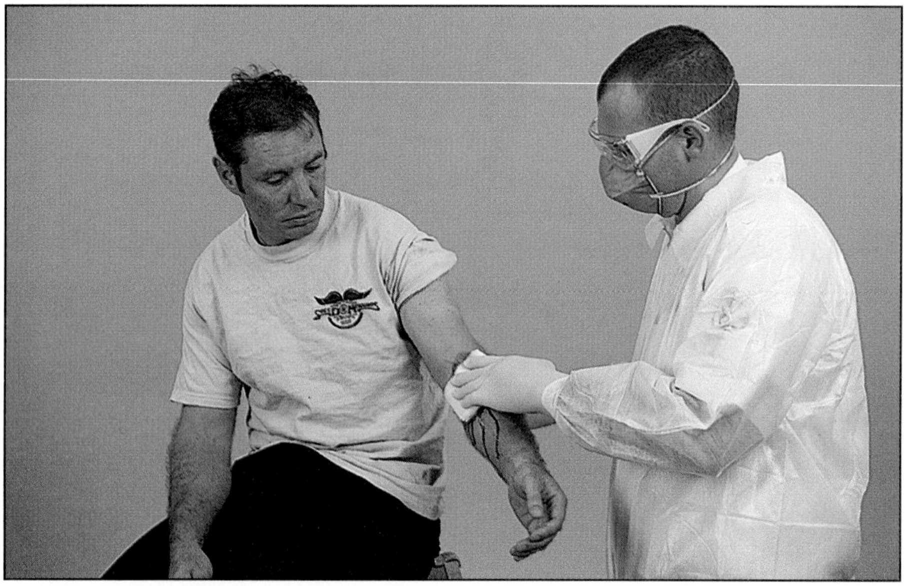

Figure 22-2

Direct pressure is the most common method to control external bleeding.

Primary Methods of Controlling External Bleeding
Most external bleeding is easily controlled using one or more of these five basic steps:

- Apply direct pressure.
- Elevate the injured area.
- Apply a pressure bandage to maintain the pressure.
- Immobilize any bleeding areas that may be associated with a bone fracture.
- Apply pressure to pressure points if other methods fail.

In rare situations, you may have to take more aggressive measures to control bleeding (see pp. 439-441).

Direct Pressure. The most common method of controlling external bleeding is to apply **direct pressure.** Place a clean gauze pad (dressing) over the wound and apply firm pressure directly on the bleeding site (Figure 22-2). If you see a deformity or other sign that there may be a bone injury, do not apply too much pressure. If the dressings become blood soaked, do not remove them. Place additional dressings on top and continue to apply pressure. Leaving the initial dressing encourages clotting.

Elevation. Elevation uses gravity to slow bleeding. Whenever possible, elevation should be done in addition to direct pressure (Figure 22-3). The bleeding site should be elevated above the level of the heart unless there are noticeable signs or symptoms of a possible fracture (for example, deformity, pain, swelling, or discoloration). If the patient is bleeding from the head or face and you do not suspect a head or spinal injury, elevate the head.

Pressure Bandage. After using direct pressure and elevation, you can apply a **pressure bandage.** This helps maintain the pressure that was initially applied by hand and frees you so that you can provide other care. A pressure bandage is applied by wrapping a roller bandage (gauze roll) securely over the top of existing pressure pads in a manner that slows but does not completely restrict blood flow (Figure 22-4). Once a pressure bandage is applied, check distal pulses to ensure that they are still present, indicating that the bandage has not been applied too tightly. Elevation should be maintained whenever possible, and a pressure dressing must be checked frequently to ensure its effectiveness. Bandages and dressings are discussed in detail in Chapter 23.

Immobilization. When bleeding is associated with a possible fracture, splinting may help reduce the bleeding. Reducing fracture movement decreases the amount and severity of soft-tissue damage and any bleeding associated with a fracture. Splinting is discussed in detail in Chapter 24.

Pressure Points. Bleeding occasionally cannot be controlled by direct pressure, elevation, or a pressure bandage. In this case, applying pressure directly over a main artery feeding the bleeding area will help control distal bleeding (Figure 22-5). Applying firm pressure on the brachial artery on the medial, upper arm will decrease circulation to the arm. Similarly, applying firm pressure to the femoral artery by pressing with the heel of your hand at the crease between the groin and the hip will reduce blood flow to the leg (Figure 22-6).

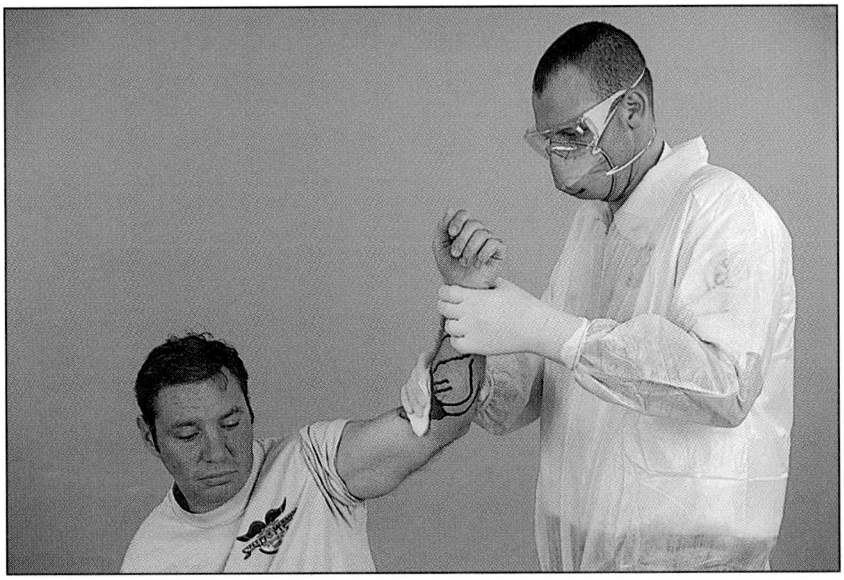

Figure 22-3

Elevation can be used in conjunction with direct pressure to slow bleeding. To elevate properly, the bleeding site should be held above the patient's heart.

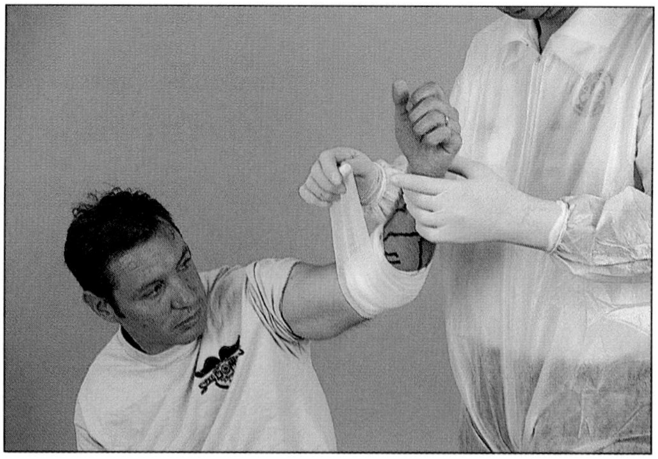

Figure 22-4

A pressure bandage is applied over pressure pads already in place. When possible, continue to keep the bleeding site elevated.

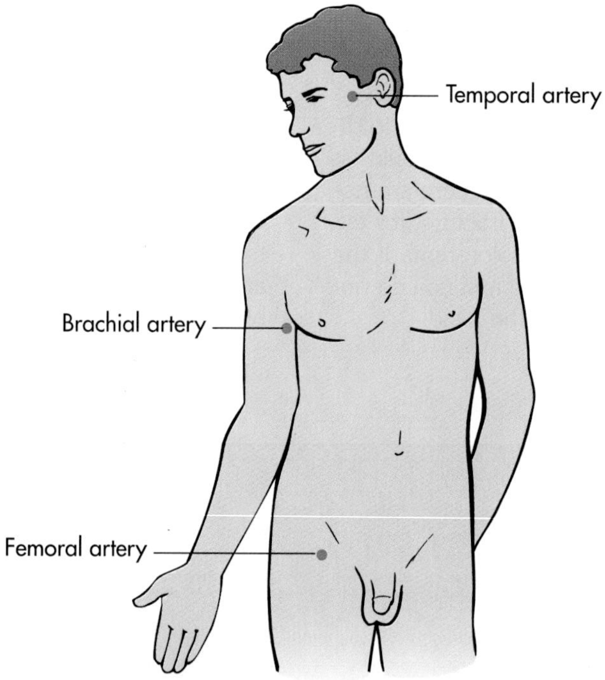

Figure 22-5

Common pressure points over main arteries.

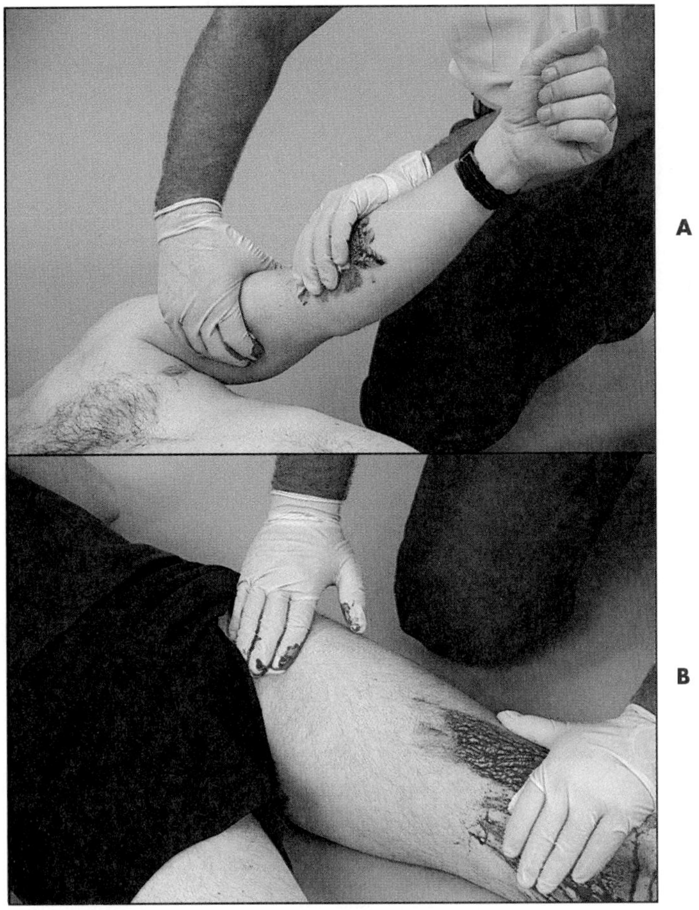

Figure 22-6

A, Pressure on the brachial artery decreases circulation to the arm. **B,** Pressure on the femoral artery decreases circulation to the leg.

Alternative Methods of Controlling External Bleeding

Two other common methods can be used to control external bleeding: the **pneumatic antishock garment (PASG)** and a tourniquet. However, each device has associated problems. Follow local protocols for applying these devices.

Pneumatic Antishock Garment. The PASG, also known as *military antishock trousers (MAST)*, may help control blood loss from the lower extremities or the pelvis (Figure 22-7). It is more commonly used to stabilize suspected fractures of the pelvis or legs. If there is injury to one leg you need only inflate that one leg compartment. If both legs are injured, you can inflate both leg compartments. If you suspect injuries to the pelvis, all three compartments can be inflated. The abdominal compartment is never used by itself, without also inflating the leg compartments. More information on the indications and contraindications for the PASG are on p. 446.

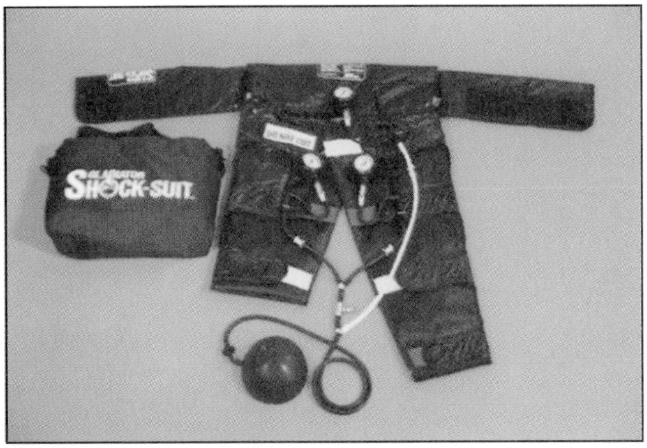

Figure 22-7

PASG can be used for stabilization of the pelvis and legs and to control bleeding in the lower extremities and pelvis.

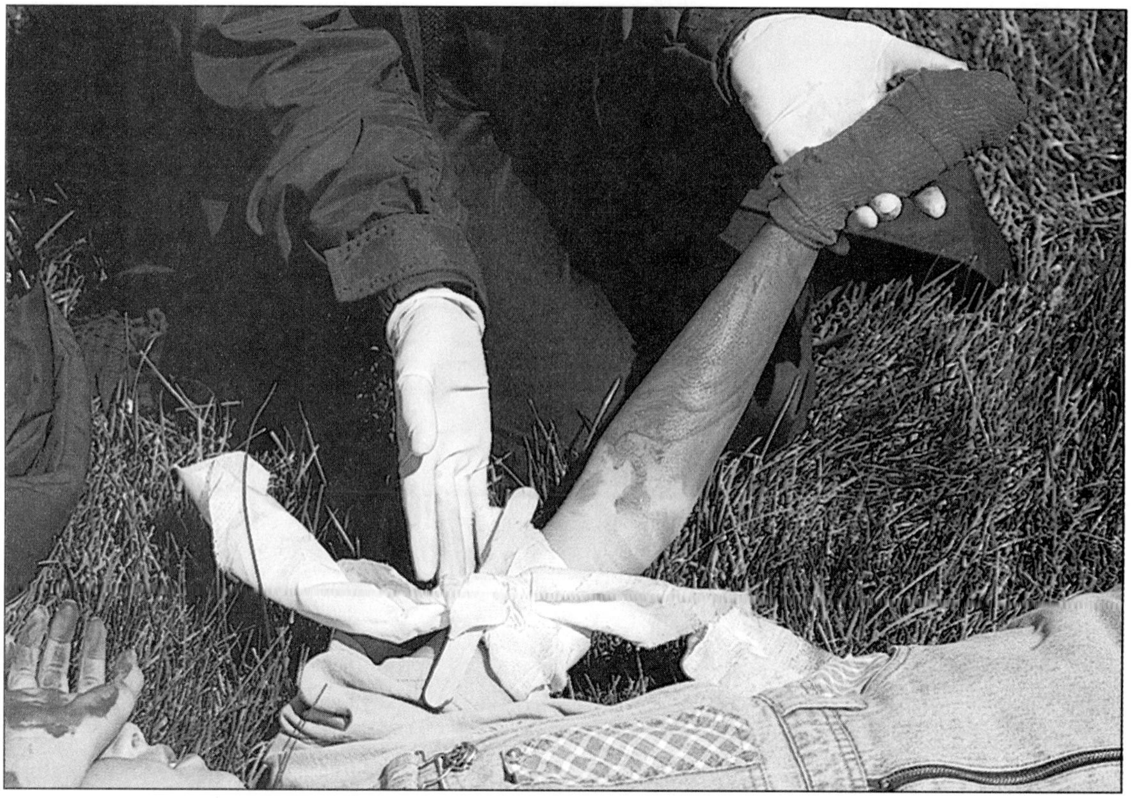

Figure 22-8

After the triangular bandage has been wrapped around the limb, tie a half knot with the ends, place a stick on the half knot, and tie a full knot over the stick.

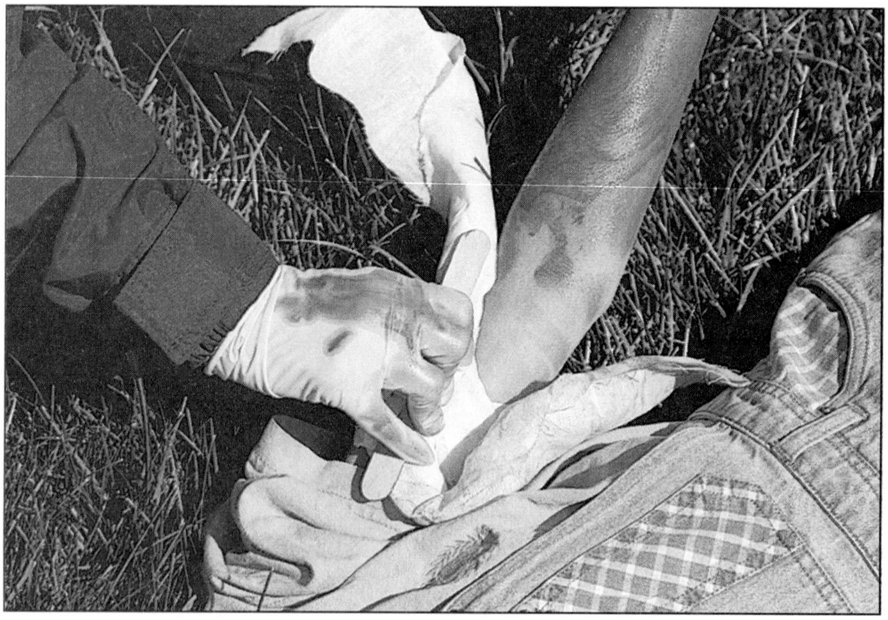

Figure 22-9

Twist the stick until the bleeding stops.

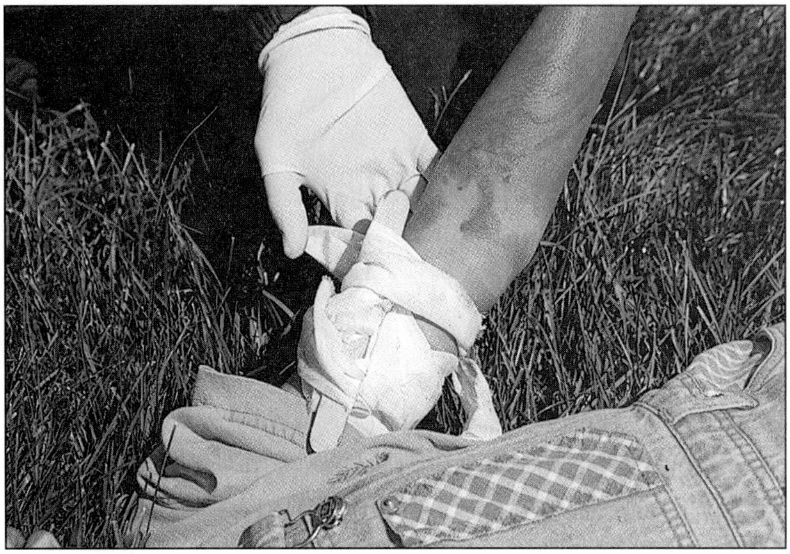

Figure 22-10

Secure the stick using either the ends of the tourniquet or another strip of cloth.

Tourniquet. As a last resort, you can consider using a **tourniquet** to control severe bleeding. A tourniquet is a wide band applied to the limb between the heart and the bleeding site. When tightened, it entirely cuts off arterial blood supply beyond that point. It can therefore cause permanent damage to nerves, muscles, and blood vessels. A tourniquet should only be used in a life-threatening situation when severe bleeding cannot be controlled with any other method. Local protocol may further define its appropriate use.

To apply a tourniquet:

- Apply a triangular bandage 2 to 4 inches wide just above the wound site. Wrap it around the limb at least twice.
- Tie a half knot, place a stick or similar object on top of the knot, and then tie a full knot over the stick (Figure 22-8). Twist the stick until enough pressure is applied to stop the bleeding (Figure 22-9).
- Once the bleeding has stopped, secure the stick in place using the end of the tourniquet or strips of cloth (Figure 22-10).
- Leave the tourniquet visible. Write the time of application and location of the tourniquet somewhere that other care givers will be sure to see, such as on a piece of tape placed on the patient's chest or forehead (Figure 22-11). Document its use on the patient-care report.

Once in place, a tourniquet should not be removed unless ordered by medical control. Never use wire, rope, or any other narrow material that may cut into the skin and underlying tissue. When applying a tourniquet it should be as close to the injury as possible, but should not be placed directly over a joint. A blood pressure cuff can be used as a tourniquet, by inflating it until the bleeding stops.

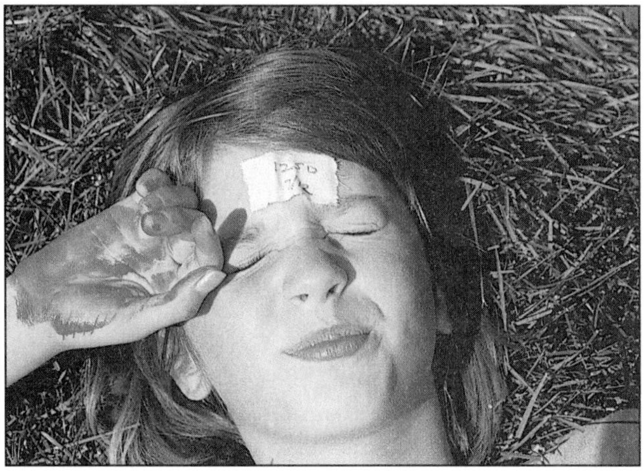

Figure 22-11

On a piece of tape, write the time of application and location of the tourniquet.

Tourniquet is also the common term for a device used to help start IV lines. This type of tourniquet works very differently. It restricts only venous, not arterial, flow and should not be confused with the method described above.

Special Situations

While treatment for most bleeding is similar, some body areas require special techniques. Bleeding from the nose, ears, or mouth is usually associated with an injury to the head, facial trauma, inserting an object into the nose, sinusitis, high blood pressure, or coagulation disorders. If

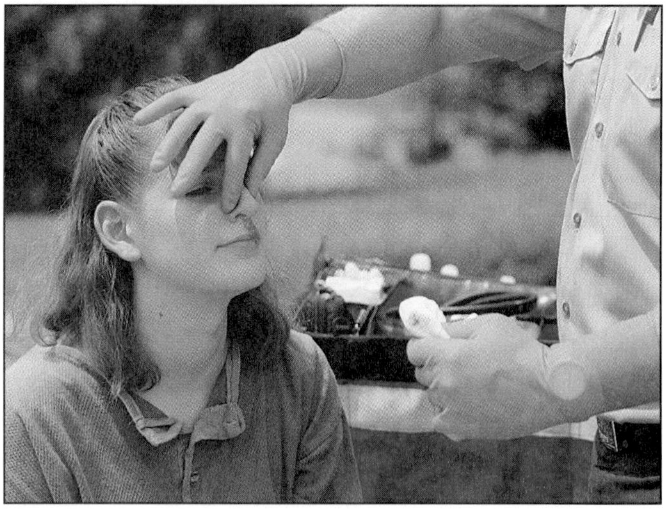

Figure 22-12

To control a nosebleed, apply pressure to the fleshy portion of the nostrils and hold that pressure for 10 to 15 minutes.

bleeding from the nose or ears is associated with significant head injury, do not attempt to stop the bleeding. This may cause an increase in intracranial pressure. Instead, stabilize the head and neck, and place a loose sterile dressing around the nose or ears to collect the blood and minimize infection.

If a trauma patient is bleeding from the nose or mouth, have suction available. The blood can drain into the back of the throat and cause an airway obstruction. If swallowed, blood can cause the patient to become nauseated and vomit.

A nosebleed usually results either from an injury to the nose or from a medical condition such as hypertension. To control a simple nosebleed, place the patient in a seated position, leaning slightly forward. Apply pressure to the nose by pinching the fleshy portion of the nostrils together, against the bone underneath, with your gloved hand (Figure 22-12). Hold that pressure for 10 to 15 minutes. This is normally all that is necessary to control the bleeding. Have the patient spit any blood into an emesis basin rather than swallowing it. Suction the airway if necessary. Nosebleeds are usually not life threatening. However, if the blood loss cannot be controlled, the patient could develop shock. These patients should be transported for further evaluation and care.

Internal Bleeding

Unlike external bleeding, where wounds are usually obvious, internal bleeding is more difficult to recognize and care for. Internal bleeding often results from trauma or some type of medical condition, such as a bleeding ulcer in the stomach or intestine. A trauma patient has a potential for significant internal blood loss from blood-rich organs such as the spleen, liver, and kidneys. The patient's condition may deteriorate rapidly from internal bleeding. Severe internal blood loss needs to be cared for in an operating room. As an EMT-Basic, your jobs are rapid identification of a patient who may have serious internal bleeding and quick transport to the hospital. Except for definitive airway control, the value of advanced life support (ALS) from paramedics is minimal in most cases of severe internal bleeding.

Severity

Internal bleeding can be as simple as a mild bruise in which the underlying capillaries burst, known as a **hematoma**. This will cause a black and blue appearance, called an **ecchymosis** (Figure 22-13). Internal organ damage, such as a ruptured spleen, commonly leads to extensive bleeding that may be concealed. Although discoloration and swelling are often not visible, you may note tenderness, pain, and rigidity in the abdomen. These can be important indicators of internal injuries. Painful, swollen, deformed extremities may also indicate serious internal blood loss. The more severe the internal bleeding, the quicker your patient's condition will deteriorate. As the patient loses blood, there will be a decrease in perfusion, ultimately resulting in shock. With the first signs of shock, you should make every effort to move quickly to the hospital.

Relationship to the Mechanism of Injury

When trying to determine the extent of internal injuries, it is important to consider the mechanism of injury. Having a basic understanding of what happens to the body when an injury occurs will help you evaluate the possible severity of injuries.

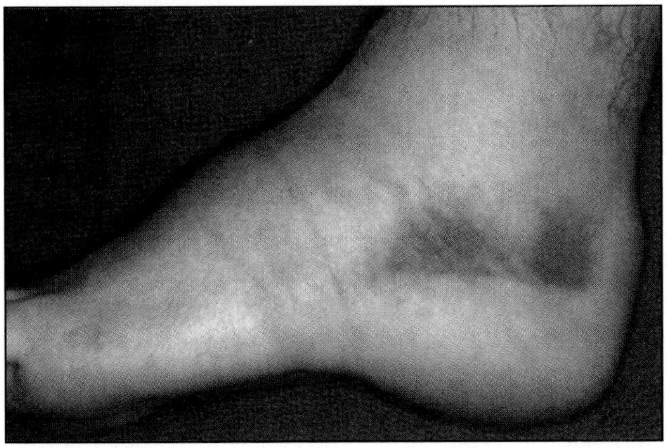

Figure 22-13

The black and blue appearance of a bruise is caused by burst capillaries.

Chapter 6 discussed the forces and motions involved in an accident and the injuries that can result based on the laws of motion. In most trauma situations, such as falls and vehicle collisions, the patient comes to a sudden stop. Any sudden deceleration will affect body organs.

The following example uses a vehicle impact to illustrate the mechanisms involved in a typical deceleration incident (Figure 22-14):

1. A vehicle hits a stationary object (pole, tree) and comes to a sudden stop.
2. The patient's body is thrown forward, then also comes to a sudden stop when it hits the vehicle interior. Consider the types of injuries that can occur if the unrestrained patient's head strikes the windshield or the patient's chest hits the steering wheel.
3. The organs inside the body continue moving forward within their respective cavities and then come to a sudden stop when they strike the rest of the body. The brain collides with the inside of the skull, for instance, and the heart hits the chest wall.

You may only see a bruise on the head or chest, but the underlying damage can be life threatening. When obtaining a general impression of your patient, it is important to consider not only the visible injuries, but also the internal injuries that could have resulted from the specific mechanism.

Any type of injury in which there is no direct penetration of the skin is called blunt trauma. This includes being struck with an object and striking an unmoving object. Blunt trauma will usually cause visible bruising, but external signs often do not reveal the full extent of any underlying internal injuries.

Penetrating trauma is the name for trauma in which the skin has been penetrated directly by an object such as a knife, bullet, or shard of glass. Penetrating trauma can puncture internal organs and cause both internal and external bleeding.

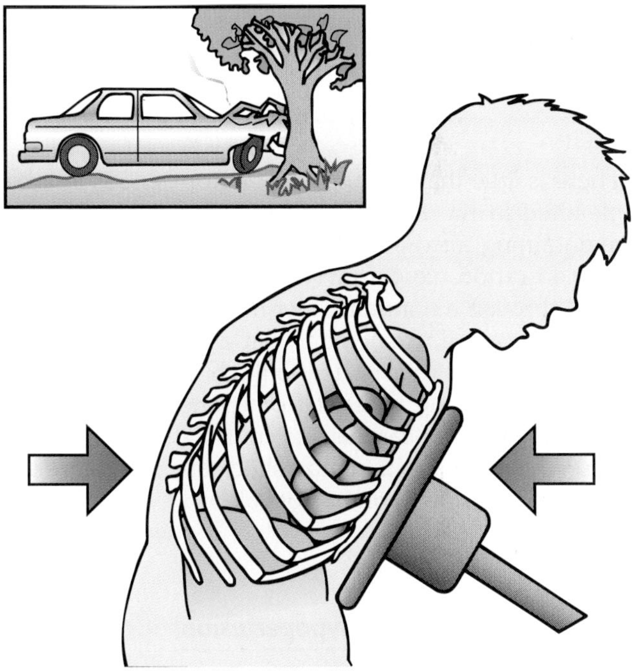

Figure 22-14

The three collisions involved in a motor vehicle collision are: 1) the vehicle hits the tree; 2) the patient's body hits the steering wheel or restraints; 3) the organs in the body strike the boundaries of their cavities.

BOX 22-1 Signs and Symptoms of Internal Bleeding

- Pain or tenderness
- Swelling or discoloration of injury site
- Bleeding from the mouth, rectum, vagina, or other orifice (ears, nose, urethra)
- Vomiting bright red blood or dark, coffee-ground–colored blood
- Dark tarry stools or stools with bright red blood
- Tender, rigid, or distended abdomen

Recognizing Internal Bleeding

Unlike external bleeding, internal bleeding is not easily visible. Look for signs and symptoms such as those listed in Box 22-1. As the patient's condition worsens, signs and symptoms of shock may appear; these are listed below.

Managing Internal Bleeding

There is little that can be done to stop serious internal bleeding in the field. Try to stabilize the patient by maintaining airway and breathing. Administer high-concentration oxygen at 10 to 15 liters per minute (lpm) through a nonrebreather mask and assist ventilations as needed. Remember that as blood is lost, less oxygen is being transported to the brain. If there is any external bleeding present from penetrating trauma, take proper BSI measures and control the bleeding. Position the patient to minimize shock and maintain comfort. Transport as soon as possible.

Shock (Hypoperfusion)

Shock develops when tissue perfusion is inadequate. If not managed early, this condition can be fatal. The best care for shock is to try to limit its progression.

Body Systems and Shock

Shock has many causes, but the end result is the same. There is a lack of oxygen and nutrients being delivered to the cells. Adequate tissue perfusion requires:

- A functioning pump (the heart)
- Adequate fluid volume (blood)
- Adequate air exchange to get oxygen into the blood
- An intact vascular system to deliver blood to the tissues

Failure of any one of these components can lead to shock. The most common cause of shock associated with trauma is loss of blood volume from disruption of the delivery system. This is called *hypovolemic (low-volume) shock*.

Severity of Shock

The longer cells go without oxygen, nutrients, and removal of metabolic waste products, the greater the chance of damage to the tissues and organs. Certain organs, such as the heart, brain, and lungs, are quicker to suffer from oxygen shortage than others.

The severity of blood loss can also be broken down into classes, as defined by the American College of Surgeons. The importance of these classes is their emphasis on the progression of shock. Shock progresses through a series of stages that are recognizable by their clinical signs. By observing these signs, alert responders can learn much about how far into shock a patient is.

- Class 1: Pulse usually <100, BP normal, respirations 14-20, slightly anxious
- Class 2: Pulse >100, BP normal, respirations 20-30, mildly anxious
- Class 3: Pulse >120, BP decreased, respirations 30-40, anxious and confused
- Class 4: Pulse >140, BP decreased, respirations >35, confused and lethargic

Signs in Classes 3 and 4 are dramatic and easy to spot, but they are late in the progression of the problem. Recognizing the more subtle signs in Classes 1 and 2 enables an EMT to move quickly to the hospital before the patient is in severe danger.

The body has many mechanisms to compensate for shock. These are what produce the early signs that the patient may be going into shock. In a more general description, the stages progress from compensated to uncompensated to irreversible shock.

Signs and Symptoms of Shock

The early signs and symptoms are indicators of compensated shock. The body is responding to blood loss well enough to maintain blood pressure. As the body loses the ability to compensate, blood pressure begins to fall. This is a relatively late sign. Only aggressive intervention will prevent this uncompensated shock from progressing to irreversible shock and death.

In the early stages, the heart tries to compensate by pumping faster. If the blood volume is low, this fast pulse will also be weak. Some patients take medications that prevent this increase in heart rate; it will be more difficult to recognize early shock in these patients.

The increased work load on the heart requires additional oxygen. To meet this oxygen demand, respirations become faster and deeper. Peripheral blood vessels constrict in an effort to raise blood pressure and force blood flow toward essential organs. This helps maintain blood pressure and also makes the skin pale and cool. Inadequate fluid in the body makes the patient thirsty.

Many of these compensatory mechanisms are caused directly by the sympathetic nervous system. Also called the *fight-or-flight response,* the action of this system releases epinephrine (adrenaline) into the body. Epinephrine has a number of effects, especially sweating, nausea, tachycardia (fast heart rate), and shunting of blood from the periphery to the core. These compensatory mechanisms and their effects explain the combination of signs seen in early, compensated shock:

- Restlessness, anxiety, altered mental status
- Cool, pale, moist skin
- Increased pulse rate; may also be weak ("thready")
- Increased breathing rate; may be shallow, labored, or irregular
- Thirst
- Nausea and vomiting
- Capillary refill greater than 2 seconds (most reliable in infants and children); cyanosis
- Normal blood pressure

When the body can no longer compensate for the blood loss, uncompensated shock develops. In this stage, the peripheral blood vessels that were initially constricted relax and dilate. This is because of the lack of oxygen, which is needed to maintain constriction. The dilation of these vessels causes blood to move away from the vital organs. Blood pressure falls. Finally, death begins to occur at the cellular level as circulation is unable to meet the perfusion demands. Wastes, especially acids, build up and contribute to the rapid deterioration.

Signs and symptoms of late (uncompensated) shock include:

- Falling blood pressure
- Decreasing pulse rate
- Decreasing respirations
- Anxiety, restlessness, combativeness, altered mental status, unconsciousness

Falling blood pressure is an even later sign in children and infants than in adults. They may maintain pressure until more than half of their small blood volume is gone. When blood pressure does drop, the change can be sudden; and they are likely to be close to death. In pediatric patients, pay special attention to earlier signs of shock.

Spinal shock is a type that differs in important ways from low-volume (hypovolemic) shock. Spinal injuries that damage nerves exiting the spine at the thoracic or lumbar levels can disrupt nervous-system control of blood-vessel constriction because epinephrine cannot exert its effect in the body. The result is widespread vascular dilation that can drop blood pressure enough to cause shock. The patient often presents with warm, flushed skin below the level of the spinal injury. Heart rate may be normal.

Caring for Shock

The objective of shock management is to maintain proper tissue perfusion and oxygenation. Care should begin during initial assessment, as soon as you have evaluated the mechanism of injury or nature of illness. This may be even before the first signs of shock are visible.

To care for shock:

- Take appropriate BSI precautions.
- Place the patient on high-concentration oxygen. If the patient is not breathing adequately, assist ventilations with a bag-valve-mask (BVM).
- Control any external bleeding.
- Elevate the lower extremities 8 to 12 inches if no lower-extremity fractures or spinal injuries are suspected (Figure 22-15). If the patient is on a backboard, raise the

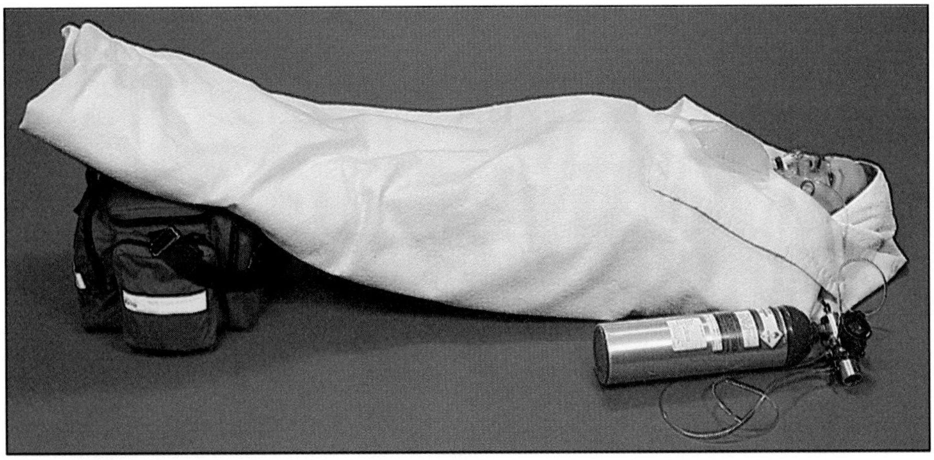

Figure 22-15

If no spinal injuries are suspected, elevate the patient's legs and feet 8 to 12 inches.

lower end of the backboard (Trendelenburg's position) (Figure 22-16).
- Apply the PASG if indicated by local protocol and medical direction.
- Maintain body temperature by covering the patient with a blanket, if appropriate.
- Transport the patient without delay.
- Request ALS assistance, if available.

During transport, continue your patient assessment. Care for any injuries. Continuously monitor the patient's airway and breathing. Note any changes in the patient's condition and notify medical direction.

IT'S YOUR CALL
CONCLUSION

Your patient is experiencing early signs and symptoms of shock. The patient does not have any obvious external bleeding, but you are concerned about internal bleeding. You immobilize the patient and place him on oxygen. Because the paramedic unit had a response time that was longer than the time needed to prepare the patient for transport, you made the appropriate decision to begin transport to the nearest hospital. You contact dispatch to advise the incoming ALS unit that you are en route. Dispatch and the ALS unit can decide if there is a location where the ALS unit can meet you during transport. Meeting during transport would allow a paramedic to get on board, or you and the paramedics may decide to transfer the patient to the other unit. Early transport is this patient's best chance for survival.

Pneumatic Antishock Garment

Bleeding that results from severe internal injuries or from a fractured pelvis or femur can cause the patient to go into shock rapidly. The PASG is an inflatable, trouserlike device with three compartments that is wrapped around the patient's lower extremities and abdomen. In the past, it was thought that this device was capable of diverting a significant amount of blood from the lower extremities into the body core for use by the vital organs. However, the true effectiveness of this device in raising blood pressure and treating shock is highly controversial. There is substantial evidence that the PASG does not shunt blood or raise blood pressure to any significant extent.[1,2]

However, the device does have potential benefits for a patient with certain injuries. The circumferential pressure applied by the device can help minimize movement of broken bone ends and control blood loss from fractures of the pelvis and the lower extremities. Even with its limitations, the PASG is still used in many EMS systems. When using it to treat a patient in shock, follow local protocols. Some protocols suggest using the PASG only with suspected pelvis or lower extremity fractures when the systolic blood pressure is less than 100 mm Hg and two or more signs of shock are present.

The use of the PASG is contraindicated in patients with: (1) pulmonary edema, (2) penetrating trauma to the chest (some protocols also include penetrating abdominal trauma), and (3) later stages of pregnancy (leg compartments may be inflated).

To apply the PASG:

1. Place the PASG on a backboard and unfasten all of the hook-and-loop closures (Figure 22-17).
2. Log-roll the patient onto the backboard. All clothing except undergarments should be removed, if possible (Figure 22-18).

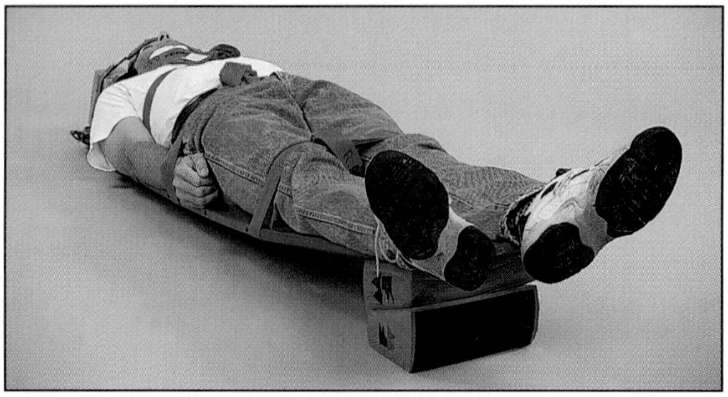

Figure 22-16

If spinal injuries are a possibility, or the patient is on a backboard, elevate the foot of the backboard 8 to 10 inches.

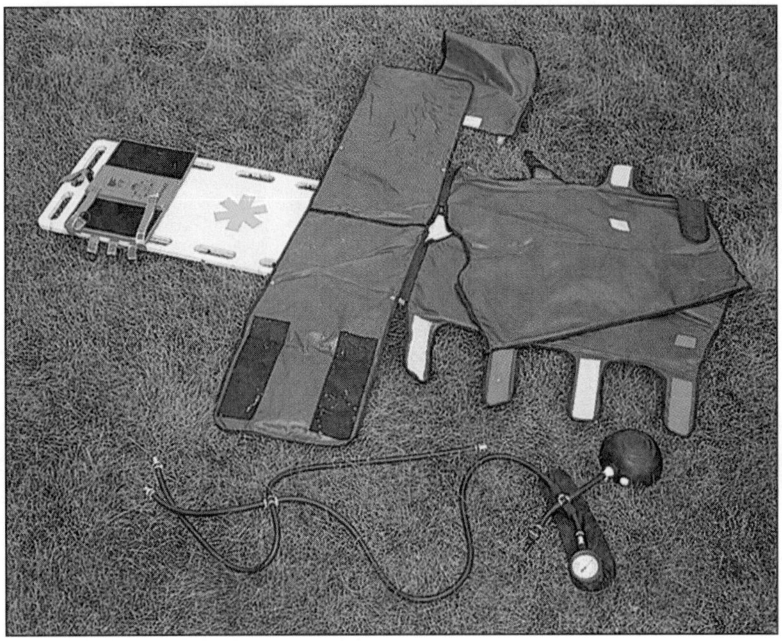

Figure 22-17

Unfasten and roll out the PASG.

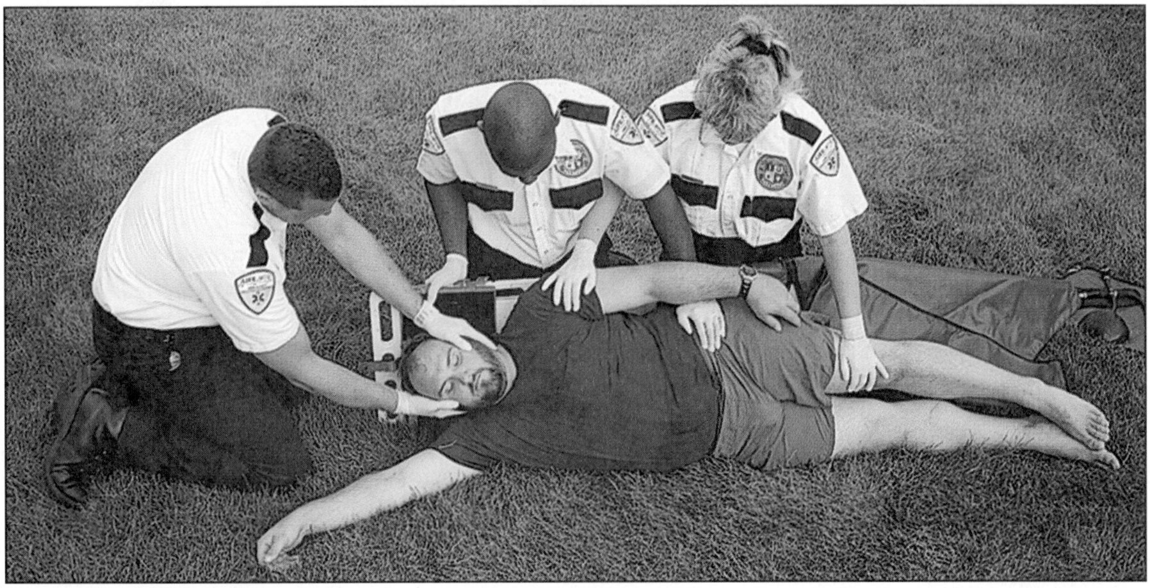

Figure 22-18

Log-roll the patient onto the backboard after removing as much clothing as possible.

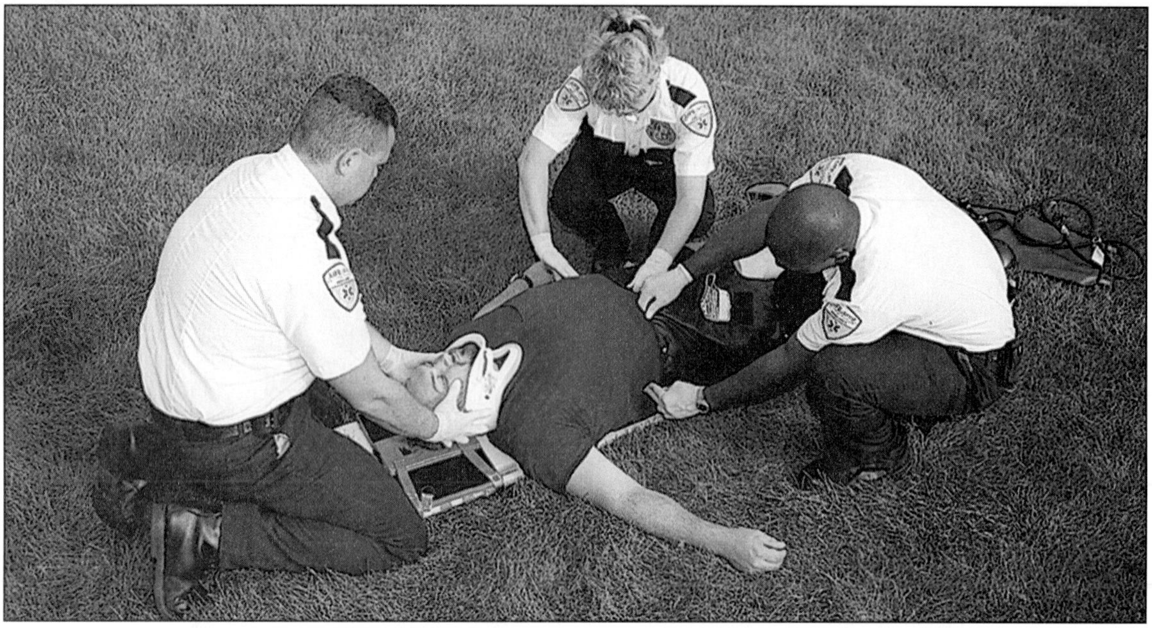

Figure 22-19

Locate the lowest ribs on the patient and adjust the PASG so that the top edge of the garment is just below them.

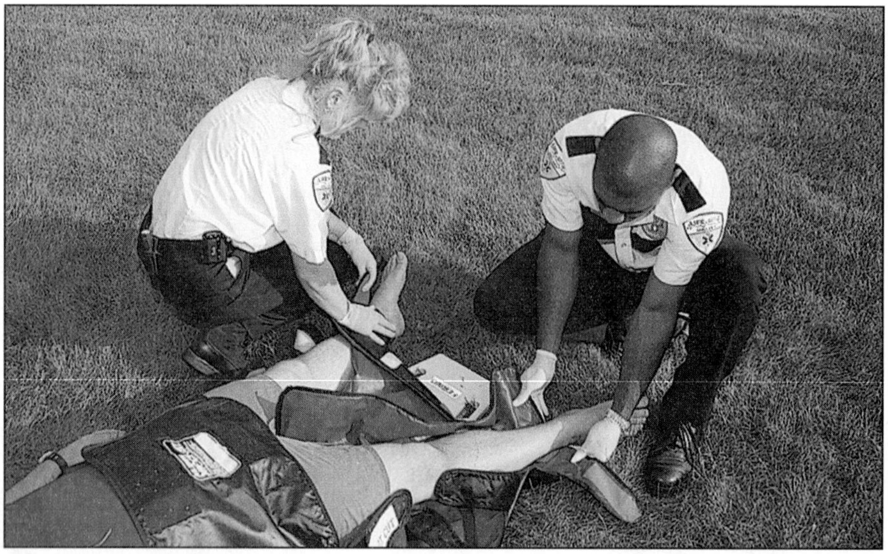

Figure 22-20

Adjust the legs of the PASG so they do not extend past the patient's ankles.

3. Adjust the PASG so that the top edge of the garment is at the level just below the lowest ribs (Figure 22-19).
4. Adjust the length of the legs to ensure that they do not extend below the ankles (Figure 22-20).
5. Wrap the PASG around the legs and the abdomen and secure the hook-and-loop closures (Figure 22-21).
6. Attach the inflation tubes to all three compartments and open the appropriate stopcocks (Figure 22-22).
7. Inflate the compartments according to your protocol, beginning with the legs and progressing to the abdomen, until adequate pressure is applied. This occurs when the hook-and-loop closures crackle or the pop-off valves release.
8. Close the stopcocks and measure blood pressure.

Once inflated, the PASG should not be deflated without approval of the medical control physician. This is usually done in the hospital once multiple intravenous lines are established. The use of a PASG on children requires a pediatric garment and special protocols.

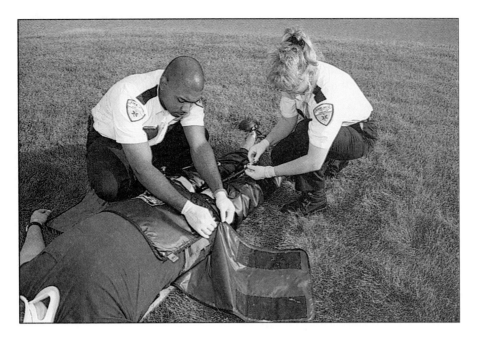

Figure 22-21

Wrap the PASG around the patient and secure the hook-and-loop closures.

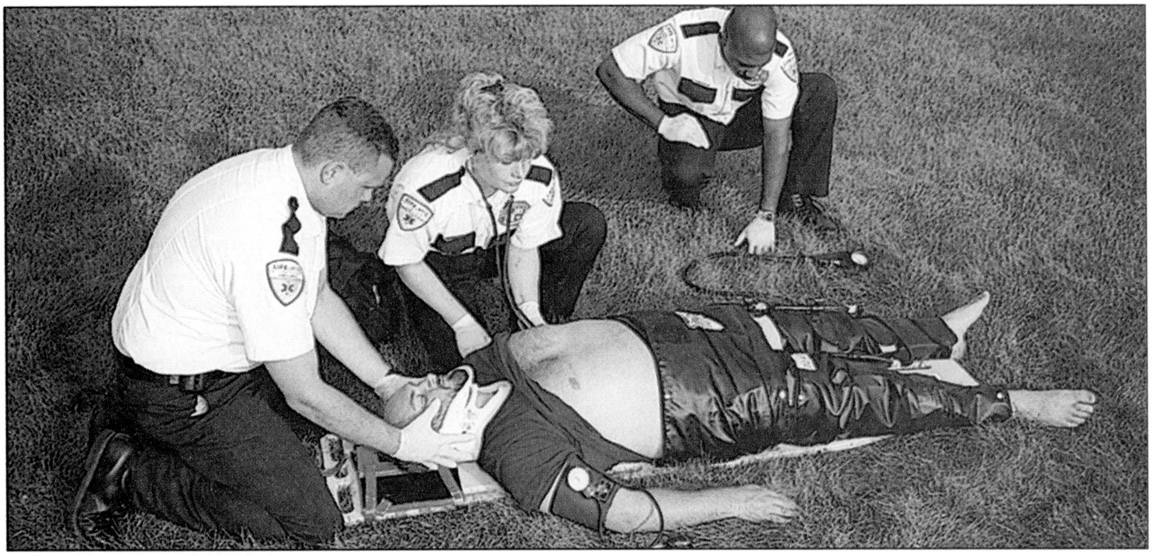

Figure 22-22

Attach inflation tubes and open the appropriate stopcocks before inflating the compartments, starting with the legs.

SUMMARY

The heart, blood vessels, and blood are the three circulatory system components that ensure perfusion of vital organs. An injury or malfunction of any of these can lead to shock.

External bleeding results when there is a break in the skin. If not controlled, the patient can lose large amounts of blood. Internal bleeding results from injuries to internal vessels and organs. Generally, internal bleeding can only be controlled by surgery.

When attempting to control external bleeding, take proper BSI precautions. Most external bleeding can be controlled by direct pressure and elevation. A pressure dressing can be applied to maintain this pressure and free you to provide other care. Alternate methods, such as pressure points and tourniquets, can be used if direct pressure and elevation do not work. When caring for internal bleeding, ensure that the patient has an open airway and is breathing adequately. Place the patient on oxygen, position the patient to minimize shock, maintain body temperature, and make the patient comfortable. If your system allows, apply a PASG. Transport immediately to a hospital.

If bleeding is not controlled, the patient will go into shock. The body has several mechanisms to compensate for inadequate perfusion. In the early stages, this is known as *compensated shock.* As these systems begin to fail, the body goes into uncompensated and finally irreversible shock.

REFERENCES

1. **Bivens HG et al:** Blood volume displacement with inflation of antishock trousers, *Ann Emerg Med* 11:409, 1982.
2. **Mattox KL et al:** Prospective randomized evaluation of antishock MAST in post-traumatic hypotension, *J Trauma* 26:779, 1986.

SUGGESTED READINGS

1. **BTLS:** Basic trauma life support for the EMT-B and first responder, ed 2. In *Basic trauma life support international*, Upper Saddle River, NJ, 1996, Brady-Prentice Hall.
2. **National Association of EMTs:** *Pre-hospital trauma life support*, ed 4, St Louis, 1999, Mosby.
3. **Stohr GM:** Pneumatic antishock garments: are the benefits overinflated? *J Emerg Med Serv* 19:34, 1996.

Chapter 23

Soft-Tissue Injuries

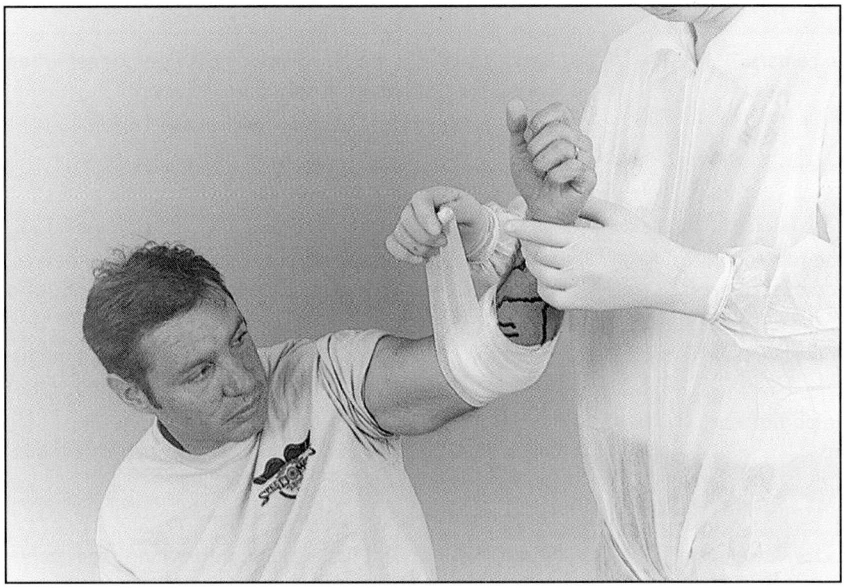

Knowledge Objectives

OBJECTIVES

As an EMT-Basic, you should be able to:

1. Describe the structure and function of the skin.
2. Describe the relationship between body substance isolation (BSI) practices and soft-tissue injuries.
3. List and describe the types of closed wounds.
4. List and describe the types of open wounds.
5. Describe how to care for a patient with closed wounds.
6. Describe how to care for a patient with open wounds.
7. List the functions of dressings and bandages.
8. Describe how to care for an amputated body part.
9. Discuss the special considerations of care for a patient with a penetrating chest trauma.
10. Describe the differences between the care for open chest wounds and that for open abdominal wounds.
11. Describe how to care for an impaled object.
12. Define the populations at risk for burns and typical patterns of burn injuries.
13. Describe the differences between thermal, electrical, chemical, and radiation burns.
14. Describe the effects of inhalation burns on the respiratory system.
15. Identify the signs and symptoms of inhalation injury.
16. Describe the factors that help determine the extent and severity of a burn.
17. Differentiate among the characteristics of superficial, partial-thickness, and full-thickness burns.
18. Describe the use of the rule of nines to determine the percentage of body surface area burned, for both adult and pediatric patients.
19. Name and describe the three classifications of burn severity.
20. Explain the difference in care for minor, moderate, and critical burns.
21. Describe the criteria for referring a patient to a burn center.
22. Describe how to care for chemical burns.
23. Describe how to care for electrical burns.

OBJECTIVES

Skill Objectives

As an EMT-Basic, you should be able to:

1. **Demonstrate how to provide care for the following soft-tissue injuries:**
   - **Closed wound**
   - **Open wound**
   - **Open chest wound**
   - **Open abdominal wound**
   - **Impaled object**
   - **Amputated body part**
   - **Superficial burn**
   - **Partial-thickness burn**
   - **Full-thickness burn**
   - **Chemical burn**
   - **Electrical burn**
2. **Demonstrate how to complete a patient-care report for a patient with soft-tissue injuries.**
3. **Given a scenario involving a burn patient, use a standard formula to determine the extent of the burn.**

Attitude Objectives

As an EMT-Basic, you should be able to:

1. **Advocate the value of transporting to burn centers.**
2. **Serve as a role model for other EMS personnel when caring for patients with soft-tissue injury.**

KEY TERMS

1. **Abrasion:** Open wound characterized by the rubbing or scraping away of the superficial layer (epidermis) of the skin.
2. **Amputation:** Open wound characterized by the complete severing of a body part.
3. **Avulsion:** Open wound characterized by the partial tearing away of soft tissue, creating a tissue flap.
4. **Burn:** An injury to the skin or other body tissues caused by heat, chemicals, electricity, or radiation.
5. **Chemical Burn:** A burn resulting from contact with wet or dry chemicals.
6. **Contusion:** A closed wound with internal bleeding resulting from contact with a blunt object; a bruise.
7. **Closed Wound:** Soft-tissue damage beneath the skin without penetration or disruption of the skin surface.
8. **Critical Burn:** A burn that is potentially life threatening or disabling, usually requiring advanced emergency care.
9. **Full-thickness Burn:** A burn that penetrates the epidermis and dermis layers of the skin and sometimes affects the underlying tissues, blood vessels, muscles, and nerves; characterized by white and charred discoloration; also called a *third-degree burn.*
10. **Hematoma:** Pooling of blood under the skin or in the tissue after the rupture of blood vessels; associated with a closed wound.
11. **Impaled Object:** A penetrating object, such as a knife, embedded in soft tissue.
12. **Laceration:** A cut or tear in the skin.
13. **Open Wound:** Soft-tissue damage resulting from penetration of the skin surface.
14. **Partial-thickness Burn:** A burn injury that penetrates the epidermis and extends into the dermis; characterized by reddened discoloration and blisters; also called a *second-degree burn.*
15. **Superficial Burn:** A burn injury that involves only the epidermis; characterized by reddened discoloration; also called a *first-degree burn.*

IT'S YOUR CALL

At 3:22 pm your unit is dispatched to a house fire with an occupant reported trapped. Upon arrival, you notice a person crawling on the ground near the house, which is fully engulfed in fire. Bystanders drag the person away from the flames and toward your unit. You begin patient assessment. Your initial impression is that he is a teenager, covered with soot from the fire, and bleeding from what appears to be wounds on his face and arms. As he lies on the ground shivering, you note that he has suffered a burn injury to his face and is having difficulty breathing. The burned area is red and charred; blisters are forming. How would you assess the extent and severity of this patient's injuries? What care are you going to provide?

Soft tissues include the various layers of skin, fat, and muscles that protect underlying body structures. When external forces contact soft tissue, the result can be as minor as a scrape or bruise or as serious as an amputated limb or critical burn. Although many soft-tissue injuries involve bleeding, most are not life threatening. It is rare to be unable to control bleeding simply by applying pressure to a wound. If external bleeding occurs, remember to follow body substance isolation (BSI) practices and to control bleeding. **Burns** are a type of soft-tissue injury caused primarily by heat. They can be painful, disfiguring, and, in some cases, life threatening. You may find that caring for a burn patient is a stressful, frightening, and even nauseating experience.

This chapter covers the various types of soft-tissue injuries, including burns and open and closed wounds. It also covers general wound care and the care for injuries affecting specific areas of soft tissue.

Reviewing Anatomy and Function of the Skin

Skin is the first line of defense against infection and injury. Skin, hair, nails, and certain glands make up the integumentary system, which protects the body from invading microorganisms and injury, helps retain body fluids to prevent dehydration, and aids in temperature regulation. The skin is the major component of the integumentary system and is extremely important because of its ability to directly repel disease-producing microorganisms. The tough, elastic fibers of the skin stretch easily without tearing, helping protect it from injury. There are three layers of skin: the epidermis, dermis, and subcutaneous tissue (Figure 23-1).

The **epidermis** is the outermost layer of skin, consisting of cells that are continually rubbed away and replaced by new cells from underneath. The epidermis is a paper thin, although tough, layer of skin that helps form a watertight covering for the body. Areas such as the soles of the feet and palms of the hand have a thicker epidermis, providing more protection to the deeper skin layers. The epidermis can be easily burned by the radiant heat of the sun, as well as hot water or other heat sources.

The **dermis** is the next layer of skin. It is thicker than the epidermis and contains nerve endings that provide sensory information about touch, temperature, pain, and pressure. This layer also contains structures such as muscle fibers, hair follicles, sweat, and sebaceous (oil) glands. The blood vessels in the dermis help supply the skin with nutrients and to some degree are responsible for changes in skin color. If the dermis is injured, the threat of infection in the skin and underlying structures increases. The larger blood vessels located in the dermis can cause significant bleeding if injured.

The innermost layer of the skin is the subcutaneous tissue. Made up partly of fat, this layer helps serve as a shock absorber, protecting underlying tissue from injury. It also insulates the body against temperature changes.

Areas of the body with openings, such as the mouth and nose, are also protected by mucous membranes,

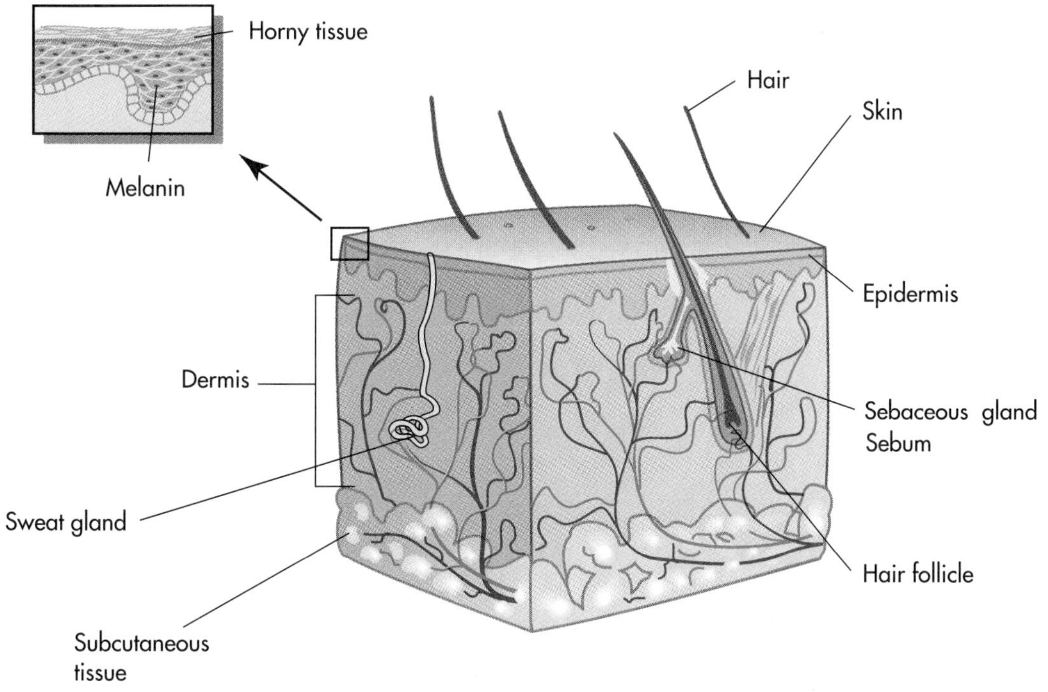

Figure 23-1

The layers and structures of the skin.

which secrete fluid to lubricate the openings and help protect against invading disease organisms.

Types of Soft-Tissue Injuries

Soft tissues are easily injured because of their direct exposure to the environment. Any injury that causes a break in the skin can result in infection. Soft-tissue injuries are called *wounds.* There are three general types: **closed wounds, open wounds,** and burns.

Closed Wounds

A closed wound is one in which the soft tissues of the skin or beneath the skin are damaged while the skin itself remains intact. Closed wounds occur as a result of blunt trauma and are characterized by swelling, discoloration, and pain at the site of the injury. The most common closed wound is a bruise, also called a **contusion** (Figure 23-2). A contusion results from the tearing of small blood vessels and damage to the cells within or below the dermis. As blood and fluid accumulate in the damaged area, the skin becomes discolored. This black-and-blue appearance is commonly called **ecchymosis.**

If a large blood vessel or many smaller blood vessels rupture and bleed rapidly, the amount of blood that pools in the area can be significant. This may cause swelling and discoloration and can be an indication of severe soft-tissue damage. The term used to describe this condition is a **hematoma** (Figure 23-3). A common example of a hematoma is the knot that forms on the forehead of a patient who is struck with a hard object. Another example occurs when a health care provider tears a vein while trying to start an intravenous (IV) line. This causes bleeding, swelling, and discoloration.

Sometimes the amount of force and the length of time the force is applied are so great that internal organs beneath the tissue are crushed or ruptured. This type of **crush injury** can potentially cause a significant amount of blood loss from solid organs such as the spleen or liver. It can also lead to inflammation and infection as food or urine seep into body cavities from a damaged hollow organ such as the stomach or bladder.

Open Wounds

Open wounds (Box 23-1) are injuries that break the skin and usually result in external bleeding:

- Abrasion
- Amputation
- Avulsion
- Laceration
- Puncture

BOX 23-1 Open Wounds

Type of Wound	Characteristics
Abrasion	Scraping or rubbing away of skin
Laceration	Smooth or jagged cut
Penetrating/ puncture	Piercing the skin with a pointed object
Avulsion	Tearing away of soft tissue, resulting in a tissue flap
Amputation	Separation of a body part from the body

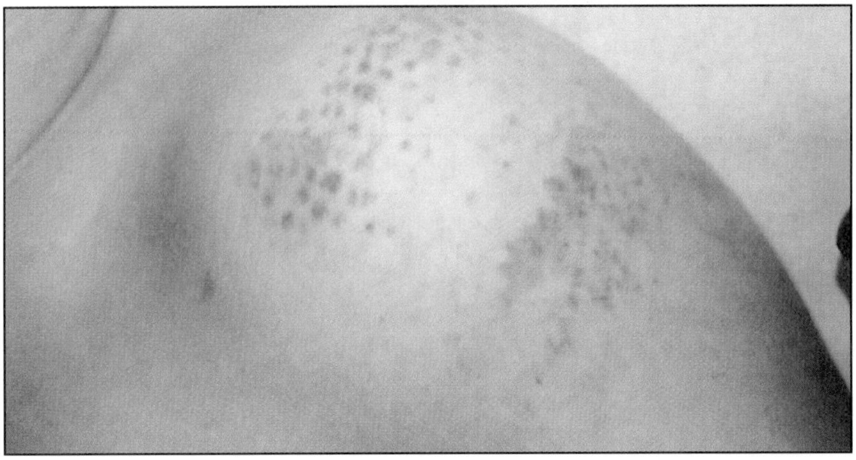

Figure 23-2

A bruise is actually the result of damage to the cells and capillaries within or below the dermis.

An **abrasion** is the most common and least serious type of open wound. It occurs as a result of friction along the outermost surface of the skin, which can cause blood to ooze from capillaries in the dermis (Figure 23-4). An abrasion commonly occurs when a child skins an elbow or knee. Abrasions may also be referred to as "road rash" and "rug" or "mat burns." Abrasions can embed dirt in the skin, which could lead to infection. Although considered a minor injury, abrasions can be painful because of the exposure of many nerve endings in the skin.

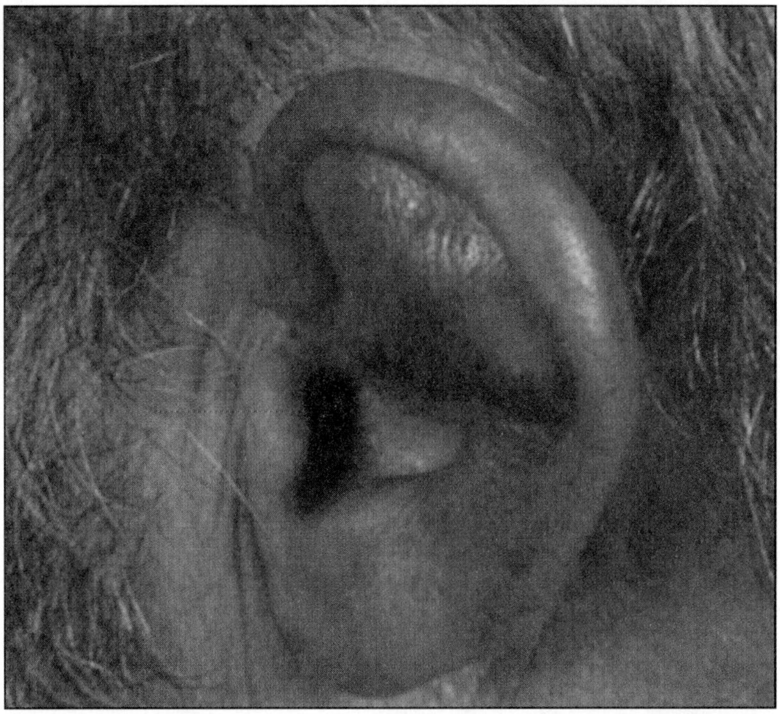

Figure 23-3

A hematoma occurs when vessels bleed rapidly, causing blood to pool under the skin. This often causes swelling and discoloration as seen here.

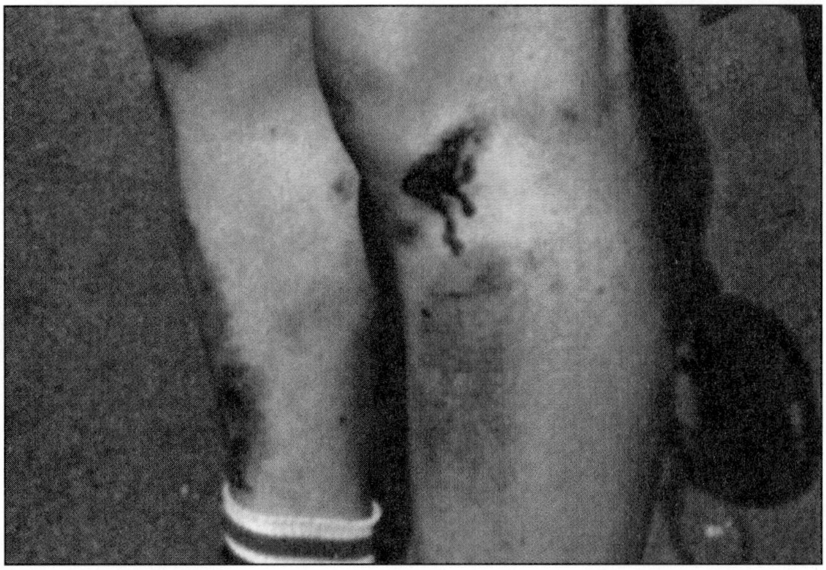

Figure 23-4

An abrasion is an injury where the outermost layers of skin are scraped away, causing blood to ooze from capillaries.

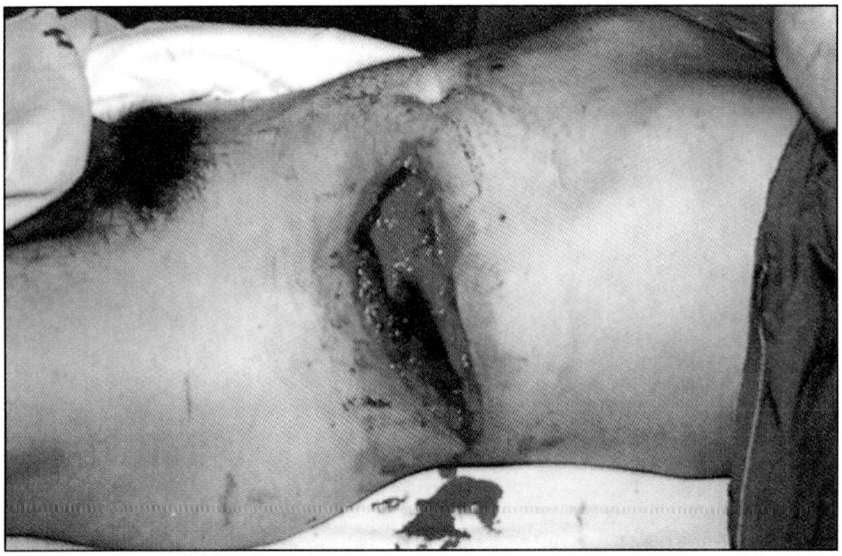

Figure 23-5

A laceration is an open wound caused by something that tears or cuts through the skin. Lacerations vary dramatically in severity.

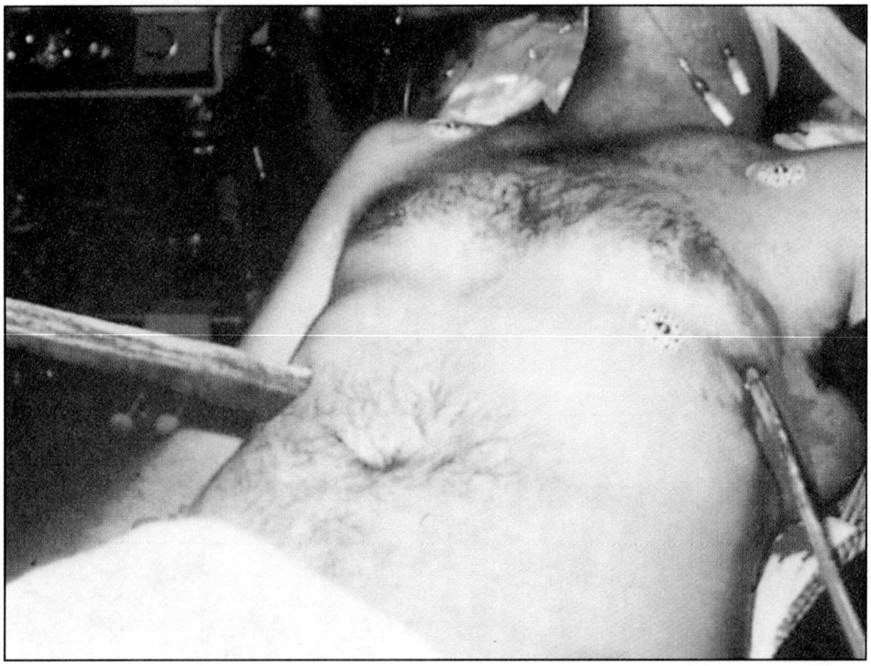

Figure 23-6

An impalement injury occurs when an object such as this piece of wood remains embedded in soft tissue.

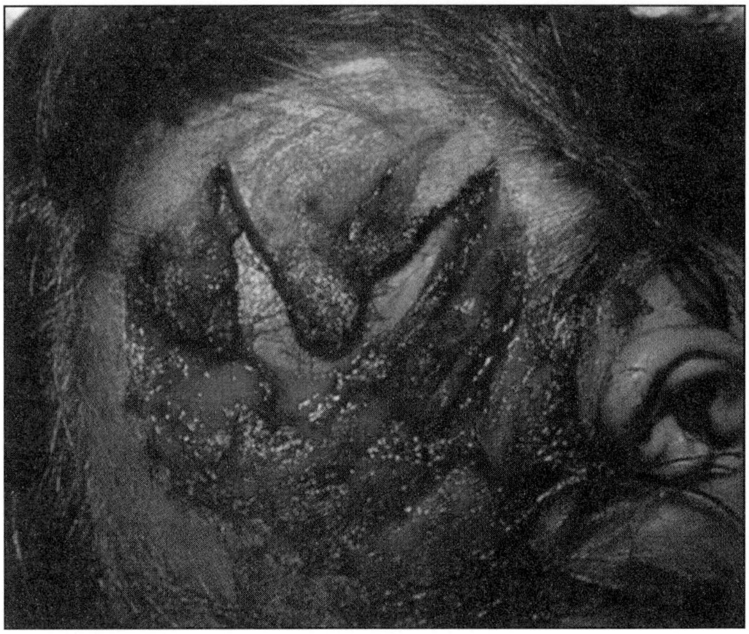

Figure 23-7

Because avulsions are tearing injuries, the skin is often jagged in appearance with noticeable tissue flaps.

Another common open wound is a **laceration.** Lacerations can be caused either by sharp objects, such as knives or glass cutting through the skin, or a blunt object tearing the skin. As a result, the wound can have either a smooth or jagged appearance and can vary in the depth and the degree of damage to underlying structures (Figure 23-5). Bleeding from lacerations can be severe, depending on the type and number of blood vessels damaged.

A penetrating or puncture wound occurs when the skin is pierced by a pointed object, such as a nail, splinter, ice pick, knife, or bullet. A penetrating wound may result in only minor external bleeding, because the skin usually closes after the object has entered the body. The amount of bleeding depends on the extent of damage to vessels and organs. If few vessels are severed, minimal bleeding will occur. If larger vessels are cut, there will be much more bleeding and it may be difficult to control. The most significant problems associated with penetrating wounds are the inability to determine the full extent of the internal damage and the high risk of infection.

The penetrating object could enter and exit the body through the same hole as a nail might. It could also pass completely through the tissue, creating an entrance and exit wound, such as a bullet through a hand. Or the object can remain lodged in the tissue, as a splinter, knife, or ice pick might. An object that remains embedded in the soft tissue is called an **impaled object** (Figure 23-6).

An **avulsion** is normally characterized by the partial tearing away of soft tissue, creating a tissue flap (Figure 23-7). This type of wound is commonly seen when the external ear or tip of the nose is torn. An avulsion in which much of the skin of a finger or hand is stripped is called a degloving injury (Figure 23-8). This type of injury often occurs when a person's hand is caught in power machinery.

An injury that completely severs a body part is called an **amputation** (Figure 23-9). Amputations are among the most serious and debilitating of injuries, although not all amputations result in major blood loss. The extent of bleeding depends on where the amputation occurs. If the arm is amputated at the elbow, there is likely to be significant bleeding because of the large blood vessels involved. If only a fingertip is severed, the blood loss will not be as great. Severed blood vessels also sometimes collapse and retract, resulting in restricted open bleeding and reduced blood loss.

Burns

Burn injuries occur when soft tissues absorb too much energy from heat sources, chemicals, electricity, or radiation. While minor sunburn damages only the outermost layers of the skin, other sources of energy, such as electricity, can cause immediately life-threatening conditions because of damage to underlying organs and tissues. The sources, recognition, and care for burns are discussed in detail beginning on p. 468.

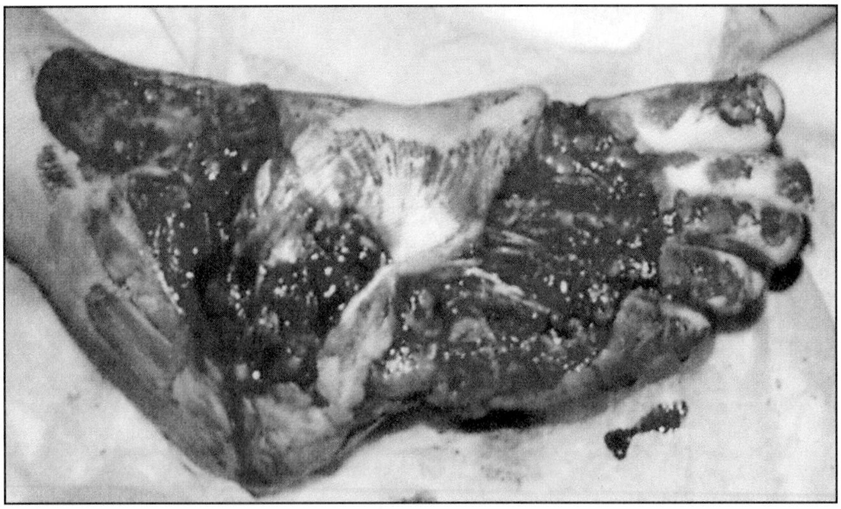

Figure 23-8

When the skin has been completely sheared away from underlying tissue, the avulsion is called a *degloving injury.*

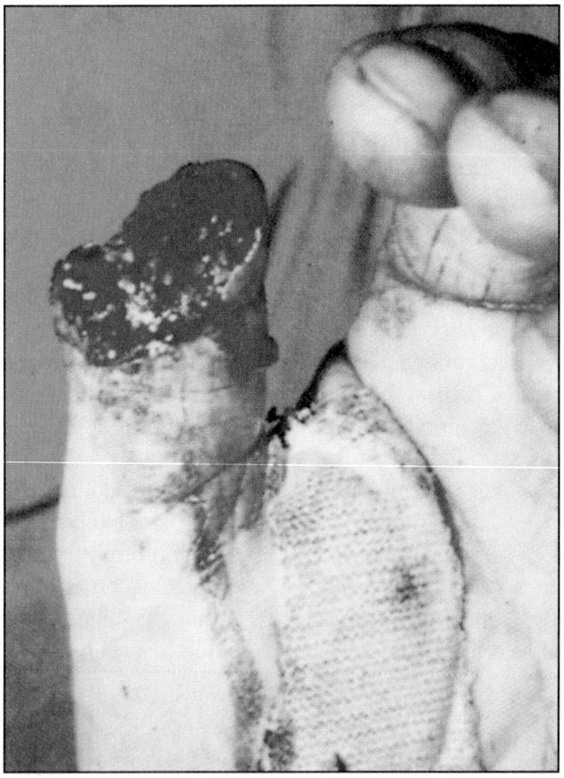

Figure 23-9

An amputation of a fingertip.

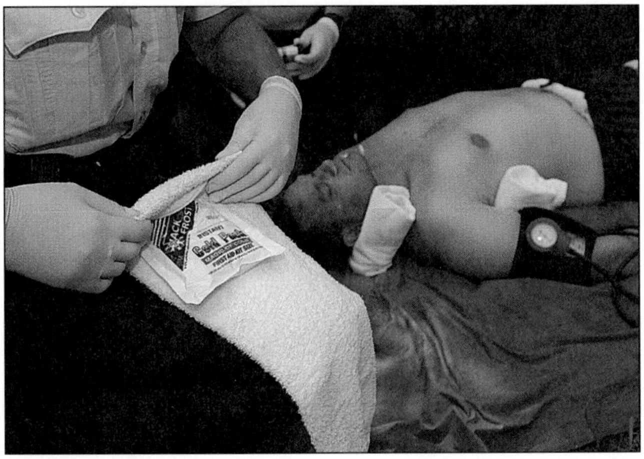

Figure 23-10

Many simple contusions can be treated with a cold compress wrapped in a towel or bandage.

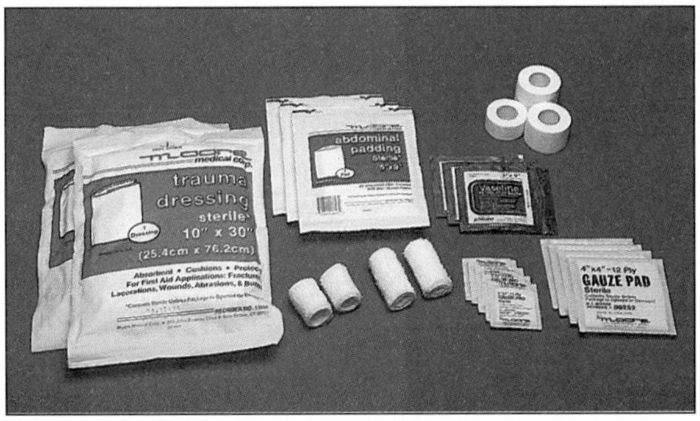

Figure 23-11

Dressings are available in a variety of sizes and types.

Caring For Closed Wounds

Most closed wounds are simple contusions that can be cared for by applying a cold compress such as an ice bag or chemical cold pack. Use of ice will help to reduce pain, constrict injured blood vessels, and reduce damage to cells, thereby reducing bleeding and swelling. Wrap the cold source in a towel or bandage to prevent it from freezing the tissue (Figure 23-10).

Applying pressure directly over a closed wound and elevating the injured area will also help reduce bleeding and swelling. Because it can be difficult to tell the extent of underlying injury in some cases, it may also be appropriate to immobilize (splint) a closed extremity wound. This minimizes movement and helps prevent further damage to the soft tissues. Splinting is discussed in detail in Chapter 24.

For more serious closed wounds, such as a crushing chest or abdominal injury from a machinery accident or overturned vehicle, conduct a rapid trauma assessment and transport the patient without delay to an appropriate trauma center. Administer oxygen at 15 liters per minute (lpm) through a nonrebreather mask. Place the patient in the shock position if it does not affect breathing. Summon advanced life support (ALS) personnel to assist, if available, and contact your medical direction physician. Minimize shock by elevating the lower extremities and maintaining normal body temperature.

Caring For Open Wounds

Caring for open wounds involves controlling bleeding. In most cases this is done simply by applying direct pressure with your hand. In more serious cases, additional methods to control bleeding must be used, as discussed in Chapter 22. Once bleeding is controlled, you will generally apply a dressing and bandage.

Dressings and Bandages

Dressings are pads placed over an open wound to help control bleeding, absorb blood, and minimize infection. The most common dressings are sterile gauze pads that come in various shapes and sizes (Figure 23-11). Universal, or trauma, dressings are large, thick dressings designed to be used on large wounds. Smaller dressings, classified according to their size in inches, are used for smaller wounds; 2×2 and 4×4 are the most common. A special type of dressing, called an occlusive dressing, is made of a nonporous material or is covered with an ointment to make an airtight seal over an open wound. In the absence of a commercially made occlusive dressing, you can use plastic wrap or aluminum foil (Figure 23-12). An occlusive dressing is used to cover open chest wounds that may have injured the lungs.

Once a dressing has been placed over the wound, a bandage is applied to keep the dressing in place and maintain pressure. Like dressings, bandages come in assorted shapes and sizes. However, bandages do not have to be sterile because they are not in direct contact with the wound. Bandages can be made of rolled gauze or cloth. Some bandages include adhesive to hold them in place, while others require you to secure the ends (Figure 23-13).

General Care Steps

1. Follow BSI practices to prevent disease transmission through direct contact with blood. This includes wear-

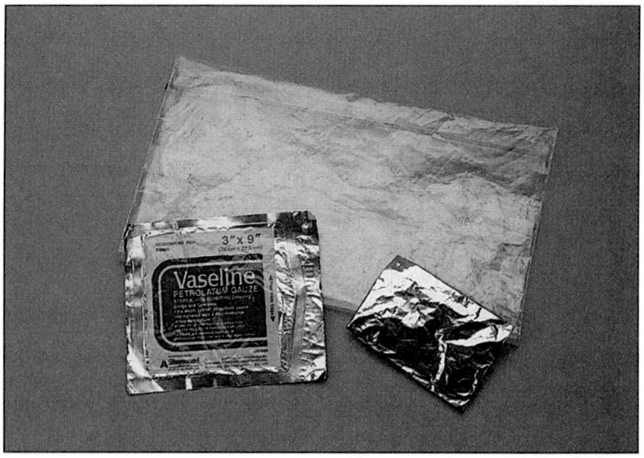

Figure 23-12

Occlusive dressings need to be able to form an airtight seal over an open wound.

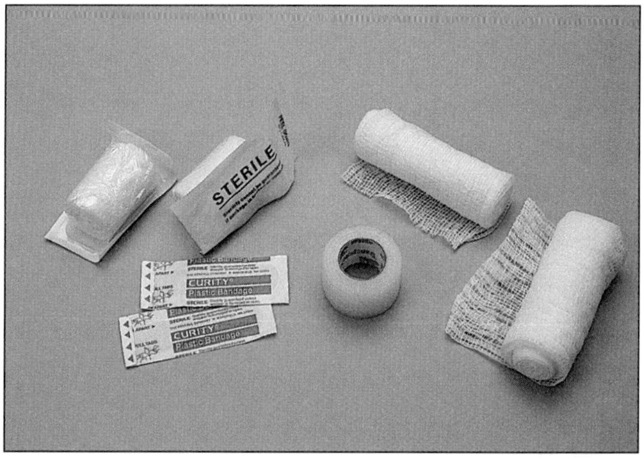

Figure 23-13

Bandages are used to secure dressings. They are not necessarily sterile and do not come in direct contact with the wound.

ing gloves when you may touch blood or other body fluids. It may also require you to wear goggles, mask, face shield, and gown to avoid splattering fluids (Figure 23-14, *A*).

2. Remove clothing or other materials to expose the wound, place a sterile dressing over it, and apply direct pressure with your gloved hand to control the bleeding (Figure 23-14, *B*). If the dressing becomes blood soaked, apply additional dressings over the top of the first one. Leaving the first dressing in place helps promote clotting.
3. Elevate the injured area above the level of the heart whenever possible (Figure 23-14, *C*). This will help slow blood flow.
4. As bleeding slows, apply a bandage to secure the dressing and maintain pressure on the wound. When using a roller gauze bandage, anchor it first and proceed with overlapping turns (Figure 23-14, *D*).
5. Immobilize the injured area if you think it may be associated with a fracture; this will help reduce pain and bleeding (Figure 23-14, *E*).
6. If bleeding is still not controlled, apply pressure to the appropriate arterial pressure point, as discussed in Chapter 22 (Figure 23-14, *F*).
7. If bleeding is severe or there are other injuries, begin to give oxygen as soon as possible.

Special Considerations

The following soft-tissue injuries require special consideration in addition to the previously mentioned General Care steps:

- Amputations
- Impaled objects
- Eye injury
- Mouth injury
- Open neck wounds
- Open chest wounds
- Open abdominal wounds

A

B

C

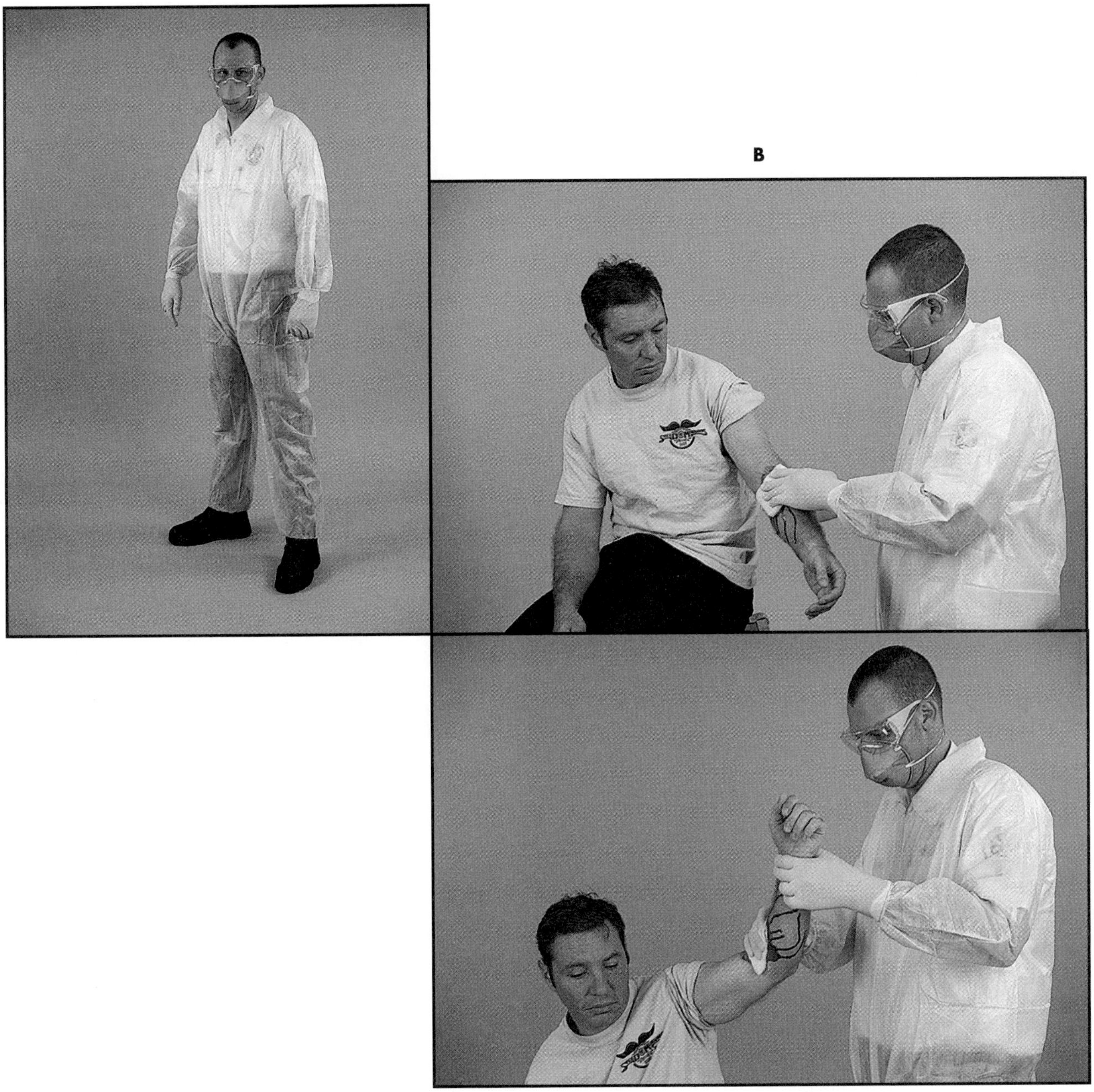

Figure 23-14

A, Complete body substance isolation procedure includes use of goggles, mask, face shield, and gown. **B,** After the wound is exposed, place a sterile dressing over the bleeding site and apply direct pressure. **C,** Elevate the bleeding site above the heart.

Continued

D

E

F

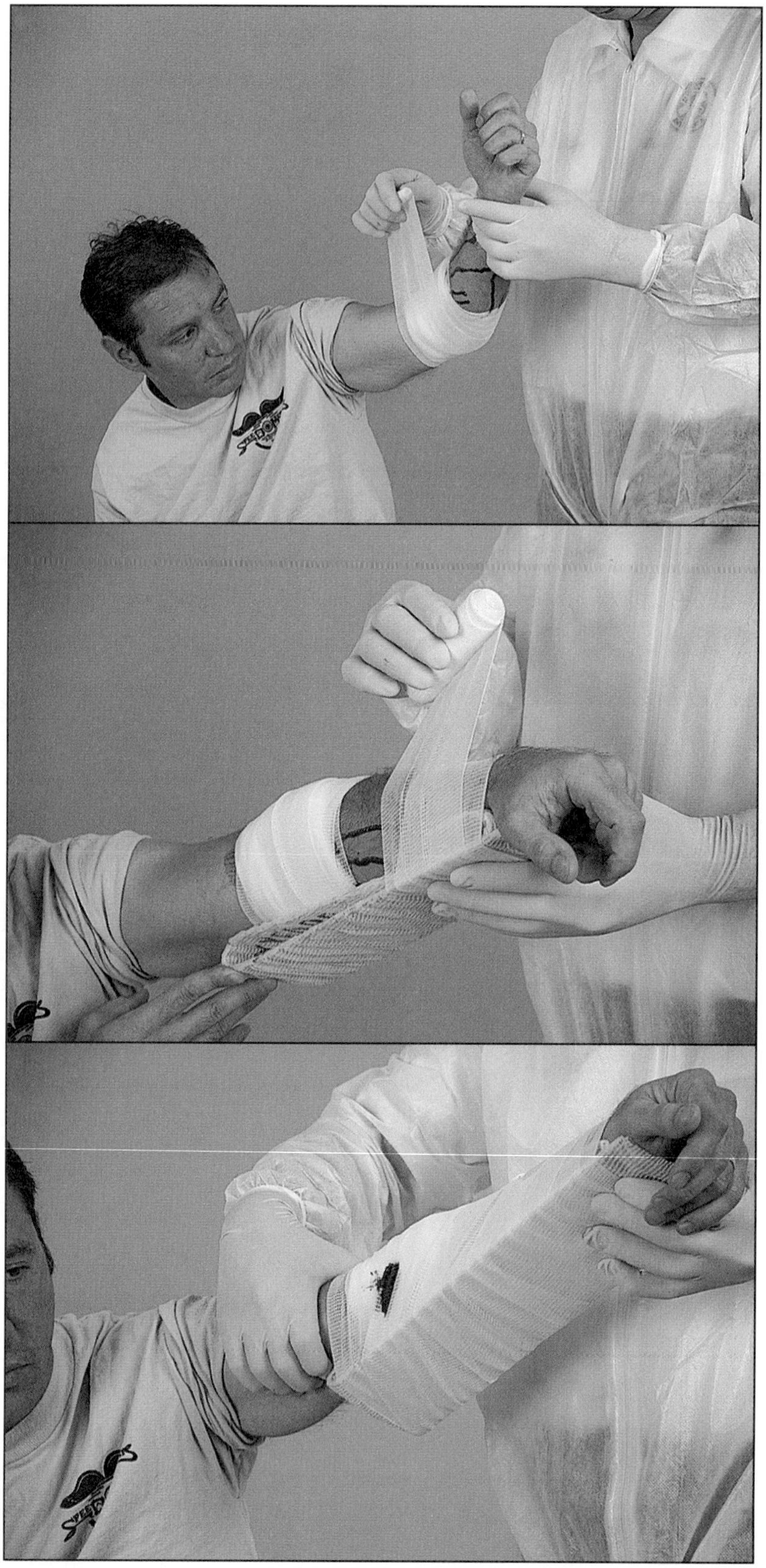

Figure 23-14, cont'd

D, Apply a bandage to secure the dressing and maintain pressure. **E,** Immobilize the area if a fracture is suspected. **F,** Apply pressure to the arterial pressure point.

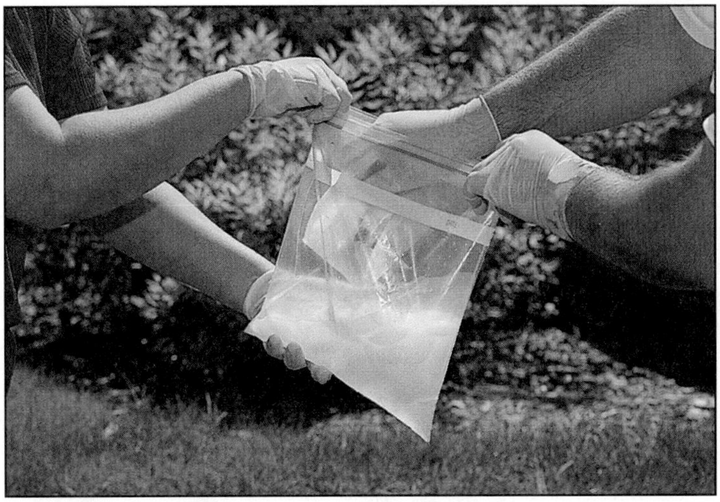

Figure 23-15

Keep the amputated part cool, but to prevent freezing it, do not place it directly on ice.

Amputations

Surgeons are more likely to be able to reattach a severed body part if it is cared for appropriately and transported with the patient. However, the success is related to the body part amputated and the extent of the damage to tissues. If you encounter a patient with an amputation, begin by controlling any bleeding from the site of the wound. Next, locate the amputated body part. Wrap that part in a sterile dressing (the dressing may be moistened with sterile saline, if available) and place it in a plastic bag or plastic wrap. Keep the wrapped amputated part cool by placing it in a cool container, but do not freeze it. Never use dry ice or place the tissue directly on ice (Figure 23-15).

Impaled Objects

An object imbedded in the body is an impaled object. The type of care needed depends on the location of the wound and object. In most situations, you will leave the object in place and stabilize it during transport to avoid movement that could cause additional damage to blood vessels, nerves, or muscles. To stabilize an impaled object, begin by applying a sterile dressing around the object (Figure 23-16, *A*). Place more dressings or bandages around the object and secure those in place (Figure 23-16, *B*). The additional bulk around the object will help keep it from moving. You may also be able to cover the object completely with a plastic, paper, or Styrofoam cup without applying any downward pressure to the top of the object. This reduces movement and helps prevent accidental jarring during transport (Figure 23-16, *C*).

Generally, impaled objects should be stabilized as found. However, there are two situations in which you might need to remove an impaled object. The first situation is when an object is impaled in the cheek that causes significant bleeding in the mouth and makes it difficult to maintain the airway. You may have to remove the object by gently pulling it back out. Use suction to keep the airway clear. If the patient is cooperative, apply pressure with sterile gauze to both the internal and external surfaces of the cheek to control bleeding. In the second situation, you may need to remove an impaled object from the chest if the object makes it impossible to perform cardiopulmonary resuscitation (CPR). Follow local protocols or contact medical direction before removing any impaled object.

Eye Injury

A penetrating injury to an eye requires care to avoid additional damage. It is extremely important not to apply any pressure to the eye while providing care. Whether the object has penetrated the eye or is still impaled in the eye, follow the steps in the previous section for stabilizing an impaled object. Very gently apply a sterile dressing over the eye. Build up padding around the object, place a cup over the object if possible, and secure the cup by bandaging it in place (Figure 23-17). Also cover the other eye to prevent movement of the injured eye.

If there is no penetration but the patient has a foreign body such as dirt or a chemical in the eye, flush the eye with sterile saline solution. This can be done by gently pouring the solution directly from the container or by using a bulb syringe. Flush the fluid from the inside corner of the eye (near the nose), outward. This keeps chemicals and foreign bodies from being washed into the other eye (Figure 23-18). Contact your medical direction physician for additional orders regarding care for a chemical in the eye, including possibly patching the eyes.

Mouth Injury

Injury to the mouth may cause bleeding that obstructs the airway or may cause the patient to swallow blood that leads to nausea and vomiting. Maintain an adequate air-

A

B

C

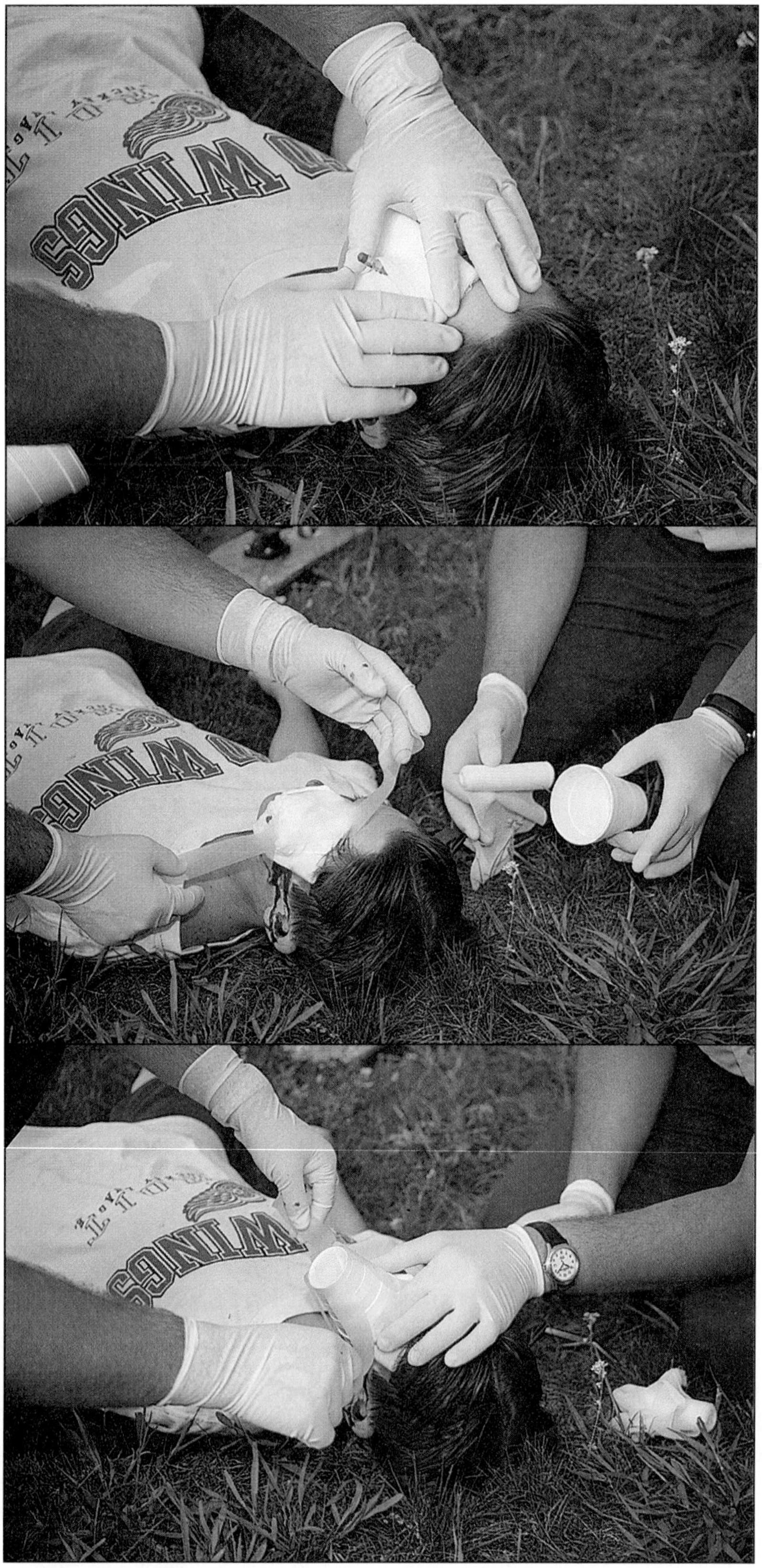

Figure 23-16

A, Apply sterile dressing around the impaled object. **B,** Build the sterile dressing up and secure it with bandages. **C,** If possible, use a cup or something similar to cover the object completely.

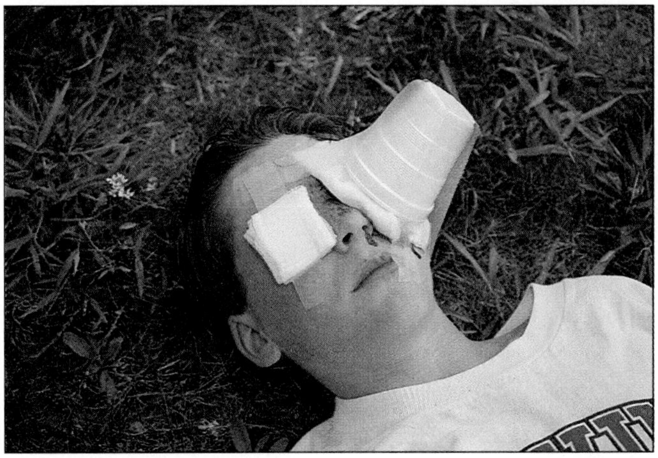

Figure 23-17
Cover the other eye to prevent movement of the injured eye.

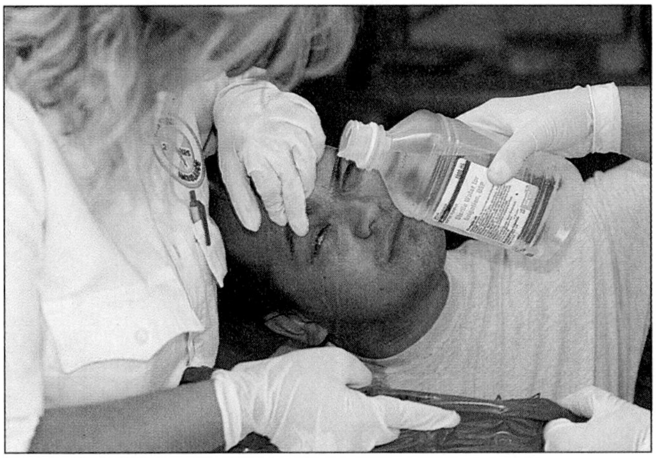

Figure 23-18
When flushing the patient's eye, pour liquid from the inside corner of the eye outward.

way with suction if needed. Look for and remove any loose objects in the mouth, such as broken teeth or loose dentures that could obstruct the airway. If a tooth has been knocked out and is intact, place the tooth in normal saline solution or milk and take it with you to the hospital. It may be possible to reimplant the tooth. If this is an isolated injury and the patient is cooperative, place a rolled gauze pad in the space where the tooth has been removed and have the patient bite down. This can help create pressure to control bleeding. If transport time will be longer than 30 minutes, contact medical direction for advice about possibly placing the tooth back in the socket after washing it with normal saline, before arriving at the hospital.

Open Chest Injury

Penetrating wounds and blunt trauma to the chest can injure the lungs and chest cavity and may cause life-threatening problems. When an object penetrates the chest, air can enter the chest cavity through the wound. This accumulation of air in the chest cavity is called a **pneumothorax** (Figure 23-19). As air continues to flow through the wound with each breath, the lung can collapse and breathing will be impaired. Blood that accumulates in the chest cavity is a **hemothorax** (Figure 23-20).

As you assess the patient, you may hear a characteristic sucking sound, commonly referred to as a **sucking chest wound.** This sound is heard as air moves through the wound into the chest cavity when the patient inhales.

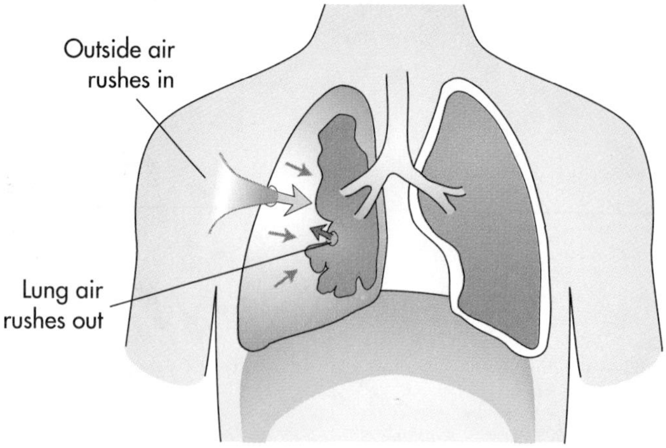

Figure 23-19

A pneumothorax occurs when air accumulates in the chest cavity.

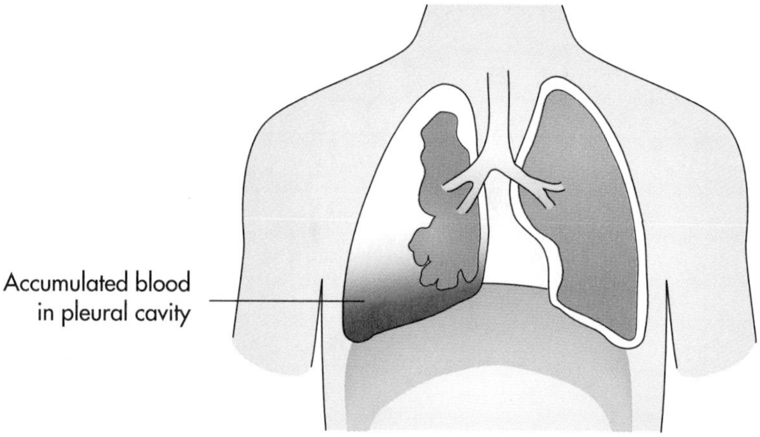

Figure 23-20

When blood gathers in the pleural cavity, it is called a *hemothorax.*

When you auscultate breath sounds, you may find diminished or absent sounds on the side of the injury. Your patient is likely to be having breathing difficulty as a result of a pneumothorax, and may be coughing up red, frothy blood.

Your goal in managing a sucking chest wound is to keep air from entering the wound during inhalation, while allowing air to escape during exhalation. This is done by applying an occlusive dressing over the wound and sealing three of the four sides with tape (Figure 23-21). Leaving the fourth side open allows air to escape during exhalation. Administer oxygen at 15 lpm through a nonrebreather mask.

If air enters the pleural space but cannot escape, pressure builds up in the chest cavity, the lung collapses, and pressure on the heart and large vessels impairs blood flow. This is a serious condition called tension pneumothorax, which requires immediate ALS intervention to relieve pressure in the chest cavity. Tension pneumothorax is also possible with blunt chest trauma that ruptures the lung or its breathing passages. Air can then escape into the pleural space with each breath. Because there is no open wound, the air has no way of exiting the chest; and pressure develops, creating the tension pneumothorax.

Open Neck Wounds

Neck injuries can cause significant bleeding and can affect the adequacy of the airway. Some injuries may also affect the airway directly. Large, open, neck wounds can expose blood vessels to the environment. If air enters

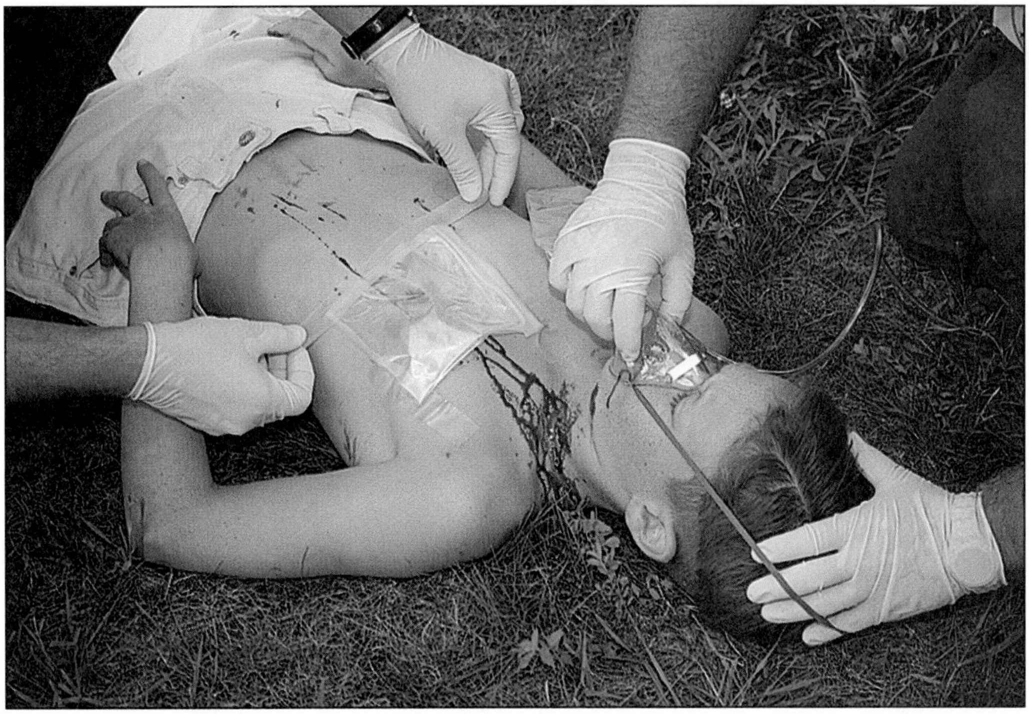

Figure 23-21

A sucking chest wound is bandaged with an occlusive dressing sealed on three sides.

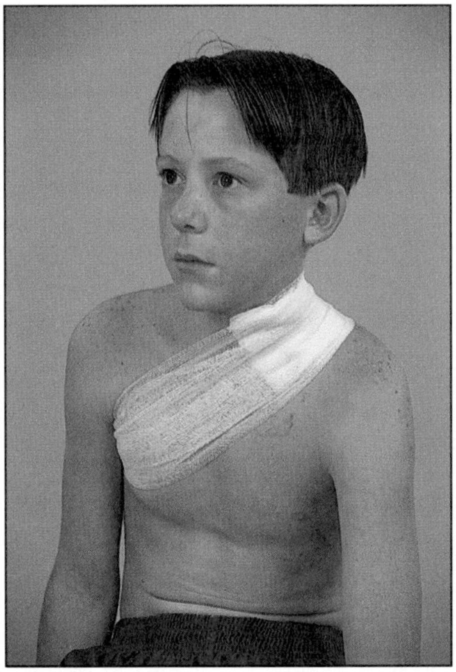

Figure 23-22

The pressure bandage on a neck wound should be wrapped under the armpit opposite the side of the injury.

these vessels, it can travel to the heart, lungs, brain, or other vital organs and cause a blockage known as an air embolism, discussed in Chapter 14.

To care for an open neck wound, apply an occlusive dressing and direct pressure. When applying pressure, be sure not to occlude the airway or compress the carotid arteries. Compressing both carotids at the same time could seriously lower blood flow to the brain. Apply a pressure bandage, wrapping it across the injured side of the neck and under the opposite armpit (Figure 23-22).

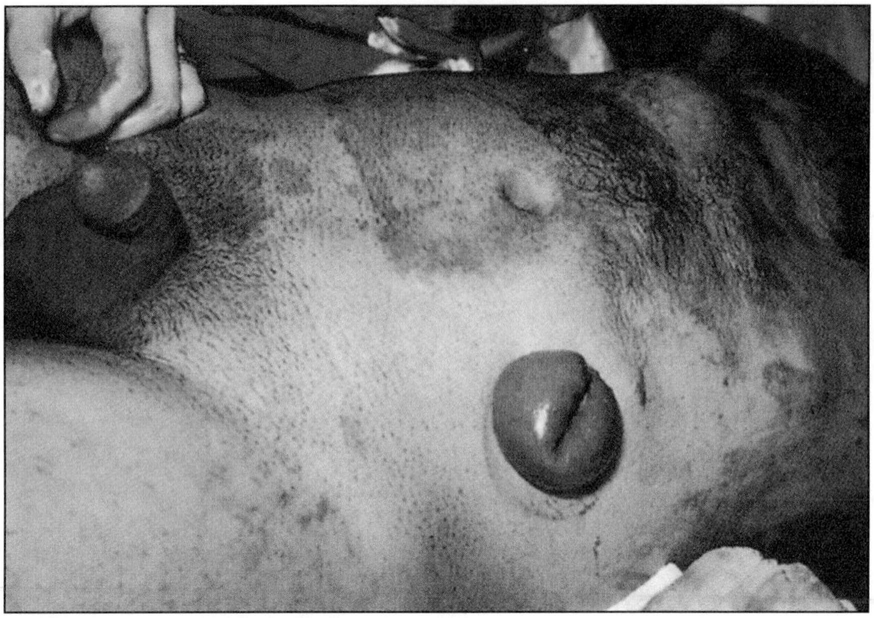

Figure 23-23

An evisceration through which the colon protrudes.

Open Abdominal Injury

An open abdominal wound can allow abdominal organs to protrude from the wound. This is known as an **evisceration** (Figure 23-23). If this occurs, place the patient in a supine position, cover the organs lightly with a moist, sterile dressing, and secure the edges of the dressing. Do not attempt to replace the organs into the abdomen. If the patient does not have any injury to the lower extremities or spine, flex the patient's legs. This will help relieve some of the pressure on the abdomen. Administer oxygen and transport the patient without delay.

Burn Injuries

The Magnitude of the Problem

Each year, more than 2.5 million Americans seek medical attention for burns. Approximately 100,000 of these burn victims require hospitalization and about 4000 people die.[1] Fire is the leading cause of burns and the fifth leading cause of accidental death in the United States.

Children and the elderly are more likely to be burned than other age groups. Among children, those under age 6 are at the highest risk. Active and curious children are unaware of the dangers associated with fires, stoves, and hot liquids. Burns to the elderly usually occur as a result of carelessness, confusion, slower reaction times, or physical infirmity (weakness, difficulty moving). Stoves, open flames, hot liquids, and radiators cause many of the injuries. People with chronic medical conditions tend to suffer more critical injuries as a result of burns.

Prevention

As with other types of injuries, some burn injuries are predictable and preventable events. In an attempt to help prevent burn injuries, the federal government has established stricter regulations regarding nonflammable textiles, flammable liquids, and the use of sprinkler systems and smoke detectors. Consumers are also encouraged by water companies and home builders to maintain lower settings on water heaters (about 120° F) to help prevent burns. Education by teachers, firefighters, EMS providers, and other health care professionals can help the public become more aware of potential dangers, and hopefully prevent thermal injuries.

Heat and the Skin

To many people, the skin's major function is that of appearance; however, the skin does much more. When heat from a burn injury breaks the integrity of the skin, the victim may suffer from pain, infection, and disturbances in fluid balance and temperature regulation.

Skin cells are sensitive to heat. The intensity of heat and the length of the exposure will determine how much damage occurs. There is usually no damage to the skin at temperatures up to 44° C (111.2° F). In fact, people immerse themselves in hot tubs at this temperature. Cellular damage will begin to occur at temperatures between 44° C (111.2° F) and 51° C (123.4° F). At higher temperatures, skin destruction will occur with even a brief exposure.

Because the dermis is covered by the epidermis, more heat or exposure is required to injure this layer. The dermis contains a specialized network of nerves and nerve endings and is therefore extremely sensitive to burn injury. Burns affecting this layer are very painful. Blister formation and weeping of fluid are also associated with dermal burns.

The subcutaneous tissue provides a layer of insulation for muscles and bones. Certain areas of the body such as fingers, toes, ears, and eyelids have much less subcutaneous tissue than other areas. In cases of electrical injury or prolonged exposure (trapped victim), burn injury may actually progress beyond the subcutaneous tissue into the muscles and bones. Injuries at this level indicate intense, severe heat exposure and injury.

Injury deep into the skin and underlying tissues can reduce the ability of tissue to heal after a burn injury. This is because of damage to specialized skin structures responsible for repair and to the blood vessels that provide vital nutrients to the healing areas.

Sources of Burns

Burns occur during contact with an energy source. Four types of energy result in four major types of burns:

- Thermal
- Chemical
- Electrical
- Radiation

Thermal Burns

Most burn injuries are caused by thermal energy, resulting from exposure to some form of heat, such as flames, steam, hot liquids, or hot solid objects. Thermal burns can also be accompanied by inhalation injury. Explosions can result in flash burns that cause a brief exposure to extremely high temperatures. With a flash burn or blast injury from an explosion, the victim may also have other trauma such as fractures or internal injuries. Scald injuries are the result of hot liquids or molten substances contacting the skin.

Bathtub accidents and overturned hot liquids account for the majority of scald burns. Children are more frequently injured by scald burns than adults. Water heaters in the United States are usually set at temperatures above 60° C (140° F). At this temperature, a serious burn can occur in as little as 5 seconds. Conversely, a water temperature of 48.8° C (120° F) would require at least a 5-minute exposure before a burn injury would occur.

Contact burns are the result of touching a hot object such as a stove or oven. Rapid reflexes often allow the victim to pull away quickly and help prevent serious injury. If the exposure is prolonged by an altered level of consciousness (LOC), poor reflexes, or inability to retreat (entrapment), deep injury can occur.

Chemical Burns

Chemical burns result from exposure to a variety of different chemicals in the form of solids, liquids, or gases. Chemical burns are most common in industrial settings but can also occur in the home. Cleaning solutions such as bleach, oven or drain cleaners, paint strippers, and lawn and garden supplies are common sources of chemicals that cause burns. Typically, strong acids and alkalis result in burn injuries. As with other types of burns, the longer the contact with the substance, the more severe the burn.

Electrical Burns

The human body is a good conductor of electricity. Whenever the body comes in conduct with an electrical source, the electricity is conducted through the body. Some body parts, such as the skin, resist the electrical current. This resistance produces heat, which can be seen as electrical burns along the path of the current. **Electrical burns** often have characteristic entry and exit wounds (Figure 23-24, *A* and *B*).

Electrical burns arise from a variety of sources. A common misconception is that low-voltage household current (120 V) is not as dangerous as high-voltage current (7620 V). Significant injury can result from either low or high voltage. Factors such as amperage, the type of current, the path of the current through the body, contact time, and resistance all influence the extent of the electrical injury.

In electrical injuries, the visible burn is often minor compared with the extensive internal damage that might occur. Electrical burns may cause cardiac dysrhythmias, ignite clothing causing associated flame injury, or result in blunt trauma during falls. Both electrical and flash burns are possible results of lightning.

Radiation Burns

Radiation burns are caused by exposure to ultraviolet (UV) radiation or ionizing radiation from a radioactive substance. UV rays are found in sunlight and are relatively harmless, although prolonged exposure produces thermal injury (sunburn) and can cause eye damage. The second form of radiant energy, ionizing radiation from radioactive materials, occurs in four forms: alpha, beta, gamma, and neutron radiation.

Alpha and beta radiation are the least dangerous of the four types of radiation. Alpha radiation is the lowest level of nuclear radiation. It is a very weak source of energy that travels only inches through the air and cannot penetrate paper, clothing, or skin. Beta radiation is medium-strength radiation that is also usually stopped by clothing, although it can penetrate the skin and create the

A

B

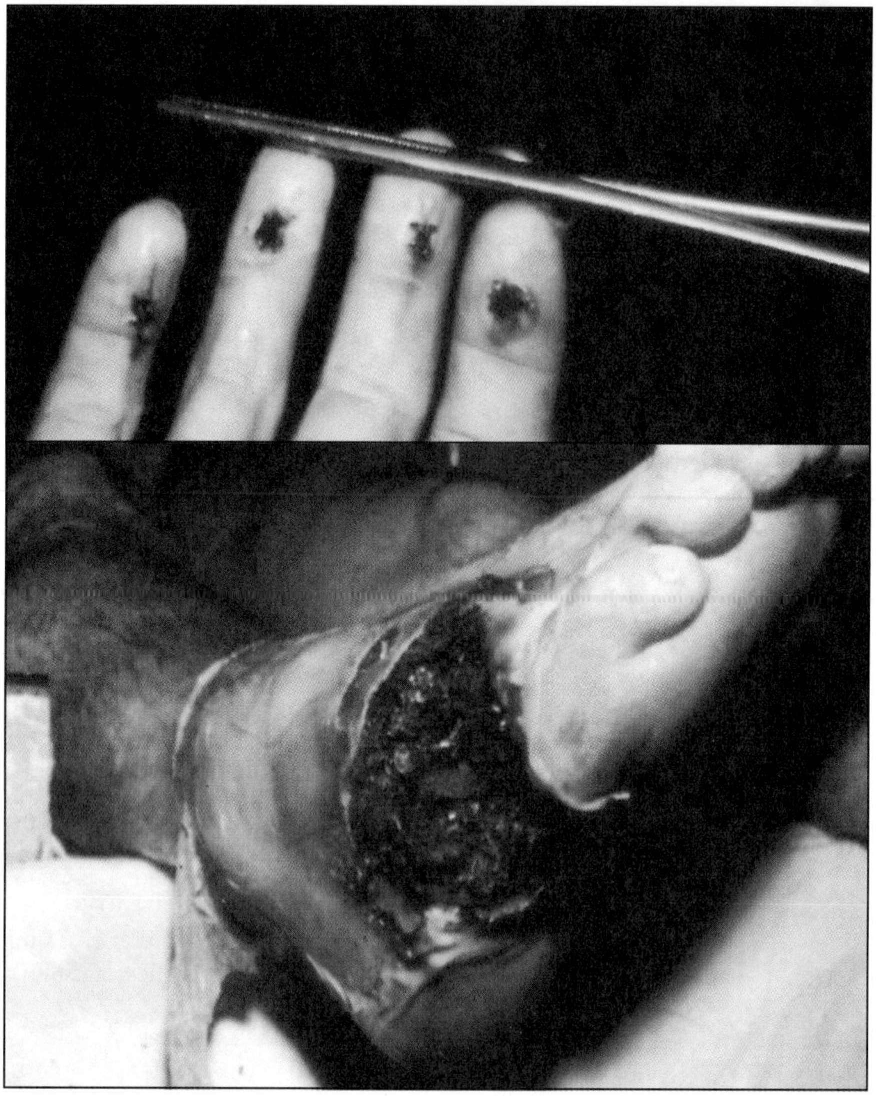

Figure 23-24

A, Entry wound from electrical burns. **B,** Exit wound from electrical burns.

potential for contamination. Gamma radiation, also known as *x-ray,* penetrates body tissue and damages cells. Neutron radiation occurs as a result of radioactive fallout.

Radiation contamination is a hazardous material exposure. Assessment and management require specialized training and equipment to protect responders from contamination. There may be a specialized response team in your area. Treat any associated injuries, consider the need for decontamination, and contact your medical direction physician. Personal precautions and special considerations in radiation accidents are discussed in Chapter 3.

Special Considerations

Inhalation Injury

Many of the fire-related deaths each year are a direct result of the inhalation of steam, smoke, superheated gas, or toxic fumes. Air that is heated to 150° F or more usually causes burns to the face and upper airway. Cooling in the upper airway protects the lower airway, unless the inspired air is very hot and cannot be cooled in the upper airway.

However, steam carries much more heat than dry air. Consequently, hot steam injury may occur to the mucous membranes, bronchioles, and alveoli. This heat results in swelling of the damaged tissues that may produce hoarseness or airway obstruction. Increasing respiratory distress can occur.

Smoke inhalation and carbon monoxide poisoning are by far the most common fire-related injuries. Carbon monoxide is a colorless, odorless gas that is produced by incomplete combustion in nearly all fires. Because carbon monoxide has an affinity for Hg 200 times greater than oxygen does, the carbon monoxide readily combines with hemoglobin and displaces oxygen. Cells throughout the body are deprived of oxygen and symptoms begin to develop.

LIGHTNING STRIKES

How much do you know about what causes lightning, how dangerous it is, and how to provide care for a patient who has been struck by lightning?

Lightning occurs when particles of water, ice, and air lose electrons while moving within storm clouds. As this happens, the cloud divides into layers of positively and negatively charged particles. The negative charge occasionally flashes toward the ground, which has a positive charge. This electrical pathway results in multiple currents running back and forth between the clouds and the ground in the split second that your eye sees only one flash.

It is estimated that lightning strikes the earth 100 times every second around the world. The current can produce 50 million volts of electricity and is five times hotter than the surface of the sun. All of this power travels through a channel that is no more than 1 inch in diameter at speeds of more than 300 miles per hour. When lightning strikes a person in its path, the results can be devastating. As the current passes through the body to the ground, tissue and organs can be damaged extensively. In some cases, obvious external burns are present. It is also possible for only small entry and exit wounds to show externally, while the path of internal destruction is severe.

Lightning claims more lives each year than any other natural disaster. Approximately 1000 people are struck by lightning in the United States annually. Surprisingly, nearly 700 of them survive the incident. Lightning strikes about 18,000 homes each year and starts approximately 7500 fires.

Contrary to popular belief, lightning can strike in the same place twice and can strike the same person more than once. Roy Sullivan, a National Park Ranger from 1942 to 1976, was struck seven times by lightning during that period.

When a storm approaches, the National Weather Service advises to:

- Seek shelter inside a building, home, or vehicle with windows rolled up.
- Avoid isolated tall structures, such as telephone poles and tall trees.
- Avoid areas that conduct electricity, such as lakes and swimming pools.
- Avoid high ground, such as hilltops.
- Avoid machinery and structures that conduct electricity, such as wire fences, rails, metal towers, etc.

If you care for a patient who is outside during a storm, try to stabilize the patient quickly and move inside a building or the ambulance to continue care. Do not try to perform a focused history or assessment while there is danger of lightning injuring you, the patient, or other providers. Wearing firefighting (turnout) gear does not provide you with any additional protection from lightning.

A small amount of carbon monoxide exists in nearly all people, especially those who smoke. When the carbon monoxide level rises, the symptoms become much more pronounced, and coma or death can follow. Carbon monoxide poisoning should be assumed in all fires, especially if a person was in an enclosed space for a prolonged period of time. Carbon monoxide inhalation can cause headaches, flulike symptoms (nausea, vomiting, body aches), and altered mental status or unconsciousness. Treatment includes maintaining the airway, giving high-concentration oxygen by nonrebreather mask, ventilating if necessary, and transporting for evaluation and treatment. The patient may also require treatment with hyperbaric oxygen.

Some of the most frequent victims of carbon monoxide poisoning are prehospital rescuers and firefighters who fail to recognize the early warning signs of smoke inhalation. Additional symptoms include difficulty breathing and cyanosis. Remember that fires produce many harmful chemicals, including cyanide gas. Anyone involved at a fire scene who experiences any signs or symptoms of distress should be relieved from duty, assessed, and treated as described above.

Associated Trauma

Additional trauma can also accompany severe burns. Depending on the specific mechanism of injury (auto accident, industrial explosion, residential fire), a patient may suffer multiple injuries such as fractures, lacerations, blunt trauma, and internal injury. The associated injuries can be more serious than the burn and sometimes require immediate attention. Management of the burn injury itself may be delayed. You will need to consider the relative priorities of associated injuries and the burn itself. This is why it is important to assess the scene and understand the mechanism of injury.

Body System Failure

One of the unique aspects of burn injury is that it affects nearly every organ system. In addition to the significant damage done to the skin, effects on other systems can compound the injury and produce fatal complications.

Shock from blood or fluid loss or from heart failure frequently accompanies major burn injuries. Shortly after a burn injury, fluids and electrolytes begin to shift within the burned tissue and elsewhere in the body. Fluid moves from blood vessels to areas inside and surrounding cells. This fluid shift is initially a compensatory mechanism that cools and hydrates the burned tissue. However, the shift reduces blood volume and therefore blood flow. This fluid shift into unburned tissue can also cause swelling that restricts the airway or affects other vital organs.

The nervous system may be damaged or compromised as a result of burn injury. Direct head and spinal trauma is common in patients burned in explosions and vehicle accidents. Hypoxia caused by shock or inhalation injury can also compromise nervous system function.

Assessing the Burn Patient

A rapid, complete assessment in the field is essential. First assess the scene for potential dangers. Determine the mechanism of injury. Complete the initial assessment and the focused history and physical examination for rapid trauma assessment. You are looking at the burn itself but also for other injuries or complications.

Always assess the potential danger before entering. When fire is present, the first personnel at the scene must determine the strategic positioning of fire apparatus and set up a triage area. Try to estimate the number of patients and their severity. Consider your agency's capabilities and those of the receiving facilities. It may be necessary to request further assistance or activate a disaster plan.

Unless you have the proper training and equipment, do not risk entering a burning building or vehicle to rescue a patient. Seemingly small residential fires can create temperatures as high as 1000° F, produce toxic products of combustion such as carbon monoxide and cyanide, and cause unstable building structures. Smoke inhalation and panic often lead to lost and disoriented rescuers.

Assessing a burn patient begins with standard trauma assessment guidelines. This includes an initial assessment of airway, breathing, and circulation that determines whether the patient has immediately life-threatening conditions, and helps make transport decisions.

Next conduct a rapid trauma assessment. Establish a baseline set of vital signs. A diminished LOC may be the result of carbon monoxide or cyanide poisoning, drug use, head trauma, shock, hypoglycemia, or hypoxia. Check breath sounds and respiratory rate for a possible inhalation injury. Blood pressure in a burned patient should initially be normal. As shock develops, a fall in blood pressure will be seen. Shock associated with burn injury is a slower process than other forms of shock. Signs and symptoms of shock within the first 30 minutes may indicate the presence of other trauma.

Obtaining an accurate history is also essential. An understanding of the mechanism of injury (house fire) and the type of injury sustained (flame, inhalation) can begin with the history. Explosions frequently cause associated injuries. Patients who were in an enclosed space for a prolonged period are at higher risk for inhalation injury.

If possible, include the patient's medical history (seizure disorder, diabetes, cardiac problems) as part of your assessment. These conditions may alter the response to standard care measures. Look for information about medications and allergies to medications. This information will be helpful as ALS providers or hospital personnel begin medication therapy.

As time and the patient's condition allow, conduct a detailed physical examination. The extent and severity of the burn will now be obvious, if it was not initially. Look more closely for signs of inhalation injury. Soot in the

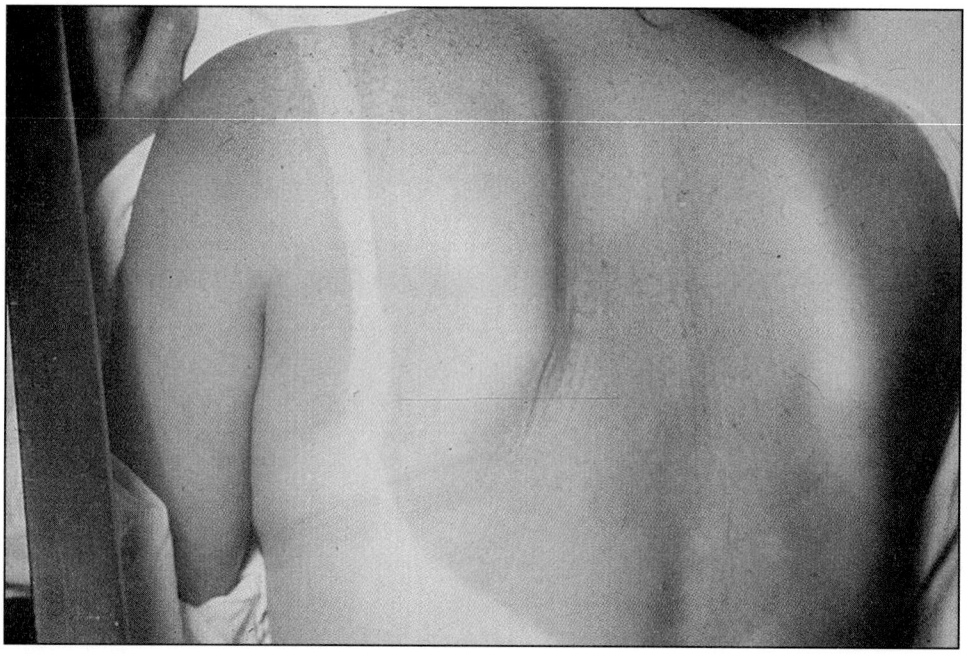

Figure 23-25

First-degree, or superficial, burn.

mouth or nose, and respiratory distress, including wheezing and raspy voice, are classic signs. Remember that the detailed examination is usually performed on the way to the hospital.

Determining the Extent and Severity of Burns

Determining the severity of a burn injury includes assessing both the source of the burn and the extent of injury. This is done by considering the depth (degree) of the burn as well as its location and size.

Burn Depth

It may initially be difficult to determine the depth of a burn. Burns have a variety of appearances and may be covered with clothing, chemicals, dirt, or other contaminants. It may be hours or days before the actual depth of a burn can be determined.

Burns are typically classified as superficial (first-degree) (Figure 23-25), partial-thickness (second-degree) (Figure 23-26), or full-thickness (third-degree) (Figure 23-27). **Superficial burns** involve only the epidermis. The skin appears red and dry, the area around the burn may swell, and the burn is usually painful. Most sunburns are superficial burns. These burns generally heal in a few days without significant intervention and without scarring.

With **partial-thickness burns,** the skin appears reddened, pink, and glistening and may have clear blisters. These burns tend to be very painful. They are sensitive to temperature changes and exposure to air and touch because of exposed and damaged nerve endings. Partial-thickness burns damage the entire epidermis and extend into the dermis. They may leave hair follicles and sweat glands intact, as well as the structures that enable the skin to regenerate. Deep partial-thickness burns may appear waxy, weep fluid, and have large blisters.

Full-thickness burns involve the entire epidermis and dermis. There is no chance of spontaneous regeneration. The area may appear dry and leathery or be covered with a charred, stiff covering. This covering, known as **eschar,** is hard, burned tissue that cannot expand as the tissue below it swells. This lack of elasticity may cause pressure to develop under the eschar that can increase to the point of impairing circulation. When eschar surrounds areas such as the chest or neck, breathing may become difficult. A procedure called an *escharotomy,* a surgical cutting of the dried tissue to allow for swelling beneath it, must be done in the hospital to relieve pressure. If a burn involves extremities, any rings, bracelets, watches, or other jewelry should be removed to prevent circulatory compromise.

Body Surface Area Involved

Several different methods can be used to determine the percentage of body surface area burned. The Rule of Nines is a popular guide for estimating the percentage of body surface area burned. Each portion of the adult anatomy is considered either 9% or 18% of the surface area, with 1% for the external genitalia. Because a small

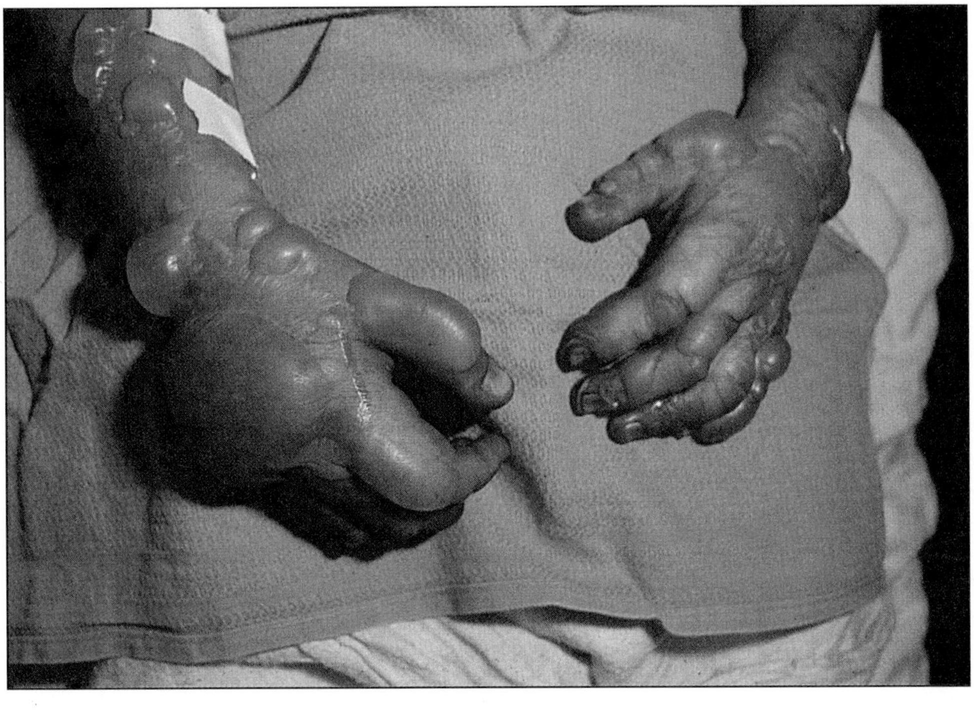

Figure 23-26

Severe second-degree, or partial-thickness, burn.

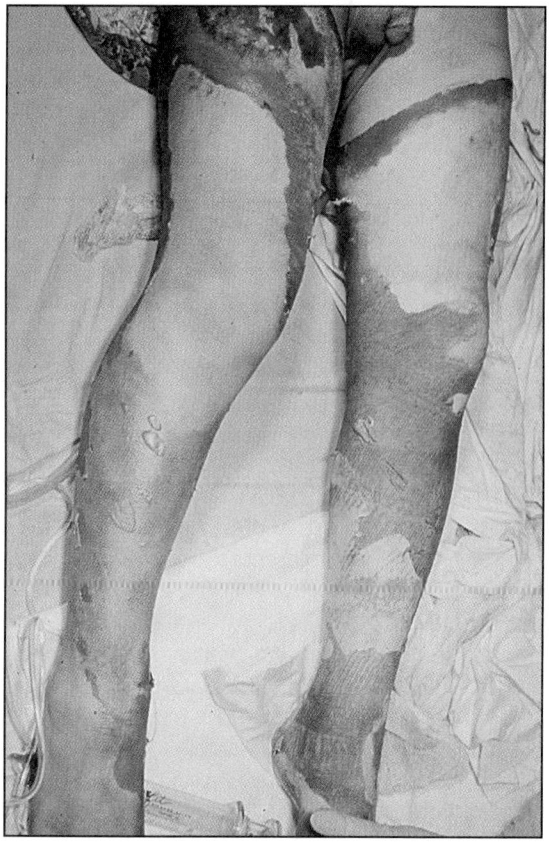

Figure 23-27

Third-degree, or full-thickness, burn.

BOX 23-2	Burn Severity

Minor Burns

- Full-thickness burns covering <2% of the body (not including face and neck, hands, feet, or genitals)
- Partial-thickness burns that cover <15% of an adult's body and <10% of a child's body
- Superficial burns that cover <50% of the body

Moderate Burns

- Full-thickness burns covering 2%-10% of the body (not including face and neck, hands, feet, or genitals)
- Partial-thickness burns covering 15%-30% of the body
- Superficial burns covering >50% of the body

Critical Burns

- Full- or partial-thickness burns of the face and neck, hands, feet, or genitals
- Full-thickness burns covering >10% of the body
- Partial-thickness burns covering >30% of the body
- Burns complicated by breathing difficulty, illness, or associated trauma
- Circumferential burns
- Moderate burns in pediatric and elderly patients

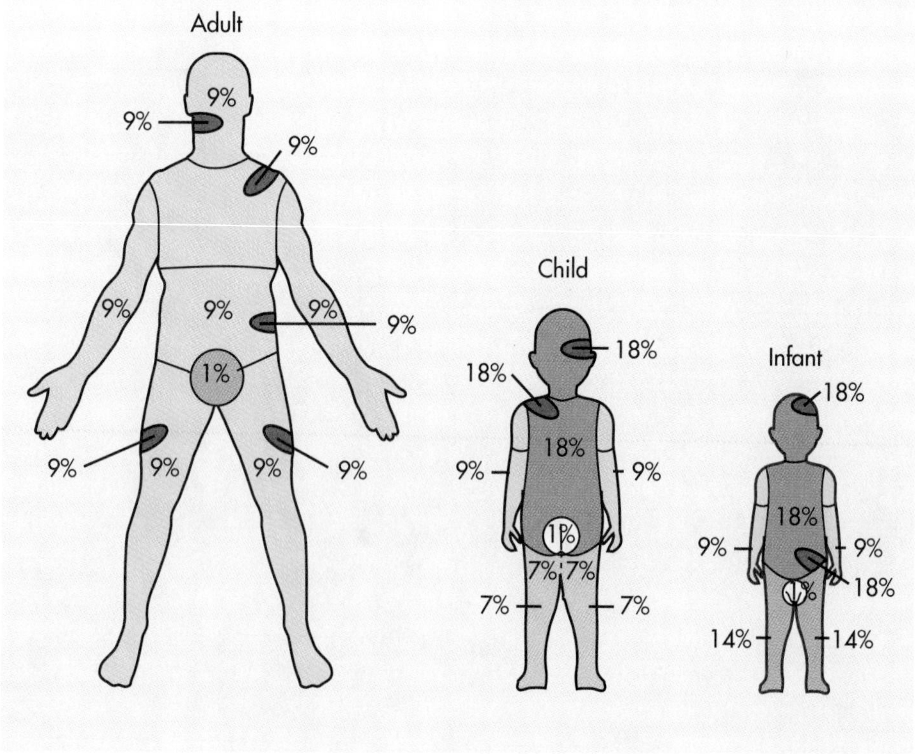

Figure 23-28

The Rule of Nines for adults, children, and infants.

child's surface area is proportioned differently, the percentages are also different. Figure 23-28 compares the Rule of Nines for adult and pediatric patients. An easy way to estimate smaller burned areas is to think of the palm of the patient's hand as 1% of the surface area.

There is controversy about whether accurate calculation is possible immediately after the injury. However, an attempt to determine the extent of the area burned is important in the field assessment, triage, and treatment of the patient.

Location of Burns

While assessing a burn patient, consider also what specific areas of the body are burned. The face, neck, hands, feet, and genitals are considered high-risk areas. Although their surface areas are small, injury to these areas is important and can be difficult to manage because of issues related to airway control, mobility, infection, and appearance. Also look for burns that extend around an entire extremity or around the chest (circumferential burns). A circumferential burn of an extremity may cause a **compartment syndrome,** a condition caused by swelling within the muscle compartments in the extremity. This swelling can exert pressure on the arteries, reducing blood supply to an area of the body. Quick identification of the potential for compartment syndrome will allow hospital care before damage sets in. Be sure to check pulses distal to severe extremity burns and reassess them frequently.

Classifying Burn Severity

The severity of a burn is determined by both affected surface area and depth. Estimating these factors will enable you to identify the severity of a burn injury according to one of the following classifications:

- Minor
- Moderate
- Major (critical)

These categories are established by the American Burn Association (ABA). Box 23-2 summarizes their characteristics.

IT'S YOUR CALL CONTINUED

You were quickly able to determine that the patient has facial burns and open wounds to the face and extremities and is having difficulty breathing.

Bystanders inform you that the patient climbed out a first floor window and fell to the ground. The patient's open wounds are minor lacerations and abrasions, with little bleeding. These probably occurred as he struggled to exit the house. During your rapid trauma assessment, you remove some of the patient's clothing and note that his neck, chest, and both arms have been burned. You observe superficial, partial-thickness, and full-thickness burns. These involve approximately 45% of the body surface area and include critical areas of the face and neck, which are contributing to his breathing difficulty. Examining his face more closely, you see soot in the mouth and nose, indicating that he inhaled smoke and possibly superheated air. You know that this patient has **critical burns.** How do you proceed to treat him?

Caring For Burns

General Burn Care

The severity of a burn is directly related to the length of exposure. It is critical that you stop the burning process as soon as possible. In most cases, the patient or bystanders will begin to stop the burning process before you arrive. If you are at the scene when a patient's clothing is still on fire, immediately put out the flames by having the patient stop, drop, and roll, wrapping the patient in a blanket, spraying the patient with water, or if no other alternatives exist, using a dry chemical extinguisher. Avoid throwing dirt or sand on the victim, or using home remedies, like butter, and topical ointments. These may aggravate the injury or hamper later care. Never place ice on burned tissue. This may cause additional tissue damage.

Clothing and accessories can retain heat and chemicals for a prolonged period, thereby increasing the length of exposure. Clothing, jewelry, shoes, and belts should always be removed. Constricting items such as rings and other jewelry can impair circulation as burned tissue swells. Remove all clothing and jewelry, even if there do not appear to be burns in that area. Full-thickness burns can occur from heated air and yet leave cotton jeans intact. If the fabric has adhered to burned tissue, cut around the fabric. Forceful removal of melted fabric will lead to increased tissue damage. Once you have removed clothing, the patient should be kept covered to maintain normal body temperature.

Caring for Minor Burns

Patients with minor burns may require the evaluation and care of both field and emergency department personnel but rarely need emergency resuscitation or prolonged hospital admission. The patient's fear and pain will require most of your attention.

Initial care for minor burns includes cooling the burned skin with room temperature water or normal saline and covering the area lightly with a sterile dressing. Elevate the affected area, if possible. These steps help alleviate pain, reduce swelling, and minimize the risk of infection. A calm and comforting attitude may also have a positive effect on the anxious patient, especially a frightened child.

Transport decisions for patients with a minor burn depend on individual circumstances and local protocols. If protocols allow, some patients may be able to have family or friends transport them to the hospital. Patients and their family should be instructed about the importance of proper treatment. If you suspect patients will not receive this care otherwise, consider transport by ambulance. Even minor burns, if they are not properly treated, can become infected and lead to disabling complications.

Caring for Moderate and Critical Burns

A moderate or critical burn is a terrifying experience for a patient and can also be emotionally difficult for responders. A calm, organized approach is essential. Stopping the burning process and managing the airway are the highest priorities. As with any major trauma, field scene times should be short (less than 10 minutes) with most treatment done during transport.

Once clothing has been removed, apply moist sterile dressings. This helps stop the heat from causing further damage and reduces fluid loss and pain. Patients with partial-thickness burns may develop large blisters. Do not break the blisters. Apply dry bandages, keeping them loose so they do not apply pressure. Some EMS agencies use burn packs with sterile sheets for covering patients with burns over large surface areas (Figure 23-29).

A patient with critical burns will begin to lose body heat rapidly. Preventing hypothermia is essential. Avoid drafts and maintain normal body temperature. This often means keeping the ambulance warm, minimizing the use of wet dressings, and covering the patient with a dry blanket.

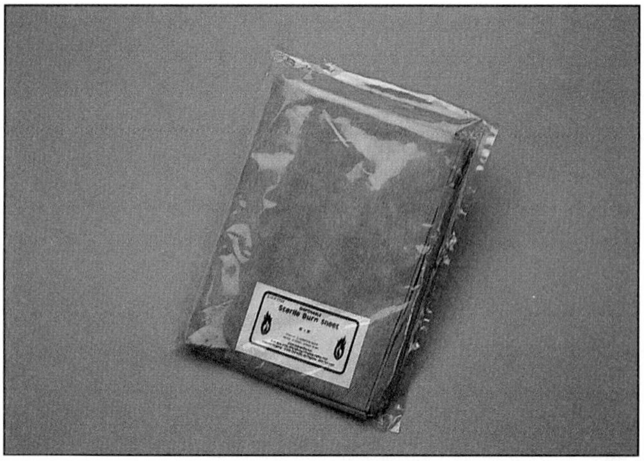

Figure 23-29
Burn pack.

Local protocols vary regarding whether to use dry or moist dressings for burns. Dry dressings do not cool the skin or help pain, and may stick to burned tissue. Applying moist dressings over large areas of the body and especially continued wetting of the dressings can lead to hypothermia. Hypothermia is not likely as a result of applying moist dressings to small areas, as long as other precautions are taken to maintain body temperature. Moist dressings are best limited to 5% to 10% of the body surface area.

As with all patients, airway management is critical. A patient may not complain of respiratory distress initially but can develop complications rapidly. Position the patient properly and maintain an open airway. Administer oxygen through a nonrebreather mask at 10 to 15 lpm. If possible, provide humidified oxygen. It may be necessary to assist the patient's ventilations. Trauma frequently accompanies major burns. Prioritize your care and follow accepted protocols for backboarding, splinting, and wound care.

Caring for Electrical Burns

To care for a patient with an electrical burn, begin by ensuring that the patient is no longer in contact with the electrical source and that it is safe for you to approach. Electrical burns often result in entry and exit wounds that indicate the points at which the current entered and left the body. Do not spend too much time caring for these two wound sites. The real concern should be for the internal damage that the electrical current caused. This can result in musculoskeletal injury or respiratory or cardiac arrest. Because of the likelihood of cardiac rhythm disturbances, summon ALS personnel, if available. Once in the hospital, the patient will be evaluated and monitored for injuries to other body systems, including the kidneys.

Caring for Chemical Burns

To care for chemical burns, remove the chemical from contact with the body. If the chemical is dry, brush away as much of it as possible, then flush with large quantities of water. If the chemical is wet, simply begin with lots of water. While flushing, remove any clothing that may be contaminated. Continue to irrigate the site of the chemical burn on the way to the hospital, if possible; however, you do not want to contaminate the ambulance or rescuers. Flushing should go on for at least 15 minutes. If you are washing a chemical out of a patient's eye, wash the affected eye from the nose outward to prevent getting any of the chemical into the uninjured eye.

Be careful not to contaminate yourself. Decontamination of large quantities of hazardous material or of multiple patients requires special training and specific equipment.

IT'S YOUR CALL
CONCLUSION

Your management of this critical burn patient includes contact with your medical direction physician, who agrees with you that the main treatment steps are as follows:

- Stopping the burning process.
- Managing the airway and immobilizing the cervical spine.
- Administering humidified oxygen.
- Controlling bleeding.
- Minimizing wound infection by dressing soft-tissue injuries.
- Summoning more advanced medical care.
- Transporting the patient rapidly to a burn center.

Transporting to Burn Centers

The decision to transport a patient to a specialized burn center is especially important. This decision may also involve an air transport decision. Local protocols should guide your decision. Guidelines for transporting patients to regional trauma or burn centers have been established by both the Committee on Trauma of the American College of Surgeons and the American Burn Association.[2] These guidelines are established according to the three classifications of burn severity, mentioned earlier in this chapter, which consider the degree of the burn, total burn surface area, and the patient's age.

Patients who have received minor burns are not likely to need the care provided at specialized burn centers and may not even require ambulance transport. These patients can use clinics, rural or community hospitals, and emergency departments. They are often treated and released for outpatient follow-up care. In some cases, they may be admitted to a hospital for a brief period (1 to 2 days).

Patients with moderate but uncomplicated burn injuries usually require ambulance transport. These patients may require hospitalization with specialized burn care.

Patients with critical burns require rapid transport to the nearest trauma center or regional burn unit. These patients usually require admission to the burn unit; hospitalization is often lengthy and complicated.

Documentation

Careful documentation will help ensure a smooth transition of patient care at the hospital. The history, mechanism of injury, findings, and treatment should be conveyed to the hospital staff verbally as well as in written documentation. Only the facts needed to establish priorities and make transport decisions should be reported by radio. When prioritizing information, include findings used to classify burns, such as their extent and severity, and any special considerations.

SUMMARY

Intact skin helps prevent infection. Skin damage weakens that protection. When various layers of skin and other tissues or organs are damaged, blood loss can be severe. Fortunately, the care is simple: use pressure and elevation to control bleeding, cover the wound with sterile dressings to help prevent infection, and bandage the wound to maintain pressure and hold the dressing in place.

Some soft-tissue injuries of the chest and abdomen and injuries involving impaled objects require special attention. Impaled objects are usually left in place and stabilized before transporting the patient. Handle abdominal eviscerations gently, covering the organs and transporting as soon as possible. Chest injuries may involve damage to the lungs. A sucking sound heard during breathing is a sign of a serious problem that can be treated by using an occlusive dressing.

Treating a patient who has suffered a major burn requires a calm and organized approach. Good patient care begins with a good assessment. Treatment of burns includes stopping the burn process, covering the burned area, maintaining the airway, administering oxygen, and transporting quickly to the appropriate facility.

REFERENCES

1. **National Safety Council:** *Accident facts,* 1995 edition, Itasca, Ill, 1995, National Safety Council.
2. **Committee on Trauma, American College of Surgeons:** Resources for optimal care of the injured patient, Chicago, 1993, American College of Surgeons.

SUGGESTED READINGS

1. **Bourne MK:** Fire and smoke: managing skin and inhalation burns, *J Emerg Med Serv* 14:62, 1989.
2. **McLaughlin E:** *Critical care of the burned patient,* Philadelphia, 1990, WB Saunders.

Chapter 24

Musculoskeletal Injuries

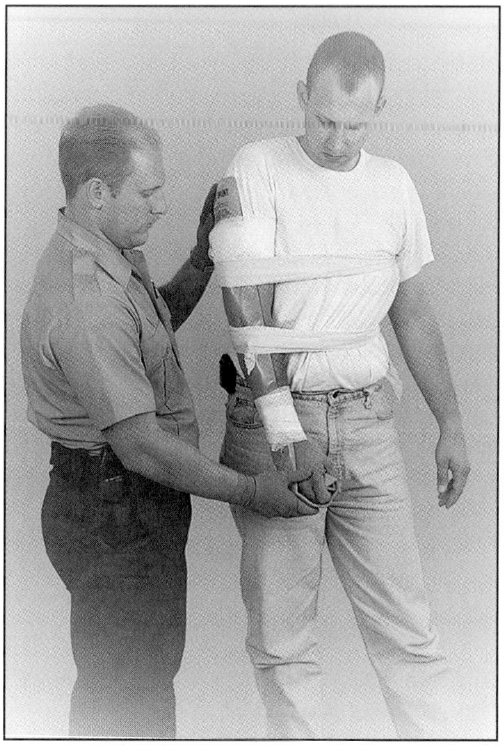

Knowledge Objectives

As an EMT-Basic, you should be able to:

OBJECTIVES

1. Review the structure and function of the musculoskeletal system.
2. Describe the role that the mechanism of injury plays in recognizing actual and potential musculoskeletal injuries.
3. List the common signs and symptoms of musculoskeletal injury.
4. Compare and contrast a fracture, dislocation, sprain, and strain.
5. Describe the purpose of splinting.
6. List the general rules of splinting.
7. Discuss the differences between care provided for open and closed musculoskeletal injuries.
8. Describe the possible complications of an improperly applied splint.
9. Describe the different types of splints.
10. Describe how to splint musculoskeletal injuries of the upper and lower extremities, including the use of the traction splint for femur injury and pneumatic anti-shock garment for pelvis and leg injuries.

OBJECTIVES

Skill Objectives

As an EMT-Basic, you should be able to:

1. **Demonstrate how to apply a splint for the following musculoskeletal injuries:**
   - **Shoulder: scapula or clavicle**
   - **Upper arm (humerus)**
   - **Elbow**
   - **Forearm**
   - **Hand or wrist**
   - **Pelvis or hip**
   - **Thigh (femur)**
   - **Knee**
   - **Lower leg**
   - **Ankle or foot**
2. **Demonstrate how to apply a traction splint for a possible broken femur.**
3. **Demonstrate how to apply a pneumatic antishock garment (PASG) for pelvis and leg injuries.**
4. **Demonstrate how to complete a patient-care report for a patient with musculoskeletal injuries.**

Attitude Objectives

As an EMT-Basic, you should be able to:

1. **Defend the need to apply a splint before transporting a patient in most situations.**
2. **Act as a role model for other EMS providers in caring for musculoskeletal injuries.**

KEY TERMS

1. **Crepitus:** A grating sound or feeling made by broken bone ends rubbing together, or by air under the skin; a probable sign of fracture when bone is involved.
2. **Dislocation:** An injury resulting from over-stretching or from severe movement in a joint that displaces the bone from the joint.
3. **Fracture:** A broken bone; can be open (break in the skin) or closed.
4. **Joint:** Area where two or more bones meet; can be movable or fixed (fused).
5. **Ligament:** Fibrous connective tissue, generally found at joints, that attaches bone to bone.
6. **Pneumatic Antishock Garment:** An inflatable garment used to immobilize an unstable pelvis or injured lower extremities.
7. **Position of Function:** The normal resting position of a limb.
8. **Splinting:** Immobilizing a painful, swollen, or deformed body part.
9. **Sprain:** An injury to tendons or the ligaments or connective tissue around a joint.
10. **Strain:** An injury caused by excessive physical effort that stretches and damages muscle fibers.
11. **Tendon:** Connective tissue that attaches muscle to bone.
12. **Traction:** The application of force along the long axis of an extremity to align bones and prevent further movement within a joint or at a possible fracture site.

IT'S YOUR CALL

You are dispatched to a local hockey rink for a shoulder injury. You arrive to find a 21-year-old male in the locker room. He tells you that he was knocked into the boards at the edge of the ice by another player and felt his shoulder pop. You carefully remove the patient's shoulder pads and assess his shoulder and arm. Your assessment reveals a swollen deformity at the shoulder. The patient complains of severe shoulder pain and numbness in his arm and hand.

The patient states that he thinks his shoulder popped out of the socket. He explains that it has happened before and that he has reset it himself. He has tried unsuccessfully to reset it before your arrival and now asks you to help him reset it. You tell him that you are not able to assist him reset it and you urge him to let you immobilize the shoulder and transport him to the hospital. The patient becomes upset, stating that he does not want to go and that he can pop his shoulder back in. After a few minutes of attempting unsuccessfully to reset the shoulder, he finally agrees to go to the hospital.

What type of injury do you think this patient has? What other injuries might he have? How should this injury be cared for during transport? Should you help him try to pop his shoulder back into place so that he will not have to go to the hospital, or should you treat the injury as if it were potentially serious?

Musculoskeletal injuries can result from falls, vehicle collisions, sporting events, and other activities that cause trauma to a bone or muscle. Most of these injuries are not life threatening. However, it is difficult to tell how serious a muscle, bone, or **joint** injury is without evaluation by a physician. In this chapter you will learn how to recognize and care for injuries to the muscle and bone. Primary care for a musculoskeletal injury involves immobilizing the injury to minimize further damage.

Reviewing the Musculoskeletal System

The musculoskeletal system allows for movement and provides the body with shape, support, and protection. It is made up of bones and muscles, and connective tissues that include tendons, ligaments, and cartilage.

Muscles

Skeletal muscles are the part of the musculoskeletal system that produce movement. Skeletal muscles are also referred to as voluntary muscles because one can consciously control them. There are more than 700 skeletal muscles in the human body (Figure 24-1, *A* and *B*). The two other types of muscles are cardiac muscle, which makes up the heart, and smooth muscle in the walls of organs such as the blood vessels, stomach, intestines, and small airways. Smooth muscle is also known as *involuntary muscle;* its movement is not under conscious control.

Skeletal muscles have three primary functions:

- Motion: Muscles contract to provide the movements of the body.
- Posture: Muscles maintain body shape and posture.
- Heat production: By contracting, muscles produce heat and help maintain body temperature.

Muscles are attached to bones by **tendons,** bands of fibrous connective tissue. This connection enables contracting muscles to move bones. Tendons may tear or pull away when a joint is injured, resulting in a sprain.

Skeleton

The skeleton provides the shape and framework of the body. It includes more than 200 bones. A basic understanding of the skeletal system enables one to use bones as landmarks and reference points for locating other structures.

The skeleton consists of two major divisions: the central (axial) and the peripheral (appendicular) skeleton. The central skeleton consists of the bones that go straight down the axis of the body. These include the skull, spinal column, ribs, and breastbone (sternum) (Figure 24-2). The peripheral skeleton includes the bones of the upper and lower extremities, and the shoulder and pelvic girdle (Figure 24-3). This chapter will deal primarily with injuries of the peripheral skeleton. Injuries of the skull and spinal column are discussed in Chapter 25.

Bones are attached to each other by bands of fibrous connective tissue called **ligaments.** When ligaments are injured, they are weakened and provide less stability and protection for joints. An injury such as a sprained ankle causes stretching and tearing of ligaments as well as tendons. (NOTE: The term *sprain* can refer to a stretching injury of either a ligament or a tendon.)

Types of Musculoskeletal Injury

Bone and Joint Injury

An injury to a bone or a joint can result in a fracture, a dislocation, or both. It can also injure surrounding connective tissues such as ligaments and tendons. The force, location, and type of injury will determine the severity of the injury.

Fracture

A broken bone is commonly called a **fracture.** It is usually not possible to diagnose a fracture in the field, but a painful, swollen, deformed area is the typical presentation for a fracture. A fracture can be open or closed. If the broken bone ends have broken the skin or if there is a laceration near a suspected fracture, it is considered to be an open fracture (Figure 24-4). In some cases, bones will protrude through the skin and then fall back inside. This is still considered an open fracture. A fracture in which the overlying skin is not broken is a closed fracture.

A fracture can also be classified as displaced or nondisplaced. A displaced fracture is one in which the bones are misaligned (Figure 24-5). A nondisplaced fracture leaves the fractured area in its normal position (Figure 24-6). A fracture can only be positively identified by x-ray. Although fractures are frequently painful, swollen, and deformed, some fractures present without deformity; and it is possible for other injuries to cause deformity when no fracture is present.

Dislocation

A **dislocation** results from over-stretching or severe movement that displaces a bone from a joint (Figure 24-7). The shoulder, knee, elbow, hip, fingers, and toes are commonly dislocated joints. Some people have joints that dislocate easily. This is especially common when a previous joint injury has weakened the surrounding connective tissues. These patients will sometimes be able to move the

Text continued on p. 486

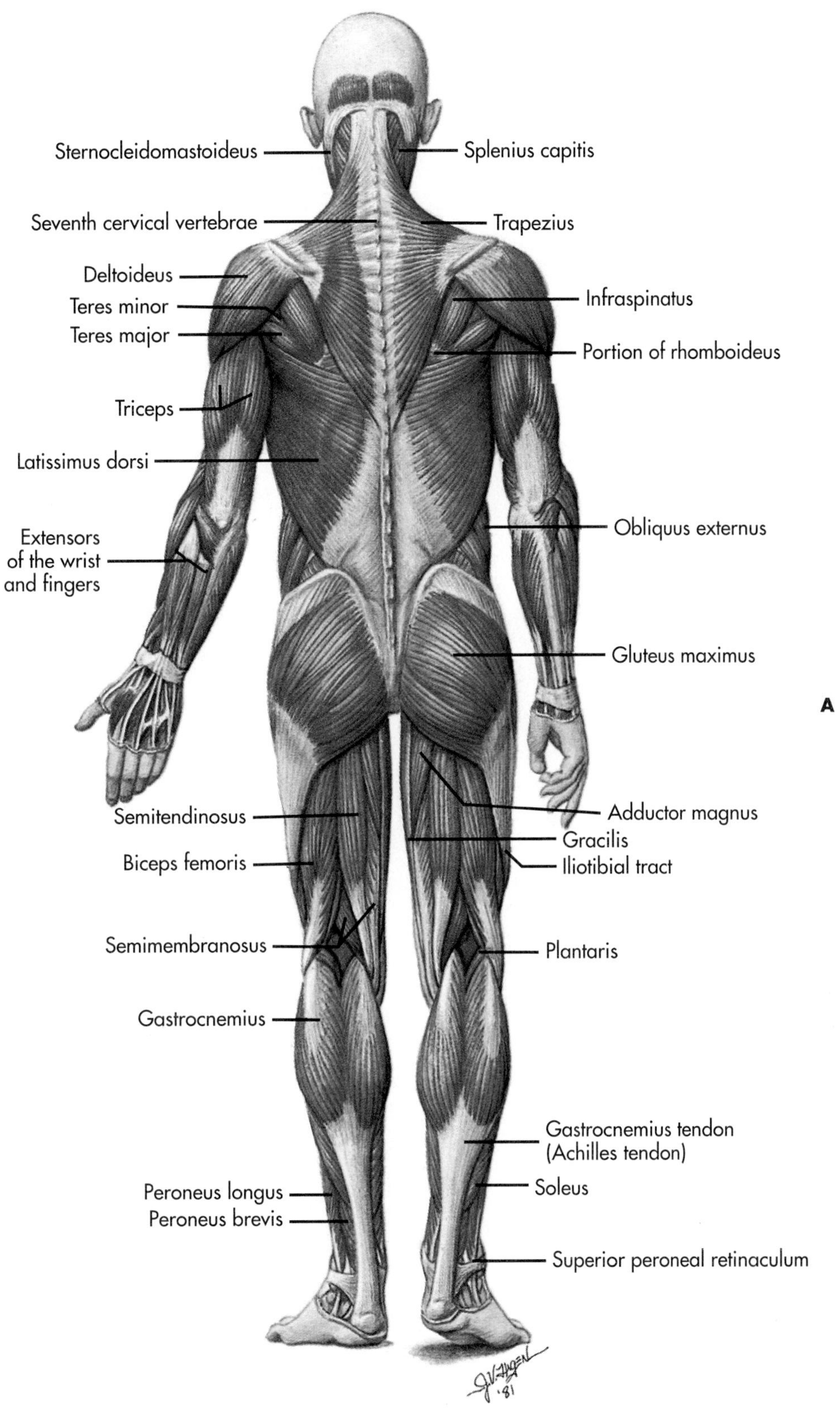

Figure 24-1

A, Posterior view of the muscular system. *Continued*

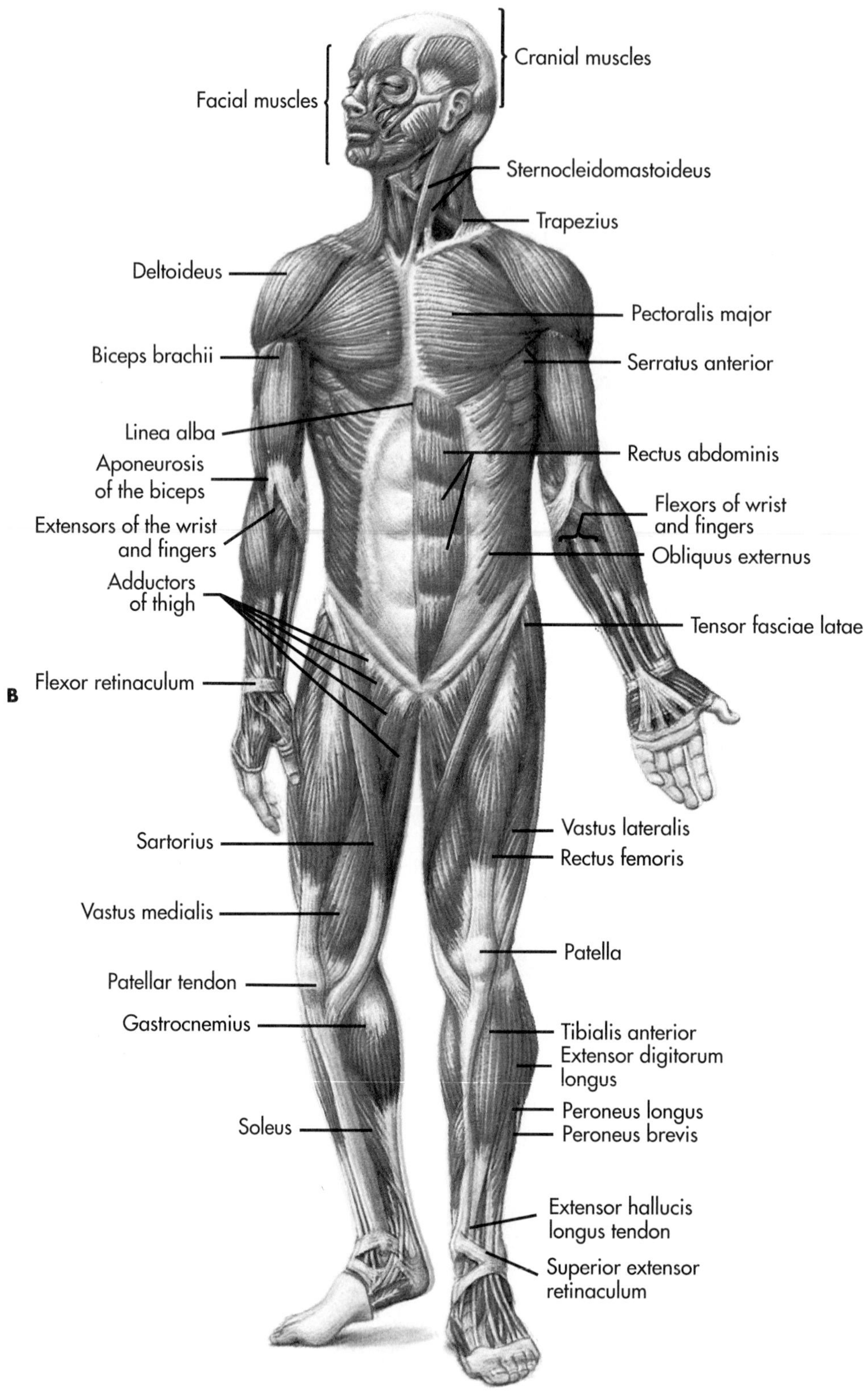
B
Cranial muscles
Facial muscles
Sternocleidomastoideus
Trapezius
Deltoideus
Pectoralis major
Biceps brachii
Serratus anterior
Linea alba
Rectus abdominis
Aponeurosis of the biceps
Flexors of wrist and fingers
Extensors of the wrist and fingers
Obliquus externus
Adductors of thigh
Tensor fasciae latae
Flexor retinaculum
Vastus lateralis
Sartorius
Rectus femoris
Vastus medialis
Patella
Patellar tendon
Gastrocnemius
Tibialis anterior
Extensor digitorum longus
Peroneus longus
Soleus
Peroneus brevis
Extensor hallucis longus tendon
Superior extensor retinaculum

Figure 24-1, cont'd

B, Anterior view of the muscular system.

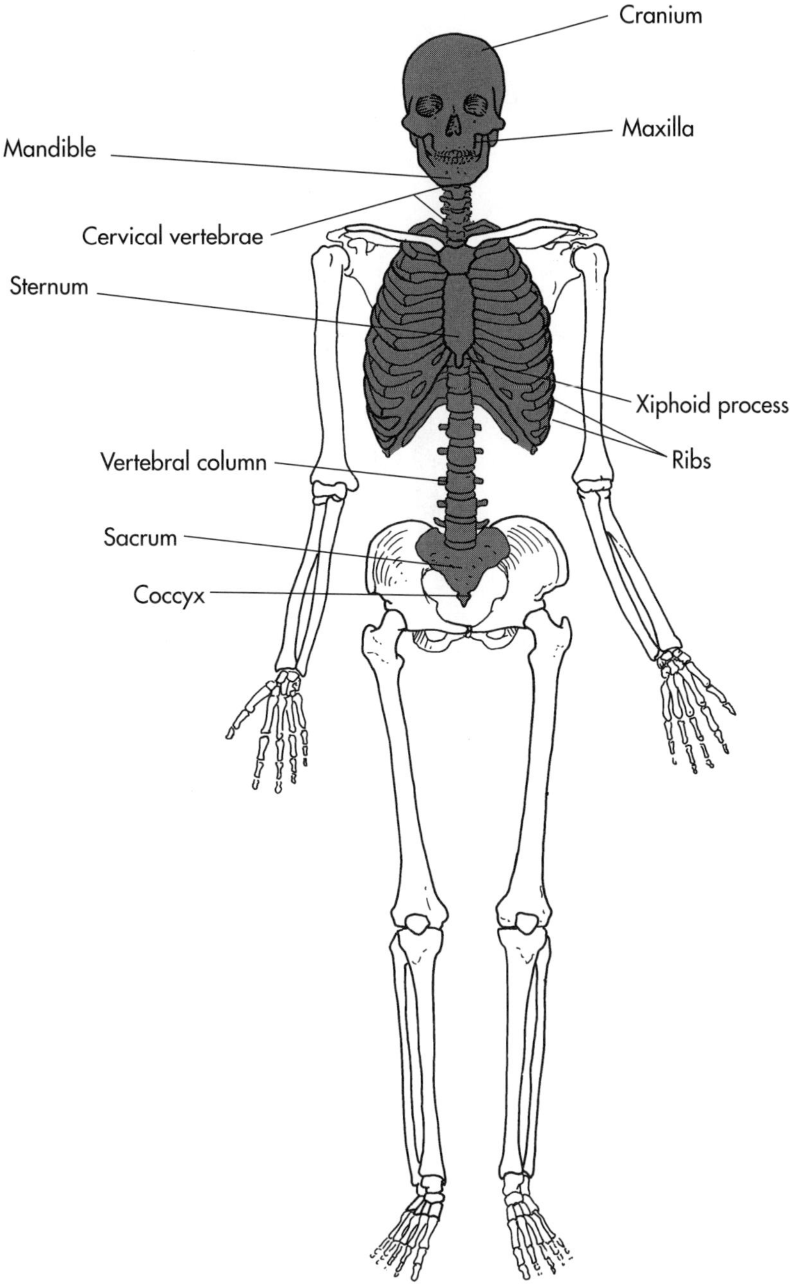

Figure 24-2

The central (axial) skeleton.

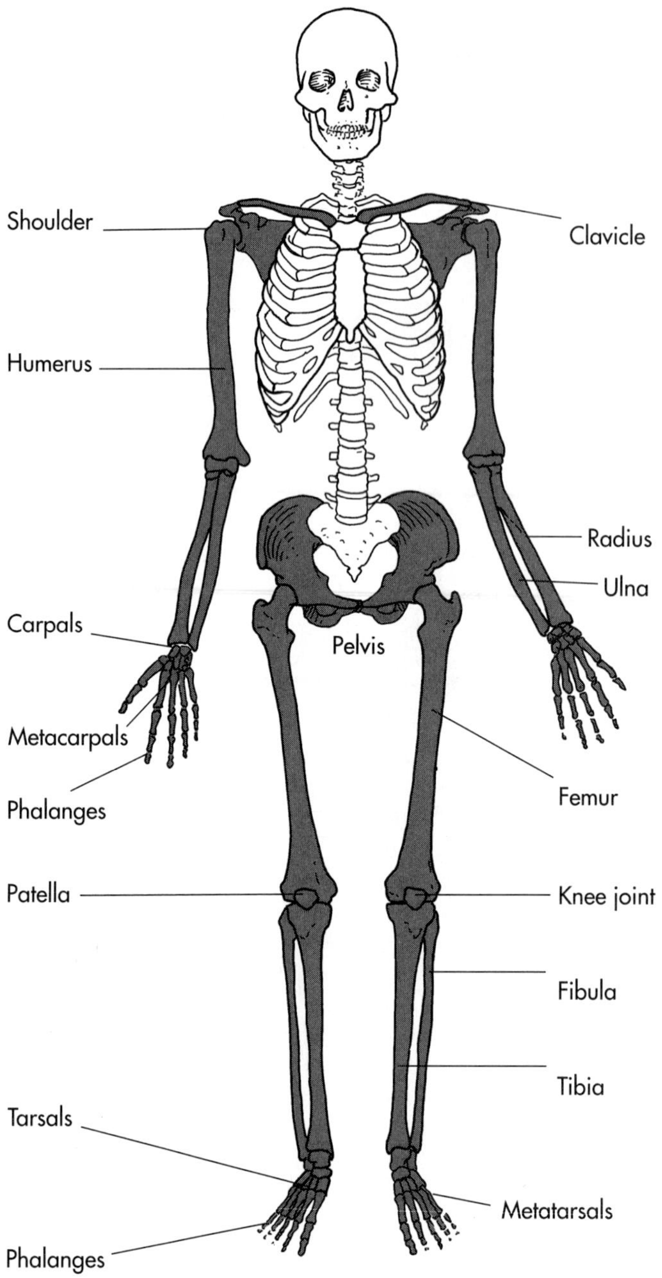

Figure 24-3

The peripheral (appendicular) skeleton.

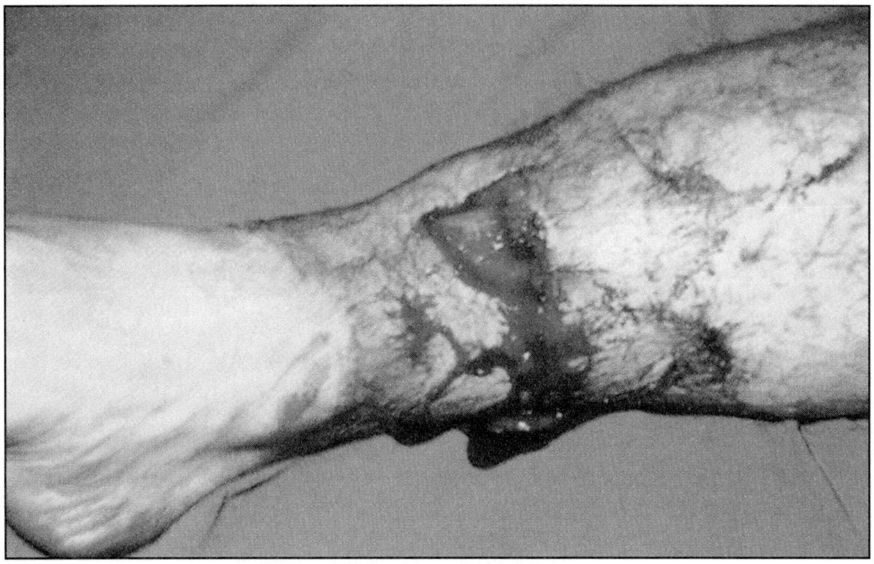

Figure 24-4
An open fracture.

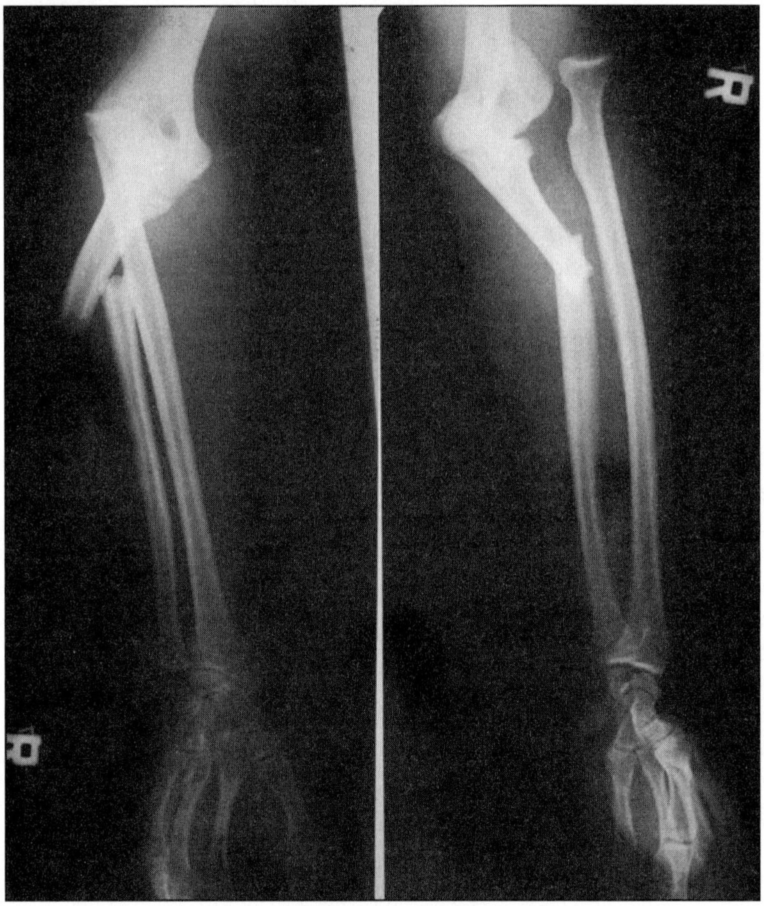

Figure 24-5
A displaced fracture.

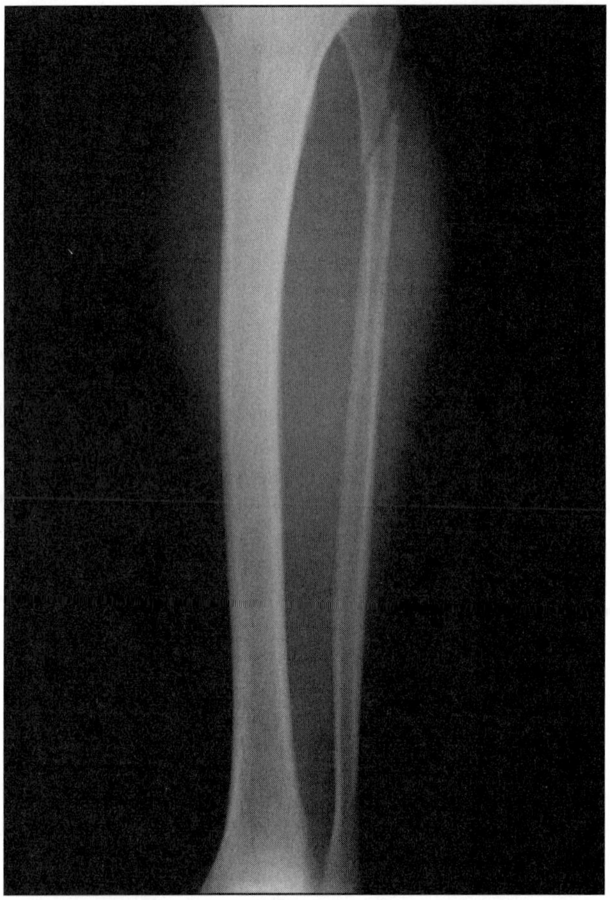

Figure 24-6

A nondisplaced fracture.

displaced bone end back into its joint on their own. As an EMT-Basic, you are not trained or permitted to replace (reduce) dislocations. You will provide basic care and transport the patient to the hospital. Joints such as the shoulder, elbow, and knee have nerves and blood vessels running through or near the joint that can be severely damaged if the joint is not reduced properly. For this reason, dislocations of the elbow and the knee (but not the kneecap) are orthopedic emergencies and should be transported immediately to the hospital.

Sprain

Sprains occur when there is an over-stretching or tearing of tendons, ligaments, or other connective tissue around a joint (Figure 24-8). A sprain may present with severe pain and swelling similar to a fracture. In many instances, a sprain can be more damaging than a fracture because stretched or torn ligaments do not regenerate as easily as bones do. As a result, the joint becomes weak and is vulnerable to repeated injury. Badly torn ligaments may need surgical repair to maintain the integrity of a joint.

Muscle Injury

An injury to a bone can also cause stretching or tearing of muscles. This is often seen when bones are fractured, although muscle injuries can also be isolated without associated fracture. A strain is a common muscle injury.

Strain

A **strain** results from over-stretched muscles caused by over-exertion or improper lifting or stretching. The neck and lower back muscles are common areas where muscles are stretched. The whiplash effect in a vehicle collision, which moves the head rapidly forward and then back, over-stretches the neck muscles. Improper lifting is a common cause of straining lower back muscles. Injuries around joints, such as dislocations, can also strain muscles. The most common sign of muscle strains is pain in the affected area.

Recognizing Common Musculoskeletal Injuries

Injuries to bones and muscles are often the result of some type of external force, such as a fall or direct trauma to the area. Awkward or inappropriate movement that puts unusual stress on the muscle, bone, or joint can also cause injuries such as a sprained ankle or strained back muscle.

Although musculoskeletal injuries are rarely life threatening, do not overlook them during assessment.

A

B

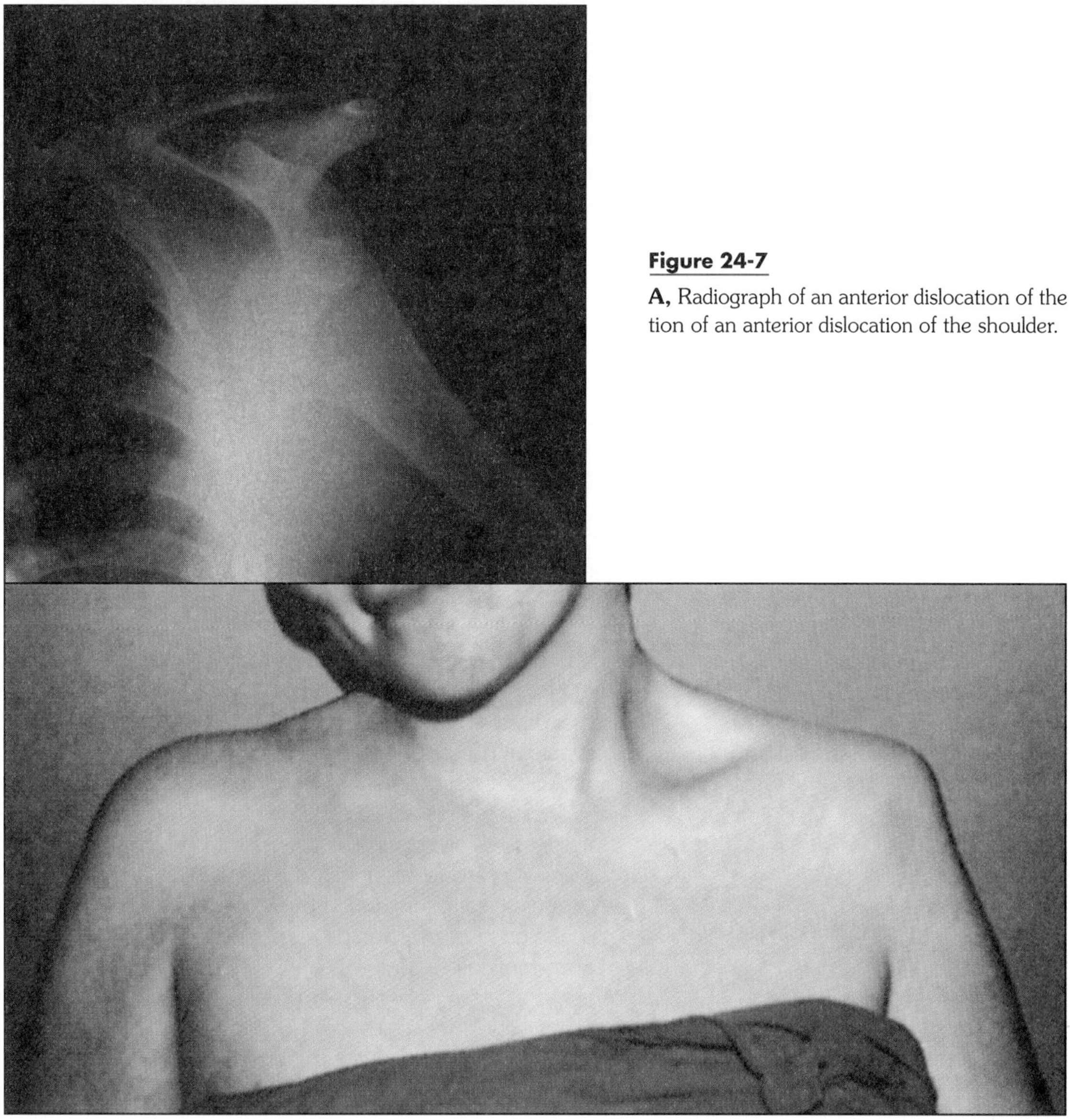

Figure 24-7

A, Radiograph of an anterior dislocation of the shoulder. **B,** Presentation of an anterior dislocation of the shoulder.

Muscle, bone, and joint injuries are often very painful. A conscious patient will usually make this clear when you arrive. Looking at the mechanism of injury and recognizing the signs and symptoms of a musculoskeletal injury will help raise your index of suspicion and determine the care needed. The few musculoskeletal injuries that can be life threatening usually involve the pelvis or femur, where there is potential for major blood loss. Because of the chance of damaging nerves in or near joints such as the knee or elbow, injuries in these areas are often considered to be possible limb threats.

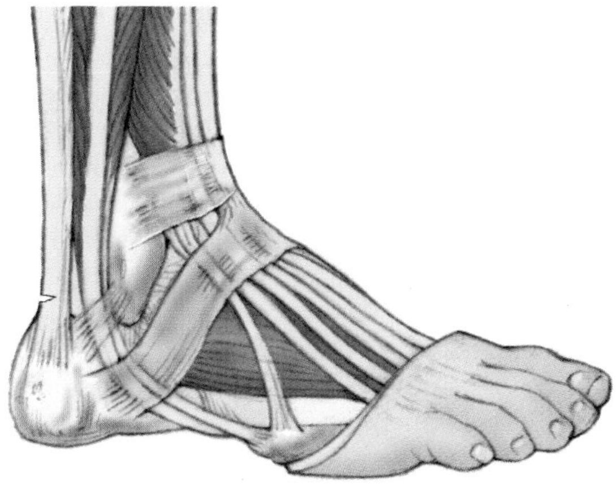

Figure 24-8

A sprain occurs when the connective tissues around a joint are torn or over-stretched.

Mechanism of Injury

Musculoskeletal injuries can result from direct, indirect, or twisting forces. As you arrive at the scene, look for clues that may indicate the mechanism of injury. Talk to the patient or bystanders whenever possible. Injuries resulting from direct and indirect force usually involve bone and muscle. An example of a direct force is a baseball that strikes a person on the head. Indirect force can be involved when a person falls from a height and lands on the feet. While the feet and ankles can be broken by the direct impact, the force of landing may also cause indirect injuries to the spine. Twisting forces usually involve the muscle and surrounding connective tissue in the joint, but can also injure the bone. This is often seen when skiers injure their knees in twisting falls.

Whenever the mechanism of injury makes you suspect significant trauma, you should also suspect and treat for musculoskeletal injury. Do not let the most obvious problems distract you from the possibility of more serious injuries that the patient may not be complaining about. For example, a person who fell off a ladder may complain of severe leg pain. But because of the mechanism of injury, you should also suspect and check for head, neck, and back injuries.

Signs and Symptoms

Signs and symptoms of musculoskeletal injuries include:

- Pain or tenderness
- Limited movement
- Deformity or angulation
- Discoloration
- Swelling
- **Crepitus**
- Bone ends protruding through soft tissue
- Absence of distal pulses
- Absence of distal motor function (movement) or sensation

One of the most significant signs of bone injury is deformity or angulation (unnatural shape or position of an extremity). Comparing the injured extremity with the uninjured side may help identify the deformity. Bones protruding through the skin (open fracture) are a sure indicator of a serious injury.

Normally, people can move limbs without pain. If the patient is unable to move or bear weight on an extremity after trauma, it is often because of the pain associated with such movement. This is another good indicator of a significant injury. Discoloration and swelling are also usually present. While these signs do not prove that a bone is broken, they do combine with other signs to suggest the need for immobilization and evaluation by a physician. The absence of distal pulses, motor function, and sensation are less common but urgent signs of serious injury.

The signs and symptoms of the various types of musculoskeletal injuries are similar. You need not, and often cannot, determine the extent or exact type of injury in the field. A positive diagnosis requires physician examination and hospital tests, such as an x-ray. To provide the proper care for the patient, treat for the worst possible injury. If this worst-case scenario turns out to be true, you have protected the patient against the major complications of musculoskeletal injuries: vessel damage and internal bleeding, nerve damage, soft-tissue injury, and damage to internal chest and abdominal organs. If the injury is less serious, there is no harm done.

General Care for Bone or Joint Injury

Your care priorities are to reduce pain and minimize further injury. Care for a bone or joint injury should focus on treating signs and symptoms rather than trying to diagnose the exact nature of the injury. You may suspect a fracture, but you are really caring for a painful, swollen, deformed area.

The mechanism of injury, the patient's chief complaint, and your focused and detailed assessments will help you identify possible musculoskeletal injuries that require care. Always begin by treating life-threatening injuries first. A patient with a possible fracture may be in severe pain but may also be bleeding severely. Address the ABCs before focusing on musculoskeletal injuries.

When you begin your assessment of a musculoskeletal injury, assess distal pulse, movement, and sensation before beginning care for that injury. The specific care needed is to immobilize the injured joint or bone to minimize movement and further damage. Once this is done, reassess pulse, movement, and sensation. Apply cold packs to the injured area and elevate it if possible to help reduce pain and swelling. Because serious musculoskeletal injuries can impair circulation, supplemental oxygen will also be helpful.

Splinting

Splinting is the process of immobilizing a painful, swollen, or deformed area. It is done to prevent movement of bone fragments, bone ends, joints, or muscles. Splinting reduces the chance of damage to muscles, nerves, or blood vessels and helps reduce pain. Splinting can also help keep a closed fracture from becoming an open fracture during movement.

Try to immobilize an injury before any movement unless life-threatening conditions require rapid movement. In this case, the musculoskeletal injury is not the primary concern. When immobilizing the injured area, ensure that it prevents movement in all directions.

Guidelines for Splinting

When splinting an injured area, follow these general guidelines:

- Expose the injury before splinting, if possible.

- Assess pulse, movement, and sensation distal to the injury before and after applying a splint.
- Stabilize and immobilize the joint above and below an injured bone, or the bones above and below an injured joint.
- Follow body substance isolation (BSI) practices, and control and bandage any external bleeding.
- Select the right size and type of splint to immobilize the injured area.
- Pad splints before application to reduce discomfort from pressure, especially near bony spots.
- Splint injured bones before moving the patient, if possible.
- Splint an injured extremity (except a hand or foot) in the position found, unless the extremity is severely angulated, cyanotic, or lacks distal pulses or sensation. In these situations, try to align the extremity by applying gentle **traction,** if allowed by local protocol or recommended by medical direction. Traction involves applying pressure above and below the site of long bone injury, but is not used if the injury involves a joint (Figure 24-9).
- Splint a hand or foot in the **position of function** whenever possible. This is the normal resting position (Figure 24-10). Do not do this if the hand or foot is found in an abnormal position that cannot be easily returned to the position of function.

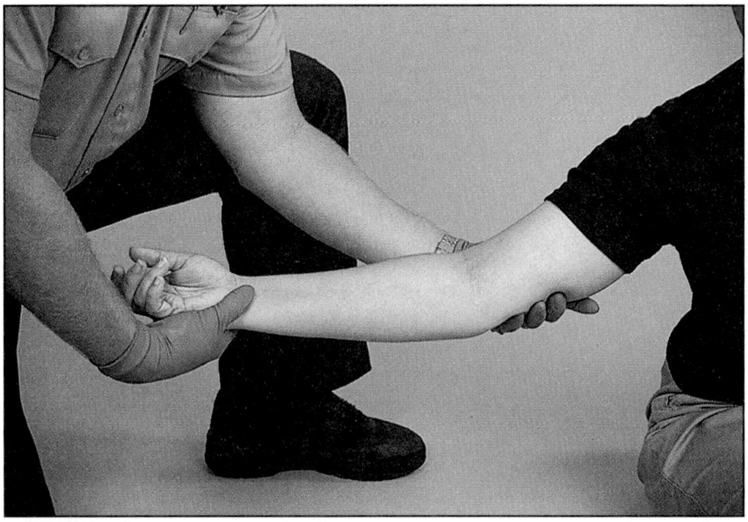

Figure 24-9

If the injury does not involve a joint and is on a long bone, gentle traction may be applied.

A 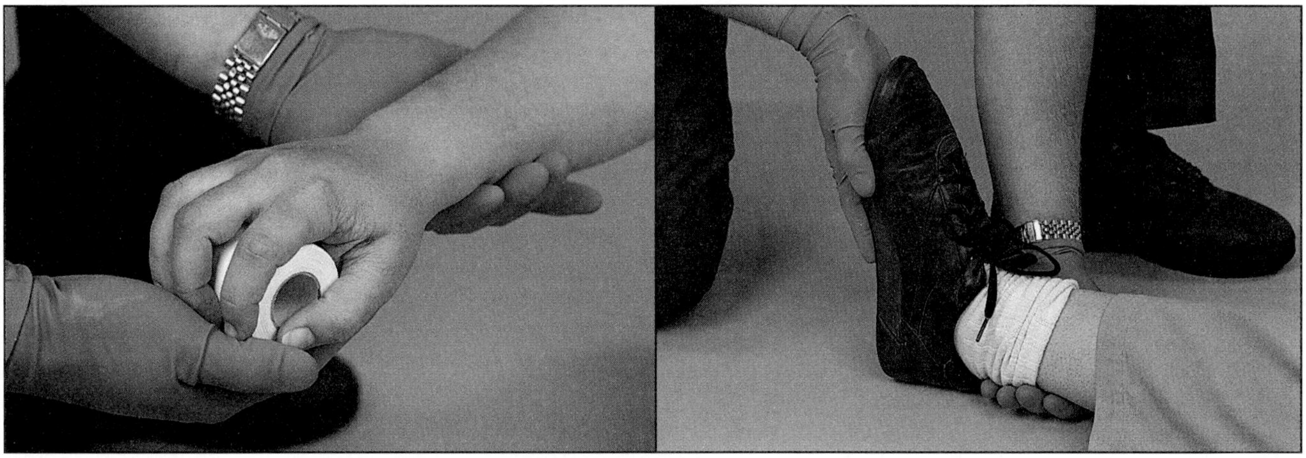 B

Figure 24-10

A, Position of function for the hand. **B,** Position of function for the foot.

A

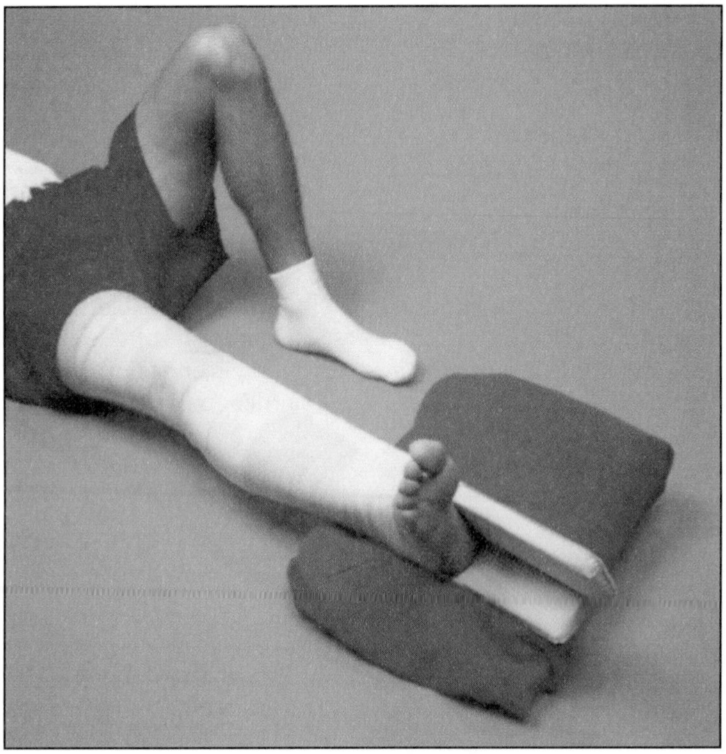

Figure 24-11

A, Rigid splint.

Splinting Precautions

Splinting is a common and effective treatment, but it does involve a few precautions:

- Straighten an angulated fracture (if allowed by local protocol) only if there is compromised circulation or nerve function. Even then, it is normally only attempted once. If you are unable to restore normal function to the extremity, transport immediately.
- If bone ends protrude from the skin, immobilize the injury in the position found and place a sterile dressing over the exposed bone. Do not try to replace the bone ends. The bone may slip back under the surface of the skin before or during splinting. If this happens, do not try to keep the wound open. If there is significant bleeding, control it. Cover the wound and splint the injured area.
- When applying a splint, avoid excessive movement that may further damage bone, nerves, blood vessels, or muscle tissue.
- Compression of nerves, muscle, and blood vessels may result from improper splinting. This is especially true if the splint is applied too tightly. Always check circulation, movement, and sensation before and after splinting. If, after applying a splint, you cannot find a pulse or the patient has lost movement or sensation, loosen the splint and adjust it. Reassess. If distal function is still not normal, transport immediately.

Types of Splints

Common Splints

There are several common types of splints. Some are rigid, such as board and cardboard splints. Others are semirigid (ladder and structural aluminum malleable (SAM) splints). Semirigid splints can be molded to the shape of the extremity, which provide the needed rigidity. Splints may also be soft, such as pillow and blanket splints (Figure 24-11).

Commercial splints are supplied in various sizes, are usually padded, and are most often rigid or semirigid. Rigid splints are typically made of wood inside a layer of foam padding and a plastic cover. They may also be made of strong cardboard or a similar, disposable material. Semirigid splints are designed to wrap or hug the injured area. They are good when dealing with a deformity. A vacuum splint is an advanced type of semirigid splint that is particularly useful for angulated extremity injuries (Figure 24-12).

Slings, pillows, and blankets are examples of soft splints that are typically used for areas where a rigid or semirigid splint cannot easily be applied, such as a foot.

There may be situations in which commercial splints are not available and you have to improvise a splint. You can do this with newspapers, magazines, umbrellas, canes, and many other materials. Another splinting method that may be helpful when the splint you want is not available is

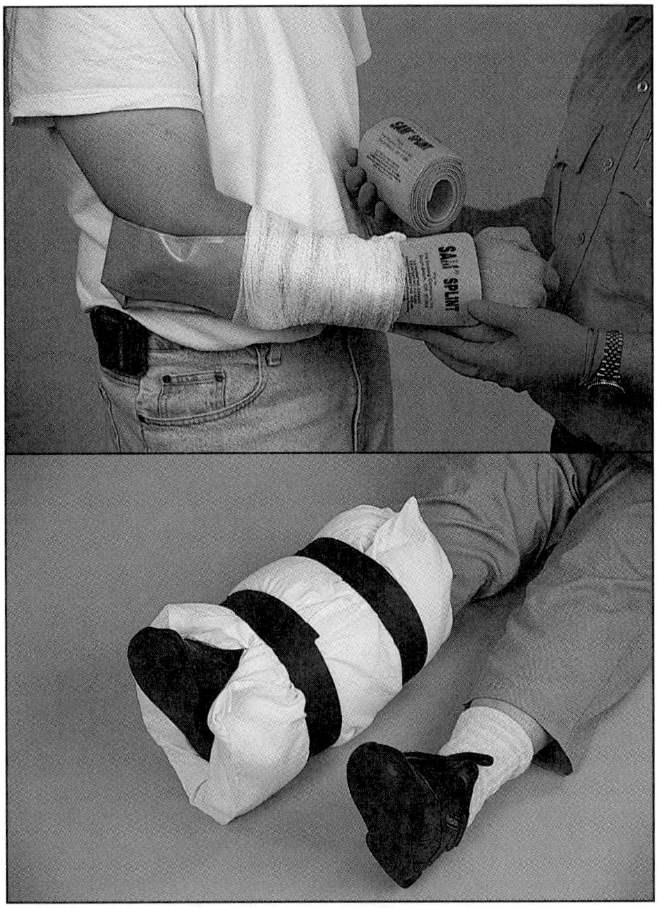

B

C

Figure 24-11, cont'd

B, Semirigid splint. **C,** Soft splint.

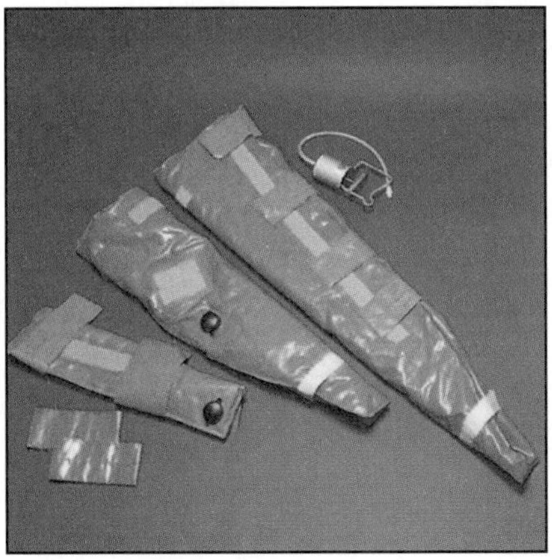

Figure 24-12

Vacuum splint.

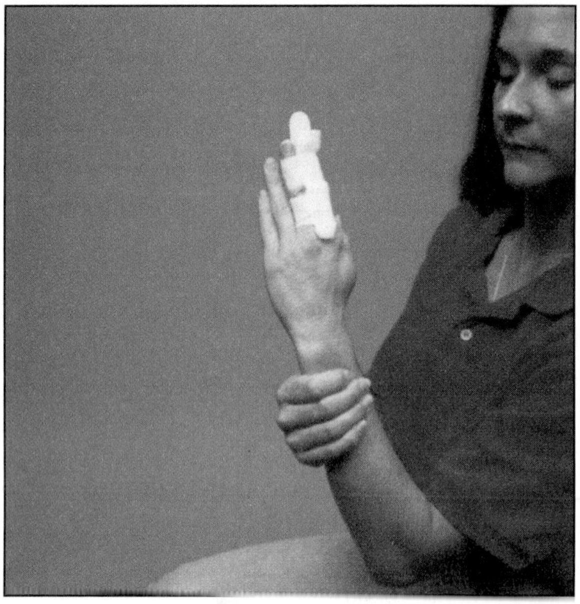

Figure 24-13
Anatomic splint.

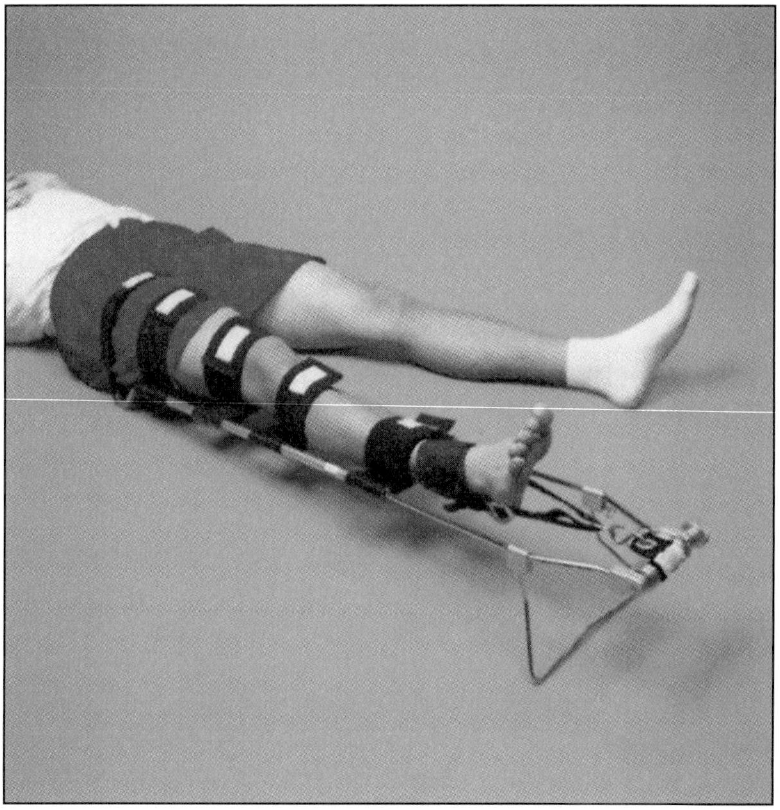

Figure 24-14
Traction splint.

BOX 24-1 Contraindications to the Use of the Traction Splint

- Injury at or near the knee
- Injury to the hip or pelvis
- Partial amputation or avulsion with bone separation
- Lower leg or ankle injury

the anatomic splint. This uses the body as a splint. Examples include securing an injured leg to the uninjured one or splinting an injured finger to the uninjured finger next to it (Figure 24-13).

Specialized Splints

Most splints are versatile and can be used to splint different areas of the body. However, there are several splints that have been designed for a specific purpose. The traction splint and the **pneumatic antishock garment** (PASG) are two of these specialized devices.

Traction Splint

The traction splint applies traction and immobilizes the injury at the same time. It is designed for mid-thigh trauma (possible femur fracture) that is not associated with joint or lower leg injuries (Figure 24-14). The traction splint helps reduce muscle spasms from the large thigh muscles. These spasms make the bone ends ride over each other, causing additional damage and pain. Box 24-1 lists contraindications to the use of the traction splint.

Pneumatic Antishock Garment

Chapter 22 explained the use of the PASG in the treatment of shock. The PASG can also splint injuries of the pelvis and lower extremities. A patient with a possible fractured pelvis or femur may go into shock because of the amount of blood loss associated with those injuries. The PASG will stabilize the fracture and may also treat the circulatory compromise.

It can be useful to place the PASG on a patient and inflate only certain compartments, depending on the type of injury. For example, if the patient has only a femur injury, then only that leg of the garment needs to be inflated. If the patient has injured the pelvis, all three compartments should be inflated to provide the best possible stabilization. Both legs should always be inflated when the abdominal compartment is inflated. Inflating only the abdomen could lead to circulatory problems by restricting venous blood return from the legs.

Two reminders are important when you use the PASG. First, if the garment will be on the patient for more than 6 hours, there is increased risk of circulation problems and resulting tissue damage in the extremities. Second, using the PASG for a possible femur fracture does not replace traction splinting. It is possible, and important, to apply a traction splint as well when the patient is stable enough that there is time to apply it. (In an unstable patient, the PASG is a good way to provide some immobilization without taking time for a traction splint.)

Caring for Specific Musculoskeletal Injuries

The following sections explain how to splint various extremity injuries. Local protocols may vary in the approach to managing specific injuries.

Upper Extremities

Injuries to the upper extremities include the shoulder, clavicle, scapula, humerus, elbow, forearm, wrist, and hand.

Shoulder: Scapula, Clavicle

The clavicle, also called the *collarbone,* is commonly injured by direct impact, a fall on an outstretched arm, or trauma to the lateral shoulder. Unlike the clavicle, which is easily injured, the scapula (shoulder blade) is much less likely to be injured. It takes extreme force to fracture the scapula. When you identify or suspect a scapula fracture, evaluate the patient carefully for injuries of the head, neck, and trunk.

The joint where the clavicle and scapula meet is called the *acromioclavicular (AC) joint.* This is a commonly injured area among athletes, such as football players who fall on the point of the shoulder. The force causes the scapula to move away from the clavicle, creating the classic shoulder separation. Sometimes the shoulder joint is injured where the head of the humerus meets it. Most often, the humerus is displaced (dislocated) anteriorly, giving the patient a "square" shoulder instead of the normal round appearance. These types of injuries can also cause a fracture of the proximal humerus or of the socket in the scapula.

You may occasionally care for an inferior shoulder dislocation in which the arm presents elevated and held away from the body. If it cannot be easily lowered without further pain or injury, you will need to splint and support the extremity in this position during transport.

Regardless of the exact injury, care is similar. To immobilize the shoulder, clavicle, or scapula, begin by stabilizing the injured area. Most patients find the most comfortable position for supporting the arm before your arrival. In many cases, this position is one in which the arm on the injured side is held close to the chest (Figure 24-15, *A*). In this case, you only need to apply a sling (Figure 24-15, *B*) and a swathe (binder) (Figure 24-15, *C*). The sling will support the weight of the arm in the most comfortable position, while the swathe limits movement by holding the arm against the chest.

A

B

C

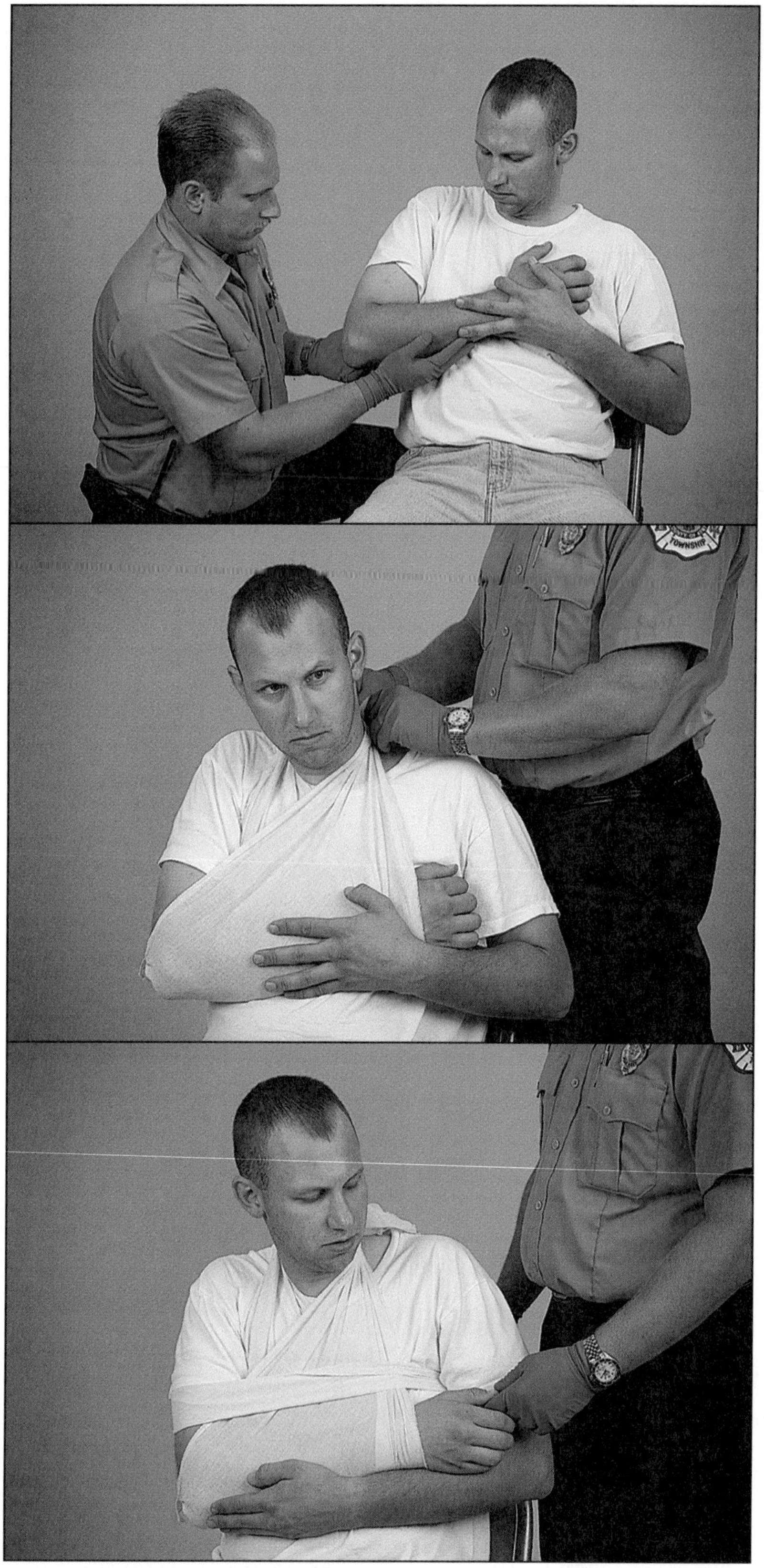

Figure 24-15

A, The patient will often have already found the most comfortable support position. **B,** Apply the sling, keeping the arm in the position of comfort. **C,** Apply the swathe to immobilize the area.

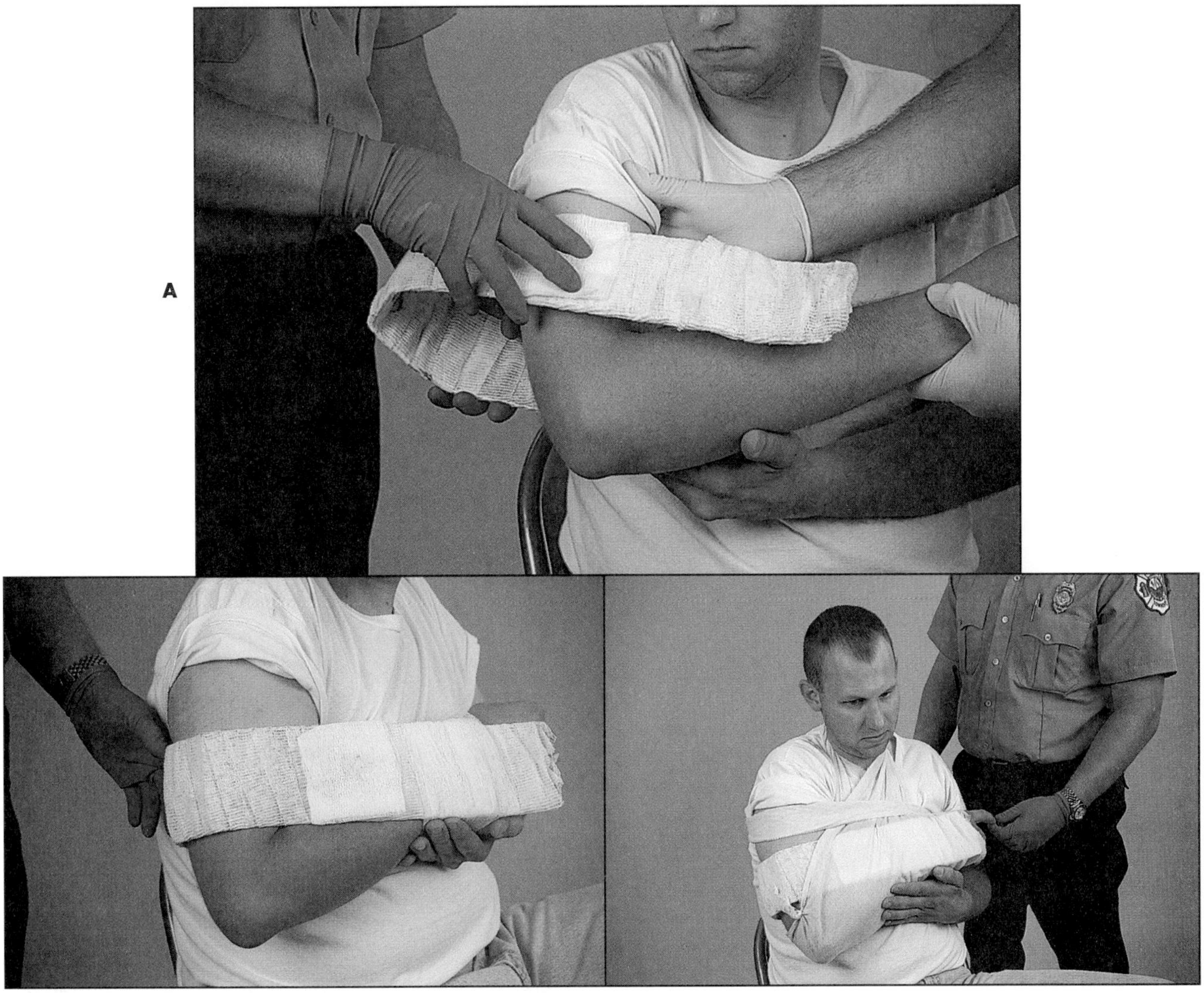

Figure 24-16

A, Place the splint on the lateral portion of the upper arm. **B,** Secure the splint with roller gauze or cravats. **C,** Apply a sling and swathe, then check for sensation and distal pulses.

Humerus

The mid-shaft and proximal humerus are the areas most commonly injured. The proximal shaft is often injured when elderly individuals fall. Mid-shaft injury is more common in younger patients as a result of violent trauma, including vehicle collisions.

Splinting a humerus injury is very similar to immobilizing the shoulder and clavicle. The injured arm is supported against the chest, and a sling and swathe are applied. Begin by stabilizing the injured area. Generally, the weight of the arm will apply gentle traction. Place a padded splint on the lateral portion of the upper arm (Figure 24-16, *A*) and secure the splint with cravats or roller gauze (Figure 24-16, *B*). Apply a sling and swathe. Mid-shaft humerus fractures can injure nerves and blood vessels easily, so make sure that distal pulses and sensation are intact (Figure 24-16, *C*).

Elbow

Because of the potential for significant nerve or blood vessel damage, all elbow injuries should be considered serious. Dislocated elbows most often occur during athletic activities. When they occur, the radius and ulna are often displaced posteriorly.

Splinting the elbow involves stabilizing the bones above and below the joint. If you find the arm in a bent position, keep it this way and apply a splint. A semirigid or vacuum splint is good for this kind of injury because it will conform to the exact shape needed. Apply a sling and swathe to further minimize movement.

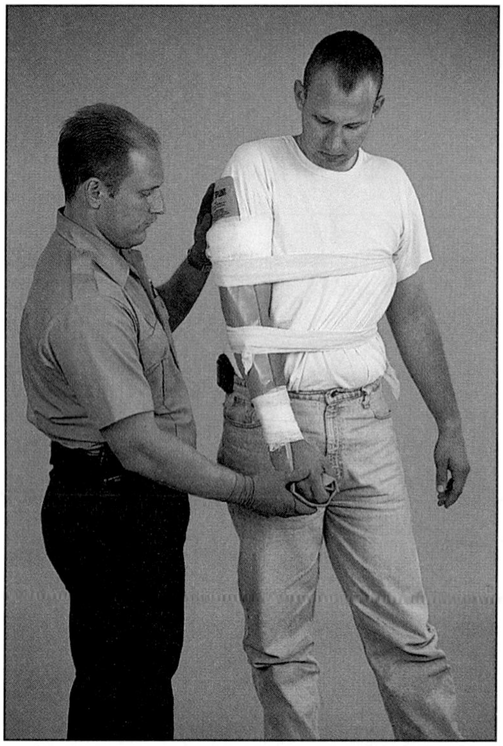

Figure 24-17

Splint from armpit to wrist, securing the injured arm to the body.

IT'S YOUR CALL
CONCLUSION

Your patient may have a shoulder dislocation. He states that he can relocate it but has not been able to after several attempts. You must also consider the possibility of a fracture. An x-ray is the only way to identify the exact nature of his injury. Your care is to immobilize the patient's injured shoulder using a sling and swathe, and provide comfortable transport to the hospital.

When the patient asks you to help him pop his shoulder back into place (reducing the dislocation), you explain that it is not part of your training. After this explanation, he accepts your offer of immobilization and transport. It is important that you document his attempts to reduce the shoulder himself just as you would have documented his refusal if he decided not to accept your help.

If the arm is in a straight position, place a splint from the armpit to the wrist and secure the splint in place. Bind the injured arm to the body using cravats or roller gauze (Figure 24-17). Elbow dislocations should be considered orthopedic emergencies. Transport without delay.

Forearm, Wrist, and Hand

Forearm injuries are common in patients of all ages. These injuries often involve both the radius (Figure 24-18, *A*) and ulna. When the distal portion of the radius is injured, usually as a result of a fall on an outstretched hand, the distal forearm or wrist may assume a curved appearance, commonly called a *silver-fork deformity* (Figure 24-18, *B*).

Begin by stabilizing the injury above and below the site. Place a splint on the underside of the forearm, extending from the elbow to the hand. Place a roll of gauze or similar padding in the palm of the hand to maintain the position of function. Secure the splint using cravats or roller gauze. If possible, apply a sling and swathe.

Injuries of the hand or fingers should generally be splinted in the position found, using small rigid or soft splints. Sensation and vascular status (pulses or capillary refill) should be confirmed.

Lower Extremities

The lower extremities include the pelvis, hip, thigh (femur), knee, lower leg (tibia and fibula), ankle, and foot. Injuries involving the pelvis and femur are less common than upper extremity injuries because the bones of the lower extremity are larger and stronger.

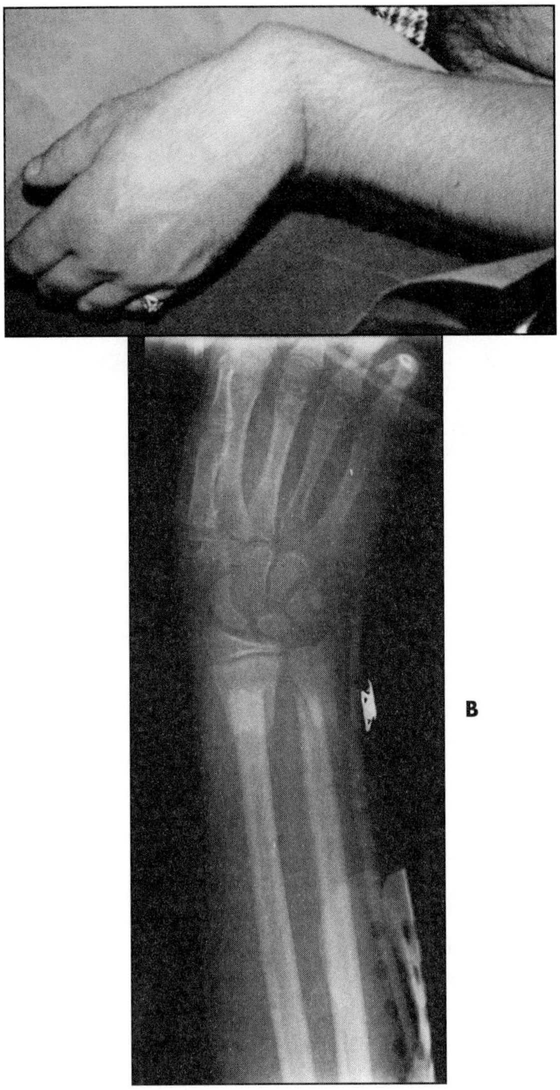

Figure 24-18

A, Fracture of the distal radius. **B,** Radiograph of a silver-fork deformity. The overlapping bone ends cause the curved appearance of the fracture.

Pelvis, Hip

The impact from a fall or vehicle collision can crush the pelvis. Because of the large blood vessels that lie near and within the pelvis, a serious pelvic injury causes major blood loss. The same trauma that crushes the pelvis can also displace the head of the femur from the hip joint (Figure 24-19). When this occurs, nerve damage can cause a loss of sensation in the leg and foot on the affected side. Because the femur is most likely to be dislocated posteriorly, the classic signs of this injury are a slightly flexed hip, flexed knee, and inward rotation of the thigh. In rare situations, the femur will be displaced anteriorly, causing the leg to be extended and rotated outward, pointing away from the body.

One of the most common methods of providing care for a pelvic or hip injury is to place a blanket between the legs, secure the injured leg to the uninjured one, and immobilize the patient on a backboard (Figure 24-20).

Femur

When the proximal head of the femur is broken, it is commonly referred to as a *hip fracture.* Osteoporosis, a degenerative bone disease, is a contributing factor in hip fractures among the elderly—even a simple fall from a chair onto a padded carpet can cause a hip fracture. Direct trauma is the most common cause of femur fractures in younger patients. Regardless of age, the injured leg is rotated and usually appears shorter than the other leg.

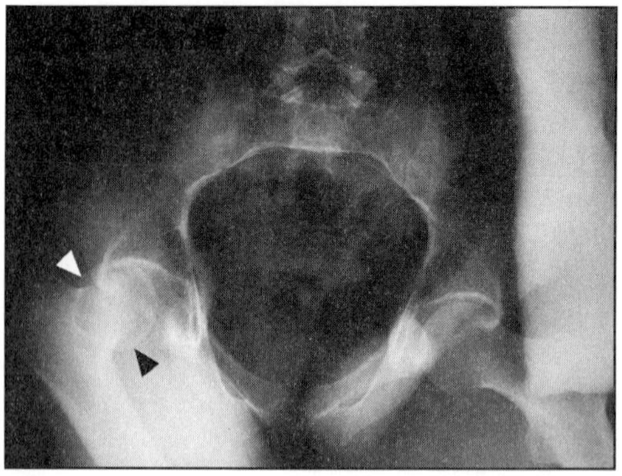

Figure 24-19

Posterior dislocation of the right femur, caused in a vehicle collision.

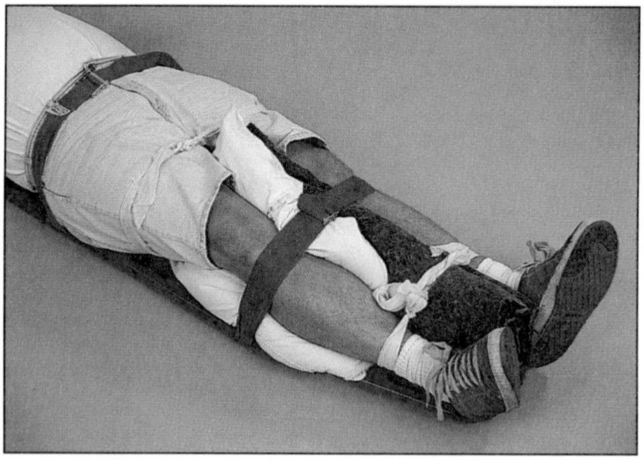

Figure 24-20

An anatomical splint of one leg to another, with the patient secured to a backboard.

If you suspect that an injury has occurred at the proximal end of the femur, treat it as you would a hip dislocation or pelvic injury. Stabilize the injured area with a PASG or secure the injured leg to the uninjured leg using a blanket between the legs, and place the patient on a backboard.

Injuries to the femoral shaft usually present with a shortened, angulated limb with swelling of the thigh. These injuries may be associated with nerve and blood vessel damage that impairs sensation and circulation. As with all potential fractures, assess the patient's pulse, motor response, and sensation distal to the injury, and record your findings. Applying gentle traction and returning the limb to its normal position often improves circulation to the foot.

The best way to immobilize this type of injury is with a traction splint. Whether you use a Hare, Sager, or other traction device, the principles are the same. The device helps stabilize the bone ends, reduce the contraction (spasm) of the large muscles of the thigh, which are causing pain and the deformity, and ensure adequate circulation and nerve function.

Working with a partner, follow these steps to apply the Hare traction splint:

1. Carefully stabilize the bone above and below the injury site.
2. Adjust the splint to the proper length, using the uninjured leg as a guide. The top of the splint should be positioned at the ischium (inferior portion of the pelvis bone), and the bottom extended 8 to 12 inches below the foot (Figure 24-21, *A*).
3. Apply the ankle hitch and begin gentle manual traction. Maintain this traction until the splint is completely secured (Figure 24-21, *B*).
4. Place the splint under the patient with the proximal end resting on the lower bone of the posterior pelvis (ischium), in the buttocks (Figure 24-21, *C*).
5. Fasten the ischial strap and the ankle hitch. Apply mechanical traction with the splint until it applies the amount of traction that the rescuer had been applying by hand (Figure 24-21, *D*).
6. Fasten the supporting straps around the leg.
7. Elevate the leg approximately 8 to 10 inches. Some splints have a built-in stand for this purpose.
8. Reassess pulses, movement, and sensation distal to the injury and record your findings. If any of these are diminished compared with the initial findings, the splint may be too tight. Adjust the tension of the traction slightly and reassess.
9. Place the patient on a backboard to immobilize the hip.
10. Secure the splint to the backboard and transport.

Knee

Abnormal movement of the knee, such as twisting, can damage the supporting ligaments. If the injury is severe enough, it can also displace the proximal end of the tibia (a true knee dislocation), or the patella (kneecap). These injuries often result in pronounced deformity of the knee. Patellar dislocations are fairly common but, although painful, are not usually serious for the patient. A dislocation of the knee, however, is an orthopedic emergency that requires immediate transport after immobilizing the extremity. Knee dislocations are serious because of the potential for associated nerve and blood vessel damage.

Care for knee injuries is similar to that for elbows: stabilize and splint the injured area in the position found. The knee will most often be found in a flexed position. In this case, place pillows under the leg to fill the area be-

A

B

C

D

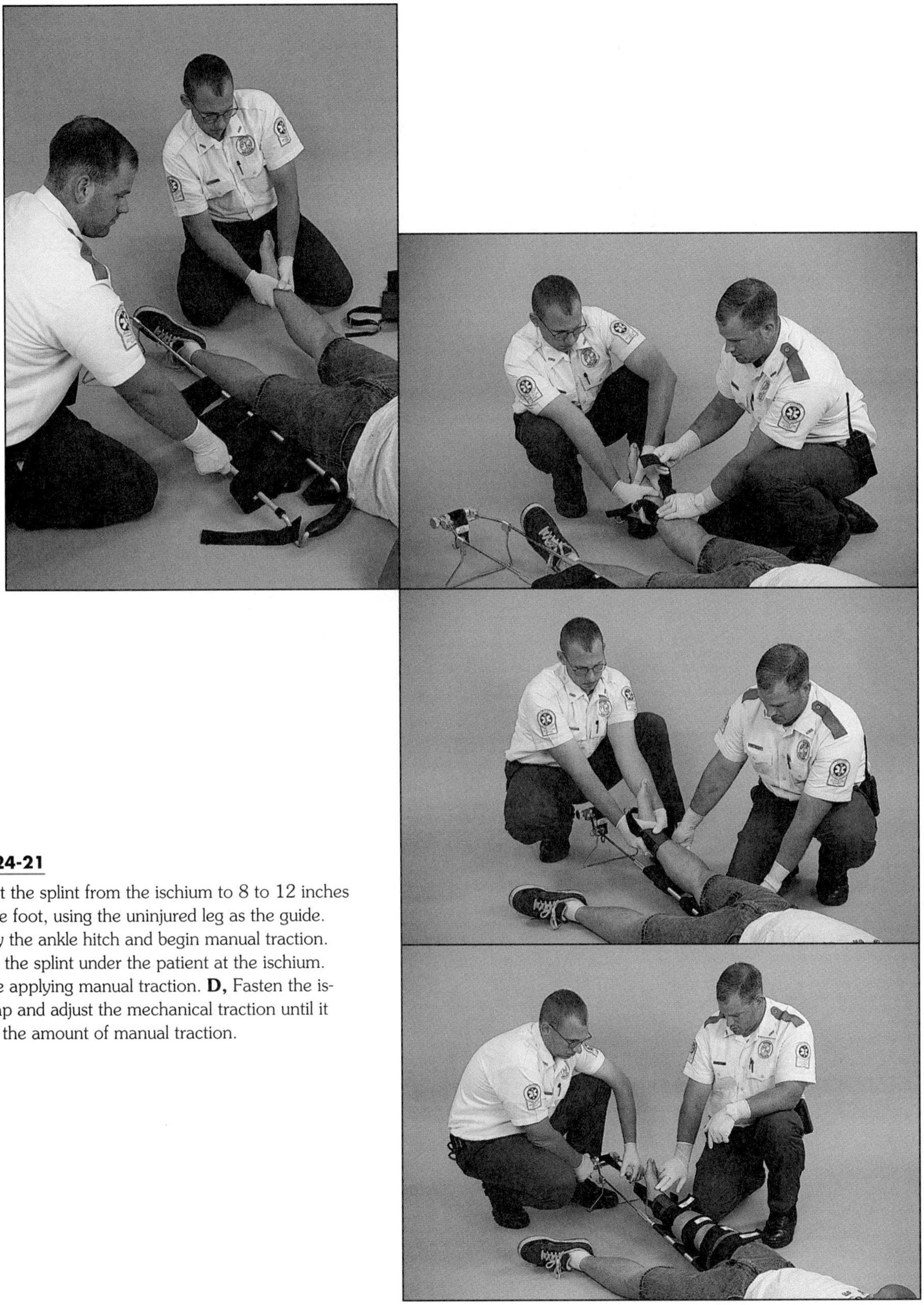

Figure 24-21

A, Adjust the splint from the ischium to 8 to 12 inches below the foot, using the uninjured leg as the guide. **B,** Apply the ankle hitch and begin manual traction. **C,** Place the splint under the patient at the ischium. Continue applying manual traction. **D,** Fasten the ischial strap and adjust the mechanical traction until it matches the amount of manual traction.

A

B

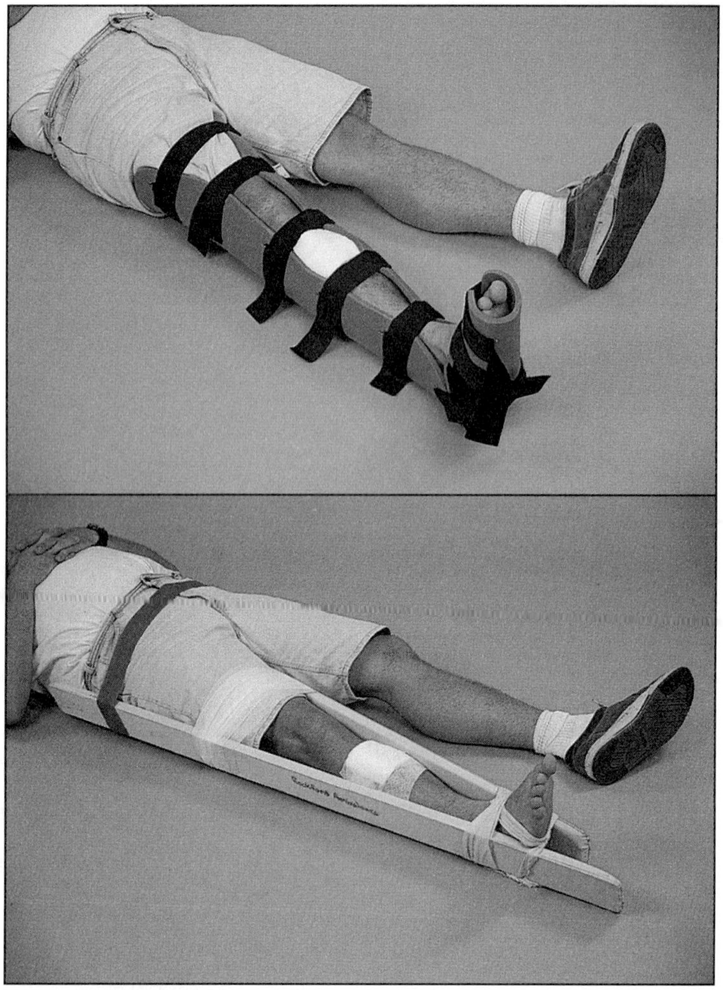

Figure 24-22

A, A semirigid splint stabilizing the joints above and below a lower leg injury. **B,** A rigid splint secured with gauze and cravats.

hind the knee. Place long, padded splints on each side of the knee, extending from the hip to the ankle. If the knee is in a straight position, place a splint underneath the injured leg from the ankle to the hip and secure it in place.

Lower Leg

The two bones of the lower leg, the tibia and fibula, may both be injured as a result of trauma to the lower leg. As with other injuries to long bones, stabilize the joints above and below the injured site. Place splints on each side of the patient's leg, from the ankle to above the knee, and secure them with cravats (Figure 24-22, *A* and *B*).

Ankle and Foot

Because of the large number of bones in the ankle and foot, there is no way to isolate an individual injured bone. It is also difficult to distinguish fractures from less serious injuries. Soft splints such as pillows and blankets work well to immobilize an injured ankle or foot. If a shoe is in place, carefully remove it from the patient's foot and check for circulation, movement, and sensation. Place a blanket or pillow around the foot in a horseshoe shape and secure it in place with tape or cravats (Figure 24-23). You can also use preformed lower-leg splints for the ankle and foot.

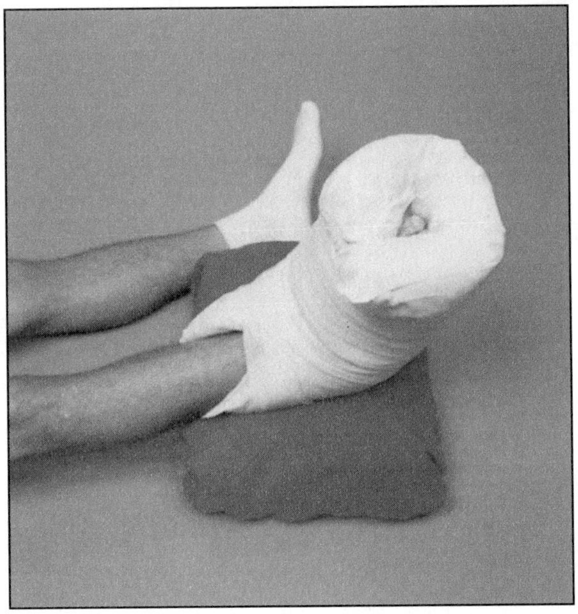

Figure 24-23

A soft splint, like a pillow splint, is most appropriate to immobilize an injured ankle or foot.

SUMMARY

This chapter discussed the care for musculoskeletal injuries. A review of the muscular and skeletal system depicted the close relationship between the bones, muscles, ligaments, and tendons that make up this system.

Trauma to the musculoskeletal system can result in sprains, strains, fractures, and dislocations. In a prehospital setting, there is no way to know the exact type or extent of the injury. All of them generally present as swollen, painful, and sometimes deformed areas. More important, it is not necessary to know the type of injury. Instead, identify the mechanism of injury and observe signs and symptoms to determine the likelihood of serious injury.

The care for bone and muscle injuries focuses on preventing further damage to the musculoskeletal system and other structures such as nerves and blood vessels. Splinting is the process used to immobilize injured areas, reducing movement. Various types of splints are available, including rigid, semirigid, and soft splints. These are commercially available or they can be improvised. Other special devices that can be used as splints include the traction splint and the PASG.

Follow the general rules of splinting and be aware of the risks of improper immobilization. Become proficient in immobilizing injuries of the upper and lower extremities. When splinting, assess distal pulses, movement, and sensation before and after applying the splint. Apply gentle traction to long bones while securing the splint. This will protect the area from further injury, reduce pain, and help restore proper circulation if it was compromised.

SUGGESTED READINGS

1. **BTLS:** *Basic trauma life support for the EMT-B and first responder,* ed 2, St Louis, 1996, Mosby.
2. **National Association of Emergency Medical Technicians, Committee on Trauma of the American College of Surgeons:** *PHTLS basic and advanced,* ed 4, St Louis, 1999, Mosby.
3. **New York State DOH EMSP:** *Critical trauma care: a student workbook,* Albany, 1990, Health Research Inc.
4. **Seeley RR, Stephens TD, Tate P:** *Anatomy and physiology,* St Louis, 1992, Mosby.

Chapter 25

Head and Spine Injuries

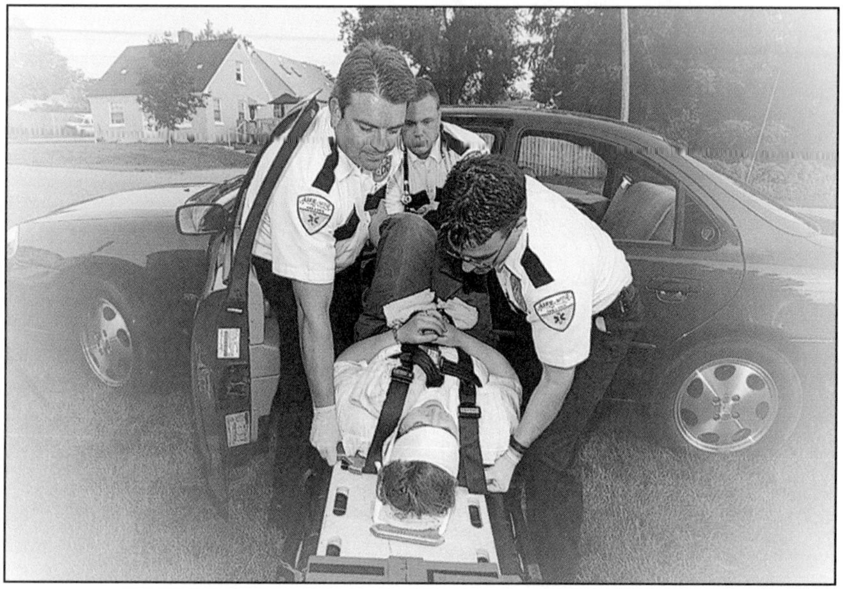

Knowledge Objectives

As an EMT-Basic, you should be able to:

OBJECTIVES

1. Identify and describe the major structures and functions of the nervous system.
2. Describe the relationship between the musculoskeletal system and the nervous system.
3. Describe how the mechanism of injury helps an EMT recognize injuries to the head and spine.
4. Describe complications of improper treatment of head and spinal injuries.
5. List the signs and symptoms of a head injury.
6. List the signs and symptoms of a spinal injury.
7. Describe how to assess a responsive or unresponsive patient with a possible head or spinal injury.
8. Describe the proper techniques for treating airway, breathing, and circulation problems in a patient with a suspected spinal injury.
9. List the indications for immobilizing a patient with a possible head or spinal injury.
10. List the indications for inline stabilization and cervical collar application.
11. Discuss the purpose and use of immobilization devices.
12. Describe how to place and secure a patient with a suspected spinal injury on a long spine board and on a short spine or extrication device.
13. Identify the special considerations for immobilizing a patient with a possible head or spinal injury.
14. List the indications and steps for performing the standing backboarding technique.
15. List the indications and steps for performing a rapid extrication.
16. Identify the circumstances in which a helmet should be removed.
17. Describe the proper technique for removing helmets.
18. Describe special considerations when dealing with a pediatric patient with a possible head or spinal injury.
19. Describe the special considerations when treating a pregnant patient with a possible head or spinal injury.

OBJECTIVES

Skill Objectives

As an EMT-Basic, you should be able to:

1. **Demonstrate how to assess a patient with a suspected head or spinal injury.**
2. **Demonstrate the technique for providing inline stabilization.**
3. **Demonstrate the measurement and application of a cervical collar.**
4. **Demonstrate how to secure a patient to a short spine or extrication device.**
5. **Demonstrate how to place and secure a patient on a long spine board.**
6. **Demonstrate how to perform the standing backboarding technique.**
7. **Demonstrate how to perform a rapid extrication.**
8. **Demonstrate how to remove a helmet.**
9. **Demonstrate how to immobilize a child with a possible head or spinal injury.**
10. **Demonstrate how to complete a patient-care report for a patient with a head or spinal injury.**

Attitude Objectives

As an EMT-Basic, you should be able to:

1. **Serve as a role model for other EMS providers when assessing and caring for patients with possible head or spinal injury.**
2. **Defend the need for immobilizing a patient who does not seem to be injured seriously, but who has a mechanism of injury suggestive of head and spinal injury.**
3. **Defend the rationale for leaving a helmet in place when transporting a patient with a head or spinal injury.**
4. **Advocate the need to take special precautions when treating a pregnant patient with a possible head or spinal injury.**

KEY TERMS

1. **Central Nervous System (CNS):** The brain and the spinal cord; the system that controls body functions.
2. **Cerebrospinal Fluid (CSF):** Clear fluid surrounding the spinal cord and brain that provides nutrients to these tissues and acts as a cushion to protect them from injury.
3. **Inline Stabilization:** Supporting a patient's head and neck in a neutral position in line with the body to prevent further movement and to minimize the chance of further injury to the head or spine.
4. **Log-roll:** A technique used to roll a patient as a unit, often for the purpose of placing the patient on a backboard.
5. **Meninges:** The three layers of protective membranes that cover the brain and spinal cord.
6. **Neurogenic Shock:** Also called *spinal shock.* Widespread dilation of blood vessels caused by a spinal injury that disrupts function of the sympathetic nervous system; presents with a different clinical picture than hypovolemic shock.
7. **Peripheral Nervous System:** The portion of the nervous system outside the central nervous system; connects the brain and spinal cord with all organs and tissues.

IT'S YOUR CALL

You are dispatched to a high school football field for an injured player. Upon arrival, you find a 15-year-old male lying on the field. A coach advises you that the patient was running at full speed when he struck another player head on. He states that the patient's head seemed to drop, so that his chin hit his chest and then he fell to the ground. To prevent further injury, the patient was kept still and his helmet was not removed.

Your partner applies inline stabilization as you begin your assessment, which reveals a chief complaint of headache with numbness and tingling in the arms and legs. The patient is breathing rapidly and shallowly, at about 38 breaths per minute.

What do these signs and symptoms suggest about the patient's condition? What questions should you ask to gather additional pertinent information? What other signs and symptoms might you expect to see?

Head and spinal injuries can result from vehicle collisions, falls, and recreational and sporting activities. These injuries can involve simple bruises to the head or face, or serious conditions such as a skull fracture or bleeding in or around the brain. Failure to recognize and properly care for a head or spinal injury may result in permanent paralysis or death.

You may be the first professional that cares for this patient, and basic care can play a big factor in the patient's outcome. Patients with severe brain or spinal injuries sometimes do not have significant signs and symptoms immediately; they may even refuse care. It is important that you review the mechanism of injury in any trauma situation. If it appears to be serious, maintain a high index of suspicion for potential injuries and try to convince the patient of the need for immobilization and transport for further evaluation.

Reviewing Body Systems

A review of the basic structure and function of the nervous system is helpful to understand the complexity and severity of spinal injuries. Although the nervous system controls actions of all body systems, it is important to understand how the musculoskeletal system integrates with the nervous system.

The Nervous System

The nervous system is the control center for body functions. It consists of two sections. The **central nervous system (CNS)** includes the brain and spinal cord and controls the entire nervous system. The **peripheral nervous system** is made up of all the nerves that connect the CNS to muscles and glands throughout the body (Figure 25-1).

The brain and spinal cord act as the command center for the entire nervous system and directly affect other body systems. Any injury to the brain or spinal cord can affect other body systems, such as the respiratory system. This could result in changes in breathing rate and quality. The brain senses, processes, and responds to every stimulus or change that occurs around the body. The spinal cord is a continuation of the brain and serves as the conduit for transmission of nervous impulses to the nerves in the body. It begins at the base of the brain and passes downward into the spinal canal.

Both the brain and the spinal cord have three protective membrane layers called **meninges.** The outer layer is the dura mater, a thick, tough layer of tissue. The middle layer is the subarachnoid layer and is very loose. The inner layer, the pia mater, is thin and adheres closely to the brain or spinal cord surface (Figure 25-2). The brain and spinal cord are also surrounded and cushioned by a clear, watery substance called **cerebrospinal fluid (CSF).** CSF protects the CNS and provides some nutrients to its tissues.

The peripheral nervous system contains thousands of nerves that sense changes, send messages to the brain, and carry brain responses back to the tissues. There are two general types of nerves in this system: motor and sensory nerves. Sensory nerves carry impulses from the sensory receptors throughout the body back to the CNS to be interpreted by the brain. Motor nerves carry responses back to the muscle or organ. This transmission of nervous impulses and reactions to them, such as pulling the hand away from a hot object, take place in fractions of a second. Injuries to the CNS may affect the ability to transmit and receive impulses between the central and peripheral nervous systems, delaying or eliminating reflexes and responses.

The Musculoskeletal System

The body depends on the combined efforts of the musculoskeletal system and nervous system for movement. The nervous system, especially the CNS, is protected by the skeleton (the skull and spinal column). The skull is made up of numerous fused bones that enclose the brain. A skull injury can result in a brain injury if the skull is compressed into the brain, if the brain is severely shaken, or if the impact causes bleeding inside the skull.

The spinal cord is protected by the vertebrae that form the spinal column. There are 33 bones that make up the spinal column, divided into five regions (Figure 25-3). The first seven vertebrae make up the **cervical spine** at the neck level. Because there is little support for these bones, they are the most commonly injured vertebrae. The next 12 vertebrae make up the **thoracic spine.** With their attachments to the ribs, they make up the thoracic cavity. Injuries to this part of the spine are less common because the vertebrae are supported by the ribs. The **lumbar spine** includes the next five vertebrae. These are commonly injured by improper lifting or direct trauma to the lower back. The next spinal column section is the **sacral spine,** or sacrum, made up of five fused vertebrae in the pelvic area. The **coccyx,** or tailbone, is the bottom of the spine and consists of four fused vertebrae. An injury to any of the vertebrae of the cervical, thoracic, or upper lumbar areas can result in injury to the spinal cord. Sacral and coccyx injuries generally do not result in nerve damage. Specific injuries are discussed later in this chapter.

Injuries to the Head

Head injuries are often the result of some type of trauma. While many can be soft-tissue injuries from bumps, cuts, and bruises, some injuries can damage the skull and the brain. Impact of the head on a windshield can cause an

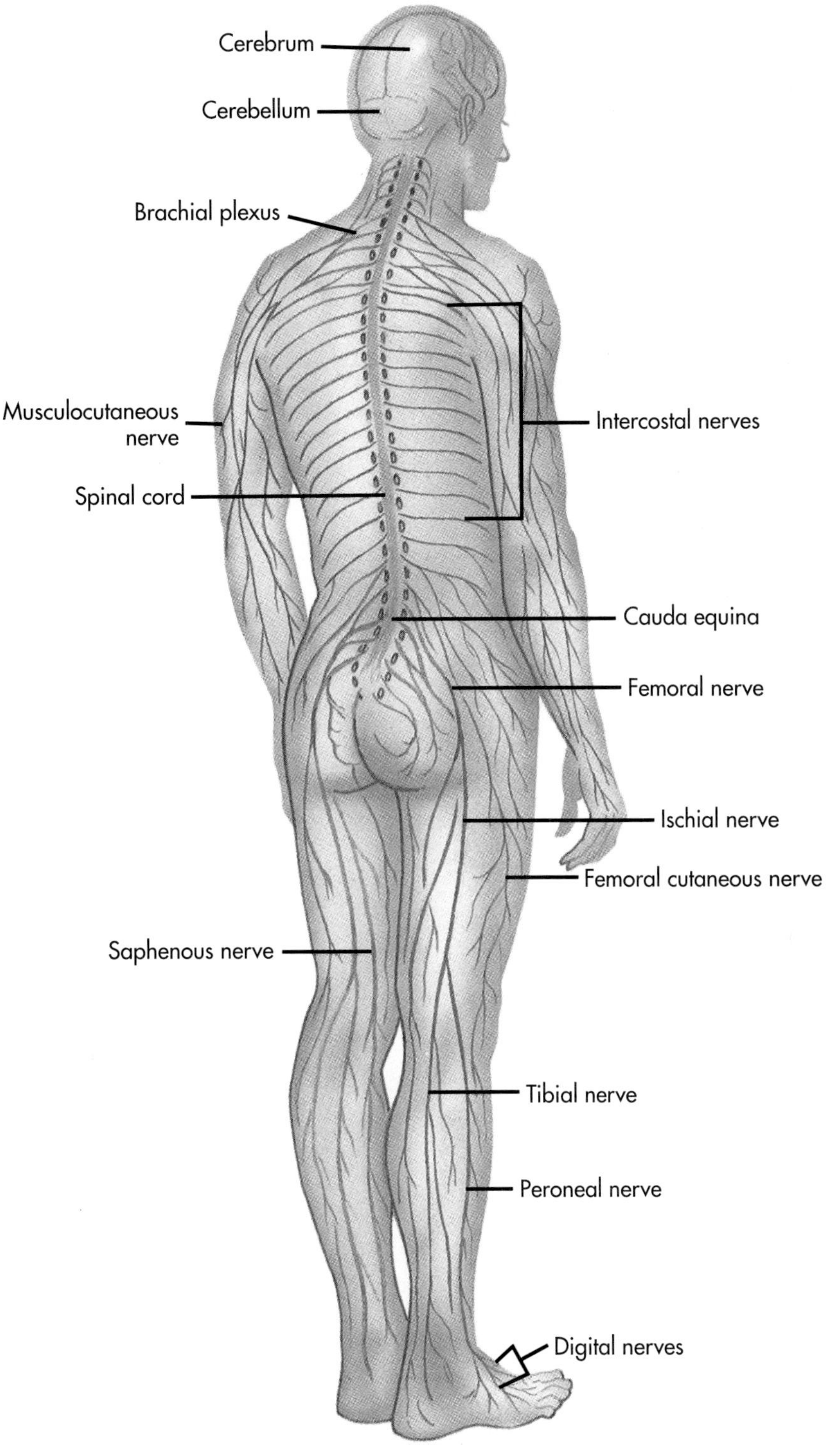

Figure 25-1

The basic components of the central and peripheral nervous systems.

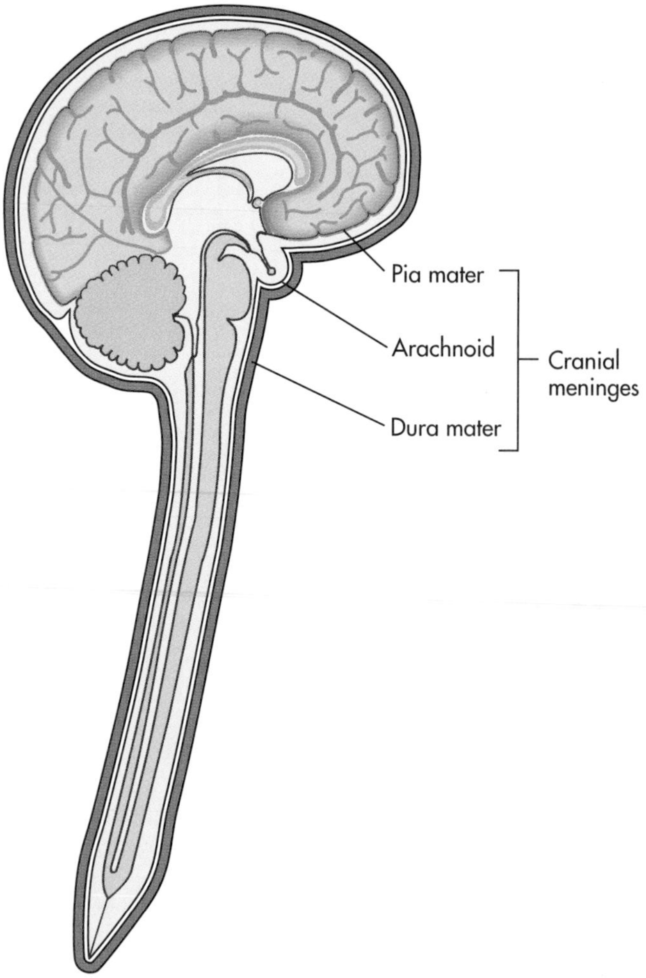

Figure 25-2

Three protective membrane layers protect the brain and spinal cord.

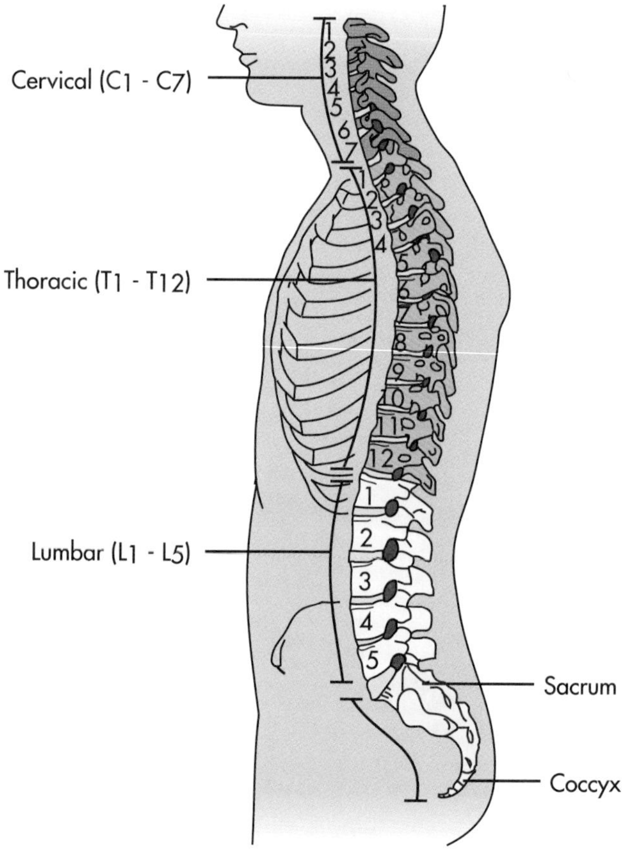

Figure 25-3

Five regions of the spinal column.

open wound, as well as a fractured skull and brain injury. Because it can be difficult to gauge the extent of underlying damage, it is important to consider all head injuries as potentially serious.

Types of Head Injuries

Head injuries range from bleeding cuts on the scalp to fatal brain injuries. Scalp injuries often bleed more than other areas of the body because the scalp is very vascular. However, this bleeding may not be serious and can usually be easily controlled with direct pressure.

Concussion

Concussion is a brain injury caused by blunt trauma that bruises the brain tissue. It causes mild confusion or temporary loss of consciousness. There is usually no permanent nervous system damage.

Intracranial Bleeding

As its name implies, intracranial bleeding is bleeding within the cranial cavity. This occurs when blood vessels in the brain or meninges are cut or torn. Because there is little space between the brain and the skull, any significant bleeding will compress the brain tissue, increase the intracranial pressure, and result in decreased brain function. There are three specific conditions associated with intracranial bleeding:

- Epidural hematoma: When blood accumulates between the skull and dura mater, the patient will often experience a brief loss of consciousness at the time of injury, regain consciousness (called a *lucid interval*), and then lose consciousness again. The onset of signs and symptoms is rapid; deterioration in the level of consciousness (LOC) sometimes occurs within minutes.
- Subdural hematoma: This occurs when blood accumulates beneath the dura mater but outside the brain. This injury often develops more slowly than epidural bleeding; LOC decreases gradually until the patient becomes unresponsive.
- Intracerebral hematoma: This bleeding within the brain itself may develop slowly or rapidly.

Because the skull cannot expand as bleeding increases, pressure on the brain increases; and circulation and oxygenation drop. Surgery is usually required for definitive treatment of these conditions.

Cerebral Edema

Swelling of the brain, commonly called *cerebral edema,* is a serious complication of head injury. When directly injured, the brain swells just as other tissues do. This swelling puts pressure on the brain cells and prevents adequate oxygenation of the brain. If there is an open wound to the head that has penetrated the brain, the brain may expand through this opening. The brain may also expand out of the cranial cavity into the spinal cavity, damaging brain tissue and compressing the spinal cord. Ventilatory support is a critical factor in treating cerebral edema. Hyperventilating the patient with a bag-valve-mask (BVM) helps reduce edema by lowering carbon dioxide levels in the blood; this results in slightly decreasing the blood flow to the brain, which decreases some of the swelling. However, this may also decrease the oxygen that gets to the brain. For this reason, all patients with head injuries must be given supplemental oxygen.

Other Conditions

Nontraumatic disturbances of the brain can result from clots or hemorrhage. These generally result in a stroke (cerebral vascular accident). The signs and symptoms are similar to those of patients with brain trauma, but there is no associated trauma or mechanism of injury. These conditions are discussed in Chapter 16.

Recognizing Head Injuries

A head injury can be present with any kind of trauma. A patient may deny a head injury when there is no pain. The mechanism of injury should raise your index of suspicion. If a person has fallen off a 10-foot ladder and has hit his head, a head injury could be present. If a football player drives his head into the ground, there may be a head or neck injury. Whenever there is a chance of major trauma, look for signs and symptoms of head injury.

Signs and Symptoms

The signs and symptoms of a head injury (Box 25-1) can be obvious or subtle. Disorientation, changes in LOC, and confusion, including repetitive questioning, are possible indicators. CSF present in the nose or ears is a sign of skull fracture. An increase in blood pressure, coupled with

BOX 25-1 Signs and Symptoms of Head Trauma

- Altered or decreasing mental status
- Contusions, lacerations, or hematomas of the scalp
- Skull deformity
- Blood or CSF leaking from the ears or nose
- Irregular breathing
- Soft area or depression upon palpation of the head
- Penetrating object in skull
- Nausea or vomiting
- Discoloration around the eyes (raccoon eyes)
- Discoloration behind the ears (Battle's sign)
- Posturing with extended or flexed extremities
- Unconsciousness

a decrease in pulse rate, is an indication of increasing intracranial pressure, called *Cushing's reflex*. This is generally only seen in unconscious patients as a late sign of a severe head injury. EMTs will often not see this combination of changes in the field and, when they do, should treat it as an immediate life threat. Other indicators of severe head injury include dilation and unresponsiveness to light in one or both pupils, and irregular respirations. Head injury can also trigger neurogenic shock (see p. 509).

It is important to detect the early signs and symptoms of a head injury and provide aggressive care without further compromising any injuries. Remember that any patient with a head injury may also have a serious spinal injury and must be immobilized.

Injuries to the Spine

Injuries to the spine can have very serious consequences. Any injury to the vertebrae may also damage the spinal cord. An injury high in the spinal cord can result in an inability to move from the neck down, called **quadriplegia.** If the spinal injury is very high in the spinal cord, it may also affect the patient's ability to breathe by paralyzing the diaphragm. An injury lower in the spinal cord can result in paralysis below the waist, known as **paraplegia.** These injuries can threaten the patient immediately if respiratory paralysis leads to apnea or if spinal cord and associated nerve damage causes spinal shock. In addition to motor function, sensation may be decreased or totally lost below the level of a spinal cord injury.

These debilitating injuries result in a total change in a person's lifestyle and are associated with other medical conditions such as bladder, bowel, and digestive disorders, as well as a reduced life expectancy. The medical costs associated with the care of these patients are very high and may impose financial hardship on the patient and family.

BOX 25-2 Signs and Symptoms of Spinal Injuries

- Pain or tenderness in the area of injury
- Pain associated with movement
- Pain along the spine, possibly spreading into the extremities
- Deformity of the spine upon palpation
- Soft-tissue bruising or discoloration
- Loss of sensation or paralysis in the upper or lower extremities
- Incontinence
- Persistent erection (priapism)

Types of Spinal Injuries

Spinal injuries result from various forces, including falls, diving accidents, vehicle accidents, and recreational and sporting activities. Some mechanisms cause compression injuries of the spine. Other injuries can cause forceful neck flexion, in which the head moves forward, almost hitting the chest. Excessive extension results in whiplash injuries, commonly seen in motor vehicle collisions. Sudden, extreme rotation and lateral bending, which are often present in sports injuries, can also damage the spine. Distraction injury is a pulling apart of the spine that is commonly seen in hangings.

Recognizing Spinal Injuries

A patient with a spinal injury will often complain of pain or tenderness in the neck or back. A patient with an injury such as a nondisplaced vertebral fracture may not present with any signs and symptoms other than pain. However, this can quickly turn into a serious emergency if movement occurs and displacement of the broken vertebrae damages the spinal cord. Occasionally, a spine-injured patient does not appear to have a serious problem at all. Mechanism of injury should lead you to suspect a spinal injury and cause you to immobilize the patient. Explain this to the patient while you are assessing for injuries. In the event that the patient refuses care, it is important to document your findings and your attempt to treat and transport the patient.

Mechanism of Injury

As an EMT-B, you have to be able to recognize patients with possible or probable spinal injuries, despite the absence of any obvious signs or patient complaints. The mechanism of injury will help. Look for clues such as a broken windshield or bent steering wheel, and check location of impact and other signs that can help determine possible injuries. Maintain a high index of suspicion when any of the following are present:

- Vehicle collisions
- Vehicle-pedestrian collisions
- Falls
- Blunt or penetrating trauma to the head, neck, or torso
- Motorcycle crashes
- Hangings
- Diving accidents and other water-related injuries
- Unconsciousness in trauma patients

In these types of situations, it is better to err on the side of caution and treat for a possible spinal injury than to risk aggravating one by moving a patient without immobilization.

Signs and Symptoms

Some of the signs and symptoms of spinal injury are the same as those for head injuries (see Box 25-1). Others include pain along the spine and any of the following problems below the point of the injury: tingling, loss of sensation, weakness, or inability to move. However, normal sensation, the ability to walk and move extremities, and lack of pain do not rule out the possibility of a serious injury. Box 25-2 provides a detailed list of the signs and symptoms of possible spinal injury.

Assessing for Spinal Injuries

In addition to immediate injury signs, watch for any changes in the patient's condition over time. Do a quick initial assessment to rule out immediate life threats such as respiratory arrest. A more extensive assessment then follows during the physical examination and detailed physical assessment. The ongoing assessment enables you to compare findings over time to determine changes in the patient's condition.

There are several major complications to watch for while assessing a patient with a possible spinal injury:

- Damage to the cervical spine above C3, the third cervical vertebra, may lead to paralysis of breathing muscles—the diaphragm and chest wall. This patient will be in respiratory arrest and will require constant ventilation.
- Spinal cord damage at the levels of C3 to C5 can paralyze chest wall muscles, but typically leaves the diaphragm functional. This patient often presents with exaggerated abdominal breathing motion, but this may not produce sufficient air movement. You may have to ventilate the patient to maintain adequate oxygenation.
- Injury or severing of the spinal cord may result in dilation of the blood vessels below the injury, causing inadequate perfusion and a drop in blood pressure. This **neurogenic shock,** also called *spinal shock,* can occur with severe head injuries as well. The mechanism disrupts nerves in the sympathetic nervous system, which is responsible for most of the normal compensatory reactions to shock. The sympathetic nerve disruption makes the body unable to respond as it normally would by increasing heart rate and constricting peripheral vessels. A spinal shock patient therefore presents with a clinical picture that is very different from hypovolemic shock. Skin is often warm, dry, and flushed below the level of injury. Heart rate may be normal or slow, even though the blood pressure is low.
- Paralysis of muscles or loss of sensation below the level of injury.

Assessing a Responsive Patient

Begin by assessing for any airway, breathing, circulation, or mental status problems. Inspect for contusions, deformities, lacerations, punctures, or swelling. Check for any tenderness or deformity. You may be able to ask questions and get accurate information. Ask the patient:

- How did this happen?
- Does your neck or back hurt?
- Where does it hurt?

Assess movement and sensation in the extremities. To do this, ask the patient to:

- Wiggle the fingers and toes.
- Push the feet against your hands.
- Pull the feet against your hands.
- Squeeze your fingers.
- Tell you which hand or foot you are touching.

Check the extremities together to compare symmetry of strength and movement. If a patient fails to perform any of the assessment adequately, a spinal cord injury is likely.

Assessing an Unresponsive Patient

Assessing for spinal injury in an unresponsive patient involves many of the same steps. The major difference is the patient's inability to answer questions and follow commands. Again, start with a check for airway, breathing, or circulatory emergencies. If the mechanism indicates possible spinal injury, immediately stabilize the head and neck; and maintain that stabilization during the remainder of the assessment. Inspect for contusions, deformities, lacerations, swelling, or puncture wounds. Palpate for any deformities or areas that elicit a pain response. Obtain information from any bystanders regarding what happened, how it happened, and what the patient's condition was before your arrival.

IT'S YOUR CALL CONTINUED

Your patient is a young football player who was injured during a game. The signs and symptoms already present indicate that serious head and spinal injuries are possible. You further assess the likelihood of serious injury by asking whether or not the patient lost consciousness and if he can remember the incident. Because it is clear that this patient's condition is serious, you request an advanced life support (ALS) unit and decide to immobilize him fully.

How would you immobilize this patient? Realizing that the patient is having slight breathing difficulty, you and your partner have also decided to administer oxygen. This requires moving the helmet. What should you consider in deciding whether to take off the helmet? What additional care should you provide?

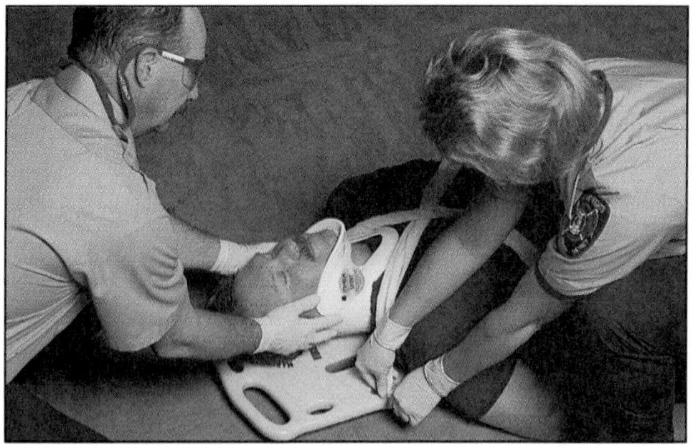

Figure 25-4
Manual stabilization of the head and neck.

Caring for Head and Spinal Injuries

Patients who have spinal pain or tenderness may try to show you where they hurt. It is important to tell patients not to move. When you ask questions, patients may also want to nod or turn their heads as a way of answering, or to look at you. To prevent this, stay in front of your patients whenever possible and give instructions not to move. Staying in front of your patients can help, but you cannot rely only on it and this is why rescuers use their hands to stabilize a patient's head and neck (manual stabilization) and prevent movement that could aggravate injuries. Any patient who has major injuries or is found unconscious for unknown reasons should be suspected to have a head or spinal injury and cared for accordingly. Any injury to the spine can also indicate a head injury, and the opposite is also true. Head and spinal injuries are therefore managed similarly.

Initial Care

Your first care priorities are to manage the patient's airway and breathing and to ensure proper circulation, all while preventing movement of the head and neck. Manually stabilize the head and neck without traction when opening the airway and assessing breathing (Figure 25-4).

Open the airway using the modified jaw-thrust maneuver (see Chapter 11). Check for adequate breathing. Any patient with a head or spinal injury should receive high-concentration oxygen through a nonrebreather mask at 15 liters per minute (lpm).

After securing the airway and ensuring adequate breathing, check that the patient has adequate circulation and is not developing signs of shock. Control any bleeding. Use body substance isolation (BSI) precautions when blood or other body fluids are present. Control bleeding by applying a sterile dressing and pressure. If the injury has caused a soft, depressed area of the skull or has exposed brain tissue, do not apply pressure directly over the wound. Instead, gently apply a dressing and secure it with a bandage (Figure 25-5).

Bleeding from the nose and ears is a possible sign of skull fracture. If a patient with a head injury is bleeding from the ears or nose, do not try to stop the bleeding. Place a gauze pad over the ears or nose to prevent infection and collect blood. CSF, a clear, watery fluid, may also be seen with a skull fracture. If CSF is present, it may separate and form a halolike circle on the gauze pad. Blood and CSF draining from the ears or nose indicate serious injury to bones of the skull. Immobilize the patient immediately and transport.

Immobilization

Immobilization is the stabilization of an injured area to prevent further movement. In head and spinal injuries, this means securing the patient on a long backboard to minimize movement of the head, neck, trunk, and limbs. This is done in five basic steps:

1. Use manual, **inline stabilization** to minimize any movement of the head and neck.
2. Apply a cervical collar to the neck to further reduce movement.
3. Place the patient on a long backboard using a method that maintains spinal stabilization.
4. Secure straps to the backboard to minimize movement of other body areas.
5. After securing the torso to the board, apply a head immobilizer to maintain the head in line with the body.

When you find a patient on the ground, immobilization is usually not a problem. The patient can often be moved easily directly onto a long backboard, using a **log-roll.** In

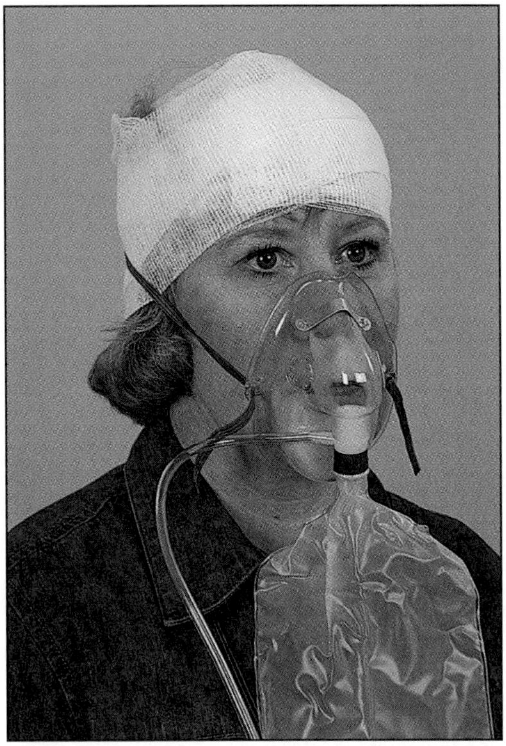

Figure 25-5

Proper bandaging for a head wound. (If the patient had a suspected spinal injury, manual stabilization or a cervical collar would have been used to immobilize the head and neck.)

situations such as those involving extrication from a vehicle or patients who are found sitting up, additional equipment such as a short backboard or extrication device may also be needed. When the patient is sitting behind a steering wheel or is on the floor of a vehicle involved in a rollover, you will not be able to move the patient directly to a long backboard. A shorter device must be used to restrict spinal movement during removal from the vehicle. To become proficient in spinal immobilization, the response crew needs to practice as a team immobilizing patients found in different positions.

Indications for Immobilization

When a patient is complaining of neck pain, has obvious tenderness or deformity of the spine, or complains of loss of movement and sensation, it will be easy to determine that the patient needs to be fully immobilized. In other situations, the mechanism of injury may be the only obvious clue of the potential for injury and the need for immobilization. Patients who have been involved in vehicle collisions—especially those who are in rollovers, are ejected from a vehicle, or have struck the windshield, rearview mirror, or steering column—are at increased risk of spinal injury. Those with altered mental status, who may be under the influence of drugs or alcohol, should be immobilized until they can be more fully assessed at a hospital. Patients with other painful injuries may be distracted from pain in the head or neck; consider immobilizing them as well.

Some EMS systems now use protocols that let field responders decide whether to immobilize a patient when the mechanism of injury does not suggest head or spinal injury. This type of protocol involves a specific set of physical examination items and an effort to ensure that alcohol and drugs are not involved. Research supporting this practice is not extensive, and many systems either do not use it or limit its use to ALS personnel. If you practice in a system that allows EMTs to make this decision, study and follow the protocol closely.

Inline Stabilization

The first step in immobilization is to establish and maintain inline stabilization, which is the maintenance of the head and neck in a neutral position in line with the rest of the body. Manual inline stabilization should be established as soon as patient contact is made and a spinal injury is suspected. If you find the patient with the head slumped forward or to the side, grasp the head and gently move it into a neutral position. Do this only if there is no resistance as you attempt movement and the patient does not complain of severe pain during movement. If the patient is standing or sitting, applying inline stabilization will also

A

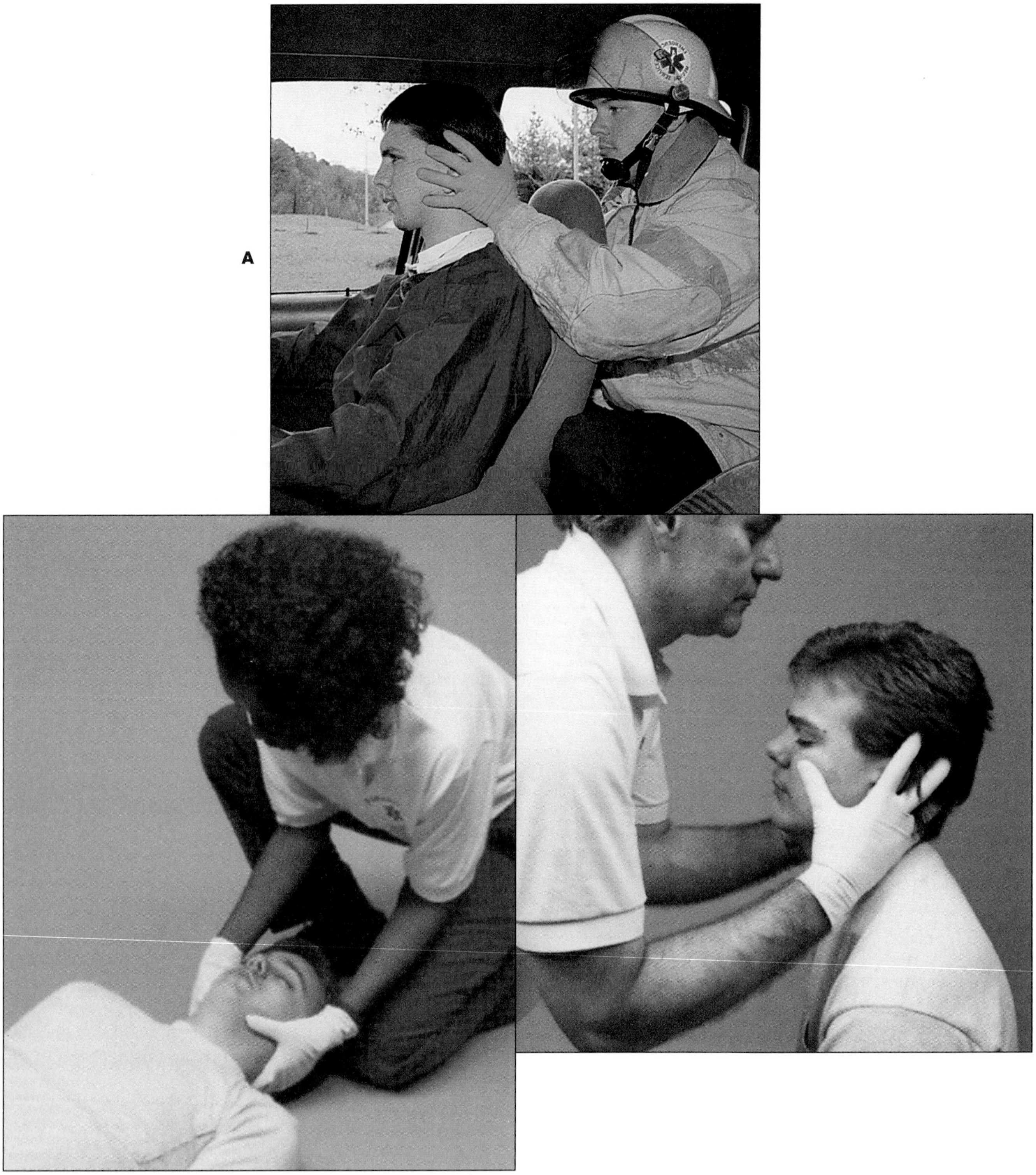

B

C

Figure 25-6

A, The rescuer is positioned behind the patient for sitting in-line immobilization. **B,** Neutral position on a supine patient. **C,** Correct position to hold inline stabilization from the front.

support the head and prevent it from pressing down on the vertebrae, because the supporting muscles around the neck may be weakened by the injury.

To establish inline stabilization for a patient found lying, sitting, or standing:

1. Get into position behind or at the top of the patient's head. Place your hands on either side of the head, with your fingers along the jaw and thumbs above the ears (Figure 25-6, *A*). Be sure to use bony prominences as resting points. Fleshy areas such as the cheeks will allow movement. If your hands are large enough, rest your fingertips or another part of the hand on top of the shoulders to increase stability.
2. Carefully place the patient's head in a neutral position (Figure 25-6, *B*).
3. If you are unable to get behind the patient, or to the top of the head, hold inline stabilization from the front (Figure 25-6, *C*).

Place the head in an inline position unless the patient complains of pain as you begin to move the head or the head is not easily moved into position. Maintain inline stabilization while the cervical collar is placed, and continue it until the torso and head are secured to the backboard. One person should be assigned to maintain stabilization throughout assessment and care, up to this point.

Cervical Collars

Cervical collars were designed to help stabilize the head and neck, minimize movement, and reduce the chance of additional injury. Collars help restrict lateral and forward/backward movement, but they do not completely prevent it. Someone must maintain manual stabilization even after the cervical collar is in place. Both one- and two-piece semirigid collars are in use (Figure 25-7). Soft collars, which have been used in the past, do not provide adequate stabilization and should not be used. It is important to apply the correct size. When properly applied, the cervical collar should:

- Maintain the head in neutral alignment (not cause significant extension or flexion).
- Provide support for the head.
- Do not interfere with airway and breathing.
- Allow the chin to rest securely on a support. If the chin extends beyond the collar, the collar is too small. If the chin can slip inside the collar, the collar is too large.

Collars that look alike may not be equivalent in function. You should know how to measure correct collar size and how to apply the brand of cervical collars your system uses.

To apply a cervical collar:

1. Have another rescuer provide inline stabilization.
2. Measure the collar according to the manufacturer's instructions. This usually means sizing the length of the patient's neck from the angle of the jaw to the trapezius muscle at the base of the neck. This measurement is then compared with landmarks on the collar (Figure 25-8, *A* and *B*).
3. Shape and assemble the collar, if necessary.
4. Apply the collar by holding the chin piece with one hand and sliding it under the patient's neck (Figure 25-8, *C*).
5. While supporting the front, wrap the rest of the collar around the back of the neck and secure it (Figure 25-8, *D*).
6. Continue to maintain inline stabilization.

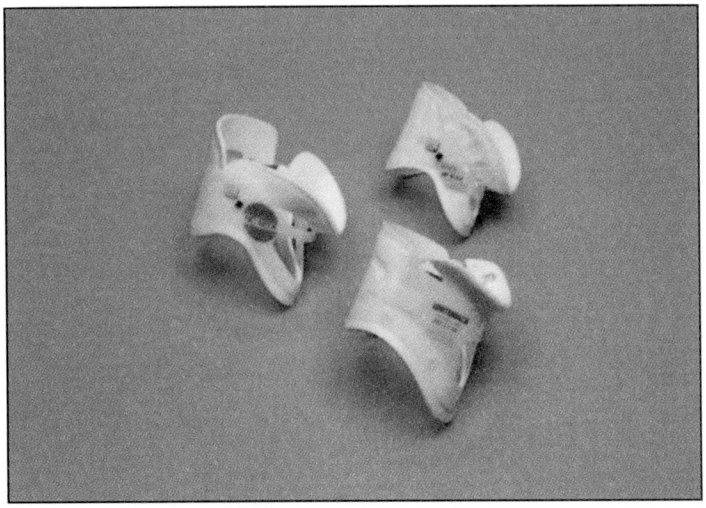

Figure 25-7

Cervical collars come in a variety of sizes.

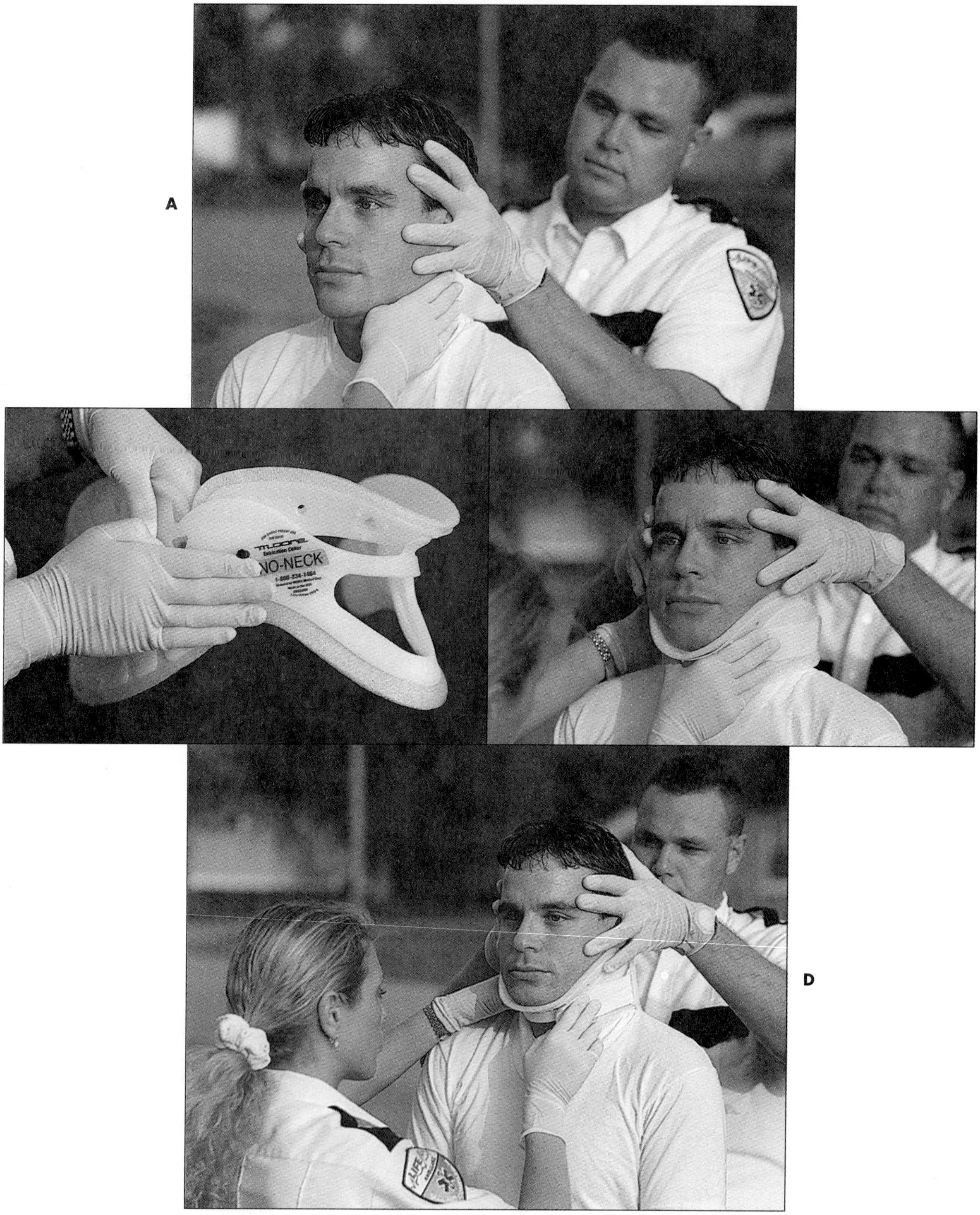

Figure 25-8

A, Use fingers to measure the patient for a cervical collar while maintaining inline stabilization. The collar is usually measured from the angle of the patient's jaw to the trapezius muscle. **B,** Compare the measurement against the collar. **C,** Hold the chin piece with one hand and apply to the front of the patient's neck. **D,** Wrap the rest of the collar around the back of the patient's neck and secure.

Immobilization Devices

Once the cervical collar has been applied, secure the patient to an immobilization device. These are designed to prevent any further movement during transport. If a patient is in a sitting position, initial immobilization should take place in that position. This is done with a short spineboard or an extrication device to immobilize the spine until the patient can be moved onto a full-length immobilization device (long backboard). Many devices and techniques are available, but the objective of immobilization is always to prevent further movement that could worsen the injury.

Short Spine Devices. The purpose of a short spine device is to help immobilize a sitting patient's head and neck and prevent it from twisting or moving while the patient is removed from the location found, usually a car, into a supine position on a long backboard. The original short spine device was known as a *short spineboard,* or *shortboard* (Figure 25-9). The shortboard is still used today but not as frequently as the extrication devices discussed later in this section. It is made of wood with hand holds cut along both sides for attaching straps and lifting the patient. The shortboard is designed to slide behind the patient and to be attached with either cravats or straps. The patient's head is secured to the board using cravats or roller gauze (Figure 25-10). This device is simple to use and slides easily between the patient and older car seats. However, changes in vehicle construction, including seat designs such as bucket seats, can make the rigid shortboard difficult to use.

As an alternative to the short backboard, a new, flexible, vest-type device, called an extrication device, was developed. The first vest-type, short immobilization devices appeared in the early 1980s. The most popular of these devices is the Kendrick Extrication Device, commonly called the *KED* (Figure 25-11). The KED has rigid slabs of wood strategically positioned throughout the vest. The vest is wrapped around the patient's torso and head and secured with straps that are already attached. This device easily fits into the smaller bucket seats found in many vehicles.

The KED is frequently used to extricate patients with possible head or spinal injuries from vehicles. Since it was developed, other similar devices have come onto the market.

To apply a short spine board:

1. Have one EMT maintain manual, inline stabilization throughout the process.
2. Apply a cervical collar.

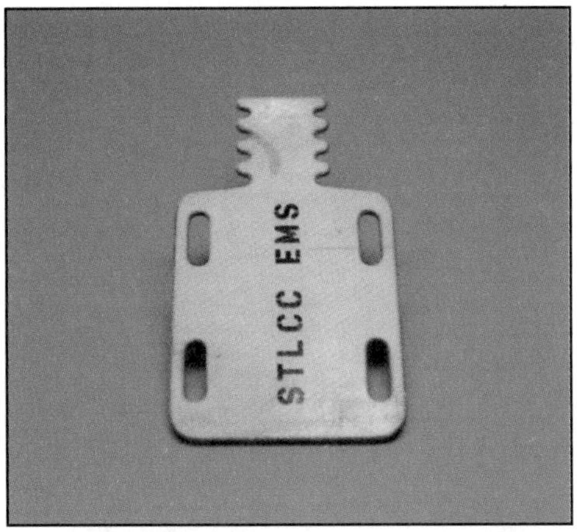

Figure 25-9

A wooden short spineboard.

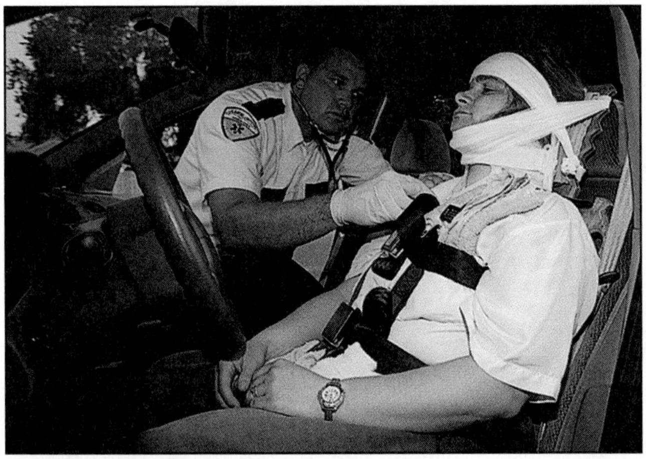

Figure 25-10

Patient secured to a shortboard with straps and cravats.

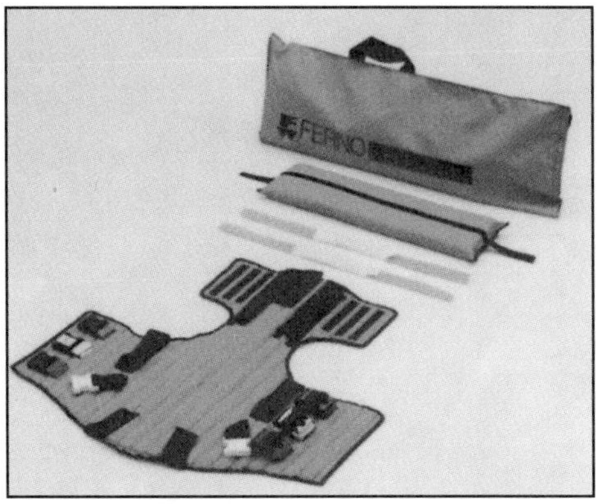

Figure 25-11

Kendrick Extrication Device.

3. Assess carotid pulse (Figure 25-12, *A*), distal pulses, and sensation and motor function of extremities.
4. While supporting the chest and back and maintaining head and neck stabilization, carefully lean the entire patient forward and slide the board behind the back, so that the top of the board is even with the top of the head (Figure 25-12, *B*).
5. Secure the pelvis to the board by wrapping two straps under the patient's thighs and buttocks and crossing them over the pelvis (Figure 25-12, *C*).
6. Secure the torso to the board with several straps.
7. Secure the head to the board using cravats, tape, or roller gauze. Try to bring the board toward the patient so that the patient's head remains in line with the body. If there is still a gap between the patient's head and the board, use a towel to pad this area. Place one cravat across the patient's forehead and tie it at an angle on the side of the board. You can place another cravat beneath the chin piece of the cervical collar for additional support (Figure 25-12, *D*). Tie the chin strap in a quick-release manner, in case of airway problems.
8. Recheck distal pulse, sensation, and motion. Note any changes since the earlier assessment.
9. Lift or slide the patient onto a long backboard. Once on the long board, release the leg straps and gently lower the patient's legs (Figure 25-12, *E*).
10. Secure the patient to the longboard (Figure 25-12, *F*).

A

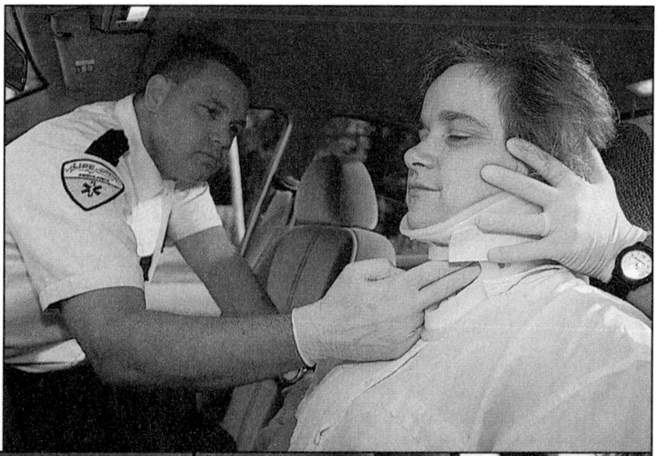

Figure 25-12

A, After the cervical collar is applied, assess the patient's carotid pulse and the extremities' distal pulses, sensation, and motor function. **B,** Lean the patient forward, being careful to maintain inline stabilization, and position the shortboard behind the patient.

B

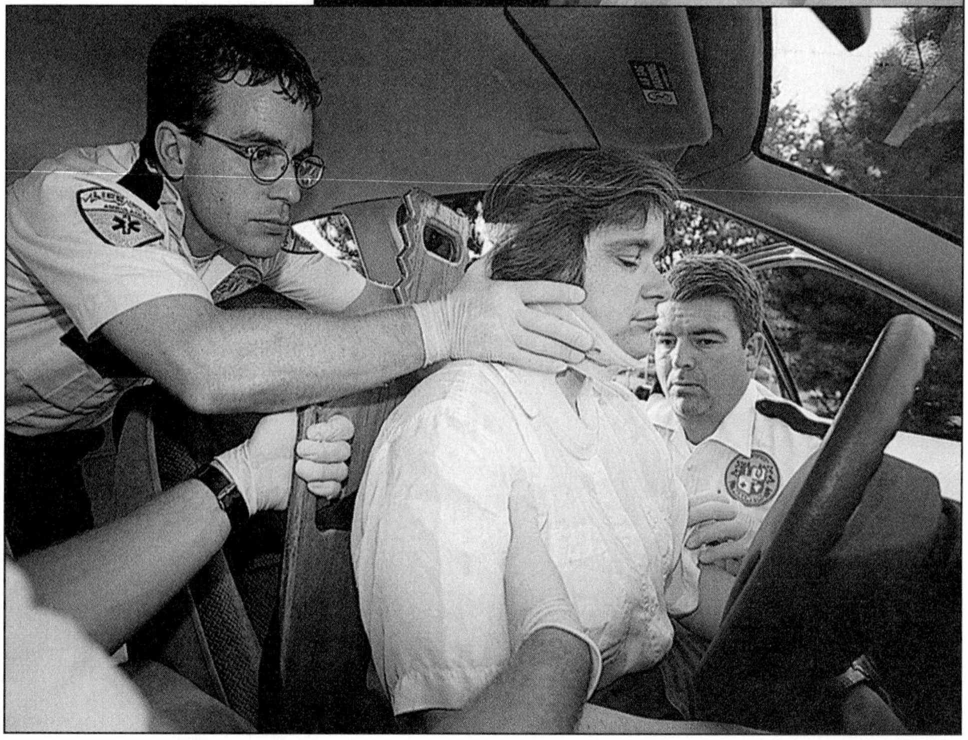

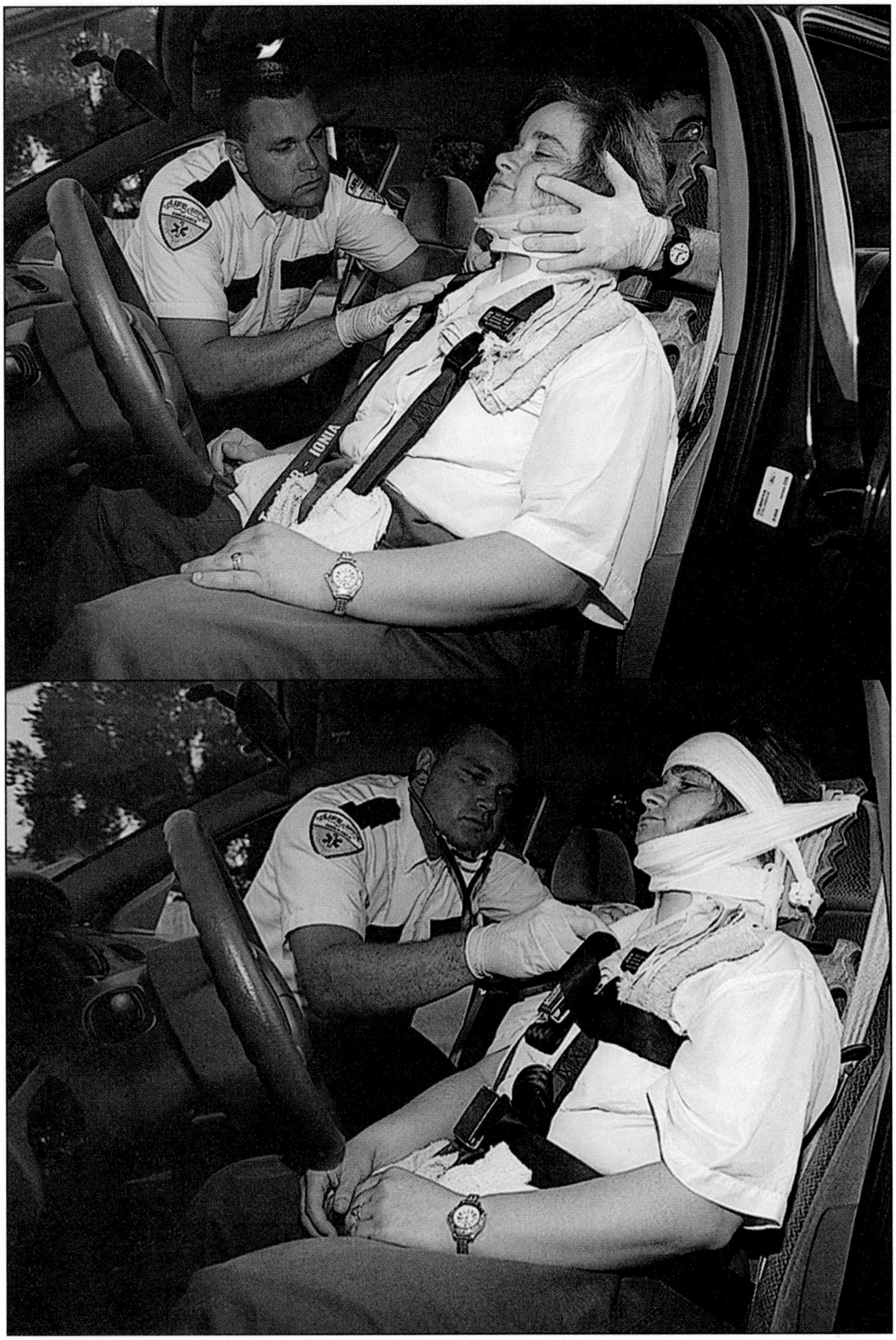

C

D

Figure 25-12, cont'd

C, Secure the patient's pelvis to the board with straps. **D,** If necessary, pad the board to prevent a gap between the patient's head and the board. Secure the patient's head to the board with cravats or roller gauze.

Continued

E

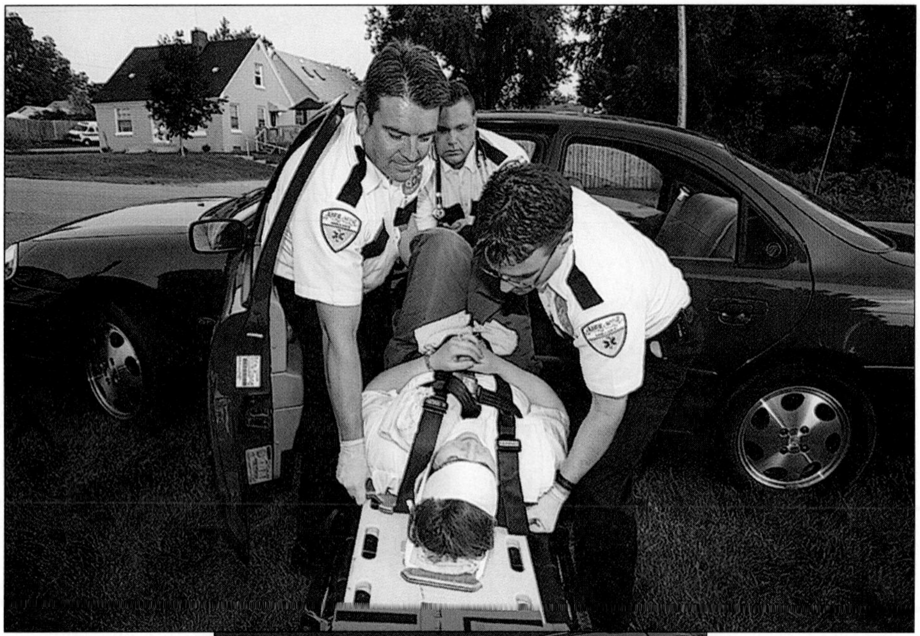

F

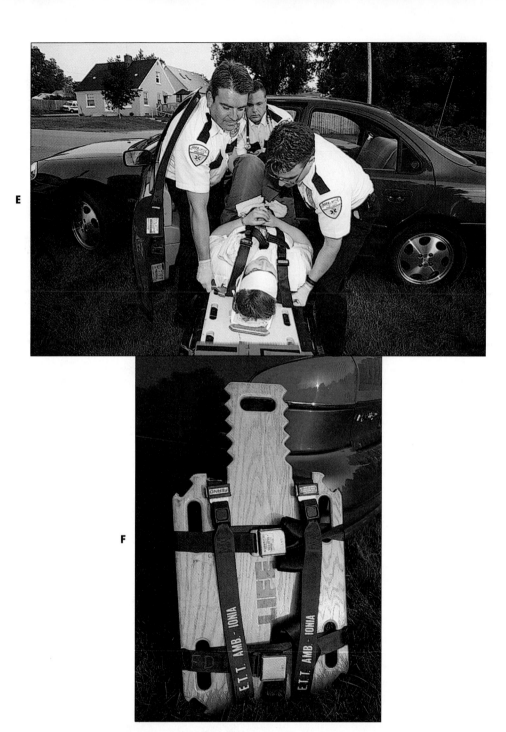

Figure 25-12, cont'd

E, Slide the patient onto a long backboard, releasing the leg straps and lowering the legs after the patient is completely on the longboard. **F,** One common strapping arrangement for the shortboard.

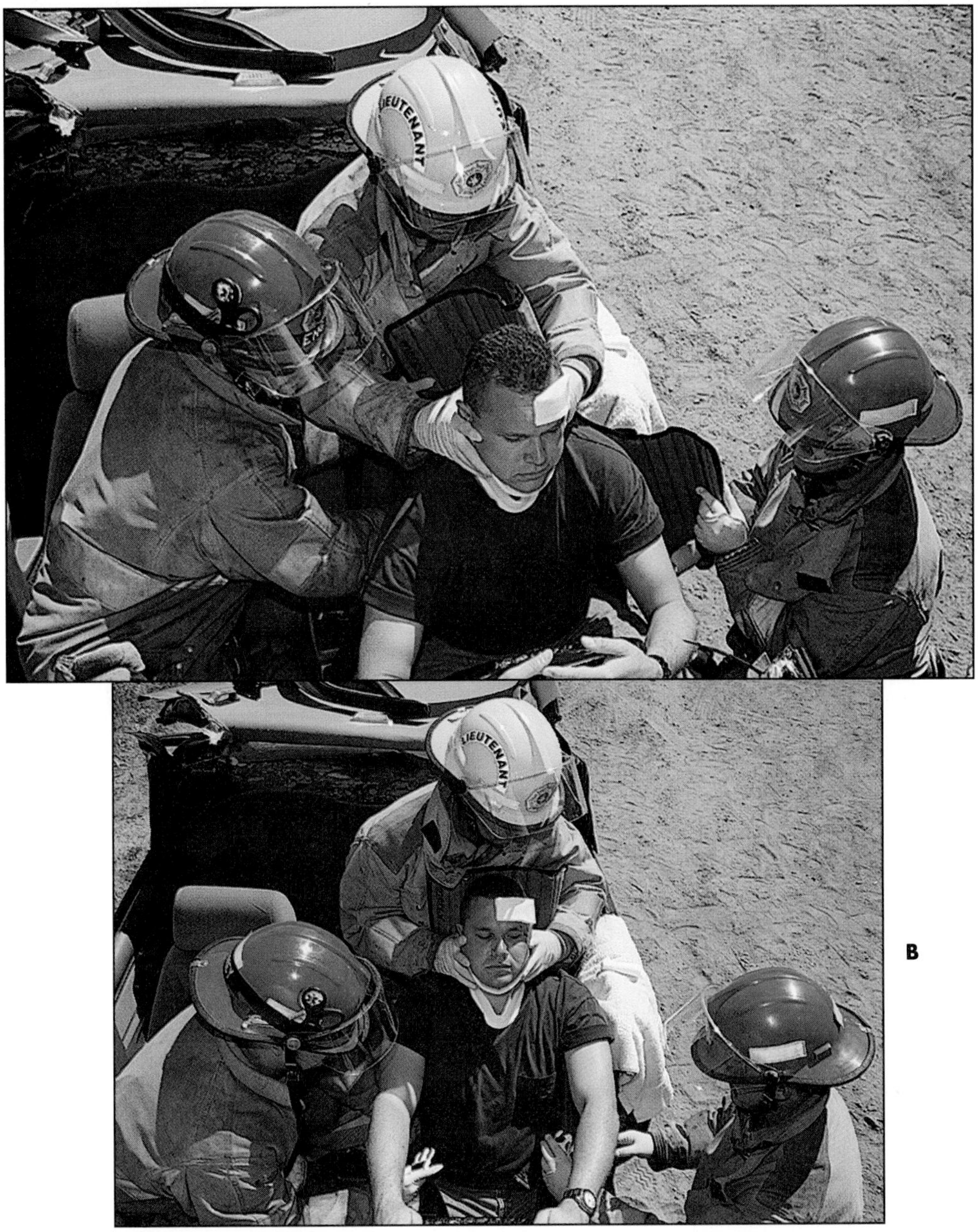

A

B

Figure 25-13

A, Position the KED behind the patient while maintaining inline stabilization. **B,** Move the patient back against the KED and wrap the vest under the patient's armpits.

Continued

There are many common points between the application of the shortboard and an extrication device. To apply a KED:

1. Begin manual, inline stabilization of the head and neck.
2. Apply a cervical collar.
3. Assess the patient's distal pulses, motor function, and sensation.
4. While maintaining inline stabilization, support the chest and back, lean the patient forward, and slide the KED behind the patient so that the top of the device is even with the top of the patient's head. Release the leg straps from the hook-and-loop attachment on the back of the KED (Figure 25-13, *A*).
5. Move the patient back, aligning the spine in a neutral, upright position. Wrap the vest around the patient's chest so that the top of the vest is positioned securely under the patient's armpits (Figure 25-13, *B*).
6. Secure the patient's torso by connecting the three torso straps. Tighten the middle and bottom straps, but keep the top strap loose temporarily (Figure 25-13, *C*).

C

D

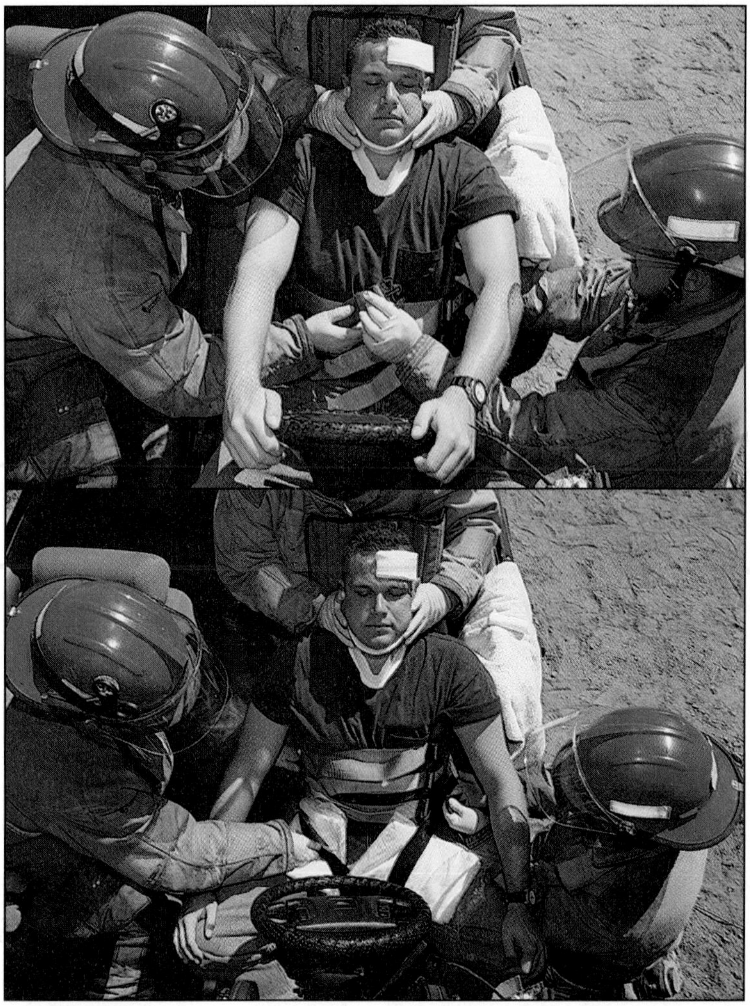

Figure 25-13, cont'd

C, Tighten the middle and bottom torso straps but keep the top torso strap loose initially. **D,** Slide the leg straps under the patient's buttocks, between the patient's legs, and secure them.

7. Slide the leg straps under the patient's buttocks and up between the patient's thighs and buckle the straps (Figure 25-13, *D*).
8. Secure the patient's head to the KED. Bring the back of the KED toward the patient. If there is still a void between the head and the device, fill it with the pad provided or with a towel. Apply the forehead and chin straps (Figure 25-13, *E*). Leave the chin strap on top for quick release, in case of airway trouble.
9. Secure the top torso strap. Have the patient inhale, then tighten the strap. Recheck all of the straps.
10. Reassess distal pulse, sensation, and movement.
11. Lift or slide the patient onto a long backboard (lift the patient, not the KED). Lay the patient down, while supporting the legs in the flexed position. Once on the longboard, release the leg straps and gently lower the legs (Figure 25-13, *F*).
12. Secure the patient to the longboard.

All stable patients found in a sitting position should be immobilized on a short spine device before being transferred to a long backboard. If the patient is not stable, you will not have time to use a short spine device. Use the rapid extrication technique for these situations (see p. 527).

Full Immobilization Devices. Full immobilization is accomplished by placing a patient on a long backboard. Backboards come in different shapes and sizes, and with differences in features such as hand holds, construction materials, and buoyancy. Traditionally, the most common construction material has been wood. Because wood is a porous material that is difficult to disinfect, many EMS agencies now prefer using plastic or fiberglass boards for immobilization.

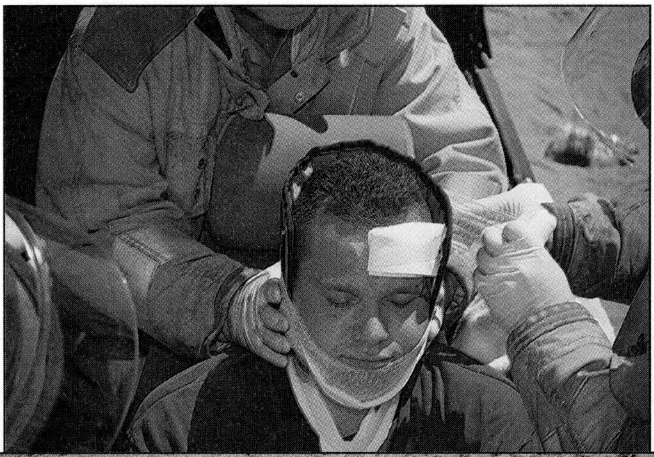

E

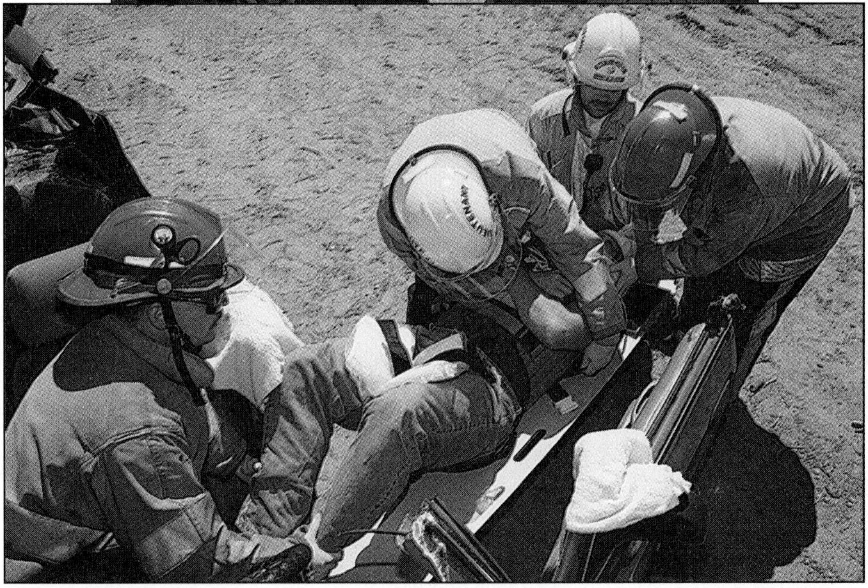

F

Figure 25-13, cont'd

E, Secure the patient's head with forehead and chin straps or roller gauze and cravats.
F, Lift the patient onto a long backboard, supporting the patient's legs in the flexed position. Once the patient is on the longboard, release the leg straps and lower the patient's legs.

The most common method for placing a supine patient on a backboard is the log-roll, a technique used to turn the patient onto the side as a unit while maintaining the head and neck in a neutral position.

To place a supine patient on a backboard:

1. While one rescuer maintains manual, inline stabilization, other rescuers kneel at one side of the patient (Figure 25-14, *A*).
2. Place the board on the opposite side of the patient. Extend the board several inches beyond the top of the head.
3. Rescuers should support the patient by the shoulders, hips, and legs while maintaining inline stabilization. Following the command of the rescuer at the patient's head, roll the patient up on one side. Maintain the head and neck in line with the body during this roll procedure (Figure 25-14, *B*). Have one rescuer do a quick examination of the back of the head, torso, and legs. This is often the only opportunity to check these areas.
4. Move the backboard so that it is positioned against the patient, and roll the patient back onto the board (Figure 25-14, *C*). If the patient is slightly off center, support the shoulders, hips, head, and neck, and slide the patient as needed (Figure 25-14, *D*).
5. Once the patient is on the backboard, maintain inline stabilization of the head and neck and secure the patient to the board.

If it is not possible to log-roll the patient, you may place the patient on a backboard using a scoop stretcher or a four-person lift. Different lifting methods are discussed in Chapter 7.

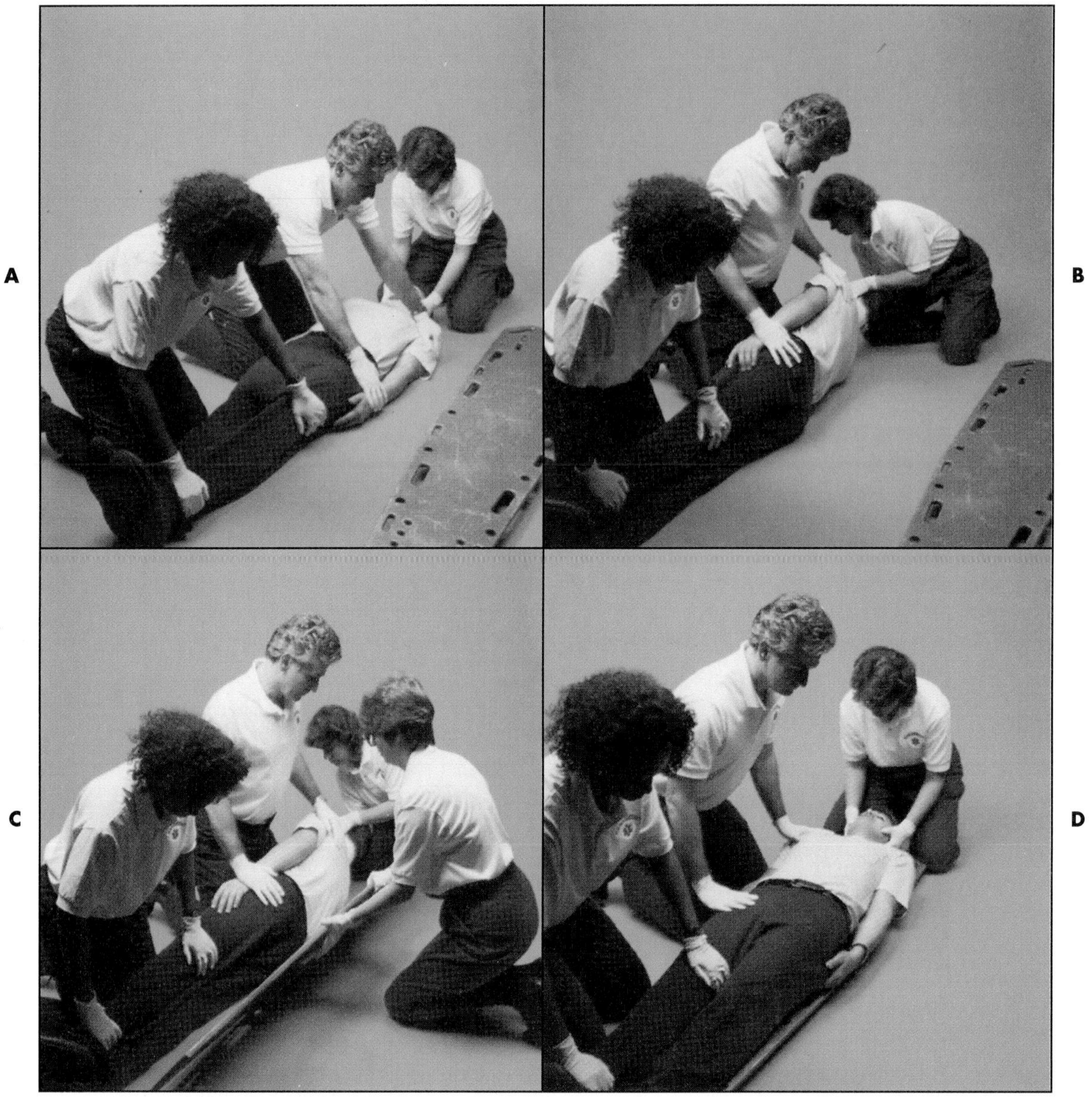

Figure 25-14

A, One rescuer maintains inline stabilization while other rescuers position themselves at the patient's side. **B,** Roll the patient up on one side, taking this opportunity to perform a back sweep. **C,** Move the board up against the patient and roll the patient back, onto the board. **D,** If necessary, longitudinally slide the patient to the center of the board.

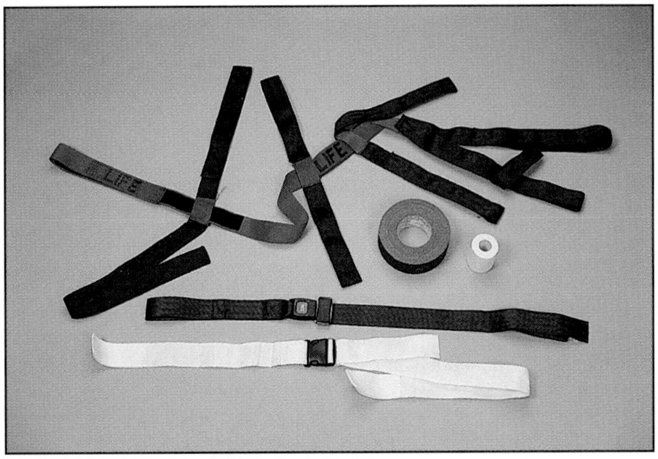

Figure 25-15
Different types of straps.

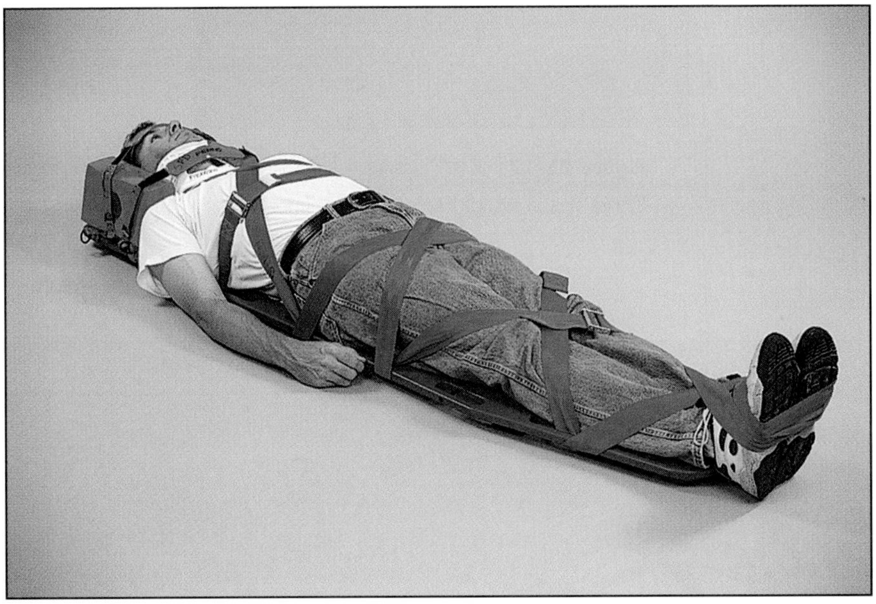

Figure 25-16
If the board will need to be handled in a vertical position, secure the patient's feet with stirrups.

Several different types of straps are available (Figure 25-15). Be familiar with those that you carry. When immobilizing a patient on a back board, straps should be secured across the chest, pelvis, thighs, and lower legs. If you will be moving the patient down stairs or will need to handle the board in a vertical position, also secure the feet with stirrups (Figure 25-16) and support the upper body with an extra strap across the chest and under the armpits.

Several strapping patterns can be used to secure a patient. Among the most common are the following:

- Three or four straps placed straight across the backboard (Figure 25-17).
- The spider strap (Figure 25-18).
- Criss-cross strapping (Figure 25-19).

Once you have secured the torso and legs to the board, you can secure the head. Always secure the body first. If you secure the head first and the patient moves, the body movement will put stress on the neck. Also, this could worsen a spinal injury if you have to roll the board when a patient vomits.

Commercial head immobilizers are available to help secure the head (Figure 25-20). Some of these devices have cushioned blocks to place at the sides of the head, and straps to secure across the head and beneath the chin

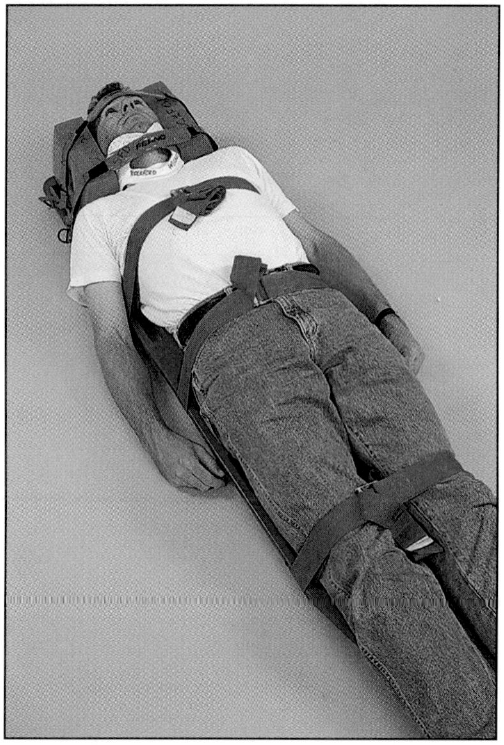

Figure 25-17

Three straps straight across the backboard.

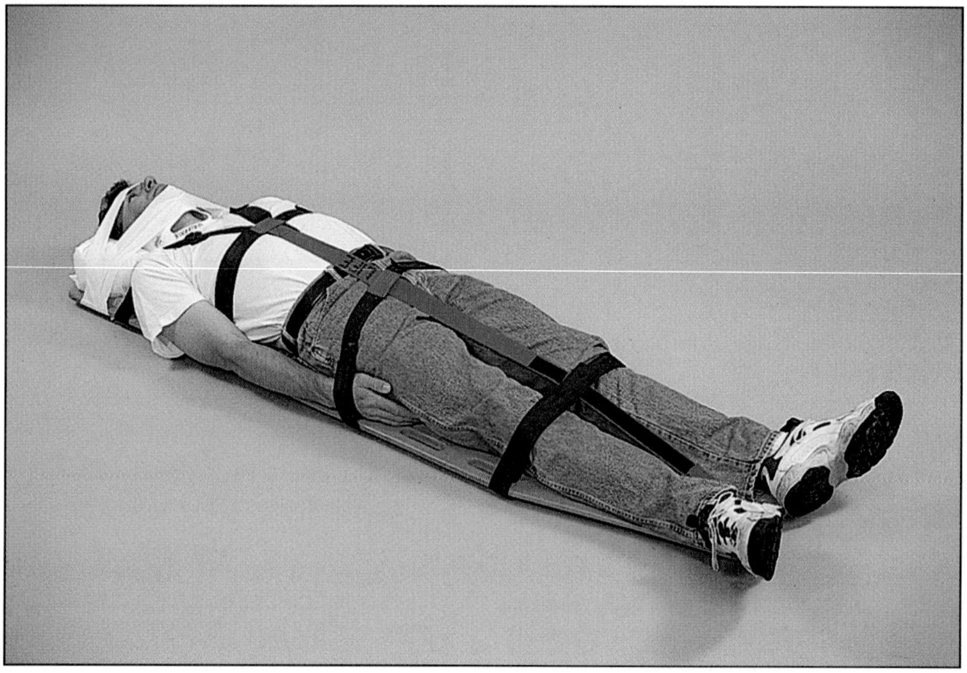

Figure 25-18

Spider strapping.

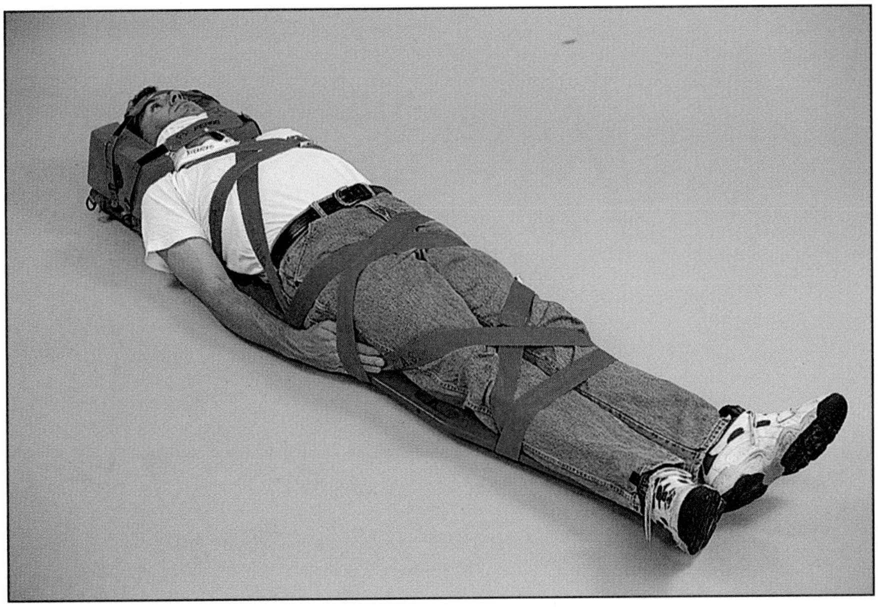

Figure 25-19
Criss-cross strapping.

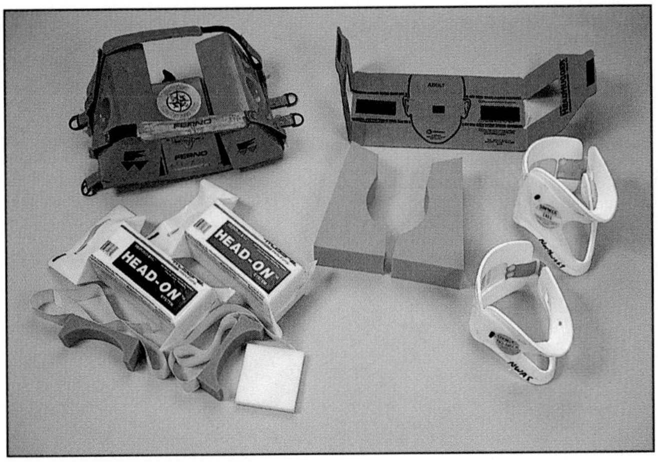

Figure 25-20
Head blocks, cervical collars, and other head immobilization devices.

of the cervical collar; or you may only have the cushioned blocks that you will tape to the backboard. Rolled blankets and towels and even the patient's clothing can be used to pad the sides of the head and help secure it to the backboard. When taping the board, use a wide tape strip across the forehead and over the eyebrows and attach it to the underside of the backboard (Figure 25-21).

In the past, sandbags or other heavy objects have been placed at the sides of the head for immobilization. However, if the patient had to be rolled to the side, the weight could move the head and apply pressure to the neck. Sandbags are no longer recommended.

Special Considerations

In certain situations, you will have to modify the usual immobilization methods. If a patient has an object impaled in the back, immobilize the patient on the side. If a pa-

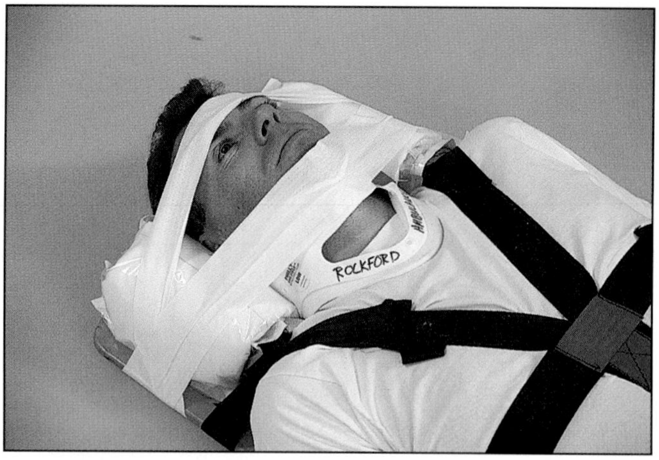

Figure 25-21

Tape across the patient's forehead and over the eyebrows, securing the tape to the underside of the board.

A

B

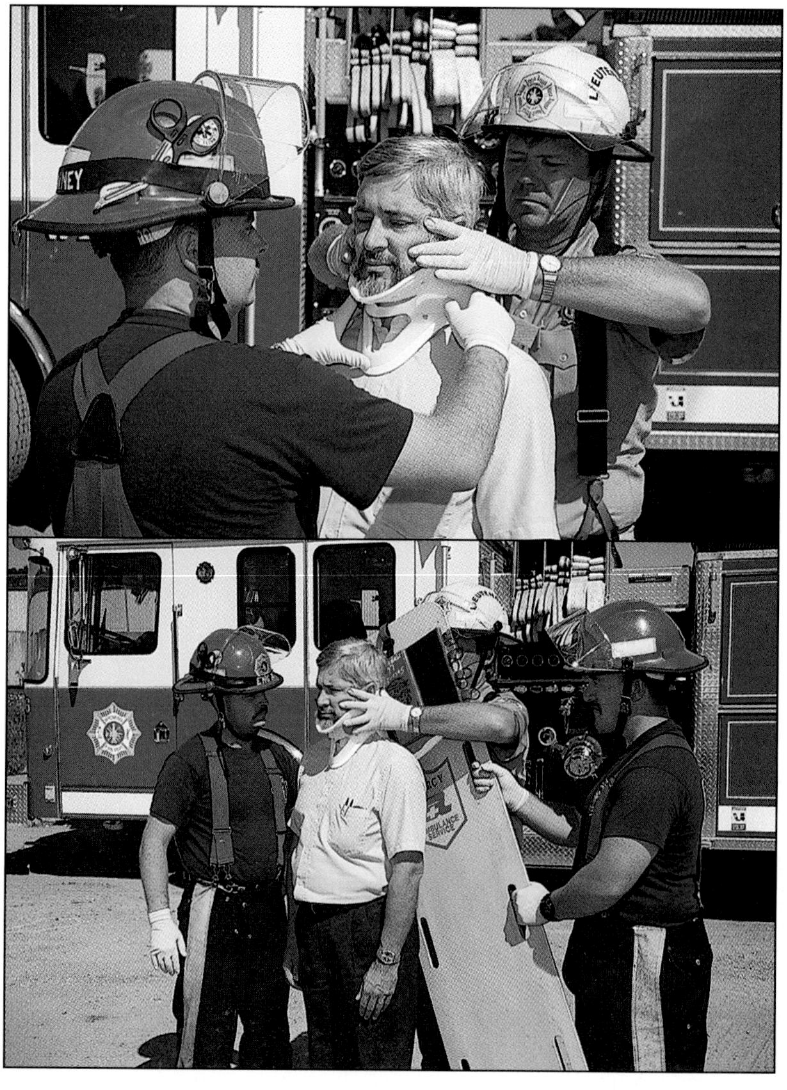

Figure 25-22

A, Apply inline stabilization, while a second EMT applies the cervical collar. **B,** Position the backboard between the patient and the rescuer applying manual stabilization.

C

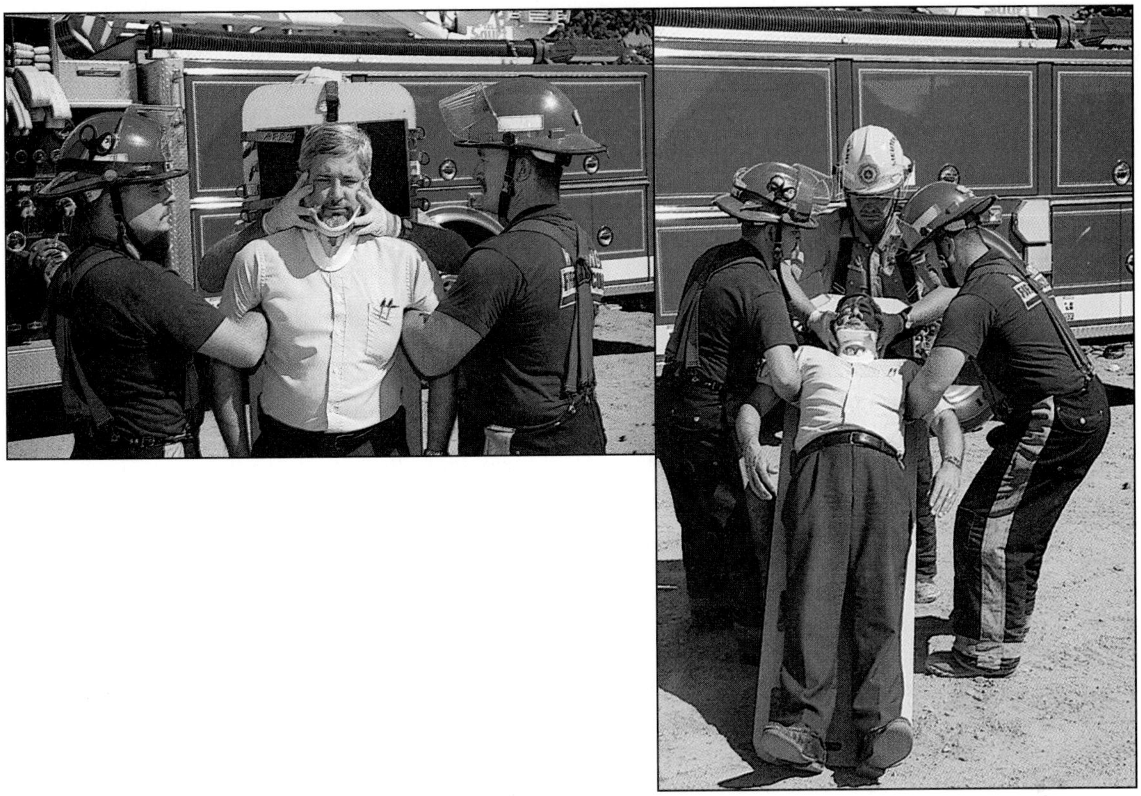

D

Figure 25-22, cont'd

C, With another rescuer, reach under the patient's armpits to grip the backboard on each side. **D,** Lower the backboard, holding the head of the board and the side grip. Maintain inline stabilization throughout the maneuver.

tient is in critical condition, you may need to remove the patient rapidly from the scene, without using devices like short backboards or extrication devices. You may find a person who is standing, complaining of neck pain. This patient must also be immobilized. If an infant or child has been involved in a vehicle collision while in a car seat, you may be able to secure the patient in the car seat and transport. Several techniques exist to help you manage these and other special situations.

Standing Backboarding Technique

The standing backboarding technique was developed to immobilize standing patients. It is not appropriate to ask the patient to move in order to lie down on the backboard. This could worsen existing injuries.

To apply a backboard to a patient who is standing, three EMTs should be available, and follow these steps:

1. One EMT stands behind the patient and applies inline stabilization while another applies a cervical collar (Figure 25-22, *A*).
2. The backboard is placed behind the patient and between the arms of the rescuer applying inline stabilization (Figure 25-22, *B*).
3. Two EMTs stand on opposite sides in front of the patient, facing each other. They reach under the patient's armpits and grasp the hand hold just above the patient's armpits (Figure 25-22, *C*). With their free hands, they grasp the head of the backboard.
4. On command from the EMT at the head, the EMTs at the sides begin to lower the patient and the board by taking one step forward and kneeling on one knee (Figure 25-22, *D*). As this is being done, the EMT at the head rotates his or her hands and arms as the board is being lowered to the ground. Once on the ground, the patient is secured to the backboard as described earlier.

Rapid Extrication

In life-threatening situations, the patient will require rapid removal. Rapid extrication is the rapid removal of a patient from a car with only a cervical collar applied and placement of the patient directly onto a long backboard. This skill is best performed with three or more trained rescuers. Chapter 7 describes rapid extrication. The basic steps are as follows:

- Applying a cervical collar.
- Turning the patient as a unit while one rescuer maintains inline stabilization.

- Extending a long backboard from a stretcher near the vehicle door, onto the edge of the patient's seat.
- Lowering the patient onto the backboard.
- Sliding the patient onto the backboard, securing the patient quickly to the board, and removing patient and board from the vehicle.

Helmet Removal

When responding to sporting events or motorcycle collisions, you may have to care for a helmeted patient with a possible head or spinal injury. The issue of removing the helmet has been a controversial topic among medical experts, and the process differs depending on the type of helmet. Sports helmets are usually open in the front and allow for easy access for managing airway and breathing problems. Some motorcycle helmets, on the other hand, are full-face (covering the jaw) and have a shield.

When caring for a patient wearing a helmet, start by determining whether the patient has any type of airway or breathing problem. Can you can gain access to the airway without removing the helmet? Also see if the helmet seems to fit the patient properly. If it does and you do not need to remove it for airway care, it can be used to help stabilize the head. This works if the helmet is still intact and you can immobilize the patient properly with the helmet in place. It will not work if it leaves a large gap behind the shoulders, which would cause the head and neck to flex when the patient is placed on a backboard. It will also not work if the helmet is loose and allows movement of the head inside the helmet.

The helmet should be left in place if:

- The helmet appears to fit well (there is little or no movement of the patient's head within the helmet).
- The helmet does not interfere with assessment of the airway or breathing and there are no airway or breathing problems.
- Removal of the helmet might cause further injury.
- Proper immobilization may be accomplished with the helmet in place.

Consider removing the helmet if:

- You are unable to assess the patient's airway and breathing.

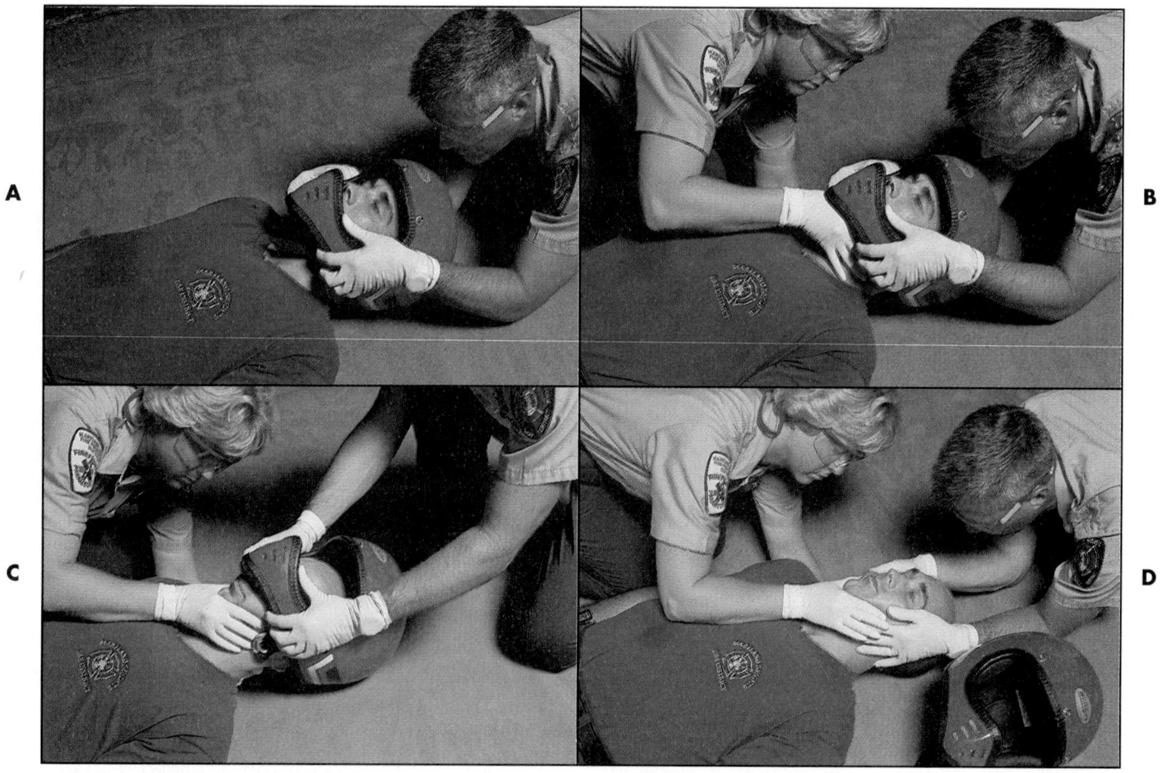

Figure 25-23

A, Kneel at the patient's head and stabilize the head and helmet. **B,** After the chinstrap is removed, slide one hand under the back of the neck and the other on the mandible.
C, While one rescuer slides the helmet halfway over the patient's head, slide the hand supporting the back of the patient's neck upward on the skull to support the patient's head.
D, Remove the helmet completely, maintaining inline stabilization.

- Airway access or breathing management is restricted.
- An improper fit allows for excessive head movement inside the helmet.
- The helmet prevents proper immobilization.
- The patient is in respiratory or cardiac arrest.

If you decide to remove the patient's helmet:

1. One EMT kneels at the head and stabilizes the helmet by placing hands on each side of the helmet, with fingers on the mandible to prevent head movement inside the helmet (Figure 25-23, *A*).
2. A second EMT removes the chin strap and places one hand on the mandible and the other on the back of the neck, as close to the **occiput** as possible (Figure 25-23, *B*).
3. The first EMT pulls the sides of the helmet apart and gently slips the helmet halfway over the patient's head (Figure 25-23, *C*).
4. The second EMT slides his posterior hand upward on the skull to support the head from falling back once the helmet has been removed.
5. The helmet is removed completely (Figure 25-23, *D*) while maintaining inline stabilization.
6. Padding is used to fill spaces under the head or shoulders and compensate for any change in spinal alignment caused by removing the helmet (a football player's shoulder pads are a common example).

This technique should be practiced using different types of helmets. Once the helmet has been removed, inspect it for cracks or other damage.

IT'S YOUR CALL
CONCLUSION

You have completed your assessment of the injured football player and have decided to administer oxygen; however, his helmet includes a cage that covers his face. You consider whether you can remove the cage by removing the screws that hold the cage in place or by using wire cutters to cut the cage away, but no tools are available. You and your partner follow the steps for a two-person helmet removal while minimizing movement of the head and neck. Once it is off, you maintain inline stabilization, ensure that the airway is clear, and administer oxygen. You are unable to apply a cervical collar with the shoulder pads in place. After immobilizing the patient on a backboard, you apply towels around the neck to help stabilize the neck, fill the void behind the head created by the shoulder pads and secure the head with a head immobilization device. You check for helmet damage and find none, information that will be helpful to the physician who will care for this patient.

Some helmets, such as those used in sports like football, hockey, and lacrosse, have cages or shields that can easily be unscrewed and removed, exposing the face. This sometimes makes it unnecessary to remove the helmet. Because these helmets do not have a lower jaw covering, helmet removal is not as complicated as removing a full-face motorcycle helmet. If you must remove a sport-type helmet, the same guidelines apply.

Infants and Children

When dealing with infants and children, the objectives of care are the same. However, you must consider several anatomic differences. The occipital area of the head is proportionately much larger than that of an adult. Placing an infant's or child's head supine will cause the neck to flex, compromising spinal position and possibly occluding the airway (Figure 25-24, *A*). To maintain a neutral posi-

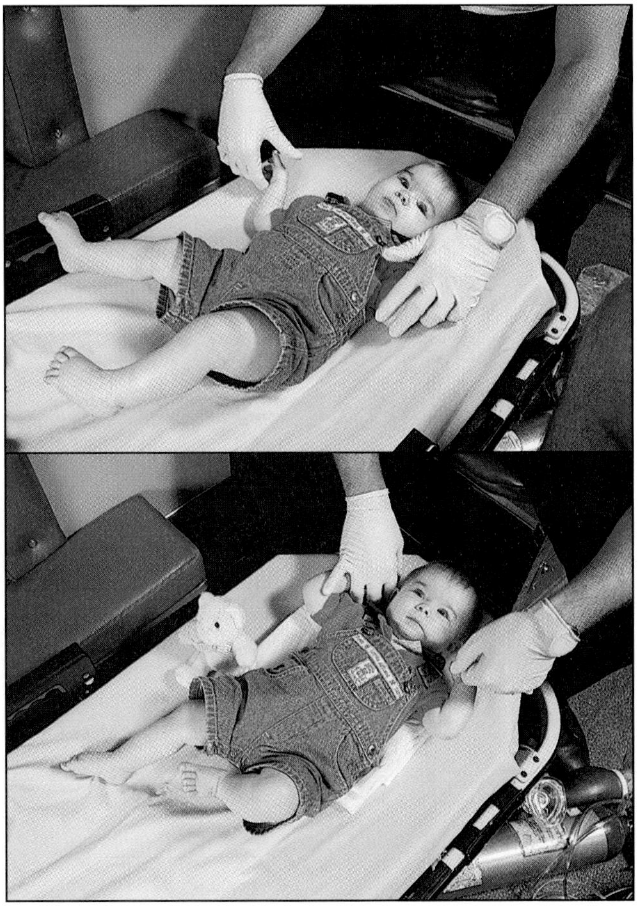

A

B

Figure 25-24

A, A supine child will have neck flexion that may compromise spinal position and occlude the airway. **B,** Placing a towel or pad underneath the upper back or shoulder blades should help to maintain a neutral position.

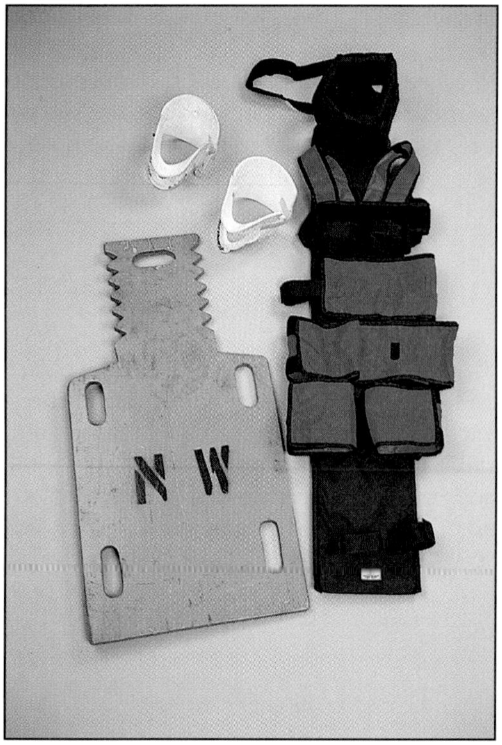

Figure 25-25

Immobilization devices sized or designed for children.

tion, you may need to place a towel underneath the upper back in the area of the shoulder blades (Figure 25-24, *B*). Your ambulance should carry collars and other immobilization equipment in sizes that will work for children (Figure 25-25).

When caring for infants or children in car seats, you may be able to immobilize the patient in that seat if the child does not appear to be seriously injured. This will often work if the seat is intact, you can gain access to and assess the patient, and you can transport the car seat to the hospital. To immobilize a child in a car seat:

1. Leave the car seat restraint in place if it is not damaged and does not interfere with assessment and immobilization.
2. Apply inline stabilization (Figure 25-26, *A*).
3. Apply a cervical collar if practical (Figure 25-26, *B*). Collars are impractical in some infants and small children because they do not fit well. In this case, you may also be able to use a towel roll in place of a cervical collar to stabilize the neck (Figure 25-26, *C*). Maintain manual, inline stabilization and secure the head in this position using a head immobilization device.
4. Immobilize the patient in the car seat by placing folded or rolled towels on the patient's lap and chest and next to the patient's head and securing these in place with tape (Figure 25-26, *D*).

A

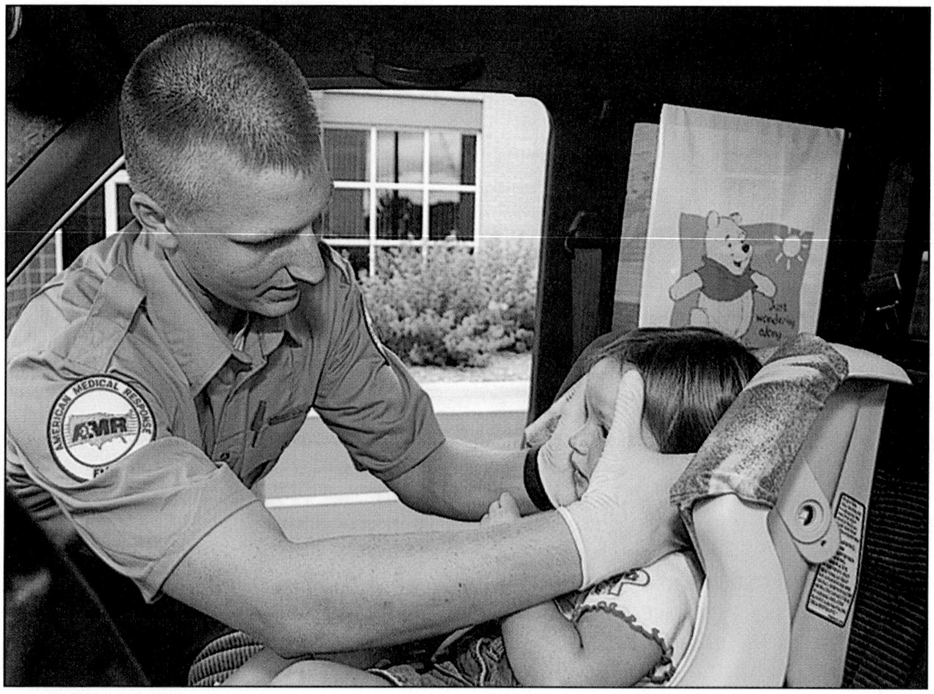

Figure 25-26

A, Applying inline stabilization to a child in a car seat. **B,** Use a cervical collar if the fit is appropriate. **C,** If a cervical collar will not fit properly, use folded and rolled towels to stabilize the head and neck. **D,** Secure the child in the car seat with tape.

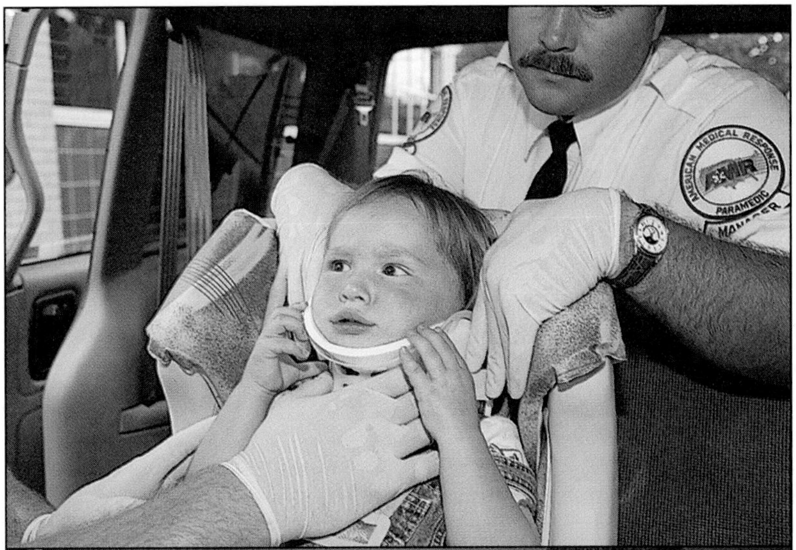

B

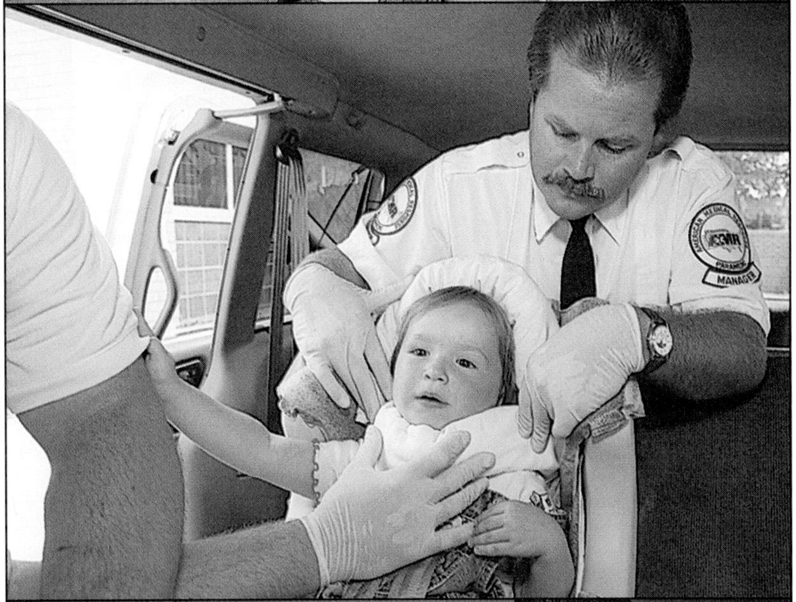

C

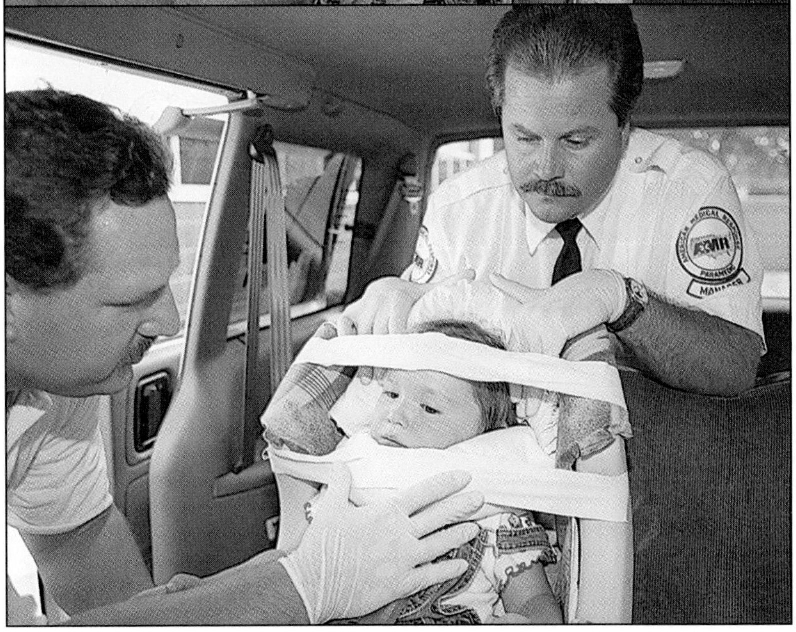

D

Figure 25-26, cont'd

For legend see opposite page.

For more seriously injured children, consider immobilizing on a backboard. This will also be necessary if the patient was riding in a child seat that was built into the vehicle.

Spinal Injury During Pregnancy

When you care for a pregnant patient, you are also caring for the developing fetus. Placing a pregnant patient who is in the third trimester of pregnancy supine may cause a drop in blood pressure **(supine hypotension).** This can be avoided, after immobilizing the mother on a backboard, by tilting the backboard approximately 30 degrees to the left. Use blankets and pillows to prop the board.

When using a KED on a patient in the late stages of pregnancy, it will probably not wrap completely around the patient's abdomen. Place the straps as you normally would, but do not make the strap tight around the patient's abdomen.

SUMMARY

This chapter discussed the recognition and care of possible head and spinal injuries. Your actions when managing a spinal injury can greatly affect the patient's outcome. When in doubt, it is better to assume that the patient has a head or neck injury. When caring for a possible head or spinal injury, begin by assessing the airway, breathing, and circulation as usual. Further assessment may reveal abnormalities in motor or sensory function. The presence of CSF in the nose or ears is a sign of serious head and possibly spinal trauma.

Proper inline stabilization and immobilization techniques are critical to the care of patients with head and spinal injuries. When immobilizing the spine, focus on the overall objective of immobilization rather than on a specific technique. You need to feel comfortable with different techniques to adapt to different situations. This requires practice with other EMS personnel. Any patient with a head or spinal injury can benefit from the administration of oxygen.

Various techniques were presented in this chapter that can help you care for patients in simple and complex situations. Techniques such as rapid extrication have been developed to help expedite the care of critical patients, but should not be used routinely. Caring for pregnant trauma patients and pediatric patients also requires special considerations.

SUGGESTED READINGS

1. **Eichelberger MR:** Pediatric trauma prevention, acute care, rehabilitation, St Louis, 1993, Mosby.
2. **National Association of Emergency Medical Technicians:** *PHTLS-basic and advanced pre-hospital trauma life support,* St Louis, 1994, Mosby.
3. **New York State DOH EMS Program:** *Critical trauma care,* Albany, 1990, Health Education Services.
4. **Ruge JR et al:** Pediatric spinal injury: the very young, *J Neurosurg* Jan:25, 1988.
5. **Suter R, Tighe T:** Thoraco-lumbar spinal instability during variations of the log-roll maneuver, *Prehosp Disaster Med* 5(3):306, 1990.

Section 8

Pediatric Emergencies

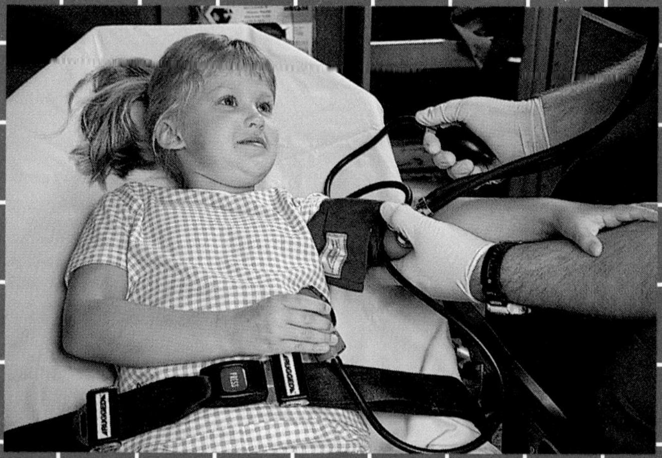

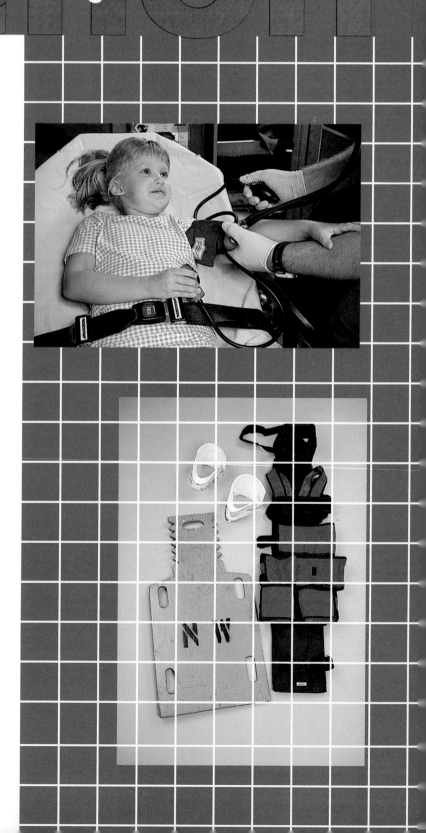

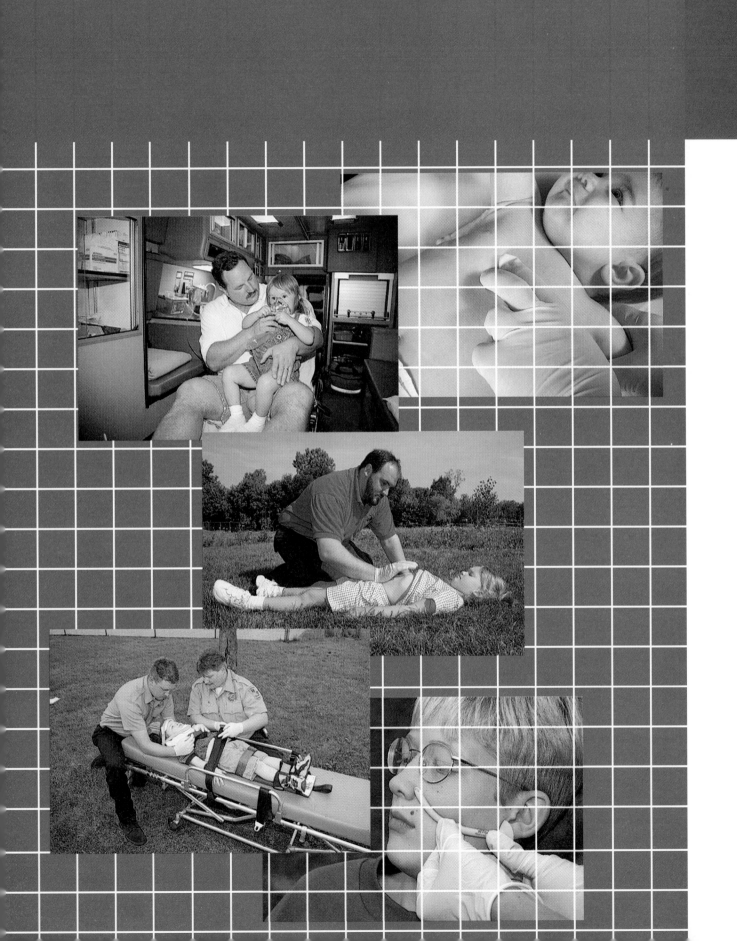
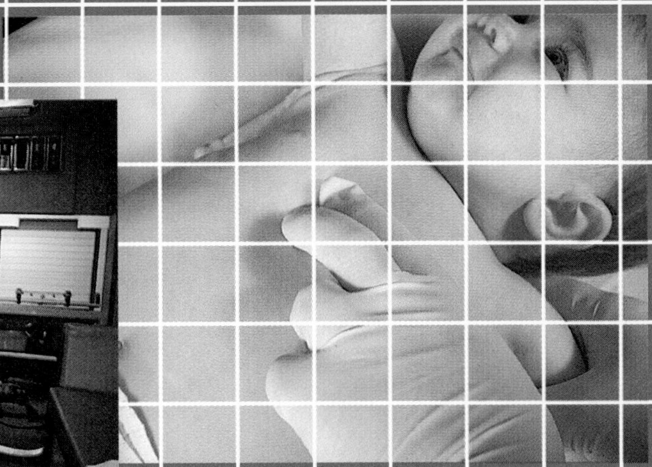
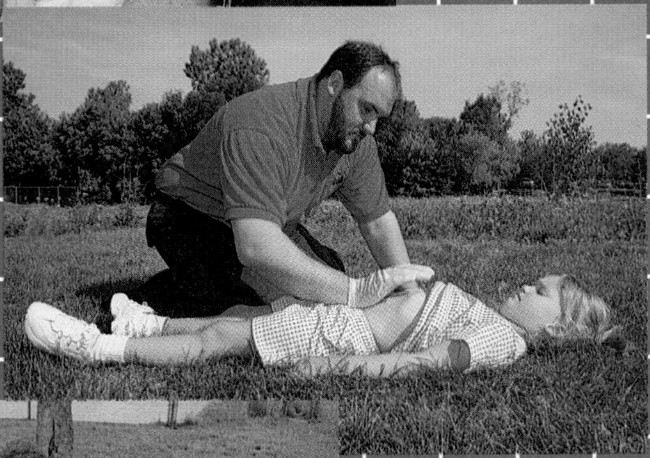
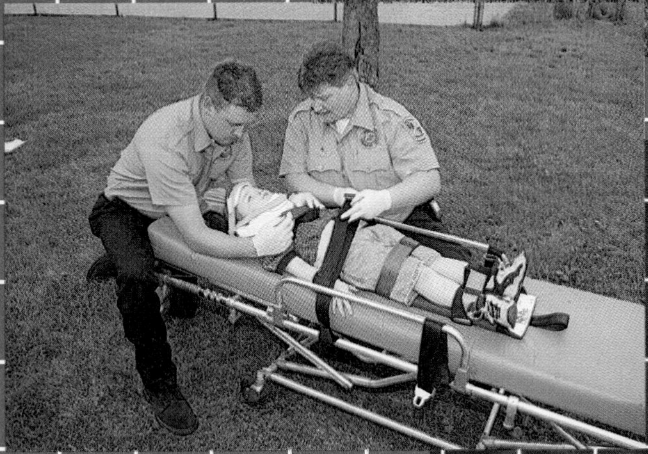
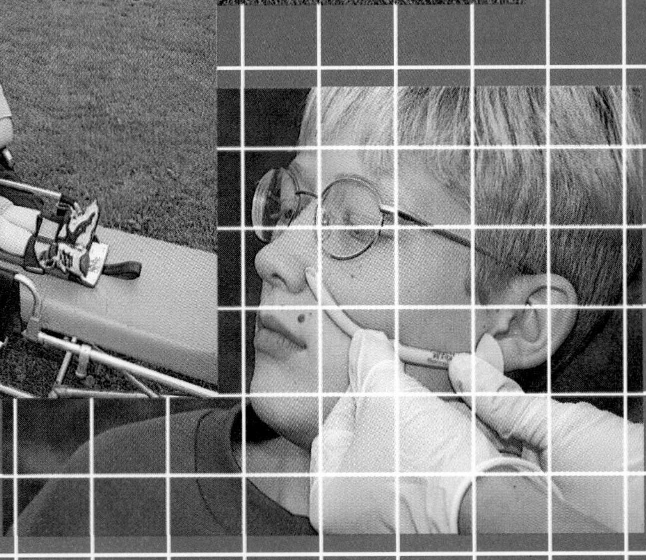

Chapter 26

Caring for Pediatric Patients

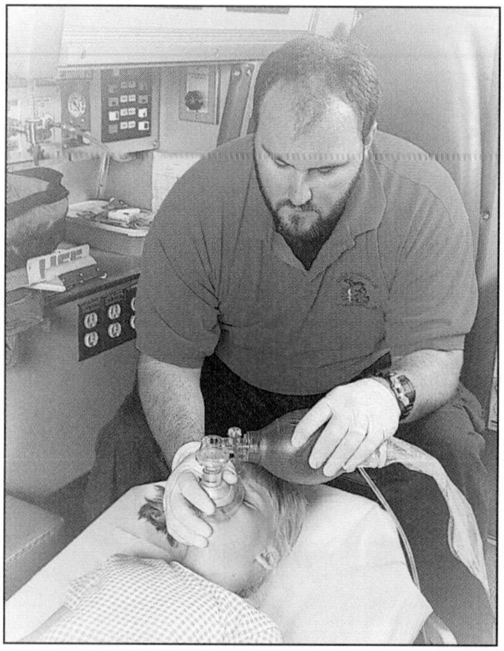

Knowledge Objectives

As an EMT-Basic, you should be able to:

OBJECTIVES

1. Describe the developmental stages of the following age groups:
   - Infant
   - Toddler
   - Preschool
   - School-age
   - Adolescent
2. Describe anatomic and physiologic differences between an adult and a pediatric patient.
3. Explain the differences between the response of an ill or injured pediatric patient and that of an adult.
4. Describe how to assess conscious and unconscious pediatric patients.
5. Identify various causes of respiratory emergencies in pediatric patients.
6. Describe how to care for a foreign body airway obstruction in pediatric patients.
7. Differentiate between respiratory distress and respiratory arrest in pediatric patients.
8. Describe how to care for respiratory distress and respiratory arrest in pediatric patients.
9. Identify signs and symptoms of shock in pediatric patients.
10. Describe methods of evaluating perfusion in pediatric patients.
11. Explain the differences between the usual causes of cardiac arrest in pediatric patients and those in adults.
12. List the common causes of seizures in pediatric patients.
13. Describe how to care for seizing pediatric patients.
14. Discuss the differences between the common injury patterns in pediatric patients and those in adults.
15. Discuss how to care for pediatric trauma patients.
16. Discuss indicators of possible child abuse and neglect.
17. Describe legal responsibilities of prehospital personnel in suspected child abuse and neglect.
18. Recognize the possible need for debriefing after a difficult response involving a pediatric patient.

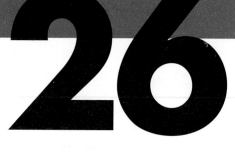

OBJECTIVES

Skill Objectives

As an EMT-Basic, you should be able to:

1. **Demonstrate how to clear foreign body airway obstructions in both infants and children.**
2. **Demonstrate how to assess a pediatric patient.**
3. **Demonstrate how to use a bag-valve-mask (BVM) to ventilate a pediatric patient.**
4. **Demonstrate how to administer supplemental oxygen to a pediatric patient.**
5. **Demonstrate how to complete a patient-care report for a pediatric patient.**

Attitude Objectives

As an EMT-Basic, you should be able to:

1. **Appreciate the feelings of family members who are involved with an ill or injured pediatric patient.**
2. **Serve as a positive role model for other EMS personnel when assessing and caring for a pediatric patient.**
3. **Value the use of debriefing after a stressful call involving a pediatric patient.**

KEY TERMS

1. **Adolescent:** A young person 12 to 18 years of age.
2. **Child Abuse:** Physical, emotional, or sexual mistreatment that causes harm to an infant or child.
3. **Infant:** A baby between birth and 1 year of age.
4. **Neglect:** Failure to provide for the essential needs of an infant or child, such as food, shelter, clothing, cleanliness, supervision, and emotional support.
5. **Newborn:** A baby between birth and 1 month of age; also called a *neonate*.
6. **Preschooler:** A child 3 to 6 years of age.
7. **School-age Child:** A child 6 to 12 years of age.
8. **Sudden Infant Death Syndrome (SIDS):** The sudden, unexpected death of an otherwise healthy infant that occurs during sleep for an unknown reason; also called *crib death*.
9. **Toddler:** A child 1 to 3 years of age.

IT'S YOUR CALL

You respond at 1:00 AM to a report of a child in respiratory distress. You are met at the door by the child's father, who appears nervous as he states that his son is having a hard time breathing. As you enter the house, you hear what sounds like a barking seal. You are escorted to the family room, where the child is seated on his mother's lap. She states that he has had a respiratory infection and a low fever for several days. He went to bed at 8:00 PM without any indication of a problem, but awoke making "funny sounds" as he coughed, and seemed to be struggling slightly to breathe.

You prepare to assess this 2-year-old. What developmental characteristics should you be aware of? How should you conduct the assessment? How would you care for this patient? What do you believe the child's problem is?

Pediatric patients differ from adults both anatomically and physiologically. They also have developmental characteristics that make them different from one another as they grow, progressing through defined stages of development from infancy to adolescence. Because of these differences, EMS educators have been stressing for years that kids are not just small adults. Assessing and caring for a pediatric patient requires you to understand how the developmental stages and differences can affect your assessment. Because EMTs only see pediatric patients in approximately 10% of their calls, a critically ill or injured child can pose a challenge to even the most seasoned responder.

This chapter presents the developmental stages of pediatric patients and the steps involved in assessing and caring for life-threatening conditions. You will also learn about the most common medical and traumatic emergencies among pediatric patients. Finally, you will learn how to recognize **child abuse** and **neglect,** serious problems that involve more than 1 million children each year.

Developmental Stages

The term *pediatrics* refers to six general age classifications (Box 26-1). Each of these stages reflects changes in a child's development: anatomically, physiologically, mentally, and emotionally. Your knowledge of these developmental stages can help you understand the normal and abnormal responses that a pediatric patient may have to injury or illness. Although the following descriptions are precisely defined by age, individual patients will not always fit them exactly. Approach each child as an individual, and use these categories as general guidelines only.

Newborns and Infants

A **newborn,** also called a *neonate,* is a baby from birth to 1 month of age. Technically, an **infant** is a baby between 1 and 12 months old, although the term is often used to describe the entire first year of life, including the first month. Infant and newborn emergencies are usually related to problems that were present at birth, such as prematurity and birth defects.

Although newborns and infants often have little anxiety when confronted by strangers, they do not like to be separated from their parents. Because they are used to being undressed, they will not usually object to this, but they do not like to be cold. Keep them warm; if using a stethoscope, warm it in your hands before placing it on the patient's chest. Newborns and infants dislike objects covering their faces, so it is common for them to object to an oxygen mask.

BOX 26-1 Developmental Stages of Pediatric Patients

Newborn (neonate)	Birth to 1 month
Infant	1-12 months
Toddler	1-3 years
Preschooler	3-6 years
School-age	6-12 years
Adolescent	12-18 years

Toddlers

A **toddler** is a child from 1 to 3 years of age. Toddlers are very active, busily learning to walk, run, and climb. Unfortunately, toddlers do not understand the concepts of danger and injury. As a result, injuries are the leading cause of death in this age group. Like newborns and infants, toddlers also dislike being separated from their parents. They do not generally like to be touched by strangers or have their clothing removed. If they are unhappy, they will express their displeasure by crying and resisting efforts to assess them. Pain and bleeding enhance a toddler's fear. They especially fear needles and resist the placement of an oxygen mask over the face. Toddlers sometimes feel as if their injury or illness is a punishment for being bad and that your presence is part of that punishment.

Using toys and play can be helpful in getting a toddler to cooperate with assessment and treatment. Many EMS services carry teddy bears to soothe a toddler in a difficult moment. It may help to suggest a "space man" game if an oxygen mask is needed, and give an adult mask to a parent so the parent can also play. Games can also help reduce fear of other equipment such as stethoscopes and blood pressure cuffs. It may be helpful to demonstrate the physical examination on the teddy bear or parent before examining the child.

Preschoolers

Preschoolers are children between the ages of 3 and 6 years. They are very similar to toddlers in many ways. Although bigger, stronger, more curious, and better able to communicate, they have similar fears about strangers, blood, pain, and separation from loved ones. These children also worry about permanent injuries. Some retain the toddler feeling that injury or illness is a punishment. They have vivid imaginations and may have frightening thoughts about what is going to happen to them. Preschoolers are aware of their bodies and are beginning to develop feelings of modesty. Therefore they dislike the idea of having their clothes removed.

School-Age Children

School-age children are between the ages of 6 and 12 years and are more developed and mobile than younger children. They take part in recreational and sports activities that result in more injuries and deaths. School-age children are the most likely to be struck by vehicles, whether on foot or on bicycles, skateboards, or roller skates.

This is the first age group in which patients are able to communicate their problems clearly and to understand what is happening to them. They also accept help from strangers more readily than younger children do. However, school-age patients are usually modest and therefore uncomfortable about undressing around strangers. They fear blood, pain, and permanent or disfiguring injuries.

Adolescents

Adolescents are young people between the ages of 12 and 18 years. As they proceed through this age range, they become increasingly independent, feel as if they are indestructible, and wish to be treated like adults. The major injuries or illnesses adolescents encounter include:

- Vehicle collisions
- Injuries associated with violence (gunshot and knife wounds)
- Alcohol or other drug misuse or abuse
- Complications associated with pregnancy

Adolescents can understand emergency situations and fear the same things as school-age children. They are often most concerned with any type of permanent or disfiguring condition because of how they will be viewed by their peers. Adolescents may be uncomfortable with the sexual changes that take place during puberty. They prefer to be treated like adults and are likely to resent being spoken to as children.

Differences in Pediatric Anatomy and Physiology

The key anatomic and physiologic differences between pediatric and adult patients occur in the following areas:

- Head
- Airway
- Respiratory system
- Blood volume

The Head

Until approximately age 4, a child's head is proportionally larger and heavier than an adult's head. Because it is heavy, the head creates a balance problem and falls more quickly than the rest of the body. A young child is therefore more likely than older children or adults to injure his or her head during a fall or other accident. The skull of an infant also has soft areas on the top, sides, and back of the head, known as *fontanelles.* These are gaps between the bones of the skull. The gaps provide the skull with some flexibility during birth and allow for the growth of the head as the child ages. The most prominent fontanelle is on top of the head (Figure 26-1). A sunken fontanelle may indicate dehydration. If it is bulging, this could be a sign of elevated intracranial pressure from infection or head trauma; it is also common to see a bulging fontanelle when an infant cries.

The Airway

Several features of infant and child airways are different from an adult's. These include:

- A smaller and more easily obstructed nose and mouth. Because infants, especially neonates, are predominantly nose breathers, they do not readily open their mouths to breathe when the nose becomes obstructed. You may need to suction secretions from an infant's nose to maintain an open airway.

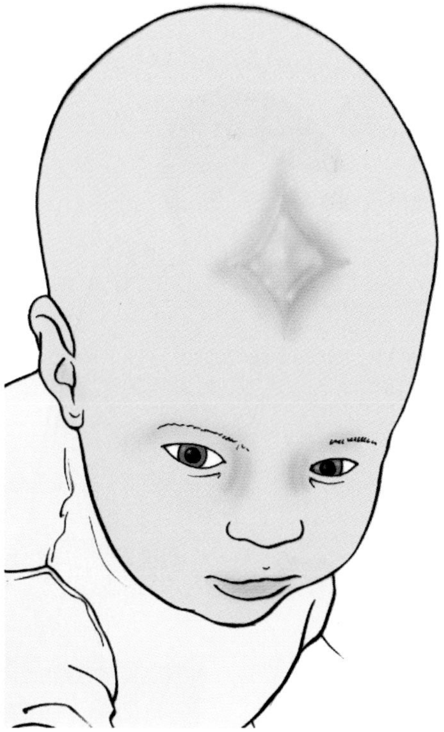

Figure 26-1

Fontanelles are soft areas on the skull, caused by gaps between the bones of the skull in a child's head.

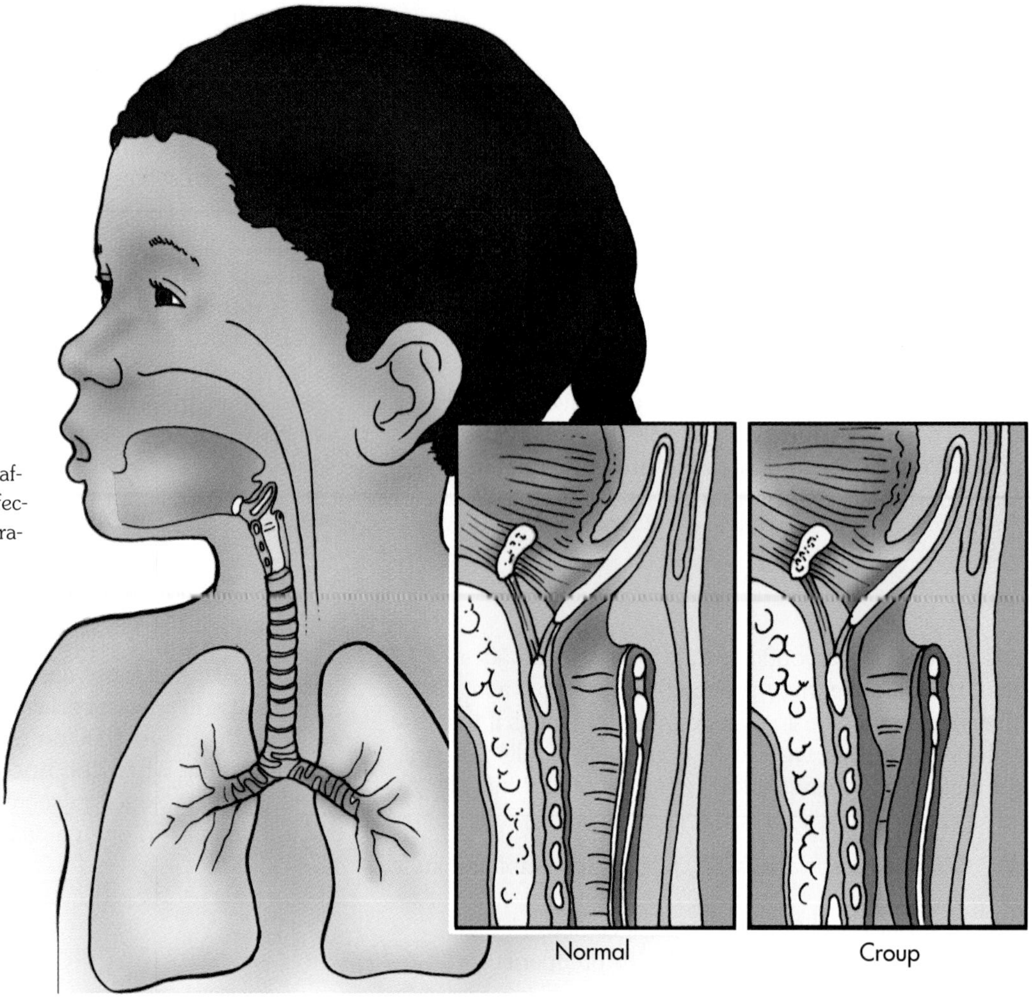

Figure 26-2

A normal child's airway and one affected by croup, an acute viral infection of the upper and lower respiratory tracts.

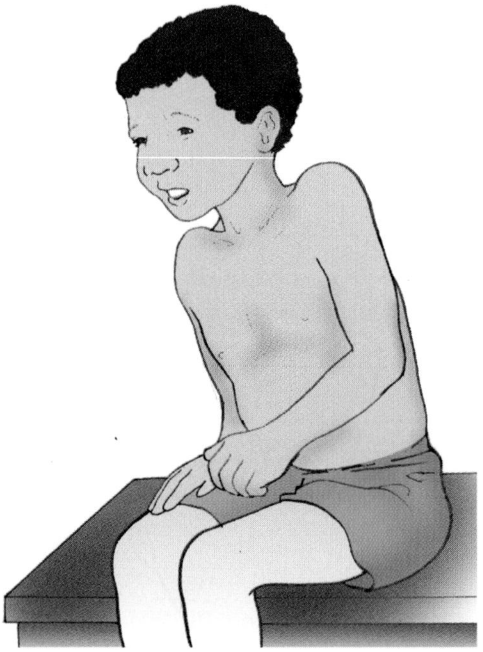

Figure 26-3

Signs of respiratory distress in a child include accessory muscle retraction and abdominal retraction.

- A proportionately larger tongue that can more easily block the airway if it swells or if the tongue falls back into the throat when the patient is unconscious and lying supine.
- A narrower and more flexible trachea that can easily be obstructed by swelling or by foreign bodies (Figure 26-2). Swelling that produces some degree of airway obstruction can be caused by common pediatric viruses. Because the airway is narrower, smaller amounts of swelling can cause airway problems. A child's neck does not have to be extended as far as an adult's when opening the airway and ventilating. Both hyperextension and flexion can obstruct the flexible pediatric trachea. Do not attempt blind finger sweeps in the mouth of an infant; it is possible to push an unvisualized object further back into the throat and block the airway.

Respiration

The chest wall of an infant or child is softer and more elastic than that of an adult. These patients also rely more on the use of the diaphragm during breathing. As a result, they are commonly said to be abdominal breathers. This is most obvious when breathing is labored because the accessory muscles between the ribs (intercostal muscles) and above the sternum pull inward (retract) (Figure 26-3). The abdomen can also retract. These retractions are not evident during normal breathing but become obvious during labored breathing. When assessing breathing, observe the abdomen as well as the chest.

Blood Volume

Blood loss can be a serious problem because infants and children have small total blood volumes. A newborn has only approximately ½ L of blood (500 ml), and an 8-year-old has about 2 L (2000 ml). A seemingly minor blood loss (when compared with an adult) can pose a significant problem for an infant.

Assessing a Pediatric Patient

Assessing a pediatric patient requires that you consider the differences in the developmental stages of infants and children, as well as the anatomic and physiologic differences between young patients and adults. How you approach and interact with a pediatric patient is very important and can set the tone for how the patient responds to you.

Conscious Patients

With a patient who is obviously conscious and breathing (crying, screaming, talking), you may be able to develop a general impression from a nearby position that does not require you to approach or touch the patient immediately. If the child is being held by a parent, gather information from the parent while observing the patient. Note the level of activity, which helps form an impression of the level of consciousness (LOC).

By watching and listening to the child breathe, you can often determine respiratory rate and quality without a hands-on examination. This helps you get an idea of the general degree of breathing distress. Noting skin color and any external bleeding gives an indication of circulatory status.

If the patient does not appear to have any immediately life-threatening conditions, approach the patient gently and casually. Explain to the parent and patient what you are going to do before you do it. Allowing young patients to touch things like the stethoscope or pen light may help make them more comfortable. If the patient has a favorite toy, offer it to him or her. Have the parent help with the physical examination, if possible. If the parent is anxious or frightened, the pediatric patient will often pick up on these feelings, which can make the situation worse. Try to calm the parent by explaining the situation.

If there are no obvious emergencies, begin your assessment by examining the patient from *toe to head.* This is different from the way you examine an adult, but it is less threatening and helps to gain the pediatric patient's trust. Immediately examining the head of a young child could increase the patient's fear and is not necessary unless there is an obvious problem in that area. It may be necessary to remove clothing to conduct a proper examination. Ask a parent to assist, if possible. Like adults, pediatric patients dislike being touched with cold hands and objects. Warm them before touching the patient's skin. You may be able to undress an infant easily by lifting a T-shirt or sleeper. Do not leave the infant uncovered for long, however; a small body loses heat quickly. If the patient is older, it is usually best to uncover and examine one area at a time, re-covering each area as you move to the next. This helps protect the patient's modesty.

To reduce fear and anxiety, reassure the patient continually. Assess breath sounds for signs of wheezing or stridor. Assess circulation by radial, brachial, or femoral pulse. Capillary refill is also an important sign to evaluate; it is a more reliable perfusion sign than it is in adults. Blood pressure is less reliable than it is in adults, although you should still assess blood pressure in children older than 3 years. Make sure to use the proper size cuff (Figure 26-4).

Altered Consciousness

As you approach a patient, it is easy to evaluate the patient's LOC. A parent can often tell you if the child has simply fallen asleep. However, you need to be certain that the patient is able to respond appropriately and is not in a comalike state. Approach the patient gently: have the par-

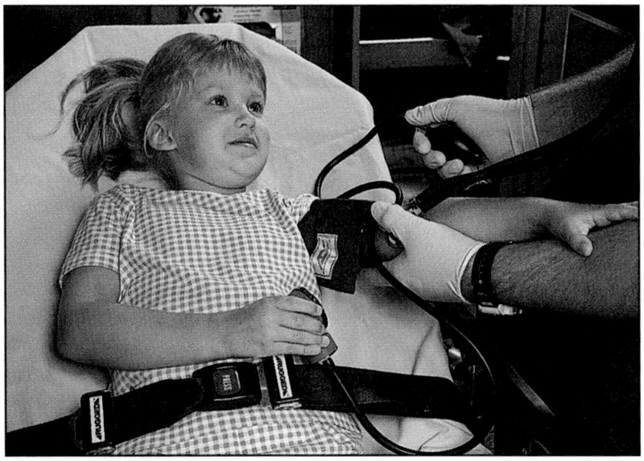

Figure 26-4

Pediatric-size blood pressure cuff.

ent try to wake the child or lightly tap and talk to the patient. If the response to verbal and physical stimulation is appropriate, the LOC is normal. A patient who fails to respond may be unconscious. Immediately assess the adequacy of the patient's airway, breathing, and circulation as described in the following sections.

Managing Immediate Life Threats

A patient who is unconscious, not breathing, pulseless, or bleeding severely has a life-threatening problem that requires immediate intervention. The basic initial assessment takes only seconds to complete, although it will take longer if you need to intervene at any point along the way.

Opening the Airway

In an unconscious infant or child, the airway should be opened and cleared of any foreign objects that could occlude it. Use the head-tilt–chin-lift method for a medical problem or the modified jaw thrust in trauma situations. If using the head-tilt–chin-lift, you will not have to tilt a pediatric patient's head back as far as an adult's. Look in the mouth for any obvious obstructions. The airway must be free of obstructions, both anatomic (the tongue) and mechanical (food, fluid, vomit, or foreign objects). Positioning the airway will resolve a problem with the tongue, but does not by itself help clear foreign objects and other materials.

Airway Obstruction

If the airway is either completely obstructed or partially obstructed with poor air exchange, you will need to clear the obstruction.

Suctioning

Vomitus, saliva, blood, and water can be removed from a patient's mouth with either a mechanical or manual suction device. A manual device such as a bulb syringe is ideal for suctioning the nose and mouth of newborns and infants up to approximately 4 months of age (Figure 26-5). Because newborns and young infants breathe primarily through the nose, it is important for the nasal passages to be kept clear. If a bulb syringe is ineffective or unavailable, a soft or French catheter can be used with a mechanical device to remove fluids.

A mechanical suction device with a rigid-tipped catheter has a wide-diameter opening that allows easier suctioning of particulate matter or large volumes of fluid from a child's mouth. Do not insert a rigid tip or a soft catheter beyond the base of the tongue, or beyond what you can see. Do not suction a breathing patient for more than 10 seconds at a time. (When using suction to clear material that completely obstructs the airway, more time may be necessary.) Provide oxygen before and after suction to compensate for hypoxia, which can be caused by the airway obstruction and suctioning air from the lungs.

Clearing a Foreign Body Airway Obstruction

Choking is a common emergency in infants and children because they often put objects in their mouths. Standard protocols for choking divide patients by age (infant or child), and according to LOC. Table 26-1 summarizes the steps for clearing foreign bodies.

If the patient is a conscious infant (less than 1 year old), use back blows and chest thrusts to clear the object. Support the patient face down on one arm and give five back blows, striking the infant firmly between the shoulder blades (Figure 26-6, *A*). Again using the arm for support, turn the patient over and use two fingers to give five chest thrusts (Figure 26-6, *B*). Check the patient's mouth and remove any obstruction that you can see. Continue these steps until the object is removed or the patient becomes unconscious.

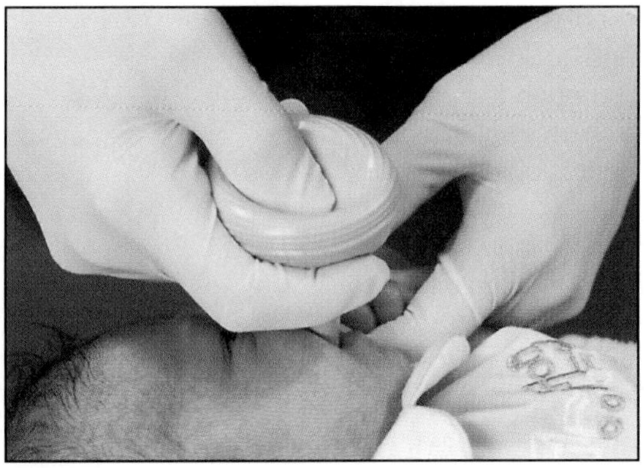

Figure 26-5

A bulb syringe can be used to suction the nose and mouth of infants and newborns.

If the infant is unconscious, open the airway and check for breathing. If there is no breathing, attempt to give two breaths. If these breaths do not go in, reposition the airway and try again. If they still do not go in, give five back blows and five chest thrusts. Look in the mouth and if you see an object, sweep it clear. Attempt to ventilate again. If this still is unsuccessful, repeat the back blows, chest thrusts, and visual checks of the mouth.

If a conscious child (1 to 8 years old) is choking, begin by administering abdominal thrusts (Heimlich maneuver). Stand behind the patient and wrap your arms around the patient's waist. Make a fist with one hand and place the thumb side in the center of the patient's abdomen, just above the navel and well below the lower tip of the sternum (xiphoid process). Grasp your fist with your other hand and give quick upward thrusts into the abdomen until the object is dislodged or the patient becomes unconscious.

To clear an obstructed airway in an unconscious child, reposition the patient's head using the head-tilt–chin-lift or modified jaw-thrust technique and attempt to ventilate. If breaths do not go in, straddle the patient's legs and deliver up to five abdominal thrusts to dislodge the object (Figure 26-7). Look in the patient's mouth; if you can see an obstruction, use a finger sweep to remove it. Attempt to ventilate again. If your breaths still do not go in, repeat these steps.

When you have dislodged an obstruction in a choking patient, it is advisable to transport the patient to the hospital for evaluation. Hospital personnel can ensure that no further obstruction exists and that no injury has been caused during removal.

Maintaining an Open Airway

Once the airway is clear, you can maintain it in an unconscious patient with either an oropharyngeal airway (OPA) or nasopharyngeal airway (NPA). To find the proper OPA size, measure from the corner of the mouth to the earlobe. Using an OPA that is too small or too large may further compromise the airway. To insert an OPA, open the mouth and insert a tongue depressor to stabilize the tongue and avoid pushing it back into the airway. Unlike the procedure for an adult, the OPA is inserted into the child's mouth right-side-up, with the tip facing the tongue (Figure 26-8). Advance it gently into place and ensure that the patient does not have a gag reflex.

An alternative to the OPA is the NPA. The advantage of the NPA is that it can be used on conscious patients; it is less likely than an OPA to stimulate a gag reflex and cause vomiting. The NPA is inserted into the nose and is slid down the back of the nasopharynx into the hy-

TABLE 26-1 Clearing Pediatric Airway Obstructions

Steps	Infant (birth to 1 yr)	Child (1-8 yrs)
Airway	Tilt head back (not as far as child) and lift chin.	Tilt head back slightly and lift chin.
Conscious patient	Use arm to support infant. Five back blows. Five chest thrusts (use two fingers). Visual check of mouth; remove object if seen. Repeat this cycle.	Abdominal thrusts until: • object is dislodged. • patient loses consciousness.
Unconscious patient	Attempt to ventilate. Reposition airway and try again. Five back blows. Five chest thrusts. Visual check of mouth; remove object if seen. Attempt to ventilate. Repeat this cycle.	Attempt to ventilate. Reposition airway and try again. Five abdominal thrusts. Visual check of mouth; remove object if seen. Attempt to ventilate. Repeat this cycle.

A

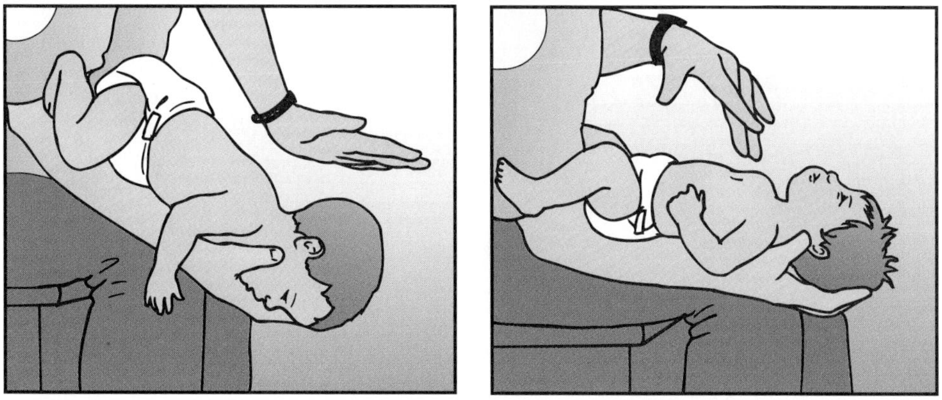

B

Figure 26-6

A, Hold the infant face down on one arm to deliver five back blows. **B,** Hold the infant face up on one arm to deliver five chest thrusts.

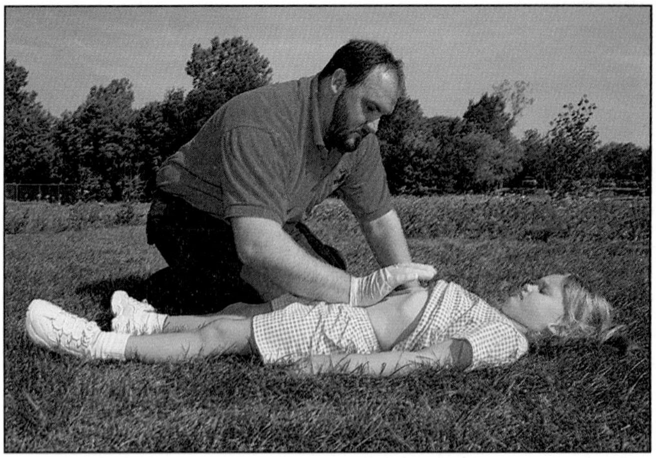

Figure 26-7

Correct hand positioning to perform abdominal thrusts on an unconscious child.

A

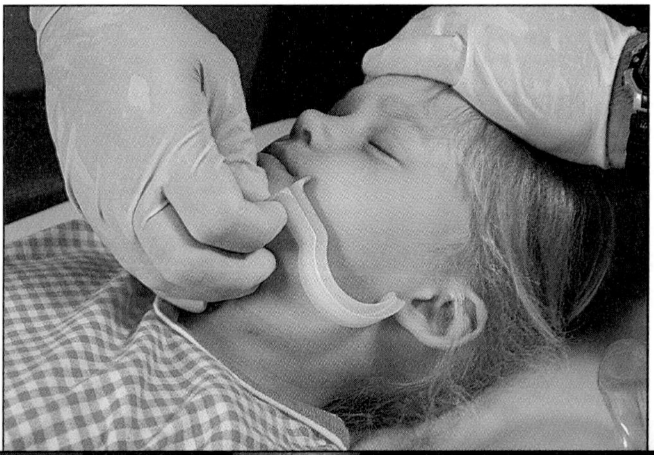

B

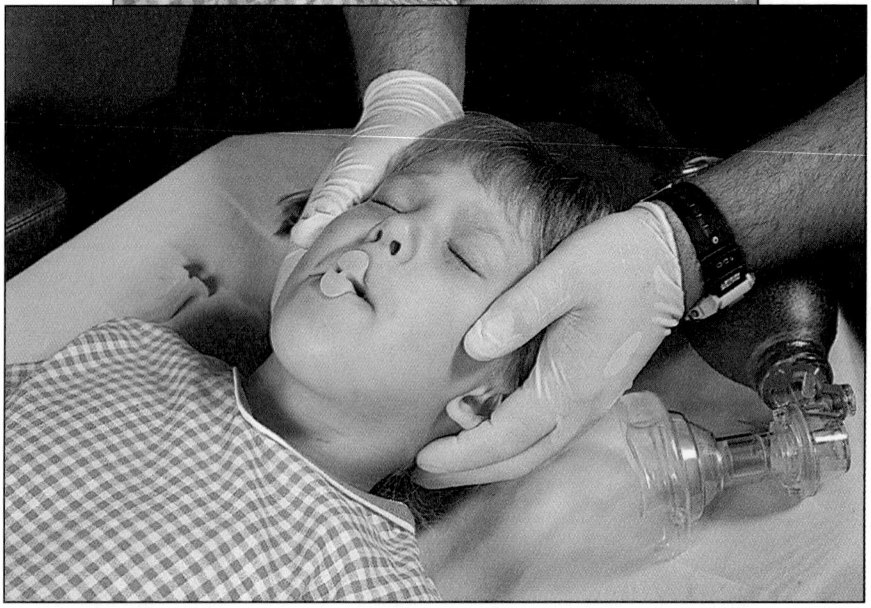

Figure 26-8

A, Sizing an oropharyngeal airway. **B,** Insert the oropharyngeal airway into a child with the tip facing the tongue.

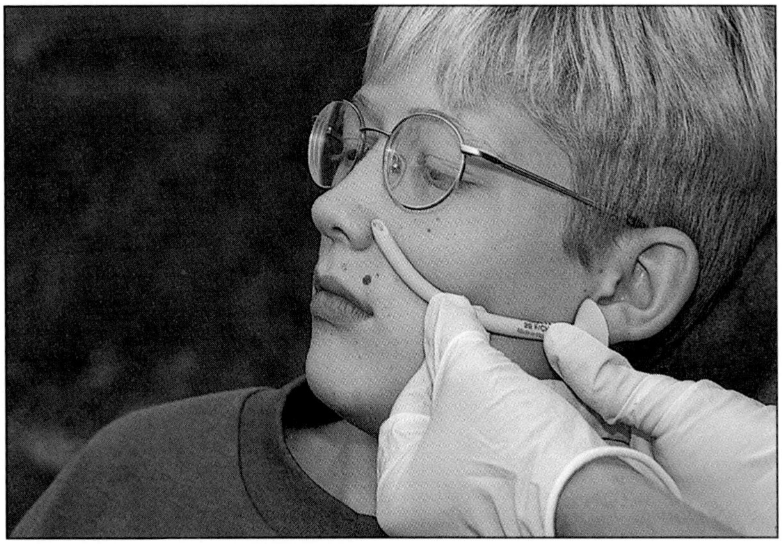

Figure 26-9

Sizing a nasopharyngeal airway.

popharynx, bypassing most of the area that stimulates gagging. It is also the adjunct of choice for patients with severe injuries to the mouth and in situations when you cannot open the mouth, such as seizures. One disadvantage of the NPA is that it is not useful in infants and very small children. The small internal size of a tube that will fit these patients does not allow adequate air flow.

Select the proper NPA size by measuring the distance from the nostril to the earlobe (Figure 26-9). Also consider the diameter of the NPA by looking at the size of the patient's nostrils. Lubricate the NPA with a water-soluble lubricant, and place the patient's head in a neutral position. Insert the airway into the nostril, with the bevel facing the midline (nasal septum) (Figure 26-10). Advance the airway until the flange rests against the nostril. If you feel resistance when inserting the airway, do not attempt to force it in. Remove the airway and try the other nostril. You may be able to suction through the NPA after insertion to remove any secretions.

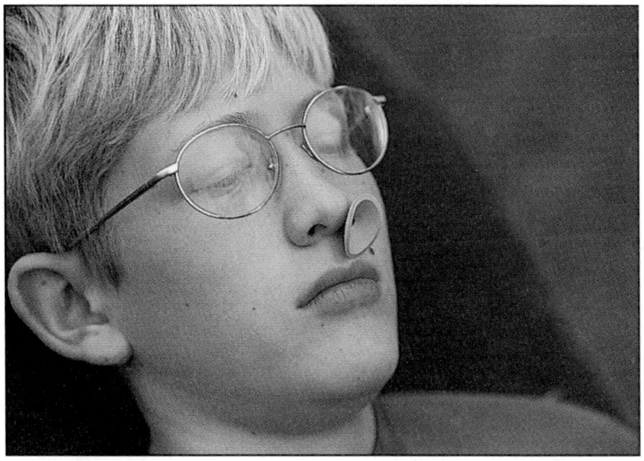

Figure 26-10

Insert the nasopharyngeal airway into a child with the bevel facing the nasal septum.

Respiratory Distress

In a breathing patient, determine if the breathing is sufficient to support life. Are the patient's respiratory rate and respiratory quality adequate? Early signs of respiratory distress in pediatric patients include:

- Increased rate
- Sounds such as stridor, grunting, and wheezing
- Use of accessory muscles to draw more air into the lungs
- Nasal flaring
- "Seesaw" breathing, in which an infant's chest falls as the abdomen rises, followed by the chest rising as the abdomen falls
- Mottled skin color

Signs of severe respiratory distress include:

- Cyanosis
- Altered LOC
- Drooling
- Slow pulse
- Significant muscle retractions

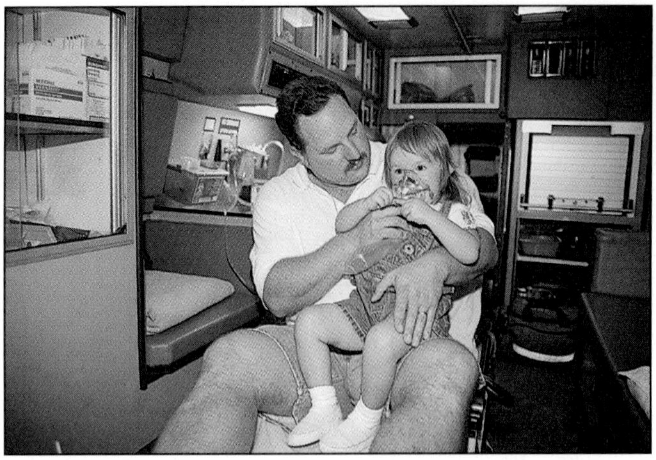

Figure 26-11

The parent may assist by holding the mask for the child.

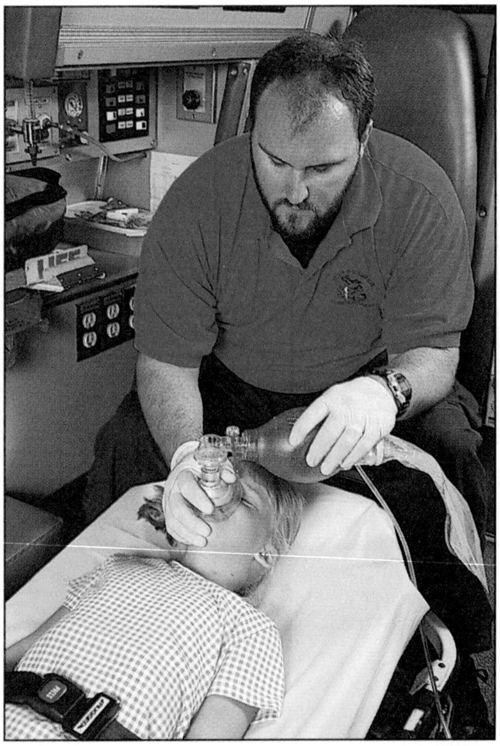

Figure 26-12

Ventilate a pediatric patient gently and evenly to prevent air from entering the stomach.

Oxygen Administration

Patients who are having difficulty breathing need supplemental oxygen. Depending on age, a pediatric patient may be able to tolerate a nonrebreather mask covering the face. If the patient will not allow this, the mask can be held near the face (blow-by administration). If possible, have a parent assist by holding the mask for the child (Figure 26-11). Deliver oxygen at a rate tolerated by the patient; 15 liters per minute (lpm) may be appropriate, but some patients will not tolerate the force of that amount of oxygen in their face. Patients having extreme difficulty moving air and breathing at a slow rate should receive assisted ventilations with a bag-valve-mask (BVM) attached to oxygen.

Respiratory Arrest

If a pediatric patient stops breathing, you will need to provide ventilations. Begin the breathing assessment by making sure the airway is open. Look at the patient's chest while placing your ear next to the mouth. Look, listen, and feel for about 5 seconds to determine if the patient is breathing. If not, provide ventilations at a rate and depth that approximates normal breathing (Figure 26-12). For infants and children, this is one breath every 3 seconds (20 per minute). Ventilate gently and evenly to ensure that the air enters the lungs and is not forced into the stomach. Gastric distention reduces the ability of the lungs to expand and may also cause vomiting. If your training and protocols allow it, insert a nasogastric tube to reduce gastric distension when ventilating.

To minimize the likelihood of disease transmission through unprotected rescue breathing, use an appropriately sized resuscitation mask or BVM to breathe for the patient. Either of these devices should be fitted for at-

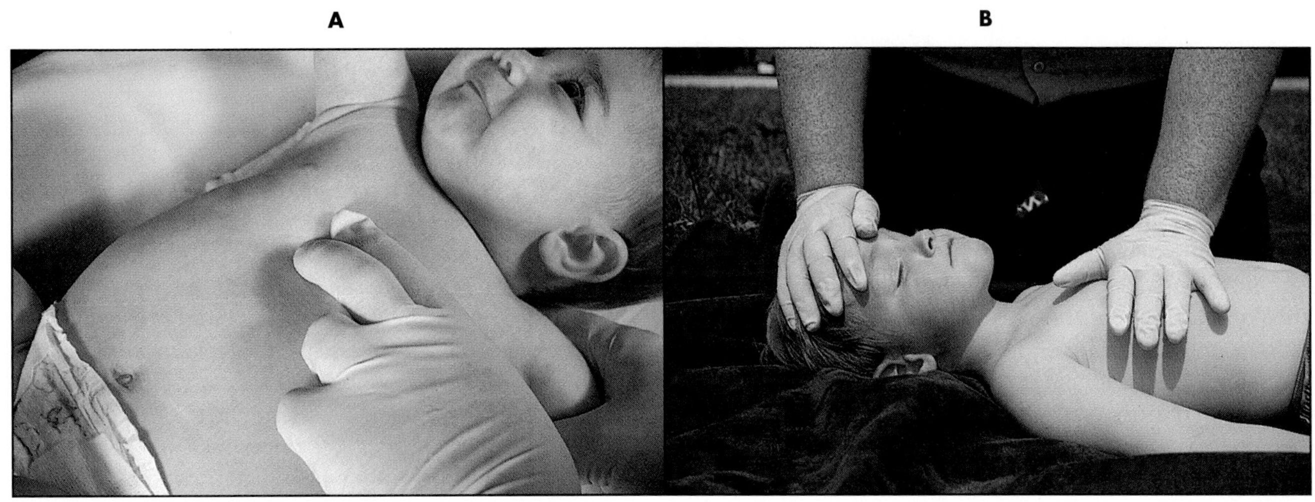

Figure 26-13

A, Use two to three fingers for chest compressions on an infant. **B,** Use the heel of one hand for chest compressions on a child.

TABLE 26-2 CPR for Infants and Children

Steps	Infant (birth to 1 yr)	Child (1-8 yrs)
Assess responsiveness	Tap and shout.	Tap and shout.
Airway	Tilt head back (not as far as child) and lift chin.	Tilt head back slightly and lift chin.
Breathing	Look, listen, feel for breathing. Cover nose and mouth. Give two slow breaths (about 1.5 seconds each).	Look, listen, feel for breathing. Pinch nose and cover mouth. Give two slow breaths (about 1.5 seconds each).
Pulse check	Check brachial pulse for 5-10 seconds.	Check carotid pulse for 5-10 seconds.
Compressions	Use two fingers to compress chest five times. Compress ½-1 inch; at least 100 compressions per minute.	Use one hand to compress chest 15 times. Compress 1-1½ inches; 80-100 compressions per minute.
Cycles	Five compressions and one ventilation.	Five compressions and one ventilation.

tachment to supplemental oxygen. The mask must fit the patient's face securely. If the pediatric BVM that you are using has a pop-off valve, you may need to disable it to deliver adequate ventilations. See Chapter 11 for detailed information about the use of these devices.

Cardiac Arrest

Sudden cardiac arrest is rare in children. Pediatric cardiac arrests generally result from respiratory problems that develop more gradually. Once you have assessed and corrected any airway and breathing problems, evaluate the adequacy of the patient's circulation, starting with the pulse. A patient who is unconscious and not breathing may be in cardiac arrest. For children, check the pulse at the carotid artery in the neck. An infant's pulse is checked at the brachial artery in the arm. If the patient does not have a pulse, begin cardiopulmonary resuscitation (CPR). Because most infants and young children do not go into cardiac arrest as a result of ventricular fibrillation, an automatic external defibrillator (AED) is not often used. AEDs are programmed with energy levels that are too high for most children. The American Heart Association recommends using an AED only for patients who are older than 12 years of age or who weigh more than 90 pounds.

If it is necessary to perform CPR on a child or infant, compress the chest less deeply but more rapidly than for an adult. Also, for the smaller chest, you will need only 2 to 3 fingers (infant) or the heel of one hand (child) for compressions (Figure 26-13, *A* and *B*). Table 26-2 provides an overview of the critical steps of CPR for children and infants. (See Chapter 21 for information on neonatal resuscitation.)

Common Medical Emergencies

Respiratory Infections

Acute respiratory infections are the most common illnesses among children. Respiratory infections can cause swelling of the mucous membranes and drainage into the respiratory passages, which in turn can lead to breathing difficulty. Because of the narrow breathing passages in children, any swelling can potentially cause severe problems. Although croup and epiglottitis are two of the more common pediatric airway infections, other viruses can also cause significant respiratory distress in children. Croup is seen quite commonly; epiglottitis is rare. While the two infections can both cause airway obstruction and difficulty breathing, they differ in several aspects. Table 26-3 provides a comparison of these differences.

Croup

Croup is a viral infection that causes inflammation and swelling in the lining of the larynx and trachea just below the vocal cords (see Figure 26-2). Because this part of the airway is normally the narrowest in children, any swelling can cause some degree of obstruction.

A patient with croup is most often between 3 months and 3 years of age. The onset of croup is usually slow, often following several days of an upper-respiratory infection with a low-grade fever. The patient typically wakes in the middle of the night with difficulty breathing and a high-pitched, barklike cough caused by swelling below the vocal cords. Breathing sometimes improves when exposed to cool, moist night air or humidified air. Transport the patient in the most comfortable position, which is often sitting upright.

Epiglottitis

Epiglottitis is caused by a bacterial infection of the epiglottis. The condition is rarely seen now because of childhood immunizations. However, when it does occur, it is extremely serious. Unlike croup, which often has a slow onset and causes partial airway obstruction, the swelling of the epiglottis may be rapid and so severe that it can cause sudden complete airway obstruction. Patients with epiglottitis are usually 3 to 7 years of age, but the disease can occur at any age. The patient often looks very ill, has a high fever and sore throat, and is drooling because of an inability to swallow. The child may be sitting up and leaning forward in an attempt to keep the airway open. To avoid aggravating the condition, do not attempt to inspect the throat. The patient should be transported rapidly in the position of comfort, with advanced life support (ALS) personnel attending if possible. Provide supplemental oxygen by whatever route the patient will tolerate. If the patient is unable to breathe well enough on his or her own, gently provide supplemental ventilation with a BVM with oxygen. This patient requires advanced medical care immediately.

TABLE 26-3 Croup and Epiglottitis Comparison

	Croup	Epiglottitis
Cause	Viral infection	Bacterial infection
Onset	Slow	Fast
Age	3 months-3 years	3-7 years
Cough	Barking cough	Not present
Drooling	Not present	Present
Fever	Low	High
Swallowing	Usually no difficulty	Difficulty

Asthma

In children, asthma is an acute condition of lower-airway constriction and inflammation. Although wheezing is a classic sign, not all wheezing is asthma. Also, patients with severe asthma may not be moving enough air to cause wheezing. However, they will demonstrate some of the other signs of severe respiratory distress. Patients with severe asthma attacks need reassurance, high-flow oxygen, and rapid transport.

Seizures

Seizures are among the most frequent pediatric emergencies. They can be either a chronic problem or the result of an acute illness or injury. Specific causes include fever, infection, poisoning, low blood sugar, head injury, hypoxia, epilepsy, and chronic conditions. As part of your assessment, consider whether the seizure is medical or traumatic in origin. This is important information for later care in the hospital, although it will not affect your initial care. In many cases, the cause cannot be determined in the field.

Many seizures, especially brief ones, are not harmful. The patient may breathe throughout the seizure, although air exchange is likely to be less than normal. Patients with known seizure disorders may seize frequently. If they have not hurt themselves physically, the most important assessment point is whether the normal seizure pattern has changed. Has the patient taken medications on schedule? Are seizures becoming more frequent or more violent or lasting longer?

Febrile seizures occur when a child's temperature changes quickly. The patient usually wakes up soon afterward and is unlikely to develop chronic seizures or epilepsy. Note, however, that febrile seizure cannot be diagnosed in the field. EMS responders must ensure that patients with apparent febrile seizures receive follow-up evaluation to avoid missing more serious causes, such as meningitis.

EMTs usually will not witness active seizing; it most often ends before ambulance arrival. If you do encounter active seizing, concentrate on preventing injury. Do not let anyone try to force objects into the mouth. This is unlikely to help protect the airway, and it often causes injury. In prolonged seizures, holding an oxygen mask near the face with oxygen running at a high flow rate may help compensate for inadequate respirations.

After the seizure, treatment is basic and supportive. Maintain a clear airway, suctioning if necessary. If you do not suspect a spinal injury, place the patient on the side. Administer oxygen and summon ALS personnel, if available. Transport the patient to the hospital for further evaluation. Although brief seizures may not be directly harmful, they can indicate a more serious underlying problem.

Watching a child seize can be terrifying, especially for someone who has not seen it before. Parents and other caregivers may need reassurance and emotional support. Explaining that seizures are common and usually not harmful should help. Inform them fully about the need for transport and evaluation.

Fever and Dehydration

Responding to a child with a high fever is a common EMS call. Often, parents will report temperature measurements that they have taken. Because it is unlikely that you will be able to identify or treat the underlying cause of the fever, the patient should be transported to the hospital for evaluation by a physician. One potentially serious cause of fever in children is meningitis, inflammation of the meninges that surround the brain and spinal cord. It can be caused by both viruses and bacteria. If left untreated, meningitis can cause complications such as cerebral edema, shock, increased intracranial pressure, permanent brain damage, or death. Any child presenting with fever accompanied by rash or a stiff neck must be transported for immediate evaluation of possible meningitis. BSI precautions are especially important in this setting.

To care for a patient with a fever, remove excess clothing but do not allow the patient to become chilled. Do not attempt to cool the child rapidly with ice water or alcohol. This can produce shivering, the body's attempt to increase temperature, and may lead to seizures. Transport the patient to the hospital for evaluation.

An ill child can sweat as a result of fever. This same illness can also result in vomiting, diarrhea, and inadequate fluid intake. The combination of these factors, particularly over a period of time, can contribute to a significant loss of body fluids known as *dehydration*. This occurs quite frequently with common childhood viruses. Dehydrated children look listless and ill. They may have dry skin and mucous membranes or they may not produce tears when crying. A dehydrated child needs ALS intervention and possibly hospitalization. Transport for further evaluation.

Communicable Diseases

Common communicable diseases in childhood include measles, chicken pox, and mumps (Figure 26-14, *A, B,* and *C*). Measles and chicken pox produce characteristic rashes, and mumps cause tenderness and swelling of the glands in front of the ears. If you have already had one of these diseases as a child, you should have immunity from further infections. Exposure to it in a child you care for does not likely pose a threat to you. However, pregnant EMS personnel should avoid exposure to these communicable childhood diseases, especially measles.

When caring for children with communicable diseases, you should use BSI measures, including gloves and a mask. Notify your supervising physician of the possibility that you are transporting a patient with a communicable disease. Whenever possible, try to minimize the number of EMS personnel that are exposed to the patient. Before returning to service, clean and disinfect the ambulance thoroughly.

Shock

Among infants and children, shock is unlikely to be the result of a heart condition. It is more often caused by infection that leads to fever and dehydration, or by blood loss. A weak, rapid pulse often indicates insufficient blood volume. Pale, cool, clammy skin and an altered LOC also indicate poor perfusion. Children can often compensate for fluid loss up to half of their total blood volume. However, they deteriorate suddenly and drastically when compensatory mechanisms fail. When assessing the need to treat shock, rely on early signs much more than on blood pressure. In addition to heart rate and skin signs, capillary refill is a reliable perfusion indicator in children.

The intervention for shock includes:

- Controlling any external bleeding
- Proper positioning of the patient by elevating the legs if there is no suspicion of spinal injury
- Administering oxygen
- Ensuring that nothing is given by mouth
- Summoning ALS personnel
- Rapid transport to the hospital

Poisoning

Poisoning is a common pediatric problem. Most unintentional pediatric poisonings are associated with ingested poisons. Children may be curious about containers that are brightly colored and hold pills that look like candy. Although usually accidental, poisonings can be associated with child abuse. Try to gather as much information as possible about the incident and the poison itself. Bring any containers with you to the hospital. Contact the su-

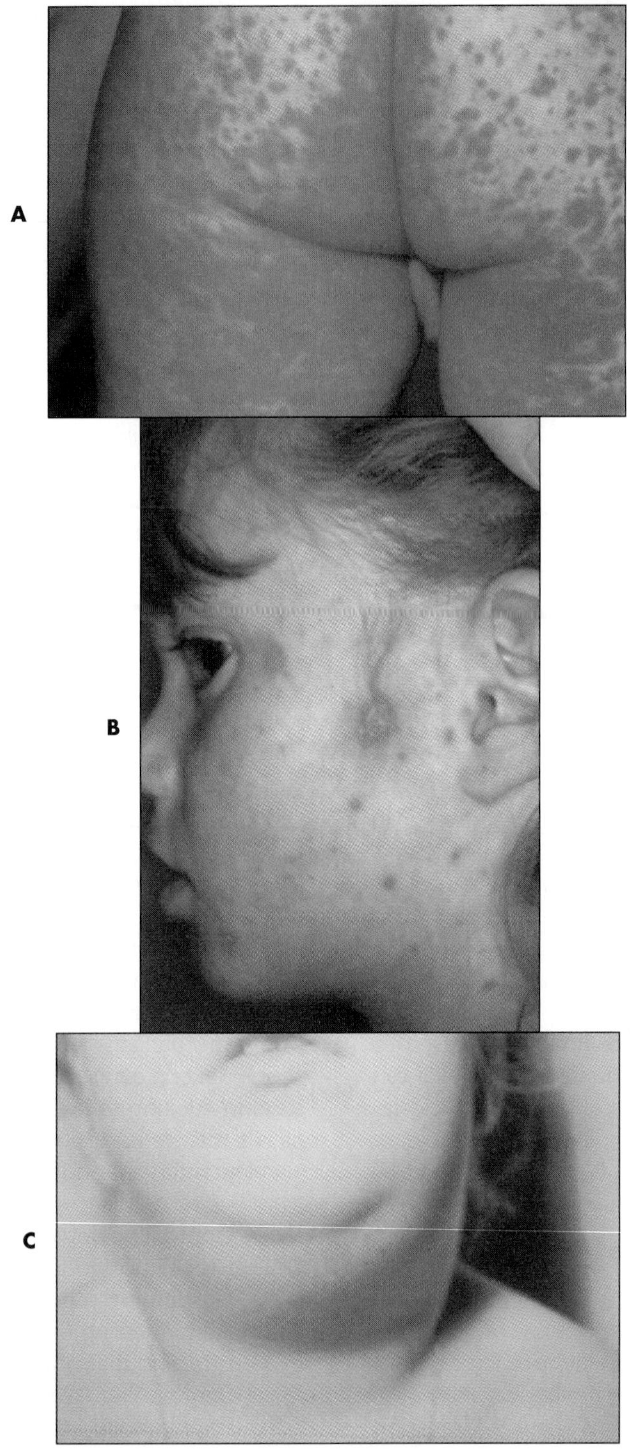

Figure 26-14

A, Measles. **B,** Chickenpox. **C,** Mumps.

pervising physician to determine whether activated charcoal should be given to a conscious patient. If the patient is unconscious, manage the airway, breathing, and circulation; and consider other possible causes of unresponsiveness. Summon ALS personnel, if available, and transport without delay. Chapter 17 provides more detailed information about poisoning.

Sudden Infant Death Syndrome (SIDS)

Sudden infant death syndrome (SIDS) is the sudden, unexpected death of an otherwise healthy infant that occurs during sleep for an unknown reason. The death is not apparently related to any previous medical history and remains unexplained after autopsy. Also referred to as *crib death,* SIDS claims between 5000 and 10,000 lives each year, making it the leading cause of death in children from 1 month to 1 year of age. The infant is often discovered in the early morning, but SIDS can occur at any time during sleep. Unfortunately, some infants who appear to be SIDS patients are actually victims of child abuse.

When you respond to an infant resuscitation, you will usually not have any way of knowing if it is a SIDS case. Unless advanced signs of death are present, you should begin CPR and try to resuscitate the infant. The most common advanced sign of death is rigid stiffening of the muscles, called *rigor mortis.* Another sign that is more difficult to assess, called *lividity,* can be confused with bruising. Do not jump to conclusions about apparent bruising. Avoid comments that might suggest the parents are at fault. Try to recall what you saw and heard and how people acted when you arrived. Relay this information to hospital staff and document it.

IT'S YOUR CALL
CONCLUSION

Your 2-year-old patient was found seated on his mother's lap. The child had obvious stridor and a barking cough. As you prepare to assess him, you consider the developmental characteristics of this toddler. These include the fear of strangers and separation from his parents. You ask the mother to keep the child on her lap while you conduct the assessment. She helps you remove the clothing covering his chest so you can assess breath sounds. You warm your hands and the stethoscope as you prepare to touch the child. Based on the child's age, the barking cough, and the history as stated by the mother, you suspect this child has croup. You treat this patient by administering humidified oxygen and allowing the patient to remain seated upright near his mother, preferably secured in a car seat, during transport.

When transport is appropriate, summon ALS personnel to assist with resuscitation. Protocols differ between systems on the issue of transporting infants with advanced signs of death. Some encourage transport for a variety of reasons related to family well-being. Others forbid transport unless resuscitation is indicated. The scene should be preserved for investigation by police or the medical examiner.

The death of a child is among the most difficult situations to handle for a parent, as well as for EMS personnel. Parents are going through the stages of grieving and will often be experiencing guilt, anger, and denial. Be sympathetic to grieving family members, but minimize their interference in your resuscitation efforts. Because this type of death can be extremely stressful, critical incident stress debriefing (CISD) may be necessary for you and other members of your crew. Family members may also need professional counseling services to help them deal with the incident. Many communities have support groups for victims of a SIDS death.

Common Trauma Emergencies

Injuries remain the number one cause of death in the pediatric age group. Vehicle collisions kill more infants and children than any other type of trauma emergency. These deaths include children struck while outside of the vehicle as well as those who are vehicle passengers. Occasionally, sport and recreational activities can also result in serious injury or death.

Children have unique anatomic and physiologic differences that lead to specific injury patterns. As mentioned earlier, the relatively large size of an infant's or young child's head in relation to the body makes this patient more susceptible to head injuries from falls. The less-developed neck muscles make the cervical spine area more prone to serious injury from sudden movement, especially in deceleration injuries such as falls and vehicle collisions. The more flexible skeleton of a child makes injury to vital organs more likely; and because of their small blood volume, children can tolerate much less blood loss than adults before progressing to shock.

Head and Spinal Injuries

Head and spinal injury in pediatric patients is usually caused by vehicle collisions, falls, or diving accidents. Head injury is the most common cause of trauma death. Any patient with an altered LOC and a mechanism that suggests injury to the head or spine should be treated as if a serious injury has occurred until the patient can be evaluated by a physician. Children are also more susceptible than adults to spinal cord injuries without having sustained an injury to the bony spinal column.

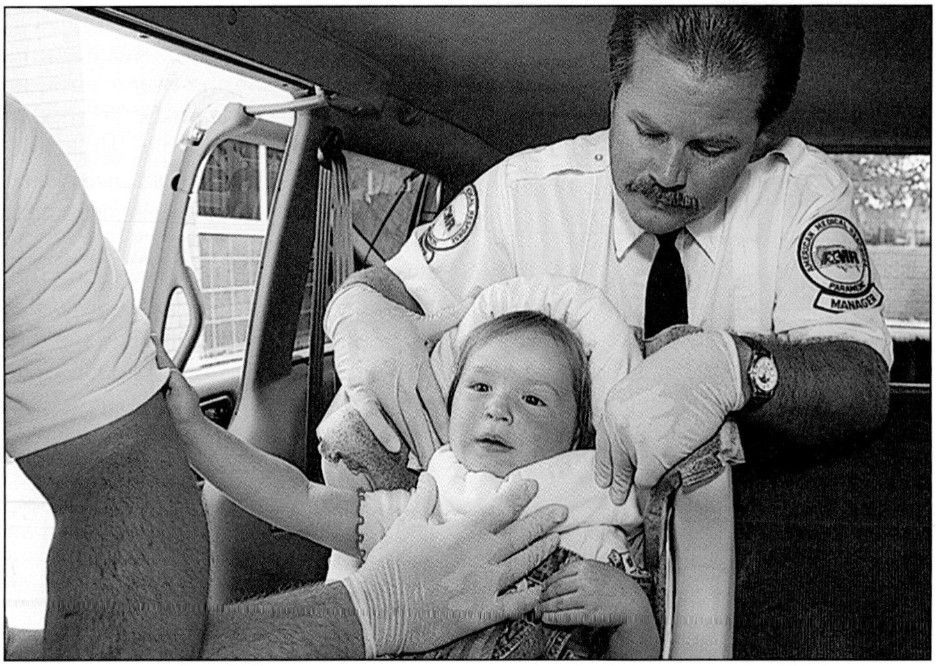

Figure 26-15

Use padding to secure the head in a neutral position and to limit movement.

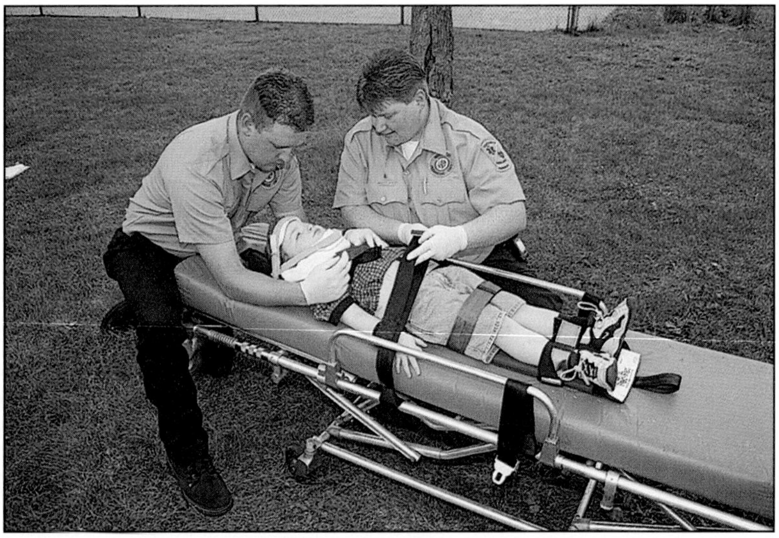

Figure 26-16

Pediatric long backboard.

If a patient is in a car seat when you arrive at a vehicle collision, leave the child in the seat whenever possible. If the car seat has not been damaged, the patient is not seriously injured, and you are able to assess the patient adequately in this position, use the car seat to help immobilize the patient. Apply a cervical collar only if you have one that fits the child properly. Pad the sides of the patient's head to minimize lateral movement. Place additional padding any place where spaces between the patient and the car seat could allow movement, especially under the neck. Secure the head in a neutral position (Figure 26-15). If the patient is not in a car seat and requires immobilization, use either a regular backboard or a special pediatric board (Figure 26-16). When on a backboard, the patient may need extra padding under the shoulders to keep the head in a neutral position.

Chest and Abdominal Injuries

The pediatric chest is more flexible than an adult's, and injury to the thoracic organs can occur without rib fractures. If ribs are broken, it is an indication of severe force that is often associated with serious or fatal injury. Children with chest or abdominal injuries often resist assessment and guard the injured area. Seat restraints often cause abdominal bruising during a vehicle collision. Attempt to identify tender areas of the trunk and look for obvious injuries. Administer supplemental oxygen and transport the patient rapidly to a hospital.

Extremity Injuries

Injuries to the extremities are the most common types of pediatric trauma. Minor cuts and bruises are commonly found on arms and legs as a result of falls. With the exception of femur or pelvis fractures, extremity injuries rarely pose a life threat. Extremity injuries in children should be immobilized in the same manner as those of an adult would be.

Near-Drowning

Drowning claims approximately 4000 lives each year, about half of which are in the pediatric population. For every drowning death, an estimated four near-drowning victims are hospitalized and survive with permanent disability. For each person hospitalized, yet another four are seen in emergency departments and released.[2,3] It has been estimated that a child under age 5 is 14 times more likely to be involved in a fatal accident in a swimming pool than in a motor vehicle.[1] While the number of drownings is decreasing, submersion accidents continue to pose significant problems for infants and children.

Children can recover after being under water for longer periods of time than adults. Many factors influence the chance of survival, including the time under water, water temperature, age of the victim, type of water, and the care provided immediately after rescue and hospital admission. Generally, younger patients who are immersed in cold water for shorter periods of time (less than 4 minutes) and receive aggressive care have the best chance of survival. If you recover a pediatric patient who has been submerged, assess the patient and care for immediate life threats: airway, breathing, and circulation. If the patient was found in cold water, remember that hypothermia may make it difficult to detect a pulse. Because these patients tend to vomit, be prepared to suction the airway.

Burns

There is a separate Rule of Nines for calculating the degree of body surface area burned in children (Figure 26-17) (see Chapter 23 for the adult rule). This is because of the anatomic differences, especially the child's relatively larger head size. When considering the severity of a burn, note the following:

- The amount of surface burned
- The specific areas burned (such as the face or neck)
- The depth of the burn
- The age of the patient
- Any additional injuries, such as possible fractures

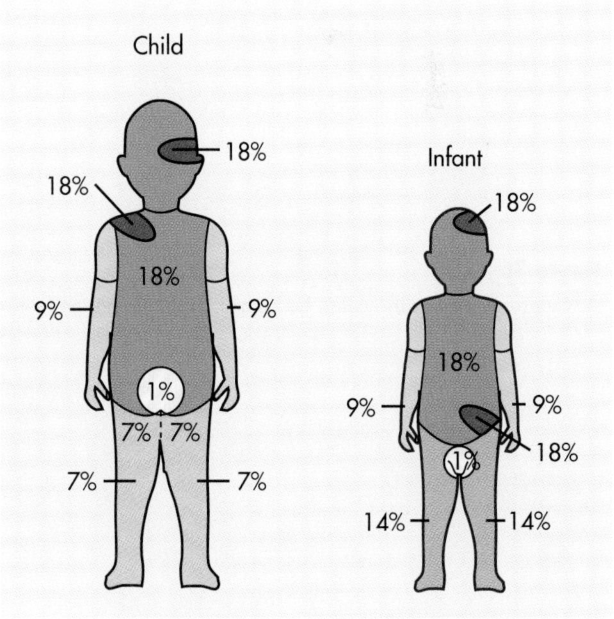

Figure 26-17
Rule of Nines for children and infants.

Respiratory problems and hypothermia are among the most serious problems associated with burns in children. Manage the airway, provide oxygen, assist ventilations if needed, and maintain body temperature. Use local protocols to decide whether the patient should be transported to a specialized burn center, if one is available. ALS care is important, particularly for IV fluid therapy. When this is not available in the field, rapid transport is important.

Child Abuse and Neglect

Child abuse and neglect are growing concerns in America. Child abuse is any physical, emotional, or sexual mistreatment. It may be inflicted by a parent, guardian, caretaker, or stranger. Potential signs include:

- Injuries inconsistent with the mechanism or description provided by the guardian
- Multiple bruises, especially in various stages of healing
- Burn marks, especially of the hands, feet, back, or genitals (Figure 26-18, *A* and *B*)
- Lack of concern on the part of the guardian
- The child's refusal to talk about the incident
- Conflicting accounts of how the incident occurred

In some situations, no visible signs of injury will be present. Injuries affecting the central nervous system (CNS), such as those inflicted by vigorously shaking an infant (referred to as **shaken-baby syndrome**), may result in an unconscious child or a cardiac arrest that appears to be a SIDS case.

Neglect is the failure to provide for a child's essential needs, including food, shelter, clothing, cleanliness, safe living conditions, health care, emotional support, and the supervision to make these available when needed. Neglect can be subtle and difficult to define exactly. Advice from child welfare authorities may be needed in some cases.

If you suspect child abuse or neglect, maintain a professional demeanor. Carefully record the information surrounding the incident, including the reported history and your assessment findings. If you believe that abuse or neglect has occurred, try to get parental permission to transport the child for physician evaluation. If the parent refuses, follow local protocols for summoning law enforcement personnel and enlisting their assistance. All states require reporting suspected child abuse and neglect to social service or law enforcement personnel (see Chapter 2). Also be sure to report your suspicions to the hospital physician. You do not need to have certain knowledge of child abuse or neglect to report it. Suspicion is an adequate reason to report your findings in good faith and in the patient's best interest.

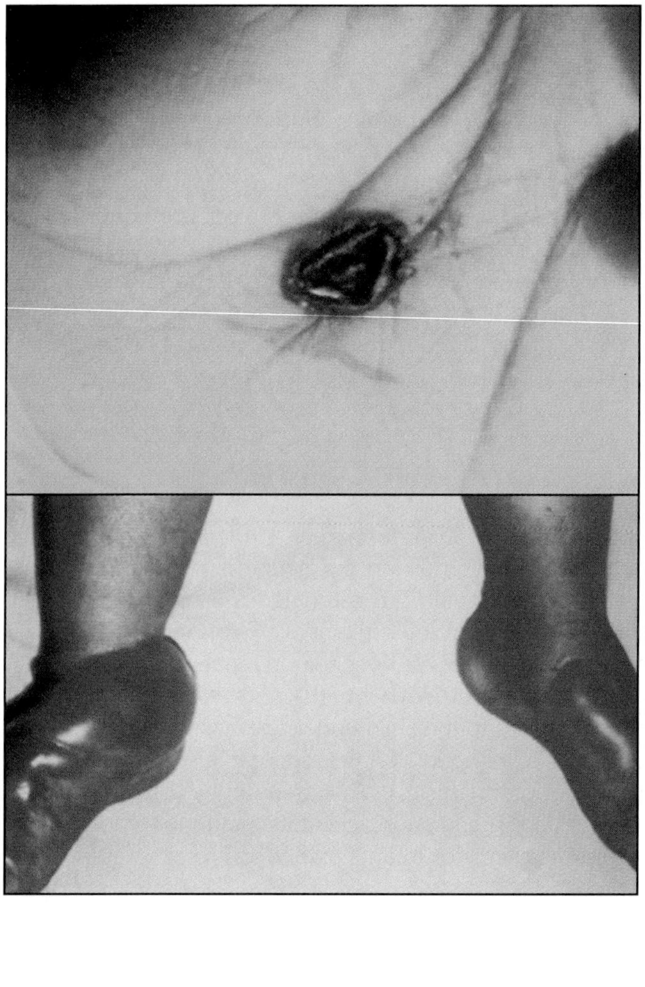

A

B

Figure 26-18

A, Cigarette burn to the palm. **B,** Immersion burns on the feet.

SUMMARY

Although pediatric patients will likely make up only a small percentage of your patients, they can be extremely stressful to care for. Pediatric patients should not be thought of as just little adults. They are anatomically, physiologically, mentally, and emotionally different from adults. A developing child progresses through defined stages from infancy to adolescence. These stages include newborn, infant, toddler, preschooler, school-age child, and adolescent. As you assess a pediatric patient, consider the developmental stage and use its characteristics to gain the patient's cooperation.

Remember that the fears typical of these stages are very real to the child. It is often difficult to calm the patient without the help of a parent. Infants and children are susceptible to many different medical emergencies, including respiratory infections, seizures, poisoning, fever, and dehydration. Falls, vehicular trauma, and sport and recreational activities are the most common causes of pediatric injuries and deaths.

REFERENCES

1. **Baxter F, O'Neill P, Karpf R:** *The injury fact book,* Arlington, Va, 1984, Insurance Institute for Highway Safety.
2. **Pearn JH et al:** Drowning and near drowning involving children, *Am J Public Health* 69(5):450-454, 1979.
3. **Wintemute J:** Preventing aquatic emergencies. In: *Good sports: preventing recreational injuries,* Baltimore, 1992, Johns Hopkins Injury Prevention Center.

SUGGESTED READINGS

1. **Hagen-Moe D:** The ABCs of pediatric physical assessment, *J Emerg Serv* 24:10, 1992.
2. **Eichelberger MR:** *Pediatric trauma: prevention, acute care, rehabilitation,* St Louis, 1993, Mosby.

Section 9

Special Populations

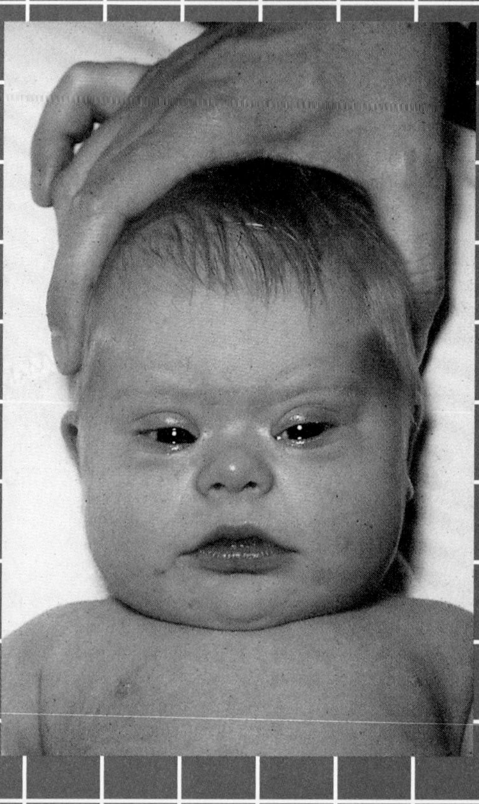

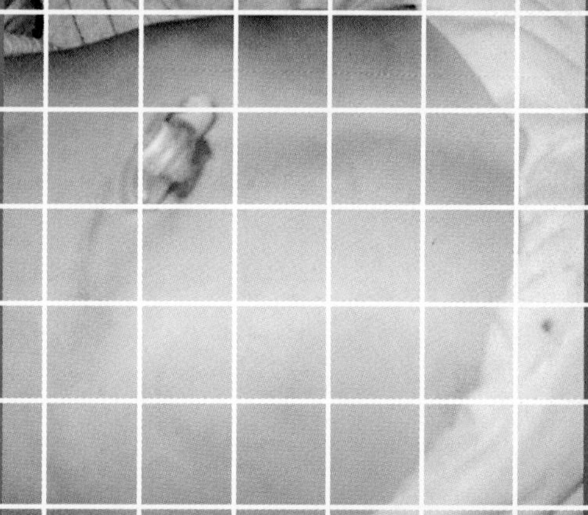

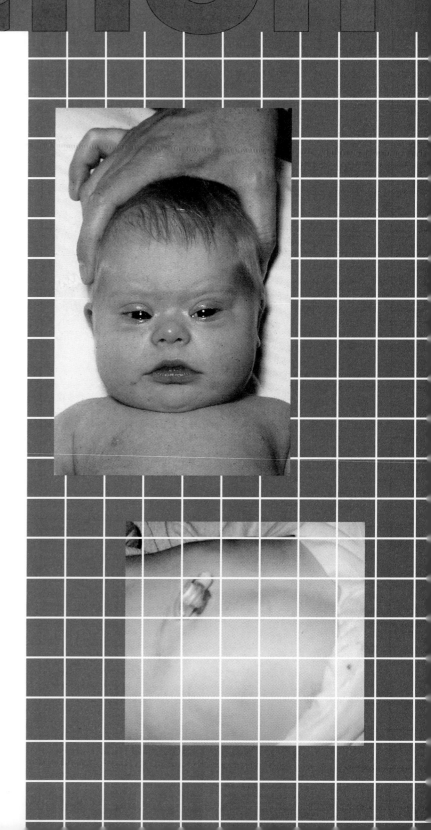

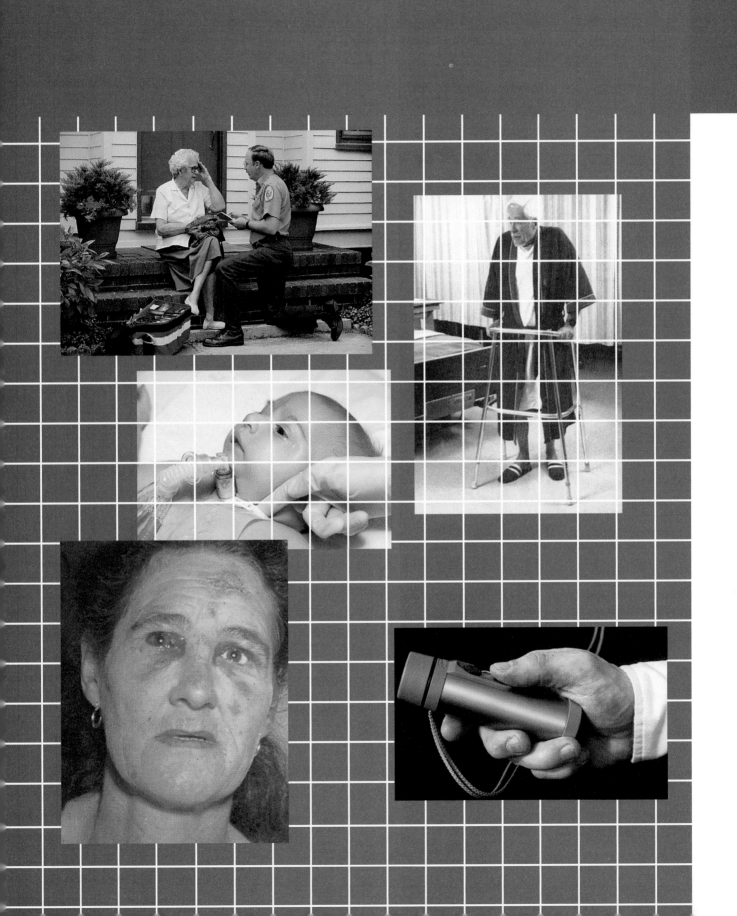
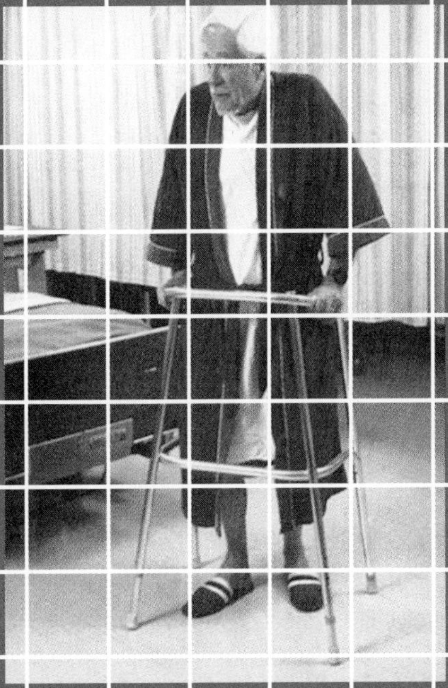
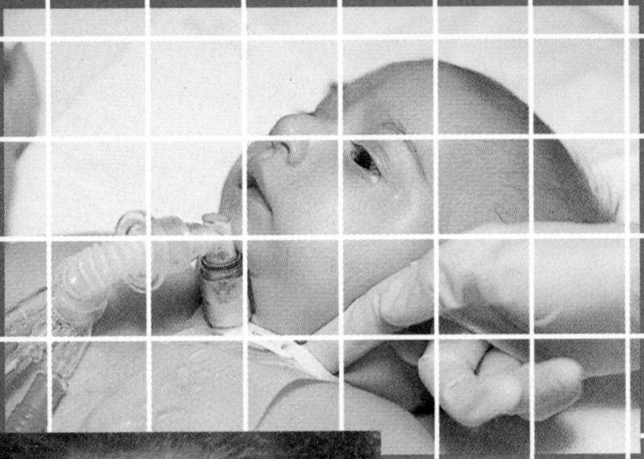
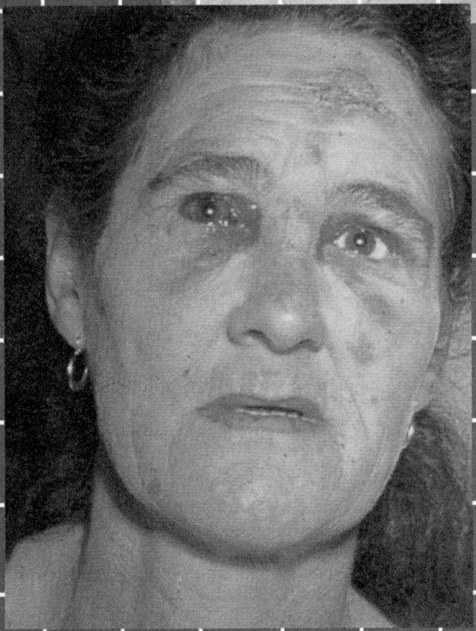
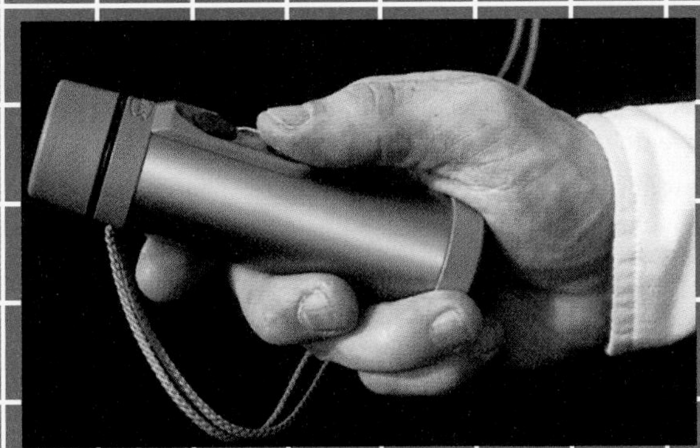

Chapter 27

The Elderly, Disabled, and Other Special Populations

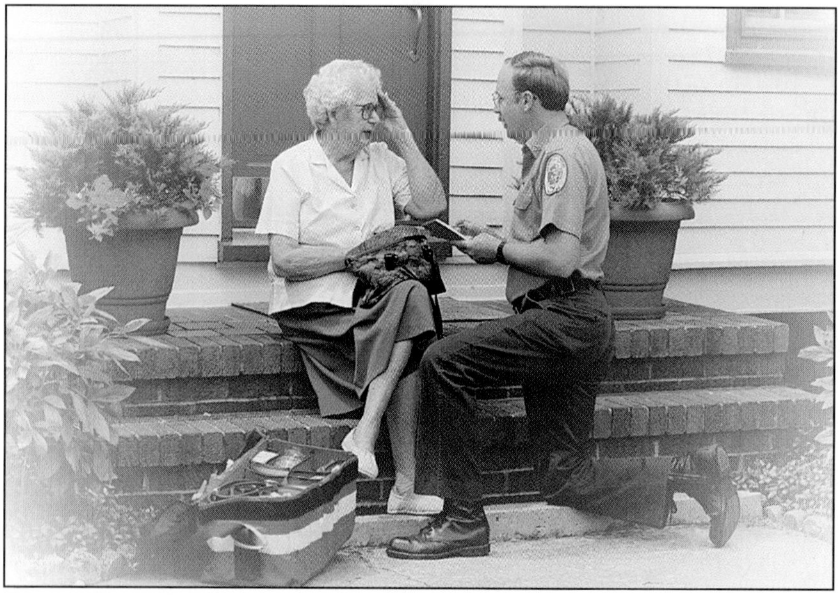

OBJECTIVES

Knowledge Objectives

As an EMT-Basic, you should be able to:

1. Describe the aging process and how it affects body systems.
2. Discuss how to assess an elderly patient and how the assessment may differ from that of a younger adult.
3. Identify common trauma and medical emergencies that affect the elderly.
4. Discuss the emotional effect a medical emergency may have on a geriatric patient.
5. Describe signs and symptoms that may be associated with elder abuse.
6. Discuss how to assess patients who are physically or developmentally disabled.
7. Identify situations that involve the use of specialized equipment for patients with special needs.
8. Describe how to use a parent during a medical emergency involving a child with special needs.
9. Name a common problem associated with tracheostomy tubes.
10. Describe how to ventilate a stoma patient who is not breathing adequately.

Skill Objectives

As an EMT-Basic, you should be able to:

1. Conduct an assessment of an elderly patient.
2. Conduct an assessment of a patient who is physically or developmentally challenged.
3. Suction a tracheostomy tube that is obstructed by mucus or other secretions.
4. Demonstrate the documentation of a patient-care report for an elderly or challenged patient.

Attitude Objectives

As an EMT-Basic, you should be able to:

OBJECTIVES

1. **Value the need for approaching and assessing a patient with special needs in a manner that may vary from other patients.**
2. **Serve as a role model for other EMS personnel when assessing and caring for special populations.**

KEY TERMS

1. **Alzheimer's Syndrome:** A degeneration of nerve cells in the brain from an unknown cause; the most common type of dementia in the elderly.
2. **Central Intravenous Line:** An intravenous line placed in a large vessel whose tip is near the heart; used for long-term administration of fluids, nutrients, and medications.
3. **Dementia:** Generalized mental deterioration caused by physical or psychologic disease.
4. **Disability:** A hereditary or acquired condition that interferes with normal functions of the body or with a patient's ability to be self-sufficient; can be either mental or physical.
5. **Down's Syndrome:** A genetic condition that causes retarded growth, facial abnormalities, and mental disabilities.
6. **Elder Abuse:** The infliction of physical pain or injury, debilitating mental anguish, or unreasonable confinement on an elderly patient.
7. **Elder Neglect:** The failure to provide for the essential needs of a dependent elderly person, such as food, shelter, health care, clothing, physical comfort, social contact, and emotional support.
8. **Elderly:** Commonly defined as persons over 65 years of age.
9. **Gastric Tube:** A tube placed into the stomach; can be used as a feeding tube.
10. **Home Ventilator:** A mechanical device often used to provide ventilation for a patient unable to breathe spontaneously; generally used together with a tracheostomy.
11. **Shunt:** A tube or device surgically placed in the body to redirect a body fluid from one area to another.
12. **Stoma:** An artificial opening from an internal organ to the surface of the body, such as a hole in the neck created by a tracheostomy.
13. **Tracheostomy Tube:** A metal or plastic tube placed through a surgical opening in the neck into the trachea (tracheostomy) to provide oxygen and ventilation.

IT'S YOUR CALL

You are dispatched to an injury from a fall at an apartment complex for senior citizens. You arrive to find an 86-year-old female sitting on the carpeted living room floor next to a chair. You question the patient about what happened, but she appears to have trouble hearing and does not respond quickly. You repeat your questions and also discuss the incident with an attendant and others present at the time of the incident. With additional questioning, you determine that she was easing herself into the chair when she misjudged the distance to the chair and fell onto her buttocks. The patient's chief complaint is pain in her right hip and numbness in her right leg.

You resurvey the scene and notice that the distance that the patient fell was no more than 1 to 2 feet. You also notice how thick and soft the new carpet is. You wonder whether the patient could be seriously injured. But the patient is complaining of pain and numbness in her leg. What is the likelihood that she has suffered a serious injury? How will you continue to assess and care for this patient?

At any time during an EMS response, you may encounter a patient or bystander who has special physical, mental, or emotional needs. These patients include the elderly, the physically, mentally, or developmentally disabled, and those who require special care because of a specific condition or need special equipment to sustain life. Such needs place these people in the category of special populations.

The **elderly** are generally considered to be those over the age of 65. This is the largest group among several types of special populations. Approximately 40 million Americans are over 65. By the year 2030, the average "baby boomer" will be 80 years old and the elderly will make up more than 20% of all Americans. The elderly population will have nearly doubled in the 50 years between 1980 and 2030.[1] Despite longer life spans, aging continues to pose many medical problems. Anatomic and physiologic changes make body systems more vulnerable to disease and injury.

Patients who are physically dependent on special equipment such as **tracheostomy tubes, home ventilators, shunts,** feeding tubes, or **central intravenous lines** also have special needs that require your attention during assessment and treatment. People disabled by the physical loss of hearing, sight, or movement, or by a mental impairment such as that associated with **Down's syndrome,** will also call for a different focus (see p. 562). Understanding patients' special needs will improve your ability to communicate with them and increase your ability to care for them appropriately.

The Elderly

The Aging Process

As aging takes place, the body's systems begin to deteriorate. This process occurs at different rates in different individuals. The effects of aging on each body system can also be variable. Generally, body system functions decrease at a fairly steady rate after age 30. In addition to cardiovascular system problems, elderly patients face declining respiratory, nervous, endocrine, and musculoskeletal system status. Aging can result in functional disabilities; performing basic daily tasks becomes more difficult, sometimes impossible. Elderly patients are also prone to malnutrition, overhydration, dehydration, heat- and cold-related emergencies, infections, and drug toxicity.

Cardiovascular System

One of the most important factors contributing to deterioration of the cardiovascular system is coronary artery disease (CAD). CAD accounts for more than 500,000 deaths each year in the United States, the majority of which occur in the elderly. In addition to CAD, cardiovascular system changes occur with aging.

- A nearly one-third decrease in cardiac output between the ages of 30 and 80.
- A diminished ability to increase the heart rate.
- Prolonged contractions of the heart chambers.
- Reduced perfusion of other organs in the body.
- A loss of cells in the cardiac conduction pathway, which can lead to cardiac rhythm problems.

Respiratory System

As a person ages, the bones of the thorax become more rigid and brittle and the lungs lose elasticity. The chest wall becomes less compliant, and the efficiency of the respiratory system decreases. The respiratory system is no longer able to work as hard or to take in as much oxygen as a younger person's can. Other changes in the respiratory system include the loss of cilia in the airways and loss of the cough reflex. Together, these make elderly patients more susceptible to respiratory disease from inhaled bacteria or particulate matter, such as smoke, pollen, and other substances in the air.

Nervous System

Nervous system function declines with age as a result of decreases in blood flow to the brain, the speed of nerve conduction in the periphery, and the number of neurons (nerve cells) in the brain. These can lead, in turn, to deteriorations in mental function, motor ability, reaction time, visual and hearing acuity, and sleep patterns. Pain perception is often altered or decreased, making your assessment of these patients more difficult. Elderly patients occasionally have "silent" heart attacks, for instance, in which they do not feel pain typical of myocardial infarctions (MI). Because the thermoregulatory center of the brain may not be functioning adequately, elderly patients are at added risk of developing hypothermia and hyperthermia.

The loss of hearing can make it difficult for the elderly to understand questions, which may make it seem as though they cannot think clearly when hearing is really the problem. Often you will have to talk more slowly and give an elderly patient more time to answer questions than you would with younger patients. Good eye contact with an elderly patient is very important.

Dementia is a loss of intellectual function (thinking, memory, and reasoning) that can be so severe that it interferes with an individual's daily function. **Alzheimer's syndrome** is the most common form of dementia.

Musculoskeletal System

Muscles become smaller with age, and both muscles and ligaments develop calcium deposits that can make them less flexible. Bone density also decreases, a condition known as osteoporosis. This is a degenerative disease that afflicts approximately one third of all people over age 65; it most often affects women. Osteoporosis occurs as a result of a significant decrease in calcium in the bones. This causes the bones to become less dense, more brittle, and less likely to repair themselves after damage. Coupled with decreased muscle mass and weakening bones, this leads to falls that can cause significant injuries, including fractures.

These problems make elderly patients more likely to break bones in seemingly minor incidents and to have prolonged healing times. It also raises potential problems during injury immobilization. Handle elderly patients gently and do not force bones or joints into alignment with the shape of a splint or backboard. Support patients' bones and spines as carefully as possible.

Aging also often results in posture and balance changes caused by increased curvature of the thoracic spine. These types of changes can make the elderly more prone to falls and can also decrease respiratory function.

Renal System

The structure and function of the kidneys also change with age. Blood flow and the ability of the kidneys to filter blood decrease significantly with aging. This can result in problems that include fluid retention (overhydration), imbalances of electrolytes such as sodium and potassium, and medication toxicity caused by reduced filtration of drugs from the blood. Overhydration can lead to further complications such as pulmonary and peripheral (extremity) edema.

Other Changes and Conditions

Aging decreases the body's ability to fight infection. This can place a patient at greater risk of many types of infection. Changes in body composition, such as the reduction of muscle mass and increase in fat tissue, can influence the effectiveness of certain medications. Proper nutrition can also become a problem for some elderly individuals because they frequently consume less than the minimum daily requirements for calories and vitamins.

Common Problems in Elderly Patients

Failing eyesight, slower reflexes, arthritis, and numbness in the extremities caused by poor circulation all contribute to common accidents, such as falls, in the elderly (Figure 27-1). Falls more frequently cause fractures because of weaker and more brittle bones. Serious injuries such as hip fractures and head injuries can occur more easily. The brain becomes smaller as it ages, and more space develops between its surface and the skull. This allows for more movement of the brain and less protection during impact; intracranial bleeding can occur more easily. Injuries may be self-inflicted in depressed patients or may be associated with **elder abuse.**

Geriatric patients have many fears that need to be dealt with. Besides the medical emergency itself, they may

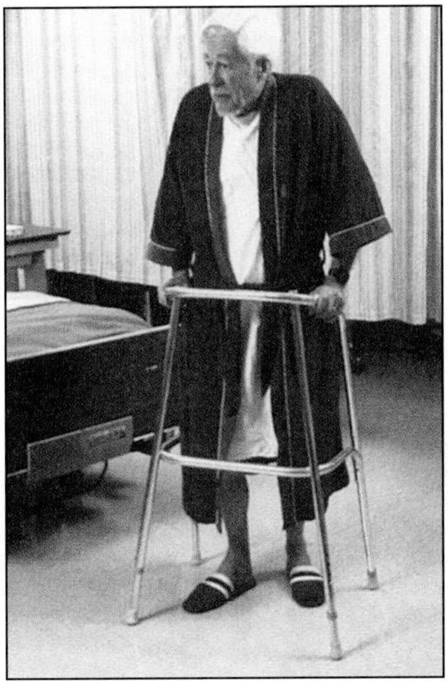

Figure 27-1

Changes that come with age, such as failing eyesight, slower reflexes, arthritis, and numbness, all contribute to common accidents.

Down's syndrome is a birth defect caused by a genetic abnormality. This condition occurs at the time of fertilization, most often in mothers over 35 years of age. Down's syndrome can be diagnosed before birth by analyzing the amniotic fluid. It is estimated that there are 200,000 older children and adults with Down's syndrome in the United States. Many fetuses with Down's syndrome die as a result of organ failure. Infants that live to birth are usually born prematurely. They often suffer from low birth weight and a variety of other problems.

Those with Down's syndrome have delayed mental development. They are slow to explore and comprehend their environment, and they are prone to injury. As they develop, they tend to be obese and short in height. Abnormal head development causes a characteristic appearance with a large forehead, slightly square head shape, and eyes set apart. The cervical spine region of the neck may be unstable, so it is important to avoid flexion and extension of the neck. The tongue of a Down's syndrome patient is usually thick, which contributes to speech difficulties. Individuals with Down's syndrome also have narrow tracheal and nasal passages. This combination of factors puts Down's syndrome patients at high risk of airway obstructions.

Down's syndrome patients frequently suffer from congestive heart failure, sleep apnea, seizure disorders, respiratory infections, and airway obstruction. Most people with Down's syndrome are open and very friendly, but this may not be the case in an emergency situation. If a patient is combative or otherwise difficult to manage, recruit the help of someone the patient knows, if possible. If the patient is unresponsive and experiencing an airway problem, opening the mouth and lifting the jaw is often all that is needed to help. Be careful not to manipulate the neck too much. Injuries or other medical emergencies such as seizures should be cared for in the same manner as for any other patient.

References

Goldberg M: Spine instability and the Special Olympics, *Clin Sports Med* 12:507, 1993.

Grennberg JA, Shannon MT: Down's syndrome: implications for emergency care, *J Emerg Med Serv* Aug. 20:38, 1995.

Wells G et al: Congenital heart disease in infants with Down's syndrome, *So Med J* 87:724, 1994.

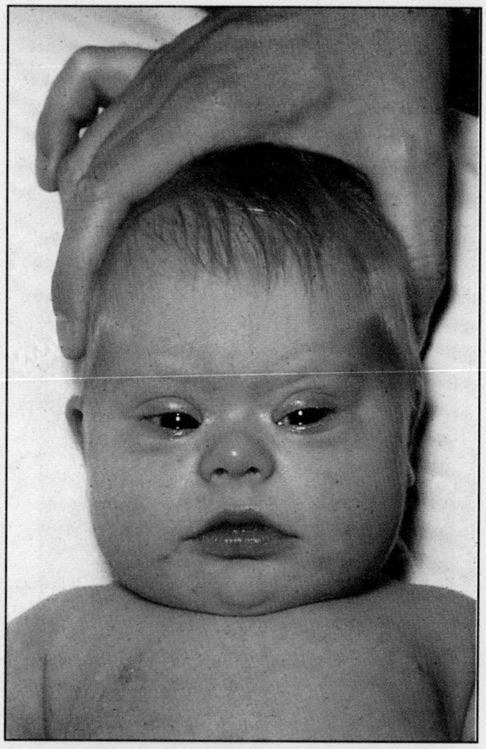

Child with Down's syndrome.

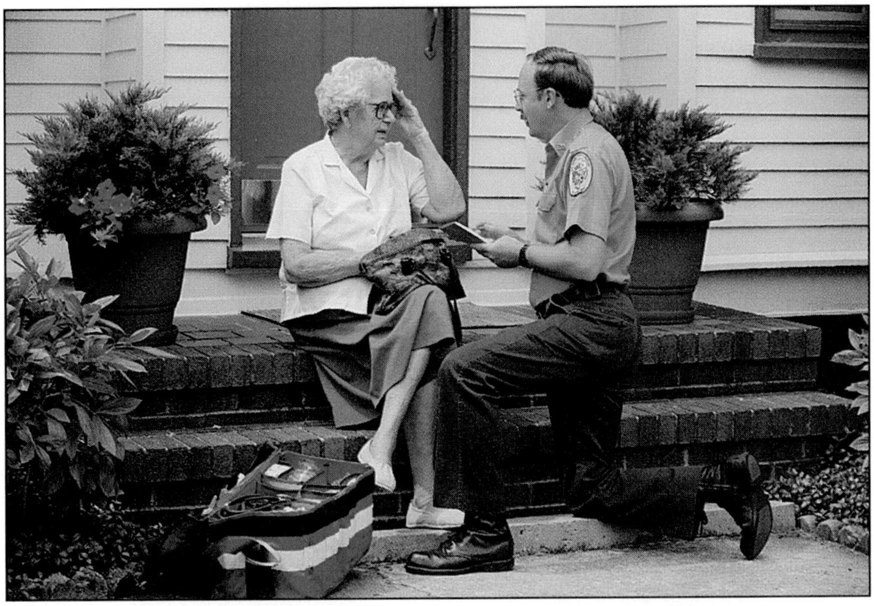

Figure 27-2
Communicate with the patient on eye-level.

be concerned about hospital costs, loss of independence, who will care for their home or pets, and whether they will be allowed to return home after the hospitalization.

Medical conditions that typically afflict the elderly include:

- Circulatory problems causing heart failure, fainting, or stroke
- Chronic lung disease, and respiratory infections such as pneumonia
- Diabetes
- Cancer
- Dementia, including Alzheimer's
- Heat-related illness, such as heatstroke
- Cold-related illness, such as hypothermia
- Depression
- Drug toxicity

Assessing an Elderly Patient

Assessment of an elderly patient is generally similar to any other assessment. However, this assessment does require special attention to the fact that the individual's sight, hearing, mental status, comprehension, and mobility may be impaired. Face the patient whenever possible, and try to get to the patient's eye level (Figure 27-2). Address the patient by name. Speak slowly and clearly. Show respect by using a title and the patient's last name, such as "Mrs. Simmons." Use open-ended questions, such as "Describe the pain in your stomach." Minimize interruptions and noise during the interview.

If the patient has difficulty communicating with you because of a hearing or speech impairment that can be corrected, help the patient locate the device needed for communication, such as a hearing aid or artificial larynx (Figure 27-3, *A* and *B*). If you still are unable to communicate, bystanders may be your only source of information.

Observe the patient's appearance, behavior, and environment. Consider the following questions:

- Is the patient dressed appropriately?
- Does the patient appear to have proper hygiene?
- Does the patient show signs of adequate nutrition?
- Does the patient appear to be in pain or discomfort, or seem withdrawn or depressed?
- Does the patient have glasses or a hearing aid that would make it easier to communicate more clearly?
- Does the patient have any obvious bruises that are not associated with the incident? (The presence of questionable bruises may be an indication of elder abuse, discussed on p. 564).
- In what daily living activities does the patient participate? Can the patient eat, wash, and attend to other aspects of self-care? To what extent does the patient have social interaction?
- Does the patient have medications; if so, what are they, and what are they for?

When performing a physical examination, consider:

- Level of consciousness (LOC): Determine if the patient is awake and oriented. Dementia typically causes disorientation; the patient may be awake and able to talk

A

B

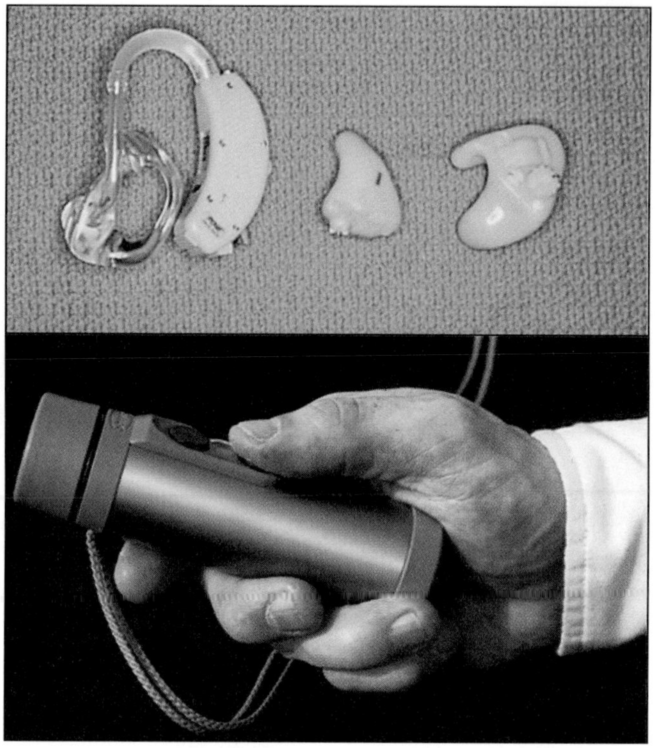

Figure 27-3
A, Hearing aids. **B,** Artificial larynx.

with you, but may say things that do not make sense. However, do not assume that all changes in mental status are caused by dementia.

- Airway: Maintain an open airway. If the patient has a possibility of spinal injury, use inline spinal stabilization.
- Breathing: Check that air exchange is adequate. If not, intervene with ventilation and oxygen. If the patient is using home oxygen, check the device for appropriate flow rate and any kinks in the tubing that could be preventing the patient from getting the correct amount. If the patient's breathing is labored and either too fast or too slow, assist ventilations. Auscultate the lungs for abnormal breath sounds.
- Circulation: Ensure that the patient's perfusion is adequate. The heart rate should be 60 to 100 beats per minute, with palpable distal pulses. Skin temperature, color, and moisture should be normal (warm, pink, and dry). Normal systolic blood pressure is between 90 and 160 mm Hg. Diastolic blood pressure should be between 60 and 90 mm Hg. (Normal blood pressure is more difficult to define in the elderly. Factors that account for the wide variation include age, body size, activity levels, medications, and current level of pain or distress.)
- Eyes: Unless affected by trauma, surgery, or medical conditions such as cataracts or glaucoma, the patient's eyes should respond to light and should track objects.
- Central nervous system (CNS): Hold the patient's hands and check for grip strength, sensation, and movement.

Complete your focused history and physical examination as appropriate for the patient's situation and complaint. If the patient is going to be transported to a hospital, explain this and move the patient gently. Ask a family member to accompany you whenever possible. Continue to be compassionate as you complete your assessment, provide care, and transport the patient. Elderly patients are often more aware of what goes on around them and how they are being treated than they sometimes appear. Care with dignity is fundamental to excellent EMS care.

Elder Abuse

Elder abuse can take many forms, including psychologic, emotional, and physical harm. By definition, elder abuse can be thought of as the infliction of physical pain or injury, debilitating mental anguish, or unreasonable confinement of an elderly patient. Most often, the abuser is a relative who is living with the patient.

There are several signs of elder abuse that you should be aware of (Box 27-1). Any injuries that are inconsistent with the nature of the call and the history require closer examination. Bruises on the arms and wrists can indicate grab marks or the use of restraints. Fractured bones in the elderly can occur from blunt injury or twisting action, such as grabbing and twisting a wrist (Figure 27-4).

Besides the patient's signs and symptoms, consider the behavior of the caregiver. If the caregiver monopo-

BOX 27-1 **Possible Signs of Elder Abuse or Neglect**

Abuse

- Bruises inconsistent with the incident or history
- Bruises on patients who are immobile
- Burn marks
- Confinement, including indications of restraint use
- Indications of intimidation or humiliation

Neglect

- Malnourishment
- Bed sores
- Unkempt appearance or poor hygiene
- Odors or soiled clothing
- Infected wounds
- Abandonment

Either Abuse or Neglect

- Inappropriate behavior of the caregiver

IT'S YOUR CALL
CONCLUSION

As an elderly female, your patient is at high risk for bone injury even though the mechanism of injury seems minor. You assess the patient and determine that pain is localized in the hip area. She does not complain of back pain. Distal pulses and sensation are normal, but she does complain of tingling in the leg.

You notice that lighting in the apartment is good. There is no loose carpet or other safety problem that might cause falls. There was an attendant available, but the patient did not call her. There are no signs of neglect, abuse, or medication problems.

You swathe both legs together for comfort and hip immobilization, then gently place the patient on a backboard so that you can move her without further discomfort. Although the attendant cannot accompany you to the hospital, she provides medications and medical records for you to take to the hospital. During transport, you talk with the patient, helping her express her concerns about the injury and how it will affect her life. X-rays in the emergency department reveal that she does have a hip fracture.

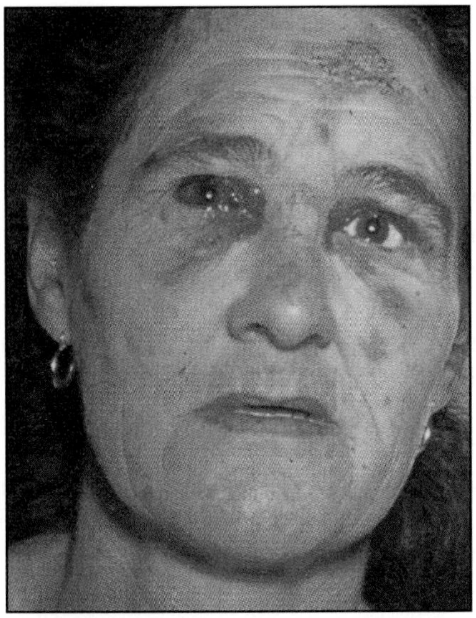

Figure 27-4
Facial bruising on an elderly woman.

lizes the conversation, not allowing the patient to speak for him or herself, this should alert you to a possible problem. Also pay special attention if the caregiver blames the patient for the problem.

As part of your care, document what you see and hear. Quote the information provided by the patient and any caregiver. Document the home surroundings. If you suspect elder abuse, you have a responsibility to report your suspicions. Follow local protocols for this situation. If you are uncertain about how to proceed, contact the medical direction physician for instructions.

As with children, the elderly can suffer from less direct forms of mistreatment than outright abuse. **Elder neglect** is the failure to provide for the essential needs of a dependent elderly person, such as food, shelter, health care, clothing, physical comfort, social contact, and emotional support. You should also know local requirements and procedures for reporting possible cases of neglect.

Patients With Special Needs

You may assist a patient who either has had special needs since birth or has developed them later as a result of a medical condition or injury. These patients may have difficulty performing even the most basic functions, but many overcome their disabilities and lead relatively normal lives. Some of these patients require specialized equipment to help them perform daily tasks or even to stay alive. This section briefly discusses the special needs of patients who depend on several types of specialized equipment:

- Tracheostomy tubes and home ventilators
- Shunts

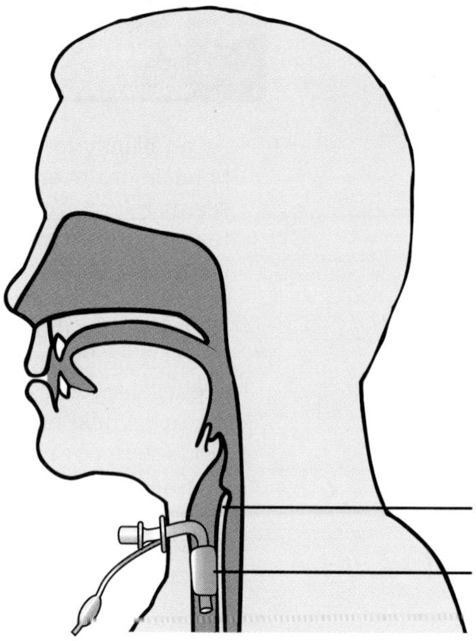

Figure 27-5
Tracheostomy tube.

- Gastric (feeding) tubes
- Central intravenous lines

Frequently, these patients are referred to as *technology-dependent patients.*

This section also covers the special needs of patients with physical and developmental disabilities.

Patients Who Depend on Special Equipment

When dealing with children who depend on special equipment, listen to what the parent has to say about what's wrong with the patient. Parents are well aware of the patient's normal status; a parent who feels something is wrong is usually correct. Parents are often the full-time caregivers, and they may understand the child better than anyone else. They may be experts when it comes to special equipment, such as airway tubes and ventilators, that are being used at home. These parents have a strong need to be involved in emergency care, and it is usually a mistake to ignore their suggestions; they are usually able to help immensely.

Tracheostomy Tubes and Home Ventilators

Some patients rely on technologic assistance from items such as tracheostomy tubes to breathe. A tracheostomy tube is a metal or plastic tube that is placed through a surgical opening in the anterior neck into the trachea (tracheostomy) in order to provide oxygen and ventilation (Figure 27-5). The hole in the neck created by the tracheostomy is called a **stoma.** The tracheostomy tube is inserted through the stoma; it is generally placed so that it can be removed if necessary. The most common problem associated with tracheostomy tubes is that they may become obstructed or dislodged. Occasionally, bleeding and infection can occur at the site of the tracheostomy.

If you are summoned to provide care for a patient with a tracheostomy tube, examine the tube to see if it is obstructed by mucus or other secretions. Suction the tube for 10 to 15 seconds if needed. If the patient is not breathing, attach 100% oxygen to your bag-valve device and attach that directly to the tracheostomy tube and ventilate the patient. If the tracheostomy tube becomes displaced and cannot be easily replaced, check to see if the patient is breathing adequately through the stoma. If not, attempt to ventilate with the bag-valve-mask (BVM) placed over the mouth and nose, and the stoma covered. If this does not work, attach a smaller mask and ventilate the patient directly through the stoma (mask-to-stoma ventilation) while sealing the mouth and nose.

A **home ventilator** is a mechanical device that is often used together with a tracheostomy tube to provide ventilation for a patient unable to breathe adequately on his or her own (Figure 27-6). If the machine fails to operate properly, the patient should be disconnected from the ventilator and ventilated as discussed above with the bag-valve device connected directly to the tracheostomy tube.

Shunts

A shunt is a tube or device surgically placed in the body to redirect a body fluid from one area to another. A **ven-**

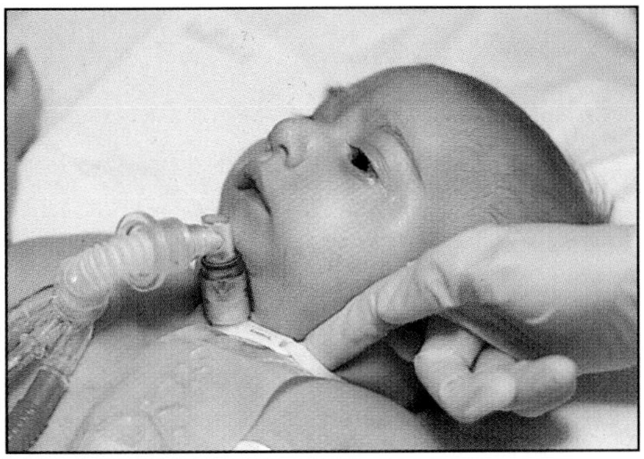

Figure 27-6

Pediatric patient with a tracheostomy tube on a mechanical ventilator.

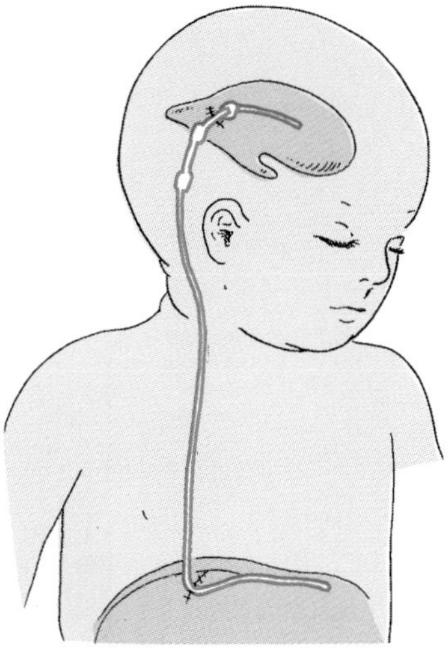

Figure 27-7

Ventriculoperitoneal shunt.

tricular shunt extends from the ventricle of the brain to the abdomen. It is designed to drain excess cerebrospinal fluid (CSF) that occurs when injury or illness prevents normal drainage (Figure 27-7). The tubing is placed below the skin, but is usually visible or palpable. If the shunt fails to work properly, the patient may complain of headache or pain, or may vomit or have a decreased mental status. You will not be able to test or find out whether the shunt is working properly. Do not touch the shunt; there is nothing you can do with it. Instead, care for your patient by treating the signs and symptoms. These patients usually have altered consciousness and are prone to respiratory difficulties, including respiratory arrest. Transport the patient to the hospital for evaluation.

Many kidney dialysis patients have venous shunts implanted in an arm. These shunts allow easy access to the circulatory system for the dialysis procedure. Do not disturb a venous shunt. If one is in place, take blood pressures on the other arm. If a patient bleeds from a shunt site, apply gentle direct pressure and transport immediately.

Gastric Tubes

Patients who cannot be fed by mouth require a gastric tube for feeding. A **gastric tube** is either placed through the nose or mouth into the stomach or is placed through a surgical opening in the left upper abdominal quadrant directly into the stomach (Figure 27-8). Gastric tubes come in various sizes. You may be summoned because a gastric tube has been dislodged. Ensure that the airway is clear, administer oxygen, and transport the patient either sitting or lying on the right side with the head elevated. This will minimize the chance of aspiration. Do what you can to maintain sterility of a dislodged tube, but do not try to replace it.

Central Intravenous Lines

A central intravenous line is an intravenous tube placed in the large blood vessels that drain close to the heart for long-term administration of fluids, nutrients, and medications.

Complications that occasionally occur with central lines include:

- A cracked or dislodged line
- Clotting
- Infection
- Bleeding
- Leakage

If bleeding is present, control it with sterile dressings and direct pressure. Try not to move or adjust the line, and do everything possible to maintain its sterility. Transport the patient to the hospital for evaluation.

A Disabled Patient

A **disability** is a hereditary or acquired condition that interferes with normal functions of the body or with a person's ability to be self-sufficient. Disabilities generally fall into two categories: mental and physical. A person unable to move normally is often said to be *physically disabled.* A person with impaired mental function is often called *developmentally disabled.* There are more than 2 million developmentally disabled people under age 21 in the United States. These terms mean different things to different people. EMTs need to look beyond the labels established by society and focus on the patient's chief complaint.

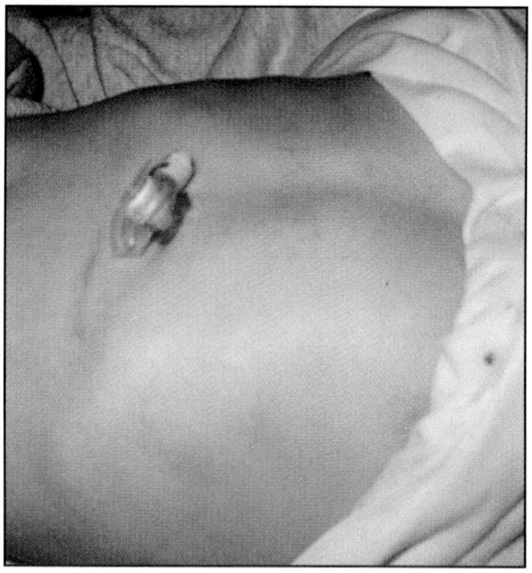

Figure 27-8

A gastric feeding tube in the upper left abdominal quadrant.

ALZHEIMER'S DISEASE AND DEMENTIA

Alzheimer's disease is named after Dr. Alois Alzheimer, who first described the condition in 1906. It is a progressive, degenerative disease that attacks the brain and impairs memory, thinking, and behavior. It is the most common form of dementia. Approximately 4 million Americans have Alzheimer's disease. One in 10 people over the age of 65 and nearly half of those over 85 have the disease. It affects men and women equally. Individuals who care for a family member with Alzheimer's often report that care consumes more time and energy as the disease progresses.

A definitive diagnosis of Alzheimer's disease is not possible; no single clinical test can identify it. Instead, patients undergo a battery of highly technical tests. These tests, in conjunction with family members' statements; help a physician reach a probable diagnosis of Alzheimer's disease. Confirmation requires examination of brain tissue, which is usually done during an autopsy after death.

Physical and social activity are important, as is proper nutrition. If you are caring for a patient with Alzheimer's, remember to speak slowly and clearly. You will likely need to repeat your questions, and the patient may repeatedly forget who you are and why you are there. Remain calm and understanding. Seek information from caregivers, such as family or nursing home staff. Because Alzheimer's patients in various stages of the disease may be frustrated or aggressive, be prepared for these behaviors. Although there is no cure for Alzheimer's, several medications are being studied; and one has been approved by the Food and Drug Administration (FDA) to help treat symptoms. For more information on Alzheimer's Disease, contact the Alzheimer's Association at 1-800-272-3900.

References

Kane RL: *Essentials of clinical geriatrics,* ed 3, New York, 1994, McGraw-Hill.

Nixon RG: Faded memories, *J Emerg Care, Rescue, Transport* 25:31, 1996.

Alzheimer's Association: Internet address: http://www.alz.org.

The causes of physical and developmental disability are many, and include:

- Cerebral palsy
- Polio
- Multiple sclerosis
- Muscular dystrophy
- Stroke
- Injury resulting in the loss of mobility
- Down's syndrome
- Infections

Approach a disabled patient as you would any other. Try to determine the patient's normal level of understanding and interaction. As you ask questions, it may become clear that the patient does not understand what you are saying. Rephrase and simplify your statements if necessary. Developmentally disabled patients usually have a structured routine to their activities. Injury or illness could upset that normal routine and cause the patient to have feelings of fear and apprehension.

When assessing a physically disabled patient for an injury, it may not always be easy to separate new injuries from preexisting conditions. This is especially true for musculoskeletal injuries. By questioning the patient and family, you may be able to determine what the patient's normal mental and physical status is. Anything beyond the "norms" for the patient should be cared for. If a caregiver is present with the patient, have the caregiver explain to the patient the care that will be provided, and accompany you during transport.

SUMMARY

You are likely to be summoned to care for a variety of patients that can be classified as belonging to special populations. Whether your patient is elderly, physically or developmentally disabled, or in need of specialized equipment to sustain life, the patient depends on you. Consider the patient's limitations and work around them. Establishing effective communication is extremely important to the care you will provide. Speak clearly and in simple terms. Rephrase questions if necessary. Be patient, understanding, and compassionate as you assess and care for the patient.

REFERENCES

1. **Schrier R:** *Geriatric medicine,* Philadelphia, 1990, Saunders.
2. **Sanders M:** *Mosby's paramedic text,* St Louis, 1994, Mosby.

SUGGESTED READINGS

1. **Janing J:** Tarnishing the golden years, *J Emerg Serv* 21:40, 1992.
2. **Nixon RG:** Faded memories, *J Emerg Care, Rescue, Transport* 25:31, 1996.
3. **Kane RL:** *Essentials of clinical geriatrics,* ed 3, New York, 1994, McGraw-Hill.

Appendix A

National Registry of Emergency Medical Technicians Skills Sheets

Patient Assessment/Management - Trauma

Start Time: ____________________

Stop Time: ____________________ **Date:** ____________________

Candidate's Name: ____

Evaluator's Name: ____

		Points Possible	Points Awarded
Takes, or verbalizes, body substance isolation precautions		1	
SCENE SIZE-UP			
Determines the scene is safe		1	
Determines the mechanism of injury		1	
Determines the number of patients		1	
Requests additional help if necessary		1	
Considers stabilization of spine		1	
INITIAL ASSESSMENT			
Verbalizes general impression of the patient		1	
Determines responsiveness/level of consciousness		1	
Determines chief complaint/apparent life threats		1	
Assesses airway and breathing	Assessment Initiates appropriate oxygen therapy Assures adequate ventilation Injury management	1 1 1 1	
Assesses circulation	Assesses/controls major bleeding Assesses pulse Assesses skin (color, temperature, and condition)	1 1 1	
Identifies priority patients/makes transport decision		1	
FOCUSED HISTORY AND PHYSICAL EXAMINATION/RAPID TRAUMA ASSESSMENT			
Selects appropriate assessment ***(focused or rapid assessment)***		1	
Obtains, or directs assistance to obtain, baseline vital signs		1	
Obtains SAMPLE history		1	
DETAILED PHYSICAL EXAMINATION			
Assesses the head	Inspects and palpates the scalp and ears Assesses the eyes Assesses the facial areas, including oral and nasal areas	1 1 1	
Assesses the neck	Inspects and palpates the neck Assesses for jugular venous distention Assesses for trachael deviation	1 1 1	
Assesses the chest	Inspects Palpates Auscultates	1 1 1	
Assesses the abdomen/pelvis	Assesses the abdomen Assesses the pelvis Verbalizes assessment of genitalia/perineum as needed	1 1 1	
Assesses the extremities	(1 point for each extremity) Includes inspection, palpation, and assessment of motor, sensory, and circulatory function	4	
Assesses the posterior	Assesses thorax Assesses lumbar	1 1	
Manages secondary injuries and wounds appropriately (1 point for appropriate management of the secondary injury/wound)		1	
Verbalizes reassessment of the vital signs		1	
	Total:	**40**	

Critical Criteria

_____ Did not take, or verbalize, body substance isolation precautions.
_____ Did not determine scene safety.
_____ Did not assess for spinal protection.
_____ Did not provide for spinal protection when indicated.
_____ Did not provide high concentration of oxygen.
_____ Did not find, or manage, problems associated with airway, breathing, hemorrhage, or shock (hypoperfusion).
_____ Did not differentiate patient's need for transportation versus continued assessment at the scene.
_____ Did other detailed physical examination before assessing the airway, breathing, and circulation.
_____ Did not transport patient within 10-minute time limit.

Patient Assessment/Management - Medical

Start Time: ____________

Stop Time: ____________

Date: ____________

Candidate's Name: ____________

Evaluator's Name: ____________

		Points Possible	Points Awarded
Takes, or verbalizes, body substance isolation precautions		1	
SCENE SIZE-UP			
Determines the scene is safe		1	
Determines the mechanism of injury/nature of illness		1	
Determines the number of patients		1	
Requests additional help if necessary		1	
Considers stabilization of spine		1	
INITIAL ASSESSMENT			
Verbalizes general impression of the patient		1	
Determines responsiveness/level of consciousness		1	
Determines chief complaint/apparent life threats		1	
Assesses airway and breathing	Assessment Initiates appropriate oxygen therapy Assures adequate ventilation	1 1 1	
Assesses circulation	Assesses/controls major bleeding Assesses pulse Assesses skin (color, temperature, and condition)	1 1 1	
Identifies priority patients/makes transport decision		1	
FOCUSED HISTORY AND PHYSICAL EXAMINATION/RAPID ASSESSMENT			
Signs and symptoms (*Assess history of present illness)*		1	

Respiratory	Cardiac	Altered Mental Status	Allergic Reaction	Poisoning/ Overdose	Environmental Emergency	Obstetrics	Behavioral
*Onset? *Provokes? *Quality? *Radiates? *Severity? *Time? *Interventions?	*Onset? *Provokes? *Quality? *Radiates? *Severity? *Time? *Interventions?	*Description of the episode? *Onset? *Duration? *Associated symptoms? *Evidence of trauma? *Interventions? *Seizures? *Fever?	*History of allergies? *What were you exposed to? *How were you exposed? *Effects? *Progression? *Interventions?	*Substance? *When did you ingest/become exposed? *How much did you ingest? *Over what time period? *Interventions? *Estimated weight?	*Source? *Environment? *Duration? *Loss of consciousness? *Effects - general or local?	*Are you pregnant? *How long have you been pregnant? *Pain or contractions? *Bleeding or discharge? *Do you feel the need to push? *Last menstrual period?	*How do you feel? *Determine suicidal tendencies. *Is the patient a threat to self or others? *Is there a medical problem? *Interventions?

	Points Possible	Points Awarded
Allergies	1	
Medications	1	
Past pertinent history	1	
Last oral intake	1	
Event leading to present illness (rule out trauma)	1	
Performs focused physical examination (*assesses affected body part/system or, if indicated, completes rapid assessment)*	1	
Vitals (*obtains baseline vital signs)*	1	
Interventions (*obtains medical direction or verbalizes standing order for medication interventions and verbalizes proper additional intervention/treatment)*	1	
Transport (reevaluates the transport decision)	1	
Verbalizes the consideration for completing a detailed physical examination	1	
ONGOING ASSESSMENT (verbalized)		
Repeats initial assessment	1	
Repeats vital signs	1	
Repeats focused assessment regarding patient complaint or injuries	1	
Total:	**30**	

Critical Criteria

_____ Did not take, or verbalize, body substance isolation precautions when necessary.
_____ Did not determine scene safety.
_____ Did not obtain medical direction or verbalize standing orders for medical interventions.
_____ Did not provide high concentration of oxygen.
_____ Did not find or manage problems associated with airway, breathing, hemorrhage, or shock (hypoperfusion).
_____ Did not differentiate patient's need for transportation versus continued assessment at the scene.
_____ Did detailed or focused history/physical examination before assessing the airway, breathing, and circulation.
_____ Did not ask questions about the present illness.
_____ Administered a dangerous or inappropriate intervention.

Cardiac Arrest Management/AED

Start Time: ________________

Stop Time: ________________ **Date:** ________________

Candidate's Name: ________________________________

Evaluator's Name: ________________________________

	Points Possible	Points Awarded
ASSESSMENT		
Takes, or verbalizes, body substance isolation precautions	1	
Briefly questions the rescuer about arrest events	1	
Directs rescuer to stop CPR	1	
Verifies absence of spontaneous pulse (**skill station examiner states "no pulse"**)	1	
Directs resumption of CPR	1	
Turns on defibrillator power	1	
Attaches automated defibrillator to the patient	1	
Directs rescuer to stop CPR and ensures all individuals are clear of the patient	1	
Initiates analysis of the rhythm	1	
Delivers shock (up to three successive shocks)	1	
Verifies absence of spontaneous pulse (**skill station examiner states "no pulse"**)	1	
TRANSITION		
Directs resumption of CPR	1	
Gathers additional information about arrest event	1	
Confirms effectiveness of CPR (ventilation and compressions)	1	
INTEGRATION		
Verbalizes or directs insertion of a simple airway adjunct (oral/nasal airway)	1	
Ventilates, or directs ventilation of, the patient	1	
Ensures that high concentration of oxygen is delivered to the patient	1	
Ensures that CPR continues without unnecessary/prolonged interruption	1	
Reevaluates patient/CPR in approximately 1 minute	1	
Repeats defibrillator sequence	1	
TRANSPORTATION		
Verbalizes transportation of patient	1	
Total:	21	

Critical Criteria

_____ Did not take, or verbalize, body substance isolation precautions.

_____ Did not evaluate the need for immediate use of the AED.

_____ Did not direct initiation/resumption of ventilation/compressions at appropriate times.

_____ Did not ensure that all individuals were clear of patient before delivering each shock.

_____ Did not operate the AED properly (inability to deliver shock).

_____ Prevented the defibrillator from delivering indicated stacked shocks.

Bag-Valve-Mask
Apneic Patient

Start Time: ____________________

Stop Time: ____________________ **Date:** ____________________

Candidate's Name: ____

Evaluator's Name: ____

	Points Possible	Points Awarded
Takes, or verbalizes, body substance isolation precautions	1	
Voices opening the airway	1	
Voices inserting an airway adjunct	1	
Selects appropriately sized mask	1	
Creates a proper mask-to-face seal	1	
Ventilates patient at no less than 800 ml volume ***(The examiner must witness for at least 30 seconds.)***	1	
Connects reservoir and oxygen	1	
Adjusts liter flow to 15 liters/minute or greater	1	
The examiner indicates arrival of a second EMT. The second EMT is instructed to ventilate the patient while the candidate controls the mask and the airway.		
Voices reopening the airway	1	
Creates a proper mask-to-face seal	1	
Instructs assistant to resume ventilation at proper volume per breath ***(The examiner must witness for at least 30 seconds.)***	1	
Total:	**11**	

Critical Criteria

_____ Did not take, or verbalize, body substance isolation precautions.

_____ Did not immediately ventilate the patient.

_____ Interrupted ventilations for more than 20 seconds.

_____ Did not provide high concentration of oxygen.

_____ Did not provide, or direct assistant to provide, proper volume/breath *(more than two ventilations per minute are below 800 ml)*.

_____ Did not allow adequate exhalation.

Spinal Immobilization Seated Patient

Start Time: ____________

Stop Time: ____________ **Date:** ____________

Candidate's Name: ____________

Evaluator's Name: ____________

	Points Possible	Points Awarded
Takes, or verbalizes, body substance isolation precautions	1	
Directs assistant to place/maintain head in the neutral inline position	1	
Directs assistant to maintain manual immobilization of the head	1	
Reassesses motor, sensory, and circulatory function in each extremity	1	
Applies appropriately sized extrication collar	1	
Positions the immobilization device behind the patient	1	
Secures the device to the patient's torso	1	
Evaluates torso fixation and adjusts as necessary	1	
Evaluates and pads behind the patient's head as necessary	1	
Secures the patient's head to the device	1	
Verbalizes moving the patient to a long board	1	
Reassesses motor, sensory, and circulatory function in each extremity	1	
Total:	**12**	

Critical Criteria

_____ Did not immediately direct, or take, manual immobilization of the head.

_____ Released, or ordered release of, manual immobilization before it was maintained mechanically.

_____ Patient manipulated, or moved excessively, causing potential spinal compromise.

_____ Device moved excessively up, down, left, or right on the patient's torso.

_____ Head immobilization allowed for excessive movement.

_____ Torso fixation inhibited chest rise, resulting in respiratory compromise.

_____ Upon completion of immobilization, head was not in the neutral position.

_____ Did not assess motor, sensory, and circulatory function in each extremity after voicing immobilization on the long board.

_____ Immobilized head to the board before securing the torso.

Spinal Immobilization
Supine Patient

Start Time: ________________

Stop Time: ________________ **Date:** ____________________

Candidate's Name: ______________________________________

Evaluator's Name: ______________________________________

	Points Possible	Points Awarded
Takes, or verbalizes, body substance isolation precautions	1	
Directs assistant to place/maintain head in the neutral inline position	1	
Directs assistant to maintain manual immobilization of the head	1	
Reassesses motor, sensory, and circulatory function in each extremity	1	
Applies appropriately sized extrication collar	1	
Positions the immobilization device appropriately	1	
Directs movement of the patient onto the device without compromising the integrity of the spine	1	
Applies padding to voids between the torso and the board as necessary	1	
Immobilizes the patient's torso to the device	1	
Evaluates and pads behind the patient's head as necessary	1	
Immobilizes the patient's head to the device	1	
Secures the patient's legs to the device	1	
Secures the patient's arms to the device	1	
Reassesses motor, sensory, and circulatory function in each extremity	1	
Total:	**14**	

Critical Criteria

_____ Did not immediately direct, or take, manual immobilization of the head.

_____ Released, or ordered release of, manual immobilization before it was maintained mechanically.

_____ Patient manipulated, or moved excessively, causing potential spinal compromise.

_____ Device moved excessively up, down, left, or right on the patient's torso.

_____ Head immobilization allowed for excessive movement.

_____ Upon completion of immobilization, head was not in the neutral position.

_____ Did not assess motor, sensory, and circulatory function in each extremity after immobilization on the device.

_____ Immobilized head to the board before securing the torso.

Immobilization Skills
Long Bone Injury

Start Time: ____________________

Stop Time: ____________________ **Date:** ______________________

Candidate's Name: ____

Evaluator's Name: ____

	Points Possible	Points Awarded
Takes, or verbalizes, body substance isolation precautions	1	
Directs application of manual stabilization of the injury	1	
Assesses motor, sensory, and circulatory function in the injured extremity	1	
Note: The examiner acknowledges "motor, sensory, and circulatory function are present and normal."		
Measures the splint	1	
Applies the splint	1	
Immobilizes the joint above the injury site	1	
Immobilizes the joint below the injury site	1	
Secures the entire injured extremity	1	
Immobilizes the hand/foot in the position of function	1	
Reassesses motor, sensory, and circulatory function in the injured extremity	1	
Note: The examiner acknowledges "motor, sensory, and circulatory function are present and normal."		
Total:	**10**	

Critical Criteria

_____ Grossly moved the injured extremity.

_____ Did not immobilize the joint above and the joint below the injury site.

_____ Did not reassess motor, sensory, and circulatory function in the injured extremity before and after splinting.

Immobilization Skills
Joint Injury

Start Time: ________________

Stop Time: ________________ **Date:** ____________________

Candidate's Name: ____

Evaluator's Name: ____

	Points Possible	Points Awarded
Takes, or verbalizes, body substance isolation precautions	1	
Directs application of manual stabilization of the shoulder injury	1	
Assesses motor, sensory, and circulatory function in the injured extremity	1	
Note: The examiner acknowledges "motor, sensory, and circulatory function are present and normal."		
Selects the proper splinting material	1	
Immobilizes the site of the injury	1	
Immobilizes the bone above the injured joint	1	
Immobilizes the bone below the injured joint	1	
Reassesses motor, sensory, and circulatory function in the injured extremity	1	
Note: The examiner acknowledges "motor, sensory, and circulatory function are present and normal."		
Total:	8	

Critical Criteria

_____ Did not support the joint so that the joint did not bear distal weight.

_____ Did not immobilize the bone above and below the injured site.

_____ Did not reassess motor, sensory, and circulatory function in the injured extremity before and after splinting.

Immobilization Skills
Traction Splinting

Start Time: ______________

Stop Time: ______________ **Date:** ______________

Candidate's Name: ______________________________

Evaluator's Name: ______________________________

	Points Possible	Points Awarded
Takes, or verbalizes, body substance isolation precautions	1	
Directs application of manual stabilization of the injured leg	1	
Directs the application of manual traction	1	
Assesses motor, sensory, and circulatory function in the injured extremity	1	
Note: The examiner acknowledges "motor, sensory, and circulatory function are present and normal."		
Prepares/adjusts splint to the proper length	1	
Positions the splint next to the injured leg	1	
Applies the proximal securing device (e.g.,ischial strap)	1	
Applies the distal securing device (e.g.,ankle hitch)	1	
Applies mechanical traction	1	
Positions/secures the support straps	1	
Reevaluates the proximal/distal securing devices	1	
Reassesses motor, sensory, and circulatory function in the injured extremity	1	
Note: The examiner acknowledges "motor, sensory, and circulatory function are present and normal."		
Note: The examiner must ask the candidate how he/she would prepare the patient for transportation.		
Verbalizes securing the torso to the long board to immobilize the hip	1	
Verbalizes securing the splint to the long board to prevent movement of the splint	1	
Total:	**14**	

Critical Criteria

_____ Lost traction at any point after it was applied.
_____ Did not reassess motor, sensory, and circulatory function in the injured extremity before and after splinting.
_____ The foot was excessively rotated or extended after splint was applied.
_____ Did not secure the ischial strap before taking traction.
_____ Final immobilization failed to support the femur or prevent rotation of the injured leg.
_____ Secured the leg to the splint before applying mechanical traction.

Note: If the Sager splint or the Kendricks Traction Device is used without elevating the patient's leg, application of manual traction is not n cessary. The candidate should be awarded one point as if manual traction were applied.

Note: If the leg is elevated at all, manual traction must be applied before elevating the leg. The ankle hitch may be applied before elevating the leg and used to provide manual traction.

Bleeding Control/Shock Management

Start Time: ____________________

Stop Time: ____________________ **Date:** ____________________

Candidate's Name: ____

Evaluator's Name: ____

	Points Possible	Points Awarded
Takes, or verbalizes, body substance isolation precautions	1	
Applies direct pressure to the wound	1	
Elevates the extremity	1	
Note: The examiner must now inform the candidate that the wound continues to bleed.		
Applies an additional dressing to the wound	1	
Note: The examiner must now inform the candidate that the wound still continues to bleed. The second dressing does not control the bleeding.		
Locates and applies pressure to appropriate arterial pressure point	1	
Note: The examiner must now inform the candidate that the bleeding is controlled.		
Bandages the wound	1	
Note: The examiner must now inform the candidate that the patient is now showing signs and symptoms indicative of hypoperfusion.		
Properly positions the patient	1	
Applies high-concentration oxygen	1	
Initiates steps to prevent heat loss from the patient	1	
Indicates the need for immediate transportation	1	
Total:	**10**	

Critical Criteria

______ Did not take, or verbalize, body substance isolation precautions.

______ Did not apply high concentration of oxygen.

______ Applied a tourniquet before attempting other methods of bleeding control.

______ Did not control hemorrhage in a timely manner.

______ Did not indicate a need for immediate transportation.

Airway, Oxygen, and Ventilation Skills
Upper Airway Adjuncts and Suction

Start Time: ____________

Stop Time: ____________ **Date:** ____________

Candidate's Name: ____________

Evaluator's Name: ____________

Oropharyngeal Airway

Oropharyngeal Airway	Points Possible	Points Awarded
Takes, or verbalizes, body substance isolation precautions	1	
Selects appropriately sized airway	1	
Measures airway	1	
Inserts airway without pushing the tongue posteriorly	1	
Note: The examiner must advise the candidate that the patient is gagging and becoming conscious.		
Removes the oropharyngeal airway	1	

Suction

Note: The examiner must advise the candidate to suction the patient's airway.		
Turns on/prepares suction device	1	
Assures presence of mechanical suction	1	
Inserts the suction tip without suction	1	
Applies suction to the oropharynx/nasopharynx	1	

Nasopharyngeal Airway

Note: The examiner must advise the candidate to insert a nasopharyngeal airway.		
Selects appropriately sized airway	1	
Measures airway	1	
Verbalizes lubrication of the nasal airway	1	
Fully inserts the airway with the bevel facing toward the septum	1	
Total:	13	

Critical Criteria

______ Did not take, or verbalize, body substance isolation precautions.

______ Did not obtain a patent airway with the oropharyngeal airway.

______ Did not obtain a patent airway with the nasopharyngeal airway.

______ Did not demonstrate an acceptable suction technique.

______ Inserted any adjunct in a manner dangerous to the patient.

Mouth-to-Mask Ventilation with Supplemental Oxygen

Start Time: ____________________

Stop Time: ____________________ **Date:** ________________________

Candidate's Name: ____

Evaluator's Name: ____

	Points Possible	Points Awarded
Takes, or verbalizes, body substance isolation precautions	1	
Connects one-way valve to mask	1	
Opens patient's airway or confirms patient's airway is open (manually or with adjunct)	1	
Establishes and maintains a proper mask-to-face seal	1	
Ventilates the patient at the proper volume and rate *(800=1200 ml per breath/10-20 breaths per minute)*	1	
Connects the mask to high concentration of oxygen	1	
Adjusts flow rate to at least 15 liters per minute	1	
Continues ventilation of the patient at the proper volume and rate *(800=1200 ml per breath/10-20 breaths per minute)*	1	
Note: The examiner must witness ventilations for at least 30 seconds.		
Total:	**8**	

Critical Criteria

______ Did not take, or verbalize, body substance isolation precautions.

______ Did not adjust liter flow to at least 15 liters per minute.

______ Did not provide proper volume per breath
(***more than two ventilations per minute were below 800 ml***).

______ Did not ventilate the patient at a rate of 10-20 breaths per minute.

______ Did not allow for complete exhalation.

Oxygen Administration

Start Time: ______________

Stop Time: ______________ **Date:** ______________

Candidate's Name: ______________________________

Evaluator's Name: ______________________________

	Points Possible	Points Awarded
Takes, or verbalizes, body substance isolation precautions	1	
Assembles the regulator to the tank	1	
Opens the tank	1	
Checks for leaks	1	
Checks tank pressure	1	
Attaches nonrebreather mask to oxygen	1	
Prefills reservoir	1	
Adjusts liter flow to 12 liters per minute or greater	1	
Applies and adjusts the mask to the patient's face	1	
Note: The examiner must advise the candidate that the patient is not tolerating the nonrebreather mask. The medical director has ordered you to apply a nasal cannula to the patient.		
Attaches nasal cannula to oxygen	1	
Adjusts liter flow to 6 liters per minute or less	1	
Applies nasal cannula to the patient	1	
Note: The examiner must advise the candidate to discontinue oxygen therapy.		
Removes the nasal cannula from the patient	1	
Shuts off the regulator	1	
Relieves the pressure within the regulator	1	
Total:	**15**	

Critical Criteria

_____ Did not take, or verbalize, body substance isolation precautions.

_____ Did not assemble the tank and regulator without leaks.

_____ Did not prefill the reservoir bag.

_____ Did not adjust the device to the correct liter flow for the nonrebreather mask *(12 liters per minute or greater).*

_____ Did not adjust the device to the correct liter flow for the nasal cannula *(6 liters per minute or less).*

Start Time: ____________

Stop Time: ____________

Ventilatory Management
Endotracheal Intubation

Candidate's Name: ______________________ Date: ____________

Evaluator's Name: ______________________

Note: *If a candidate elects to initially ventilate the patient with a BVM attached to a reservoir and oxygen, full credit must be awarded for steps denoted by " ** " provided the first ventilation is delivered within the initial 30 seconds.*

		Points Possible	Points Awarded
Takes or verbalizes body substance isolation precautions		1	
Opens the airway manually		1	
Elevates the patient's tongue and inserts a simple airway adjunct (oropharyngeal/nasopharyngeal airway)		1	
Note: The examiner must now inform the candidate "no gag reflex is present, and the patient accepts the airway adjunct."			
** Ventilates the patient immediately using a BVM device unattached to oxygen		1	
** Hyperventilates the patient with room air		1	
Note: The examiner must now inform the candidate that ventilation is being properly performed without difficulty.			
Attaches the oxygen reservoir to the BVM		1	
Attaches the BVM to high-flow oxygen (15 liters per minute)		1	
Ventilates the patient at the proper volume and rate *(800-1200 ml/breath and 10-20 breaths/minute)*		1	
Note: After 30 seconds, the examiner must auscultate the patient's chest and inform the candidate that breath sounds are present and equal bilaterally and medical direction has ordered endotracheal intubation. The examiner must now take over ventilation of the patient.			
Directs assistant to hyperoxygenate the patient		1	
Identifies/selects the proper equipment for endotracheal intubation		1	
Checks equipment	Checks for cuff leaks	1	
	Checks laryngoscope operation and bulb tightness	1	
Note: The examiner must remove the OPA and move out of the way when the candidate is prepared to intubate the patient.			
Positions the patient's head properly		1	
Inserts the laryngoscope blade into the patient's mouth while displacing the patient's tongue laterally		1	
Elevates the patient's mandible with the laryngoscope		1	
Introduces the endotracheal tube and advances the tube to the proper depth		1	
Inflates the cuff to the proper pressure		1	
Disconnects the syringe from the cuff inlet port		1	
Directs assistant to ventilate the patient		1	
Confirms proper placement of the endotracheal tube by auscultation bilaterally and over the epigastrium		1	
Note: The examiner must ask, "If you had proper placement, what would you expect to hear?"			
Secures the endotracheal tube *(may be verbalized)*		1	
	Total:	21	

Critical Criteria

______ Did not take or verbalize body substance isolation precautions when necessary.
______ Did not initiate ventilation within 30 seconds after applying gloves or interrupts ventilations for greater than 30 seconds at any time.
______ Did not voice or provide high-oxygen concentrations (15 liters/minute or greater).
______ Did not ventilate the patient at a rate of at least 10 breaths per minute.
______ Did not provide adequate volume per breath (maximum of two errors per minute permissible).
______ Did not hyperoxygenate the patient prior to intubation.
______ Did not successfully intubate the patient within three attempts.
______ Used the patient's teeth as a fulcrum.
______ Did not assure proper tube placement by auscultation bilaterally over each lung and over the epigastrium.
______ The stylette (if used) extended beyond the end of the endotracheal tube.
______ Inserted any adjunct in a manner that was dangerous to the patient.
______ Did not immediately disconnect the syringe from the inlet port after inflating the cuff.

Ventilatory Management
Dual Lumen Device Insertion Following an Unsuccessful Endotracheal Intubation Attempt

Start Time: ________

Stop Time: ________

Candidate's Name: ____________________ **Date:** ____________

Evaluator's Name: ____________________

		Points Possible	Points Awarded
Continues body substance isolation precautions		**1**	
Confirms the patient is being properly ventilated with high-concentration oxygen		**1**	
Directs the assistant to hyperoxygenate the patient		**1**	
Checks/prepares the airway device		**1**	
Lubricates the distal tip of the device (*may be verbalized)*		**1**	
Note: The examiner should remove the OPA and move out of the way when the candidate is prepared to insert the device.			
Positions the patient's head properly		**1**	
Performs a tongue-jaw lift		**1**	
☐ **Uses Combitube**	☐ **Uses the PTL**		
Inserts device in the midline and to the depth so that the printed ring is at the level of the teeth	Inserts the device in the midline until the bite block flange is at the level of the teeth	**1**	
Inflates the pharyngeal cuff with the proper volume and removes the syringe	Secures the strap	**1**	
Inflates the distal cuff with the proper volume and removes the syringe	Blows into tube #1 to adequately inflate both cuffs	**1**	
Attaches/directs attachment of BVM to the first (esophageal placement) lumen and ventilates		**1**	
Confirms placement and ventilation through the correct lumen by observing chest rise, auscultation over the epigastrium and bilaterally over each lung		**1**	
Note: The examiner states, "You do not see rise and fall of the chest and hear sounds only over the epigastrium."			
Attaches/directs attachment of BVM to the second (endotracheal placement) lumen and ventilates		**1**	
Confirms placement and ventilation through the correct lumen by observing chest rise, auscultation over the epigastrium and bilaterally over each lung		**1**	
Note: The examiner states, "You see rise and fall of the chest, there are no sounds over the epigastrium, and breath sounds are equal over each lung."			
Secures device or confirms that the device remains properly secured		**1**	
	Total:	**15**	

Critical Criteria

_____ Did not take or verbalize body substance isolation precautions.
_____ Did not initiate ventilations within 30 seconds.
_____ Interrupted ventilations for more than 30 seconds at any time.
_____ Did not hyperoxygenate the patient prior to placement of the dual lumen airway device.
_____ Did not provide adequate volume per breath (maximum two errors/minute permissible).
_____ Did not ventilate the patient at a rate of at least 10 breaths/minute.
_____ Did not insert the dual lumen airway device at a proper depth or at the proper place within three attempts.
_____ Did not inflate both cuffs properly.
_____ Combitube - Did not remove the syringe immediately following the inflation of each cuff.
_____ PTL - Did not secure the strap prior to cuff inflation.
_____ Did not confirm, by observing chest rise and auscultation over the epigastrium and bilaterally over each lung, that the proper lumen of the device was being used to ventilate the patient.
_____ Inserted any adjunct in a manner that was dangerous to the patient.

Appendix B
Cardiopulmonary Resuscitation

Karen Snyder, RN, CEN, EMT-P
EMS Coordinator
Fire Training Center
Cincinnati Fire Division
Cincinnati, Ohio

Cardiopulmonary resuscitation, or CPR, is one of the most common skills for Emergency Medical Technicians (EMTs), particularly if EMTs serve a dense urban population. Unfortunately, CPR is one of the skills most often poorly performed on skills examinations. EMTs fall into a false sense of security believing that they can perform the skill just because they are EMTs. Unfortunately, many EMTs do not take the time to refresh their CPR skills, and as with any other skill, the practitioner may become rusty over time.

Sudden cardiac death is the sudden and unexpected loss of heart function (cardiac arrest) that appears abruptly in a person who may or may not have been diagnosed with previous cardiovascular disease. Sudden cardiac death occurs instantly or shortly after the onset of symptoms, usually with little or no warning. According to the American Heart Association (AHA), sudden cardiac death occurs approximately 250,000 times per year, or 700 to 1,000 times per day. That number is equivalent to losing a city the size of Cincinnati every year. If a bacteria, virus, or chemical compound were causing this kind of loss of life, authorities would be scrambling to defeat it. However, we have not really accepted sudden cardiac death as the plague it is.

The most common cause of sudden cardiac death comes from underlying *cardiovascular disease,* particularly coronary artery disease. According to the AHA, about half of all deaths from coronary artery disease are sudden and unexpected. To break it down further, 50% of deaths from *atherosclerosis* and 50% of deaths from degeneration of the heart muscle or cardiac enlargement in patients with high blood pressure, are defined as sudden cardiac death.

Many other maladies may cause sudden cardiac death, such as drug overdose, electrical shock, or trauma. Although the victim of sudden cardiac death due to one of these causes may have underlying coronary artery disease, the victim suffers an aberrant heart beat causing rerouting of electrical impulses and ultimately cardiac arrest.

Sudden cardiac death is the result of cardiac arrest. This arrest may or may not be caused by any known heart disease. Most cardiac arrests are due to the rapid or chaotic activity of the heart, commonly referred to as *ventricular fibrillation* or pulseless *ventricular tachycardia.* When this rhythm occurs in the heart, blood cannot be pumped adequately through all four chambers of the heart and the lungs. In ventricular fibrillation, the heart "quivers," which does not allow adequate blood pumping. It is estimated that ventricular fibrillation is the presenting rhythm in 80% of cardiac arrests and lasts approximately 8 minutes. Ventricular fibrillation then develops into *asystole,* or lack of any heart rhythm. This rhythm is most often irreversible.

Commonly, the term *massive heart attack* is used to describe sudden cardiac death. Heart attack or *myocardial infarction* refers to death of heart muscle tissue that occurs due to loss of blood supply to the muscle. Although a heart attack may be the cause of a cardiac arrest and sudden cardiac death, many people suffering myocardial infarction do not experience a cardiac arrest. The terms *massive heart attack* and *sudden cardiac death* are not synonymous.

Cardiac arrest is treatable and reversible in victims if it is recognized and treated within a few minutes. This conclusion became evident in the early 1960s with the advent of coronary care units. Both research and anecdotal evidence have shown greatly improved success rates for sudden cardiac death since the institution of CPR and early defibrillation.

CPR partially maintains blood flow to the heart and brain through compressions and ventilations. Although most sudden cardiac death victims require early defibrillation, CPR provides a bridge until that becomes available. To be even marginally successful, CPR must be started immediately upon recognition of cardiac arrest through the absence of respiration and pulse. There are no reliable national statistics on CPR because no single agency collects information pertaining to the arrest event, such as how many people receive CPR, how many people are trained in CPR, and the effectiveness of CPR. Studies have been done at local levels, and according to the AHA, the following statements are fair generalizations:

- "Right now early CPR and rapid *defibrillation* combined with early advanced care can result in long-term survival rates for witnessed *ventricular fibrillation* as high as 40%."[1]
- "The value of early CPR by bystanders is that it can buy time by prolonging ventricular fibrillation. Early bystander CPR is less helpful if EMS personnel equipped with a defibrillator arrive later than 8 to 12 minutes after the collapse."[1]

There needs to be adequate numbers of trained personnel to intervene when the time is appropriate to perform CPR. To meet these needs, the AHA supports the concept of the need for a *chain of survival* to rescue the person who suffers cardiac arrest in the community. The chain consists of the following:

- Early access
- Early CPR
- Early defibrillation
- Early advanced care

Early Access

Although we as prehospital care providers are used to handling *emergency* situations, the average lay person is not. According to Dr. Jeffrey Clawson and the Medical Priority Group, it takes average citizens approximately 90 seconds to 2 minutes to mentally process that an emergency exists. It is only after they decide they cannot handle the situation that they place the call to the universal number 9-1-1. After that call is received, another 45 to 90 seconds may lapse until emergency units are dispatched. With a minimal response time of 4 minutes added to the time since cardiac arrest, it is easy to understand why so few cardiac victims survive without intervention early in the process.

This is significant because at the time heartbeat and breathing stop, the victim is suffering *clinical death.* The brain begins to die within 4 to 6 minutes without oxygen. This statistic is important if you think about the 2 minutes that it takes the person calling 9-1-1 to recognize there is an emergency. Immediately, we have lost 2 minutes of *brain time. Biological* or *irreversible* brain death occurs within 6 to 10 minutes after loss of oxygen.

Early CPR

CPR is essentially a holding pattern that maintains minimal perfusion to organs during a cardiac arrest, prolonging ventricular fibrillation. CPR, in and of itself, is not definitive treatment; it only buys the rescuer time until definitive treatment can be rendered with defibrillation. Without early CPR, a victim is more likely to die, and if the victim does survive, often the brain has been severely damaged. The longer the body remains in cardiac arrest, the more acids build up in the body, making *lethal arrhythmias,* such as ventricular tachycardia or fibrillation more difficult to correct. The AHA puts it this way: "The timely application of CPR has been credited with helping save thousands of lives each year in the United States. Better understanding of CPR and refinements in its use can help save more lives."

Early Defibrillation

Providing the patient in cardiac arrest with defibrillation offers the best remedy to ventricular fibrillation. Because statistics prove that an adult cardiac arrest patient is most likely to be in ventricular fibrillation at the time of cardiac arrest, application of defibrillation increases the liklihood to correct this lethal arrhythmia. The advent of newer, lighter, and smarter automated defibrillators allows defibrillation to be provided by basic prehospital providers and lay rescuer personnel. This link has become so critical in the chain of survival, it is now common to see defibrillators on commercial aircraft and other public locations.

Early Advanced Care

Early advanced life support plays a critical role in cardiac arrest management. With the advent of early defibrillation, many cardiac arrest victims can be converted to a perfusing rhythm prior to advanced life support arrival. This is not to downplay advanced life support's (ALS) role in cardiac arrest situations. It is ALS that provides advanced airway management, appropriate prehospital pharmacology, and treatment such as external pacemakers.

How CPR Works

CPR works as a stopgap until more definitive care can be provided to the cardiac arrest victim. In reality the physics of CPR are very simple. Think about how simply a turkey baster works.

You are baking your Thanksgiving turkey and because you do not want the turkey to be dry, you will baste the bird at regular intervals. You begin by squeezing the large plastic bulb at the end of the baster. Then you stick the open end into the juices in the pan to collect the juices. When you release your grip on the bulb of the baster, fluid quickly pours out and onto the turkey.

The same principle works with CPR. By creating both negative and positive pressures within the chest cavity, blood enters the heart, is circulated through the lungs for oxygenation, is sent back to the heart, and ultimately to the heart muscle and brain. Normally the heart only has about 2½ oz of blood in the left ventricle at any given moment and CPR provides only 25% to 33% as much contraction force as the normal heart. Therefore even with properly applied CPR, only a small amount of blood is circulated with each compression cycle.

Special Considerations in CPR

How Do You Know CPR is Effective?

"How do you know CPR is effective?" is often a difficult question, especially because we may work for long periods doing CPR without seeing immediate results. There are several ways we can determine if CPR is being applied properly.

First, the patient's skin color gets better or the patient *pinks up.* Initial cyanosis indicates a body that has been without oxygen for a significant period and has used all available oxygen. By breathing for the patient, particularly with high concentrations of oxygen via a bag-valve-mask, we provide higher oxygen levels to the body.

A second way to tell if CPR is being appropriately applied is to have another rescuer gently palpate a carotid pulse. If the pressure generated by chest compressions is adequate, a second rescuer should be able to feel a carotid pulse. Take adequate time to feel for the pulse; the pulse check should last between 5 and 10 seconds.

Another way to determine if CPR is effective is by watching for subtle changes in the patient's pupils. When a person suffers a cardiac arrest the body goes without oxygen and in response the pupils will dilate. If CPR is being done properly, you may see a change in pupillary reaction after the body has received improved oxygen. Pupillary reaction is not a good test once ALS arrives on the scene. Some of the medications used in resuscitating a cardiac arrest victim will cause the pupils to dilate and become nonreactive.

The final way to tell if CPR is effective is if the patient awakens. This is a rare and uncommon occurrence. It usually indicates that the patient had a pulse that was too weak to be palpated. CPR was probably not needed in that patient.

When May You Terminate CPR?

There are four general times when you may terminate CPR. The first is when the patient recovers from the cardiac arrest. This means the patient awakens and regains a pulse. The second is when another rescuer appears and takes over the resuscitation effort. The third time is when the rescuer is too fatigued to continue and there is no possibility another rescuer will arrive. Finally, you may terminate CPR when the physician tells you to cease resuscitation efforts.

When Do You Not Have to Start CPR?

Generally, you do not have to begin resuscitation efforts if there is obvious death by evidence of *rigor mortis* and *lividity.* This often causes confusion for rescuers. Both rigor mortis and lividity are dependent on several factors, including body temperature, ambient temperature, and activity at the time of death.

Lividity can become evident within 30 minutes of death and is demonstrated by pooling of blood in dependent body positions. However, depending on numerous variables, lividity may not be evident for up to 4 hours after death. After approximately 6 hours, lividity fixes and attempts to blanch; the skin will reveal nothing. Because we do not strip our cardiac arrest victims of their clothes, lividity may go unnoticed.

A better parameter for checking death is the presence of rigor mortis. In order for rigor mortis to be present, the body must have a supply of an enzyme called *adenosine triphosphate (ATP).* If ATP has been depleted prior to death, such as from a fight or seizure, rigor mortis will be slower to begin. Rigor mortis is characterized by the extreme stiffening of the body after death. This is the reason, in our gallows humor, we refer to the dead as *stiffs.*

At 24 hours after death, decomposition of the body occurs. Because the bowel is full of bacteria, the abdomen is the first place to show decomposition by turning green. After decomposition, the body will swell and skin tissue will slough. After 24 hours, the body also becomes fair game for flies, and as a rescuer you may notice maggots. It takes approximately 24 hours for their eggs to hatch.

Do not resuscitate (DNR) orders may be followed if the order is established by recognized protocol and policy. Usually a person who wants a DNR order has a terminal illness and is in an extended care facility, hospice, or has come home to die. Honoring DNR orders may be very difficult when the family has not resolved issues with the impending death and has not come to the stage of acceptance. Follow your local protocols in those situations.

Another time you may not have to start CPR is in the event that the victim has suffered obvious injuries that are incompatible with life, such as decapitation, the body being burned beyond recognition, or other obviously fatal injuries.

How Long May You Interrupt CPR When Necessary?

CPR should generally not be stopped except in very few circumstances. First, you may stop CPR for up to 90 seconds to deliver three defibrillation shocks. Second, you may stop for up to 30 seconds to move a patient to a better or different location. Third, you may stop for up to 15 seconds to change positions with another rescuer.

How Do You Move a Patient During CPR?

Obviously, you must move a patient very carefully during CPR. When transporting a patient who is under CPR down a flight of stairs or into the ambulance, it is important for you not to stop CPR for longer than 30 seconds. That may mean that you will have to stop at stair landings and do CPR for 1 minute prior to proceeding.

What are the Complications of CPR?

Despite our best efforts, complications can occur even when CPR is done properly. Some of the more common complications are fractured cartilage and ribs, punctured lung, and lacerated liver. Although these injuries seem like horrible complications, they can be fixed. A patient's major problem is no respirations or pulse—the complications of which far outweigh a few broken ribs.

Checking Responsiveness

Checking responsiveness may seem obvious, but it is amazing how many rescuers fail to check this important component. A person responding to either verbal or painful stimulus does not need CPR.

Opening the Airway

Opening the airway properly is one of the most important techniques we have when rendering CPR. Everything hinges on the airway being opened and the patient being properly ventilated. While remembering the simple mnemonic ABCs, you should keep in mind that it does not matter what "C" is if "A" is not patent.

The most common methods used for opening the airway of the unresponsive cardiac arrest victim are the *head-tilt and chin-lift* maneuver for the nontraumatized patient and the *jaw-thrust* maneuver for the traumatized patient. Never begin chest compression until an airway has been established and the patient is oxygenated.

Beginning CPR

When beginning CPR, you should keep a couple of facts in mind. First, the patient should be lying in the supine, or face up position, on a firm, flat surface (the floor or the ground). The patient should not be lying in a regular bed, a waterbed, a hammock, or a sofa. The firm surface is necessary for compressions to be effective.

As stated before, it is important to make sure the victim is *pulseless* and *apneic.* A person who exhibits a pulse and who is breathing does not need CPR. One of the most common mistakes made by rescuers is not evaluating these two parameters adequately. A breathing check should last at least 5 to 10 seconds, with the rescuer's head facing the patient's chest, feeling, looking, and listening for air exchange. A pulse check should last 10 to 15 seconds and should be done carefully and gently at the carotid pulse on the adult and the brachial pulse on the infant.

How To Do CPR

CPR is a process that includes assessment and appropriate intervention. Important components of CPR include proper positioning of the patient, determination of absence or presence of breathing and pulse, providing adequate ventilations and compressions, and timely and adequate reassessment at frequent intervals.

Finding the appropriate compression site can be accomplished a couple of different ways. First, the rescuer may feel for the bony prominence that lies at the end of the breastbone or sternum. This little prominence is called the *xiphoid process,* and compressing here during resuscitation events may cause damage. Once the xiphoid process is located, the rescuer may then place a hand approximately two finger-widths above this point and begin compressions.

An alternative to this method is to use the lower half of the sternum. Using the normal nipple line as the midpoint of the chest, compressions are applied just below this point. This means the normal nipple line, not the one created by old and pendulous breasts.

Correct CPR incorporates alternate ventilations with chest compressions. The age and size of the patient will determine what ratios will be used. Generally, one-rescuer adult CPR uses a compression/ventilation ratio of 15:2. The professional rescuer, who has two capable people, will usually use a 5:1 compression/ventilation ratio. A 5:1 compression/ventilation ratio should always be used in infants and children regardless of the number of rescuers.

One-Rescuer CPR

Usually reserved for the lay rescuer, one-rescuer CPR incorporates compressions and ventilations at a ratio of 15 compressions for every two breaths and is used solely on the adult patient. Ventilations should last 1½ to 2 seconds, allowing for deep inflation of the lungs as well as passively allowing full exhalation. Chest compressions should be on the lower half of the sternum, and depth should be 1½ to 2 inches. Compressions should be applied at a rate of 80 to 100 times per minute.

Two-Rescuer CPR

The *professional rescuer* usually uses the two-rescuer CPR technique, which incorporates five chest compressions for every ventilation. The technique provides a little more oxygen than one-rescuer CPR and allows CPR to be continued for longer periods without fatigue because the rescuers can switch places when the compressor becomes tired. When this change occurs, the rescuer doing compressions should call for the change in positions. The change should occur at the end of a 5:1 cycle, ending and beginning with ventilation.

Another advantage to this technique is that the rescuer maintaining the airway and providing ventilations can check the adequacy of the CPR being performed by checking a carotid pulse during compression. Although AHA standards state that the compression depth should be 1½ to 2 inches, in reality, compression depth should be deep enough to generate a carotid pulse with compressions. Just as with one-rescuer CPR, the compression rate should be 80 to 100 times per minute.

Not only should the professional rescuer check a pulse during compressions but also the professional rescuer should check a pulse frequently without compression to ascertain if a spontaneous pulse has returned. This is generally done after the first minute (usually about four cycles of five compressions to every ventilation) and every few minutes thereafter.

CPR Techniques for Infants and Children

The AHA has standardized CPR techniques for infants and children. According to the AHA, an infant is classified in age as any child from day 1 to year 1. A child falls into the category of ages 1 through 8.

There are a few important things to remember about rescucitating children. Their heads are generally larger in proportion to the rest of their bodies, and their tracheas are smaller and more pliable. By hyperextending the neck of an infant or child, as you would with an adult, you may actually block the airway. It is important to maintain a child's or infant's airway in the *neutral* or *sniffing position*. To find the correct position, think of walking into your house and smelling a pan of brownies baking. Immediately your head moves into the *sniffing* position.

Checking a pulse on an infant or child is also a little different. Just like the adult, the child's pulse may be checked at the carotid artery. It is generally recommended that the infant's pulse be checked at the brachial artery because it is difficult to feel a carotid artery on a fat, little neck. The brachial pulse is located just proximal to the elbow on the medial portion of the upper arm. However, you may find it more reliable to place your stethoscope on the infant's chest over the heart to determine the presence of an apical pulse. It is important that the pulse check be completed for a full 10 seconds to determine the presence of a pulse. Keep in mind that most children have cardiac arrests from respiratory events, and the usual mechanism in children is that they will drop their pulse rate when in respiratory compromise.

Although it may be predictable that the respiratory rate will drop in a child in distress, this does not preclude performing CPR when necessary. It becomes important to intervene, especially in infants, when their pulse drops below 60 beats per minute. At this level, perfusion is not adequate and intervention must be swift.

Both infants and children are resuscitated with five chest compressions for every one ventilation, despite the number of rescuers. Compression rates should be at least 100 times per minute. Compression depth on infants is ½ to 1 inch and 1 to 1½ inches on children. Just as with the adult, compressions should be deep enough to produce a palpable pulse during compressions.

Hand placement is important when performing CPR on infants and children. Their chests are bonier and more compliant than the adult's chest. In the infant, hand placement is usually recommended at one finger width below an imaginary line at the nipples. This should give the rescuer a landmark to identify the lower half of the sternum. Compressions should be provided with two fingers.

Because a child's chest is a little bigger than an infant's chest but not as large as an adult's chest, we must modify our techniques a bit. Generally, compressions on children are done with one hand on the lower half of the sternum. It is possible for the rescuer to maintain the head in neutral position with one hand while providing compressions with the other hand.

Rescue Breathing

Compressions and ventilation ratios were discussed previously, but we have not looked at various rescue breathing techniques. It is possible for a victim to stop breathing but maintain a pulse. In these cases it is incumbent upon the rescuer to ventilate the patient. The following techniques are not limited to the patient with a pulse but may be incorporated as ventilation techniques during CPR.

Artificial ventilation is important because the brain will begin to die within 4 to 6 minutes without oxygen. The normal oxygen content supplied in room air is approximately 21%. The oxygen percentage in normal exhaled air is approximately 16%. This means that every time we breathe, our bodies use about 5% of the oxygen available. Because 16% is greater than 5%, it makes sense that ventilating a nonbreathing person with our expired air will provide enough oxygen to sustain life.

When performing artificial ventilations, it is important to provide the victim with enough air to cause the chest to rise and then fall. By breathing too deeply, air may enter the stomach causing gastric distention, particularly in infants and children. Gastric distention does not allow ventilations to be adequate and may lead to regurgitation. Should the victim vomit, vomitus may be aspirated into the lungs hindering the absorption of oxygen into the blood or cause pneumonia.

Early in CPR, mouth-to-mouth and mouth-to-nose ventilations were taught to both professional and lay rescuers. However, as we have learned more about infectious diseases, these techniques have fallen out of favor unless an appropriate barrier device is used.

It is very easy for a professional rescuer to see a child who is not breathing and want to immediately begin mouth-to-mouth resuscitation. This is not a good idea. Not only do you run the risk of the patient vomiting in your mouth but also most pediatric communicable diseases are spread through oral and nasal secretions. Pediatric communicable diseases in adults usually run a more severe course than they do in the child or infant.

Mouth-to-mask ventilations have become the recommended standard when providing artificial ventilation to the nonbreathing patient. This technique provides many advantages that conventional mouth-to-mouth or mouth-to-nose resuscitation do not.

First, by using a pocket mask, a barrier device has been placed between the rescuer and the patient. Most masks have a one-way valve that does not allow expired air to return to the rescuer, which decreases the possibility of transmission of diseases.

By using the pocket mask, the rescuer can also judge the amount of air entering the victim's lungs. During ventilation, the rescuer can feel *lung compliance* or how adequately ventilations are being delivered. This decreases the possibility of gastric distention and its subsequent problems.

Ventilating Neck Breathers

Some people do not breathe through their mouth and nose like other people do; they breathe through a surgical opening in their neck called a *stoma*. Because these openings can be unsightly, many people cover them up with scarves, ties, or turtlenecks. It is important that the rescuer identify neck breathers promptly. Unfortunately this may not be recognized until the rescuer attempts to ventilate the stoma patient normally. Either during or after blowing into the patient's lungs, the rescuer will feel or hear a rush of air escaping from the stoma.

There are a couple of different techniques used to ventilate stoma patients. The most common technique used is to ventilate the patient through the stoma, sealing the mouth and nose so that air does not escape.

The easiest technique is to cover the stoma with a *nonporous occlusive* dressing and ventilate the patient normally through the nose and mouth. The occlusive dressing seals the stoma, preventing air from escaping.

Ventilating Infants and Children

As discussed before, ventilating infants and children differs somewhat from ventilating an adult. Remember that the infant's or child's head should always be kept in a neutral position.

The Recovery Position

The recovery position is now recommended for unconscious patients who have a spontaneous pulse. This position is accomplished by placing patients on their left side without a pillow under the head. By placing patients in this position, the rescuer facilitates drainage of secretions as well as protection of the airway. Three patient populations that benefit from this position include the postseizure patient, the stroke patient, and the overdose patient.

Clearing the Airway

Ensuring a clear and patent airway is of utmost importance to maintain life for any patient. An obstructed airway can happen for a variety of reasons. Obstruction may occur from something as simple as the tongue falling back against the soft palate or pharynx occluding the airway, the victim may have foreign material caught in the trachea as seen with foreign body airway obstruction, or the airway may close due to swelling from trauma or inhalation injury. Whatever the mechanism, the airway must be clear for adequate ventilation of the patient to occur.

The most common cause of airway obstruction is by a flaccid tongue when a victim loses consciousness. If the person remains breathing, snoring will be evident. *Remember that noisy breathing is obstructed breathing.* If the person is not breathing, no sounds will be heard. Clearing a tongue obstruction is one of the easiest procedures to perform and is accomplished by using the head-tilt and chin-lift or jaw-thrust maneuvers.

If the victim is not suspected of having sustained any trauma (meaning the victim has not dropped from a vertical to a horizontal position) the airway may be opened easily by placing one hand on the forehead of the victim and the other hand at the bony portion of the jaw and simply lifting the victim's head backward. This maneuver displaces the mandible forward, lifting the tongue out of the way. Remember that if the patient is unresponsive there is not ability to protect the airway, and we should intervene by insertion of an oropharyngeal airway or nasopharyngeal airway.

If the rescuer suspects that the patient may have sustained any trauma, it is important *not* to perform the head-tilt and chin-lift maneuver because this requires extension of the cervical spine and may exacerbate any spinal injury. In these cases, the rescuer should place one hand on each bony prominence of the mandible of the patient and gently lift it forward without moving the head backward. This will allow the tongue to be lifted from the palate without the patient sustaining movement of the neck. Once again, when the patient cannot protect the airway, an appropriate airway adjunct should be used.

Procedures for Clearing the Airway

Not all people with airway obstructions are unresponsive. Many people suffer foreign-body airway obstruction and are still awake, which commonly occurs while people are eating. Talking with the mouth full, alcohol consumption, not chewing properly, and eating too fast can all contribute to the patient choking.

If you have ever really choked, you know how scary it can be. All too often, well-meaning rescuers step in and try to help the victim without really knowing how.

A person who is choking should be asked if choking is taking place. Although this may seem silly, it is important to determine the patient's precise problem. Universally, choking victims will clasp a hand around their neck indicating they are choking. In assessing the victim, you may hear high-pitched inspiratory sounds called *stridor* or you may hear nothing. However, the victim may still be coughing.

When this victim is still awake and coughing, it is important to encourage continuation of coughing in an attempt to dislodge the object. Never smack the patient on the back. This may cause the obstruction to lodge even further into the airway. Also, do not give the patient anything to drink.

If the victim is making no noise while breathing, odds are the airway is completely occluded. The person with a completely occluded airway will be unable to speak. It is of vital importance for the rescuer to determine this fact immediately and intervene swiftly and appropriately. The most common intervention is the *Heimlich maneuver.* You may also hear this called the *abdominal thrust* or *upward thrust.*

The principle behind the Heimlich maneuver is very simple. By applying pressure below the diaphragm, the rescuer creates an *artificial cough,* helping the victim to expel the occluding object. This maneuver may be repeated until the object becomes dislodged or the patient loses consciousness.

In a conscious patient, the Heimlich maneuver is performed with the rescuer standing behind the victim. The rescuer's arms should be around the victim's waist. With the fist pressed into the abdomen just above the umbilicus, the rescuer should deliver quick inward and upward thrusts aiming the fists toward the label in the back of the patient's shirt.

Should the victim be grossly obese or pregnant, the Heimlich maneuver should be modified some. In these cases, chest thrusts are going to be performed. The rescuer stands behind the victim and places their arms under the armpits of the victim, encircling the chest. Quick backward thrusts should be delivered to the lower half of the sternum.

If during your intervention of the obstructed airway the victim becomes unresponsive, gently lay the victim on the floor and perform a finger sweep to clear the airway of anything that might have become dislodged.

Open the airway with the maneuvers previously described, either by using the head-tilt and chin-lift or jaw-thrust maneuvers. Try to give the victim two full breaths. Successful breaths are demonstrated by a significant rise and fall of the chest as well as hearing air escape from the mouth and nose during inhalation. If these two breaths are not successful, reposition the head and try again.

If you are unable to successfully ventilate the patient, you will have to perform the Heimlich maneuver. To do this, kneel astride the victim's thighs. Carefully place the heel of one hand on the victim's abdomen (in the midline just above the navel but well below the xiphoid). The second hand should be placed on top of the first hand. Using the weight of your body, press into the patient's abdomen with quick upward thrusts.

This sequence should be repeated until the airway is successfully cleared, using the finger sweep, rescue breathing attempt, and abdominal thrusts.

Treating an obstructed airway in children 1 to 8 years of age is very similar to treating adults and older children. It is important to remember not to perform blind finger sweeps on children because this may actually force the object back into the airway in the event it is dislodged. Instead of performing blind finger sweeps on children, lift the jaw forward and look into the airway. If you see the object you may sweep the mouth with your fingers but only if you can remove the object easily.

Obstructed airway in the infant is different than in an adult. Although an adult with an obstructed airway will not be able to talk, an infant will display the inability to cry. It is important to remember that the following should not be performed on a conscious infant unless a complete airway obstruction is present, as evidenced by serious breathing difficulty, ineffective cough, or no cry. The following should also be performed only due to a witnessed or strongly suspected obstruction by a foreign object. If the obstruction is due to swelling from an infection, the infant should be swiftly taken to the nearest advanced life-support facility, and the rescuer should not intervene, particularly by placing anything, including the fingers, into the throat.

To determine airway obstruction, observe for breathing difficulties, ineffective cough, weak or absent cry, and dusky color. Remember that an infant's pulse slows in response to inadequate oxygenation.

Carefully place the infant face down and over your nondominant arm. Support the neck with one hand, and place the infant face down with the head lower than the trunk. Using your dominant hand, quickly deliver up to five back blows forcefully between the shoulder blade using the heel of the hand.

When this is accomplished, turn the infant face up, sandwiching the infant between your arm. Deliver five chest thrusts, using two fingers on the lower half of the sternum, using the same landmarks as those you would normally use for chest compressions. Remember to deliver chest thrusts a little more slowly than you would chest compressions. You should repeat the back blow and chest thrusts until the object is expelled or the infant becomes unresponsive.

If the infant becomes unresponsive, or you find the infant in this condition, gently shake the shoulder in an attempt to arouse the infant. Place the infant on a firm and hard surface while supporting the head and neck. Open the airway taking care not to tilt the head too far back. The head must remain in a neutral or sniffing position.

Determine by looking, listening, and feeling for air exchange. While maintaining an open airway, place your ear over the patient's mouth with your face toward the chest. While listening for air exchange at the nose and mouth, look for chest rise and fall. Attempt to ventilate the infant twice, making sure to seal both the mouth and nose. If this attempt is unsuccessful, reposition the head and try again.

Cautiously lift the mandible and look for a foreign object. Carefully remove the object only if it is seen.

Treat the airway obstruction in the infant as described earlier using a combination of back blows and chest thrusts until the airway is clear, checking the mouth often for evidence of a dislodged obstruction.

Common Mistakes in Performing CPR

Common Resuscitation Mistakes

- Not maintaining an adequate head tilt
- Not pinching the nose
- Not making an adequate seal
- Not pausing between the first two breaths
- Checking the pulse with the wrong hand
- Not checking the pulse long enough
- Incorrect timing of breaths

Mistakes in One-Rescuer CPR

- Pivoting at the knees instead of the hips
- Bending at the elbows
- Shoulders not above the sternum
- Fingers touching the chest
- Heel of bottom hand not in line with sternum

Mistakes in Two-Rescuer CPR

- Not pausing for the breath after each five compressions
- Inhaling too soon or too late in preparation to deliver breaths
- Waiting through the entire cycle of five compressions if one breath is missed, instead of giving the breath at the soonest possible moment

Mistakes in CPR for Infants and Small Children

- Giving jerky, stabbing compressions
- Not supporting the back with the noncompressing hand
- Improper finger placement
- Holding the child's head higher than the body
- Not pausing after compressions to give breaths
- Not timing breaths well
- Breathing too deeply

REFERENCES

1. From American Heart Organization, www.amhrt.org, October 2, 1998.

Appendix C

Baseline Vital Signs

Average Vital Signs

	Newborn	1-12 mo	1-3 yr	4-5 yr	6-10 yr	11-15 yr	16 and up	Quality
Pulse	120-150	100-130	90-130	80-120	70-100	70-90	60-80	Steady, regular, strong
Average systolic blood pressure/average diastolic BP = approximately ⅔ SBP	80 + twice age (yr) (systolic)	80 + twice age (yr) (systolic)	80+ twice age (yr) (systolic)	90/60	100/60	110/64	120/80	Watch for trends; use initial reading as baseline
Respirations	30-60	25-40	20-30	20-30	15-24	15-20	12-20	Virtually silent and effortless
Pupils	Symmetrical	Symmetrical	Symmetrical	Symmetrical	Symmetrical	Symmetrical	Symmetrical	Respond to light
Skin	Normal color, capillary refill <2s	Normal color, capillary refill <2s	Normal color, capillary refill <2s	Normal color, capillary refill <2s	Normal color, capillary refill <2s	Normal color	Normal color	Warm and dry to the touch
Level of consciousness	Awake, may be crying	Awake, interacts	Alert, oriented	Alert, oriented	Alert, oriented	Alert, oriented	Alert, oriented	Level of orientation will vary based on maturity

Note: The above vital signs ranges are general. Vital signs should always be evaluated in the context of the patient's overall condition.

Glossary

Abandonment Terminating patient care without the patient's consent, at a time when there is a need for continued care by an EMT.

Abortion Delivery of an embryo or fetus before it is able to live on its own, usually in the first trimester of pregnancy; spontaneous abortion is often called *miscarriage.*

Abrasion Open wound characterized by the rubbing or scraping away of the superficial layer (epidermis) of the skin.

Abruptio placentae A condition in which the placenta separates from the uterine wall, resulting in significant bleeding (either internal or external).

Absorbed poison A toxic substance that enters the body through the skin, eyes, or mucous membranes.

Acquired immune deficiency syndrome (AIDS) The end condition resulting from infection with the human immunodeficiency virus (HIV) characterized by opportunistic infections.

Activated charcoal A medication that is taken orally for the management of certain ingested poisonous substances; charcoal adsorbs (sticks to) the substance and prevents its absorption by the digestive system.

Acute myocardial infarction Death of an area of heart muscle; commonly called a *heart attack.*

Adolescent A young person 12 to 18 years of age.

Advance medical directive A person's written statement of preference relative to receiving medical care (e.g., do not perform CPR).

Aerobic metabolism The process of converting glucose to energy for body use, in the presence of adequate oxygen; opposite of anaerobic metabolism.

Airborne transmission A route for disease transmission that results from inhaling infected droplets that become airborne when an infected person coughs or sneezes.

Airway The structures of the respiratory system through which air travels to the lungs; divided into the upper and lower airways.

Allergen A foreign substance that produces an allergic reaction.

Allergic reaction An immune response to contact with a foreign substance (allergen).

Altered level of consciousness A condition in which a patient is not appropriately oriented to elements such as person, place, time, or recent events; an abnormal state of mind.

Alveoli The microscopic air sacs of the lungs where oxygen and carbon dioxide are exchanged.

Alzheimer's syndrome A degeneration of nerve cells in the brain from an unknown cause; the most common type of dementia in the elderly.

Ambient temperature The environmental temperature to which the body is exposed; the surrounding air or water temperature.

Ambulance Emergency vehicle used to treat and transport ill or injured patients to medical facilities.

Amniotic sac A thin membrane surrounding the fetus, containing up to 2 L of amniotic fluid that helps cushion and protect the developing fetus.

Amputation Open wound characterized by the complete severing of a body part.

Anaerobic metabolism The process of converting glucose to energy for body use, in the absence of adequate oxygen. The oxygen shortage results in the production of excess acids. It is the opposite of aerobic metabolism.

Anaphylaxis A severe, potentially life-threatening, allergic reaction.

Anatomic position An imaginary position, used as standard for consistent references to locations on a patient's body and directions in relation to the body. The position is standing, facing the observer, with the arms at the sides, and the palms facing forward. Also called *standard anatomic position.*

Anemia Term for a number of blood conditions in which either less hemoglobin or fewer red blood cells than normal are present in the blood.

Aneurysm Dilation or ballooning of a blood vessel, resulting from high blood pressure or a weak area of vessel wall.

Angina pectoris Chest pain associated with a cardiac emergency. The pain is caused by inadequate blood supply to the heart muscle.

Anterior The front of the body or body part; opposite of posterior.

Antibodies Protein complexes released by select white blood cells to weaken or destroy an invading pathogen.

Antigens Proteins on the surface of many bacteria and viruses that trigger an immune response by white blood cells in the body.

Antivenin A commercially produced substance that counteracts the effect of an animal or insect venom.

Aorta A large artery that is the main trunk of the systemic arterial system.

Artificial ventilation The process of ventilating a nonbreathing or inadequately breathing patient; can be done with mouth-to-mask breathing or breathing adjuncts such as a bag-valve-mask (BVM) (see *ventilation*).

Aspiration The inhalation of foreign matter such as blood, water, or vomitus into the trachea and lungs; a life-threatening problem that the EMT tries to anticipate and prevent.

Assault An act that intentionally places a person in fear of immediate bodily harm without consent.

Asthma A condition that results in excessive mucus production, inflammation, and narrowing of the bronchiolar air passages.

Asystole The absence of electrical activity in the heart; electrical flat line.

Aura A sensation of light, color, warmth, smell, flickering lights, or other abnormal sensation that sometimes precedes the onset of a seizure.

Auscultation Evaluation by listening; usually through a stethoscope.

Autoinjector A sealed, plastic-encased syringe that automatically injects medication when pressed against the injection site, usually the thigh.

Automated external defibrillator (AED) An automated device used to recognize lethal dysrthymias and to defibrillate (shock) a patient's heart (see *defibrillation*).

AVPU A four-point assessment of level of consciousness (LOC) based on patient response: *A*lert, *V*erbal, *P*ainful, *U*nresponsive.

Avulsion Open wound characterized by the partial tearing away of soft tissue, creating a tissue flap.

Backboard (long spineboard) A rigid device used to support patients suspected of having head, spine, pelvic, or extremity injury.

Bacteria One-celled microorganisms responsible for spreading disease. They are not dependent on other organisms for life, so they can live outside of the human body. Bacteria cause diseases such as meningitis and tuberculosis. Antibiotics are used to help destroy bacteria.

Bag-valve-mask (BVM) A device that can be attached to supplemental oxygen and used for artificial ventilation; consists of a self-inflating bag, a one-way valve, and a face mask.

Barotrauma Tissue damage that results when a person is exposed to increased environmental pressure; commonly associated with scuba diving injuries.

Base station A fixed station such as a hospital or dispatch center containing equipment necessary for radio transmission and reception; equipment includes at least a transmitter, transmission lines, antenna, and receiver.

Basket stretcher Commonly called a *Stokes litter;* a basket-shaped device with high sides, used to move a patient in technical rescue situations, such as mountain, cave, or water rescues.

Battery Unconsented or unlawful contact with a person.

Behavior How a person acts, including mental and physical activities.

Behavioral emergency A situation in which a patient exhibits abnormal behavior that places the patient or others in danger.

Bilateral On both sides; opposite of unilateral.

Bloodborne pathogens Microorganisms present in human blood and body fluids that can cause disease in humans. Infectious materials contained in other body fluids (saliva, tears, etc.) are generally included in this grouping.

Blunt trauma External impact to the body by a mass that does not penetrate internal body areas.

Body mechanics The way the body works when lifting and moving patients and equipment. Knowledge about body mechanics helps prevent injury.

Body substance isolation (BSI) practices A form of infection control practice designed to prevent infections that are transmitted by direct or indirect contact with infected blood of body fluids. It assumes that all body fluids and substances are potentially infected.

Botulism Potentially-fatal neurologic condition caused from eating improperly canned food in which clostridium spores grow and produce.

Breach of duty One of four elements needed to prove negligence. A breach occurs if a person had a duty to another person and breached this duty by failing to act as a reasonable person would have acted under the same or similar situation, resulting in injury (damage) to the person.

Bronchial inhaler A device used to administer inhaled, aerosolized medication that dilates bronchial tubes, reducing the effects of respiratory distress in patients with asthma, chronic bronchitis, and emphysema; called *bronchodilators* because they dilate bronchial passages.

Burn An injury to the skin or other body tissues caused by heat, chemicals, electricity, or radiation.

Capillary refill The time required by a capillary bed to refill after the application and release of pressure in an area such as the nailbed or finger pad. Refill time of 2 seconds or less is considered normal.

Carbon monoxide Invisible, tasteless, odorless gas produced by incomplete combustion of fuel that kills by taking the place of life-giving oxygen in the bloodstream.

Cardiac arrest A condition in which the heart has stopped or is beating too weakly to pump blood effectively; absence of a pulse.

Cardiogenic shock A type of shock in which the pump (heart) is unable to deliver adequate circulating blood volume to maintain tissue perfusion.

Carina The point at which the trachea divides into the two mainstem bronchi.

Cell The basic unit of life.

Central intravenous line An intravenous line, placed in a large vessel whose tip is near the heart; used for long-term administration of fluids, nutrients, and medications.

Central nervous system (CNS) The brain and the spinal cord; the system that controls body functions.

Cerebrospinal fluid (CSF) Clear fluid surrounding the spinal cord and brain that provides nutrients to these tissues and acts as a cushion to protect them from injury.

Cervical spine The spine in the neck area; made up of the first seven vertebrae.

Cervix The lower, necklike portion of the uterus.

Chemical burn A burn resulting from contact with wet or dry chemicals.

Chief complaint The most important, current problem as stated by the patient; often the reason EMS personnel were summoned.

Child abuse Physical, emotional, or sexual mistreatment that causes harm to an infant or child.

Chock A block of wood, commercially made metal device, or improvised object that can be wedged directly in front or back of a vehicle tire to prevent the vehicle from rolling.

Chronic Occurring repeatedly or continually over time; ongoing.

Chronic bronchitis A form of chronic obstructive pulmonary disease (COPD) that causes an increase in mucus production, primarily in the bronchioles; limits adequate ventilation and gas exchange.

Chronic obstructive pulmonary disease (COPD) A chronic condition in which air is trapped behind obstructions, including secretions, in the bronchioles; emphysema and chronic bronchitis are two forms of COPD.

Cilia Hairlike structures lining the bronchi that help expel foreign particles and mucus from the respiratory tract.

Circulatory system The organs and structures that transport oxygen and other nutrients in the blood to all parts of the body.

Closed wound Soft-tissue damage beneath the skin without penetration or disruption of the skin surface.

Clostridium Bacteria that can grow in food and produce a toxin that can cause botulism.

Coccyx The bottom four fused vertebrae; the tailbone.

Common law The body of principles and rules of action derived from society's acceptance of customs and norms over time, which are reflected in the decisions of judges.

Communicable disease An infectious disease that can be transmitted from person to person; also called a *contagious disease.*

Conduction The direct transfer of heat from a warm object to a colder object or fluid.

Confidentiality The duty owed to the patient by the EMT not to disclose information revealed by the patient while receiving care.

Congestive heart failure (CHF) The backup of venous blood returning to the heart when the heart fails to pump as much as it receives; raises venous pressure, which can force fluid into the lungs (see *pulmonary edema*).

Consent The verbal or written acceptance of medical treatment.

Constitutional law A form of law based on the Constitution of the United States and individual states.

Contraction A rhythmic tightening of the muscles in the uterus, often indicating labor.

Contraindication Situation in which a medication should not be used because it may harm the patient.

Contusion A closed wound with internal bleeding resulting from contact with a blunt object; a bruise.

Convection The transfer of heat from the body to colder-moving air or water vapor.

Convulsions Uncontrolled muscular movement of the body; another term for tonic-clonic seizure activity.

Coronal An imaginary plane through the midaxillary lines separating the body into front and back.

Crepitus The grating vibration made by bone fragments rubbing together, or by air under the skin (subcutaneous emphysema); also referred to as *crepitation.*

Cribbing Material used to stabilize a vehicle or a loose object threatening rescuers or the patient; often consists of wooden blocks propped under the vehicle or object.

Cricoid cartilage Cartilage ring just inferior to the larynx.

Critical burn A burn that is potentially life threatening or disabling, usually requiring advanced emergency care.

Critical incident stress debriefing (CISD) A team approach to counseling individuals who have been involved in a particularly stressful incident.

Critical trauma Life-threatening injury; the result of blunt or penetrating trauma.

Croup A respiratory infection that causes inflammation and swelling of the laryngeal lining and narrowing of the trachea below the vocal cords; usually seen in younger children.

Crush injury A type of closed or open wound resulting in tissue or organ damage from severe blunt trauma.

Cyanosis Bluish discoloration of the skin caused by inadequate oxygenation of the blood.

Damages One of four elements of negligence, requiring that some type of injury (physical, mental, or emotional) must have occurred.

Decompression sickness An illness that occurs when nitrogen bubbles expand in the tissues in which they have dissolved; usually caused by ascending too rapidly during scuba diving; also called the *bends*.

Decontamination The process of cleaning a person's body, equipment, or other materials after exposure to hazardous materials.

Defendant A person named in a lawsuit as having caused damages to another (plaintiff).

Defensive driving Driving in a manner that considers factors that affect safe vehicle operation and incorporates practices that will minimize the likelihood of a collision.

Defibrillation The process of delivering an electric shock to the heart in order to restore normal electrical and mechanical (pumping) activity.

Delivery The process in which the baby is expelled from the uterus.

Depression An emotional state in which there are extreme feelings of sadness, dejection, lack of worth, and emptiness.

Dermis The layer of skin directly beneath the epidermis containing nerves, glands, hair follicles, and blood vessels.

Detailed physical examination A thorough, methodic assessment of a patient after completion of the focused history and physical examination, looking for secondary conditions.

Diabetes mellitus A disease associated with inadequate insulin production; commonly called *diabetes* or *sugar diabetes*.

Diaphragm The dome-shaped breathing muscle that separates the thoracic and abdominal cavities.

Digestive system The organs and structures that digest food and eliminate waste.

Direct ground lift Technique requiring two or more rescuers to lift a patient, who does not have a suspected spinal injury, from the ground onto a stretcher.

Direct pressure The first step in controlling external bleeding, by using the hand (with appropriate protective barriers) to apply pressure directly to the wound.

Direct-contact transmission The transmission of disease by touching another person's infected blood or other body fluids, or inhaling airborne particles infected with a disease-causing agent.

Disability A hereditary or acquired condition that interferes with normal functions of the body or with a person's ability to be self-sufficient.

Disaster An incident of such great magnitude that it exhausts all local resources and requires the assistance of several other jurisdictions; includes natural and man-made disasters.

Disaster plan A predetermined set of activities that identifies how a community will deploy its resources in the event of a disaster.

Dislocation An injury resulting from over-stretching or severe movement to a joint, which displaces the bone from the joint.

Disproportion A condition in which the infant's head is too large to fit through the mother's pelvis; caused by a small pelvis, or by fetal abnormalities.

Distal Further away from the trunk; opposite of proximal.

Distal pulse A pulse site away from the center of the body; the radial pulses in the wrists, and pedal or tibial pulse in the feet.

DNR order DNR stands for "do not resuscitate"; a written directive that indicates situations in which resuscitation efforts are to be withheld or stopped.

Dorsal The back of the hand or top of the foot; opposite of palm of hand or planter surface of foot.

Dose The correct amount of medication to administer.

Draw sheet method A technique used to transfer a patient between a stretcher and a bed using the bed sheet that the patient is lying on.

Drowning Death resulting from submersion in fluid, most commonly water.

Drug A chemical substance that alters the body's function when introduced into the body.

Duplex A mode of radio transmission in which simultaneous two-way communication takes place using two separate frequencies to transmit and receive.

Duty to act One of four elements of negligence, in which it must be proven that a person was required to provide for the well-being of another.

Dyspnea Difficulty breathing; shortness of breath.

Dysrhythmia Abnormal electrical rhythm in the heart.

Ecchymosis Damage to the blood vessels underneath the skin resulting in discoloration; a bruise.

Eclampsia The progression of preeclampsia to include seizures; a threat to both mother and fetus.

Edema Swelling produced by fluid (plasma) seeping from capillaries into surrounding tissues.

Elder abuse The infliction of physical pain or injury, debilitating mental anguish, or unreasonable confinement on an elderly patient.

Elder neglect The failure to provide for the essential needs of a dependent elderly person, such as food, shelter, health care, clothing, physical comfort, social contact, and emotional support.

Elderly Commonly defined as persons over 65 years of age.

Electrical burn A burn resulting from contact with low- or high-voltage electricity, including lightning.

Emancipation Special situations in which the courts have determined a person, who is otherwise a minor, to be considered an adult for purposes of medical treatment (e.g., a 16 year old who is an unmarried mother is considered an adult for the purpose of accepting or refusing medical treatment).

Embryo The developing baby inside the uterus, during the first 2 months of pregnancy.

Emergency medical services system A network of resources, including medical facilities, personnel, and equipment necessary to provide care to victims of injury or illness. Includes five basic elements: patient and bystander access, emergency medical dispatch, first responder care, emergency medical technician care, and hospital care.

Emergency medical technician A person who has successfully completed a state-approved training program consistent with the Department of Transportation's (DOT) National Curriculum and successfully passed the certification examination. The three recognized levels of EMTs are Basic, Intermediate, and Paramedic.

Emergency vehicle operator training Specialized training for persons who will be driving emergency vehicles, such as an ambulance, to assist them in operating the vehicle in a safe manner.

Emesis Vomiting.

Emphysema A form of chronic obstructive pulmonary disease (COPD) that results in the destruction of the alveoli and the bronchioles; occurs more commonly in adults than children.

EMT-Basic A person trained with a minimum of 110 hours of classroom, clinical, and field experience to provide basic emergency patient care according to local EMS protocols.

EMT-Intermediate A person trained at the next level above EMT-Basic. At this level, additional training is provided in advanced life-support skills such as intravenous (IV) access, advanced airway skills, and medication administration.

EMT-Paramedic A person with the highest level of EMT training, including all of the skills found in the Basic and Intermediate levels of training and even more advanced skills, such as interpreting difficult heart-rhythm disturbances, administering additional medications, and performing invasive airway and resuscitation procedures.

Endocrine system The organs and structures that produce chemicals to help regulate the activities of other body systems.

Endotracheal intubation The process of inserting an endotracheal tube into a patient's trachea to maintain an open airway and provide effective oxygenation and ventilation.

Enhanced 9-1-1 An advanced form of telephone communication that routes emergency calls to the appropriate answering point; it enables a call taker to immediately know the phone number and location of the caller and to identify the appropriate response units (e.g., police, fire, rescue) to send to the emergency scene.

Envenomation Venom deposited in a wound.

Epidermis Outermost layer of the skin comprised of dead or dying cells.

Epigastrium Area of the abdominal surface directly anterior to the stomach and just inferior to the xiphoid process.

Epiglottis A small flap of tissue that covers the trachea during swallowing to prevent foreign matter such as food and fluid from entering the lungs.

Epiglottitis A severe infection causing swelling of the epiglottis that can lead to complete airway obstruction.

Epilepsy A chronic nervous system disorder with characteristic seizure patterns; the type and duration of seizures varies.

Epinephrine A medication commonly used to relieve the signs and symptoms of a severe allergic reaction; constricts blood vessels, dilates bronchial passages, and helps block histamine response. A hormone secreted by the adrenal glands in response to stressful situations; also known as *adrenaline.*

Eschar A charred, stiff skin covering associated with full-thickness burns.

Esophagus The tube leading from the pharynx to the stomach.

Evaporation The process in which a liquid changes to a gas; also involves transfer of heat, and can thus be a mechanism of heat loss.

Evidence Anything that has a bearing on or establishes an issue in a legal proceeding.

Evisceration An open wound in which organs protrude through the skin; associated with abdominal organs.

Expressed consent A patient's verbal or written consent to accept treatment; requires informed consent.

Extremity Limb; arm or leg.

Extremity lift A lifting and moving technique for a patient without spine or extremity injury that requires two rescuers to grasp the patient under the arms and legs.

Extrication The removal of a patient from a building, vehicle, or area of danger to a location more suitable for care and preparation for transport. The term can refer more specifically to removal from a damaged vehicle, collapsed structure, or other position of entrapment.

False imprisonment Detention of a person, without consent or lawful justification, so as to substantially interfere with the person's liberty.

Fetus The developing baby inside the uterus, during the third and following months of pregnancy.

First responder Usually the first medically-trained person to respond to an emergency situation, such as law enforcement personnel and firefighters.

Flexible stretcher A carrying device capable of being rolled or folded' commonly called a Reeve's or SKED stretcher.

Focused history and physical examination The second phase of the patient-assessment process, which includes gathering pertinent information, obtaining vital signs, and completing a physical examination, while focusing on the chief complaint.

Fontanelle Soft spot on an infant's head; line where skull sections grow together.

Fowler's position A semisitting position; also described as *semireclining.*

Fracture A broken bone; can be open (break in the skin) or closed.

Frostbite A cold-related emergency in which body tissues freeze.

Full-thickness burn A burn that penetrates the epidermis and dermis layers of the skin and sometimes affects the underlying tissues, blood vessels, muscles, and nerves; characterized by white and charred discoloration; also called a *third-degree burn.*

Fungi A type of disease-causing agent that include molds and yeast that cause diseases such as athlete's foot.

Gag reflex A reflex that causes a patient to gag when the back of the throat is stimulated; a protective mechanism designed to protect the airway from aspiration.

Gastric distension Inflation of the stomach with air, often by using too much force or volume when ventilating a patient; can make ventilations less effective, or cause vomiting.

Gastric tube A tube placed into the stomach; can be used as a feeding tube.

Generic name A medication's noncommercial name, which is often an abbreviated version of the chemical name (see *trade name*).

Glottis The opening between the vocal cords, leading to the trachea.

Glucose A simple form of sugar found in foods and produced by the digestion of carbohydrates; serves as the body's primary source of energy.

Golden hour The first 60 minutes after the onset of a critical injury or illness in which the patient requires definitive care in a hospital.

Good Samaritan Laws Limited type of protection afforded EMTs; derived from the Bible and designed to offer protection to those rendering care in good faith, a reasonable manner, and usually without compensation for their acts.

Governmental immunity A form of protection against liability that is afforded to public employees that is actually designed to protect state or other governmental entities from any negligent acts by an employee.

Gynecology The branch of medicine dealing with women's health care.

Halo test A test used to determine the presence of cerebrospinal fluid (CSF) in blood. Blood placed on a gauze pad may separate into a halolike shape if CSF is present.

Hazardous materials incident An incident involving the release of hazardous substances into the environment.

Head-tilt–chin-lift Technique used to open a patient's airway by tilting the head back and lifting the chin forward.

Hematoma Pooling of blood that results when blood vessels rupture. It may be under the skin or in an organ.

Hemoglobin A blood protein that carries oxygen and changes color depending on the amount of oxygen that it carries.

Hemophilia A bleeding disorder in which blood fails to clot.

Hemorrhage The loss of blood internally or externally.

Hemothorax The accumulation of blood in the chest cavity.

Hepatitis A serious viral infection of the liver; caused by several different viruses, of which Hepatitis B virus (HBV) is potentially the most serious.

Hepatitis A A common type of hepatitis infection in the United States; transmitted through contaminated food or drink or the oral-fecal route.

Hepatitis B A serious viral infection of the liver that poses a significant threat to EMS personnel. It is transmitted through blood and other body fluids.

Hepatitis C A serious viral infection of the liver similar to hepatitis B, that is primarily transmitted through blood transfusion.

Herpes simplex A highly contagious virus transmitted through direct contact. The virus enters the body through breaks in the skin or mucous membranes. One type of the virus causes cold sores or fever blisters; another type causes genital lesions.

High-altitude illness Illness associated with insufficient oxygen from decreased atmospheric pressure at high altitude.

Histamine A chemical released by the immune system in response to exposure to an allergen.

History Subjective information about the patient's condition, as reported by the patient.

History of present illness (or incident) Information provided by the patient about the current event; begins with the chief complaint and proceeds to questions that gather more information about it.

Hives (urticaria) A type of rash produced by an allergic reaction; characterized by itching and raised (swollen) areas of skin.

Home ventilator A mechanical device often used to provide ventilation for a patient unable to breathe spontaneously; generally used together with a tracheostomy.

Hormones Chemicals secreted by glands; hormones influence body activities and functions.

Host An organism in which another, usually parasitic, organism is nourished and harbored.

Human immunodeficiency virus (HIV) The virus that destroys the immune system (the body system used to fight off infections) and causes AIDS.

Hyperbaric Related to atmospheric pressures greater than that of the earth's atmosphere at sea level; hyperbaric therapy takes place in a recompression chamber.

Hyperglycemia A condition in which there is too much sugar (glucose) in the blood.

Hyperthermia A condition in which the body retains more heat than it loses, causing body temperature to rise above normal levels.

Hypoglycemia A condition in which there is too little sugar (glucose) in the blood; associated with a diabetic emergency.

Hypoperfusion Inadequate blood flow through the tissues, which results in inadequate delivery of oxygen and nutrients to the cells and inadequate removal of waste products; also known as *shock*.

Hypothermia A condition in which the body loses more heat than it retains, causing body temperature to fall below normal levels.

Hypoxia Inadequate oxygenation of the tissues; can be localized in one area, or body-wide (systemic).

Iliac crests The anterior, superior portions of the pelvis.

Immobilization The process of securing an injured area to prevent further movement.

Immune system The organ system that protects the body from infection, and invasion by foreign substances.

Impaled object A penetrating object, such as a knife, embedded in soft tissue.

Implied consent Consent granted by virtue of law for a patient who is unconscious or otherwise unable to communicate his or her desire to receive medical care, or who is a minor.

Incident command system (ICS) A system used to manage a disaster or multiple casualty incident (MCI). This system defines a chain of command beginning with the overall scene commander and includes others responsible for functions such as triage, treatment, and transportation.

Indication A situation in which a specific medication should be given because of its potential ability to improve a condition; the condition for which a drug is prescribed.

Indirect-contact transmission The transmission of disease through indirect contact, such as contact with an object that was contaminated by an infected person.

Infant A baby between birth and 1 year of age.

Infectious disease Any disease that invades the body as a result of a pathogen.

Inferior Away from the head; opposite of superior.

Informed consent Patient consent indicating that he or she has been informed of, understands, and agrees to receive the care to be rendered.

Ingested poison A toxic substance that enters the body through the mouth and is absorbed in the digestive tract.

Inhaled poison A toxic substance that enters the body through the lungs during inhalation.

Initial assessment The first phase of the patient-assessment process, used to rapidly identify and correct immediate threats to life that include consciousness, airway, breathing, and circulation problems.

Injected poison A toxic substance that enters the body through a puncture in the skin.

Inline stabilization Supporting a patient's head and neck in line with the body to prevent further movement and minimize the chance of further injury to the head or spine.

Insulin A hormone produced in the pancreas, crucial to the body's effective use of glucose (sugar).

Insulin-dependent diabetic A diabetic patient who requires insulin injections for proper sugar metabolism.

Integumentary system The organs and structures, especially components of the skin, that cover the body, help establish identity, retain fluid, and prevent infection.

Interpersonal communication skills Skills used to enhance verbal communication, including the proper use of eye contact, body language, verbal language, and attentive listening.

Invasion of privacy Disclosing information about a patient that results in harm to the patient.

Involuntary consent Consent obtained by a person other than the patient, usually only as allowed by a statute, such as in the case of a prisoner or other person whom the court has determined to be legally incompetent.

Ischemia Lack of oxygen in an area of tissue.

Joint Area where two or more bones meet; can be movable or fixed (fused).

Jugular vein distention (JVD) Engorged veins on the sides of the neck, indicating a backup of blood in the venous system.

Kinetic energy The energy an object has while it is in motion. It is related to the velocity and size (mass) of the object.

Labor The process of childbirth; proceeds from the beginning of contractions, through delivery of the newborn, to delivery of the placenta.

Laceration A cut or tear in the skin.

Laryngectomy A surgical procedure in which the larynx is removed (see *stoma*).

Laryngoscope An instrument that allows one to see the vocal cords directly before inserting an endotracheal tube during orotracheal intubation.

Laryngospasm The closing of the vocal cords in response to stimulation, such as contact with food or fluid.

Larynx The portion of the upper airway that joins the pharynx to the trachea and houses the vocal cords.

Lateral recumbent position A horizontal position, lying on the side; also known as the *recovery position*.

Lateral Toward the side or away from the midline; opposite of medial.

Level of consciousness (LOC) The patient's state of awareness and orientation. Initial assessment may be done on a four-point scale (see *AVPU*).

Ligament Fibrous connective tissue, generally found at joints, that attaches bone to bone.

Log-roll A method of rolling a supine patient onto the side with a minimum of spinal movement; usually performed in order to place a backboard under the patient.

Long bone A long, straight bone such as the humerus, femur, tibia, or fibula; the main part of the bone is called the *shaft*.

Lumbar spine The spine in the low back area; made up of five vertebrae.

Lyme disease Caused by bite of deer ticks; causes memory loss, arthritis, and vision and hearing problems.

Lymphatic system A system within the body that aids in the elimination of dead pathogens and in the production of antibodies.

Mainstem bronchi The two main airway branches that lead from the trachea to the lungs.

Mania A state in which a patient is severely agitated, often marked by rapid speech or constant physical activity such as pacing.

Mechanism of action The manner in which a medication works in the body; also simply called its *action.*

Mechanism of injury The manner in which an injury has occurred, including the forces, directions of force, and areas of impact involved.

Med channels Channels dedicated by the Federal Communications Commission (FCC) for the exclusive use of emergency medical service systems.

Medial Toward the midline; opposite of lateral.

Medical direction (medical oversight) Oversight by a supervising physician of all patient-care–related activities provided by EMTs. This oversight has two forms: on-line (direct or concurrent), and off-line (indirect), also described as prospective, concurrent, and retrospective. Another common previously used term is *medical control.*

Medical director A physician who has accepted the responsibility to oversee the patient-care–related activities provided within an EMS system. This person is responsible for developing the standards (policies, procedures, and protocols) for system operation.

Medication A drug used in patient care to treat or prevent a specific disease or condition.

Medulla The lower portion of the brainstem; controls respiration.

Meninges The three layers of protective membranes that cover the brain and spinal cord.

Meningitis Inflammation of the membranes surrounding the brain and spinal cord, caused by either bacteria or viruses. Meningitis can cause serious consequences, including death, if not treated promptly.

Menstruation The periodic discharge of blood, mucous, and tissue from the lining of the uterus; associated with normal function of the uterus and ovaries.

Midaxillary An imaginary vertical line through the middle of the armpit.

Midclavicular An imaginary vertical line through the center of the clavicle.

Midline An imaginary vertical line running through the center of the body, dividing the body into right and left halves.

Military antishock garment (MAST) See *pneumatic antishock garment.*

Miscarriage Another term for spontaneous abortion.

Modified jaw thrust Technique used to open the airway of a patient with suspected spinal injury, keeping the head in a neutral position while lifting the jaw forward.

Multiple casualty incident (MCI) An incident, sometimes called a *disaster,* where the incident and number of victims overwhelms the capabilities of the EMS service or system.

Multiplex A mode of radio transmission that enables voice and other data to be transmitted simultaneously on the same frequency.

Musculoskeletal system The organs and structures that provide support and structure for the body, protect internal organs, and manufacture blood cells.

Myocardial infarction (MI) Death of cardiac muscle; a heart attack.

Myocardium A thick layer of muscle cells that makes up the majority of the heart wall.

Nasal cannula A flexible tube used to administer oxygen through the nostrils of a breathing patient.

Nasogastric tube A tube passed through the nose and esophagus into the stomach, to relieve the pressure that causes gastric distention.

Nasopharyngeal airway A flexible rubber tubelike device inserted into one of the patient's nostrils and nasopharynx to keep the tongue from obstructing the airway.

Nature of illness The general type of illness, often described by the patient's initial complaint or the primary physical examination finding.

Near drowning A submersion incident in which the patient survives.

Neglect Failure to provide for the essential needs of an infant or child, such as food, shelter, clothing, cleanliness, supervision, and emotional support.

Negligence Failure to act in a reasonable manner, resulting in harm to another person.

Neonate A newborn baby.

Nerve A channel for the transmission of information, in the form of electrical impulses, from one area of the body to another.

Nervous system The organs and structures that coordinate the function of body systems by generating and transmitting electrical impulses throughout the body over the nerves.

Neurogenic shock Also called *spinal shock;* widespread dilation of blood vessels by a spinal injury that disrupts function of the sympathetic nervous system; presents with a different clinical picture than hypovolemic shock.

Newborn A baby between birth and 1 month of age; also called a *neonate.*

Nitroglycerin A medication taken sublingually to help reduce chest pain of cardiac origin.

Nonrebreather mask A mask covering the patient's mouth and nose, used to administer oxygen to a breathing patient.

Normal sinus rhythm The normal electrical activity of the heart.

Obstetrics The branch of medicine dealing with pregnancy and childbirth.

Occiput The posterior area of the skull, just above the top of the neck.

Off-line medical direction Also called *indirect medical direction,* it refers to the medical oversight of EMS patient care, which occurs before and after the care of the individual patient.

Ongoing assessment The final step of the patient-assessment process, which repeats the initial assessment and the focused history and physical examination.

On-line medical direction Also called *concurrent medical direction,* it refers to direct communication with a physician, usually at a hospital, to receive orders for patient care.

Open wound Soft-tissue damage resulting from penetration of the skin surface.

Opportunistic infections An infection that strikes a person with a weakened immune system, such as that caused by HIV.

OPQRST Abbreviation to help remember questions for gathering the history of present event (or illness); stands for *O*nset, *P*rovokes, *Q*uality, *R*adiation, *S*everity, and *T*ime.

Oral glucose An oral sugar medication administered for the treatment of altered consciousness that may have resulted from low blood sugar during a diabetic emergency.

Organs A group of similar tissues.

Oropharyngeal airway A curved plastic tube inserted into the mouth and oropharynx of a patient without a gag reflex to keep the tongue from obstructing the airway.

Orotracheal intubation The primary type of endotracheal intubation, in which the tube is passed through the mouth into the trachea.

Overdose Intentional administration of a toxic quantity of a medication or other substance(s) that is not harmful in smaller amounts.

Ovulation The release of an egg (ovum) from one of the ovaries; occurs approximately 14 days after the beginning of the previous menstrual cycle.

Oxygen saturation The percentage of available hemoglobin-binding sites that are carrying oxygen (see *pulse oximeter*).

Oxygenation The process of bringing oxygen into the body and delivering it to the tissues.

Palmar surface The palm side of the hand.

Paradoxical movement Movement of one part of the chest wall in opposition to the remainder of the chest during breathing; may occur when multiple consecutive ribs have been broken in more than one place (flail chest).

Paranoia Irrational fear that others intend to harm or kill one.

Paraplegia Paralysis of the lower extremities resulting from an injury to the spinal cord at the mid- or lower-back level.

Parasites One-celled disease-causing organisms that range in size from as small as bacteria to much larger intestinal worms.

Partial-thickness burn A burn injury that penetrates the epidermis and into the dermis; characterized by reddened discoloration and blisters; also called a *second-degree burn.*

Pathogen A microorganism, such as bacteria or virus that causes disease.

Patient-care report A written report summarizing vital patient administrative information; a medical-legal document.

Penetrating trauma Penetration of the body by a projectile such as a bullet, or by a knife or other sharp instrument.

Perfusion The circulation of blood to all the organs of the body, carrying oxygen and other nutrients to the cells and removing waste products.

Perineum The skin area between the vagina and anus; can be torn during delivery or damaged in straddle injuries.

Peripheral nervous system The portion of the nervous system outside the central nervous system (CNS); connects the brain and spinal cord with all organs and tissues.

Pharmacology The study of drugs and how they affect the body.

Pharynx The throat.

Placards Signs placed on vehicles, railroad cars, and storage facilities indicating the presence of hazardous materials.

Placenta The structure that develops during pregnancy and attaches to the wall of the uterus; delivers oxygen and other nutrients from the mother to the fetus, and receives carbon dioxide and other wastes back from the fetus.

Placenta previa A condition in which the placenta implants in the lower portion of the uterus, covering the opening of the cervix.

Plaintiff A person filing a lawsuit in an effort to recover damages as a result of the actions of another.

Plantar surface The bottom or sole of the foot.

Pleura Thin membrane linings of the lungs and thoracic cavity; the visceral and parietal pleura.

Pleuritic chest pain Chest pain associated with breathing movement or other motion; usually caused by an injury or infection of the pleural membranes or chest wall.

Pneumatic antishock garment (PASG) Inflatable garment used as a pressure splint to stabilize pelvic or lower extremity fractures; may assist in the treatment of shock; also called *MAST* (military antishock trousers) or *MAST pants.*

Pneumonia An infection that results in the accumulation of fluid, bacteria and inflammatory cells between the alveoli and the capillaries.

Pneumothorax The accumulation of air in the chest cavity that leads to collapse of a lung.

Poison Any substance that produces adverse effects when it enters the body through absorption, ingestion, inhalation, or injection; also called a *toxin.*

Portable radio A handheld, low-power device that allows for radio communications when responders are away from the ambulance.

Portable stretcher A lightweight folding device used to carry a patient.

Position of comfort The position in which the patient states he or she is most comfortable being transported.

Position of function The normal resting position of a limb.

Posterior The back of the body or a body part; opposite of anterior.

Power grip Technique used to securely grip an object such as a stretcher with both hands.

Power lift The preferred lifting position, in which the rescuer squats near the object to be lifted, keeps a straight back, and uses the legs to lift. This technique reduces the chance of back injury.

Preeclampsia A condition of pregnancy associated with high blood pressure, fluid retention, and edema (see *eclampsia*).

Preschooler A child 3 to 6 years of age.

Pressure bandage A bandage applied to control external bleeding.

Prone Position of the body being in a horizontal position when lying on the stomach.

Protocols Written directives from a medical director that provide a standardized approach to common patient problems and a consistent level of care for different levels of EMTs. They include standing orders.

Protozoa Disease-causing agent responsible for malaria and dysentery.

Proximal Closer to the trunk; opposite of distal.

Proximate cause A legal concept of negligence that links the action or omission and the damages suffered by another.

Psychosis A severe mental disorder that involves a distorted sense of reality; may include hallucinations (false impressions of the senses) or delusions (imaginary ideas or beliefs).

Pulmonary edema The collection of fluid in the lungs, often caused by rising venous pressure in congestive heart failure (CHF).

Pulmonary embolism The blockage of a pulmonary artery by foreign matter, such as a blood clot, fat, tumor tissue, or air.

Pulse The wave of pressure in the blood generated by the pumping of blood from the heart.

Pulse oximeter An electronic device that uses colored-light technology to measure the percentage of blood hemoglobin that is saturated with oxygen.

Quadriplegia Paralysis of all four extremities resulting from a spinal cord injury at the neck level.

Quality assurance A process designed to continually monitor and measure the quality of clinical care provided within a system. Objective data such as response times, adherence to protocols, and survival rates are used to document the effectiveness of the care provided.

Quality improvement A process that continually reevaluates the EMS system. It takes the information obtained through the quality-assurance process, analyzes it, makes and implements corrections, and reevaluates to determine if the corrections were effective.

Rabid animal An animal infected with rabies, a frequently fatal disease (if untreated) that affects the nervous system.

Radiation The transfer of heat from a warm surface to the cooler environment.

Rapid extrication Technique used to move a patient rapidly from a sitting position in a vehicle to a spineboard for immobilization; generally used only in critical situations involving immediate danger to the patient or rescuers.

Rapid trauma assessment Another term for the physical examination portion of the focused history and physical examination, when performed on a trauma patient.

Reasonable force The minimal force necessary to keep a patient from injuring self, rescuers, or bystanders.

Recovery position Also known as *left lateral recumbent position*, the placement of an unconscious patient without suspected spine injury on the left side to maintain an open airway and allow drainage of blood or vomitus.

Regulations A rule or order having the force of law, issued to guide the activity of those subject to the agency and the governmental officers who enforce the agency's authority.

Regulator Device attached to an oxygen cylinder that reduces the pressure within the cylinder to an amount that can be safely administered to a patient.

Repeater A radio base station that receives a low-power radio transmission on one frequency and retransmits it over another higher-power frequency in order to increase the range of the broadcast.

Respiration The exchange of oxygen and carbon dioxide between the cells and the blood, and between the lungs and the environment; breathing.

Respiratory arrest Cessation of breathing.

Respiratory distress Difficult or inadequate breathing.

Respiratory system A system comprising the lungs and a series of tubes and passageways that provide the body with oxygen from the air breathed during inhalation and remove carbon dioxide, a waste product, during exhalation.

Rickettsia Disease-causing agent responsible for typhus and Rocky Mountain spotted fever.

Route The way in which a medication enters the body; oral, sublingual, intramuscular, and inhalation are examples.

Ryan White Comprehensive AIDS Resources Emergency Act Federal legislation that allows EMS personnel to determine if they have been exposed to an infectious disease while providing care.

Sacral spine The spine in the pelvic area; made up of five fused vertebrae.

Sagittal An imaginary plane through the body from anterior to posterior.

Salmonella A bacteria that causes food poisoning.

SAMPLE history Abbreviation used to gather pertinent medical information from a patient; it stands for *S*igns and symptoms, *A*llergies, *M*edications, *P*ast history, *L*ast oral intake, and *E*vents leading to the incident.

Scanner A radio receiver that continually searches multiple frequencies for transmissions.

Schizophrenia A form of mental illness in which a patient loses touch with reality and is no longer able to think or act normally (rationally).

School-age child A child 6 to 12 years of age.

Scoop stretcher A rigid carrying device that is split lengthwise into two sections; used to lift and move a patient while minimizing movement of the spine and other areas of possible injury.

Scope of practice Defined medical actions that are allowed to be performed by a licensed or certified health care provider.

Sector One of seven divisions within the incident command system; a specific area of responsibility assigned to a group of rescuers and a sector officer to help ensure a smooth operation.

Seizure A disorder of the electrical activity in the brain that causes sudden changes in level of consciousness (LOC) or behavior, and sometimes causes uncontrolled muscle movement.

Self contained breathing apparatus (SCBA) A specialized air cylinder and mask used for entering toxic environments, such as smoke and fire and confined spaces.

Sellick maneuver Pressure applied to the cricoid cartilage to prevent passive aspiration and assist in visualizing the vocal cords; also called *cricoid pressure.*

Sensation A feeling or awareness in an area of the body.

Shaken-baby syndrome Injuries inflicted to the central nervous system (CNS) as a result of vigorously shaking an infant.

Shock Inadequate perfusion of the cells and tissues; see *hypoperfusion.*

Shunt A tube or device placed in the body to redirect a body fluid from one area to another.

Side effect Any action that a medication causes, other than the desired action.

Sign An objective indicator that can be readily observed about the patient's condition, such as sweating or vomiting (in contrast to subjective elements; see *symptom*).

Simplex A mode of radio transmission in which transmission and reception occur on the same frequency, limiting communications to one direction at a time.

Splinting Immobilizing a painful, swollen, or deformed body part.

Sprain An injury to tendons or to the ligaments or connective tissue around a joint.

Stair chair A lightweight carrying device used to transport a seated patient up or down stairs.

Standard of care The level of care expected of an EMT based on education, laws, court decisions, local protocols, policies, and procedures.

Standing orders The portion of protocols issued by a medical director that authorize EMTs to perform certain patient-care activities in specific situations without communicating directly with a physician for further medical direction.

Staphylococcus A type of bacteria normally found on skin; can produce a toxic effect when food contaminated with the bacteria is kept at too warm a temperature.

Status epilepticus Prolonged or repetitive seizure activity during which the patient does not regain consciousness.

Stoma A surgical opening in the neck; the primary (or only) breathing opening for a person whose larynx has been removed.

Strain An injury caused by excessive physical effort that stretches and damages muscle fibers.

Stridor High-pitched sound indicating a narrowing or obstruction of the upper airway.

Stroke A disruption of blood flow to the brain caused by an occluded or ruptured artery; also called a *cerebrovascular accident (CVA).*

Stroke volume The amount of blood ejected from each of the ventricles with each contraction of the heart.

Stylet A semiflexible device placed in an endotracheal tube to help hold the tube's shape to assist during endotracheal intubation.

Substance abuse The deliberate, excessive use of a substance without regard for the health consequences.

Substance misuse The use of a substance for unintended purposes or for appropriate purposes but at an improper dose.

Sucking chest wound An open chest injury that creates a sucking sound with each breath.

Suction The use of manual or mechanical devices to draw vomitus and secretions, such as saliva and blood, from a patient's mouth and throat.

Sudden infant death syndrome (SIDS) The sudden, unexpected death of an otherwise healthy infant that occurs during sleep for an unknown reason; also called *crib death.*

Suicide The act of taking one's own life.

Superficial burn A burn injury that involves only the epidermis; characterized by reddened discoloration; also called a *first-degree burn.*

Superior Toward the head; opposite of inferior.

Supine Lying on the back.

Supine hypotension Drop in blood pressure in a pregnant patient, especially during the third trimester, when in a supine position; caused by compression of the inferior vena cava by weight of the uterus.

Surfactant A chemical that helps prevent the alveoli from collapsing.

Symptom Subjective (history) factor that is not readily observable and must be described by the patient, such as the presence and location of pain (in contrast to subjective elements; see *sign*).

Syncope A sudden, temporary loss of consciousness; a fainting episode.

Telemetry Radio or telephone transmission of converted electronic signals; sometimes used by advanced life support (ALS) personnel to transmit heart rhythm findings.

Tendon Connective tissue that attaches muscle to bone.

Thoracic spine Part of the spine made up of 12 thoracic vertebrae, to which the ribs are attached.

Thyroid cartilage Cartilage covering most of the larynx; the Adam's apple.

Tidal volume The amount of air taken in with each breath.

Tissue A collection of similar cells.

Toddler A child 1 to 3 years of age.

Tourniquet A device used to control bleeding, made of a wide strip of cloth and a stick; completely stops the arterial blood flow to an extremity.

Toxin A poison.

Trachea The tubelike structure, located in front of the esophagus, that carries oxygen to the lungs; commonly called the *windpipe.*

Tracheostomy tube A metal or plastic tube placed through a surgical opening into the trachea (tracheostomy) to provide oxygen and ventilation.

Traction The application of force along the long axis of an extremity to align bones and prevent further movement within a joint or at a possible fracture site.

Trade name The commercial brand name under which the manufacturer of a medication markets the product (see *generic name*).

Trendelenburg's position A position in which the patient's legs and feet are higher than the head.

Triage A systematic process of establishing treatment and transportation priorities according to the severity of the patient conditions.

Trimester One of the three approximately 13-week intervals in a normal pregnancy.

Tuberculosis A respiratory system infection caused by bacteria.

Ultra high frequencies (UHF) Radio frequencies that perform well in the presence of large physical obstacles such as city skyscrapers, but are not as effective as very high frequencies (VHF) over long distances.

Umbilical cord The "supply line" between the fetus and placenta through which nourishment of the fetus and removal of fetal wastes take place.

Unilateral On one side only; opposite of bilateral.

Universal precautions A form of infection-control practice that assumes that all human blood and certain body fluids are handled as if they were known to be infectious for human immunodeficiency virus, hepatitis B and other bloodborne pathogens.

Urinary system The organs and structures that filter and excrete waste products in the form of urine from the body.

Uterus The hollow, muscular organ within which the fetus develops; the womb.

Vaccination A specific substance containing weakened or dead pathogens that is introduced into the body to build resistance against a specific infection.

Vallecula A space between the base of the tongue and the epiglottis, into which the tip of a curved laryngoscope blade is inserted during endotracheal intubation.

Vasodilators A class of medications that dilates blood vessels; nitroglycerin is an example.

Ventilation The movement of air between the lungs and the environment.

Ventricular fibrillation A state of disorganized electrical activity in the heart that results in quivering of the heart chambers and loss of effective pumping activity; can sometimes be corrected by defibrillation.

Ventricular shunt A tube extending from the ventricle of the brain to the abdomen, to drain excess cerebrospinal fluid (CSF) from the brain.

Ventricular tachycardia A very rapid contraction of the ventricles that often does not allow heart chambers to fill completely with blood; can sometimes be corrected by defibrillation.

Vertebrae Thirty-three bones that comprise the five regions of the spinal column: cervical, thoracic, lumbar, sacral, and coccygeal. The spinal column protects the spinal cord.

Very high frequencies (VHF) Radio frequencies that perform well over a long range, but are more prone than ultra high frequencies (UHF) to interference from large physical obstacles.

Virus Microorganisms responsible for spreading many diseases, including the common cold. They depend on other organisms to live and grow. Hepatitis B virus and human immunodeficiency virus are the two most serious viruses of concern to EMTs.

Vital signs Signs that indicate the level of function in vital body systems. Usual vital sign measurements include level of consciousness (LOC), respirations, pulse, blood pressure, skin signs, and pupils.

Vocal cords The two folds of tissue at the entrance to the larynx that vibrate and produce sounds as air passes between them.

Wheeled ambulance stretcher A device with wheels and a collapsible undercarriage used to transport patients.

Wheezing A musical breathing noise caused by air flowing through narrowed airway passages in the lungs (the lower airways); commonly associated with asthma.

White blood cells Part of the body's immune system that fights infection; also called *leukocytes.*

Photo and Illustration Credits

Figure 21-12: From Aehlert B: *PALS pediatric advanced life support study guide,* ed 1, St Louis, 1994, Mosby.

Figures 1-5, 1-8, F, 2-2, 2-5, 2-8, 3-9, 3-15, 3-17, A-B, 3-19, 4-3, 4-4, 4-5, 4-10, 4-11, 5-10, 5-13, 6-10, 7-1, 7-3, 7-4, 7-7, 7-38, 7-41, 7-42, 8-3, 8-4, 8-14, A-B, 9-1, 9-4, 9-5, 10-9, 10-10, 10-12, 10-13, 10-14, 11-12, 12-3, 12-4, 12-7, 12-10, 12-11, 12-19, 12-20, 12-25, 13-4, 14-10, 15-10, 17-15, 17-16, 17-20, 17-21, 17-22, A-C, 20-6, B, 21-5, 22-12, 23-25, 23-26, 23-27, 25-6, A, 27-2: From American College of Emergency Physicians: *Paramedic field care: a complaint-based approach,* ed 1, St Louis, 1997, ACEP.

Figures 17-14, 17-19, A, 23-3, 27-1, 27-3, A, 27-5, unnumbered 27-1: From Anderson KN, Anderson LE, Glanze WD: *Mosby's medical, nursing & allied health dictionary,* ed 5, St Louis, 1998, Mosby.

Figures 17-3, 17-6, 17-7, 17-9, A-D, 17-10, 17-12, 17-19, B: From Auerbach PS: *Wilderness medicine: management of wilderness and environmental emergencies,* ed 3, St Louis, 1995, Mosby.

Figures 18-3, 24-7, A: From Barkin RM: *Pediatric emergency medicine,* ed 2, St Louis, 1997, Mosby.

Figures 21-7, A-D, 21-7, F: From Bobak IM et al: *Maternity nursing,* ed 4, St Louis, 1995, Mosby.

Figure 1-6: From Gurley LT: *Introduction to radiologic technology,* ed 4, St Louis, 1996, Mosby.

Figures 8-7, 8-9, 8-10, 8-13, 8-16, 8-17, 8-25, 8-26, 8-27, 8-28, 8-29, 11-1, 11-2, 15-1, B, 15-2, 21-1, A-B, 23-1, 24-1, A-B, 24-2, 24-3, 25-1: From Brooks ML: *Exploring medical language,* ed 4, St Louis, 1998, Mosby.

Figures 2-6, 27-3, B, 27-9: From Lewis SM, Collier IC, Heitkemper MM: *Medical-surgical nursing: assessment and management of clinical problems,* ed 4, St Louis, 1996, Mosby.

Figures 14-6, 24-5, 24-6, 24-18, B, 24-19: From Mace JD, Kowalczyk N: *Radiographic pathology for technologists,* ed 3, St Louis, 1998, Mosby.

Figures 1-8, E, 1-9, 1-11, 7-21, 7-30, 7-31, 7-32, 7-36, 7-37, 7-43, 7-44, 7-45, 10-3, 10-6, 10-7, 11-14, 17-17: From McSwain NE et al: *The basic EMT: comprehensive prehospital care,* ed 1, St Louis, 1997, Mosby.

Figures 2-1, 3-11, 3-13: From Moore RE: *Vehicle rescue and extrication,* ed 1, St Louis, 1991, Mosby.

Figures 6-6, D, 10-11, 11-10, 25-4, 25-23, A-D, 27-4: From NAEMT: PHTLS: *Basic and advanced prehospital trauma life support,* ed 4, St Louis, 1999, Mosby.

Figures 1-7, A-B, 10-18, 10-19, 11-19, 11-21, 11-38, 11-45, 11-47, 12-5, 12-6, 12-12, 12-16, 12-17, 12-18, 17-2, 17-13, 21-2, 21-7, E, 22-7, 23-2, 23-5, 23-6, 23-8, 23-9, 23-24, 24-7, B, 24-11, A, 24-13, 24-14, 24-18, A, 24-23, 25-6, B-C, 25-7, 25-9, 25-11, 25-14, A-D, 26-14, A-C, 26-18: From Sanders MJ: *Mosby's paramedic textbook,* ed 1, St Louis, 1994, Mosby.

Figures 3-4, 3-5, 3-6, 10-16, B, 10-17, 17-8, 18-2: From Seidel HM et al: *Mosby's guide to physical examination,* ed 4, St Louis, 1999, Mosby.

Figures 5-20, B, 10-15, 10-19, 10-20, 11-6, 11-8, 11-13, 11-15, 11-16, 11-17, 11-22, 11-23, 11-26, 11-27, 11-28, 11-31, 11-32, 11-33, 11-34, 11-35, A, 12-21: From Shade B et al: *Mosby's EMT-intermediate textbook,* ed 1, St Louis, 1997, Mosby.

Figures 6-3, 6-4, 7-2, 7-5, 7-10, 7-11, 7-12, 10-1: From Smith BD: *Rescuers in action,* ed 1, St Louis, 1996, Mosby.

Figures 1-3, 3-16, 5-1, 5-2, 5-17, 5-22, 7-39, 7-40, 7-46, 8-5, 10-5, 12-22, 13-3, 13-8, 13-9, 13-11, A-B, 15-11, A-B, 17-11, 19-3, 19-4, 22-13, 22-15, 23-4, 23-7, 23-11, 23-23, 24-4, 24-12, 26-5: From Stoy WA: *Mosby's EMT-Basic Textbook,* ed 1, St Louis, 1996, Mosby.

Figures 11-7, 11-9, 11-11: From Stoy WA: *Mosby's first responder textbook,* ed 1, St Louis, 1997, Mosby.

Figure 3-2: From Thibodeau GA, Patton K: *The human body in health and disease,* ed 2, St Louis, 1997, Mosby.

Figures 27-6, 27-7, 27-8: From Wong DL: *Nursing care of infants and children,* ed 6, St Louis, 1999, Mosby.

Index

A

C

D

F

G

H

I

N

Q

R

U

V

W

X

Y

Z